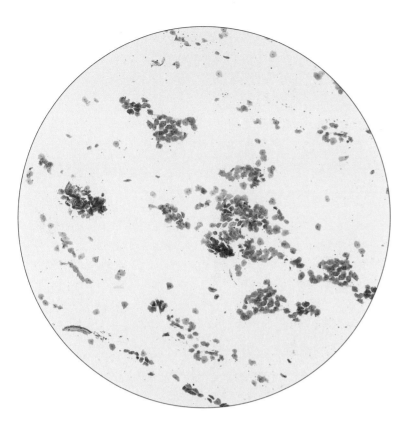

~500 cells. Adequate if at least 16 fields have similar (or greater) cellularity. (4× field, CPS) [Courtesy of Dr. George Birdsong, Atlanta]

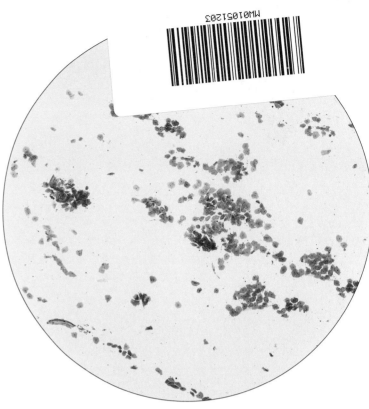

~666 cells. Adequate if at least 12 fields have similar (or greater) cellularity. (4× field, CPS) [Courtesy of Dr. George Birdsong, Atlanta]

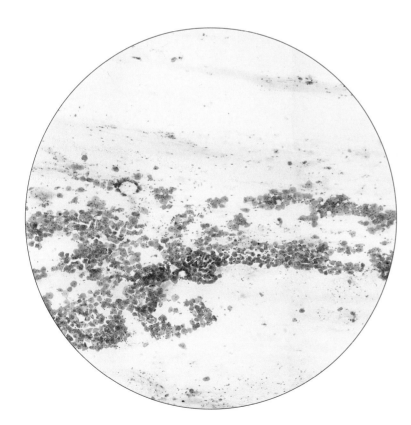

~1000 cells. Adequate if at least 8 fields have similar (or greater) cellularity.(4× field, CPS) [Courtesy of Dr. George Birdsong, Atlanta]

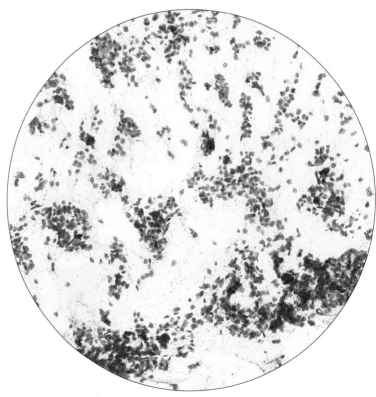

~1400 cells. Adequate if at least 6 fields have similar (or greater) cellularity. (4× field, CPS) [Courtesy of Dr. George Birdsong, Atlanta]

The Pap Test

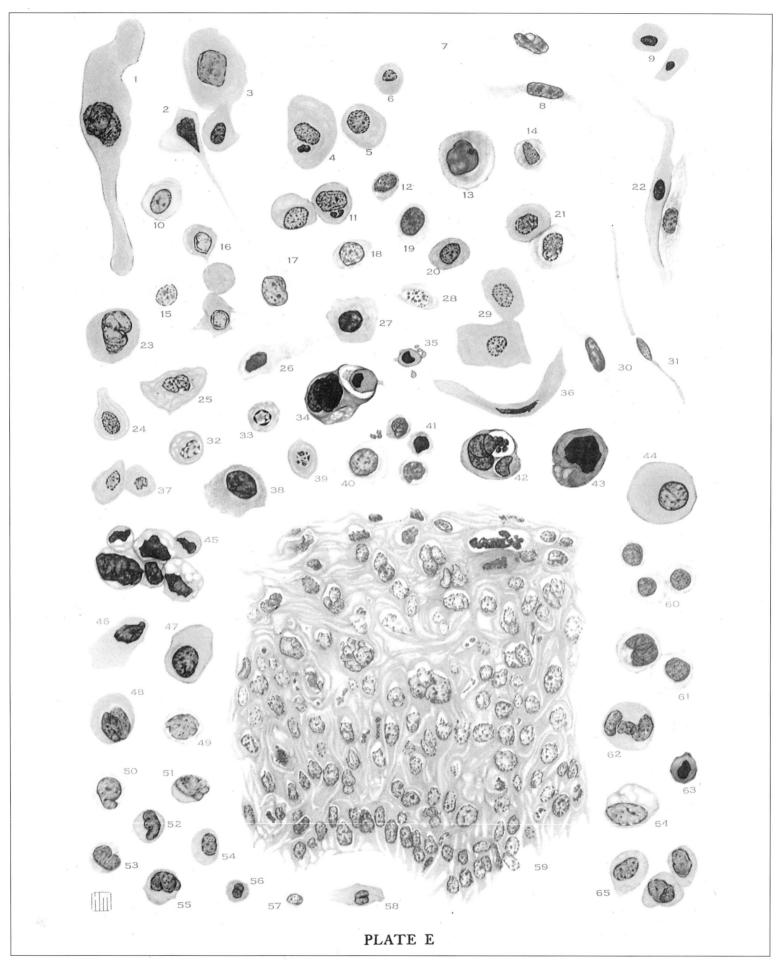

PLATE E

Cancer cells found in vaginal smear. Reprinted from Papanicolaou GN, Traut HF: *Diagnosis of Uterine Cancer by the Vaginal Smear*. New York. The Commonwealth Fund, 1943.

The Pap Test

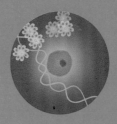

Richard Mac DeMay, MD
Professor of Pathology
Director of Cytopathology
University of Chicago

ASCP Press
American Society for Clinical Pathology
Chicago

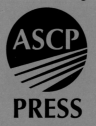

ASCP

PRESS

Publishing Team

Erik Tanck (production manager/designer)
Joshua Weikersheimer (publisher)
(with assistance of Adam Fanucci, Terri Horning and Jeffrey Carlson, production/design)

Printed in Singapore

06 05 04 03 02 01   6 5 4 3 2 1

Table of Contents

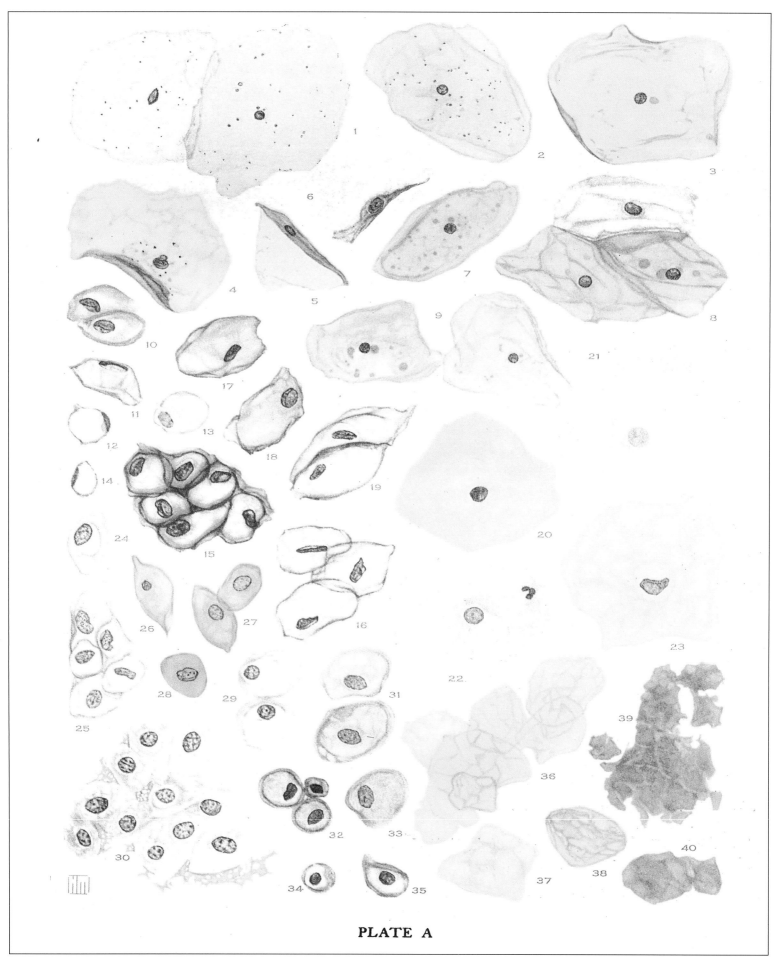

PLATE A

Normal cells found in vaginal smear. Reprinted from Papanicolaou GN, Traut HF: *Diagnosis of Uterine Cancer by the Vaginal Smear*. New York. The Commonwealth Fund, 1943.

Preface

This book began life as a chapter in *The Art & Science of Cytopathology*. But the contents of that original chapter have been greatly revised, updated, and expanded to include liquid-based cytology, new concepts of human papillomavirus in cervical carcinogenesis, HPV-DNA testing, the latest Bethesda System changes, new management guidelines from the ASCCP, lessons from litigation over the past 10 years, and much more. Even the title, *The Pap Test*, recognizes a "paradigm shift" from predominance of the conventional Pap smear to liquid-based cytology, which now accounts for most cervicovaginal cytology in America. Some may want this book for the atlas of liquid-based cervicovaginal cytology alone....

The audience for this book is students, residents, fellows, cytotechnologists, pathologists, gynecologists, and in fact, anyone involved with Pap testing. Obviously, this will include a wide range of readers, from beginners in the field to advanced practitioners to those subjected to mandatory proficiency testing. Therefore, the work is offered as something of a smorgasbord, with a good helping of something for everyone. Acknowledging that not everyone will read the book "cover-to-cover," each section is a complete discussion—those who do read all of it, bless them, will naturally find some redundancies in the text. The presentation is comprehensive, but mindful of providing practical information useful in daily practice. Liquid-based cytology is compared and contrasted with conventional Pap smears throughout the text. In addition, a synoptic *Liquid-Based Cytology Atlas* (aka LBC Fun Park) is included in chapter VIII for your viewing pleasure. Of course, most of the information about cervical disease applies to both technologies.

All together, there are well over 500 images, all but 1 in full color. Important criteria for cytologic interpretation are emphasized at every useful turn in the text. Synoptic lists, tables, and illustrations are applied liberally to summarize key information and make it easier to remember. Clinical correlation is stressed because it is vital in formulating a cytologic interpretation. References are included as an academic exercise, and boy-howdy there sure are a lot of them (>4000). In addition, the history of the Pap test and the discovery of the role of human papillomavirus in cervical carcinogenesis, as well as other historical tidbits, are offered for the reader's enjoyment. The reader might also get a kick out of the new DeMay Classification System, which really gets down to brass tacks. Philosophically, a spoon full of sugar helps the medicine go down.

Finally, chapters on the *Failure of the Pap Test* and *Lessons from Litigation* are included, in recognition that the Pap test is not perfect. But, it's still the best test ever invented for cancer prevention! And we all thank Dr Papanicolaou every time we mention it by name.

Mac DeMay
Author

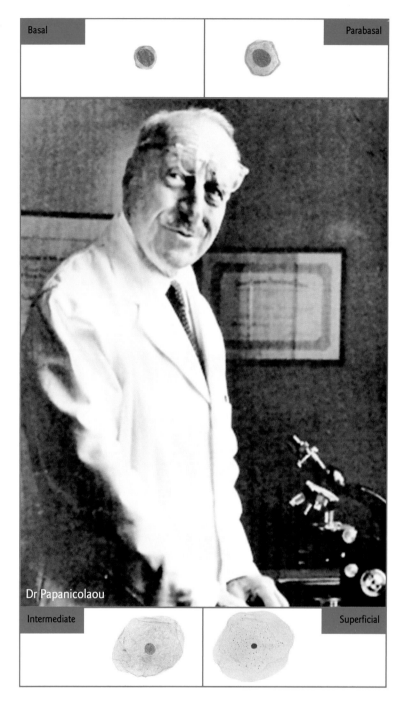

Basal

Parabasal

Dr Papanicolaou

Intermediate

Superficial

Abbreviations

AdCA:	adenocarcinoma
αFP:	alpha-fetoprotein
AGC:	atypical glandular cells
AGUS:	atypical glandular cells of undetermined significance
AIDS:	acquired immunodeficiency syndrome
AIS:	adenocarcinoma in situ
ALTS:	ASCUS / L SIL triage study
ASC:	atypical squamous cells
ASC-H:	atypical squamous cells-cannot exclude H SIL
ASCUS:	atypical squamous cells of undetermined significance (pre 2001)
ASC-US:	atypical squamous cells-undetermined significance (post 2001)
ASCCP:	american society for colposcopy and cervical pathology
BCC:	benign cellular changes
BCP:	birth control pill
βHCG:	beta–human chorionic gonadotropin
[C]:	conventional Pap smear, *see also* CPS
CA:	carcinoma
CD:	cluster designation
CDC:	centers for disease control
CEA:	carcinoembryonic antigen
CGIN:	cervical glandular intraepithelial neoplasia
CIN:	cervical intraepithelial neoplasia
CIS:	carcinoma in situ
CK:	cytokeratin
CLIA:	clinical laboratory improvement act
CMV:	cytomegalovirus
CPS:	conventional Pap smear, *see also* [C]
CT:	cytotechnologist
DDx:	differential interpretation
DES:	diethylstilbestrol
DNA:	deoxyribonucleic acid
EBV:	Epstein-Barr virus
EC:	endocervical
EC/TZ:	endocervical cell/transformation zone
eg:	exempli gratia
EGD:	endoglandular dysplasia
EGN:	endocervical glandular neoplasia
EM:	endometrial
etc:	et cetera
FDA:	Food and Drug Administration
FLC:	funny looking cell
FN:	field number
FNA:	fine needle aspiration
FSH:	follicle stimulating hormone
GI:	gastrointestinal
H SIL:	high-grade squamous intraepithelial lesion
H&E:	hematoxylin and eosin
HCGs:	hyperchromatic crowded groups
HG:	high grade
HIV:	human immunodeficiency virus
HK:	hyperkeratosis
HLA:	human leukocyte antigen
HPV:	human papilloma virus
HRT:	hormone replacement therapy
HSV:	herpes simplex virus
ICL:	intracytoplasmic lumen
ie:	id est

ISH:	in situ hybridization
IUD:	intrauterine device
K SCC:	keratinizing squamous cell carcinoma
[L]:	liquid-based cytology, *see also* LBC
L SIL:	low-grade squamous intraepithelial lesion
LBC:	liquid-based cytology, *see also* [L]
LCA:	leukocyte common antigen
LCR:	long control region
LEEP:	loop electrosurgical excision procedure
LG:	low grade
LH:	luteinizing hormone
LHAs:	lymphohistiocytic aggregates
LLETZ:	large loop excision transformation zone
LN:	lymph node
MG bodies:	Michaelis-Gutmann bodies
MI:	maturation index
MicroCA:	microinvasive carcinoma
MMMT:	malignant mixed müllerian tumor
MSBR:	multiple slide blinded rescreening
N/C:	nuclear/cytoplasmic
N-C:	nucleocytoplasmic
NCR:	noncoding region
NILM:	negative for intraepithelial lesion or malignancy
NOS:	not otherwise specified
ORF:	open reading frame
PAS:	periodic acid-Schiff
PBC:	pale bland cell
PC:	politically correct
PCR:	polymerase chain reaction
pg:	page
PK:	parakeratosis
PPK:	pseudoparakeratosis
PMNs:	polymorphonuclear neutrophils
PNET:	primitive neuroectodermal tumor
RB:	retinoblastoma
RBC:	red blood cell
RCH:	reserve cell hyperplasia
RNA:	ribonucleic acid
RV:	recto-vaginal
Rx:	therapy
SBLB:	satisfactory but limited by
SCC:	squamous cell carcinoma
SIADH:	syndrome of inappropriate antidiuretic hormone secretion
SIL:	squamous intraepithelial lesion
SRC:	sarcoma
TBS:	the Bethesda System
TGF:	transforming growth factor
TM:	tubal metaplasia
TTF1:	thyroid transcription factor one
TZ:	transformation zone
URR:	upstream regulatory region
VCE:	vaginal cervical endocervical
WHO:	World Health Organization
WBC:	white blood cell
WNL:	within normal limits
YY1:	ying yang one

Acknowledgements

Joan Hives, factotum and library
researcher extraordinaire,
without whom this work would
not be possible

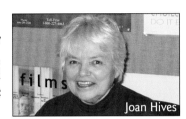

Joan Hives

Gregory Spiegel, for careful review of manuscript
and numerous helpful suggestions

Jim Linder, for generous contribution of glass slides

Joshua Weikersheimer, because he's the best

Also wish to acknowledge bureaucratic red tape, busy work, and meetings, without which this work would have been completed a lot sooner.

To my Father, Richard, my Sister, Laurie, and the memory of my Mother, Gloria.

The Pap Test

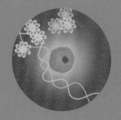

Richard Mac DeMay, MD

Introduction

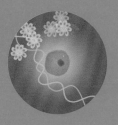

ap tests save lives! The Pap test is one of the greatest success stories in the history of medicine. Before the era of the Papanicolaou smear, now commonly known as the Pap test to include liquid-based cytology, carcinoma of the uterine cervix was a leading cause of cancer-related deaths in American women [Janicek 2001] (and remains a leading cause where Pap tests, and appropriate clinical follow-up, are not widely available [Parkin 1999a,b, Pisani 1999, 2002, Robles 1996, V Schneider 2001]). By detecting cervical abnormalities that can be treated *before* they develop into invasive cancer, Pap test screening has correlated with a remarkable reduction in the morbidity and mortality of this disease [Adami 1994, JL Benedet 1992, Cannistra 1996, Christopherson 1970a,b, 1976, 1977b, Devesa 1989, J Dunn 1981, Herbert 2000, Hernandez–Avila 1997, Janicek 2001, Koss 1989a, G-K Nguyen 1996, van der Graaf 1990]. Cervical cancer has been knocked out of the top ten and now accounts for less than 2% of all malignancies in American women [Jemal 2005]. *No other test—indeed no other public health measure—has been as successful in stamping out cancer!*

Because of its undeniable success, certain myths have developed about the Pap test. Many people believe that Pap tests provide a fail-safe system for prevention of malignancy [Frable 2004]. Unfortunately, this is not true. Many people also believe that Pap tests screen for every kind of gynecologic cancer, including ovarian, uterine, and all cervical cancers [Roach 2003,CL Woodman 1998]. In fact, Pap test screening is primarily effective in preventing only squamous cell carcinoma of the cervix in middle aged women [Solomon 2002]. The Pap test has never been proven effective in preventing adenocarcinoma, the second most common form of cervical cancer, which has increased in incidence despite widespread screening [Andersson 2003, Austin 2003b,c, A Benoit 1984, Bergström 1999, Bjersing 1991, Boddington 1976, Boon 1987, Brinton 1987b, J Burk 1974, Canavan 2000, Christopherson 1979, Colgan 2001a, Crum 2002, Erzen 2002, Etherington 2001, Franco 2003, Fry 1969, Fu 1987, Hayes 1997, Herbert 2001, Herrero 1992, Janerich 1995, Jaworski 1990, Keyhani–Rofagha 1995, H-S Kim 1991, Kinney 2003, Krane 2002, K Lee 1997b, 1998, 1999, 2002, S Liu 2001, Makino 1995, A Miller 1995, H Mitchell 1988, 1990c, 1993a, 1995a, Mody 1999, Moriarty 2003a, G-K Nguyen 1993, Nieminen 1995, Ollayos 1997, Parkin 1985, R Peters 1986a, Renshaw 2004c, Ruba 2004, Sasieni 2001, Schoolland 2002a,b, H Smith 2000, Stockton 1997, Vizcaino 1998, SS Wang 2004, Zappa 2004, T Zheng 1996]. Extraordinarily, the Pap test can lead to detection of malignancies of the uterus, fallopian tubes, ovaries, or even distant sites; however, Pap tests are not reliable in screening for these cancers [M Sasagawa 2003, Solomon 2002]. Under appreciated is that Pap test screening is less effective in preventing cancer in young women (<35 years of age) and postmenopausal women [Colgan 2002, Gustafsson 1995, 1997, Macgregor 1994, Morrow 1995, Parkin 1985, Sasieni 1999, M Quinn 1999].

Furthermore, the conventional Pap smear is, in fact, a rather crude screening test with poor sensitivity (as low as ~50%) [Fahey 1995, Franco 2000, Giard 2001, Hartman 2001, ML Hutchinson 1999, Martin–Hirsch 2002, Nanda 2000, Renshaw 2002b], although liquid-based cytology seems to improve on that sensitivity [McCrory 1999, Nanda 2000]. And, of course, new lesions can develop at any time. Therefore, regular screening is crucial for cancer prevention: precursor lesions missed in one screening can usually be found in the next few screenings. Limitations of the Pap test include problems with sampling, interpretation, and clinical follow-up. Also, a few cancers apparently can develop rapidly in the interval between Pap test screenings, precluding prevention. Because of these inherent limitations, unfortunately, but

---

Important Points About the Pap Test

Excellent—but not perfect—test
  to prevent cancer
Mostly for squamous cell carcinoma
  ...of cervix in middle-aged women
Not proven to prevent adenocarcinoma
No effect for any other cancer
Detects treatable precursor lesions
Regular screening crucial!

---

inevitably, some women develop cervical cancer even though they have been screened [Kurman 1994, Wied 1981]. Yet, *by far* the most important reason for failure of the Pap test in cancer prevention is failure to get women adequately screened in the first place [Janerich 1995, Kinney 1998a, Sung 2000].

The cause of cervical cancer is no longer a mystery [Crum 2000]. Cervical cancer is a rare outcome of a common venereal disease caused by human papillomavirus, the lowly wart virus [Helmerhorst 2002]. Two ways to reduce the risk of developing cervical cancer include minimizing exposure to the virus (primary prevention) and testing for presence of the virus or precursor lesions. A third preventative method, vaccination, is on the horizon [Coursaget 1999, Duggan–Keen 1998, Galloway 1998, Hines 1995, 1998, Koutsky 2002, Lowy 1998, Sherman 1998, P Stern 2001, Suzich 1995, Tindle 1996]. Although inadequate Pap test screening is customarily considered a major risk factor for cervical cancer [Brinton 1987a, Christopherson 1976, E Clarke 1979, Herrero 1992], the risk is probably more closely related to sexual practices than to differences in screening [de Vet 1994, Kjaer 1989, H-q Li 2000a]. (In fact, cervical cancer is theoretically almost entirely preventable, even without Pap tests, by controlling risk factors [Braun 1998, H-q Li 2000a, H Mitchell 1990c].) And today, much more sensitive screening tests, such as HPV-DNA testing, are available for cervical cancer detection and prevention [Austin 2003a,b, T Wright 2003b]. The combination of a liquid-based Pap test with an HPV-DNA test (the "HPV-Pap test") can achieve sensitivity to clinically significant cervical lesions approaching perfection (>95% sensitivity) [Belinson 2001, Hutchinson 1999, K-J Lee 2004, Renshaw 2002a, Schiffman 2000b].

Historical Perspective

Of all the plagues and miseries which any demon ever invented, cancer is surely among the most ancient. The earliest known unequivocal neoplasm occurred in a fossilized fish, *Phanerosteon mirabile,* about 300 million years ago [Capasso 2005]. Malignant tumors have been found in dinosaurs, on the order of 100 million years old [Svitil 2003]. By comparison, the earliest hominids are only about 5 million years old and evidence of malignancy has been found in the remains of prehistoric hominids [Capasso 2005]. So, cancer has been a part of the human experience since the very beginning of our evolution. Cervical cancer is probably also primeval, because the papillomavirus that causes it co-evolved with humans over a span of millions of years [Bernard 1994, Ong 1993].

Early evidence of cancer is also found in fossilized bone tumors, mummies in ancient Egypt and Peru, and ancient manuscripts [Capasso 2005]. The oldest extant description of malignant tumors is recorded in the *Ramayana*, a great epic poem from ancient India dating from c 2000 BCE (before the common era). The poem comments on the treatment of cancer by excision or application of ointments containing arsenic [Diamandopoulos 1996].

Egyptians started practicing medicine around 4000 BCE. Knowledge of human anatomy was obtained through the practice of mummification, which removed and examined parts of the body after death. Cancer is described in the Edwin Smith papyrus, an ancient Egyptian medical text that dates from the 17th century BCE, and is itself is a copy of an older, but now lost, papyrus estimated to date from the 30th century BCE. The Edwin Smith papyrus tells of eight breast tumors or ulcers that were treated by cauterization, with an instrument called "the fire drill" [Kardinal 1979]. Peseshet is the first known woman physician. She practiced at the time of the building of the great pyramids in Egypt, about 2500 BCE [Harer 1989]. The oldest known text on gynecology, the Kahun papyrus, dates to 1825 BCE. The Ebers papyrus, from 1552 BCE, contains a chapter on diseases of women (it depicts the uterus as a separate animal, often a tortoise, newt, or crocodile) as well as descriptions of tumors (ie, swellings, which lumped inflammation and neoplasia), including cancer of the uterus (described as an eating of the uterus with vaginal ulcers) [Diamandopoulos 1996]. The ancient Egyptians were the first to recognize that there were different types of tumors and that they had to be treated differently. For example, a red, hot tumor (ie, an abscess) should be treated by incision to drain the pus, while a firm, solid tumor should be treated by excision (using opium as an anesthetic) or with "chemicals" extracted from the earth [Diamandopoulos 1996]. (Plutarch [66-120 CE] notes the word, chemistry, derives from the Egyptian word, chemi, which means "black land" and refers to the original name of ancient Egypt, so called because of its fertile black soil [Diamandopoulos 1996].) Tumors of the breast are mentioned briefly in cuneiform tablets from the library of Nineveh in Babylonia, c 800 BCE [Diamandopoulos 1996].

Hippocrates of Cos (460-370 BCE), a contemporary of Socrates (469-399 BCE) and Plato (427-347 BCE), is the ancient Greek physician known as the father of medicine. Before Hippocrates, disease was believed to be punishment brought on by the wrath of the gods, who had to be appeased through prayer, ritual, or sacrifice. Hippocrates separated medicine from religion, superstition, and magic, and established it as a natural science based on critical observation and logical thinking [Hajdu 2004a]. Hippocrates wrote extensively about tumors, or oncoi (singular, oncos), from which the word, oncology, is derived. He was the first to distinguish benign (innocuous) tumors from malignant (malicious) ones. He coined the word, carcinoma (from the Greek, for crab [probably referring to distended veins surrounding breast cancer]), to describe malignant tumors.

Following the lead of the Greek natural philosopher (ie, scientist) Empedocles (495-435 BCE), who taught that air (gas), water (liquid), earth (solid), and fire (energy) were the four cardinal elements of the universe, Hippocrates theorized that disease was an imbalance of the biological counterparts, or body humors, ie, blood (air), phlegm (water), black bile (earth), and yellow bile (fire). He hypothesized that an excess of black bile, melancholy (Greek: melan, black; chole, bile), caused cancer, and prescribed the use of garlic fumes (a treatment known as "fumigation") to combat uterine cancer [Orr 1998]. Although his beliefs were attacked in his lifetime, Hippocrates has been revered through the ages as the "Ideal Physician." The principles of the Hippocratic Oath, based on respect for human life and helping without harm, are still held sacred today [Diamandopoulos 1996].

Soranus of Ephesus (98-138 CE) is considered the foremost authority on gynecology from antiquity. He performed the first hysterectomy (for prolapse), and was also the first to recognize the cervix as a separate portion of the uterus [Krantz 1967]. His writings formed the foundation of gynecology until the 17th century. The Roman physician, Celsus (25 BCE-50 CE), described different stages of evolution of cancer and, like today, said that therapy depends on the stage of the disease. Another early writer on cancer was Aretaeus the Cappadocian (81-138? CE), who described malignancies of the uterus and distinguished between malignant ulcerations and malignant tumors.

Six centuries after Hippocrates, the humoral theory of disease was embraced by the Roman physician, Galen (131-201 CE). Possibly the most influential physician ever, Galen's views became medical dogma for 1300 years, through the Middle Ages, until the Renaissance. Galen taught that the early diagnosis of cancer is based on probability, while the definitive diagnosis is determined by its eventual effect on the patient. Galen used the word, cancer (from cancrum, Latin for crab), and coined the word, sarcoma (from the Greek for flesh). Galen was celebrated for his surgical skills, perfected by treating gladiators, and became the personal physician to the Roman Emperor, Commodus [Diamandopoulos 1996].

Following the fall of the Roman Empire in the west in 476 CE, scientific knowledge migrated to the eastern, or Byzantine Empire, where it flourished. The Byzantine period is characterized by collecting, cataloging, and commenting on scientific information in the form of encyclopedias. Although not original, these writings were of great value because they preserved knowledge that otherwise might have been lost. Oribasius (325-403) compiled all medical knowledge gained before his time and added his own observations. He used a knife to excise anogenital condylomas. He noted that cancers were not red, like inflammation, but contained coarse black bile, and that early forms could be cured [Hajdu 2004b]. Aetius of Amida (527-565), physician to Emperor Justinian, described ulcerated and nonulcerated cervical cancers and recommended cautery to treat nonulcerated tumors [Hajdu 2004b]. Papanicolaou and Traut cite Paul of Aegina (625-690) as the first expert in the diagnosis and treatment of cancer, particularly of the uterus and breast, in their famous monograph, *Diagnosis of Uterine Cancer by the Vaginal Smear* [Papanicolaou 1943].

In 431, the Christian Orthodox Patriarch, Nestorius, was banished from Constantinople for heresy. He and his followers, many of whom were physicians, emigrated to Syria, and from there to Persia, because of religious persecutions. The Nestorian Christians translated many Greek and Latin medical texts into Persian. These texts were rediscovered when the Arabs invaded Persia in the 7th century and were retranslated into Arabic. Ibn Sina (980-1037), Latinized as Avicenna, was the most famous physician of the era. He noticed that tumors grow slowly, invade neighboring tissues, resulting in the loss of sensation in the affected parts. His *Canon of Medicine*, although not original because it was based on Hippocrates and Galen, nevertheless was one of the most famous medical texts ever written, remained an authority on medicine until the 19th century, and contributed to a Golden Age of Arab Medicine (850-1050), which only ended with the Crusades.

The Crusades were largely responsible for the return of the "lost knowledge" of antiquity to Europe, with the end of the Dark Ages, where it inspired a revival of the scientific approach to medicine. Abu al-Qasim (Albucasis [936-1013]) of Cordova, Spain, known as the father of surgery, recommended excision of early stage cancers and cauterization of the tissue around the area of the tumor. Another famous physician of the era was the Rabbi Moses ben Maimon (Moses Maimonides, 1135-1204), who was born in Cordova, studied medicine in Morocco, migrated to Egypt, and eventually became court physician to the Sultan Saladin. He wrote that the physician should treat the patient, not the illness [Diamandopoulos 1996].

The Middle Ages are the period 476-1453, from the fall of Rome to the Goths, to the fall of Constantinople to the Turks. Before the founding of independent universities during the 10th-13th centuries, members of religious orders, who called themselves Doctors (Latin, docere, to teach), taught the dogma of the Catholic church and suppressed free and independent thought. As a result, astrology, alchemy, and magic gradually replaced the rational approach to diagnosis and therapy of human diseases including cancer. Once universities began to be established, however, study of ancient texts, especially those of Galen, was reinstituted and practical experience was gained by clinical evaluation of patients [Diamandopoulos 1996]. Galen dominated medical thought until the 17th century and any challenge to his authority was considered heresy [Kardinal 1979].

The Renaissance, 14th-17th centuries, saw the beginning of the scientific study of the human body and disease, a change from Aristotelian-Galenic rationalism based on metaphysics to Baconian-Newtonian empiricism based on experiment [Kardinal 1979]. Leonardo da Vinci (1452-1519) initiated modern anatomical illustration, including pelvic anatomy and the earliest accurate drawings of the fetus in utero, but unfortunately, his sketches were seen by only a few of his contemporaries. Andreas Vesalius (1514-1564), the great Flemish anatomist, taught "authority must yield to original investigation" [Diamandopoulos 1996]. In 1543, at the ripe old age of 28, Vesalius had the audacity to challenge the god-like Galen and show him in error. Vesalius's book, *De humani corporis fabrica libri septem* ("The Seven Books on the Structure of the Human Body"), was based on human dissections, while Galen's anatomy was based on animals. Vesalius provided the first accurate descriptions of the entire female genital tract. Sir William Osler (1849-1919) called the *Fabrica* "the greatest medical book ever written—from which modern medicine starts."

William Harvey (1578-1657) discovered the circulation of blood in 1628, and compared the heart to a mechanical pump, proving that the human body could be studied scientifically. He shares with William Gilbert, investigator of magnetism, credit for initiating accurate experimental research that gave birth to modern science. Four years after Harvey's death, Marcello Malpighi (1628-1694), an Italian biologist and physician, provided proof of Harvey's theory by discovering capillaries using a microscope. Malpighi is regarded as the father of microscopic anatomy and his discovery was another fundamental advance in the history of science.

Giovanni Morgagni (1682-1771) applied the scientific method to the study of disease by relating the pathologic findings after death to the patient's illness. This laid the scientific foundation for oncology, the study of cancer. John Hunter (1728-1793), the London surgeon known as the founder of scientific surgery ("don't think, try"), wrote that if a tumor were "moveable" (had not invaded locally) "there is no impropriety in removing it." Apparently not benign himself, Hunter died after suffering a fit while arguing with a colleague.

In the 17th and 18th centuries, cancer was thought to be caused by parasites and as contagious as phthisis (tuberculosis). (As late as 1926, the Nobel Prize was awarded for the "discovery" that worms [nematodes] caused cancer. But, we now know that certain infectious agents can cause cancer, and so–perversely–it's true, "cancer can be caught.") René Descartes (1596-1650), among others, theorized that benign tumors developed from coagulating lymph, which could ferment and turn malignant [Diamandopoulos 1996]. This theory was not doubted for nearly 150 years, despite lack of conclusive evidence.

By the end of the 18th century, the old humoral theories (black bile, lymph) were being replaced with the modern idea that cancer represents a change in cells. Improvements in the microscope, such as the invention of achromatic lenses in the 1830s, allowed these changes to be studied. In 1838, the German pathologist, Johannes Müller (1801-1858), demonstrated that cancer is made of cells, not lymph. However, he thought that cells arose from blastema (budding noncellular germinal elements) between normal tissues [Kardinal 1979]. His student, Rudolph Virchow (1821-1902), determined that all cells, including cancer cells, derive from other cells ("omnis cellula e cellula"). As Morgagni before him had related gross autopsy findings to the patient's disease, Virchow related microscopic findings to disease. This ushered in the era of microscopic analysis of tumors. Müller, Virchow, and others who studied tumors gradually formulated a classification system still in use today, based on the type of cells composing tumors (eg, epithelial-carcinoma, mesenchymal-sarcoma) and their behavior in a living organism (ie, benign-innocuous, malignant-malicious). Note that this "morphological-behavioral" classification system is not so different from Hippocrates and Galen, except that it is based on microscopy rather than gross observation [Diamandopoulos 1996].

In the 19th century, when anesthesia became available (1846), surgery began to flourish, and classic cancer operations were developed by such eminent figures as Billroth in Germany, Handley in London, and Halsted at Johns Hopkins in America. Although the French surgeon, Amboise Paré, recommended amputation of the cervix as therapy for cervical cancer as early as 1575, Sauter performed the first successful total vaginal hysterectomy as cancer treatment in 1822. Building on the work of Emil Ries, John G. Clark, and Heinrich T. M. Rumpf, Ernst Wertheim proceded to perform his improved radical hysterectomy in 1898. As the 19th century drew to a close, Wilhelm Roentgen discovered x-rays, in 1895, and Marie and Pierre Curie isolated radium, in 1898. Shortly thereafter, in 1903, M. A. Cleaves first described the use of radiation to treat cervical cancer [Cleaves 1904, Orr 1998, S Rubin 2001]. By the dawn of the 20th century, the mainstays of cervical cancer therapy, surgery and radiation, were already in use, although improvements continue to evolve.

In the 19th century, it was believed that cervical cancer started as a tiny node in the stroma, which arose from stromal cells, displaced epithelial cells, embryonal rests, or even "wandering" blood cells [L Johnson 1969]. As early as 1852, however, writing in a French journal, Charles Robin recognized the epithelial nature of carcinoma [L Johnson 1969, Robin 1852]. Sir John Williams was practically clairvoyant in recognizing the origin of cervical carcinoma in stratified epithelium in the marginal surface or transitional zone at the external cervical os [L Johnson 1969]. In his 1886 lectures, he noted noninvasive epithelial abnormalities related to cervical cancer [J Williams 1888]. In the early 20th century it was proposed that some cancers, including cervical cancer, have an incipient or noninvasive stage [Pronai 1909, I Rubin 1910, Schauenstein 1908]. T.S. Cullen described "suspicious changes in the epithelium along the outer margin of a squamous cell carcinoma of the cervix" in his textbook, *Cancer of the Uterus*, in 1900 [Te Linde 1973, Woodruff 1981]. Julius Schottlaender and Fritz Kermauner observed carcinoma confined to the epithelium at the periphery of invasive squamous cell carcinoma of the cervix in 1912 [Footer 1944, I Rubin 1957, Schiller 1933, Schottlaender 1912]. They called it "Zuckerguss" (sugar icing), believing it to be a method by which cervical cancer spread in some cases [Te Linde 1973]. John T. Bowen reported "precancerous dermatosis" and credited Grover W. Wende with demonstrating that noninvasive cancers could progress to true malignancy [Bowen 1912, Wende 1908]. In the 1930s, Albert C. Broders stated that a lesion composed of undifferentiated, atypical cells, which he called "carcinoma in situ," was a precursor of squamous cell carcinoma [Broders 1932]. Later, Charles S. Stevenson and Elemer Scipiades reported that two of their 18 cases of noninvasive cervical carcinoma became invasive after 3 and 8 years [Stevenson 1938].

Although the concept of precancerous lesions was slow to be accepted, it gradually became known that cervical cancer could be cured, if it were found early. In those days, cervical cancer was a scourge, all too often killing women in the prime of their lives [Footer 1944]. The challenge was to find early cancers, or even precursor lesions, assuming they existed.

In 1925, Hans Hinselmann invented the colposcope, in Germany, as a way of detecting early invasive cancer. The colposcope illuminates and magnifies the cervix, making early cancer visible as either a small ulcer or a small exophytic lesion. In 1928, Walter Schiller, a student of Schottlaender, devised a test for cervical cancer that involved painting the cervix with an iodine solution [O Petersen 1955, Schiller 1938]. In theory, healthy cells stain dark owing to glycogen content, while abnormal cells remain unstained. Unstained ("Schiller positive") areas were biopsied [Graves 1933, Henriksen 1935]. Unfortunately, in practice, the test was painful, costly, and not foolproof, with numerous false-positive results [Martzloff 1938]. Nevertheless, Schiller proved that carcinoma of the cervix could be diagnosed before invasion occurred and that when adequately treated, preinvasive cancers were nearly always (96%) curable [Schiller 1927, 1933, 1937, 1938]. William P. Graves agreed that cervical cancer had an early phase, detectable with the Schiller test, when it was completely curable [*Graves 1933*]. He also recognized that asymptomatic women would have to be examined *repeatedly* to detect these lesions.

Before the era of the Pap test, carcinoma of the cervix was documented by either full thickness biopsy or curettage [*Footer 1944*]. A. Wollner detected unsuspected early carcinomas by removing the entire cervical mucosa [*Wollner 1939*]. R. Meyer reported that cervical cancer could be diagnosed from tissue fragments of superficial epithelium, removed using a curette, without observing its relation to the underlying stroma [*Meyer 1941*]. R. Knight described 17 cases of noninvasive carcinoma, among 406 primary squamous cancers of the cervix, 11 of which were unsuspected. He concluded that treatment for the noninvasive form of the disease should be just as thorough as for invasive cancer [*Knight 1943*]. However, general application of tissue biopsy was problematical owing to risks of surgery, time and expense, as well as patient acceptance, which precluded use as a screening test. By the 1940s, the groundwork was laid for an early cancer detection test that was easy to perform and that women would accept. But, the road was long and winding.

Schleiden and Schwann proposed the cell theory in 1838. By 1858, Rudolph Virchow focused the study of disease, including cancer, on the cellular level in his textbook, *Cellular Pathology*. Yet, even Virchow taught that the only reliable means of proving a tumor malignant was by demonstrating invasion into surrounding tissue. Not until the 20th century was it learned there is a preinvasive phase in the life of malignant neoplasms that can be recognized by minute changes in the cells themselves [*Papanicolaou 1943*].

In the 1920s, George Nicholas Papanicolaou, MD, PhD (1883-1962) made the discovery that eventually made him famous [*J Barter 1992, Berkow 1960, D Carmichael 1973, E Carmichael 1984, Jin 2001, TS Kline 1997, Koss 1977, 2000c, Kyle 1977, Naylor 1988, Valente 1999, Vilos 1998, Zachariadou–Veneti 2000*]. Papanicolaou held a medical degree from the University of Athens (1904) and a doctorate in zoology from the University of Munich (1910). In 1913, he emigrated from Greece to America with his wife, Andromache (Mary). After a two-day stint as a carpet salesman at Gimbals Department Store and brief service as an assistant in the department of pathology at New York Hospital, Papanicolaou found work at Cornell University in the department of anatomy, beginning in 1914 (where he remained for 47 years).

Charles R. Stockard, then chairman of anatomy at Cornell, was studying the effects of alcohol on chromosomes and the genetic transmission of any acquired defects, a subject of great popular interest just prior to Prohibition in America (1920-1933) [*Berkow 1960*]. The study involved a large guinea pig colony, and Papanicolaou saw an opportunity to use these animals for his research on reproductive endocrinology. He wanted to test the theory of sex determination by X and Y chromosomes in spermatozoa and ova [*Berkow 1960*]. For this, he needed to obtain ova at the time of polar body formation, which occurs near ovulation, but removing the ovaries or sacrificing the animals was not acceptable because that would conclude the observations [*Koss 2000c*]. The dilemma seemed insoluble, but in 1916, the solution came in the middle of the night, as if in a dream, which he recorded the next morning: "The females of all higher animals have a periodic vaginal menstrual discharge; so lower animals, such as rodents, should also have one, but one probably too scanty to be evidenced externally" [*Berkow 1960*]. The thing to do was to examine the female guinea pigs, daily, for a vaginal discharge. For this examination he used a nasal speculum. Papanicolaou later decided to obtain vaginal smears to examine microscopically. Eventually, it became possible to predict ovulation in these animals by studying their "cast off" vaginal cells.

In 1917, Papanicolaou (and Stockard) published two landmark papers on the use of vaginal cytology as an indicator of the stage of the estrous cycle in guinea pigs [*Stockard 1917a,b*]. Because the chairman's name was placed first on these

scientific reports, Stockard initially received credit for Papanicolaou's work. Papanicolaou's cytologic method allowed the effects of hormones to be assessed without ending the experiment. His biological assay spread like wildfire and helped spark a golden age in the study of reproductive endocrinology in the 1920s and 1930s [*M Casper 1998, A Clarke 1996, Vilos 1998*]. Innumerable scientific papers were published on sex hormones and their relation to amenorrhea, functional uterine bleeding, and sterility [*Berkow 1960*]. Although the importance of Papanicolaou's endocrinological research is now overshadowed by his work on cancer, at the time he was known as the "father of modern endocrinology" [*Berkow 1960*].

Papanicolaou next transferred his cytological method from zoology to medicine [*M Casper 1998*]. In 1923, he began studying the hormonal maturation of the human vaginal mucosa [*Berkow 1960*]. Because uterine cancer was so common then, it was inevitable that one day, Papanicolaou would chance upon some malignant cells. As he himself admitted, his great discovery was an example of "serendipity," but as Louis Pasteur said, "In the field of observation, chance favors the prepared mind." Papanicolaou later wrote, "the first observation of cancer cells in a smear of the uterine cervix was one of the most thrilling experiences of my scientific career" [*Papanicolaou 1955a*]. It is likely that the eminent pathologist, James Ewing, of New York's Memorial Hospital (which was, and still is, associated with Cornell), played an important role in helping Papanicolaou recognize cancer cells, because at that time, Papanicolaou had no familiarity with cancer [*Koss 2000c*]. In the beginning it was not clear whether endometrial cancers could be separated from cervical cancers or if it would be possible to diagnose cancer at an early, asymptomatic stage before it was visible clinically [*Papanicolaou 1949*].

Papanicolaou presented his *New Cancer Diagnosis* at the Third Race Betterment Conference, held in Battle Creek, Michigan, on January 4, 1928 [*Papanicolaou 1928*]. Dr. John Kellogg, brother of the cereal tycoon, hosted the Conference, which aimed at promoting eugenics. Stockard and Kellogg had both served on the advisory council of the American Eugenics Society [*Eugenics Watch 2003*]. Ironically, American eugenicists supported restrictions on immigration from nations with "inferior stock," such as Greece. Papanicolaou's contact with German biologists, while studying for his doctor of philosophy, may also have exposed him to eugenics. Kellogg was medical director of the Battle Creek Sanitarium (the "San"), where the meeting was held, and President of the Race Betterment Foundation, which he founded. The San was a world-renowned health spa for the rich and famous. Kellogg was a skilled surgeon and an early advocate of exercise and preventive medicine, or "biologic living." He also engaged in practices that were, at best, eccentric, including an obsession with the bowel, elimination, and enemas as well as the benefits of sexual abstinence (the subject of a treatise written on his honeymoon) and medical applications of electricity. (*The Road to Wellville* is based on Kellogg and the San.)

As frequently happens in science, Papanicolaou was not alone (nor even the first) in this discovery. Papanicolaou had important predecessors in the 19th century. In 1843, Gottlieb Gluge described and illustrated the cytology of scrapings of many tumors, including uterine cancer. In 1844, Alfred Donné, and in 1847, Félix-Archimède Pouchet described the cytology of vaginal secretions, although not in the context of cancer diagnosis [*Papanicolaou 1952, Spriggs 1977*]. Pouchet was apparently the first to study hormonal cytology, ie, vaginal epithelial cells in relation to the menstrual cycle [*Hajdu 1977, Koprowska 1985*]. In 1854, Lionel Smith Beale, in his book, *The Microscope, and Its Application to Clinical Medicine*, described subjecting vaginal discharge to microscopy: "In cases of cancer of the uterus, we should expect to meet with cancer cells" [*Beale 1854*]. Hermann Lebert illustrated cells exfoliated from a cervical carcinoma in his *Atlas of 1861* [*Lebert 1861, Naylor 2000*]. WH Dickenson, in 1869, examined discharges from women with cervical cancer, but failed to find diagnostic cells: "In case of carcinoma of the uterus I have often examined the discharge but never succeeded in finding anything diagnostic of the disease" [Hajdu 1977]. In 1871, JG Richardson advocated cytologic examination of patients clinically suspected of having uterine cancer [Richardson 1871, Spriggs 1977]. In 1886, C Friedlaender used the cytologic method to diagnose cervical cancer, but recommended confirmation by examination of a small piece of excised tissue (which a decade later became known as a "biopsy") [Friedlaender 1886, Spriggs 1977]. Thus, vaginal smears had been examined, and exfoliated cancer cells had been detected, long before Papanicolaou [Koprowska 1985].

In the 20th century, F. Lehmann made a study of the value of the human vaginal smear, from a pathologic and diagnostic point of view in 1921 [F Lehmann 1921]. Then, Aurel A. Babès (1886-1962), a Romanian pathologist, published a paper entitled, in translation, "The possibility of diagnosing uterine cancer by the smear technic" in the Proceedings of the Conference of the Gynecologic Society of Bucharest of January 23, 1927 [Koprowska 1985, Naylor 1988, 2002, Tasca 2002, Wied 1964]. Babès elaborated on his findings in another paper, translated, "Diagnosis of Cancer of the Uterine Cervix by Means of Smears," in April 1928 in *La Presse Medicale* [Babès 1928, Douglass 1967, Grosskopf 1978]. Babès examined 20 biopsy proven cases of invasive squamous cell carcinoma of the cervix. The material was obtained with a platinum bacteriologic loop, spread on a glass slide, fixed in methanol, and stained with Giemsa. He compared these findings with those in a number of benign conditions [Tasca 2002]. Babès proposed that a cytologic diagnosis of preinvasive carcinoma was possible many years before this concept was generally accepted [Koss 2002]. Later, in a 1931 paper, Babès wrote that Kermauner and Schiller had used a modified vaginal smear method for the diagnosis of cervical cancer on a large scale with very good results [Babès 1931, Koprowska 1981]. However, Babès apparently had no thought of applying this technique to *asymptomatic* women; indeed this idea seemed revolutionary even when Papanicolaou introduced it nearly 20 years later [Naylor 2002]. Despite having published nearly 300 scientific articles and books during his career, Babès wrote little else on cytopathology [Naylor 2002].

Another early player in the cytologic detection of cervical cancer was Odorico Viana (1877-1942), an Italian gynecologist [Douglass 1970]. In 1928, influenced both by his countryman, Scalabrino, and by Babès, Viana reported favorably on his own experiences with smear diagnosis, stressing the importance of the new technique, which he considered a type of biopsy [Viana 1928, 1933].

By the late 1920s, incipient carcinoma had been described, and efforts, including the colposcope and the Schiller test, were underway to diagnose cancer in an early, curable stage. It would seem that the time was ripe for the cytologic method of early cancer diagnosis, but the time was out of joint, at least in America. Papanicolaou's findings had practically no impact at the time. A transcript of his address appeared in the *Proceedings* of the Third Race Betterment Conference, but was apparently not approved by Papanicolaou, because it contained critical stenographic errors (eg, repeatedly transcribing "cancerous cells" as "conscious cells"). In addition, Papanicolaou claimed that specific changes in monocytes "makes possible the diagnosis of cancer morphologically in cases where cancer cells are not present" [Papanicolaou 1928]. A colleague recollected that Papanicolaou's "presentation was weakly received and almost rebuffed by many especially the pathologists" [Marchetti 1969]. Indeed, it must have been practically incomprehensible to the few who read it. The *New York World* newspaper carried a short article on his presentation the following day, but the only other reference to his cancer detection technique (and, indeed, the *only* publication ever actually written by Papanicolaou himself on this subject until 1941 [*New*

Cancer Diagnosis was a poor transcription of an oral presentation]) was a brief mention in his 1933 monograph, *The Sexual Cycle in the Human Female as Revealed by Vaginal Smears* [Papanicolaou 1933].

Why Papanicolaou chose not to report his cytologic cancer detection method in a recognized medical journal before 1941 is an enigma, but he may have been discouraged by James Ewing, whose dogmatic opinion was that since the uterine cervix was accessible to biopsy, the use of the cytologic examination was superfluous [Papanicolaou 1955a]. Moreover, Papanicolaou's work came at a time when histologic techniques were being perfected and cytologic methods were on the wane. The idea of diagnosing cancer on exfoliated cells was absurd, if not horrifying, to pathologists (who asked, "How can one expect to interpret changes in single cells when there is still much confusion about the histologic diagnosis of tissue specimens containing thousands of cells?" [R Scott 1962]), and moreover, Papanicolaou was an outsider, an anatomist, not a pathologist. Martin and Ellis's landmark paper on needle aspiration biopsy, published at nearly the same time, in 1930 (and from the same place, Memorial Hospital, where Ewing practiced), also met with little enthusiasm at first [H Martin 1930]. Papanicolaou's own view was that his work was poorly received owing to technical problems (including his early fixation and staining method), pathologists' preference for tissue biopsies, and gynecologists' interest in the menstrual cycle per se rather than cancer [M Casper 1998, Papanicolaou 1958]. In short, Papanicolaou was in the wrong place at the wrong time [V Schneider 1995].

Disappointed by the lack of support for his *New Cancer Diagnosis*, Papanicolaou continued his study of reproductive endocrinology [Michalas 2000, Papanicolaou 1958]. Then, in 1939, Joseph C. Hinsey, the new chairman of anatomy at Cornell, urged Papanicolaou to return to his work on cancer detection via the vaginal smear [Hinsey 1962, Marchetti 1969]. Hinsey thought there might be more merit (not to mention more money) in research into cancer of the female genital tract than in the menstrual cycle [Koss 2002]. Together, they outlined a three-step program, first to establish the validity of the cytologic method, then to train others to use it, and finally to educate the medical profession and the public concerning what the method had to offer [D Carmichael 1973]. Hinsey also arranged collaborations with Herbert F. Traut, a gynecologist trained in pathology, and Andrew Marchetti, who later became chairman of the department of obstetrics and gynecology at Cornell. This collaboration provided Papanicolaou with a wealth of material to study: every woman admitted to the gynecology service was required to have a vaginal smear.

Papanicolaou applied to three societies for funding for cancer research, but was turned down [Berkow 1960]. Then, in 1940, Lester Evans, medical director of the Commonwealth Fund, began supporting Papanicolaou's research, providing a total of $124,000 over the next decade, a sizable sum in those days [M Casper 1998]. Papanicolaou first focused on development of a new staining technique, which included wet fixation in an ether-alcohol solution [Papanicolaou 1942]. Papanicolaou's research showed that the vaginal smear permitted a much earlier cancer diagnosis than would have been possible by biopsy (which was still preferred by pathologists) and that the diagnosis was made only because vaginal smears had been taken *repeatedly* [D Carmicheal 1973]. Papanicolaou later said, "by far the most important feature of Exfoliative Cytology is that it has furnished us with the means of detecting cancer in its incipiency" [Papanicolaou 1958]. (The word, exfoliative, was coined by Papanicolaou and derives from Greek, *ex*-away, and Latin, *follium*-leaf; hence, the meaning is similar to leaves falling away from a tree [Koprowska 1977].) Diagnosis of small, localized tumors meant that surgical and radiation therapies available at the time could not only cure the cancer in an individual woman, but might even eradicate the disease from the human race.

In 1941, Papanicolaou and Traut published their historic paper, *The Diagnostic Value of Vaginal Smears in Carcinoma of the Uterus*, in the American Journal of Obstetrics and Gynecology [Papanicolaou 1941]. Their classic monograph, *Diagnosis of Uterine Cancer by the Vaginal Smear*, was underwritten by the Commonwealth Fund and published in 1943 [Papanicolaou 1943]. Hashime Murayama, an artist who had worked for National Geographic, illustrated the manuscript with beautiful camera lucida watercolor drawings. This short monograph (48 pages of text plus 11 color plates with descriptions) introduced the technique of diagnosing uterine cancer by cytology, as well as the possibility of detecting early cervical cancer, to a broad audience [S Long 1991]. Publication of this monograph marked the turning point in the attitude of the medical profession [Ayre 1946, Foote 1948a,b, Fremont–Smith 1947, CA Jones 1945, Pund 1947]. Even Ewing became a proponent of the cytologic method before he died (of bladder cancer detected cytologically) [D Carmichael 1973].

A substantial practical problem was the overwhelming amount of work that cytologic screening of the entire adult female population for cancer represented. Furthermore, most women were expected to be normal, so the number of smears that had to be reviewed to find a positive case seemed daunting. In response, a new profession was born, cytotechnology. But, many difficulties remained, including educating a host of professionals to acquire and read Pap smears as well as convincing the public of the value of the test.

The Pap smear was given a tremendous boost in 1945, by the newly renamed and restructured American Cancer Society (ACS). Begun in 1913 to warn women of the danger signs of uterine cancer, by 1943 the ACS had a "Women's Field Army" of 350,000 volunteers. The ACS was transforming itself from an educational organization into a major sponsor of biomedical research. In 1943, the annual budget was $102,000; by 1945, it was over $4 million and rising [M Casper 1998].

In 1945, Charles Cameron, the director of the ACS, became a major advocate of the Pap smear as a core focus for research, cancer prevention, and early intervention. At about the same time, the US Public Health Service was revitalizing the National Cancer Institute (NCI). The Pap smear fit well with the goal of early intervention promulgated by the ACS and the NCI. It was a simple technique that could help fulfill their slogan, "Every Doctor's Office a Cancer Detection Center," without the need for elaborate or expensive new technologies [M Casper 1998]. At last, Papanicolaou was in the right place at the right time, and nothing is so powerful as an idea whose time has come (Victor Hugo).

Shortly after Papanicolaou's publications, more studies confirmed the value of the cytologic method [Ayre 1944, CA Jones 1945, Meigs 1943, 1945]. It also was confirmed that the test could detect precancerous changes still confined to the epithelium of the cervix [Ayre 1948, Foote 1948a, Pund 1947]. The Pap test was hailed as the ultimate tool in cancer detection and prevention [Koss 1989a]. In 1947, Papanicolaou began offering cytology-training courses at Cornell. Another milestone for the cytologic technique was reached in 1948, when at the urging of Cameron, the ACS sponsored the First National Cytology Conference in Boston [Papanicolaou 1958]. More and bigger conferences followed. Cameron asked Arthur Holleb, a recent medical graduate who later became a renowned surgical oncologist [Hutter 2000], to persuade pathologists and gynecologists to embrace Pap testing, which he did with great success [M Casper 1998, A Clarke 1996]. The Inter-Society Cytology Council, the forerunner of the American Society of Cytology (now the American Society of Cytopathology) was founded in 1951. Joe Meigs, doyen of American gynecologists, was the first president; later, Papanicolaou became president [Naylor 1988]. The first International Cancer Cytology Congress was held at the Drake Hotel in Chicago in 1956. The International Academy of Gynecologic Cytology, later known as the International Academy of Cytology,

was founded in 1957 with 56 members from 21 countries [Naylor 1988]. Ruth M. Graham published the first modern comprehensive cytology text, *The Cytologic Diagnosis of Cancer*, in 1950. The first issue of *Acta Cytologica* appeared in 1957, with George L. Wied as editor-in-chief.

Physicians were now enthusiastic about the possibility of completely conquering cervical cancer. By the late 1940s, cytology laboratories were opening, and by the 1950s, Pap test screening was becoming widespread, even before clinical trials could be performed to prove its value [Koss 1993a]. In the 1950s, the ACS and the NCI initiated major public health screening studies involving tens of thousands of women in multiple locations [A Clarke 1996, R Nelson 1951, Sandmire 1976]. In the early 1960s, 30% of women had at least one Pap test, but by the 1990s, more than 90% of adult women had been screened at least once [CDC 1999, Holmquist 2000, Pretorius 1991]. In the 1970s and 1980s, reports on large-scale screening programs from several countries confirmed the value of mass screening for precancerous lesions of the cervix [JL Benedet 1981, Christopherson 1976, Hakama 1988, Johannesson 1982, Lääri 1987, Macgregor 1976, 1978b, A Miller 1976]. For example, the mortality rate of cervical cancer fell by more than two-thirds following introduction of screening programs in regions of the United States [Christopherson 1977b] and Canada [G Anderson 1988]. Furthermore, the reduction in mortality was directly related to the level of screening [D Cramer 1974a, Lääri 1987, Macgregor 1978b, A Miller 1976]. Unexpectedly, however, in the late 1980s, the incidence, and then the mortality, of cervical cancer climbed slightly, before resuming a downward trend in the 1990s (see below).

Papanicolaou's original method acquired vaginal pool secretions using a pipette and rubber suction bulb: these samples were easy to obtain, but difficult to screen. It was also recognized that there were relatively few cervical cells present in vaginal smears and that spontaneously exfoliated cells were often poorly preserved. In 1947, J. Ernest Ayre introduced the method known today as the conventional Pap smear, in which a simple device, the Ayre spatula, was used to scrape cells directly from the cervix, which were then literally smeared on a glass slide [Ayre 1947, 1948].

By the time Papanicolaou published his *Atlas of Exfoliative Cytology* in 1954 [Papanicolaou 1954], it was clear that the cytologic technique could be extended to virtually any body site [Papanicolaou 1949, Breathnach 1983]. The *Atlas* was considered the bible of cytology and earned Papanicolaou the honor of being known as "the father of modern cytology." Papanicolaou was repeatedly nominated for the Nobel Prize in Medicine, and although he was not chosen, many thought he deserved the award [Broso 1993, Koss 2000c, 2002, Koprowska 1985, Naylor 1988, Tasca 2002]. By 1961, doctors were nearly ready to write the epitaph for cervical carcinoma, thanks to Papanicolaou [Lund 1961]. In 1978, the United States honored him with a postage stamp. Papanicolaou's name became had become a household word. But then, clouds gathered on the horizon [Boronow 1998].

In theory, cervical cancer should be completely preventable, but in practice, cervical cancer has never been completely eradicated, even where there are well-organized screening programs [Fidler 1968, Koss 1989a]. This was a bitter disappointment. Unfortunately, some problems proved insurmountable, including: reaching all women, including high-risk, low income women; consistently obtaining satisfactory, representative samples; achieving and maintaining high laboratory standards; and providing appropriate clinical follow-up of women with abnormal results [Koss 1989a]. Furthermore, because the mortality of cervical cancer had been falling even before the Pap test was introduced, some questioned its effect on preventing this disease [Pontén 1995]. Indeed, screening programs seemed ineffective because the number of precancerous lesions of the cervix actually *increased* dramatically, following the "sexual revolution" in the late 1960s (after "the pill" became available). It also turned out that the microscopic assessment of cervical cancer precursor lesions was difficult, subjective, and irreproducible [Holmquist 1967b, A Robertson 1989b, Seybolt 1971, Siegler 1956]. And even if it were possible to diagnose lesions, it was impossible to predict their behavior in individual women: the lesions could progress, persist, or regress [Boyes 1962, Koss 1963, M Jordan 1964, K Nasiell 1983, 1986, Richart 1968].

By the 1970s, it was becoming apparent that the Pap test was not a panacea for cervical cancer. Failure of the Pap test to discover all precursor lesions before cancer developed was well documented in the scientific literature [Adcock 1982, Berkowitz 1979, Cecchini 1985, Fetherston 1983, Foltz 1978, Gompel 1974, Gunn 1973, Rylander 1976, van der Graaf 1987a,b]. In fact, from the earliest days there were concerns about the problem of false diagnoses [Isbell 1947, Papanicolaou 1943]. Although the first Pap test-related lawsuit dates from the late 1960s (filed in California), probably the first public alarm involving Pap test failures was sounded by the United States Air Force in 1977. A former employee made allegations of inaccuracies against a laboratory the Air Force had contracted for reading Pap tests, charging that technologists were given screening quotas and that too many slides were being read. The Air Force eventually turned the matter over to the Federal Bureau of Investigation. The laboratory's slides (some 700,000) were seized, a batch of 1200 "normal" slides was reviewed, and "a 3 percent discrepancy rate" was found, which "consisted mainly of slides which were of too poor a quality to be read at all" and "a small number" that were suspicious [Anonymous 1978]. It is left to the reader to judge these results.

In the early days, there was no quality control, rescreening, histologic correlation, or proficiency testing, and results were reported using the then-accepted Papanicolaou classification system [Frable 1995]. At that time, however, the service was being provided to the public inexpensively, often as a "loss leader" to attract other laboratory business, a practice now regarded as questionable by some [Pelchich 1997, Perey 1998]. (This practice also made it more difficult to collect reasonable fees for Pap tests in later times, because they were offered so cheaply in the past [Dupree 1998].) However, providing low cost Pap tests was viewed as a public service [Lund 1961]. In the early days, it took an average of 15 to 20 minutes to read a slide, and up to two hours for a particularly difficult case [Isbell 1947]. Papanicolaou himself would sometimes spend hours studying a slide.

Then, in late 1987, the Wall Street Journal published a front page, two-part investigative report by Walt Bogdanich, which won the Pulitzer Prize for journalism, and generated considerable "bad press" for the Pap test. Bogdanich described the deaths of young women from cervical cancer, citing "lax laboratories" and "physicians' carelessness" with Pap tests as the cause [Bogdanich 1987a,b]. Sensational copycat stories soon appeared in weekly news magazines and on television. The Pap test was denounced on prime time television for its "failure" to prevent cancer in a woman who turned out to have endometrial, not cervical, carcinoma and, in any event, was cured of her disease. Over the next several years the incidence *and the mortality* of cervical carcinoma increased in the United States before resuming a downward trend. Could the media frenzy have caused a loss of faith in the Pap test so that, for a time, more women failed to get tested regularly and died?

In response to public outcry, the United States Congress hastily passed the Clinical Laboratory Improvement Act of 1988 (CLIA '88), which President Reagan signed on Halloween of that election year. CLIA '88 imposed severe—and expensive—restrictions on the practice of gynecologic cytology in the United States. With the Wall Street Journal articles providing a blue print for litigation, Pap test-related lawsuits became a growth industry for crusading trial lawyers who were out to do good (and not coincidentally, to do well) [Briselli 1995]. In a decidedly modern twist, malpractice lawyers solicited "victims" on the Internet. Multimillion-dollar malpractice awards became common. By the 1990s, Pap test-related litigation accounted for 40% of pathology malpractice claims

[Skoumal 1997]. And, in a chilling development, *homicide* was charged against a laboratory for misreading a Pap smear [Voelker 1995]. This story was carried on the front page of newspapers nationwide, as well as on television, and according to the plaintiff's attorney, "every women's magazine." But, at the end of the day, no plaintiff's attorney ever saved a woman's life [D McCoy 2000].

The year 1988 also saw the first of a series of consensus conferences, convening in Bethesda, Maryland, which developed a standardized protocol for reporting of gynecologic cytology, known as the Bethesda System. The Bethesda System introduced the terminology of "squamous intraepithelial lesion" (SIL) and "atypical squamous cells of undetermined significance" (ASCUS), among other innovations. Also beginning in the late 1980s, a new industry was born, devoted to cervical cancer screening. Advances included liquid-based processing, computer-assisted screening, and human papillomavirus-testing. As always, costs must be weighed against benefits. Cervical cancer screening tests, which were once offered for as little as one dollar [Lund 1961], could now cost 50 to 100 *times* as much. The reality is that cervical cancer occurs primarily in the underscreened population. Improving the test provides no benefit to women who are not tested, but increasing the cost makes it more likely that more will go unscreened [Janicek 2001]. On the other hand, a better test could make less frequent screening more cost-effective and reduce the risk of cancer in those who are tested.

There is nothing more difficult in pathology than the interpretation of the cytology of the uterine cervix [Koss 2000a]. To say the least, the current medicolegal and regulatory environment has not made the practice of cytology any easier. But, thanks to the remarkable diligence of dedicated professionals, cytology has become, and remains, a dominant force in cancer detection and prevention. The mortality of cervical cancer has fallen by at least 70%-80% since the introduction of the Pap test. Keep in mind that this figure includes all women; counting only those who are screened regularly, the mortality of cervical cancer has fallen more than 90%! The Pap test has saved many women's lives and prevented untold human suffering [Vilos 1998]. We can be proud of this!

Anatomy and Embryology of the Female Genital Tract

The female genital tract comprises the vulva, vagina, uterus including the cervix, fallopian tubes, and ovaries [F1]. Embryologically, the primordial ovarian germ cells arise in the wall of the yolk sac and migrate into the urogenital ridge. Mesothelium of the urogenital ridge proliferates, incorporating the germ cells, eventually producing the epithelium and stroma of the ovary. So, the germ cells are of endodermal origin and the remainder of the ovary is of mesodermal origin. The fallopian tubes, uterus, and upper vagina develop from the Müllerian (para-mesonephric) ducts [Krantz 1967, E Stern 1973]. The lateral Müllerian ducts develop as an invagination and fusion of the coelomic lining epithelium (mesothelium). The caudal portions fuse, forming the uterus and upper vagina. The unfused portions form the fallopian tubes, or oviducts. The fused duct contacts the urogenital sinus, which forms the lower vagina and vestibule. The linings of the uterus (endometrium) and fallopian tubes (endosalpinx), as well as the ovarian surface, are all derived from coelomic epithelium. Tumors of these sites are morphologically similar. The lining of the upper vagina is of Müllerian origin and is originally a glandular epithelium, but normally changes in utero to squamous epithelium. If this process is interrupted, eg, by diethylstilbestrol (DES), remnants of glandular tissue may persist in the vagina (vaginal adenosis) [Herbst 1972]. The lower vagina, of urogenital sinus origin, is lined by squamous epithelium.

F1 Drawing of Female Genital Tract

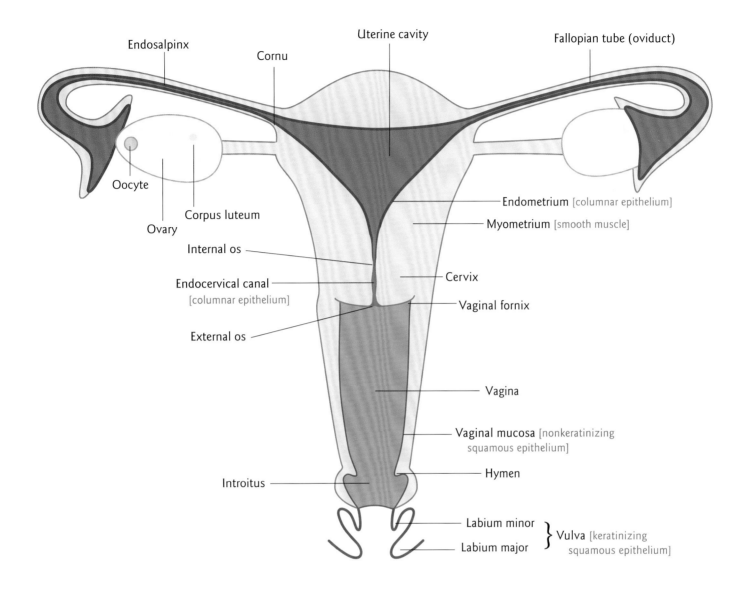

The ovaries each measure about 3 x 2 x 1 cm in women of reproductive age, but increase in size during pregnancy and atrophy after menopause. A single layer of serosal cells, which originate from coelomic epithelium, and are continuous with mesothelium, covers the ovary. The ovary itself is divided into three poorly defined layers: an outer cortex, an inner medulla, and a central hilus. The outer portion of the cortex is a poorly cellular collagenous zone, sometimes known as the tunica albuginea. The inner cortex and medulla are continuous and composed of ovarian stromal tissue. The ovarian stroma consists of densely packed bundles of spindle-shaped stromal cells that secrete androgens, primarily androstenedione, and lesser amounts of testosterone, as well as other hormones. Ovarian follicles, located predominantly in the cortex, produce estrogen. Each menstrual cycle, one follicle usually develops into a bright yellow body, or corpus luteum, which produces progesterone. It eventually scarifies into a white body, or corpus albicans, that usually disappears. Luteinized stromal cells usually occur in the medulla; these are sources of androgens. Hilus cells are epithelioid cells surrounded by loose mesenchymal tissue; they primarily secrete androstenedione.

Every menstrual cycle, under the influence of pituitary follicle stimulating hormone (FSH) and luteinizing hormone (LH), many primordial follicles begin to ripen, but usually only one follicle becomes dominant and ripens completely, releasing an oocyte (ovulation). Estrogen production from the ovarian follicle peaks sharply just before ovulation, and then falls [F2]. After

F2 Daily Variation of Ovarian Hormones

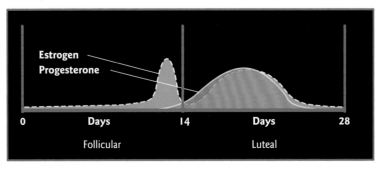

9

ovulation, around day 14, the estrogen levels slowly rise again, to a plateau around day 21, then fall again, beginning 3 or 4 days before the next menstruation. The level of progesterone, produced by the corpus luteum, increases through the second half of the cycle, and falls just before menses.

The fallopian tubes (oviducts, named for the Italian anatomist, Gabriel Fallopius, d 1562) are lined by three cell types, ciliated columnar cells, secretory columnar cells, and intercalated cells. On cross section, the mucosa is thrown into a series of folds, or plicae, that resemble papillae.

The uterus (womb) is a pear-shaped organ that measures about 8 x 5 x 3 cm during the reproductive years, and ranges from 50 g (nulliparous) to 100 g (multiparous). After menopause, the uterus atrophies. The uterus comprises the body (corpus), the lower uterine segment, and the cervix (neck).

The uterine corpus is made mostly of smooth muscle, but has a cavity lined by glandular tissue, the endometrium. Endometrium undergoes cyclic changes during the reproductive years that are governed by ovarian hormones, which in turn are under control of the hypothalamic-pituitary axis.

The cervix has an outer, vaginal portion (portio vaginalis, or ectocervix), visible during vaginal examination, an external os and internal os ("mouth" or opening), and the endocervix, a canal lined predominantly by glandular tissue. The protrusion of the cervix into the vagina creates folds of tissue, known as fornices (singular, fornix), with anterior, lateral (two), and posterior folds. Exfoliated cells tend to pool in the fornices. At birth, the portio vaginalis is covered by stratified squamous epithelium. In the endocervix, deep infoldings of the mucosa tunnel into the endocervical stroma, forming crypts that histologically look like branching glands, but are not true glands [E Stem 1973]. A simple columnar epithelium lines these mucosal folds, which are known as plicae palmatae.

The squamocolumnar junction is the point at which the cervical squamous and glandular epithelia meet. Before puberty, the squamocolumnar junction is normally at the external os: this is known as the original squamocolumnar junction. However, after puberty, the cervix changes configuration, and endocervical mucosa is exposed on the portio vaginalis, where it is visible as a red zone (properly called ectropion or eversion, but often incorrectly referred to as an erosion) [Briggs 1979]. Ectropion can also occur as a result of hormonal influences, including some oral contraceptives, and in particular, pregnancy. The acidic environment of the vagina then causes the glandular epithelium to transform into a squamous epithelium (squamous metaplasia). This transformation, or metaplasia, is accomplished by reserve cells of the endocervix differentiating into squamous cells instead of glandular cells [R Carmichael 1941, Krantz 1967]. The "transformation zone" is of particular interest because it is the area in which most cervical neoplasia develops. After menopause, the cervix atrophies and the squamocolumnar junction retreats into the endocervical canal.

The vagina (and also, the urethra) opens into the vestibule of the vulva. The vaginal introitus contains mucin-secreting glands, including Bartholin glands, in the lower vaginal wall. The vagina is normally lined by nonkeratinized squamous epithelium. It is sensitive to estrogen and progesterone, undergoes cyclic changes in women of reproductive years, and then atrophies.

The vulva comprises the labia majora and minora, both covered with keratinizing, stratified squamous epithelium. The outer surface of labia majora is hair bearing. The inner surface of the labia majora contains numerous sebaceous and apocrine sweat glands. The labia minora and the clitoris are devoid of hair and skin appendages, but have numerous sebaceous glands. The degree of keratinization of the epithelium diminishes from the outer to the inner aspect of the labia, which has only a thin layer of keratin. This epithelium covers the vestibule, as far as the hymen.

I. Cytology of the Squamous Epithelium

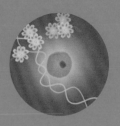

A Simplifying Synopsis of Pap Test Interpretation

The Pap test is the "bread and butter" of clinical cytology, and because of its remarkable success in cancer prevention, the general perception of the uninformed is that Pap test interpretation is easy. But it isn't. Pap test interpretation is difficult and subjective—one of the most mentally challenging chores in all of pathology. To most people—and this includes most health care providers—the Pap test is a black box: put cells in one end and a result comes out the other. The simplicity of the conventional method—smear some cells on a slide and take a look under the microscope—reinforces this misconception that the Pap test is simple. But, if you lift the lid to peak inside the box, instead of a well-oiled machine humming away, you find a sputtering Rube Goldberg contraption.

The technoscience of the Pap test includes women, cytologists, pathologists, an array of medical and technical practices, clinical infrastructure, including obstetrician/gynecologists, other physicians, nurses, and other health care providers, family planning clinics, community and other hospitals, public health departments, laboratories, shipping facilities, computers, and so on—in short, all the people, places, and things, that ultimately crank out a Pap test result [A Clarke 1996]. Moreover, the Pap test exists not only in a medical-scientific-technical context, but also in social, historical, economic, political, cultural, and of course, legal contexts as well [M Casper 1998, V Lane 1997, Plaut 1959]. Most of this is well beyond the scope of the present work.

This section will briefly explain the workings of the black box: to dissect, analyze, and simplify the underlying concepts of interpreting the Pap test. Like dismantling a clock, there are lots of small parts, and it may be not be obvious how they go back together again. The following synopsis illustrates how the major parts fit together (applies only to squamous cell carcinoma).

At the most basic level, in carcinogenesis, for some reason the tissue goes haywire, and changes from *normal* to *abnormal* to *cancer*. Human papillomavirus is now known to be the monkey wrench in the works (the "works" being the cell cycle machinery). The abnormalities, or precursor lesions, are not cancer, but sometimes develop into cancer if left untreated. Precursor lesions are named and graded. Various names have been used over the years. The traditional nomenclature is dysplasia/carcinoma in situ; this was followed by cervical intraepithelial neoplasia (CIN); and most recently, the Bethesda System, with its squamous intraepithelial lesion (SIL). Precursor lesions are also graded: in theory, the higher the grade, the higher the risk of cancer.

There are three key points about the progression from normal to abnormal to cancer. First, progression *takes time*: usually several years, sometimes even decades. Second, progression is *not inevitable*: millions of women have lesions, but relatively few develop cancer. Third, progression is *unpredictable* in individual women, leading to a dilemma regarding the cost of treating all lesions vs the risk of not treating all of them [Cuzick 1994, Herbst 1990a, 1992, JM Hunt 1994, Koss 1993b, Kühler–Obbarius 1994a, Kurman 1994, Richart 1993].

In theory, the Pap test works by its ability to *detect* the abnormalities preceding cancer, which usually develops slowly. Once detected, the abnormalities can then be *destroyed* (using loop electrocautery excision procedure [LEEP], cryotherapy, laser vaporization, or excision), thereby preventing cancer. Two additional important points: first, no one ever died of precursor lesions. In fact, precursor lesions are usually asymptomatic [C Mao 2003]. In a way, this is unfortunate because if precursor lesions were symptomatic, women would seek treatment, and the Pap test would be unnecessary. Second, because progression usually takes years, there is usually a "long window of opportunity" to detect precursor lesions. But, we cannot be complacent about Pap test screening, because the Pap test is not perfect.

In practice, the Pap test is a complex system and complex systems are subject to failure, particularly when they depend upon perfect human performance. The sensitivity of the conventional Pap smear may be as low as 50% [Fahey 1995, Franco 2000, Giard 2001, Hartman 2001, ML Hutchinson 1999, Martin–Hirsch 2002, McCrory 1999, Nanda 2000, Renshaw 2002b]. Limitations include problems with sampling ("no cells, no diagnosis") and microscopy. Microscopy limitations include problems with screening (failure to find abnormal cells) and interpretation (failure to properly categorize cells). To put it bluntly, the Pap test simply *cannot* detect all significant abnormalities: lesions come, lesions go, but may come back again. Some lesions evade cytologic detection (owing to few, small, or bland cells; hyperchromatic crowded groups; adenocarcinomas; obscuration [eg, excess blood or exudate, degeneration]; etc). Still, most women who get cervical cancer never had a Pap test, or haven't had one recently. Unfortunately, however, some women develop cancer even though they have been regularly screened.

Introduction to Intepretation

Many of the concepts, as well as the morphometry, to be discussed are based on Stanley Patten's classic monograph, *Diagnostic Cytopathology of the Uterine Cervix* [Patten 1978]. This monograph is highly recommended reading [Bonfiglio 1997]. (***Important note: the morphometric measurements presented in this text were made on cells from conventional Pap smears, not liquid-based cytology, unless otherwise stated.**)

During normal maturation, the squamous epithelium of the uterine cervix can be conceptualized as differentiating from *basal cells* to *parabasal cells* to *intermediate cells* to *superficial cells*. These four cell types, the "Icons," are the keys to the most common daily problem in Pap test interpretation, ie, "Is it is, or is it ain't, dysplasia?" (Note: Other terms for dysplasia, cervical intraepithelial neoplasia [CIN] and squamous intraepithelial lesion [SIL], will be used interchangeably, as appropriate

---

Pathogenesis of Cervical Cancer

Normal → Abnormal* → Cancer

*Abnormalities (precursor lesions)

  Not cancer, but can develop into cancer

  Named: Dysplasia/CIS; CIN; SIL

  Graded: Higher grade ⟹ higher risk

Key points about progression:

  1. Usually takes several years

  2. Not inevitable: Millions of SILs; <1% CA

  3. Unpredictable: Cost Rx vs Risk No Rx

How the Pap Test Works: Theory

Cervical CA usually develops slowly

Normal → Abnormal → Cancer

1. Pap test detects abnormalities

  preceding cancer

2. Abnormalities destroyed (LEEP, etc)

  preventing cancer

No one ever died of precursor lesions

  Usually asymptomatic

Long "window of opportunity"

  But cannot be complacent, because...

How the Pap Test Works: Practice

...the Pap test is not perfect!

  Complex system, subject to failure

  Miss lesions in sampling and microscopy

Works by doing it over & over again

  Lesions missed in one screening usually

  picked up in the next 1 or 2

Regular screening crucial

Most failures: inadequate screening

---

to their definitions, throughout the text.) [T1.1]. Dysplasia mimics these four iconic cell types.

T1.1 Rosetta Stone for Deciphering Various Diagnostic Terminologies

Traditional Nomenclature	CIN	The Bethesda System
(Condyloma)	(Condyloma)	L SIL
Mild dysplasia	CIN 1	L SIL
Moderate dysplasia	CIN 2	H SIL
Severe dysplasia	CIN 3	H SIL
Carcinoma in situ	CIN 3	H SIL

CIN, cervical intraepithelial neoplasia; L SIL, low-grade squamous intraepithelial lesion; H SIL, high-grade squamous intraepithelial lesion

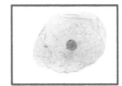

The intermediate cell, or more precisely, its nucleus, is of particular interest because it serves as a benchmark for nuclear size and chromatin quality (texture and staining). Nuclear features are critical in interpreting cells in the Pap test.

There are two questions to answer vis-à-vis dysplasia. The first question is: "Is the cell dysplastic?" Compare the nucleus of the cell in question with an intermediate cell nucleus; in essence, *"if it's big and it's dark—it's dysplasia."* The area of an intermediate cell nucleus is about 35 μm^2, which is about the size of a red blood cell. Dysplastic nuclei range from 120 μm^2-200$^+$ μm^2, or more than three times the area of an intermediate cell nucleus [Patten 1978].

Next, if—and only if—the cell is dysplastic, the second question is: "How dysplastic is it?" Evaluate the nuclear /cytoplasmic (N/C) ratio. The higher the nuclear/cytoplasmic ratio, the more advanced the dysplasia [Maeda 1997]. Carcinoma in situ exfoliates hyperchromatic crowded groups of undifferentiated abnormal cells with very high N/C ratios [DeMay 2000].

Now, to make an oversimplification [T1.2]: mild dysplasia (CIN 1, low-grade squamous intraepithelial lesion) usually resembles mature cells (ie, intermediate to superficial cells with "big, dark" nuclei); moderate dysplasia (CIN 2, low end of spectrum of high-grade squamous intraepithelial lesions) usually resembles metaplastic cells (parabasal-sized cells with "big, dark" nuclei); and severe dysplasia/carcinoma in situ (CIN 3, high end of spectrum of high-grade squamous intraepithelial lesion) usually resembles basal cells (with "big, dark" nuclei). High-grade dysplastic lesions can also be characterized by pleomorphic, abnormally keratinized cells. Koilocytes (ie, mature squamous cells with large,

well-defined cytoplasmic vacuoles, or halos, and atypical—big, dark—nuclei) are pathognomonic of condyloma/human papillomavirus (HPV) infection, a form of low-grade squamous intraepithelial lesion.

Perhaps surprisingly, the largest nuclei in the whole spectrum of carcinogenesis, ranging from normal squamous cells to invasive squamous carcinoma, are found in mild dysplasia (CIN 1, low-grade SIL). Hence, low-grade SILs have the biggest, "ugliest" nuclei, occur in the largest (most mature) cells, and tend to be conspicuous. On the other hand, high-grade dysplasias can sometimes shed teeny-tiny little cells, which make them difficult to detect ("no-see-ums," Ruth Graham's third type cells [R Graham 1961]), with subtle cytologic abnormalities, which can make them difficult interpret (look like squamous metaplasia or even histiocytes [Montes 1999, PA Smith 1997]).

Carcinoma in situ (CIS), the most advanced form of high-grade SIL (H-SIL), characteristically exfoliates crowded groups of cells with hyperchromatic nuclei ("hyperchromatic crowded groups" or HCGs [DeMay 2000]) classically described as syncytial aggregates (though they are not true syncytia). Unfortunately, there are many morphologically similar HCGs (ranging from benign endometrial cells to invasive cancers) that can cause interpretive problems [Boon 1991, DeMay 2000, Goff 1992, K Lee 1995, MV Harris 2000, Stanbridge 1980].

In liquid-based cytology, the cytologic features of dysplasia/carcinoma in situ are essentially similar to those in conventional Pap smears. The findings in low-grade SILs are practically identical to those in conventional Pap smears and in fact, if anything, the abnormal cells tend to stand out even more conspicuously in LBC. However, high-grade SILs can be even more subtle in LBC. Nuclear hyperchromasia can be minimal and the nuclei tend to be smaller and more uniform. Therefore, other interpretive criteria, such as irregular nuclear membranes (nuclei that look like brains in bottles), assume increased importance. Interpretation of hyperchromatic crowded groups can be more difficult in LBC, because it can be harder to examine the cells at the edges, which is often the best clue to the nature of the groups.

Two Basic Concepts: Squamous Differentiation & Carcinogenesis

Simplification is the secret to understanding the bewildering array of benign, premalignant, and malignant conditions that can affect the uterine cervix. Using just two basic concepts, squamous differentiation and carcinogenesis, a simple chart that illustrates the fundamental principles of Pap test interpretation can be constructed. The cytologic manifestations of squamous differentiation and carcinogenesis are seen primarily in the cytoplasm and nucleus of the cell, respectively.

> *Two Fundamental Concepts*
> *1. Squamous differentiation (Cytoplasm)*
>   *Dense cytoplasm, distinct cell borders*
>   *Cells: Basal, parabasal, intermediate, superficial*
> *2. Carcinogenesis (Nucleus)*
>   *Size, outline, chromatin, nucleoli, N/C*
>   *Lesions: Dysplasia, CIS, MicroCA, SCC*

The *cytoplasm* provides information about the origin and functional differentiation of a cell. Accordingly, cytoplasmic features are evaluated to determine the degree of squamous differentiation. Dense cytoplasm and distinct cell boundaries are the hallmarks of squamous differentiation.

The *nucleus* provides information about the state of health of the cell (ie, whether it is normal, inflamed, hyperplastic, neoplastic, etc). Accordingly, nuclear features are evaluated to help determine where in the spectrum of neoplastic transformation, or carcinogenesis, the cell may be. Nuclear size,

T1.2 Synoptic Oversimplification for Understanding the Pap Test

Low-Grade SIL		High-Grade SIL		
HPV/ Condyloma	Mild dysplasia	Moderate dysplasia	Severe dysplasia	Carcinoma in situ
Koilocytes (cytoplasmic halos, nuclear atypia)	Mature (intermediate to superficial) cells	Metaplastic (parabasal-sized) cells also pleomorphic, abnormally keratinized cells	Basaloid cells;	Hyperchromatic crowded groups, associated dysplasia

REMEMBER; IF THE NUCLEUS IS BIG AND DARK, IT'S DYSPLASIA

outline, chromatin (staining and texture), and nucleoli are key features of carcinogenesis.

Nuclear and cytoplasmic changes each form continuous threads, without obvious breaking points or divisions. Unfortunately, the warp and weft of these changes weave an infinitely fine fabric of findings in cervicovaginal cytology. Therefore, to be practical, the two basic concepts of squamous differentiation and carcinogenesis must be further simplified into manageable units. Squamous differentiation (cytoplasmic changes) can be arbitrarily divided into four cell layers, which are epitomized by the four iconic cell types: *basal, parabasal, intermediate,* and *superficial cells* [F1.1]. Carcinogenesis (nuclear changes) can also be divided into four stages, starting with *normal* and proceeding to *benign proliferative reactions,* then *intraepithelial neoplasia* (dysplasia/carcinoma in situ), and finally, *carcinoma* (microinvasive and fully invasive) [F1.2]. (Note: The discussion of cytologic changes involved in carcinogenesis is presented here primarily as a morphologic "construct" to help teach the microscopic appearance of the lesions. Carcinogenesis per se is complex and incompletely understood, and will be discussed later [see pgs 75, 83].)

Now, putting the two arms, squamous differentiation and carcinogenesis, together a simple chart can be devised, creating interpretive categories [F1.3]. The cytologic interpretation is made by analyzing nuclear and cytoplasmic features, and using them to map the cell to a place in the chart. For example, if a cell has metaplastic cytoplasm and a dysplastic nucleus, it will map to an interpretation of metaplastic dysplasia. Although simple in theory, this can be difficult in practice, in part because there are no sharp divisions between categories. Even between in situ and invasive cancer, a seemingly clear-cut distinction, there is a gray area of microinvasive carcinoma. There are also confounding variables, such as inflammation, that bedevil interpretation.

Each category will be examined in detail as the interpretive chart is constructed step by step. The normal maturation of the squamous epithelium and its orderly progression from basal cells, to parabasal cells, to intermediate cells, and finally, superficial cells (the Icons), as well as hormonal and Barr body cytology will be discussed. Then, carcinogenesis, beginning with the benign proliferative reactions, will be considered. Benign proliferative reactions mimic normal maturation and recapitulate, with slight perturbation, the sequence of events epitomized by the Icons. Next dysplasia and carcinoma in situ (also known as cervical intraepithelial neoplasia [CIN], and more recently as squamous intraepithelial lesions [SILs]), which arise in and reflect, in a distorted, disorderly way, the benign proliferative reactions will be addressed. Finally, carcinoma, which arises from intraepithelial neoplasia (or SILs) and imitates in a chaotic way the Iconic cell types, will be analyzed.

Squamous Differentiation

Squamous differentiation represents a spectrum of cytoplasmic changes ranging from undifferentiated, basal cells to mature fish-scale-like squamous cells. The primary purpose of the squamous epithelium is to protect the cervix and vagina from various physical, chemical, and microbiologic assaults. The squamous mucosa may also be important in providing glycogen, and perhaps other nutrients, for sperm. The cell's journey from base to surface normally takes about 5 days [Averette 1970, Bulten 2000b, Mittal 1999a, Payne 1996].

The Cells

The mucous membrane that normally covers the vagina and vaginal portion of the uterine cervix (portio vaginalis) is a nonkeratinizing, stratified squamous epithelium [I1.1a]. This nonkeratinizing epithelium can be conceptually—and somewhat arbitrarily—divided into four cell layers (germinal, deep spinous, superficial spinous, and superficial) based upon histologic features. These four histologic cell layers correspond to the cytologic nomenclature of basal, parabasal, intermediate, and superficial cells, respectively [F1.1]. This widely used cytologic nomenclature was recommended, in 1958, by the International Academy of Cytology based on opinion polls of leading experts [IAC 1958a,b]. Note that the names derive from their histologic counterparts in a fully mature epithelium.

Basal Cells

Basal cells are small, undifferentiated cells that measure about 10 μm to 12 μm in diameter [I1.1b] [R Carmichael 1939]. They resemble small histiocytes, particularly when occurring singly. Basal cells have a central, round to oval, vesicular nucleus and a small amount of delicate cytoplasm. Isolated basal cells are rarely, if ever, recognized specifically in Pap tests. However, basal cells can be identified in severe atrophy, as syncytial-like aggregates or hyperchromatic crowded groups of small cells with

Basal Cells
Small undifferentiated cells
Resemble small histiocytes
Seldom identified in Pap tests
Except in severe atrophy
Parabasal cells usually present
Germinative cells

F1.1 Normal Squamous Differentiation in Histology and Cytology

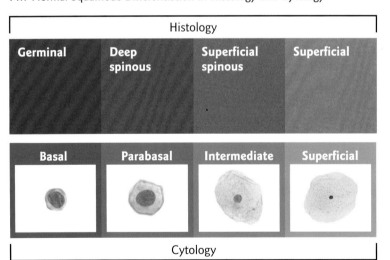

Histology			
Germinal	Deep spinous	Superficial spinous	Superficial
Basal	Parabasal	Intermediate	Superficial

Cytology

F1.2 Sequence of Events in Carcinogenesis

Normal	Proliferation	Dysplasia	Cancer
Order	Perturbation	Disorder	Chaos

F1.3 Matrix of Interpretive Categories

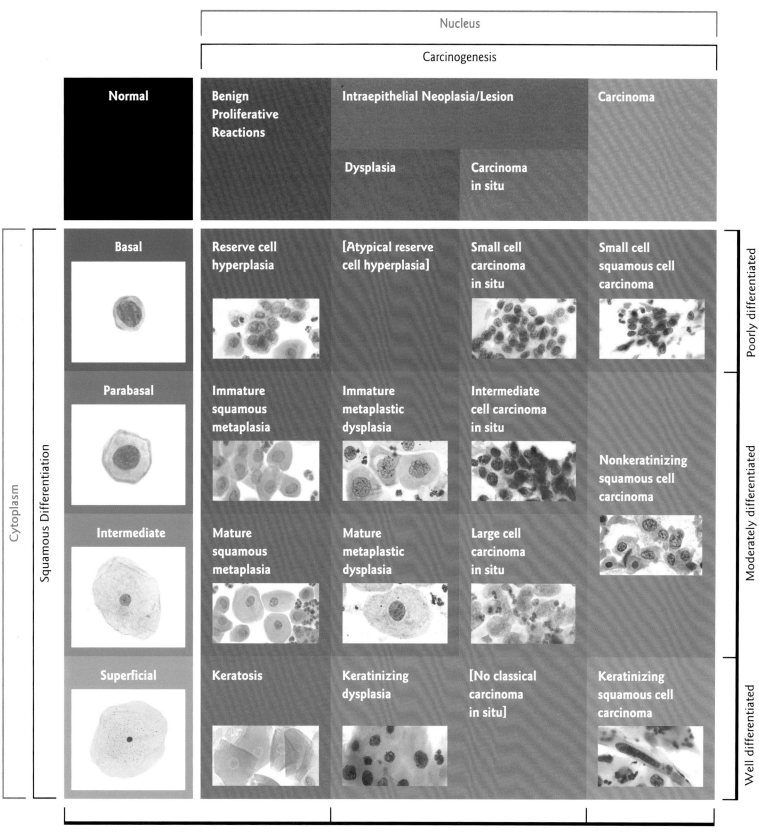

	Normal	**Benign Proliferative Reactions**	**Intraepithelial Neoplasia/Lesion**		**Carcinoma**
			Dysplasia	**Carcinoma in situ**	
Basal		Reserve cell hyperplasia	[Atypical reserve cell hyperplasia]	Small cell carcinoma in situ	Small cell squamous cell carcinoma
Parabasal		Immature squamous metaplasia	Immature metaplastic dysplasia	Intermediate cell carcinoma in situ	Nonkeratinizing squamous cell carcinoma
Intermediate		Mature squamous metaplasia	Mature metaplastic dysplasia	Large cell carcinoma in situ	
Superficial		Keratosis	Keratinizing dysplasia	[No classical carcinoma in situ]	Keratinizing squamous cell carcinoma

Nucleus

Carcinogenesis

Cytoplasm — Squamous Differentiation

Poorly differentiated — Moderately differentiated — Well differentiated

Benign — Premalignant — Malignant

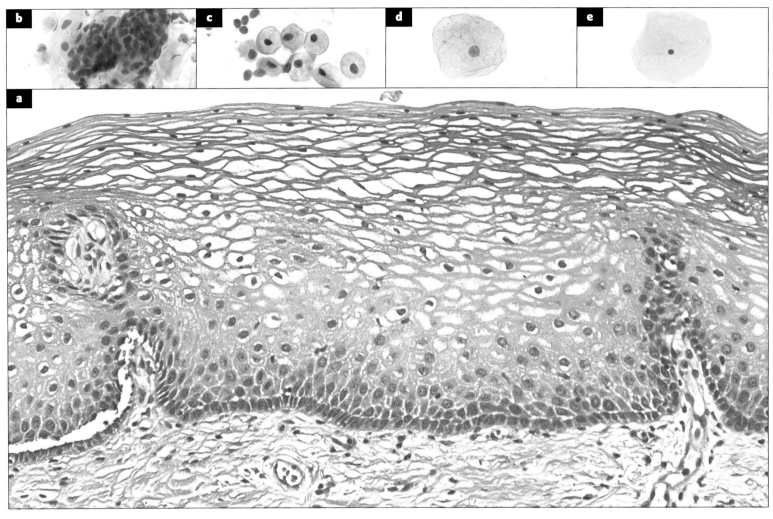

11.1
a, Normal histology; **b**, Basal cells [C]; **c**, Parabasal cells [C]; **d**, Intermediate cell [C]; **e**, Superficial cell [C]

uniform nuclei and scant cytoplasm. Basal cells can also be seen in a sample taken from the edge of an ulcer or if a tissue fragment is evulsed by an excessively hard scrape. When basal cells are present in a Pap test, they are usually associated with the next larger cell type, parabasal cells.

Basal cells serve several important functions. They are the cells that anchor the epithelium to the basement membrane by hemidesmosomes. They also are the germinative cells responsible for continually renewing the epithelium, because they are the only cells in the squamous mucosa that normally undergo cell division. When the basal cell divides, one of the daughter cells commits itself to squamous differentiation, manifested by dense, protective cytoplasm that gives it distinct cell boundaries. This selfless daughter cell eventually dies and is exfoliated: it serves to protect the underlying tissue from trauma and inflammation. The other daughter cell, which remains attached to the basement membrane, is an "immortal" cell (lasting for the life of the woman herself). The basal cell may also participate (by sending a signal to the stroma?) in producing a basement membrane, which separates the epithelium from the underlying mesenchyme.

Parabasal Cells

Parabasal cells, the next larger cell type, are commonly observed in Pap tests [11.1c]. When parabasal cells are found in the Pap test, this implies that they were present on the mucosal surface, where the sample was taken. Parabasal cells at the mucosal surface indicate that the epithelium is incompletely or "poorly" differentiated, ie, atrophic. Atrophy is a common finding during childhood, post-menopause, and postpartum.

In histology, parabasal cells have definite squamous features, including dense cytoplasm, distinct cell boundaries, and intercellular bridges. Intercellular bridges, which are the spinous processes of the histologic stratum spinosum, correspond ultrastructurally to long microvilli (which are attached to one another by intercellular junctions known as desmosomes) [Ashworth 1960]. Intercellular bridges can be difficult to identify in cytologic preparations.

Parabasal cells exfoliate singly or in sheets, or commonly, are present as aggregates of cells with indistinct cell borders, often referred to as "syncytia" (although they are not truly syncytial). Parabasal cells are moderately large, ranging from 15 μm to 30 μm in diameter. They have round to oval outlines. The nuclei are round to oval with finely granular, evenly distributed chromatin and occasional chromocenters. Nucleoli are inconspicuous or invisible, unless the

Parabasal Cells

1st to acquire squamous features
 ie, dense cytoplasm, distinct cell borders
Cytoplasm: Moderately abundant
Nucleus: Round-oval, fine chromatin
 Nuclear area ~ 50 μm²
Associated with atrophy

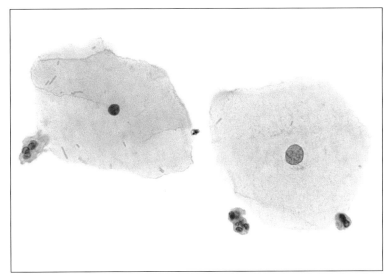

I1.2
Superficial, intermediate cell [L]

I1.3
a, Navicular cells [C]; **b**, Cytolysis [C]

cells are reactive or inflamed. The nuclear area averages about 50 μm², or 8 μm to 9 μm in diameter, which is slightly larger than a red blood cell. The N/C ratio varies, averaging about 20%. Parabasal cells have moderately dense cytoplasm and typically stain blue-green or gray, sometimes pink, and, rarely, orange.

Intermediate Cells

The ovoid parabasal cells flatten and mature into intermediate cells [I1.1d]. Intermediate cells exfoliate singly, or in sheets or clusters. They range from about 35 μm to 50 μm in diameter, ie, from about the size of parabasal cells (low intermediate cells) to the size of superficial cells (high intermediate cells) [I1.2]. The cytoplasm also changes from somewhat thick with rounded outlines, like that of parabasal cells, to thin with polygonal outlines, like that of superficial cells.

Intermediate Cells

Cells: Parabasal to superficial size

Nucleus is key reference

   Size: averages 35 μm² (~ RBC)

Chromatin quality:

   Staining: Normochromatic

   Texture: Fine, even

"If it's big and it's dark, it's dysplasia"

Associated with progesterone

Intermediate cells may contain glycogen, depending on the woman's hormonal status [Chowdhury 1981]. Glycogen appears golden-yellow with the Papanicolaou stain, but does not stain with hematoxylin and eosin. Marked accumulations of glycogen sometimes result in elongated cells with prominent cell borders, that are shaped like little boats, hence, navicular cells (Latin *navis* = ship, as in the navy) [I1.3a]. Navicular cells may be present in the Pap test late in the menstrual cycle and, in particular, during pregnancy.

The vaginal fluid is normally slightly acidic (pH 4 ± 0.5) owing to the presence of lactic acid that is produced from metabolism of glycogen by lactobacilli, the organisms originally observed by Döderlein in vaginal secretions [Döderlein 1894]. Acidity inhibits growth of most bacteria, including pathogens, as well as *Candida*. The action of the Döderlein bacillus causes cells to lyse (a process known as cytolysis), leaving naked nuclei (cells stripped of their cyto-

plasm), strewn in the background of the slide [I1.3b]. Cytolysis is essentially limited to intermediate cells: superficial cells rarely cytolyse and parabasal cells almost never do, although they may undergo other degenerative changes. Also, dysplastic cells typically lack significant glycogen (the basis of the Schiller iodine test [Richart 1964b, Schiller 1938]) and, therefore, rarely undergo cytolysis.

The nucleus of an intermediate cell is in the center of the cell, which is characteristic of squamous cells in general. The nuclear area averages about 35 μm², or 7 μm-8 μm in diameter, which is about the size of a red blood cell, and somewhat smaller than the parabasal nucleus (50 μm²). The N/C ratio is very low (about 3%-5%). The nucleus of an intermediate cell is round to oval. The nuclear membrane is smooth, or may have a neat longitudinal fold or groove [S Gupta 2000, Kaneko 1998, Payandeh 2003, Tahlan 2001]. The chromatin is finely divided and evenly distributed, with occasional chromocenters. This chromatin pattern is frequently described as "open and vesicular." Barr bodies (sex chromatin), though normally present in all female nuclei, can only be identified in some. Nucleoli normally are invisible.

The nucleus of an intermediate cell is a benchmark reference in cytopathology. It is used to gauge nuclear size, intensity of chromatin staining, and chromatin texture. It also serves as an internal control for staining and fixation artifacts. The intermediate cell nucleus is a key reference in evaluation of dysplasia. Dysplastic nuclei are characteristically three to six times the area of an intermediate cell nucleus. Hyperchromasia is judged relative to the staining of an intermediate cell nucleus. Chromatin is coarse compared with the fine texture of an intermediate cell's chromatin.

Superficial Cells

Superficial cells are the most differentiated squamous cells in a normal, nonkeratinizing squamous mucosa [I1.1e]. They usually occur singly, and rarely form clusters. Superficial cells measure about 45 μm-50 μm in diameter and look almost identical to the most mature intermediate cells, *except* that superficial cell nuclei are small and pyknotic, or dense structureless masses of chromatin [I1.2] [Wied 1955a]. They look like little dots of India ink; such nuclei are nonfunctional (dead). There may be a small, clear halo around the pyknotic nucleus as a reminder of its former size. The nucleus of a superficial cell is normally smaller than a red blood cell (ie, 5 μm-6 μm in diameter, or about 15 μm²-20 μm²); if it is larger than a red blood cell, suspect dysplasia.

The N/C ratio is about 2%-3%. The cytoplasm is abundant, thin, delicate, and transparent. The cell borders are well defined and have polygonal outlines. There is a tendency for superficial cells to stain pink and intermediate cells blue, but color is an unreliable criterion for distinguishing the two cell types. The nuclear change from vesicular (intermediate cell) to pyknotic (superficial cell) is the key to differential interpretation.

Superficial Cells
  Resemble mature intermediate cells
    Except nuclei pyknotic (ink dots)
  Cytoplasm: Tends to stain pink
    (Intermediate cells: blue)
  Nucleus, not color, for identification
  Associated with estrogen

Hormonal Cytology

The cervicovaginal squamous epithelium responds to a wide variety of stimuli, particularly hormones [Rakoff 1961a,b, Wied 1968]. [Note: Glandular cell changes are discussed in section II. Cytology of the Glandular Epithelium.] Félix-Archimède Pouchet was the first to describe, in 1847, epithelial cell changes in vaginal secretions related to ovulation. In 1925, Papanicolaou reported his findings on cytohormonal evaluation, the work that eventually led to his most important discovery [Papanicolaou 1925]. After Papanicolaou, investigators claimed that hormonal cytology could play a significant role in the diagnosis and management of conditions as diverse as infertility, pregnancy, polycystic ovarian disease, functioning ovarian tumors, fetal death in utero, postmaturity, threatened abortion, and premature onset of labor [Birtch 1961, Holmquist 1967a, W Johnston 1971, Papanicolaou 1925, Puttarajurs 1959, V Schneider 1995, Wachtel 1966]. Although cellular changes in response to hormones can be seen in Pap tests, these changes vary from woman to woman, and are affected many factors other than hormones. Today, direct measurement of hormones is routine, and hormonal cytology as a diagnostic technique is outmoded. Nevertheless, some knowledge of these changes is important for proper evaluation of Pap tests.

The squamous mucosa, especially the vaginal mucosa, is highly sensitive to estrogen and progesterone. It is varyingly sensitive to a host of other factors, including retinoids (such as vitamin A), androgens, corticoids, thyroxin, vitamins, antibiotics, digitalis, mechanical stimulation, and inflammation. There is about a five day delay between the time the hormonal signal is received by the basal cell and the time the mature cell is formed at the surface.

During the first half of the menstrual cycle, the follicular phase, the squamous mucosa is primarily under the hormonal influence of estrogen, which promotes full maturation of the epithelium to the level of the superficial cell. Estrogen receptors are present in nuclei of basal cells, diminish in concentration as the cells mature, and are lost in superficial cells; receptors show some cyclic variation. Endocervical cells also have estrogen receptors. Estrogen receptor concentration is reduced in atrophy [Kanai 1998, Nonogaki 1990].

During the second half, or luteal phase, of the menstrual cycle, and also during pregnancy, the epithelium is primarily under the hormonal influence of progesterone. Progesterone inhibits full squamous differentiation, with maturation only to the intermediate cell, rather than the superficial cell, layer. Normal mucosal thickness, which ranges from about 26 to 28 cells, is maintained by functional hyperplasia of the intermediate zone [D Patton 2000]. Progesterone is produced by the corpus luteum of the ovary, which develops after ovulation.

During pregnancy, progesterone is produced first by the corpus luteum, and later by the placenta. Progesterone receptors in cervical epithelial cells are at a minimum during the follicular phase of the cycle, but increase in the luteal phase and during pregnancy [Konishi 1991].

The Pap test is a biologic assay that correlates with ovarian function, time of ovulation, placental function, and hormonal therapy. A Pap test that is dominated by intermediate cells (ie, intermediate predominant maturation) is characteristic of the late luteal and early follicular phases of the cycle. Superficial cell predominance reaches its peak at the time of ovulation. Between ovulation and the late luteal phase, there is a change from the superficial to the intermediate cell pattern. Obtaining parabasal cells from the scraped surface indicates that the epithelium is thin and atrophic, and has not matured even to the intermediate cell layer.

There are several different ways to express the degree of maturation of the vaginal epithelium, including the folded cell, crowded cell, eosinophilic, and karyopyknotic indices. Because the Maturation Index, or MI, is the most reproducible and best known, it will be discussed in detail [McEndree 1999].

For hormonal evaluation, the sample is taken as a *gentle* scrape (to obtain naturally exfoliated surface cells) about two thirds of the way up the lateral wall of the vagina. (Note: The sample is taken *firmly* for an ordinary Pap test.) This site is chosen because the vaginal epithelium is most sensitive to hormonal changes; samples from this area are usually clean (ie, free of inflammation, bacteria, debris, or other contaminants); and other types of cells are usually absent. Cyclic changes, including ovulation, can be appreciated only when samples are taken daily for at least one full cycle, and to minimize technical artifacts, the cytologic samples should be batched and stained together, and screened by one cytologist.

Hormonal Cytology
  Sample gently upper mid-vagina
  Count 300 single cells
  Maturation Index (MI) = PIS Ratio
    Parabasal %: Intermediate %: Superficial %
    eg, 0: 80: 20, Intermediate predominant MI
  To be valid:
    •No inflammation or dysplasia
    •Only 2 cell types (3 ⟹ inflammation)
  Pertinent clinical history required
  Report: MI is, or is not, compatible c̄ age, hx
  Numbers are secondary

A satisfactory specimen for hormonal evaluation has no evidence of inflammation, since inflammation can cause nonhormonal maturation of the epithelium. Cervical (as opposed to vaginal) samples are unsatisfactory for hormonal analysis owing to the frequent presence of inflammation and other confusing cell types, eg, squamous metaplasia, which can mimic ordinary parabasal cells.

Three hundred single (not clustered) cells are counted, and the relative percentages of parabasal, intermediate, and superficial cells are calculated as a ratio: Parabasal %: Intermediate %: Superficial %, eg, 0: 80: 20. Basal cells are counted with parabasal cells as one cell type in a maturation index. Normally, only one or two cell types are represented. If all three types of cells are seen, inflammation usually is present or the sample was taken from the cervix. Such samples are unsatisfactory for hormonal evaluation. Exceptions to the "two cell rule" may occur when the epithelial maturation is changing, eg, prior to puberty or as menopause progresses, when cells from all three layers can be present normally.

The general pattern of maturation is more important than the actual numbers. For example, there is no significant difference between an MI of 0: 60: 40 and one of 0: 70: 30, both of which represent intermediate cell predominance. On the other hand, two women with identical MIs may have completely different explanations for them. What may be normal for one woman, might be abnormal for another (eg, a maturation index of 80: 20: 0 would be normal in late postmenopause, but would suggest intrauterine fetal demise in a pregnant woman). The two most characteristic maturation patterns are atrophy, with a predominance of parabasal cells, and high estrogen-like effect, with a predominance of superficial cells.

Two Most Characteristic Maturation Patterns

1. *Atrophy: Parabasal predominance, without superficial cells*
2. *Estrogen effect: Superficial predominance, without parabasal cells*

In summary, a MI specimen should be free of inflammation, glandular cells, metaplastic cells, hyperkeratosis, and parakeratosis, as well as evidence of dysplasia; usually no more than two cell types should be present [T1.3]. The cytology can be properly interpreted only in the light of adequate clinical history. This includes age, menstrual history, last menstrual period, past menstrual period, pregnancy, hormone therapy, surgery, all drugs, and radiation or chemotherapy. Finally, what is of primary importance is whether the MI is, or is not, compatible with the woman's history; the actual numbers are secondary.

T1.3 Representative Maturation Patterns

	Parabasal %	Intermediate %	Superficial %
Newborn	0	90	10
Child	80	20	0
Preovulatory	0	40	60
Postovulatory	0	60	40
Pregnancy	0	100	0
Postmenopause	80	20	0

Parabasal Predominant Maturation Index (Atrophy)

Parabasal Predominant MI

Atrophy

- *Late postmenopause (classic)*
- *Postpartum/Lactation*
- *Childhood (>1 month)*
- *Other, eg, progestin contraception*

The parabasal predominant maturation pattern ("shift to the left") indicates a poorly-differentiated, or atrophic, epithelium. Atrophic epithelium is thin and does not provide adequate protection, which may lead to bleeding and inflammation.

The parabasal cells may be single [I1.4b,i] or, in long-standing atrophy, in sheets [I1.4a]. Sheets of atrophic parabasal cells often appear syncytial (fused) [I1.4c,e], because the intercellular space is too small to be resolved in the light microscope. Occasionally, the cells actually do fuse. Because atrophic cells are fragile, naked nuclei, often in clumps resembling endometrial cells, may be present in the background [I1.1c, 1.4d]. (For differential, see Endometrial Cells, pg 116, and Tamoxifen, pg 163) Occasionally, the parabasal cells have a spindle configuration [I1.4e] (see also transitional cell [urothelial] metaplasia, pg 48).

The nuclei are generally as described for parabasal cells. However, airdrying artifact is common in conventional Pap smears in atrophy. This leads to nuclear enlargement, usually without hyperchromasia, although degenerative changes can cause hyperchromasia. Basophilic bodies, so-called "blue blobs,"

which are basically mummified parabasal cells with a strong affinity for hematoxylin stain, can be alarming looking [I1.4f] (see pg 67) [Milligan 1959]. Variable nuclear enlargement, pleomorphism, and hyperchromasia can make screening of these cases challenging (see atypia of atrophy, pg 66).

The squamous features of these atrophic cells, including keratin formation and intercellular bridges, are also poorly developed. The cytoplasm appears delicate rather than dense, and the cells usually lack glycogen, which is important in maintaining normal vaginal flora and pH [Chowdhury 1981]. Lack of glycogen makes the mucosa more susceptible to various assaults (see androgenic atrophy, below). In some cases, random parabasal cells degenerate, the cytoplasm becomes orangeophilic and the nuclei become pyknotic, mimicking parakeratosis (pseudokeratosis) [I1.4g,h] [G Acs 2000, C Buckley 1994, Saminathan 1994, Weintraub 1987]. The background commonly shows granular debris and inflammation [I1.4b,f,g,h,i], sometimes including multinucleated giant cell histiocytes (see "atrophy with inflammation," pg 68).

In liquid-based cytology (LBC), parabasal cells have bland nuclei, predominantly smooth nuclear borders, with occasional grooves. Because airdrying artifact is eliminated, nuclear enlargement is minimized. However, N/C ratios may increase, because cells "round up" in fluids. This, together with slight nuclear enlargement, nuclear grooves, and hyperchromasia, could lead to overinterpretation of H SIL [Wilbur 1996b]. Three-dimensional clusters of these somewhat atypical basal/parabasal cells ("hyperchromatic crowded groups") plus naked nuclei could also mimic a neoplastic process. Absence of marked nuclear membrane irregularities, abnormal chromatin patterns, and mitotic figures favors a benign intepretation. The background is cleaner in liquid-based cytology; granular debris, if present, tends to cling to the cells [I1.4b,h].

The postmenopausal state, with its attendant decrease in sex hormones, is typically associated with a parabasal predominant, or atrophic, pattern [Batrinos 1975a,b]. However, the postmenopausal MI varies significantly from woman to woman. A mature maturation pattern may persist for many years, possibly maintained by peripheral conversion of adrenal or ovarian stromal androgens [Efstratiades 1982, Meisels 1966a] or exposure to semen, which is high in estrogen [Hess 2001, Luboshitzky 2002]. Long-acting progestin-only contraceptives (eg, depomedroxyprogesterone acetate, Depo-Provera® and levonorgestrel, Norplant®) can cause atrophy in some women. The atrophic pattern is also normal during childhood. Various of other conditions, including starvation and anorexia nervosa, with decreased pituitary gonadotropins resulting in ovarian failure, can also be associated with an atrophic pattern. Gonadal dysgenesis, Turner syndrome, severe hypothyroidism/cretinism, and prolactin are other possible causes of atrophy. Cigarette smoking is associated with earlier menopause and atrophic changes in vaginal epithelium [Karamanidis 2001]. An atrophic pattern postmenopause predicts reduced bone mineral density (positive predictive value ~85%); hence, the Pap test could provide in an inexpensive screening test for osteoporosis [Repse-Fokter 2004].

During the postpartum period, the epithelium may become atrophic, secondary to the withdrawal of placental progesterone, until the ovaries begin to cycle again hormonally. Postpartum atrophy is more common with lactation and usually lasts about 3 to 6 weeks, but can persist several months, or until the infant is weaned [Butler 1973, McLennan 1975b]. An atrophic pattern occurring *during* pregnancy is abnormal and suggests fetal death in utero.

In postpartum and lactational Pap tests, the parabasal cells are typically heavily glycogenated. Similarly, in response to androgens, the mucosa may become atrophic, with glycogenated parabasal cells found in the specimen [Batrinos 1975a, Papanicolaou 1939]. This pattern, atrophy with glycogenated parabasal cells, is

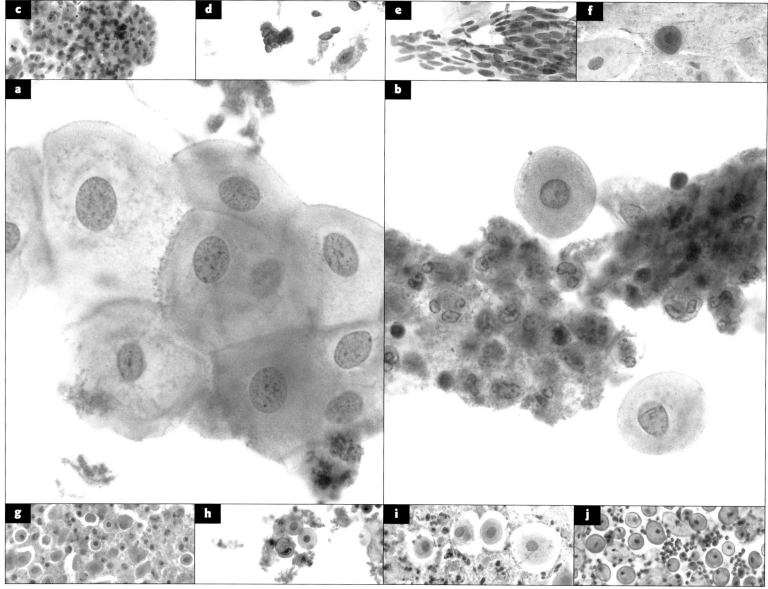

11.4
a, Atrophy, parabasals [L]; **b**, Atrophy, inflammation [L]; **c**, Atrophy, syncytium [L]; **d**, Atrophy, naked nuclei [L]; **e**, Atrophy, spindle cells [C];
f, Atrophy, blue blob [C]; **g**, Atrophy, pseudokeratosis [C]; **h**, Atrophy, pseudokeratosis [L]; **i**, Atrophy, inflammation [C]; **j**, Atrophy, androgenic [C]

known as androgenic atrophy [11.4j]. The source of the androgen can be either exogenous (eg, testosterone given for treatment of lichen sclerosis) or endogenous. In a postmenopausal woman, the adrenal glands and, to a lesser extent, the ovarian stroma, are the primary sources of androgen [R Chang 1981]. Rarely, androgenic atrophy may be caused by virilizing functional ovarian tumors (eg, Sertoli-Leydig, Leydig, lipid cell tumors, or ovarian stroma reactive to primary or metastatic carcinomas). Glycogenated parabasal cells can mimic koilocytes in both conventional Pap smears and LBC; however, the nuclei are not abnormal and the glycogen vacuoles are not as sharply defined as compared with koilocytes.

Intermediate Predominant Maturation Index

The intermediate predominant maturation pattern ("shift to the middle") is characteristic of progesterone effect, which inhibits complete matura-

tion to the superficial cell layer [Heber 1975] [11.5]. Progesterone production is associated with the postovulatory, luteal phase of the menstrual cycle as well as pregnancy. The normal, pure intermediate pattern (0/100/0) characteristic of pregnancy may take a trimester or more to develop. Progesterone also facilitates glycogen accumulation and, particularly during pregnancy, navicular cells may be present [11.6a].

The cytologic sample is dominated by intermediate cells (shift to the middle), which often have folded or curled edges, arranged in compact clusters. The background typically has many lactobacilli; leukocytes may also be present. Cytolysis, characterized by naked squamous nuclei, may be prominent.

Intermediate Predominant MI
Progesterone
· *2nd half of menstrual cycle*
· *Pregnancy*
· *Newborn (< 1 month)*
· *Other*

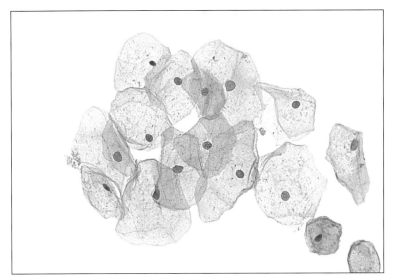

II.5
Intermediate predominant MI [C]

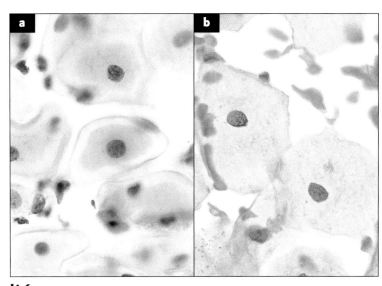

II.6
a, Navicular cells [C]; **b**, Newborn girl [C]

In liquid-based cytology, the typical picture of intermediate cell predominance is similar: intermediate cells, numerous bare nuclei (cytolysis), and lactobacilli (often overlying cells or trapped in mucus).

For about a month following birth, a newborn girl's vaginal mucosa will be under the (transplacental) influence of her mother's hormones, and will have intermediate cell predominance [II.6b]. As the maternal hormones are metabolized, the newborn's vaginal mucosa atrophies [Fraenkel 1938, Wied 1967]. It remains atrophic until a few years before menarche, when a noncycling intermediate predominant MI gradually replaces the atrophic pattern [Sonek 1969]. About a year or so before actual menarche, the mucosa begins to undergo cyclic changes [Krantz 1967, Tambouret 2003].

Loss of ovarian function (postmenopause, surgery, radiation, etc) is usually associated with atrophy. However, some postmenopausal women never develop an atrophic pattern and maintain an intermediate predominant maturation, perhaps sustained by peripheral conversion of adrenal or ovarian stromal androgens by adipose tissue [McLennan 1971]. Some postmenopausal women on long-term, low-dose estrogen replacement also maintain an intermediate, rather than superficial, predominant pattern. In addition, several drugs, including digitalis [Britsch 1963, Navab 1965] and broad-spectrum antibiotics, can influence the maturation of the cervicovaginal epithelium. Other possible causes of an intermediate predominant MI include: progesterone therapy, cortisone therapy, adrenocortical hormones, premenarche, androgens including tumors, luteinized follicles, and corpus luteum cyst.

Superficial Predominant Maturation Index

Estrogen stimulation, either endogenous or exogenous, usually produces a superficial predominant maturation pattern ("shift to the right" or "estrogen effect"), which is characteristic of the first half, or follicular phase, of the menstrual cycle. Superficial cell predominance normally reaches its peak at ovulation [II.7].

The cytologic sample is dominated by mature superficial cells, which lay flat, and usually occur singly. The background is clean.

Sensitivity to estrogen varies greatly, but a mature maturation pattern can occur with minimal estrogen [Nilsson 1995]. Superficial predominance in postmenopause indicates estrogen stimulation, which is a risk factor for endometrial hyperplasia and carcinoma. In postmenopausal women, estrone is the chief estrogen, and is derived predominantly from peripheral tissue conversion of androstenedione. About 80% of circulating androstenedione in postmenopausal women comes from the adrenal gland; the ovarian stroma also makes a contribution [R Chang 1981]. Adipose tissue is a major source of aromatase, an enzyme that converts androgens (eg, androstenedione) into estrogens (particularly estrone) [Sherman 2000].

Superficial Predominant MI

Estrogen

- *1st half of menstrual cycle*
- *Postmenopausal causes include:*
  - *Obesity (androstenedione → estrone)*
  - *Cirrhosis (↓ hepatic estrogen catabolism)*
- *Inflammation (pseudomaturation)*
- *Other: Drugs (digitalis, vitamins);*
  - *Radiation/ChemoRx*

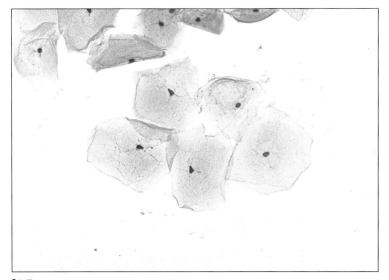

II.7
Superficial predominant MI [C]

Consequently, obesity can result in increased maturation and is a risk factor for endometrial pathology. Theoretically, psychological stress, with its attendant rise in adrenal hormones, could cause an estrogen effect. Cirrhosis of the liver can interfere with degradation of estrogen, resulting in relative estrogen excess. Rarely, a mature maturation pattern in a postmenopausal woman may be associated with ovarian stromal luteinization induced by a primary or metastatic ovarian tumor. As mentioned, semen is rich in estrogen [Hess 2001, Luboshitzky 2002]. Paradoxically, tamoxifen, an estrogen antagonist used in the treatment of breast cancer, can cause an estrogen-like effect in postmenopausal women with atrophy, owing to a weak estrogen effect [Athanassiadou 1992, Edis 1990, Friedrich 1998, Ganesan 1999, Rayter 1994, Shiota 2002]. Estrogen containing drugs or cosmetics can produce an estrogen effect. Some pharmaceuticals may also have an estrogen effect. For example, digitalis, which is chemically similar to steroid hormones, may lead to maturation of the squamous mucosa in postmenopausal women [Navab 1965]. (For you worry-warts, the environment is heavily contaminated with a wide range of industrial waste products, many of which have estrogenic activity [not to mention estrogens in products not originally intended to have estrogenic activity, such as soy based infant formula [Burton 2002]; this could be contributing to everything from male infertility to epidemic obesity to cancer: no word yet on their effect on the maturation index.)

Summary of Changes During Menstrual Cycle, Menopause, Pregnancy

The Menstrual Cycle

The first day of menstrual bleeding is defined as the first day of the menstrual cycle (menses: Latin, for months). All other days are approximate and can vary somewhat from cycle to cycle among individual women [Papanicolaou 1943].

The menstrual phase of the cycle typically ranges from the first to the fifth days. During this time, there is a predominance of intermediate squamous cells in the Pap test, but superficial cells are also present. There are also endometrial glandular and stromal cells, blood, inflammatory cells, and debris, but endocervical cells may be sparse in samples obtained with an Ayre spatula.

During the proliferative phase of the cycle, also known as the follicular or estrogenic phase, days 6 through 14, the maturation pattern gradually shifts from an intermediate predominant pattern [II.5] to a superficial predominant pattern [II.7]. During exodus, days 6 through 10, many histiocytes are present. Endometrial cells are most characteristically present in "double contour" cell balls (endometrial wreaths), but decrease in number by day six, and normally disappear by day 10 to 12 (rare beyond day 14). The cytoplasm of endocervical cells is relatively dense and basophilic. The background of the slide becomes clean by ovulation.

At ovulation, about day 14, superficial cell predominance reaches a peak. Endocervical cells become secretory and remain so until the end of the menstrual cycle. Leukocytes are rare, bacteria are few, and the background is clean. Ferning of endocervical mucus may be seen in conventional Pap smears near ovulation. However, the Pap test can only *approximate* the time of ovulation [Papanicolaou 1943].

The secretory phase of the cycle, also known as the luteal or progestational phase, ranges from days 14 to 28. Superficial cell predominance changes to intermediate cell predominance after ovulation. A few navicular cells may be present. Toward the end of the menstrual cycle, marked cytolysis occurs, resulting in naked nuclei and cytoplasmic fragments, which together with an increase of leukocytes and bacteria, contributes to a "dirty" background. Just

before menstruation, the maturation index begins to shift toward the right (ie, superficial cell predominance), and the cycle begins again. Some women shed endometrial cells a few days before the onset of menses.

Pregnancy, Post-Partum, and Lactation

When pregnancy occurs, the corpus luteum of the ovary does not involute, but grows and produces more progesterone. Around the end of the first trimester, the placenta takes over responsibility for producing this hormone. During the first few weeks of pregnancy, there is a premenstrual maturation pattern that may show a slight estrogen effect. As pregnancy progresses, the maturation index changes to a pure intermediate cell pattern that does not cycle [II.5]. By the third trimester, numerous navicular cells (heavily glycogenated intermediate cells) [II.6a], lush lactobacilli, and extensive cytolysis are the most characteristic pregnancy findings. Endocervical cells are secretory; Arias-Stella reaction may be present (ie, hypersecretory endocervical cells, see pg 166). In some women, in the week preceding delivery, there is an increase in superficial cells possibly reflecting a change in placental function; however, this is not a reliable indicator of impending delivery [Lencioni 1969].

In the postpartum period, with the loss of the placental hormones, navicular cells and cytolysis are rapidly replaced with a predominance of parabasal cells that often contain glycogen ("androgenic atrophy") [II.4j]. Normal maturation gradually returns with the onset of regular menstrual cycles. Immediately post-partum, and for several weeks thereafter, the sample may show marked inflammatory and reparative changes, including reactive/atypical glandular cells, as a reflection of damage to the cervix incurred during delivery, which can cause problems in cytologic interpretation.

If the mother nurses her child, postpartum atrophy usually changes gradually to a mature pattern, but atrophy may persist as long as the ovarian cycle is suppressed by lactation [McLennan 1975b]. Be aware that many women do not have typical postpartum patterns.

Other pregnancy-associated changes, such as Arias-Stella reaction, decidual cells, and trophoblasts, are discussed in section IV. Cytology of Pregnancy (beginning on pg 165).

Menopause

Shortly before menopause, the menstrual cycle often becomes irregular. Although the ovarian follicle may persist, ovulation does not occur. These anovulatory cycles are characterized by unopposed estrogen production, which replaces the cycling of estrogen and progesterone. Estrogen withdrawal after variable intervals may lead to breakdown hemorrhage of the endometrium (withdrawal bleeding), but not true menstruation. Anovulatory cycles are usually associated with a superficial cell predominant maturation index (owing to continued production of androgens by the ovary that are converted peripherally to estrone). When ovarian cycles stop completely at menopause, the vaginal mucosa no longer undergoes cyclic changes, although the maturation pattern is highly variable from woman to woman. Surgical removal or radiation damage of the ovaries may cause changes similar to those of menopause.

In early menopause, there is typically an intermediate predominant maturation pattern [II.8a]. This may persist for a relatively long time, particularly if the woman remains sexually active. With time, the exact length of which is quite variable from woman to woman, the maturation pattern gradually shifts to a parabasal predominant maturation index, ie, gradually becomes atrophic [II.8b]. Cells from all three cell layers may be present for a time, a pattern which is seldom seen normally, and glycogenated cells may also be present.

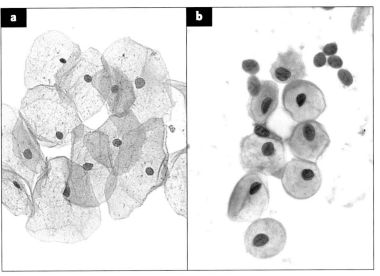

II.8
a, Intermediate predominant MI [C]; **b**, Parabasal predominant MI [C]

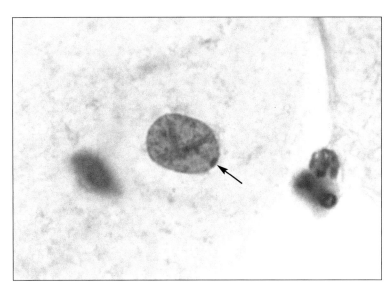

II.9
Barr body (arrow) [C]

Barr Bodies

The Barr body is a mass of condensed sex chromatin in the nuclei of normal female somatic cells due to inactive X chromosome. Murray L. Barr and E. George Bertram showed that it is possible to determine the (female) sex of an individual by identifying this chromatin mass [Barr 1949]. The term Barr body was introduced by Mary Lyon. According to the Lyon hypothesis, one of the two X chromosomes in each somatic cell of the female is inactivated. The Barr body represents the inactivated X chromosome. X inactivation occurs around the 16th day of embryonic development.

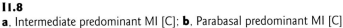

Barr Bodies
  Inactivated X chromosomes
  Normal maturation
    (+) BBs: Normal
    (−) BBs: Testicular feminization (XY)
  Abnormal maturation
    (+) BBs: Ovarian failure
        Down syndrome (trisomy 21)
    (−) BBs: Turner (XO) syndrome

Barr body count is a now outmoded genetic test; however, some familiarity with it can be useful [Moore 1962]. In every female somatic cell there is normally one Barr body. Barr bodies are normally present as dense, triangular or rectangular bits of heterochromatin, about 1 μm in width, attached at random to the inner aspect of the nuclear membrane [II.9]. Barr bodies can usually be seen microscopically only when present on the lateral margin of a nucleus; therefore, they are identified in only 20% to 60% of cells, even in normal females. Multiple Barr bodies occur not only in genetic diseases, but also in intraepithelial and invasive neoplasia due to chromosomal abnormalities. Hormonal status and Barr bodies can be evaluated together [T1.4]. (Note: When counting Barr bodies, a buccal specimen is preferred: easier to obtain, has fewer artifacts.)

Finally, in longstanding atrophy, intermediate and superficial cells practically disappear. Syncytial-like aggregates of basal-parabasal cells are common. The parabasal cells are commonly accompanied by inflammation ("atrophy with inflammation"). Blue blobs and pseudokeratinized cells may be present (see pg 67). Endocervical cells are usually sparse. Cytologic atypia may occur ("atypia of atrophy" see pg 66).

T1.4 Hormonal Status and Barr Bodies

Normal hormonal status, (+) Barr bodies
  Normal female
  Congenital atresias of genital tract (except ovaries)
  Disease/endocrinopathy (insufficient for abnormal hormonal pattern)
Note: Very few, or small, Barr bodies may indicate mosaicism or translocation.

Abnormal hormonal pattern, (+) Barr bodies
  Dysfunction of endocrine organs
    Ovary
    Other (eg, pituitary, adrenal, thyroid [marked hypofunction])
  Dysfunction of chromosomes
    Down syndrome, somatic trisomy
    XXX (double Barr body)
Note: Rule out hormone therapy, inflammation, cervical or vulvar contamination.

Normal hormonal pattern, (−) Barr bodies
  Testicular feminization (androgen insensitivity syndrome)
  (= XY with feminizing male pseudohermaphroditism)

Abnormal hormonal pattern, (−) Barr bodies
  Turner syndrome (XO)
  Other gonadal dysgenesis (XY)

Carcinogenesis

Cancers generally follow a recognizable pattern of development, which has been extremely well studied in the uterine cervix. The discussion of carcinogenesis begins with the benign proliferative reactions, including metaplasia and keratosis, which are not precancerous, but provide the soil in which the seeds of cancer may be sown. Next, dysplasia/carcinoma in situ is taken up, followed by microinvasive and finally, fully invasive squamous cell carcinoma [F1.3].

Benign Proliferative Reactions

In response to a wide variety of stimuli, ranging from pH changes to hormonal alterations to inflammation to trauma, the delicate glandular epithelium of the cervix changes into a protective squamous epithelium, by a process known as *metaplasia* (ie, one adult, or fully differentiated, type of tissue replaces another). When the stress is particularly severe, the nonkeratinizing squamous epithelium of the cervix and vagina can also undergo *keratosis,* becoming hyperplastic and keratinized, providing a tough, skin-like epithelium. Metaplasia and keratosis are the two basic benign proliferative reactions. Although not premalignant, these epithelial proliferations, particularly metaplasia, are the milieu in which cervical carcinogenesis may begin [E Stern 1973]. *Proliferation is the force that drives carcinogenesis.*

Benign Proliferative Reactions

   •*Squamous Metaplasia*

    Immature to mature

   •*Keratosis*

    Hyperkeratosis

    Parakeratosis

  Not premalignant, but milieu for

    precursor lesions

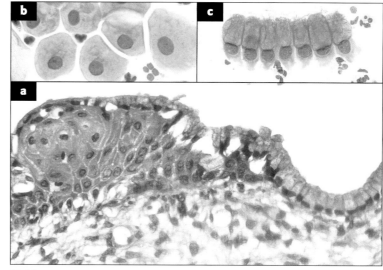

II.10
a, Squamocolumnar junction; **b**, Metaplastic cells [C];
c, Endocervical cells [C]

Metaplastic Reactions

During fetal development most of the vagina is lined by columnar (endocervical-like) glandular epithelium of Müllerian origin. Squamous epithelium normally grows in from the urogenital sinus lining the vagina and the ectocervix, and replaces the columnar epithelium through the process of metaplasia. (Diethylstilbestrol [DES] interferes with this normal process and may leave islands of glandular epithelium in the vagina, a condition known as vaginal adenosis.) At birth, the glandular and squamous epithelia meet at the external os of the cervix. The site where they meet is designated the "original" squamocolumnar junction, and the squamous mucosa is known as the "native" squamous epithelium.

At puberty and during pregnancy, the cervix increases in size and changes in shape, resulting in eversion of the endocervical glandular epithelium onto the portio vaginalis of the cervix, properly termed ectropion (Greek: outturning), but commonly and erroneously called an erosion (because the underlying red, vascular stroma can be seen through the delicate columnar epithelium [Briggs 1979]). Ectropion is more common and more extensive on the anterior lip than on the posterior lip of the cervix (the same is true of the distribution of dysplasia [Richart 1965a]).

In response to the normal acidity of the vagina, as well as a host of other possible factors, including inflammation, polyps, and oral contraceptives, the everted columnar epithelium is replaced by metaplastic squamous epithelium, forming a new squamocolumnar junction. Squamous metaplasia is at its peak during fetal development, puberty, pregnancy (particularly the first), and postpartum. (There is a significant increase in the vaginal acidity at puberty, resulting in extensive metaplasia [Briggs 1979], and possibly, increased susceptibility to carcinogenic agents, including human papillomavirus.) Because of this metaplasia, instead of a squamo-columnar junction, there may now be a squamo-metaplastic-columnar junction or "zone." The metaplastic zone between the native squamous and glandular epithelium is known as the transitional zone (also known as the transformation zone in colposcopy, or simply the "T zone") [Fluhmann 59] **[II.10a]**. *The T zone is the usual site of origin for both squamous and adenocarcinoma of the cervix* [Ehrmann 1996, L Johnson 1969, Matsukuma 1989, Noda 1983, Reagan 1953a, Teshima 1985].

The T zone is the critical area to sample for optimal cancer surveillance by the Pap test. Due to squamous metaplasia, the location of the T zone changes during a woman's lifetime: the squamocolumnar junction gradually recedes proximally (ie, upward, into the endocervix). During the reproductive years, the squamocolumnar junction is usually distal to the external cervical os, and is easy to sample. However, later in life, especially postmenopause, the T zone may be within the endocervical canal, where it can be difficult to sample. Endocervical cells **[II.10c]**, and to some degree metaplastic cells **[II.10b]**, are the best evidence that the T zone is represented in a Pap test.

There is a gradient of maturity of the metaplastic process. Squamous metaplasia is less mature proximally and more mature distally, toward the site of the original squamocolumnar junction on the ectocervix. Indeed, squamous metaplasia on the ectocervix may be so mature as to be cytologically indistinguishable from the native squamous epithelium.

Squamous metaplasia is so common that it is considered a normal physiologic process. It is thought to begin with the endocervical reserve cell, the precise origin of which is still controversial, but ultimately agreed to be Müllerian [L Howard 1951, Reagan 1962a]. Endocervical reserve cells are morphologically similar to squamous basal cells. However, the reserve cell has the capacity to differentiate into either a glandular or a squamous cell, unlike the basal cell (squamous only). When the reserve cell receives the signal to undergo squamous metaplasia, the first step is for the reserve cells to proliferate, which is known as reserve cell hyperplasia. Then, squamous differentiation begins (immature, followed by mature, squamous metaplasia). The undifferentiated reserve cell is also thought to be the ultimate source of most cervical carcinomas, including squamous cell carcinoma, adenocarcinoma, and mixed adenosquamous carcinoma **[F1.4]**.

Squamous Metaplasia

  Begins with Reserve Cell

    → *Gland or Squamous Cell*

    •*Reserve cell hyperplasia (RCH)*

      Earliest change

      Rarely recognized in Pap tests

    •*Immature Squamous Metaplasia*

      Parabasal-sized cells

      Begin to acquire squamous features

    •*Mature Squamous Metaplasia*

      Intermediate-sized cells

      Eventually looks like native cells

F1.4 Reserve Cell Differentiation

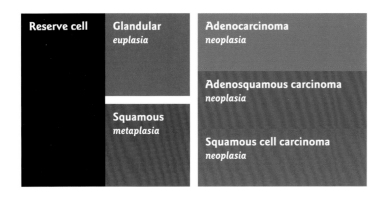

Reserve cell	Glandular *euplasia*	Adenocarcinoma *neoplasia*
		Adenosquamous carcinoma *neoplasia*
	Squamous *metaplasia*	Squamous cell carcinoma *neoplasia*

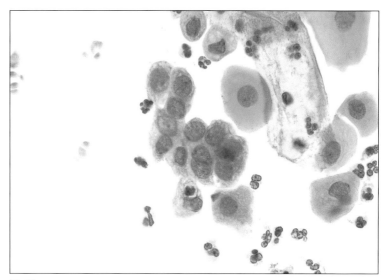

II.II
Reserve cell hyperplasia [C]

Reserve Cell Hyperplasia

In the earliest phase of nascent metaplasia, the reserve cells begin to proliferate along the basement membrane, underneath the endocervical-type glandular epithelium. This is reserve cell hyperplasia (RCH).

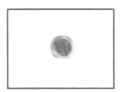

Histologically, this single row of reserve cells is the first recognizable stage of reserve cell hyperplasia. Next, the reserve cells begin to pile up, forming two to five poorly defined layers of undifferentiated small cells, before they start to acquire definite squamous features, such as dense cytoplasm, distinct cell boundaries, intercellular bridges, and stratification, that is, before true squamous metaplasia begins. Reserve cell hyperplasia usually remains covered by glandular epithelium.

Reserve Cell Hyperplasia
Icon: Basal cell
Histology: commonly observed
Cytology: rarely recognized
Syncytial-like aggregates
Histiocyte-like cells
(+) endocervical cells; squamous metaplasia

Although commonly observed in histology, reserve cell hyperplasia is rarely recognized specifically in gynecologic cytology. Reserve cells closely resemble basal cells (therefore, the basal cell is the iconic cell type). Individual reserve cells are indistinguishable from small histiocytes or superficial endometrial stromal cells. Reserve cell hyperplasia can be recognized most reliably in cytology when occurring in aggregates of undifferentiated, small cells lined on one surface by endocervical cells.

Reserve cells are small and have scant cytoplasm [II.II]. The cytoplasm is delicate, finely vacuolated, and cyanophilic, with poorly defined cell borders, resulting in a syncytial appearance. A honeycomb pattern is never seen. The single, central nucleus may be round to oval, or sometimes bean-shaped, and may have a fold or groove in the nuclear membrane. The nucleus averages about 50 µm^2 in area and the N/C ratio is high. The chromatin is fine, with occasional chromocenters, similar to that of a normal endocervical cell nucleus. Neither hyperchromasia nor conspicuous nucleoli are present. Extensive immature squamous metaplasia usually accompanies reserve cell hyperplasia, and provides supporting evidence for a cytologic interpretation of RCH.

Because reserve cell hyperplasia is composed of primitive cells, it can be mistaken for carcinoma in situ in either cytologic or histologic studies [de Brux 1961]. In cytology, reserve cell hyperplasia can exfoliate syncytial-like

aggregates of undifferentiated cells with immature nuclei, features shared with carcinoma in situ. However, aggregates of reserve cells are more uniform and orderly, and the nuclei appear bland and benign. Carcinoma in situ, on the other hand, exfoliates disorderly, hyperchromatic crowded groups, with abnormal nuclei.

Immature Squamous Metaplasia

Squamous metaplasia begins when the reserve cells start to acquire squamous features (ie, differentiate into squamous cells). Squamous differentiation is recognized, cytologically, by the presence of dense cytoplasm and distinct cell borders.

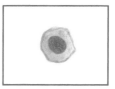

These features begin to develop as the cells start to lay down intermediate-sized tonofilaments in their cytoplasm. Immature metaplastic cells become packed with tonofibrils (bundles of tonofilaments, the keratin apparatus) and "round up" (ie, become more spherical, to achieve maximal volume in minimal space), resulting in moderate N/C ratios.

Histologically, the metaplastic cells begin to stratify and develop a well-defined basal layer, two features that help distinguish squamous metaplasia from reserve cell hyperplasia. Intercellular bridges are not conspicuous at this point, but become prominent as the metaplasia matures. The immature

Immature Squamous Metaplasia
Icon: Parabasal Cell
Cells: Cobblestone pattern
Cytoplasm: Thick, dense
Nuclei: 50 µm^2, vesicular
8–9 µm diameter

metaplastic epithelium is composed of two zones, basal and parabasal. Consequently, the cells at the surface are the size and shape of parabasal cells, which the immature metaplastic cells closely resemble (hence, the icon). The border between the immature metaplastic epithelium and the native squamous epithelium is sharply defined histologically.

Immature squamous metaplasia usually is easily recognized in the Pap test as parabasal-sized cells with dense cytoplasm and rounded cell borders. They are characteristically arranged in a cobblestone pattern, and tend to be single or only loosely aggregated [II.12]. The cytoplasm usually stains

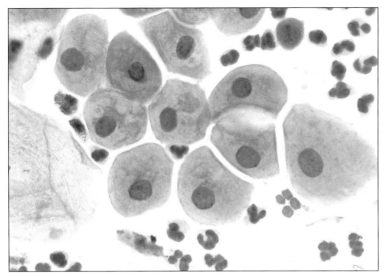

11.12
Squamous metaplasia [C]

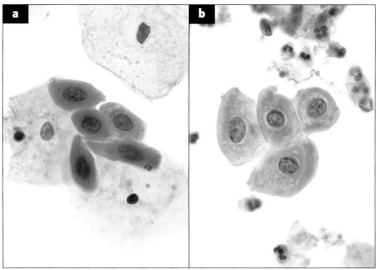

11.13
a, Squamous metaplasia [L]; **b**, Squamous metaplasia [L]

blue-green and usually does not contain visible glycogen. The cytoplasm is notably thick and dense and the cell borders are sharply defined ("cookie cutter" look). There often is a dense zone just underneath the cell membrane, known as the ectoplasmic rim, which is distinct from the endoplasm of the cell. Cytoplasmic vacuolization is common.

The nucleus is round to oval and has a smooth membrane, fine chromatin, and rare chromocenters. Although nucleoli are not seen normally, they may be present in reactive change, which commonly affects metaplastic cells. The nucleus measures about 50 μm², about 8 μm in diameter, which is slightly larger than either a red blood cell or an intermediate cell nucleus.

Squamous metaplastic cells can be fairly variable in size and shape, depending upon the degree of maturation [11.13a,b]. If the cells have been forcibly scraped, rather than spontaneously exfoliated, from the mucosal surface, they may also show thin, spidery legs extending from the main body of the cell [C Buckley 1994]. These are called spider cells [11.14a].

In liquid-based cytology, squamous metaplastic cells are similar to those in conventional Pap smears, including loose sheets of cells with dense cytoplasm in cobblestone arrangements or single cells [11.13a,b]. However, the metaplastic cells tend to appear smaller and rounder, have higher nuclear/cytoplasmic ratios, and cell clusters round up. This can mimic dysplasia, including H SIL. Hyperchromasia and nuclear membrane irregularities favor an interpretation of SIL. The differential of squamous metaplasia also includes high endocervical cells and histiocytes, either of which can have dense, squamoid cytoplasm in LBC.

Histologically, layers of pleomorphic, immature squamous cells with high N/C ratios and nuclei showing reactive changes ("atypia") can be difficult to distinguish from dysplasia. Cytologically, distinguishing immature metaplastic cells from dysplasia is a common dilemma that is sometimes very difficult to resolve in Pap tests. Critical examination of the nucleus, particularly its size and the quality of the chromatin, is the ultimate key to the proper classification of the cells (see pgs 34,57 for more discussion).

Immature metaplastic cells are frequently vacuolated. Vacuolated metaplastic cells with active nuclei can suggest adenocarcinoma [11.14b]. Vacuolated cells in a Pap test are far more likely to be benign metaplasia than glandular cancer. The vacuoles of metaplastic cells can be of three types: (1) degenerative (hydropic

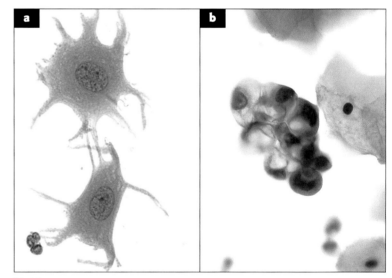

11.14
a, Spider cells [C]; **b**, Vacuolated metaplastic cells [C]

degeneration, the vacuoles contain only water and electrolytes, and appear crystal clear), (2) secretory (vacuoles contain mucin, which stains lightly), or (3) phagocytic (vacuoles contain stainable debris or cells).

Differentiating parabasal-sized cells of squamous metaplasia (a quality indicator for Pap tests) from those of atrophy (as can be seen in menopause, postpartum, or progestational therapy) is another common dilemma that may not always be possible to resolve. Robust, actively proliferating metaplastic cells differ from delicate atrophic cells by the thickness and density of metaplastic cytoplasm, the presence of an ectoplasmic rim, and the cobblestone arrangement of the cells. Mucin vacuoles may be present in metaplastic cells, but not in atrophic parabasal cells. Spidery forms are more frequent in metaplasia, while syncytial-like aggregates are common in atrophy. The company the cells keep is also helpful: parabasal-sized immature metaplastic cells are often accompanied by intermediate-sized mature metaplastic cells, while parabasal-sized atrophic cells are often accompanied by undifferentiated basaloid cells. Also, atrophic cells tend to dominate the slide, while metaplastic cells are more limited.

Mature Squamous Metaplasia

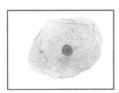

As the cytoskeleton (keratin) and cell membrane continue to develop, the metaplastic cell becomes a shield-like scale. The epithelium now comprises three histologic layers: basal, parabasal, and intermediate. This stage is known as mature squamous metaplasia.

Histologically, a good clue to the metaplastic origin of a mature squamous epithelium is the presence of underlying endocervical glands, indicating its endocervical source. Endocervical glands do not occur directly beneath the native squamous epithelium.

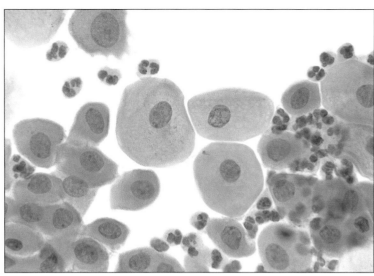

II.15
Mature, immature metaplasia [C]

Mature Squamous Metaplasia

  Icon: Intermediate Cell
  Like native epithelium
  Overlies endocervix
  Rounded cell outlines
  Slightly dense cytoplasm
  Remnants of cobblestone

The cells at the surface of the epithelium closely resemble normal intermediate cells (hence, the icon), except that their cell outlines may be a little more rounded than polygonal and the cytoplasm may be slightly denser than mature intermediate cells [II.15]. Remnants of a cobblestone arrangement of the cells may be seen cytologically. Eventually, the squamous metaplasia matures completely and becomes cytologically indistinguishable from the native squamous epithelium, including its response to cyclic hormonal changes.

Keratotic Reactions

Estrogen stimulates complete maturation of the nonkeratinizing squamous epithelium to the superficial cell layer, represented by the final icon, the superficial cell. Under certain circumstances, the normally nonkeratinizing squamous epithelium, whether native or metaplastic, can undergo further differentiation into a keratinized, skin-like squamous epithelium. This "hyperdifferentiation" is called keratosis, and it can take two forms, hyperkeratosis and parakeratosis. Keratosis can be caused by marked irritation of the mucosa, eg, due to uterine prolapse, inflammation/infections, pessaries, radiation, or DES exposure in utero, but in many cases the cause is unknown. In addition, keratosis can be related to condyloma or dysplasia. In the Pap test, anucleate superficial cells characterize hyperkeratosis, while miniature superficial cells characterize parakeratosis. Note that "hyperkeratosis" and "parakeratosis" are not specifically listed in the Bethesda System terminology, but can be used to describe the morphologic findings.

Keratosis

  Icon: Superficial cell
  Due to irritation, eg, prolapse, inflammation,
    radiation, DES in utero; also SIL, CA
  Hyperkeratosis: Anucleate superficial cells
    Also, spiegelosis (hypergranulosis)
  Parakeratosis: Miniature superficial cells
    Single, layered strips, pearls
  Benign, but can mask underlying lesion!

Keratosis usually is associated with a fully mature epithelium, but it can also be found on the surface of an atrophic epithelium or, more ominously, a neoplastic epithelium. The keratotic surface looks white, which is termed leukoplakia (Greek: white plaques) clinically, or white epithelium, colposcopically. In addition to hyperkeratosis and parakeratosis, various conditions, including warts (condyloma), dysplasia, and even cancer can have a white appearance. Glycogen is minimal and cytologic atypia is absent in keratotic reactions.

Keratosis is benign; there is no evidence that it is a precursor to cervical neoplasia. However, keratinization may figure prominently in some cases of dysplasia or cancer, particularly keratinizing types. Also, as a surface reaction, keratosis can cover an underlying abnormality, including cancer, which consequently may not be detected by the Pap test, because it samples the mucosal surface. Women with extensive hyperkeratosis or parakeratosis, in otherwise normal Pap tests, may be at increased risk of dysplasia (usually low-grade), particularly if they are younger than 50 years of age [S Andrews 1989b, Brotzman 1996, Cecchini 1990c, Sorosky 1990, Williamson 2003, Zahn 2002]. In women with a history of dysplasia, hyperkeratosis or parakeratosis may correlate with persistence of the lesion or HPV infection, even if no other abnormality is detected cytologically [Kern 1991b]. If keratosis is combined with inflammatory changes and, particularly, atypical squamous cells, there is a definite risk of dysplasia [Hudock 1995]. Management options include colposcopy/biopsy, repeat Pap testing, and HPV-DNA testing [Zahn 2002].

Hyperkeratosis

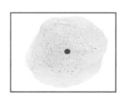

Hyperkeratosis is a proliferative process that usually is characterized by overall thickening of the epithelium with elongation of the rete pegs (acanthosis) and formation of an additional two layers of cells at the surface: the stratum granulosum and the stratum corneum. In some cases, keratosis occurs on an atrophic epithelium (atrophy with keratinization).

In the stratum granulosum, or the granular cell layer, the prekeratin of the superficial cell forms small, darkly staining granules of dense keratin, known as keratohyalin granules. Commenting on the presence a granular layer in a tissue biopsy (hypergranulosis or spiegelosis [II.16b]) can explain the presence of white epithelium that may have been seen colposcopically. In the stratum corneum, the degenerated, pyknotic nucleus of the superficial cell dissolves completely (a process known as karyolysis), forming a layer of anucleate squames.

The cytologic feature most characteristic of hyperkeratosis is the presence of anucleate squames, particularly when occurring in clusters [I1.16a]. Anucleate squames resemble superficial cells (note the icon), but lack a nucleus. However, there may be a pale area in the space that was occupied by the nucleus before it lysed. This has been termed the nuclear ghost (boo!). Anucleate squames of hyperkeratosis usually stain yellow, orange, or pink. Nucleated cells from the granular cell layer also may be present. These cells resemble normal superficial cells, but have small, dark blue cytoplasmic keratohyalin granules, which corresponds to hypergranulosis or spiegelosis [I1.17a]. The characteristic findings in liquid-based cytology are essentially identical to those in conventional Pap smears, ie, anucleate squames, with or without keratohyaline granules.

A few uniform, polygonal anucleate squames in a Pap test have little clinical importance. However, hyperkeratosis and parakeratosis are common findings in women with condylomas or SILs. Women with extensive clusters of anucleate squames should be followed closely to rule out a hidden underlying dysplasia or cancer, particularly if there is no obvious explanation for the hyperkeratosis (eg, uterine prolapse). If the squames have irregular or pleomorphic outlines (tadpole, spindle, etc), colposcopy is suggested, because these abnormal cellular shapes are more likely to be associated with a significant keratinizing dysplasia or even carcinoma [Nauth 1983].

The Pap test may be contaminated with anucleate squames from the skin (of the vulva or fingers). In contrast to the squames of hyperkeratosis, which stain pretty in pink, yellow, and orange, these contaminant squames are coated with oils from the skin and stain an ugly ocher or rust. In pregnancy, poorly stained anucleate squames could possibly derive from fetal skin cells in amniotic fluid in cases of ruptured fetal membranes.

Keratohyalin granules look something like the brown artifact known as cornflakes [T1.5] [I1.17b]. Cornflakes are caused by tiny air bubbles trapped on top of the cell, which occur where xylene evaporated before coverslipping. These air bubbles are seen as refractile, dark golden-brown, relatively uniform, tiny speckles that cover the squamous cell, giving it the appearance of a brown cornflake. The bubbles focus above the plane of the cell. Keratohyalin granules are blue-black, somewhat larger, variable in size, and focus inside the cell [I1.17a]. Cornflakes can obscure cellular detail; recoverslipping the slide may help reduce the artifact.

Parakeratosis

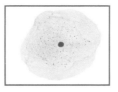

Parakeratosis is another surface keratotic reaction. Parakeratosis is benign, but like hyperkeratosis, it can conceal a significant underlying lesion, including dysplasia or cancer. Parakeratosis is brought on by the same factors that stimulate hyperkeratosis, but parakeratosis is more frequently associated with condyloma or SIL.

Parakeratosis is composed of small polygonal or rounded cells resembling miniature superficial cells (note the icon) forming layers on the epithelial surface. It is not obvious why parakeratotic cells are small.

Parakeratosis, in cytology, appears as single flat cells [I1.18a], layered strips of cells [I1.18b], or concentrically arranged "pearls" [I1.18c]. The cells usually stain orange (but may also be yellow, red, or even blue) and typically have centrally placed, pyknotic nuclei, although some nuclei may be more open. The findings are similar in liquid-based cytology, except that the parakeratotic cells tend to stain more eosinophilic than orangeophilic. Parakeratosis and hyperkeratosis frequently co-exist.

Degeneration of any cell type can cause cytoplasmic orangeophilia (a staining artifact) and nuclear pyknosis. Therefore, not every small orange cell with

T1.5 Differentiation of Keratohyalin Granules From "Cornflakes"

Keratohyalin	Cornflakes
In cell	Above cell
Fewer (granules)	More (bubbles)
Blue-black	Golden brown
Slightly larger, variable	Minute, uniform
Indicates keratosis	May obscure cell detail

T1.6 Differentiation of Pseudokeratosis and Parakeratosis

	Pseudokeratosis	Parakeratosis
Milieu	Atrophy (or birth control pills)	Mature
	Signs of degeneration	Clean, keratosis
Cell	Rounded (or columnar)	Polygonal
Cytoplasm	Granular	Waxy
Distribution	Spotty (or linear)	Groups

an ink-dot nucleus indicates parakeratosis. For example, degenerative changes can occur in endocervical cells of some women taking oral contraceptives [I1.18d]. These "pseudoparakeratotic" endocervical cells typically are found in linear arrangements in conventional Pap smears (see "Microglandular Endocervical Hyperplasia," pg 113). Look for better preserved glandular cells nearby as a clue [T1.6] Parabasal cells of atrophy also commonly undergo similar pseudokeratotic degenerative changes ("pseudo-pseudoparakeratosis"?). These degenerated atrophic cells are randomly scattered in the sample in a background of atrophy. Atypical parakeratosis, or pleomorphic parakeratosis, is a form of atypical squamous cells [I1.18e] (see pg 65).

Summary of Benign Proliferative Reactions

There are two basic benign proliferative reactions, metaplasia and keratosis, which are classically associated with the endocervix and ectocervix, respectively. Squamous metaplasia begins with reserve cell hyperplasia, which is composed of undifferentiated, basal-like cells that resemble histiocytes (generally covered by small endocervical cells). This begins to differentiate into immature squamous metaplasia with dense, rounded parabasal-like cells typically occurring in a cobblestone arrangement. These cells then differentiate to mature squamous metaplasia, with cells resembling normal intermediate cells at the surface. Under the influence of estrogen, superficial cells differentiate, indicative of a fully mature nonkeratinizing squamous epithelium, identical to the native squamous epithelium of the ectocervix. The mucosa may also "hyperdifferentiate," resulting in hyperkeratosis or parakeratosis, represented in the Pap test by anucleate or miniature superficial cells, respectively. [F1.5] recaps the benign proliferative reactions.

Dysplasia and Carcinoma In Situ (CIN, SIL)

This section takes a fairly traditional approach to recognition of preinvasive lesions, emphasizing the familiar terminology relating to dysplasia/carcinoma

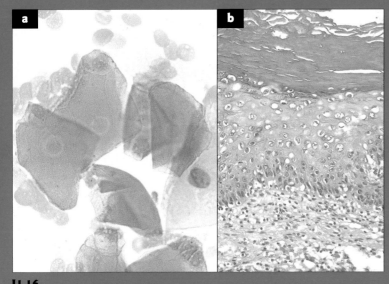

11.16
a, Anucleate squames [C]; **b**, Hyperkeratosis

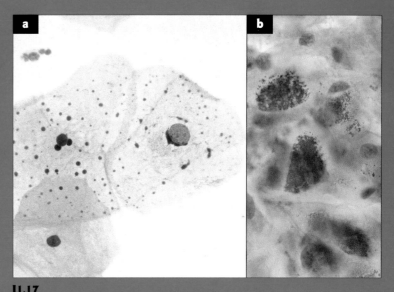

11.17
a, Spiegelosis, hypergranulosis [C]; **b**, Cornflakes [C]

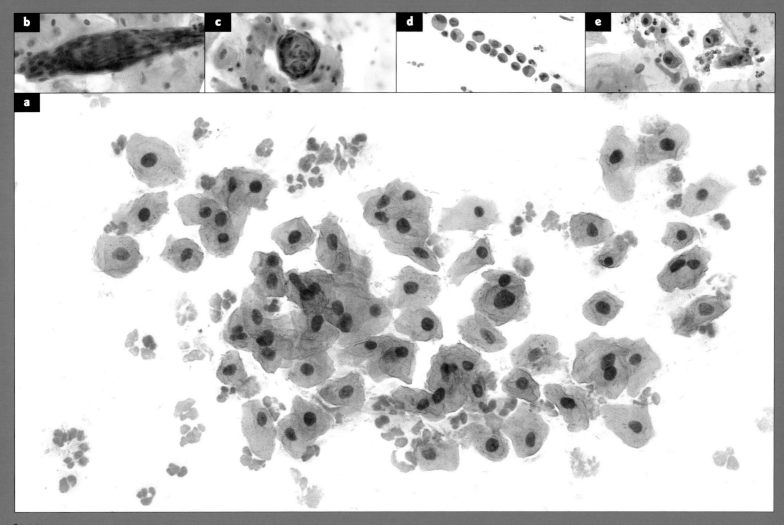

11.18
a, Parakeratosis, single cells [C]; **b**, Parakeratosis, strips [C]; **c**, Parakeratosis, pearl [C]; **d**, Pseudoparakeratosis [C]; **e**, Atypical parakeratosis (in SCC) [C]

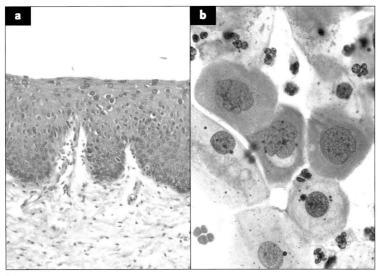

11.19
a, Squamous dysplasia; **b**, Squamous dysplasia [C]

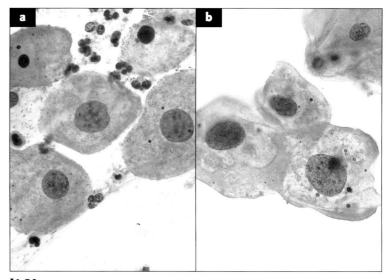

11.20
a, Mild dysplasia (L SIL) [C]; **b**, Mild dysplasia (L SIL) [L]

F1.5 Benign Proliferative Reactions

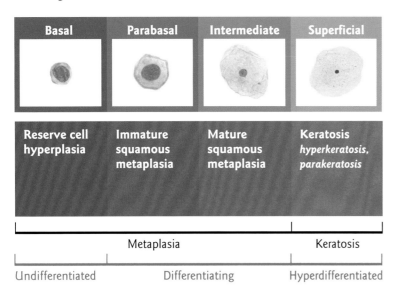

Basal	Parabasal	Intermediate	Superficial
Reserve cell hyperplasia	Immature squamous metaplasia	Mature squamous metaplasia	Keratosis *hyperkeratosis, parakeratosis*

Metaplasia		Keratosis
Undifferentiated	Differentiating	Hyperdifferentiated

in situ. Dysplasia and carcinoma in situ form a morphologic spectrum known as cervical intraepithelial neoplasia (CIN), although whether these lesions are truly neoplastic is controversial [MC Anderson 1985]. In part because of this controversy, in the late 1980s another terminology, squamous intraepithelial lesion (SIL), was introduced as an element of the Bethesda System. *The various terminologies all describe essentially the same abnormalities.* (See "Nomenclature" pg 53)

Morphogenesis

Benign proliferation indicates that the cell's machinery for division (the cell cycle) has been "revved up." Although the biologic system is perturbed, it is still under control, and can revert to normal if the inciting stimulus is removed or neutralized. Cell division is normally confined to a single layer of basal cells attached to the basement membrane. The daughter cells blossom and mature in an orderly fashion.

However, if something (eg, a virus) causing genetic injury deranges the proliferating cells, they may gradually lose control of basic cellular functions, like division and differentiation, and become neoplastic. The abnormal cells continue to divide, but fail to differentiate completely, as they rise in the epithelium, ie, the proliferation is disorderly. *Disordered proliferation is the essence of dysplasia* ("Dysplasia" derives from the Greek: bad molding, ie, abnormal development.) [11.19a].

As the abnormality progresses, the cells differentiate less and less, gradually losing their squamous features, until eventually the full thickness of the epithelium is made up of *undifferentiated*, atypical, basaloid cells. This stage is known as carcinoma in situ [11.22a].

The essential difference between dysplasia and carcinoma in situ is the presence or absence, respectively, of any visible sign of squamous differentiation in the abnormal cells (discounting surface keratotic reactions). The morphology of the squamous lesion depends on the maturity of the epithelium in which the abnormal process occurs [Patten 1978]. Stated simply: *dysplasias essentially resemble the benign proliferative reactions*, just as, in turn, the benign proliferative reactions resemble normal maturation and the icons. For example, a dysplasia may arise in, or mimic, immature squamous metaplasia. The dysplastic cells resemble ordinary immature metaplasia, but have abnormal ("big, dark") nuclei, in other words, parabasal-like cells with dysplastic nuclei.

Morphology of Dysplasia and Carcinoma In Situ

Because carcinoma in situ is often described as a "full thickness abnormality" of the epithelium, a common misconception is to think that dysplasia is not a "full thickness" epithelial abnormality [c Walsh 1995]. Here are two key concepts. First, the abnormal process involves the full thickness of the epithelium in *both* dysplasia and carcinoma in situ, as it must in

Normal, Dysplasia, CIS
  Grade ~ differentiation in tissue
    Mild, Moderate, Severe Dysplasia;
    Carcinoma in situ
  Undifferentiated basaloid cells:
    Normal: Confined to single layer
    Dysplasia: Above basal layer
    CIS: Through full thickness

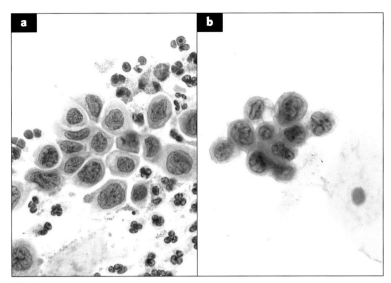

11.21
a, Severe dysplasia (H SIL) [C]; **b**, Severe dysplasia (H SIL) [L]

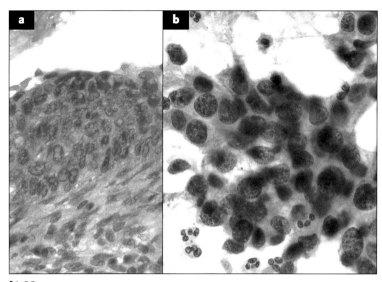

11.22
a, Carcinoma in situ; **b**, Carcinoma in situ (H SIL) [C]

order for the abnormal cells to be sampled at the mucosal surface where the Pap test is taken. Second, the essential difference between dysplasia and carcinoma in situ is whether squamous differentiation is present (dysplasia) or completely absent (carcinoma in situ). Dysplasias are graded, histologically, based on how high in the epithelium the undifferentiated basaloid cells ascend in the epithelium.

Normal and dysplastic cells have been studied by electron microscopy [Hafez 1982, Ito 1982, J Murphy 1975, 1977, Ruiter 1979]. Ultrastructural examination of dysplastic cells shows progressive loss of differentiation at the ultrastructural level with increasing severity of the lesion. There is a progressive decrease in cytoplasmic glycogen, tonofilaments, and desmosomes [Shingleton 1968, 1974]. In cell cultures, there is progressive decrease in cellular adhesion, basal pseudopodia, and cell contact inhibition [Richart 1967]. Changes in the cell surface also occur, with reduction or absence of surface microridges, but presence of abundant microvilli [Rubio 1976, Shingleton 1968, AE Williams 1973, Younes 1969].

Both dysplasia and carcinoma in situ (CIS) are characterized by abnormalities of the nucleus, including its size, shape, and outline, as well as chromatin texture and staining. (Irregular chromatin distribution is associated with invasive cancer.) Nucleoli are rare in dysplastic cells and uncommon in CIS, particularly in conventional Pap smears; their presence suggests either a reactive condition or invasive carcinoma. However, in liquid-based cytology (also histologic sections), small or indistinct nucleoli occur more commonly in dysplasia and CIS. Mitotic activity is associated with undifferentiated cells. Therefore, mitotic figures at the mucosal surface (where the cytologic sample is taken) imply a full thickness of undifferentiated cells, and hence are associated with CIS, rather than with dysplasia, in Pap tests. The background is either clean or inflammatory; a tumor diathesis (adverse host response) is associated with infiltrating cancer (see pg 42).

(see pg 42)

Cytology of Dysplasia

Cells: Single or loose sheets
Nuclei: Big, dark, ↑ N/C ratios
Cytoplasm: Squamous, dense
Background: No diathesis

Dysplasia

Dysplasia is characterized, cytologically, by the presence of at least some squamous features in the cytoplasm of the abnormal cells [11.19b]. The hallmarks of squamous differentiation are dense cytoplasm and distinct cell boundaries. Dysplastic cells frequently are single or occur in loose, flat sheets, and the cells have sharply demarcated edges [Reagan 1956a]. Nuclear features are paramount in determining whether a cell is dysplastic. Nuclear enlargement and hyperchromasia are critical in this determination (remember, compared with the intermediate nucleus, "if it's big and it's dark, it's dysplasia") [11.19b]. Dysplasias can be cytologically graded in severity depending, in essence, on how closely the abnormal cells resemble the corresponding type of benign proliferative reaction (and its icon). The N/C ratio is a measure of the degree of maturity of a cell. The higher the N/C ratio (compared with its appropriate iconic cell type), the more advanced the dysplasia. Cells that closely resemble their icon, but have abnormal ("big, dark") nuclei and mildly increased N/C ratios, indicate mild dysplasia (CIN 1, L SIL) [11.20a,b]. (Note: Although the largest nuclei are found in mild dysplasia, mildly dysplastic cells have relatively abundant cytoplasm, which tends to preserve the N/C ratio.) Cells that barely resemble their icon, with very abnormal nuclei and very high N/C ratios, but still retain some squamous cytoplasmic features, indicate severe dysplasia (CIN 3, H SIL) [11.21a,b]. The chromatin in dysplasia is usually hyperchromatic,

Determining Dysplasia

First: Evaluate nucleus

Dysplasia → nuclear enlargement, hyperchromasia

Compare with intermediate cell nucleus:
"if it's big, and it's dark, it's dysplasia"
Intermediate cell nucleus = 35 μm²
Dysplasia = 120-200+ μm² (> 3X)
Largest nuclei: Mild Dysplasia, L SIL, CIN 1 (!)

Grading Dysplasia

Then: Evaluate N/C ratio
Measure of cell maturity
Higher N/C, less mature
Mild Dysplasia: Low N/C ratios
Well-differentiated cells
Largest nuclei, abundant cytoplasm
Severe Dysplasia: High N/C ratios
Poorly-differentiated cells
Small, "raisinoid" nuclei, scant cytoplasm
Carcinoma in situ: Highest N/C ratios
Undifferentiated cells
Hyperchromatic crowded groups

evenly distributed, and relatively finely granular, although chromatin clumping may occur [Reagan 1956a]. Nuclear membrane irregularities become more pronounced with advancing degrees of dysplasia, and so, severely dysplastic cells typically have irregular, "raisinoid" nuclei [González–Oliver 1997]. High-grade dysplastic cells tend to be small, making them more difficult to spot, and chromatin abnormalities may be *less* conspicuous than in low-grade lesions, making them more difficult to interpret. Small, bland dysplastic cells are particularly likely in liquid-based cytology; therefore, nuclear membrane irregularities assume increased importance in LBC. The background is clean or inflammatory, with no tumor diathesis.

Carcinoma In Situ

Carcinoma in situ is the final stage of intraepithelial neoplasia [II.22a,b]. At this stage, the abnormal cells shed all visible signs of squamous differentiation [Reagan 1956b, 1961b]. The cells of CIS devote themselves to cell division, rather than differentiation. In contrast with dysplasia, the cytoplasm of CIS is characteristically undifferentiated (vs squamous differentiation) and appears delicate (vs dense), with ill-defined (vs distinct) cell borders [T1.7]. Three-dimensional syncytial-like aggregates, or hyperchromatic crowded groups, which are crowded clusters of disorderly, abnormal cells with hyperchromatic nuclei, are particularly characteristic of CIS (vs flat sheets of cells in dysplasia) [Reagan 1956a,b]. The hyperchromatic crowded groups typically have "chaotic architecture" (loss of nuclear polarity), coarse, dark chromatin, and mitotic figures [DeMay 2000]. Ultrastructurally, the aggregates are not true syncytia; the cells are closely spaced, but remain separate [Rubio 1976, Shingleton 1968, Stanbridge 1980, AE Williams 1973, Younes 1969].

Cytology of Carcinoma in situ

Cells: Hyperchromatic crowded groups

Nuclei: Like high-grade dysplasia

Cytoplasm: Undifferentiated, delicate

Background: No diathesis

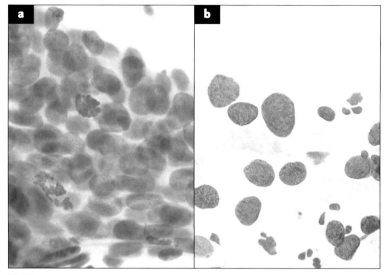

I1.23
a, CIS, mitotic figures [C]; **b**, CIS, naked nuclei [C]

Mitotic figures, including prophase nuclei (in which the nuclear envelopes have dissolved for impending cell division) are commonly seen in the cytology of CIS (but not dysplasia) [I1.23a]. Naked abnormal nuclei, which escape from the delicate, undifferentiated cytoplasm, provide a clue to the presence of CIS [I1.23b]. Oval or spindle-shaped cells may occur in CIS and are apparently caused by rapid proliferation and mechanical pressure. Rudimentary features of glandular differentiation (eg, nuclear palisading, columnar cells, microacini or rosette-like structures, feathering) are *commonly* present in the syncytial-like aggregates of squamous CIS [I1.24a]. This is said to be related to endocervical glandular extension, but is not specific, and may well reflect the ability of the neoplastic reserve-like cells to differentiate along glandular or squamous lines [W Andersen 1988, DeMay 2000, Drijkoningen 1996, K Lee 1995, P Levine 2002, Mattosinho 2003, Nasu 1993, Raab 2000, Selvaggi 1994, Siziopikou 1997, Solomon 1998, Valente 2001, van Hoeven 1996b, Wilbur 1995]. Nucleoli are not a typical feature of CIS in conventional Pap smears [Reagan 1956b], but can occur, and are more commonly observed in liquid-based cytology [I1.24b]. (Nucleoli are more closely associated with reactive conditions or invasive carcinoma, rather than in situ lesions [dysplasia, CIS].) The background may be clean or inflammatory, but there is no tumor diathesis.

There are morphologic similarities between CIS and reserve cell hyperplasia as well as between dysplasia and squamous metaplasia. In reserve cell hyperplasia, the cells are undifferentiated and often appear as syncytia. Undifferentiated cells and syncytia-like aggregates are also characteristic of CIS. In dysplasia and squamous metaplasia, the squamous features are more obvious, resulting in numerous isolated cells with dense cytoplasm and distinct cell boundaries.

T1.7 Differentiation of Dysplasia From Carcinoma In Situ

Dysplasia	Carcinoma In Situ
Histology	
Well-defined basal cell layer	Loss of basal palisade
Squamous differentiation toward surface	No differentiation
Horizontal layering (stratification)	± Vertical orientation
Increasing number mitotic figures	More abnormal mitotic figures
Mitotic figures above basal layer	Mitotic figures at surface
Cytology	
Distinct cell boundaries	Syncytial appearance
Dense cytoplasm	Delicate cytoplasm, naked nuclei
Flat sheets, single	Hyperchromatic crowded groups, ± spindle, microacini
Increasing nuclear/cytoplasmic ratio	Maximum nuclear/cytoplasmic ratio
Less irregular nuclear membrane	More irregular nuclear membrane
Finer chromatin	Coarser chromatin
Indistinct/absent nucleoli	Indistinct/absent nucleoli

The cells of CIS usually are relatively small, with scant cytoplasm. The highest N/C ratios occur in CIS: the cells are composed almost entirely of their nuclei [Reagan 1956b]. Nuclear abnormalities, including membrane irregularity and chromatin coarseness, tend to be more pronounced than in dysplasia [I1.22b].

Metaplastic and Keratinizing Lesions

There are two basic morphologic types of dysplasia, metaplastic and keratinizing, just as there were two basic types of benign proliferative reactions. Metaplastic and keratinizing dysplasias arise in, or mimic, the respective benign proliferative reactions

---

Types of Dysplasia

Two basic morphologies:

•Metaplastic Dysplasia

•Keratinizing Dysplasia

Mimic Benign Proliferative Reactions

For pattern recognition, not prognosis

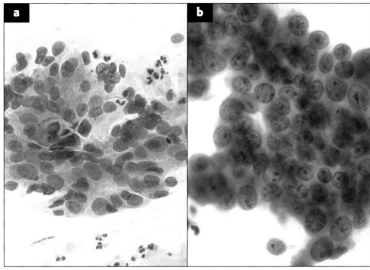

II.24
a, CIS, "glands" [C]; **b**, CIS, nucleoli [L]

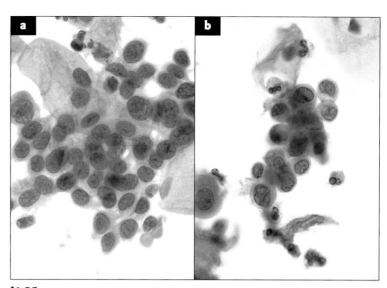

II.25
a, CIS, small cell [C]; **b**, CIS, small cell [L]

(ie, metaplasia and keratosis), which in turn imitate their corresponding icons (basal, parabasal, intermediate, and superficial cells). Metaplastic dysplasia, which is more common than the keratinizing form, can be further subdivided into immature and mature types. The morphology of carcinoma in situ is simple and based on cell size: small, intermediate, and large cell types. Microinvasive and fully invasive squamous cell carcinomas are considered later.

Metaplastic Dysplasia

Icons: Parabasal & Intermediate cells
Mimics ordinary squamous metaplasia
Except nuclei "dysplastic" (ie, big, dark)
· (Immature) Metaplastic Dysplasia
~Parabasal-like cells
...More often high grade
· (Mature) Metaplastic Dysplasia
~ Intermediate-like cells
...Usually low grade

Metaplastic Lesions
CIN Mimicking Reserve Cell Hyperplasia
Atypical Reserve Cell Hyperplasia

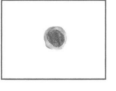

Atypical reserve cell hyperplasia, or reserve cell dysplasia, is more of a philosophical concept than an actual diagnosis [F1.6]. Reserve cell hyperplasia occurs before the onset of squamous differentiation. Therefore, an epithelial abnormality recapitulating this early stage of development would not be true squamous dysplasia, since no squamous differentiation occurred. What's more, a lesion composed of atypical, undifferentiated reserve cells would be indistinguishable from carcinoma in situ (see below) [Beyer-Boon 1978, Boon 1995]. (Atypical reserve cell hyperplasia is sometimes also used as a term for a lesion that suggests small cell carcinoma, but lacks complete diagnostic features.)

Small Cell Squamous Carcinoma In Situ

Small cell squamous carcinoma in situ is composed of atypical, undifferentiated, relatively small cells [II.25a,b]. These atypical, reserve-like cells average 11 μm in diameter. They may be present singly or in characteristic "syncytia" (hyperchromatic crowded groups). The nuclei are usually oval to spindle shaped, with a high mitotic rate. Prophase nuclei are common. The nuclear area averages ~68 μm^2 (range, 60 μm^2-80 μm^2), which is about twice the area of an intermediate cell nucleus (35 μm^2) [Patten 1978]. The chromatin is hyperchromatic and evenly distributed. It is usually coarse, but may be fine, with variable chromocenter formation. Nucleoli are absent, or rare and small in conventional Pap smears.

When small cell squamous carcinoma in situ progresses to invasive cancer, it is associated with small cell, poorly-differentiated, nonkeratinizing squamous cell carcinoma, an aggressive malignancy. (Small cell *squamous* carcinoma is not the same as small cell *neuroendocrine* carcinoma, see pg 173.) Only a minority of cases of CIS are small cell type [Patten 1978].

CIN Mimicking Immature Squamous Metaplasia
Immature Metaplastic Dysplasia

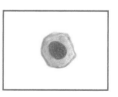

A squamous abnormality that manifests a bit further down the road of proliferative reactions from reserve cell hyperplasia, ie, after the advent of squamous differentiation, is the beginning of true squamous dysplasia. This abnormality is known as immature metaplastic dysplasia, or simply, metaplastic dysplasia [F1.7]. Although immature metaplastic dysplasia represents only 10% to 15% of all cases of dysplasia, it is particularly significant because it is

F1.6 Morphologic Range of the Basal/Reserve Cell

Basal	Reserve cell hyperplasia	[Atypical reserve cell hyperplasia]	Small cell carcinoma in situ	Small cell squamous cell carcinoma

F1.7 Morphologic Range of the Parabasal Cell

Parabasal	Immature squamous metaplasia	Immature metaplastic dysplasia	Intermediate carcinoma in situ	Non-keratinizing squamous cell carcinoma

the type most likely to progress to classical carcinoma in situ [Patten 1978]. Immature metaplastic dysplasia characteristically arises proximal to the external cervical os, in the endocervical canal.

In essence, immature metaplastic dysplasia resembles immature squamous metaplasia, except that the abnormal cells have dysplastic nuclei [II.26a,b]. The dysplastic cells usually occur singly in the Pap test, but can also be found in loose sheets or cobblestone arrangements, like ordinary immature metaplasia. Also like benign immature metaplasia, the dysplastic cells are predominantly round to oval, but may be polygonal. They are parabasal-sized and usually stain blue-green (cyanophilic). The cytoplasm is also typical of immature squamous metaplasia (ie, very dense, with very distinct cell boundaries, the "cookie cutter" look). In contrast with benign metaplasia, however, the nuclei are enlarged and hyperchromatic ("big and dark"). The dysplastic nuclei average $156 \pm 35 \ \mu m^2$, which is about 2.5 to 4 times the size of a normal immature metaplastic cell's nucleus ($50 \ \mu m^2$) or about 3 to 6 times an intermediate nucleus ($35 \ \mu m^2$) [Patten 1978]. The chromatin is generally moderately granular—finer than in small cell lesions, but coarser than mature metaplastic dysplasia. In general, the more advanced the dysplasia: the smaller the nucleus; the more irregular the nuclear membrane; the coarser the chromatin (including chromocenter formation); the scantier the cytoplasm; and the higher the N/C ratio [Sheils 1997]. Nucleoli are usually absent or indistinct.

The differential of metaplastic dysplasia can be challenging, to say the least[D Gupta 2001a,b, Zuna 2002]. The first interpretive problem is distinguishing ordinary metaplasia, particularly inflamed, degenerated metaplasia [II.27a], from metaplastic dysplasia [II.27b]. Both are composed of metaplastic cells that can be pleomorphic, with increased N/C ratios, and atypical nuclei (reactive versus dysplastic). Nuclear enlargement can occur in either reactive or dysplastic metaplastic cells, but is typically more marked in dysplasia. Although nuclear abnormalities can be subtle, hyperchromasia, coarse chromatin, or chromocenter formation favor dysplasia, while pale, fine chromatin, and prominent nucleoli favor a benign, reactive process. The presence of irregular nuclear membranes is an important sign that points to dysplasia.

Differential of Metaplastic Dysplasia

Low Grade: vs Reactive changes

High Grade:

• Small cells: Difficult to spot
  "no-see-ems," 3rd cell type

• Bland cells: Difficult to interpret
  ~ very immature metaplasia, histiocytes

  Raisinoid nuclei clue to dysplasia

Another interpretive problem is distinguishing high-grade immature metaplastic dysplastic cells from histiocytes [Sherman 2001]. When the dysplastic cells are very small and immature ("very immature metaplastic dysplasia" aka Ruth Graham's "third type cells," ie, small basaloid dysplastic cells), they can closely resemble small histiocytes [II.28a,b]. In conventional Pap smears, the dysplastic cells sometimes hide in strands of mucus with inflammatory cells, which they may resemble, and can be so well camouflaged that they are easily missed in screening ("no-see-ums"). (It's like hunting for mushrooms; once you find one, stop and look around, because there are probably others nearby.) Also in conventional Pap smears, the atypical cells often are present in a streak; therefore, look carefully at strings of cells in mucus ("follow the yellow brick road…"), as one does for small "oat" cell carcinoma in sputum [Wilbur 1997b]. (The differential of strings of cells includes: dysplasia, squamous metaplasia, histiocytes, endometrial stromal cells, endocervical cells, and pseudoparakeratosis.) Unfortunately, this helpful feature is lost in liquid-based cytology, in which the cells are randomly scattered [Solomon 1998]. Another interpretive clue is "like accompanies like." Benign immature metaplasia will usually be accompanied by benign mature metaplasia. High-grade dysplasia is usually accompanied by low-grade dysplasia. Low-grade dysplastic cells not only

tend to be larger than high-grade dysplastic cells, and therefore easier to find, but their nuclei also tend to be easier to evaluate (ie, bigger, darker, "uglier"). High-grade lesions sometimes have subtle nuclear abnormalities (look for "raisinoid nuclei" and speckled chromatin patterns [II.28a]). This brings us to an unfortunate paradox of Pap test interpretation: *the higher the grade of the dysplasia, the more difficult it can be to detect the abnormality*. Some women have severely dysplastic lesions that shed little tiny cells, which can hide in mucus, and have subtle cytologic abnormalities. Needless to say, this can make cytologic recognition difficult or impossible, particularly when the abnormal cells are sparse.

Grading of immature metaplastic dysplasia can also be difficult [II.29a,b,c]. The N/C ratio is a measure of cell maturity and is a key factor in assessing the grade of dysplasia. However, since these metaplastic cells are, by definition, immature, *the N/C ratio is elevated in both ordinary and dysplastic metaplastic cells*. Therefore, critical evaluation of nuclear features is particularly important in grading immature metaplastic dysplasia. Unfortunately, as discussed above, as the degree of dysplasia progresses, the nucleus becomes smaller and may be more difficult to evaluate. Nevertheless, the key is that the N/C ratio increases in concert with the nuclear features of advancing dysplasia. Irregular nuclear membranes favor dysplasia; smooth nuclear membranes favor a reactive process.

Intermediate Cell Carcinoma In Situ

Immature metaplastic dysplasia may progress to carcinoma in situ composed of cells intermediate in size between small cell and large cell squamous carcinoma in situ [II.30a,b]. Intermediate cell carcinoma in situ is the most common type, accounting for more than half of all cases [Patten 1978]. As usual, syncytia-like aggregates (hyperchromatic crowded groups) are characteristic. The nuclei are round to oval and average about $95 \ \mu m^2$ (range, $80 \ \mu m^2$-$120 \ \mu m^2$), about 2 to 3.5 times the size of an intermediate cell nucleus ($35 \ \mu m^2$), or about twice the size of an ordinary metaplastic cell nucleus ($50 \ \mu m^2$) [Patten 1978]. The chromatin is hyperchromatic with variable texture (usually relatively fine, but occasionally coarse). Chromocenters are variable, too, ranging from few to many. Nucleoli are usually absent or indistinct, but may be more conspicuous in some cases. Intermediate cell carcinoma in situ may progress to nonkeratinizing squamous cell carcinoma.

CIN Mimicking Mature Squamous Metaplasia

Mature Metaplastic Dysplasia

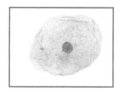

Mature metaplastic dysplasia, also known as large cell or nonkeratinizing dysplasia, arises in or mimics a mature squamous metaplastic process or the native nonkeratinizing squamous epithelium [F1.8] [Patten 1978]. The icon for this type of dysplasia is the intermediate cell, which the dysplastic cells resemble [II.31a,b]. Mature metaplastic dysplasia is usually found near the cervical os, in or near the T zone of the cervix. It is one of the most common patterns of dysplasia in the Pap test, but as might be expected from its high degree of differentiation, this

F1.8 Morphologic Range of the Intermediate Cell

Intermediate	Mature squamous metaplasia	Mature metaplastic dysplasia	Large cell carcinoma in situ	Non-keratinizing squamous cell carcinoma

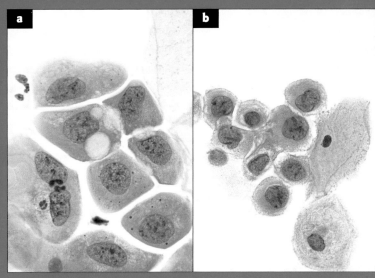

I1.26
a, Metaplastic dysplasia [C]; **b**, Metaplastic dysplasia [L]

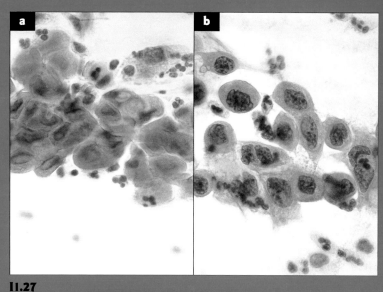

I1.27
a, Inflamed, degenerated metaplasia [C]; **b**, Metaplastic dysplasia [C]

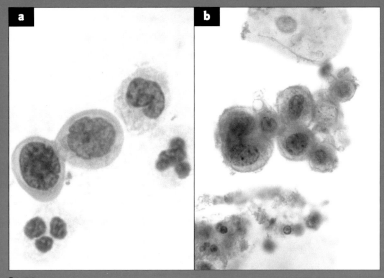

I1.28
a, Very immature metaplastic dysplasia [C, oil]; **b**, Very immature
metaplastic dysplasia [L]

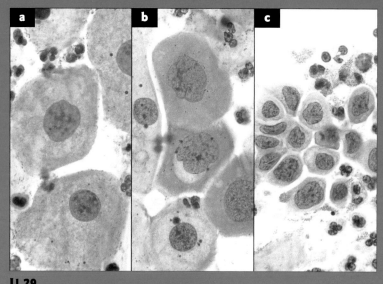

I1.29
a, Mild dysplasia [C]; **b**, Moderate dysplasia [C]; **c**, Severe dysplasia [C]

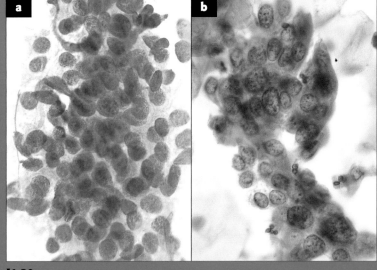

I1.30
a, Carcinoma in situ [C]; **b**, Carcinoma in situ [L]

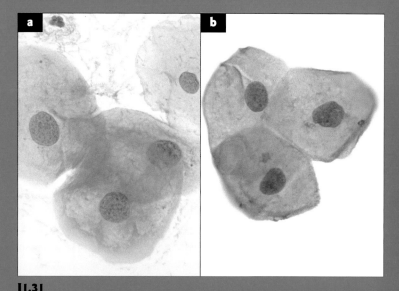

I1.31
a, Mature metaplastic dysplasia [C]; **b**, Mature metaplastic dysplasia [L]

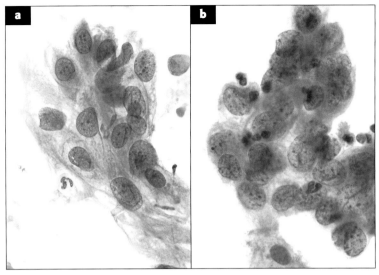

II.32
a, CIS, large cell [C]; **b**, CIS, large cell [L]

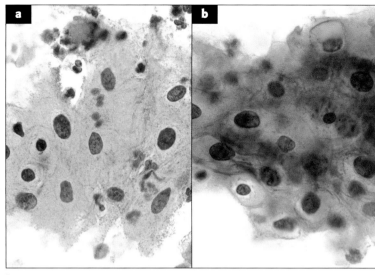

II.33
a, Keratinizing dysplasia (L SIL) [C]; **b**, Keratinizing dysplasia (L SIL) [L]

type of dysplasia is usually low-grade, often regresses spontaneously, and is unlikely to progress to carcinoma in situ or cancer, although it can.

Mature metaplastic dysplasia is composed of cells that resemble normal intermediate cells, except that their nuclei are dysplastic ("big and dark," compared with an intermediate cell nucleus). Nearly all of the cells are single and they usually have polygonal outlines, with well-defined cell borders. Most of the cells stain blue, and a few stain pink, like normal intermediate cells. However, the cytoplasm is somewhat immature and appears slightly thick and dense, and less abundant, compared with normal intermediate cell cytoplasm. The nuclei are usually only slightly hyperchromatic, but can be dark. The chromatin is usually fine, reminiscent of the normal intermediate cells, with occasional chromocenter formation. Nucleoli are usually absent or indistinct. The nuclei average $178 \pm 32 \ \mu m^2$, which is 4 to 6 times the size of a normal intermediate cell nucleus ($35 \ \mu m^2$) [Patten 1978].

When dysplasias progress, the cells become more immature. Therefore, as mature metaplastic dysplasia becomes more advanced, it begins to resemble immature metaplastic dysplasia. Because the lesions represent a morphologic spectrum, a merging of features is expected. (This spectrum of morphology is emphasized by the terminology, immature and mature metaplastic dysplasia, as opposed to metaplastic dysplasia and large cell, nonkeratinizing dysplasia, respectively.) The more or less theoretical divisions between the "two" forms of metaplastic dysplasia are presented to teach morphology and to develop the fine observational skills necessary for the cytologist [Wilbur 1997a]. However, in practice, it is not always possible, nor is it necessary, to distinguish immature from mature metaplastic dysplasia. The important things are first to recognize the cells as dysplastic, and second to grade the lesion, which in the Bethesda System, is only low-grade vs high-grade SIL.

Large Cell Carcinoma In Situ

Large cell carcinoma in situ (CIS) [II.32a,b] is the least common type of CIS [Patten 1978]. Like other kinds of classical carcinoma in situ, and in contrast with dysplasia, large cell carcinoma in situ lacks features of squamous differentiation. Although the N/C ratios are elevated, these cells can have more abundant cytoplasm and do not appear as crowded as other forms of CIS, which can lead to interpretive difficulties. The cytoplasm is usually cyanophilic, relatively delicate, and

appears syncytial (ie, not dense with well defined cell borders as is typical of squamous differentiation). Single CIS cells are rare in the large cell type, although naked nuclei may occur. The nuclei are abnormal (irregular membranes, loss of polarity, etc) and the chromatin is hyperchromatic, but rather fine, with variable chromocenter formation. The nuclei average about $164 \ \mu m^2$ (range, $150 \ \mu m^2$-$200 \ \mu m^2$) or about four to six times the size of an intermediate cell nucleus ($35 \ \mu m^2$) [Patten 1978]. Nucleoli are usually absent or indistinct. Both intermediate and large cell CIS can progress to nonkeratinizing squamous cell carcinoma.

Keratinizing Lesions
CIN Mimicking Keratosis
Keratinizing Dysplasia

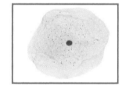

Keratinizing dysplasia, and keratinizing squamous cell carcinoma which is associated with it, arises in or mimics the hyperdifferentiated benign proliferative reaction, keratosis [F1.9]. Keratinizing dysplasia tends to arise distal to the cervical os, in the ectocervical epithelium. It is less common than the metaplastic types of dysplasia, at least in its more advanced forms [Patten 1978].

The morphology of keratinizing dysplasia echoes the morphology of the normal superficial cell, consisting of cells with dense, sometimes orangeophilic cytoplasm, and very hyperchromatic, sometimes pyknotic, nuclei [II.33a,b, I.34a,b]. Despite the image conjured up by the word "keratinizing," orangeophilic cells may be a minor, albeit characteristic, component of keratinizing dysplasia. Blue, pink, or polychromatic cells also occur. The cells are mostly single, with occasional sheets or clusters. Many of the cells, particularly in low-grade lesions,

---

F1.9 Morphologic Range of the Superficial Cell

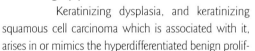

| Superficial | Keratosis *hyperkeratosis, parakeratosis* | Keratinizing dysplasia | No classical carcinoma in situ — *severe keratinizing dysplasia is equivalent* | Keratinizing squamous cell carcinoma |

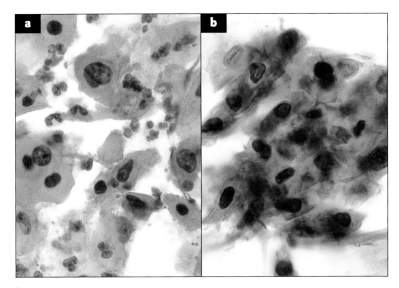

II.34
a, Keratinizing dysplasia (H SIL) [C]; **b**, Keratinizing dysplasia (H SIL) [L]

sometimes be cytologically indistinguishable from invasive keratinizing squamous cell carcinoma. In such cases, an interpretation of "H SIL with features suspicious for invasion" can be used.

Keratinizing Carcinoma In Situ

By definition, the cytoplasm of keratinizing neoplastic lesions is always keratinized. Since keratinization is the *sine qua non* of squamous differentiation, there cannot be a classical keratinizing CIS, because classical CIS requires undifferentiated cells. Therefore, in theory, severe keratinizing dysplasia is the direct precursor lesion of invasive keratinizing squamous cell carcinoma and this lesion can invade directly without going through a classical CIS stage. In practice, invasive cancer can arise from any degree, or type, of dysplasia, including low-grade lesions, but it is much more likely to arise from high-grade lesions. Severe keratinizing dysplasia can be considered the equivalent of classical CIS and both are grouped as cervical intraepithelial neoplasia, grade three (CIN 3).

Various types of dysplasia can coexist. The more serious lesions tend to occur farther up in the endocervical canal, especially in postmenopausal women, where the dysplasia identified in the Pap test may be only the "tip of the iceberg" of a more advanced lesion, including invasive cancer.

Microinvasive Squamous Cell Carcinoma

G. Mestwerdt first introduced the concept of microinvasive carcinoma in 1947 [Mestwerdt 1947]. Microinvasive carcinoma is a gray area between carcinoma in situ and fully invasive squamous cell carcinoma. As the name implies, microinvasive carcinoma is an invasive tumor, unlike carcinoma in situ, which is noninvasive. But, unlike frankly invasive cancer, microinvasive carcinoma seldom metastasizes and has a very low mortality rate (0%-5%). Therefore, microinvasive carcinoma can be treated more conservatively than frankly invasive carcinoma.

> *Microinvasive Carcinoma*
> *Gray area between CIS & SCC*
> *Invasive cancer,*
> *but curable with conservative Rx*
> *(eg, cone biopsy with adequate margins)*
> *Definition: < 3 mm of invasion*

As intraepithelial neoplasia progresses, the nucleus and cytoplasm are reverting to a more primitive state, the cells abandoning the commitment to mature and succumbing to the urge to reproduce. As the abnormal cells break through the basement membrane into the cervical stroma, which is the definition of invasion, both nuclear and cytoplasmic changes occur [Richards 1990] [T1.8]. As one of the earliest visible changes that occurs with invasion, a prominent nucleolus develops

> *Keratinizing Dysplasia*
> *Icon: Superficial cell*
> *Milieu: Abnormal keratinization*
> *HK, PK, Atypical PK*
> *Low-grade: ~ Superficial cells*
> *with dysplastic (big, dark) nuclei*
> *As grade increases: More pleomorphic*
> *including spindle & bizarre cells*
> *aka "Pleomorphic Dysplasia"*
> *Background: No diathesis*

> *Keratinizing Dysplasia*
> *Low-grade:*
> *Associated with flat condyloma*
> *Dysplastic cells = "dyskeratocytes"*
> *In essence, koilocytes without halos*
> *High-grade:*
> *DDx = Invasive Keratinizing SCC*

have well-defined, polygonal outlines, similar to normal superficial cells [II.33a,b]. Low-grade keratinizing dysplasia is closely associated with flat condyloma; the dysplastic cells are sometimes referred to as dyskeratocytes (see pg 50). As the degree of dysplasia advances, the cells become more pleomorphic (a characteristic feature), with tadpole, spindle, and irregularly shaped cells, eventually resembling keratinizing squamous cell carcinoma [II.34a,b]. A synonym for keratinizing dysplasia is pleomorphic dysplasia.

Most nuclei have relatively fine, but very hyperchromatic, uniform chromatin. Perhaps surprisingly, very coarse chromatin is not a common feature of keratinizing dysplasia. Pyknotic nuclei are characteristic, but are present in only a minority (~15%) of the cells [Patten 1978]. Other signs of nuclear degeneration (eg, karyorrhexis or lysis) also may occur. The nuclei average about 169 ± 42 µm^2 or 3.5 to 6 times the area of an intermediate cell nucleus (35 µm^2) [Patten 1978].

Keratinizing dysplasia, which arises in the milieu of keratosis, is usually accompanied by hyperkeratosis, parakeratosis, and atypical parakeratosis [Navarro 1997]. Benign keratinization features many anucleated squames, bland nuclei, uniform cells, and an organized growth pattern. In contrast, keratinizing dysplasia has abnormal keratin formation, and is associated with nuclear atypia, pleomorphic cells, and a disorganized growth pattern [Navarro 1997]. However, degenerated or pyknotic nuclei can mask the typical nuclear features of cancer and a tumor diathesis may be lacking in a keratinizing squamous cell carcinoma, which tends to grow exophytically [P Levine 2003]. Therefore, high-grade keratinizing dysplasia can

T1.8 Differential Features of Carcinoma In Situ, Microinvasive Carcinoma, and Squamous Cell Carcinoma

	Nucleus		Cytoplasm	Background
	Prominent nucleoli	Irregular chromatin distribution	Squamous differentiation	Tumor diathesis
Carcinoma in situ	−	−	−	−
Microinvasive carcinoma	+	+	±	±
Squamous cell carcinoma	++	++	++	++

in carcinoma in situ-like cells—a nonspecific marker of increased protein synthesis. Nucleoli herald the beginning of invasion (microinvasion) as the cells gear up to make proteins, possibly including a "basement membranase." Then the chromatin, which has been becoming progressively coarser during the intraepithelial phase, begins to break up into shards, changing from regular to irregular in distribution. Irregularly distributed chromatin, with parachromatin clearing, is the first truly malignant morphologic change that can be recognized in the cell.

The cytoplasm is also undergoing changes with incipient invasion. Recall that as the abnormal cells progress from dysplasia to carcinoma in situ, they *de*-differentiate. Paradoxically, as the cells progress from carcinoma in situ to invasive cancer, they *re*-differentiate: this is termed "paradoxical maturation." The cytoplasm "plumps up" a little, reacquiring squamous features. The cellular changes can be viewed as a blossoming from carcinoma in situ to microinvasion to frank carcinoma: invasive cancer germinates from seeds of carcinoma in situ. As invasion progresses, the cells differentiate to varying degrees, ranging from poorly-differentiated or small cell squamous cell carcinoma, to moderately differentiated or nonkeratinizing squamous cell carcinoma, to well-differentiated or keratinizing squamous cell carcinoma. With deep invasion, the stroma is broken down, the surface ulcerates, and bleeding occurs, which results in protein, fibrin, fresh and old blood, dead cells, and debris in the background. This "dirty" background, known as a tumor diathesis, is highly characteristic of invasive cancer (see pg 42 for more discussion of tumor diathesis).

The exact definition of microinvasive carcinoma remains controversial, with both its beginning and end points in dispute. Some make a distinction between early stromal invasion and microcarcinoma [Lohe 1978a,b,c]. The Society of Gynecologic Oncologists suggests that questionable stromal invasion be regarded as carcinoma in situ [Seski 1977]. Various authors arbitrarily set the deepest limits of microinvasion of the stroma between 1 and 5 mm, or even deeper [G Larsson 1983]. Lymph node metastases are rare to nonexistent with less than 1 mm of invasion, but occur in proportion to greater depth of invasion, reaching as high as 11.1% at 5 mm of invasion [Creasman 1998, A Ng 1969, van Nagell 1983].

The two most widely used definitions of microinvasive carcinoma are those of the Society of Gynecologic Oncologists (SGO) and the International Federation of Gynecology and Obstetrics (FIGO) [W Benson 1977, Burghardt 1991, Creasman 1985, Robert 1990]. The SGO limits depth of penetration to 3 mm or less, with no vascular space involvement by tumor [Seski 1977]. FIGO divides microinvasive carcinoma into two groups, stage IA1 and IA2 [JH Benedet 2000, FIGO 1986]. FIGO Stage IA1 exhibits "minimal" or "early" stromal invasion; the maximum depth of stromal invasion is less than 3.0 mm [JH Benedet 2000]. There is no evidence that tumors with less than 1 mm of invasion carry any more risk than carcinoma in situ; in fact, tumors with less than 3 mm have less than 1% risk of lymph node metastases even with vascular space invasion [Ehrmann 1996, A Ng 1969]. FIGO Stage IA2, measurable lesions, limits invasion to 5.0 mm or less; vascular invasion is noted, but does not exclude a diagnosis of microinvasion. However, vascular invasion is a negative prognostic factor for any tumor that is more advanced than stage IA1. For stage IA1 or IA2 tumors, the maximum horizontal spread is 7.00 mm [JH Benedet 2000].

Invasion is measured from the base of the epithelium, at the basement membrane, where invasion begins, which could be from a gland [JH Benedet 2000, Östör 1993b]. (Note: This is in contrast to melanomas, which are measured from the granular cell layer of the overlying epithelium.) Histologic features that help to determine prognosis are: depth of invasion, lateral extent, extension into vascular spaces, growth pattern (pushing vs spray),

and host immune response (inflammation, including eosinophils in the stroma [G Spiegel 2002]). Confluence of tumor growth is important insofar as it affects the overall extent of the tumor. Confluence generally correlates with the depth of invasion [Robert 1990].

Clinical Features

As part of the general trend in earlier cervical cancer detection, microinvasive carcinoma is being recognized with increasing frequency. Currently, as many as a quarter of all squamous cell carcinomas are microinvasive when first diagnosed, depending upon the patient population and whether the 3 mm or 5 mm criterion is used. Cytology is critical in the detection of this disease because up to two thirds of the patients are asymptomatic, many symptoms are nonspecific, and more than half of the patients have a grossly normal appearing cervix. However, about one third of the patients present with more specific symptoms, eg, abnormal bleeding or vaginal discharge [Kolstad 1989, G Larsson 1983, A Ng 1969].

The mean age at diagnosis of microinvasive carcinoma is midway between that of CIN 3/CIS and fully invasive cancer, with each step taking nearly a decade to evolve (eg, average ages for CIN 3–30 years, microinvasive squamous carcinoma–39 years, frankly invasive squamous carcinoma–47years) [A Ng 1969, Paraskevaidis 1992]. (Note that in an individual patient, the progression can occur faster, slower, or not at all [Christopherson 1964].) More than half the cases of microinvasive carcinoma occur in the anterior portion of the cervix, another third involve both the anterior and posterior cervix, while the posterior cervix alone is involved in only about 10% of cases, a distribution similar to CIN [A Ng 1969].

Histology

Just as when Julius Caesar crossed the Rubicon, when neoplastic cells cross the basement membrane, invasion has begun: *Alea jacta est*, the die is cast [II.35a]. There are three histologic clues to early invasion, pertaining to the lesion contour, the host response, and paradoxical maturation. Early invasion actually begins when a single cell or cell cluster enters the stroma from the overlying neoplastic epithelium [Marcuse 1971], dissolving the basement membrane as it pushes out a few microns, forming a "microinvasive bud" [Ehrmann 1988, Fennell 1955, Fidler 1959]. As the tumor invades a little deeper into the stroma, the contour of the lesion becomes irregular or raggedy. The basement membrane is disrupted and tongues of tumor infiltrate the stroma. A host response to the infiltrating tumor is usually present histologically and includes local desmoplasia with edematous, young collagen (which is metachromatic) and a chronic inflammatory reaction, which may include granuloma formation and eosinophils [Östör 1993b, Leman 1976, Rubio 1974, Santo 1987, G Spiegel 2002]. Paradoxical maturation refers to squamous maturation occurring at the base of the lesion [Burghardt 1973]. The infiltrating cells begin to differentiate and accumulate eosinophilic cytoplasm. Squamous pearls may be seen at the base of the epithelium. Observing keratinized cells directly abutting stroma is an important histologic clue to invasion. Giant bizarre cells, large keratinized cells, keratin pearls, and necrosis also suggest invasion [Leung 1994]. Microinvasion usually (90% of cases) arises from the surface epithelium, with or without involvement of the glands [A Ng 1969]. There are usually (>90% of cases) two or more foci of invasion [A Ng 1969]. The epithelial surface may be ulcerated.

Most (~80%) cases of microinvasive carcinoma are nonkeratinizing squamous cell carcinoma, some are keratinizing (~15%), and a few are small cell

(~5%) [G Larsson 1983, A Ng 1972, Tweeddale 1969]. Keratinizing microinvasive carcinoma may have the best prognosis [G Larsson 1983].

The larger the size of the CIN lesion, the greater the risk of microinvasion [Tidbury 1992]. In nearly 95% of cases in which a determination can be made, the origin of the invasion is carcinoma in situ with or without dysplasia. *Invasive carcinoma almost always arises from the most advanced intraepithelial abnormalities, usually classical carcinoma in situ.* Only a few cancers seem to arise from dysplasia, and in very rare cases, the overlying epithelium is histologically normal [Burghardt 1976, A Ng 1969]. Therefore, classic CIS, rather than squamous dysplasia, would seem to be the critical lesion in cervical carcinogenesis, since CIS is almost always the immediate precursor lesion of cervical squamous cell carcinoma. (It would appear that the "old guys" [Reagan, Patten, et al] were basically right: CIS is the true precursor lesion, with squamous dysplasia of any grade being much less risky. It is unfortunate that both the CIN and SIL terminologies fail to account specifically for classic CIS. While acknowledging the difficulties of separating severe dysplasia from carcinoma in situ, without a specific interpretive category for CIS, it seems more likely that CIS will be overlooked, but I digress...)

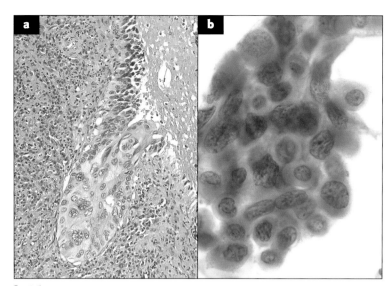

II.35
a, Microinvasive carcinoma; **b**, Microinvasive carcinoma [L]

Cytology

Microinvasive carcinoma is the bridge between in situ and fully invasive squamous cell carcinoma. The cells are changing from being merely neoplastic to frankly malignant. As an evolving process, microinvasive carcinoma presents a spectrum of morphologic findings. As invasion begins, the cells closely resemble carcinoma in situ, but the deeper the invasion, the more microinvasive carcinoma resembles frank cancer [F1.10, 1.11]. There are four key cytologic clues to microinvasive carcinoma, regarding: nucleoli, irregular chromatin, squamoid cytoplasm, and tumor diathesis [T1.8].

Microinvasive carcinoma commonly exfoliates hyperchromatic crowded groups, or syncytial-like aggregates, of cells that look like those of classic carcinoma in situ [II.35b]. Single cells are more common than in CIS. The nuclei average about $88 \pm 39.2 \ \mu m^2$ in area, or about 1.5 to 3.5 times the size of an intermediate cell nucleus ($35 \ \mu m^2$) [Patten 1978]. The N/C ratio is high. The nuclear membrane is focally thickened. The nuclear outline is irregular and may have sharp, jagged angles. Another clue is molding of a nucleus in one cell around the cytoplasm of another ("bird's eyes") [II.36a] [Ehrmann 1996].

The earliest, though non-specific, cytologic change in microinvasive carcinoma is the development of prominent nucleoli that are the harbingers of microinvasion [II.36b,c] [Patten 1978]. True nucleoli are circumscribed masses that have a distinctly acidophilic staining reaction; circumscribed basophilic masses are classified as chromocenters ("false nucleoli") [Reagan 1961b]. In conventional Pap smears, true nucleoli are unusual in carcinoma in situ, and when present, are usually small; however, chromocenters are common in CIS [Reagan 1961b]. In contrast, in microinvasive carcinoma, prominent nucleoli are found in up to 25%

Cytology of Microinvasive Carcinoma

Key clues: Nucleus, Cytoplasm, Background

Evaluate HCGs of CIS
 · *Prominent nucleoli?*
 · *Irregular chromatin?*
 · *Squamoid cytoplasm?*
 · *Tumor diathesis?*

Deeper invasion ⇒ more like SCC

In practice: histologic, not cytologic, diagnosis

F1.10 Nucleoli Related to Depth of Stromal Invasion

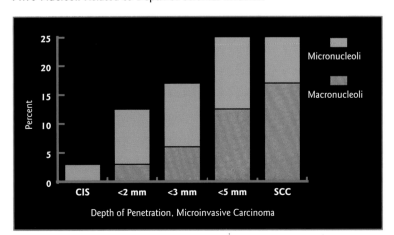

[A Ng 1969]

F1.11 Cytologic Findings Related to Depth of Stromal Penetration

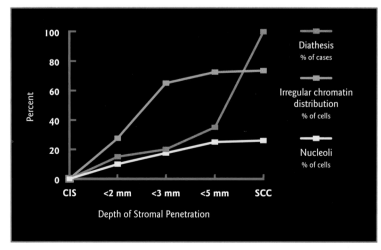

Features of squamous differentiation also develop [A Ng 1969, 1972]. At <1 mm, microcarcinoma resembles CIS [Nguyen 1984a], and at >5 mm, frank SCC. A diathesis is not always present in invasive SCC.

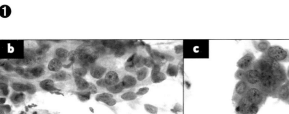
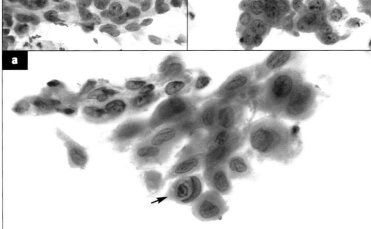
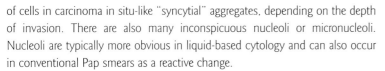

II.36
a, Microcarcinoma, bird's eye (arrow) [L]; **b**, Microcarcinoma, nucleoli [C];
c, Microcarcinoma, nucleoli [L]

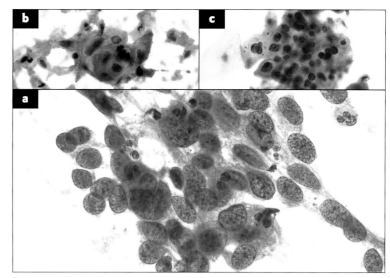

II.37
a, MicroCA, irregular chromatin [C]; **b**, MicroCA, squamous differentiation [C];
c, MicroCA, squamous differentiation [L]

of cells in carcinoma in situ-like "syncytial" aggregates, depending on the depth of invasion. There are also many inconspicuous nucleoli or micronucleoli. Nucleoli are typically more obvious in liquid-based cytology and can also occur in conventional Pap smears as a reactive change.

The chromatin texture varies from fine to coarse, and chromocenter formation is variable. Irregular chromatin distribution, with clear space between the granules (parachromatin clearing), is the first truly malignant feature of the nucleus, but may be very subtle in the beginning [II.36b, I.37a]. To judge chromatin texture, think of ice cream. Fine, even chromatin, such as in normal intermediate cell nuclei, is smooth and uniform, like chocolate ice cream (smooth chromatin texture). Coarse, evenly distributed chromatin, as may be seen in dysplasia/carcinoma in situ, is like chocolate chip ice cream (uniform chromatin chips, evenly distributed). Coarse, irregularly distributed chromatin, as seen in invasive carcinoma, is like chocolate chunk ice cream (irregular chromatin chunks, randomly distributed—chunky monkey chromatin).

The first cells that invade the stroma acquire dense, acidophilic cytoplasm (apparent keratinization), ie, they "redifferentiate" from the undifferentiated state of carcinoma in situ (paradoxical maturation) [II.37b,c]. Differentiation is minimal at first, but becomes progressively more prominent with deeper invasion. The differentiated malignant cells are larger than those of carcinoma in situ, with more abundant cytoplasm, and lower N/C ratios. They are also more pleomorphic and may have abnormally heavy keratinization. Excessive keratinization, keratin clumps, concentric keratin rings, pearls, snake or tadpole cells speak not only for invasion, but also say that the carcinoma is squamous cell type [Ehrmann 1996].

The deeper the invasion and the greater the horizontal spread, the more the cytologic picture looks like frank cancer [Sugimori 1987]. A tumor diathesis begins to appear, reflecting the host response, which is characteristic of fully invasive carcinoma. Fiber-like cells in this setting make squamous cell carcinoma likely [Ehrmann 1996]. Cancer cells tend to lose their cohesion and scatter individually in the sample. The cytologic features of microinvasive carcinoma are the most distinctive at 3 mm of invasion. Shallower invasion resembles carcinoma in situ, but by 5 mm of penetration, microinvasive carcinoma may be cytologically indistinguishable from deeply invasive cancer.

A cytologic interpretation of microinvasive carcinoma should *not* be considered definitive [Covell 1992]. Although some retrospective cytologic studies have reported remarkable accuracy (nearly 90%) [W Johnston 1982, A Ng 1972, G-K Nguyen 1984a], microinvasive carcinoma is ultimately a histologic, not a cytologic, diagnosis. In practice, in a substantial number of cases, there is neither cytologic nor colposcopic suspicion of invasion ("occult carcinoma") [MC Anderson 1995, Paraskevaidis 1992]. Conversely, virtually any of the features of microinvasive carcinoma, including prominent nucleoli, irregular chromatin, and a necrotic background, can be present occasionally in noninvasive lesions, particularly when obtained by the endocervical brush [Covell 1992]. For staging purposes the diagnosis must be based, at a minimum, on thorough examination of an adequate excisional specimen (with the margins being free of disease). The most important contribution of the cytology of microinvasive carcinoma is to detect the presence of a possibly invasive lesion. When microinvasion is suspected, a useful cytologic interpretation is "carcinoma in situ, invasion not excluded" or, to use Bethesda System language, "H SIL, with features suspicious for invasion." (The term, microinvasive carcinoma, is not included the Bethesda System lexicon.) When microinvasive carcinoma is suspected cytologically, colposcopy and biopsy are the next appropriate steps in clinical management. The diagnosis of microinvasive carcinoma always requires histologic assessment of the entire lesion.

Differential

The differential of microinvasive carcinoma includes carcinoma in situ and frankly invasive squamous cell carcinoma. Prominent nucleoli, occurring in carcinoma in situ-like aggregates, are the most sensitive feature to the presence of invasion. However, *nucleoli are not specific for invasion*. For example, carcinoma in situ can have prominent nucleoli as a reactive change [II.38a]. High-grade CIN involving glands may also have micronucleoli, falsely suggesting microinvasive carcinoma [Covell 1992]. The presence of both prominent nucleoli and irregular chromatin distribution is more specific for invasive malignancy than either one alone. In most cases, frank squamous cell carcinoma has more abnormal cells, with more pleomorphism, more irregular chromatin, and more prominent nucleoli, as well as a tumor diathesis.

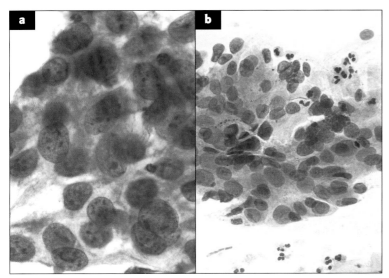

11.38
a, CIS, nucleoli [C]; **b**, CIS, "glands" [C]

Microinvasive carcinoma typically exfoliates three-dimensional groups of cells with relatively delicate (nonkeratinized) cytoplasm and prominent nucleoli. These features may resemble those of adenocarcinoma. Furthermore, squamous carcinoma in situ commonly has rudimentary glandular features (eg, palisading, columnar cells, microacini, rosettes, feathering), which further heighten the resemblance to adenocarcinoma [11.38b] [*W Andersen 1988, DeMay 2000, Drijkoningen 1996, K Lee 1995, P Levine 2002, Mattosinho 2003, Nasu 1993, Raab 2000, Selvaggi 1994, Siziopikou 1997, Solomon 1998, Valente 2001, van Hoeven 1996b, Wilbur 1995*]. Well-formed glands, columnar cells, and evidence of mucin production indicate true glandular differentiation. Rare tumors may be mixed adenosquamous microinvasive carcinoma.

Since squamoid features of the cytoplasm are relatively common in microinvasive carcinoma, ordinary squamous dysplasia also enters into the differential. However, in dysplasia, the chromatin is regularly distributed and nucleoli are usually absent or indistinct. Furthermore, evidence of *heavy* cytoplasmic keratinization, which can be present in either microinvasive carcinoma or frankly invasive cancer, is not a usual feature of dysplasia. (Let it also be noted that some cases of high-grade keratinizing dysplasia are difficult to distinguish from invasive squamous cell carcinoma.) Finally, an inflammatory background (inflammatory diathesis) can closely mimic a tumor diathesis, in which case the key to the correct interpretation is the presence (or absence) of definitive tumor cells. (For further discussion of diathesis, see "Squamous Cell Carcinoma.")

Biology

According to an older study, the average age of women with stromal penetration of <1 mm is 42.8 years; for 1 mm to <3 mm, 46.7 years; and for 3 mm to <5 mm, 50.3 years [*A Ng 1969*]. This suggests that the tumor infiltrates at the rate of roughly about 0.5 mm per year, at least in the beginning. Early invasion may be reversible in some cases, possibly because the immune system may work to eradicate foci of invasive carcinoma [*Patten 1978, Reagan 1967, Wentz 1962*].

A characteristic feature of invasion is cytoplasmic differentiation of the invasive cells. The differentiation of the invasive vanguard of cells resem-

bles keratinization, but is actually due to increased production of contractile protein filaments consistent with actin and myosin [*Genadry 1978*], which like keratin filaments, are acidophilic. These contractile proteins are important in cell motility, hence, they could also be significant in invasion of the stroma. However, after invasion has been established, the cells undergo true squamous differentiation to varying degrees, although the invasive vanguard continues to make contractile proteins.

Therapy

Therapy for microinvasive carcinoma is as controversial as its definition. [T1.9] gives a general idea of the extent of surgery. Depth of stromal penetration is but one aspect of complete evaluation of the lesion. Other important factors to be considered in recommending appropriate therapy include horizontal extent or volume, confluence, vascular invasion, histologic type, and margins of the excisional specimen (eg, cone biopsy). Although LEEP is now commonly used in diagnosis and therapy of microinvasive carcinoma, some authors have suggested it should be avoided when invasive carcinoma is suspected [*G Eddy 1994*].

Relative indications for more extensive surgery in microinvasive carcinoma include: (1) extensive or apparently multifocal disease, (2) extensive tumor confluence, (3) unequivocal vascular involvement, especially away from the tumor, (4) positive margins in excisional specimen, (5) cell type (small cell, adenosquamous, etc), and (6) tumor differentiation (especially poorly-differentiated adenocarcinoma or mixed).

Conization is acceptable management for stage IA1 tumors. For stage IA2 tumors, primary therapy may consist of radical hysterectomy and bilateral pelvic lymphadenectomy. Squamous cell carcinoma is not a hormonally dependent tumor; therefore, oophorectomy is optional. Radiation therapy is another management alternative [*JH Benedet 2000*].

T1.9 Therapy for Microinvasive Carcinoma

	Extent	(+) LN	Therapy	Mortality
FIGO Ia1	<1 mm*	<1%	Cone biopsy	0
SGO	≤3 mm	<2%	Hysterectomy†	1%
FIGO Ia2	≤5 mm	<7%	Individualized	5%

[*W Benson 1977, Burghardt 1991, Creasman 1985, Robert 1990*]
*Not defined—see text.
†Simple hysterectomy; also cone biopsy with margins.

Squamous Cell Carcinoma

In the past, when people spoke of cervical cancer, they were speaking almost exclusively of squamous cell carcinoma, because 95% of cervical cancers were squamous type. Squamous cell carcinoma is the cancer that Pap tests are primarily effective in preventing. Because of the Pap test, the incidence of squamous cancer has fallen dramatically, although it still remains the most common form of cervical cancer. (In stark contrast, glandular cancers are on the rise despite extensive Pap test screening.) Squamous cell carcinoma is also being detected at earlier stages today than in the past, thanks to the Pap test [*J Carmichael 1984, Pretorius 1991*]. Cervical squamous cancers in asymptomatic women presenting with abnormal Pap tests are usually (> 90% of cases) stage I or stage II at the time of discovery, with as many as 25% being only microinvasive [Pretorius 1991]. Today, many are either asymptomatic or have only nonspecific symptoms, an ominous one being abnormal bleeding (eg, postcoital, intermenstrual, postmenopausal). Pain, weight loss, anemia, etc, are usually late symptoms. Cytology plays an important role in detecting cervical cancer, but unfortunately, by the time the invasive cancer has developed, the battle of preventing cancer by detecting preinvasive disease has already been lost.

The gross appearance of squamous cell carcinoma is variable. The tumor can grow exophytically, having a polypoid or papillary pattern reminiscent of venereal warts, or it can be flat or ulcerating. In any case, the tumor usually infiltrates as cords of cells into the stroma and surrounding tissues. There is often chronic inflammation, composed predominantly of lymphocytes and plasma cells, surrounding the infiltrating tumor. Papanicolaou mentions eosinophils being associated with invasive carcinoma [Papanicolaou 1941]; eosinophils may be a marker of invasion in cervical squamous neoplastic lesions [G Spiegel 2002].

Squamous cell carcinomas are traditionally divided into three major categories: large cell keratinizing, large cell nonkeratinizing, and small cell nonkeratinizing types [Reagan 1957, 1961b]. These three categories encompass most squamous cancers, although there are also rare types, such as verrucous, papillary, lymphoepithelioma-like, and spindle cell squamous carcinomas. The WHO classification recognizes only keratinizing and nonkeratinizing types. The Bethesda System does not specifically distinguish among types of squamous cell carcinoma.

Squamous Cell Carcinoma

· *Poorly Differentiated (Small Cell)*

· *Moderately (Nonkeratinizing)*

· *Well Differentiated (Keratinizing)*

Other: Verrucous, Warty, Papillary,

Urothelial, Lymphoepithelioma-like,

Spindle squamous cell carcinomas

Keratinizing SCC was formerly the most common cervical cancer, and remains common in countries without screening programs, but nonkeratinizing SCC is now more common in the United States. Although reported rates vary, up to one third of cases of cervical carcinomas either have a glandular component (adenosquamous carcinoma) or are pure adenocarcinomas (see "Cervical adenocarcinoma") [C Buckley 1989]. Keratinizing SCC is well to moderately differentiated and composed of large cells. Nonkeratinizing SCCs are usually moderately to poorly-differentiated, but essentially all small cell squamous carcinomas are poorly-differentiated. Note also that other types of small cell carcinomas, including poorly-differentiated neuroendocrine carcinomas, occur in the cervix and that not all poorly-differentiated squamous carcinomas are small cell type. These and other rare tumors are discussed separately.

The prognosis of squamous cell carcinoma depends primarily upon the stage of the tumor, but age is also important. The survival rate for younger women, especially those younger than 30 years of age, is generally poorer than for older women, particularly if there is lymph node involvement [Fenton 1990, Maddux 1990]. In other words, squamous cell carcinoma tends to be more aggressive in young women. Regardless of age, lymph node involvement and distant metastases are poor prognostic factors. The effect of histologic type and grade of squamous cell carcinoma on prognosis is controversial. Small cell squamous carcinoma is probably more aggressive than other squamous cancers, although once small cell neuroendocrine carcinomas are excluded, the differences diminish. In most body sites, keratinizing squamous cell carcinoma is associated with better differentiation and therefore, a better prognosis. However, because the cervical epithelium is normally nonkeratinizing, an argument could be made that nonkeratinizing squamous cell carcinomas are the better differentiated at this site [Wentz 1959, 1965]. In summary, it has yet to be conclusively proven that histologic grading or typing of squamous cell carcinoma reliably predicts prognosis of cervical squamous cell carcinoma [Goellner 1976, Crissman 1985]. However, mucus secretion, indicating glandular differentiation, may portend a worse prognosis (see discussion under adenocarcinoma, pg 125) [C Buckley 1988].

Prognostic Factors

Stage

Local extent

Vascular invasion

Metastases

Cell type and subtype

Squamous (large or small)

Adenocarcinoma (origin)

Sarcoma (type)

Broders grade

Age

Cytology

The cellular characteristics of squamous cell carcinoma are similar to those of microinvasive carcinoma, but more developed, and feature classical malignant criteria [Reagan 1957, 1961b]. These include nuclear enlargement, irregular membranes, variable hyperchromasia, abnormal chromatin structure, prominent nucleoli, and squamoid (dense) cytoplasm; the findings are similar in both conventional Pap smears and liquid-based cytology, with only minor differences [T1.10]. A tumor diathesis reflects the host response to the invading tumor, as the stroma breaks down and bleeds. ("Diathesis" is an odd choice of words; it means susceptibility to a disease, rather than a reaction to it, but the word is here to stay.) A tumor

---

Tumor Diathesis

Host response to tumor

Degenerated cells, debris

Fibrin, protein

Fresh & old blood

Necrosis

CPS: Granular "dirty" background

LBC: Fibrillar/granular, "clings" to cells

T1.10 General Cellular Features of Squamous Cell Carcinoma

Single cells, loose aggregates

Variation of features from cell to cell

Tadpole, spindle, or heavily keratinized cells

Nuclei

  Average smaller than in dysplasia

    (50 –120 μm^2 for SCC vs 120–210 μm^2 for dysplasia)

  Pleomorphic (size/shape)

  Irregular membranes

  Chromatin abnormalities

    Irregular distribution

    Increased coarseness

    Parachromatin clearing

  Nucleoli

    Increased size and number

    Irregular shapes

Tumor diathesis

Often associated with dysplasia/carcinoma in situ

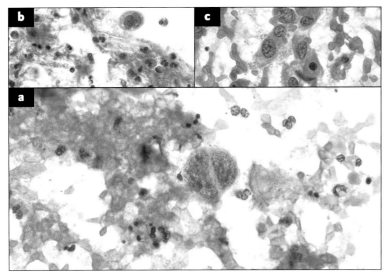

II.39
a, SCC, diathesis [C]; **b**, SCC, diathesis [L]; **c**, SCC, diathesis [C]

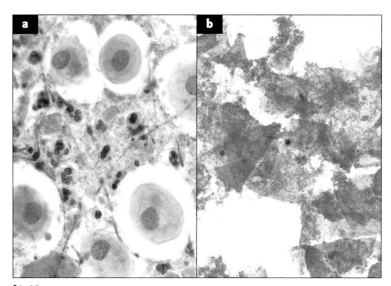

II.40
a, Atrophy, benign diathesis [C]; **b**, Cocci, mimic diathesis [C]

diathesis consists of degenerated cells and debris, fibrin (fine threads or fragments), old blood (finely granular pinkish material or RBC stroma), and necrosis [II.39c]. The diathesis may be spread diffusely in the background or may only be focally present around tumor cells. In liquid-based cytology, the diathesis usually occurs as clumps of dense fibrillar to granular material with a "ratty" appearance, but sometimes is seen as a thin "tissue paper-like" sheets of proteinaceous material with well-defined edges, that may contain entrapped tumor cells, cell debris, inflammatory cells, and red blood cells. The necrotic material tends to adhere to cells ("clinging diathesis"), rather than being dispersed in the background of the slide as in conventional Pap smears [II.39a,b].

Tumor diathesis is a key cytologic feature of frankly invasive carcinoma that is, in and of itself, a suspicious finding [von Haam 1954, Patten 1978]. Complete absence of blood or diathesis is rare in cervical cancer [Papanicolaou 1943]. However, not all cancers are accompanied by a tumor diathesis [Rushing 1997]. Microinvasive carcinomas, exophytic tumors, and metastases are more likely to have a clean background, while deeply invasive tumors are more likely to have a diathesis. Tumor diathesis can be subtle in some cases. In other cases, the diathesis may be so extensive that it dilutes or obscures diagnostic cells. Also, a tumor diathesis alone is insufficient for an unequivocal interpretation of cancer: *cancer cells must also be identified*. Several different benign processes can be associated with a background that looks like a tumor diathesis ("benign diathesis"). For example, an inflammatory, dirty background is frequently present in severe infections, particularly due to *Trichomonas* or herpes. A granular background resembling a tumor diathesis is also common in severely atrophic samples from postmenopausal women [Selvaggi 2002b] [II.40a]. Some other possible explanations for a "benign diathesis" include: cervical stenosis, abscess, necrotic polyp, and radiation therapy. Inspissated mucin from a nabothian cyst can have a granular character similar to a tumor diathesis. In situ lesions in a gland

can break down and result in comedo-like necrosis, mimicking a tumor diathesis [P Levine 2003, Leung 1994]. Also, abundant bacteria, especially cocci, can produce a blue, granular background, mimicking a tumor diathesis (look for bacteria-coated "clue cells," see pg 100) [I.40b]. The absence of cancer cells, despite careful search, favors a benign interpretation. However, tumor cells may be sparse or absent in liquid-based cytology, eg, owing to clogging of filters with necrotic material and blood [Chacho 2003, S Clark 2002]. Furthermore, tumor diathesis and other invasive features may be subtle in LBC, resulting in some cancers being misinterpreted as dysplasia. The various types of squamous cell carcinomas are discussed below [T1.11].

Benign Diathesis

Severe infection, eg, Trichomonas, herpes

Pyometra, Abscess

Cervical stenosis

Necrotic, ulcerated polyp

Severe atrophy

Coccoid bacteria

Key: presence or absence of cancer cells

T1.11 Characteristic Features of Squamous Cell Carcinomas

	Small Cell	Nonkeratinizing	Keratinizing
Arrangements			
Single cells	+	+	++
Hyperchromatic crowded groups	+	++	+
Cells			
Size	Small	Medium	Large
Variance	Uniform	Relatively uniform	Pleomorphic
Shape	Oval	Round/polygonal	Spindle or bizarre
Cytoplasm			
Density	Delicate	Moderate	Dense
Stain	Basophilic	Cyanophilic	Orange
Nucleus			
Chromatin*	Coarse	Moderately coarse	Pyknotic
Macronucleolus	+	++	±
Background			
Diathesis	+	+	±

*irregularity distributed in SCC

±, may be present; +, present; ++, conspicuous

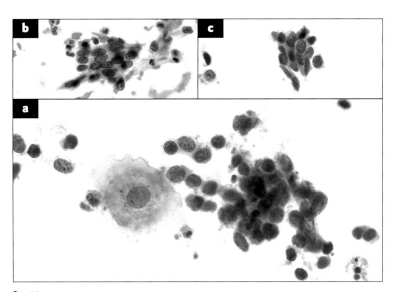

II.41
a, SCC, small cell type [L]; **b**, SCC, small cell type [C];
c, SCC, small cell type [L]

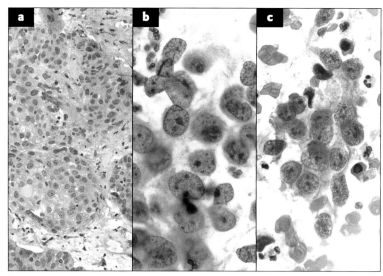

II.42
a, Nonkeratinizing SCC; **b**, Nonkeratinizing SCC [C]; **c**, Nonkeratinizing SCC [C]

Small Cell Squamous Carcinoma

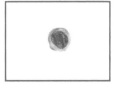

Small cell squamous carcinoma is a form of poorly-differentiated nonkeratinizing squamous cell carcinoma with small cells [II.41a,b,c]. (Note: not all poorly-differentiated squamous cell carcinomas are small cell type and not all small cell carcinomas are of squamous origin.) It is a rare, but potentially aggressive, tumor that may be increasing in incidence, particularly in younger women. It tends to arise high in the endocervical canal (difficult to sample), may shed only a few, small cells (difficult to detect), and may develop rapidly in the interval between Pap test screenings, any of which can make early (preinvasive) detection difficult or impossible.

Small Cell SCC

   Icon: Basal cell

   Cells: Small, with high N/C ratios

   Nuclei: Dark, coarse chromatin

     Small nucleoli

   Cytoplasm: Scant, delicate

     Squamous features subtle

   Background: Tumor diathesis

   Aggressive behavior

Histologically, small cell squamous carcinoma infiltrates in a diffuse pattern of sheets and nests of small neoplastic cells with high N/C ratios and poorly defined cell borders. Pearls are usually not present and there is little or no evidence of keratinization. Mitotic figures and necrosis may be prominent.

Cytologically, syncytial-like aggregates are common, but isolated cells also are present [Patten 1978]. Single, small, undifferentiated cells, which are characteristic of this tumor, may be particularly difficult to locate and interpret. The cells appear relatively uniform owing to their overall small size. The mean cell area is 169 ± 37 μm² [Reagan 1957]. Characteristically, many cells are oval or spindle shaped.

The cytoplasm is scant and basophilic, with poorly defined cell borders. Evidence of cytoplasmic keratinization is absent or minimal. The N/C ratio is very high; the cell is composed almost entirely of its nucleus.

The average nuclear area is 65 ± 13 μm², which is about 1.5 to 2 times the size of an intermediate cell nucleus (35 μm²) [Reagan 1957]. The chromatin is usually coarse and very hyperchromatic to pyknotic, although occasional cases have fine chromatin. Nucleoli may be difficult to appreciate due to the small size and dense chromatin structure of the nucleus. Naked nuclei are commonly

present and mitotic figures may be numerous. A tumor diathesis is characteristically present.

In liquid-based cytology, the findings are similar to those in conventional Pap smears. The cells are small, relatively uniform, with high N/C ratios, and scant cytoplasm. Syncytial-like aggregates and naked nuclei are common. The nuclei have fairly smooth membranes, and coarse, dark chromatin. Nucleoli may be more apparent in LBC. Cell clusters tend to round up; these can mimic endometrial cells, carcinoma in situ, or small cell neuroendocrine carcinoma.

The differential includes other benign and malignant conditions exfoliating small cells. Benign conditions include endometrial cells, basaloid cells in severe atrophy, and follicular cervicitis. Malignant conditions include lymphoma and small cell neuroendocrine carcinoma. These entities are discussed in their appropriate sections.

Nonkeratinizing Squamous Cell Carcinoma

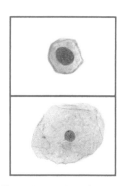

Large cell nonkeratinizing squamous cell carcinoma, or simply, nonkeratinizing squamous cell carcinoma, is associated with the pathways of either immature or mature metaplastic dysplasia (and intermediate and large cell carcinoma in situ, respectively). Nonkeratinizing squamous cell carcinoma is now the most common type of cervical cancer in the United States.

Histologically, nonkeratinizing squamous cell carcinoma invades as sheets, nests, cords, or trabeculae. The invasive pattern, particularly the leading edge, may be either pushing or diffusely infiltrating [II.42a]. Although focal areas of keratinization and dyskeratosis can be seen, the tumor lacks prominent keratinization and there are no keratin pearls. The stroma has an inflammatory response or a fibroblastic reaction.

Cytologically, syncytial-like aggregates, as well as naked nuclei, are common [Patten 1978]. Nonkeratinizing squamous cell carcinoma is composed of medium to large cells: the size of the cells varies from case to case, but in any

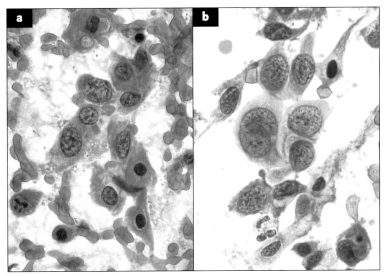

II.43
a, Nonkeratinizing SCC [C]; **b**, Nonkeratinizing SCC [L]

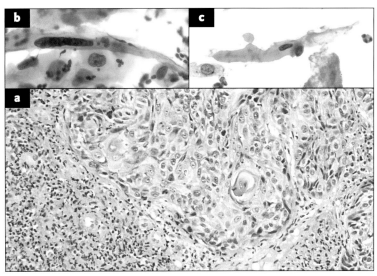

II.44
a, Keratinizing SCC; **b**, K SCC, bizarre cell [C];
c, K SCC, bizarre cell, bleb [L]

given case, they are relatively uniform [II.42b,c II.43a,b]. Marked cellular pleomorphism, including bizarre cells, is more characteristic of keratinizing squamous cell carcinoma. The mean cell size is 256 ± 69 μm² [Reagan 1957].

The nuclei are round to irregular in outline, and relatively large. The nuclear area averages 88 ± 30 μm², which is about two to three times the size of an intermediate cell nucleus (35 μm²) [Reagan 1957]. The hallmark of malignancy in these cells is the coarse, irregularly distributed chromatin. The chromatin particles vary considerably in size. Nucleoli are frequent and large, and some are irregular. Mitotic figure may be present. The cytoplasm of most cells is cyanophilic. A few individual cells may keratinize (dense orangeophilic "dyskeratotic cells"). However, keratin pearls are, by definition, absent in nonkeratinizing squamous cell carcinoma. A tumor diathesis is usually present, and often more pronounced than in keratinizing squamous cell carcinoma.

In liquid-based cytology, the findings are similar to those in conventional Pap smears. The cells are relatively uniform, medium to large, present singly, in small sheets, or syncytial-like aggregates. The nuclei typically have irregular membranes, coarse, irregular chromatin, prominent or irregular nucleoli, and moderately elevated N/C ratios. The cytoplasm is dense and cyanophilic. A tumor diathesis is usually present.

The differential of nonkeratinizing squamous cell carcinoma includes a benign reparative process (regeneration/repair). Both have large cells, with altered N/C ratios, and macronucleoli, which can be multiple and irregular. However, in contrast with cancer, reparative cells occur in flat, cohesive, well-ordered sheets, with few single cells. The chromatin of repair is neither hyperchromatic nor coarse, and a tumor diathesis is not present, although evidence of inflammation is common (see pg 95 for more discussion). Cytoplasmic vacuolization and prominent nucleoli in nonkeratinizing squamous cell carcinoma can mimic adenocarcinoma, particularly in LBC, where cell clusters tend to round up.

Nonkeratinizing SCC
Icons: Parabasal &Intermediate cells
Cells: Relatively uniform, medium-sized
  HCGs, loose clusters, single cells
  Moderate N/C ratios
Cytoplasm: Dense, distinct cell borders
Nuclei: Coarse, irregular chromatin,
  prominent nucleoli
Background: Tumor diathesis

Keratinizing Squamous Cell Carcinoma

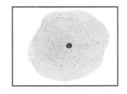

Keratinizing squamous cell carcinoma is associated with the pathway of keratinizing dysplasia. Keratinizing squamous cell carcinoma is characterized by presence of bizarre keratinized cells. [II.44a,b,c] and keratin pearls [II.45a,b]. The cancer may form grossly visible wart-like lesions resulting from exophytic growth.

Histologically, in contrast to the pushing invasion characteristic of nonkeratinizing squamous cell carcinoma, keratinizing squamous cell carcinoma commonly, but not always, invades with finger-like projections and incites a desmoplastic stromal reaction. In addition to keratin pearls, sheets and nests of cells with dense pink to orange cytoplasm, and single keratinized cells (dyskeratotic cells) are typical. The stromal response has an acute and chronic inflammatory infiltrate that may contain foreign body type giant cells in response to keratin that has "leaked into" the stroma.

Keratinizing SCC
Icon: Superficial cell
Cells: Spindle to bizarre shapes
  Single > aggregates
Cytoplasm: Densely keratinized
  Typically orangeophilic
Nuclei: Markedly pleomorphic;
  Low-to-high N/C ratios
Chromatin: Coarse to pyknotic
Nucleoli: Present, not prominent
Pearls: Pathognomonic (of keratinization)
Background: Variable diathesis (exophytic)

Cytologically, most of the cells are single, with occasional sheets and syncytia [Patten 1978]. Keratinizing squamous cell carcinoma usually is accompanied by evidence of hyperkeratosis, parakeratosis, atypical parakeratosis, and keratinizing dysplasia. The mean cell size is 275 ± 107 μm², which is larger and more variable than the nonkeratinizing type [Reagan 1957].

Keratinization and pleomorphism are hallmarks of keratinizing squamous cell carcinoma [II.44b,c]. However, these features, while characteristic, may represent a minor component of the tumor.

Keratinization manifests as squamous pearls, cytoplasmic density, and orangeophilia. Squamous pearls or squamous eddies ("whorls and pearls") are

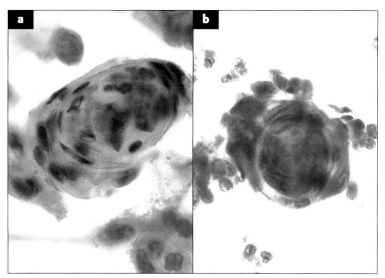

11.45
a, Keratinizing SCC, pearl [C]; **b**, Keratinizing SCC, pearl [L]

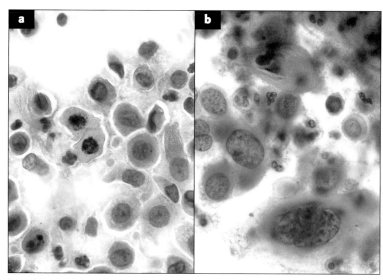

11.46
a, K SCC, orangeophilia [C]; **b**, K SCC, orangeophilia [L]

three-dimensional clusters of concentrically wrapped squamous cells, occasionally containing a central core of keratin [11.45a,b]. The size, number, and maturation of the pearls vary from case to case. Although pearls are pathognomonic of keratinization, they can be present in either benign or malignant keratinizing conditions. Individual dyskeratotic cells may also be present.

Intracellular keratin deposition causes cells to have dense cytoplasm and distinct cell boundaries, the hallmarks of squamous differentiation. Keratin expression may be appreciated as concentric rings, resulting in a thick, dense endoplasm and a thin outer rim of ectoplasm. Herxheimer spirals and keratohyaline granules are some other expressions of keratinization. Cytoplasmic keratin blebs may be seen in liquid-based cytology [11.44c].

Orangeophilia (associated with dense keratinization) is also characteristic of keratinizing carcinoma [11.46a,b]. Abnormal cells with *highly* keratinized, glassy, bright orange cytoplasm are usually not present in dysplasia; their presence suggests invasive cancer. However, orangeophilia is not necessarily extreme in keratinizing squamous cell carcinoma: eosinophilia may be more prominent and many cells are cyanophilic. The cytoplasm may also contain phagocytosed leukocytes or debris.

Pleomorphic cells with bizarre configurations (snakes, tadpoles, etc) are characteristic of keratinizing squamous cancer; however, bizarre cells account for only a minor, albeit important, component of the tumor [11.44b,c]. Tadpole cells consist of a spherical head and a tail-like prolongation; the head contains the nucleus [Papanicolaou 1943]. Snakes, or fiber cells, are spindle-shaped cells with the nucleus in the center, that resemble smooth muscle cells [R Graham 1958b, Papanicolaou 1943]. Angular, polygonal, and amoeboid forms may also be present [Papanicolaou 1943]. Nuclear/cytoplasmic ratios are variable, and range from low to high.

The nuclei are usually rounded, but can be spindle-shaped or irregular. Most cells have one nucleus, but some have multiple nuclei and others have none. The nuclear area averages 77 ± 28 µm², which is 1.5 to 3 times the size of an intermediate cell nucleus [Reagan 1957]. Nuclear membrane irregularities, including sharp angulations, are common. The chromatin is typically coarse to pyknotic (ink dot), but some nuclei have fine chromatin. Macronucleoli may be present, but are rare. Mitotic figures are variable, but tend to be less prominent than in nonkeratinizing squamous cell carcinoma.

The presence of highly keratinized anucleate squames with irregular outlines is a suspicious finding; in some cases, these pleomorphic squames predominate. Keratinizing squamous cell carcinoma is frequently accompanied by atypical parakeratosis (a possible warning sign) [Vela Velasquez 1997], but atypical parakeratosis can also occur in condyloma, dysplasia, and even inflammation. A tumor diathesis is less common and less pronounced in keratinizing, as compared with nonkeratinizing, squamous cell carcinoma.

In liquid-based cytology, the findings are similar to those in conventional Pap smears; in fact, keratinization (dense orangeophilia, pearls, and keratin blebs [blebs are rare in conventional Pap smears]) [11.44c] and pleomorphism (including bizarre cells [spindle, tadpole, etc]) tend to stand out in LBC. Single abnormal cells are prominent. Nuclear hyperchromasia, ink dot nuclei, and nuclear ghosts occur in LBC, but tumor diathesis is minimal.

The differential between severe keratinizing dysplasia and keratinizing squamous cell carcinoma can be difficult [P Levine 2003] [11.47a,b]. Theoretically, there is no intervening stage of classical carcinoma in situ (see "Keratinizing Carcinoma In Situ" pg 37). The background of all dysplasias, as well as some exophytic keratinizing squamous cell carcinomas, is clean or inflammatory, but lacks a tumor diathesis. Although the presence of a tumor diathesis suggests invasive carcinoma, the absence of a diathesis does not exclude invasive cancer. Malignant nuclear features, eg, nucleoli and irregular chromatin clumping, can also be difficult to detect in keratinizing squamous cell carcinoma due to nuclear pyknosis. In practice, a cytologic sample in which more than 15% of the total cellularity has high-grade "keratinizing dysplasia" is suspicious for keratinizing squamous cell carcinoma [Patten 1978]. In summary, factors favoring an interpretation of keratinizing squamous cell carcinoma over keratinizing

> *Differential of Squamous Carcinomas*
> *Small Cell SCC vs Neuroendocrine CA*
> *SCC: Less molding, coarser chromatin,*
> *more prominent nucleoli, denser cytoplasm,*
> *no crush artifact*
> *Nonkeratinizing SCC vs Adenocarcinoma*
> *SCC: Denser chromatin, denser cytoplasm*
> *less prominent nucleoli*
> *AdCA: Acini, secretory vacuoles, mucin*
> *Keratinizing SCC vs High-grade dysplasia*
> *SCC: More cells, keratinization, abnormal*
> *nuclei (+) tumor diathesis*

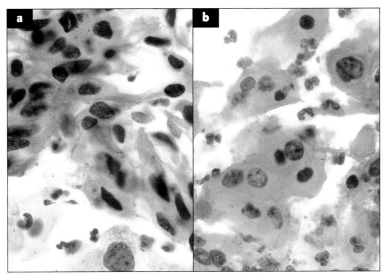

II.47
a, Keratinizing SCC [C]; **b**, Keratinizing dysplasia [C]

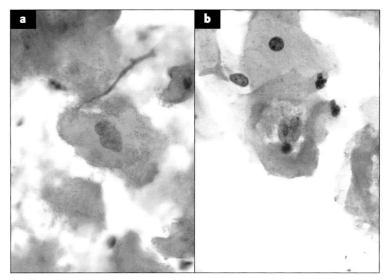

II.48
a, Verrucous carcinoma [C]; **b**, Condylomatous carcinoma [C]

dysplasia include: more cells; more pleomorphism and keratinization; coarse, irregular chromatin; macronucleoli; syncytial-like aggregates; and a tumor diathesis.

Rare Variants of Squamous Cell Carcinoma

Verrucous (Squamous Cell) Carcinoma

Verrucous carcinoma was first described in the oral cavity by Lauren Ackerman in 1948 [Ackerman 1948]. Formerly known as "giant condyloma acuminatum of Buschke and Lowenstein" (misleading because it is not a condyloma), verrucous carcinoma is a rare type of squamous carcinoma in the genital tract, that usually involves the vulva, but can occur in the cervix or vagina [Crowther 1988, Isaacs 1976, Japaze 1982, F Kraus 1966, Lucas 1974, Powell 1978]. Although HPV is not always identified (particularly in vulvar lesions), this tumor has been associated with HPV type 6, a "low risk" viral type rarely found in cancer [Okagaki 1984].

Histologic features of this tumor include "papillary" (wart-like) growth pattern and infiltration with rounded, pushing borders, which makes invasion difficult to appreciate on histologic section [Ramzy 1976]. Fibrovascular cores are poorly developed compared with benign genital warts (condylomas). Koilocytosis is minimal or absent. By definition, the tumor is very well-differentiated and deceptively benign appearing. Therefore, this lesion can be very difficult to diagnose histologically. Because the histology is similar to condyloma acuminatum, it is frequently misdiagnosed as a benign wart.

The cytology can be even more difficult to interpret than the histology and false-negative interpretations are common [Degefu 1986, De Jesus 1990, Kashimura 1984, Rorat 1978, Spratt 1977, Wood 1978]. Hyperkeratosis and parakeratosis may be the only findings, or the cellular pattern may be suggestive of only a low-grade CIN, in a pattern of keratinizing dysplasia, or ASC-US [II.48a] [Barua 1983, DeTorres 1981, Inaba 1992, C Morrison 2001, G-K Nguyen 1996, Pantanowitz 2003]. The cytoplasm tends to be thick and eosinophilic and the nuclei pyknotic [Fontanes De Torres 1981]. Koilocytes are sparse or absent. Pearls may be present, indicative of keratinization. Spindle cells may occur.

This cancer is characterized by slow, but relentless growth, does not metastasize, but frequently recurs. Because the diagnosis comes late, the tumor has a poor prognosis. Traditionally, radiotherapy was considered contraindicated owing to possible anaplastic transformation [Damian 1973, Isaacs 1976, Richart 1987].

Warty (Condylomatous) Carcinoma

Warty carcinoma is a variant of squamous carcinoma with marked condylomatous changes (aka condylomatous carcinoma). It differs from verrucous carcinoma in that the tumor infiltrates like ordinary squamous carcinoma and koilocytotic changes are prominent [II.48b]. Cytologically, the combination of koilocytes with marked nuclear atypia, vague papillary-like aggregates, and other features typical of squamous carcinoma (tadpoles, diathesis, etc) are characteristic findings [W-K Ng 2003b]. Both low-risk (6, 11) and high-risk (16, 18) human papillomavirus has been identified [Cho 1998].

Papillary Squamous Cell Carcinoma

The growth pattern of papillary squamous cell carcinoma is similar to that of verrucous squamous cell carcinoma, but exhibits significant nuclear atypia, resembling carcinoma in situ [Qizilbash 1974c]. Condylomatous changes are absent. HPV cannot be detected in many cases [Mirhashemi 2003]. Some cases resemble papillary urothelial (transitional cell) carcinoma and some authorities consider these tumors synonymously (see below). The cytology of papillary adenosquamous carcinoma has also been described [W-K Ng 2003c]. This tumor has a propensity for late recurrence and metastases [M Randall 1986].

The differential of papillary squamous lesions of the cervix includes: benign lesions such as papilloma, papillary immature metaplasia, urothelial (including inverted) papilloma, inverted condyloma, and exophytic condyloma, and malignant lesions such as urothelial carcinoma and papillary squamous carcinoma [Trivijitsilp 1998]. In some biopsy specimens, papillary carcinoma may be difficult to distinguish from tangentially sectioned carcinoma in situ.

Transitional Cell (Urothelial) Carcinoma

Transitional cell (urothelial) carcinoma is rare in the female genital tract, where it occurs most commonly in the ovary, but has also been described in the adnexa, endometrium, fallopian tube, and cervix [Lininger 1997]. It closely resembles papillary transitional cell carcinoma of the bladder and is also similar to papillary

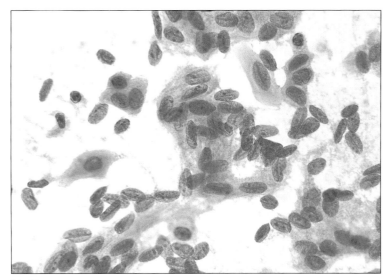

II.49
Urothelial metaplasia [C]

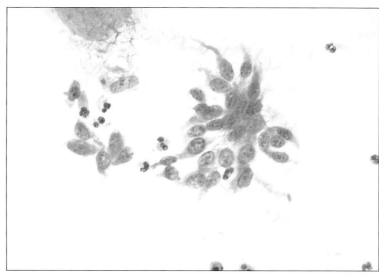

II.50
Spindle cell carcinoma [C]

squamous cell carcinoma [W–K Ng 2003d, Ortega–González 2002, Tardio 2001, Vesoulis 2001]. The cells have urothelial features, form cohesive, multilayered groups, and are oval to spindle shaped. The nuclei range from bland to hyperchromatic with granular chromatin, and typically have nuclear grooves. Nucleoli are small or absent. Tumor cells with squamous features are usually present.

Whether this tumor is truly urothelial in origin or a metaplastic variant of squamous cell carcinoma is unresolved. However, both tumors share epidemiologic risk factors and both are commonly associated with HPV 16 [Lininger 1998, Matthews–Greer 2004]. Cytokeratin reaction pattern (typically CK7 positive; CK20 negative) is similar to squamous cell carcinoma of the cervix and different from ordinary transitional cell carcinoma of the bladder (CK7 and CK20 positive) [Ortega– González 2002].

Transitional Cell (Urothelial) Metaplasia

Transitional cell, or urothelial, metaplasia of the cervix occurs predominantly in postmenopausal women [Duggan 2000, A Egan 1997, MA Jones 1998, Lawrence 1991, Weir 1997, 1998] [II.49]. Whether it represents a unique entity, is merely a variant of another entity (especially, atrophy), or even exists at all, is controversial. Its primary importance is that it can be confused with high-grade dysplasia or carcinoma in situ [Ambros 1990, Weir 1997]. However, some women have a previous history of dysplasia, and it is possible that some cases represent high-grade dysplasia in atrophy [Koss 1998a,b].

Transitional cell (urothelial) metaplasia is characterized by cohesive sheets of relatively monotonous, bland, parabasal-like cells with high N/C ratios and elongated or spindle-shaped nuclei that "stream" [Duggan 2000, Weir 1998]. Characteristically, the nuclear membrane has a prominent fold or groove, or is wrinkled. The chromatin is powdery fine, nucleoli are inconspicuous, and mitotic figures are absent or rare. Perinuclear cytoplasmic clearing (ie, a small halo) is common. The expression of cytokeratins (CK 13, CK 17, and CK18) is identical to the pattern observed in normal urothelium [Harnden 1999]. HPV-DNA, particularly type 58, has been reported to be present in some cases [W–K Ng 2002b].

The differential includes atrophy, high-grade dysplasia/carcinoma in situ (CIN 3), and tubal metaplasia. Streaming, spindled, wrinkled nuclei with halos in transitional cell metaplasia contrast with overlapping, rounded, smooth nuclei in atrophy [Weir 1998]. Tubal metaplasia most characteristically displays cilia. In contrast

with CIN 3, crowding, nuclear atypia (irregular membranes, hyperchromasia), and mitotic figures are absent in urothelial metaplasia. However, in practice, this differential may be difficult or impossible [Koss 1998a,b, 1999]. Whether transitional cell metaplasia is a risk factor for transitional cell carcinoma of the female genital tract is unknown [Weir 1998].

Lymphoepithelioma-like Squamous Cell Carcinoma

First described in 1968 as medullary carcinoma with lymphoid infiltration [Hamazaki 1968], lymphoepithelioma-like squamous cell carcinoma is extremely rare in cervix [Hafiz 1985, Halpin 1989]. It is morphologically similar to lymphoepithelioma-like carcinomas of the nasopharynx [Iezzoni 1995, Mills 1985, Proca 2000]. Like its counterpart, it seems to be more common in Asia and, in Asia, is often associated with Epstein-Barr virus (EBV) [Tseng 1997]. In Western women, at least some cases are associated with HPV 16 and 18, rather than EBV [López–Rios 2000, Noel 2001, Weinberg 1993]. The tumor is radiosensitive, there is a low rate of metastases, and the prognosis is favorable [Hafiz 1985, Hasumi 1977, McCluggage 2001a].

In cytologic preparations, there are syncytial-like aggregates and single anaplastic cells. The nuclei are relatively uniform, round to irregular, hyperchromatic, and contain macronucleoli. The cytoplasm is delicate to finely granular with indistinct cell borders. There is a lymphoplasmacytic infiltrate. No keratinization, dysplasia, or gland formation is present [G–K Nguyen 1996, Proca 2000, Reich 1999].

The tumor cells express cytokeratin; the lymphoid cells express CD45 (leukocyte common antigen, LCA). The differential includes poorly-differentiated squamous cell carcinoma or adenosquamous carcinoma ("glassy cell carcinoma") with marked inflammation, and malignant lymphoma.

Spindle Squamous Cell Carcinoma

Spindle squamous cell carcinoma, or sarcomatoid carcinoma, is characterized by spindly, nonkeratinized cells, high nuclear grade, and numerous mitotic figures. The tumor may resemble a spindle cell or pleomorphic sarcoma [G–K Nguyen 1996] or spindle cell melanoma [II.50]. Cytokeratin expression can be helpful in this differential (neither sarcoma nor melanoma express cytokeratin). The stroma may be heavily fibrotic or hyalinized (also known as scirrhous carcinoma). Despite the aggressive appearance, the tumor is reported to metastasize infrequently [M Harris 1982].

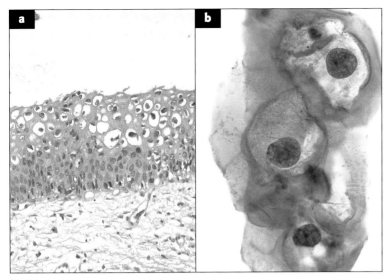

I1.51
a, Flat condyloma; **b**, Koilocytes [L]x

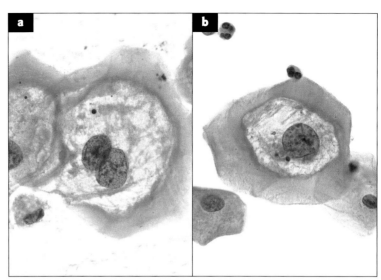

I1.52
a, Koilocyte [C]; **b**, Koilocyte [L]

Condylomata Acuminata (Genital Warts)

Condylomata acuminata, or genital warts (condyloma acuminatum is singular), are caused by human papillomavirus (HPV). Condylomas, as they are often called, are contagious (more than half of sexual partners contract disease), have an incubation period ranging from 3 weeks to 8 months or more (average, 3 months), and tend to be multifocal [Oriel 1971]. However, they have a high regression rate: at least one-half to two-thirds resolve spontaneously without therapy [A Evans 1985, Meisels 1981a]. Condylomas are more common in younger women (especially <30 years) [Meisels 1992]. Women with visible external genital warts are at high risk of having cervical lesions (SIL, CIN) [M Howard 2002].

There are two basic histologic growth patterns of condyloma: acuminatum (cauliflower-like, warty) and planum (commonly called flat). Although warty condylomas have been known since ancient times, flat condylomas were first described in 1977 [Meisels 1977b, Purola 1977]) **[I1.51a]**. There is also an endophytic variety of condyloma, but this may simply represent endocervical glandular extension of the lesion. Spike condyloma is a variant of condyloma acuminatum that has a multitude of spike-like projections, known as "asperites," that look like velvet when viewed colposcopically.

Whether a condyloma is warty or flat depends on the maturation of the infected epithelium [Meisels 1982, Crum 1984a, Handsfield 1997]. If a *keratinized* epithelium is infected, typical cauliflower-like venereal warts, condylomata acuminata, are the likely result. If a *mature metaplastic* epithelium is infected, flat condylomas usually occur **[I1.51a]**. Most condylomas of the cervix are flat. Flat condylomas are usually inconspicuous or invisible to the naked eye, but can be seen during colposcopy using acetic acid to enhance their visibility. Both types of condylomas yield abnormal cells on cytology, but the histologic growth pattern (warty, flat) cannot be predicted by cytology. HPV can also infect an *immature metaplastic* epithelium, causing a noncondylomatous lesion known as atypical immature metaplasia [Crum 1983b, Geng 1999, JJ Park 1999].

Finally, only a minority of women with HPV infection have lesions. HPV infection is most often present without any clinically or morphologically detectable lesion. This is known as latent infection; these infections can only be detected by sensitive techniques such as DNA Hybrid Capture and PCR. (Some authors use "subclinical infection" to include *lesions* invisible to the naked eye, ie, flat condyloma or atypical immature metaplasia.) Women with latent infections have colposcopically normal cervices, normal Pap tests, and normal biopsy specimens, but evidence of HPV infection can be detected using special tests (discussed below). Despite the absence of detectable lesions, these women are at risk of developing cervical neoplasia.

The word, condyloma, is frequently used unmodified to refer to a lesion without specifying whether it is flat or warty. Condyloma, or more precisely, HPV infection, is important in the pathogenesis of cervical neoplasia [R Reid 1982, 1983]. Condyloma is classified, along with ordinary CIN I (mild dysplasia), as a low-grade squamous intraepithelial lesion in the Bethesda System.

Condyloma in the Pap Test

The Pap test cannot detect the vast majority of HPV infections because they are latent (ie, there is no lesion to detect). However, when an HPV-associated lesion is present, the abnormality (ie, condyloma) can often be detected by cytology. Koilocytes, dyskeratocytes, macrocytes, etc, are some of the cytologic findings that are characteristic of condylomas.

Criteria for Condyloma, HPV
> *Koilocytes (pathognomonic)*
> *Dyskeratocytes*
>> *Atypical parakeratosis*
>> *Keratinizing dysplasia*
> *Minor (nondiagnostic) criteria:*
>> *Cells: Macrocytes, kites, balloons*
>> *Cytoplasm: Polka dots, cracks, two-tone*
>> *Nuclei: Binucleation, spindling, smudging*

Koilocytes

Human papillomavirus causes a cytopathic effect in some cells, resulting in the formation of a halo cell known by the rather intricate name, koilocyte (Greek, koilos = hollow; kytos = cell) [Koss 1956] **[I1.52a,b]**. Koilocytes are pathognomonic of condyloma and HPV infection, *if* strict criteria are used to identify these cells [Boras 1989, Koss 1987b, 2000b, Meisels 1979, 1981a, 1982]. However, koilocytes are not very sensitive in the cytologic detection of condyloma and HPV infection. (See Methods of detection of HPV infection pg 79.)

The koilocyte is a mature (intermediate or superficial) cell that has a characteristic large halo, or vacuole, surrounding an abnormal nucleus [De Girolami 1967, Koss 1956, Mayelo 1994, Meisels 1976a, Recher 1981, Saigo 1986a]. (Koilocytes have halos, but they're not angels.) The edge of the halo is very distinct and sharply defined, and surrounded by a wall of dense, often hyalinized, cytoplasm. Condensation of cytoplasmic fibrils causes the density.

Koilocytes
Cytoplasmic vacuoles
* Sharp, dense periphery*
Nuclear dysplasia
* Big, dark*
Background
* Dyskeratocytes*

The cytoplasm stains pink, or blue, or both (polychromasia). Sometimes a few tiny dots of degenerated cytoplasm float in the space, but the halo usually is otherwise clear. Glycogen is rarely present in the vacuole. Koilocytes can be found singly or in small clusters in cytologic specimens. Koilocytes often stand out like **STOP** signs in liquid-based cytology.

To be specific for condyloma and HPV infection, the nucleus of the koilocyte must be abnormal: enlarged and hyperchromatic (big and dark). The nuclear membrane is frequently wrinkled and the chromatin is usually dark, distinct, and granular. In a word, the nucleus looks dysplastic—usually of mild or moderate degree. Sometimes, the nuclei degenerate, and have "smudgy," pyknotic, fragmented, or marginated chromatin. Nucleoli are absent or indistinct. Although virus may be present in the nucleus [Casas–Cordero 1981], neither intranuclear nor intracytoplasmic viral inclusions are seen with the light microscope. Binucleation is common, multinucleation less frequent, and giant nuclei are rare [Koss 1956, Mayelo 1994, Meisels 1977b].

Differential of Koilocytes: Koilocytes are not the only cells in the Pap test that can have "halos" [De Girolami 1967].Perinuclear halos are frequently seen in squamous cells as a consequence of inflammation, especially due to *Trichomonas* infection ("trich halos") [II.53a].

Differential of Koilocytes
Glycogenated Cells
* Normal vs dysplastic nuclei*
Inflammatory "Trich" Halos
* Inflamed vs dysplastic nuclei*

However, the two types of halos form differently, and knowing how they form, makes them easier to distinguish. The koilocyte halo is caused by *destruction* of the cytoplasm; it is relatively large, with peripheral cytoplasmic condensation. Inflammatory perinuclear halos are caused by *shrinkage* of an enlarged, edematous, inflamed nucleus when fixed in alcohol. This leaves a small clear space, usually with little or no damage or condensation of the peripheral cytoplasm. As a rule of thumb, inflammatory halos are usually less than the width of an intermediate cell nucleus and koilocyte halos are usually larger (ie, >7 μm-8 μm).

Squamous cells sometimes contain abundant glycogen in their cytoplasm (eg, navicular cells or androgenic atrophy cells), which forms a perinuclear vacuole ("halo"). This glycogen vacuole can look a bit like a koilocyte halo [II.53b,c]. Koilocyte halos only rarely contain visible glycogen, which is golden-yellow in the Pap stain, although the periodic acid-Schiff (PAS) stain may highlight glycogen deposits [Recher 1981]. Moreover, the edge of the koilocyte halo is dense and sharply defined, and the nucleus is abnormal, while the edge of a glycogen vacuole is usually hazy or indistinct, and the nucleus is normal.

Immature squamous metaplastic cells may have an attenuated, pale staining endoplasm with a relatively dense ectoplasmic rim, but lack the sharp demarcation and marked peripheral cytoplasmic density characteristic of koilocytes. Also, immature metaplastic cells are parabasal-sized cells, while koilocytes resemble intermediate or superficial cells. Both immature metaplastic cells and koilocytes usually lack visible glycogen. The nuclei are normal or reactive in metaplastic cells (vs dysplastic in koilocytes).

In summary, if the nucleus is not abnormal ("big and dark"), then the halo cell is not a *definitive* koilocyte [Koss 1987b, P Ward 1990]. Based on HPV-DNA analysis, cells with perinuclear cytoplasmic halos, but without nuclear atypia, are nonspecific findings [Franquemont 1989, Mittal 1990, Nuovo 1988, BE Ward 1990]. Abnormal nuclei are also diagnostically important in histopathology, where they help differentiate normal glycogenated epithelium ("basket-weave pattern") from koilocytosis. One final note: although koilocytes indicate a low-grade squamous intraepithelial lesion, they do not exclude a co-existing high-grade lesion—or even invasive carcinoma [Dudding 1996b].

Dyskeratocytes

Dyskeratocytes are "abnormally keratinized (squamous) cells," hence the term "dys-kerato-cytes." Dyskeratocytes occur on the surface of the condyloma. In the Pap test, dyskeratocytes are characteristically found in dense clusters of haphazardly arranged cells, with loss of nuclear polarity, but they can also occur singly.

Dyskeratocytes are pleomorphic in size and shape. [II.54a,b]. Small dyskeratocytes have orange cytoplasm and dense to pyknotic, atypical nuclei. Small dyskeratocytes are similar, or identical, to atypical parakeratosis [II.54a]. Large dyskeratocytes have dense, orange cytoplasm, and contain one or more enlarged, atypical nuclei, with coarse, dark, smudgy, or pyknotic chromatin. Large dyskeratocytes are similar, or identical, to keratinizing dysplasia [II.54b]. They are essentially koilocytes without halos. Asperites suggest condyloma and tend to be more conspicuous in liquid-based preparations [II.55].

The presence of thick, disorganized clusters of bright orange dyskeratocytes strongly suggests condyloma, even in the absence of typical koilocytes [Boras 1989, Mayelo 1994, Meisels 1976a]. Although ordinary hyperkeratosis and parakeratosis commonly occur in condyloma, they are not pathognomonic of HPV infection (see minor criteria, below).

Macrocytes

Macrocytes are commonly found in condylomas, but are not specific findings. The macrocytes of condyloma are morphologically similar to those occurring in response to radiation, chemotherapy, or vitamin deficiency (folate or B_{12}) [van Niekerk 1966]. Macrocytes are literally "large cells," often several times the size of intermediate or superficial cells [II.56a,b]. The cytoplasm is abundant, and stains pink or blue or, frequently, polychromatic (a cell of many colors). Cytoplasmic vacuolization is common and the vacuoles may contain particles or neutrophils, or even other squamous cells. The nuclei are frequently enlarged and hyperchromatic ("big and dark," ie, "dysplastic"), and often multiple. However, the N/C *ratio* is relatively unaltered or within normal limits.

Minor Cytologic Criteria for Condyloma

Hyperkeratosis occurs in about two-thirds of cases of condyloma, and parakeratosis in about one-third of cases [Burrows 1990]. However, hyperkeratosis and parakeratosis are non-specific findings. There are several other cytologic features that are more suggestive, but not pathognomonic, of condyloma. These nonclassic signs (or minor criteria) include not only cytomegaly (macrocytes, discussed above), but also kite cells (stretched out cells with long tails [II.57a,b]), polka dot cells (cells with numerous small globules of condensed cytoplasm [II.58a]), balloon cells (clear cytoplasm, peripheral nucleus, resemble lipocytes [II.58b]),two-tone (polychromatic) cells, cracked cells (condensed cytoplasmic filaments give the impression of cracks), and hyalin cytoplasmic inclusions (condensed intermediate

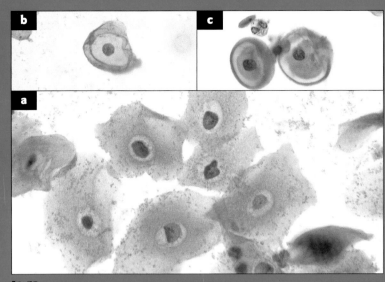

I1.53
a, "Trich" halos [C]; **b**, Glycogen vacuole [C]; **c**, Glycogen vacuoles [L]

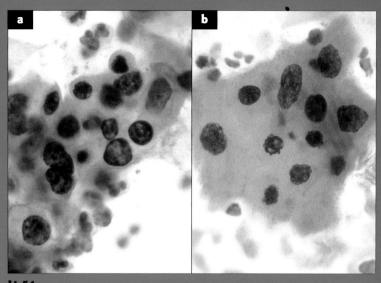

I1.54
a, Small dyskeratocytes [C]; **b**, Large dyskeratocytes [C]

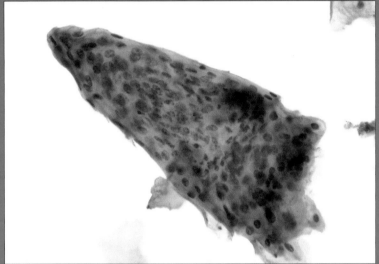

I1.55
Asperite [L]

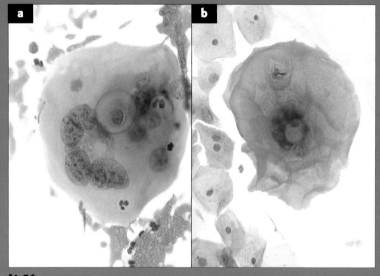

I1.56
a, Macrocyte [C]; **b**, Macrocyte [C]

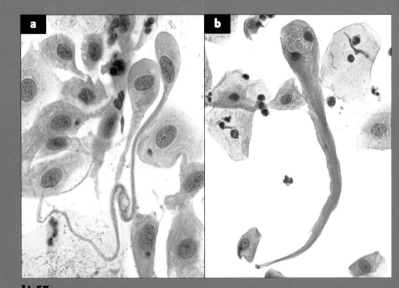

I1.57
a, Kite cells [C]; **b**, Kite cell [L]

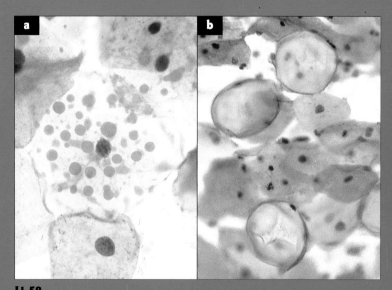

I1.58
a, Polka dot cell [C]; **b**, Balloon cells [C]

filaments), as well as binucleation or multinucleation, spindle nuclei, chromatin smudging, and karyorrhexis [Cecchini 1990b, H Cramer 1997, de Borges 1989, Mayelo 1994, R Nayar 1999, Schlaen 1988, A Schneider 1987b, V Schneider 1989, Shroyer 1990, Sidawy 1992, Spitzer 1990, Tanaka 1993].

Although these minor ("soft" or nonclassic) criteria are nonspecific, they can still be helpful in evaluating Pap tests. For example, binucleation is present in 95% of condylomas, but is also common in inflammatory reactions [Prasad 1993]. Thus, binucleation is highly sensitive, but poorly specific, for condyloma. Polka dot cells are also non-specific findings, but double the risk of condyloma compared with cases that do not have these cells [Shiffer 2001]. Minor criteria provide clues to search carefully for more specific findings; when these cannot be found, the interpretation of "atypical squamous cells-undetermined significance (ASC-US)" can be used as appropriate. Many women (up to 65% to 85%) with these "nonspecific" findings are HPV positive [R Nayar 1999, A Schneider 1987b]

Atypical Immature Metaplasia

Atypical immature metaplasia is a lesion, distinct from condyloma, caused by HPV infection of immature metaplastic cells [Crum 1983b, Geng 1999]. Like condyloma, atypical immature metaplasia is thought to be part of the spectrum of squamous intraepithelial lesions [Crum 1984a]. However, koilocytes are not present in atypical immature metaplasia, unless it coexists with typical (flat or warty) condyloma. Atypical immature metaplasia resembles immature metaplastic dysplasia, with parabasal-sized cells and minimally atypical nuclei. In practice, atypical immature metaplasia is difficult to distinguish from both benign metaplasia and H SIL, and so it may be interpreted as "atypical squamous cells—cannot exclude H SIL" (ASC-H).

Differential of Condyloma

Condylomas exfoliate cells that look (or are) dysplastic. When strict criteria are used, koilocytes are pathognomonic of condyloma and HPV infection (low-grade squamous intraepithelial lesion). Dyskeratocytes are cells that resemble keratinizing dysplasia, often low-grade, and can be thought of as koilocytes without halos. Koilocytes/dyskeratocytes frequently correlate with the interpretive "trifecta" of L SIL, condyloma, and mild dysplasia. Macrocytes are often present in condyloma, and although nonspecific, when occurring in a background of dysplasia, they usually correlate with condyloma. Minor criteria for condyloma are nonspecific, but alert the cytologist to search carefully for more convincing evidence of condyloma or dysplasia.

Occasionally, the cells exfoliated from a condyloma have markedly atypical or malignant appearing ("butt ugly") nuclei: very big, with very coarse, dark chromatin. However, despite the marked atypia, there can still be a high degree of squamous differentiation in the corresponding tissue (ie, a low-grade lesion on biopsy). In the past, such cases were sometimes designated "atypical condyloma" [Meisels 1981b]. Owing to the strikingly abnormal appearance of the cells, the Pap test can overestimate the histologic grade of the lesion, and can even be misinterpreted as H SIL or squamous cell carcinoma [Koss 1956, Meisels 1981b]. However, some authorities use severe nuclear atypia to "boost" the grade of a CIN lesion and this may justify the interpretation of a high-grade SIL [Kadish 1992, Kurman 1992, Ziol 1998].

The best clue to the grading of a squamous lesion is the N/C ratio. Although the nuclei of condyloma are enlarged, they are typically found in relatively abundant cytoplasm, so that the N/C ratio is little altered or only slightly increased, indicating a low-grade lesion. The chromatin in condylomatous lesions is hyperchromatic, and either coarse or smudgy, but regularly distributed.

Features favoring an interpretation of squamous cell carcinoma include abnormal nuclei with frankly malignant appearing, irregularly distributed chromatin, prominent nucleoli, bizarre shaped cells, and a tumor diathesis. Note, again, that condyloma (L SIL) can coexist with H SIL or even invasive cancer.

Condyloma Redux

Condyloma has been a subject of controversy. There are two basic schools of thought about it. One school makes a distinction between condyloma and dysplasia, maintaining that condyloma is only a viral infection that can cause cellular changes that mimic dysplasia, but is not genuine dysplasia. The other believes that condyloma *is* dysplasia, or at least, that it is *indistinguishable from* dysplasia. There is also a middle ground, those who believe that condyloma is a *precursor to* dysplasia. A related debate, taken up later, is whether L SIL and H SIL are distinct entities or a spectrum of lesions.

The Bethesda System includes mild dysplasia (CIN 1) and HPV effect (condyloma) in the same interpretive category, low-grade squamous intraepithelial lesion (L SIL). Reasons for the grouping of these "two" lesions are summarized below:

There is high interobserver variability in interpretation, ie, the two lesions cannot be differentiated by light microscopy with much more accuracy than flipping a coin [DM Evans 1986, Ismail 1989, 1990, Kurman 1991, K Lee 1997a, A Robertson 1989a,b, Sherman 1992c, Tabbara 1992].

DNA ploidy levels are similar in CIN 1 and condyloma. The majority of lesions classified histologically as flat condyloma and CIN 1 lesions are diploid or polyploid [Fu 1983, Jakobsen 1983], although either lesion can demonstrate aneuploidy [Watts 1987].

The molecular virology of the two lesions is similar or identical, ie, they are associated with the same HPV types [Crum 1984a, 1985, Dürst 1983, Gissmann 1982, Kadish 1986, Kurman 1991, Lörincz 1987a, Mitao 1986, R Reid 1987, Richart 1987, Schiffman 1991, Tabbara 1992, G Willett 1989].

The lesions have similar or identical clinical behavior, ie, they have a low progression rate [Campion 1986, MH Jones 1992, Kataja 1989, Kurman 1991, K Nasiell 1986, K Syrjänen 1988, G Willett 1989].

Therefore, mild dysplasia (CIN 1) and condyloma are now viewed as essentially the same thing, designated low-grade squamous intraepithelial lesion. There is no reason to attempt to separate these "two" lesions, and in fact, you can't. Histopathologists who diagnose "Condyloma, no evidence of dysplasia" are not only deceiving themselves, but also misleading and confusing clinicians. Low-grade SIL is thought to be the morphologic manifestation of productive HPV infection. Productive infection yields abundant viral particles, which can be demonstrated using in situ hybridization, in the intermediate to superficial cell layers. Infected cells usually have viral cytopathic effects, ie, koilocytosis. Koilocytosis consists of perinuclear cytoplasmic cavitation and nuclear atypia, including anisonucleosis, enlargement, irregular membranes, and hyperchromasia. Mitotic spindle abnormalities occur in productive infection that interferes with mitosis and cytokinesis. This leads to the polyploidy and binucleation or multinucleation characteristic of condyloma.

In summary, *if it looks like dysplasia, it is dysplasia* [Fletcher 1983]. Dysplasia (or CIN, SIL), with or without koilocytes, is interpreted using standard morphologic criteria. The lesions are graded according to the degree of abnormality of the nucleus and the N/C ratio, regardless of whether HPV is thought to be present or not. Importantly, the presence of koilocytes does not exclude the possibility of a co-existing high-grade lesion or even cancer, and in fact, increases the risk. A statement regarding evidence of HPV infection can be added to the report, but women with condyloma should receive the same clinical management as those with conventional forms of cervical intraepithelial neoplasia (see discussion of clinical management) [Bajardi 1986, R Kaufman 1983a,b, Raymond 1987, Richart 1987].

A Final (?) Word on Nomenclature

Schottlaender-Kermauner phenomenon; unruhige (restless) epithelium; unquiet epithelium; leucohyperkeratosis; irregular epithelium; atypical epithelium; atypical hyperplasia; basal cell–hyperactivity, hyperplasia, or anaplasia; precancerous metaplasia; metaplasia with atypicality; metaplasia with anaplasia; prickle cell hyperplasia; spinal cell atypia; leukoparakeratosis, leukohyperkeratosis, dyskaryosis; dissociated intraepithelial anaplasia; atypical epithelial hyperplasia; noninvasive atypical epithelium; aggravated atypical epithelium; surface cancer; dysplasia; carcinoma in situ; cervical intraepithelial neoplasia; squamous intraepithelial lesion [Bottles 1991, T Wright 1994b]. What's next? [F1.12]

Noninvasive epithelial abnormalities related to cervical cancer have been commented on since at least 1886 (in lectures by Sir John Williams [J Williams 1888]), and the controversy surrounding the best terminology to use in diagnosis of the "Schottlaender-Kermauner phenomenon" [Schottlaender 1912] has been raging ever since [Bottles 1991, Briggs 1979, Crum 1989a, 2002, Drake 1984, Giacomini 1983, 1991, Herbst 1990a, NCI 1989a,b,c, Kurman 1994, Llewellyn 2000, Reagan 1953a, 1956a, Richart 1973, V Schneider 2003a, Selvaggi 1999b], creating a veritable Tower of Babel [Selvaggi 2001]. In the 1930s, Broders found that a lesion composed of undifferentiated, atypical cells, which he called "carcinoma in situ," was a precursor of invasive squamous cell carcinoma [Broders 1932]. It later became apparent that a similar, but less abnormal (or more differentiated) lesion also occurred [Reagan 1955]. This was designated "dysplasia" by Papanicolaou at the suggestion of William B. Ober of the National Cancer Institute, in 1949 [Papanicolaou 1949]. The term, dysplasia, was popularized by James Reagan. Reagan and his colleagues described the histologic and cytologic features of dysplasia in 1953, and reported that the majority of dysplastic lesions regressed or remained unchanged for many years, if left untreated [Reagan 1953b, 1956a]. They stressed the importance of squamous differentiation in dysplasia, which was lacking in carcinoma in situ, and thereby introduced the concept of a "two disease system." This had important prognostic implications, ie, carcinoma in situ was considered a definite precursor lesion, while dysplasia was more unpredictable in its behavior. Later, Reagan and Patten subdivided dysplasia was into slight (mild), moderate, and severe [Reagan 1962a]. The dysplasia/carcinoma in situ nomenclature was published in a World Health

F1.12 Comparison of Nomenclature Systems

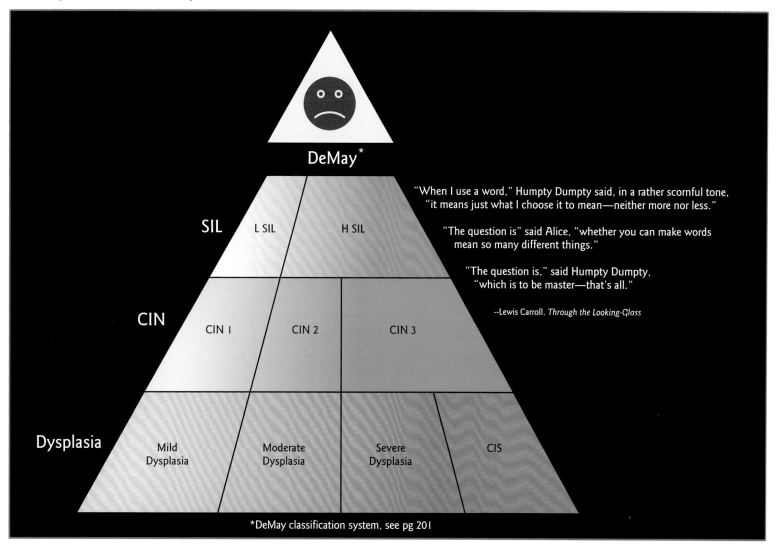

DeMay*

"When I use a word," Humpty Dumpty said, in a rather scornful tone, "it means just what I choose it to mean—neither more nor less."

"The question is" said Alice, "whether you can make words mean so many different things."

"The question is," said Humpty Dumpty, "which is to be master—that's all."

--Lewis Carroll, *Through the Looking-Glass*

SIL — L SIL — H SIL

CIN — CIN 1 — CIN 2 — CIN 3

Dysplasia — Mild Dysplasia — Moderate Dysplasia — Severe Dysplasia — CIS

*DeMay classification system, see pg 201

Organization monograph that was widely distributed internationally [Riotton 1973]. Generations of cytologists were brought up using this system (who would now probably be considered "tribal elders" [aka old farts] by young whippersnappers). However, young or old, practically everyone in the field understands the dysplasia/carcinoma in situ terminology, which can be applied without modification to any body site, not just the uterine cervix.

The Papanicolaou Classification System for cytologic diagnosis was introduced in the 1950s [T1.13] [Papanicolaou 1954]. Prior to this, there was no generally accepted cytology reporting system and this one was intended to encompass all types of cytologic specimens, not limited to cervicovaginal smears. Papanicolaou, not being a pathologist, was reluctant to use pathologic terms, and substituted a system of "classes" instead. He emphasized that Class V is actually the only conclusive category. Papanicolaou seldom used the Class V category and warned that because abnormal cells could be rare, a negative diagnosis should always be made with extreme caution [Papanicolaou 1943].

T1.13 Papanicolaou Classification System

Class I: Absence of atypical or abnormal cells
Class II: Atypical cytology, but no evidence of malignancy
Class III: Cytology suggestive of, but not conclusive for, malignancy
Class IV: Cytology strongly suggestive of malignancy
Class V: Cytology conclusive for malignancy

Although the Papanicolaou Class was never intended to substitute for a narrative diagnosis, this unfortunately became common practice [Maguire 1988]. In its original form, the Papanicolaou Class was used to indicate the degree of certainty that cancer was present or absent. However, as the concept of precursor lesions became more widely accepted, the emphasis shifted from degrees of *certainty* to degrees of *abnormality*. Consequently, the Papanicolaou system suffered modifications too numerous to count, in essence trying to fit square pegs into round holes. Moreover, the Papanicolaou Class has no correlation with histopathology, and had been considered outmoded for decades [Reagan 1965]. But, everything old is new again: it has been proposed to combine the old Papanicolaou classification with the new Bethesda System to facilitate triage [K Frankel 1994]. In fact, its very lack of correlation with histopathology has even been viewed as a possible benefit of the "Pap Class" in the current medicolegal environment. Using histologic terminology for reporting Pap tests may mislead those unfamiliar with the limitations of cytopathology into believing that the Pap test is as definitive as a tissue biopsy. (On the other hand, the Pap test can more accurately reflect what is happening with the patient than a tissue biopsy; ultimately, there is no gold standard.)

In the late 1960s and early 1970s, prospective clinical studies and DNA ploidy analysis proved that dysplasia and carcinoma in situ were closely related; therefore, a new terminology, cervical intraepithelial neoplasia, was proposed by Ralph Richart to encompass both lesions [Richart 1968, 1973, T Wright 1990]. Prior to that time, dysplasia was too often undertreated clinically, while a diagnosis of carcinoma in situ could lead to unnecessary hysterectomy, sometimes even radical hysterectomy; in short, overtreatment [Przybora 1959, Richart 1973]. The primary purpose behind the introduction of the cervical intraepithelial neoplasia terminology was to emphasize that these lesions represent a continuum of change [Richart 1968], that all grades are important, and should be treated, but by the most conservative method indicated [Richart 1973].

Cervical intraepithelial neoplasia was initially divided into five grades (very mild dysplasia, mild dysplasia, moderate dysplasia, severe dysplasia, and carcinoma in situ), which later was reduced to three grades (mild dysplasia, moderate dysplasia, and severe dysplasia/carcinoma in situ corresponding to CIN 1, 2, and 3, respectively). The word, carcinoma, was eliminated from CIN because of its connotation of established malignant disease [A Clarke 1996]. The concept of a continuum diminishes the importance of grading. What is most important is to distinguish cervical intraepithelial neoplasia from benign, reactive changes, on the one hand, and invasive carcinoma on the other [Crum 1984a]. Nevertheless, cervical intraepithelial neoplasia, with good evidence of squamous differentiation, statistically behaves better than poorly-differentiated CIN lesions. In 1990, after the first Bethesda conference (see below), Richart again modified the grading of CIN, dividing it into low-grade and high-grade CIN, analogous to low-grade and high-grade squamous intraepithelial lesions [Richart 1990].

More recent information pointing to an apparent biologic dichotomy between mere "infection" and genuine "neoplasia" has resulted in the latest entry, the Bethesda System [Kurman 1994, NCI 1989a,b,c]. The Bethesda System terminology suggests that the disease is not a continuum after all, but rather a discontinuous, two-disease system, emphasized by the terminology of low-grade and high-grade squamous intraepithelial lesions. Low-grade squamous intraepithelial lesion, L SIL, is caused by a heterogeneous group of viruses, including both low-risk (eg, 6 and 11) and high-risk (eg, 16 and 18) viral types, which can produce morphologically indistinguishable, well-differentiated lesions. Low-grade SIL is expected to have an unpredictable clinical behavior, but is less likely to progress than the other category, high-grade squamous intraepithelial lesion, H SIL. High-grade SIL is predominantly caused by high-risk virus and is expected to behave as a precursor lesion [Richart 1990]. The two-tier Bethesda System terminology has also been adopted for histopathology [Crum 2002b, 2003, T Wright 2002b]. (The Bethesda System, a complete scheme for reporting Pap tests, is discussed in more detail beginning on pg 235.)

So, return with us now to the days of yesteryear, when precursor lesions were a two-disease system (ie, dysplasia and carcinoma in situ)! The gurus (Reagan, Patten, et al) were right after all. Though the concepts have now been refined to include our understanding of DNA ploidy and low-risk and high-risk HPV, the morphology still roughly corresponds to dysplasia and carcinoma in situ, and the degree of risk of invasive cancer correlates with the morphologic grade of the lesion.

With each new nomenclature, there has been a "frame shift" in the line of division (see [T1.12]). At first, the split was between carcinoma in situ and severe dysplasia, then cervical intraepithelial neoplasia incorporated these two lesions into one category, CIN 3. Next, the Bethesda System amalgamated moderate dysplasia and CIN 3 into one category, high-grade squamous intraepithelial lesion, H SIL. These changes may be, at least in part, a reflection of an increasingly risk-averse population, not to mention aggressive malpractice lawyers. Nevertheless, most invasive cancers arise from high-grade dysplasia and particularly, classical carcinoma in situ [A Ng 1969]. A concern is that women will be overtreated because the threshold has been lowered [K Syrjänen 1992]. Estimates indicate that the change from the old Pap Classification System to the new Bethesda System, when coupled with the increased fear of litigation, has resulted in a doubling or even tripling of colposcopy referrals [Cox 2001].

An alleged advantage of diminishing the number of diagnostic or interpretive categories is increased reproducibility. But, critics might scoff that all you're doing is manipulating the data, or "cooking the books." The apparent benefit may really be more of a cosmetic effect achieved by lumping categories than a genuine improvement in reproducibility [MC Anderson 1991]. Some actual reported data are shown in T1.14 [Boon 1996]. The accuracy, defined as exact match between cytology and histology, was 42% for a cytologic interpretation of mild dysplasia; 32% for moderate dysplasia; 33% for severe dysplasia; and 45% for CIS. When reported in Bethesda System terminology of L SIL (mild dysplasia) and H SIL (lumping moderate dysplasia, severe dysplasia, and carcinoma in situ), the accuracy of an L SIL interpretation remains the same, but the accuracy of H SIL increases to 51%, higher than any individual category! Nothing changed, except the way the data were manipulated.

Which system(s) of nomenclature to use is left to the reader. Although now widely employed, the Bethesda System does not *require* the "squamous intraepithelial lesion" terminology [Solomon 2002]. All three systems can, in fact, be used together, providing the clinician with a veritable smorgasbord of interpretations. Note that the dysplasia/carcinoma in situ terminology can always be translated into the other systems, but the reverse is not true. When other systems of nomenclature are described, they are almost invariably compared with the dysplasia/carcinoma in situ scheme. This simple fact speaks volumes. Dysplasia/carcinoma in situ remains a widely used terminology (squamous intraepithelial lesion has increased, cervical intraepithelial neoplasia diminished) [Davey 1992b]. Dysplasia/carcinoma in situ can be utilized for tissues throughout the body, and the concept of dysplasia/carcinoma in situ is covered in standard textbooks of pathology [V Kumar 2005]. The morphologic appearance of precursor lesions corresponds better to grades of dysplasia/carcinoma in situ, than to grades of SIL, eg, moderate dysplasia looks nothing like carcinoma in situ, yet both are H SIL [C Buckley 1982]. Only with adherence to standard nomenclature will it be possible to study the natural history of disease and communicate in one language [Christopherson 1977a]. For example, some believe that carcinoma in situ is the true precursor lesion of squamous cell carcinoma and that all grades of dysplasia are less risky; however, if a specific interpretation of CIS is no longer made, it will be difficult to collect data. And, if history holds any lesson, other terminologies will be introduced in the future. The lesions do not change, only the names do. Of course, in the future, interpretation may be totally based on molecular biology, or other technology, and it is at least possible that morphology will no longer be relevant. (Although the death of morphology has been predicted for decades, it is not likely to occur anytime soon, but if I'm wrong, look for me with my cardboard sign, "Will interpret for food.")

Histology and Cytology: Yin and Yang

Definitions

Carcinoma In Situ

Carcinoma in situ is defined as "an abnormal [neoplastic] reaction of the squamous mucosa which, in the absence of invasion, through the full thickness of the epithelium, no squamous differentiation takes place."

Dysplasia

Dysplasia is defined as "all other similar abnormal reactions, but which show some squamous differentiation toward the surface." (Modified from an International Agreement made in Vienna in 1961 [Wied 1962a].)

T1.14 Histo-Cyto Correlation Data

| CYTOLOGY | HISTOLOGY | | | | | | |
	Neg	Mild	Moderate	Severe	CIS	Cancer	Total
Mild dysplasia	22	31	10	9	1	0	73
Moderate dysplasia	8	8	13	4	7	0	40
Severe dysplasia	3	4	5	11	10	0	33
CIS	1	2	3	4	10	2	22
Total	34	45	31	28	28	2	168

[Boon 1996]

Justification Sola Fide

Pap test interpretation is justified based on the belief that the cells exfoliated from the mucosal surface faithfully reflect the morphology of the hidden underlying epithelium—to hold, as 'twere, the mirror up to nature. Squamous dysplasia is a spectrum of morphologic abnormalities, bookended by normal at one end and carcinoma in situ at the other, with grades of dysplasia in between [F1.13]. The cytoplasm and nucleus manifest squamous differentiation and carcinogenesis, respectively, as previously discussed. In theory, the spectrum of nuclear and cytoplasmic changes in the cells observed in the Pap test accurately indicates the spectrum of changes in the tissue, from normal to dysplasia to carcinoma in situ and finally cancer [Reagan 1956a].

F1.13 Precursor Lesions of Cervical Squamous Cell Carcinoma

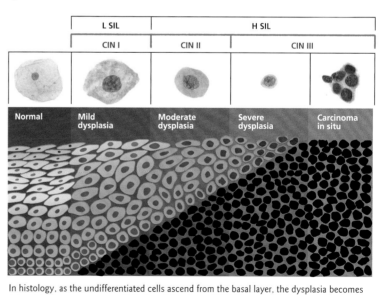

In histology, as the undifferentiated cells ascend from the basal layer, the dysplasia becomes progressively more severe, until finally, at the stage of CIS, the entire thickness of the epithelium is replaced with undifferentiated cells. In cytology, as the dysplasia becomes more advanced, the cell exfoliated at the surface become progressively less differentiated, until finally, at the stage of CIS, the surface cells are undifferentiated. Of important note is that even in mild dysplasia, the entire thickness of the epithelium is abnormal, but differentiates toward the surface; in CIS, the entire thickness is both abnormal and undifferentiated. Invasive cancer usually arises from most advanced lesions, particularly classical CIS. [Modified from Wright 1994]

Histology

In essence, grade of the dysplasia depends on how high undifferentiated cells rise in the epithelium before squamous differentiation, if any, begins. The transition between the undifferentiated and the differentiated cells is usually fairly well demarcated. Undifferentiated cells have delicate cytoplasm and indistinct cell boundaries; differentiated cells have dense cytoplasm and distinct cell boundaries.

Traditionally, in mild dysplasia, the undifferentiated, abnormal, basaloid cells are confined to the lower third of epithelium; considerable squamous differentiation occurs before the cells are exfoliated at the surface [F1.13]. In moderate dysplasia, the undifferentiated abnormal cells occupy at least the lower one third, but no more than two thirds, of the thickness of the epithelium. In severe dysplasia, at least two thirds of the thickness of the epithelium is composed of undifferentiated, abnormal cells, but some squamous differentiation still occurs near the surface.

The final stage of intraepithelial neoplasia is carcinoma in situ. In CIS, the full thickness of the epithelium is made up of undifferentiated abnormal cells, although the cells at the surface may flatten a little, due to surface tension effects, or there may be a keratinized surface reaction (hyperkeratosis, parakeratosis, atypical parakeratosis).

Mitotic figures correlate with undifferentiated cells. Normally, mitotic figures are confined to a single layer of undifferentiated cells in the basal layer of the epithelium. In dysplasia, mitotic figures ascend above the basal layer, while in carcinoma in situ, they can be found at all levels of the epithelium, including the surface. Although abnormal mitotic figures have been reported in mild dysplasia, they are usually associated with more advanced dysplasia and carcinoma in situ [D Jenkins 1986]. Abnormal mitoses are abortive and correlate with aneuploidy.

Some authorities use severe nuclear atypia or abnormal mitotic figures in the tissue to "boost" a CIN 1 lesion to a higher grade (CIN 2) [Kurman 1992]. Because these abnormalities may occur below the epithelial surface, the grade of such "boosted" lesions may be underestimated by the Pap test.

The severity of the lesion often varies from area to area. Surface keratotic reactions (hyperkeratosis, parakeratosis) are not included in the histologic assessment of the grade of the lesion, including carcinoma in situ. In dysplasia, a certain amount of order remains in the epithelium. In carcinoma in situ, there is no order left at all. So, in contrast with even severe dysplasia, there is no palisading of the basal layer of cells in carcinoma in situ. However, in carcinoma in situ, the cells may proliferate so rapidly they crowd each other into vertical spindle shapes. Since there is no maturation in carcinoma in situ, the epithelium looks about the same right side up as upside down, when viewed histologically. In some high-grade lesions, in which the epithelium matures poorly, the abnormality may be only a few cells thick (known as "thin CIN"). Although these lesions can exfoliate highly abnormal cells, the danger of "thin CIN" is that it may be underdiagnosed or overlooked altogether in histologic studies [MC Anderson 1991]. Thin CIN is a high-grade lesion.

Cytology

Because carcinoma in situ is defined in terms of a "full thickness" abnormality of the epithelium, a common misconception is that dysplasia is not a full-thickness abnormality [MC Anderson 1991]. But—this is crucial—dysplasia represents a profound biologic upheaval and derangement of epithelium, and the entire epithelial thickness is abnormal, even in mild dysplasia (CIN 1, L SIL). Otherwise, abnormal cells would not appear at the surface. If abnormal cells were not present at the epithelial surface, the Pap test could not detect dysplasia, because only the surface is sampled cytologically. (In fact, if abnormal cells are not present at the surface, there is no dysplasia in the first place.) The important concept is that in

dysplasia, there are abnormal cells through the full thickness of the epithelium, but they differentiate toward the surface, while in carcinoma in situ, the full thickness of the epithelium is made up of undifferentiated cells.

Histologically, the fraction of the whole epithelium that is composed of *undifferentiated* abnormal cells determines the degree of dysplasia. Cytology has a different perspective: it looks at differentiated cells exfoliated from the surface. The two perspectives are complementary: as the undifferentiated level ascends from the basal layer (viewed histologically), there is a corresponding decrease in the degree of squamous differentiation at the surface (viewed cytologically). By analogy, a glass that is "more full" (histology) is correspondingly "less empty" (cytology).

In low-grade dysplasia, considerable maturation occurs before the cells exfoliate, and therefore the abnormal cells at the surface appear fairly mature. In high-grade dysplasia, the undifferentiated cells ascend high in the epithelium, and little squamous maturation occurs before the cells exfoliate. Therefore, the abnormal cells at the surface of high-grade dysplasia appear quite immature. In carcinoma in situ, the full thickness of the epithelium is undifferentiated; therefore, undifferentiated cells are found at the mucosal surface.

Cellularity, Nucleus, Cytoplasm, and N/C Ratio

An underlying principle of Pap test interpretation, indeed, to interpretation of exfoliative cytology in general, is that cancer cells are less adherent to one another compared with normal cells [Coman 1944]. This facilitates sampling of abnormal cells in the first place. In general, the more advanced the lesion, the more cells that are exfoliated, but cellularity alone is not reliable in grading lesions (eg, sampling could be a problem). Lesions are graded in the Pap test—not by the number of abnormal cells, nor by the predominant cell type—but rather by the most abnormal (worst) cells present, even if there are only a few of them. However, the more cells that are present, the more likely the cytologic interpretation will be confirmed on biopsy [S Hall 1994]. Similarly, the worse the cells look (ie, the higher the grade), the more likely that the biopsy will show a correlating abnormality (lower grade, less likely).

> *Advancing Dysplasia*
>
> More advanced dysplasia →
>
> More cytologic abnormalities:
>
> ·More (number) abnormal cells
> ·More nuclear irregularities
> ·More chromatin abnormalities
> ·Decreased cell & nuclear size
> ·Increased N/C ratios

Squamous differentiation is manifested principally by the presence of dense cytoplasm and distinct cell boundaries. In fact, these are the hallmarks of squamous differentiation. Nuclear changes correlate with the degree of epithelial abnormality, or carcinogenesis.

Nuclear size, shape, outline, chromatin texture and distribution, and nucleoli, all follow a more or less predictable pattern of development in carcinogenesis. The nucleus of an intermediate cell serves as the reference. Its mean nuclear area is 35 µm^2, about the size of a red blood cell. By definition, the chromatin of an intermediate cell nucleus is finely granular and evenly distributed. The nuclear membrane generally is smooth, or it may have a neat fold or groove [S Gupta 2000, Kaneko 1998, Payandeh 2003, Tahlan 2001].

Important changes occur as cells progress from metaplastic to dysplastic to neoplastic [Wied 1962b]. The nucleus of a metaplastic cell enlarges to about 50 µm^2, but is otherwise similar to an intermediate cell nucleus in terms of its nuclear membrane and chromatin quality.

F1.14 Nuclear Areas in µm² (vs Intermediate Cell Nucleus)

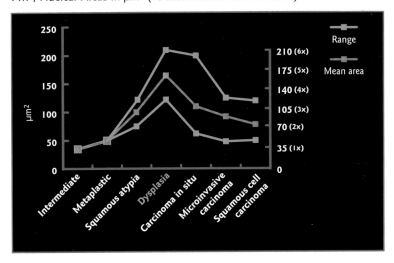

Nuclear area peaks at dysplasia (mild); x = intermediate cell nuclear area [Patten 1978].

F1.15 Nuclear/Cytoplasmic Ratios (Relative Nuclear Area in %)

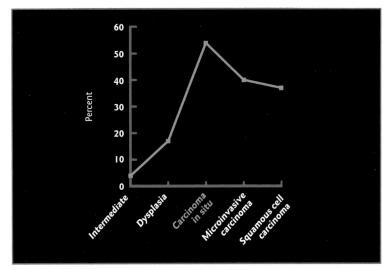

The nuclear/cytoplasmic ratio peaks at carcinoma in situ [Patten 1978].

At the next stage, dysplasia, profound changes are occurring in the nucleus. Perhaps most surprising is that the nuclei of dysplasia are, on average, the largest nuclei in the whole chain of events from normal to cancer, and the largest of all are found in mild dysplasia (CIN 1), a low-grade squamous intraepithelial lesion. From this point, average nuclear size diminishes [F1.14].

Dysplastic nuclei average about 165 µm² (range, ~120 µm²-210 µm²), which is 3.5 to 6 times the size of an intermediate cell nucleus [Patten 1978]. The nuclei of dysplasia are on average larger than those of invasive cancer [Patten 1978]. The mean nuclear area of squamous cell carcinoma is only about 85 µm² (range, ~50 µm²-120 µm²), or about 1.5 to 3 times the size of an intermediate cell nucleus. Compared with the life of a star, dysplasia is a red giant (in which viruses may be multiplying) and cancer a white dwarf (in which the viruses are integrated). T1.15 is an aid to juding relative nuclear sizes.

T1.15 An Aid to Judging Nuclear Areas and Relative Sizes

Coin	Area, µm²	
Dime	35	Intermediate cell nucleus
Nickel	50	Squamous metaplastic nucleus
Quarter	70	Beginning squamous atypia
Half-dollar	100	Average of squamous atypia
Silver dollar	150	Range of dysplasia

On the other hand, there is almost complete overlap in the range of nuclear areas of carcinoma in situ, from ~60 µm²-200 µm², with both squamous cell carcinoma (~50 µm²-120 µm²) and dysplasia (~120 µm²-210 µm²) with an average of about 155 µm² [Patten 1978, Reagan 1962b]. This suggests that carcinoma in situ is a dynamic process in which the cells are changing from merely dysplastic to frankly malignant. The nuclei of microinvasive and fully invasive squamous cell carcinoma are nearly identical in size.

At the stage of mild dysplasia, with its big, bad nuclei, the nuclear membranes may be more or less smooth and the chromatin is often relatively fine. Hyperchromasia is an important feature of dysplasia; however, the degree of hyperchromasia is variable from case to case, and is minimal to absent in some cases, particularly in liquid-based cytology. In fact, a common mistake is to expect all dysplastic nuclei to be practically "pitch black," when in reality, hyperchromasia can be very subtle in some cases, and particularly in liquid-based cytology, may be lacking altogether. The British use the term "pale dyskaryosis" for hypochromatic dysplasia [C Buckley 1994, Dudding 1996a, PA Smith 1997]. To recognize pale, bland cells (PBCs) indicative of high-grade dysplasia (or cancer), particular attention must be paid to the abnormalities of the nuclear outline (like brains in bottles), the depth of focus of the nucleus (great), and the N/C ratios (increased). The pale chromatin is characteristically "speckled," ie, finely and irregularly clumped. In practice, neoplastic PBCs can be difficult to distinguish from reactive/inflammatory changes [PA Smith 1997].

Fortunately, however, the nuclei are usually at least somewhat hyperchromatic, compared with an intermediate cell nucleus, even in liquid-based cytology. As the dysplasia progresses, the chromatin "precipitates," and tends to become coarser and darker, with chromocenter formation. At the same time, the nuclear envelope becomes wrinkled or crinkled as the nucleus crumples (like wadding up a ball of paper). By the stage of CIN 3, the nuclei are typically small and irregular, or "raisinoid." Single cells out of context (common in liquid-based cytology) can be particularly difficult to interpret: benign cells such as endometrial cells, immature metaplasia, or histiocytes can be overcalled as H SIL, or more ominously, H SIL can be undercalled as benign cells [PA Smith 1997].

In histology, the degree of dysplasia is diagnosed by the ratio of the thickness of the undifferentiated layer to the thickness of the whole epithelium (an undifferentiated/mucosal thickness ratio). In cytology, an analogous ratio is the N/C ratio: the higher the N/C ratio, the less differentiated the cell [F1.15]. Therefore, in both cases, the higher the ratio, the more advanced the dysplasia.

Intermediate cells are mature; their N/C ratios are low. Metaplastic cells are relatively immature, their N/C ratios are higher. Low-grade dysplasia has low N/C ratios; high-grade dysplasia has high N/C ratios. Cellular immaturity, measured by N/C ratio, reaches its peak at the stage of carcinoma in situ (completely undifferentiated cells), after which the cells "redifferentiate" as they become invasive cancer, and the N/C ratio falls. Poorly-differentiated cancer cells have higher N/C ratios than well-differentiated cancer cells. In summary, although the largest nuclei are found in dysplasia, the highest N/C ratios are found in carcinoma in situ.

When invasion begins, the chromatin falls apart, separating into irregular, pointed shards, with areas of clearing. A prominent nucleolus develops. The cell acquires more cytoplasm, and redifferentiates, though abnormally. A matrix simplifies these features for easy comparisons [T1.16].

T1.16 Cytologic Features Compared for Squamous Lesions

	Dysplasia	Carcinoma In Situ	Microinvasive Carcinoma	Squamous Cell Carcinoma
Nuclear size	Maximum	Variable	Minimum	Minimum
Nuclear/ cytoplasmic ratio	Increases	Maximum	Decreases	Decreases
Chromatin	Finer	Coarser	Irregular distribution	Irregular distribution
Prominent nucleoli	Rare	Rare	Herald invasion	Invasion
Cytoplasm	Dedifferentiates	Undifferentiated	Abnormal differentiation	Abnormal differentiation

The Secret of Dysplasia Revealed

There are really only two steps to recognizing dysplasia in Pap tests. The first step is to determine whether or not the cell is dysplastic. Then, if the cell is dysplastic, the second step is to grade the degree dysplasia.

First, a cell is determined to be dysplastic by virtue of its nuclear features. Dysplastic nuclei are *big* (nuclear enlargement >120 μm² or >3 times intermediate cell nucleus) and they're *dark* (hyperchromatic compared with an intermediate cell nucleus). So, it's simple—compare the nucleus in question with that of an intermediate cell: *If it's big and it's dark, it's dysplasia.*

Second, if—and only if—the cell is determined to be dysplastic, then the N/C ratio is assessed to grade the dysplasia. The N/C ratio is a measure of cellular maturity. The higher the N/C ratio (relative to its icon), the higher the grade of dysplasia [Ehrmann 1996].

Nuclear changes characteristic of advancing dysplasia occur in concert with N/C ratio alterations. For example, if a cell has a high N/C ratio, but the nucleus has a smooth, regular membrane, it is probably not CIN 3, which usually has irregular, "raisinoid" nuclei but may be, for example, an immature metaplastic cell. (Unfortunately, CIN 3 cells sometimes do have smooth nuclear membranes, which can lead to interpretive problems.) Single cells, or small groups of cells, are easier to evaluate than cells found in thick groups, especially with respect to the N/C ratio. Although binucleated or multinucleated cells can certainly be dysplastic, they are less helpful in evaluation of degree of dysplasia, because the N/C ratio is distorted when there is more than one nucleus. Dysplastic cells usually form a separate population of cells that tends to stand out from the background of normal or inflamed cells. Also, there is usually a spectrum of abnormality, eg, in high-grade dysplasia, there are usually also low-grade dysplastic cells.

The Secret of Carcinoma In Situ Revealed

Carcinoma in situ is characterized by the presence of three-dimensional syncytial-like aggregates of abnormal cells, with indistinct cell borders, and chaotic architecture ("loss of nuclear polarity"). These cellular aggregates can be seen at low scanning power in the microscope as "hyperchromatic crowded groups" (HCGs). It is important to look for hyperchromatic crowded groups and to examine them carefully, because these may represent serious lesions, such as squamous carcinoma—in situ or invasive [DeMay 2000, Koike 1994]. However, many other benign and malignant conditions can be associated with hyperchromatic crowded groups, including endometrial cells and severe atrophy, as well as reactive endocervical cells and endocervical glandular neoplasia [Boon 1991, DeMay 2000, Goff 1992, K Lee 1995]. Mitotic figures and chromatin abnormalities in HCGs are clues to the possibility of a significant lesion. Another clue is that "like accompanies like." As a rule (probably >90% of cases), squamous carcinoma in situ is accompanied by squamous dysplasia, forming a spectrum of abnormality (grades of dysplasia plus carcinoma in situ). This spectrum indicates that the HCG in question really is carcinoma in situ and not a benign mimicker [T1.17]. Exceptionally, when the cervix is extensively involved by a pure carcinoma in situ lesion, an accompanying dysplasia will not be found, and a valuable interpretive clue is lost. This situation is more likely to occur in postmenopausal women, who may also have CIS cells with bland nuclei and rare mitotic figures, compounding the interpretive problems. Because the syncytial cytoplasm is delicate, atypical naked nuclei are common in carcinoma in situ, another interpretive clue [Boon 1995]. (See pg 182 for further discussion of HCGs.)

Summary: 2 Key Questions

1st: Is the cell dysplastic?

Compare with intermediate cell nucleus

"If it's big and it's dark, it's dysplasia"

2nd: How dysplastic is it?

Evaluate N/C ratio:

Higher N/C ⇒ more advanced dysplasia

Carcinoma in situ exfoliates HCGs

T1.17 Benign Conditions Mimicking L SIL, H SIL, and Cancer

Mimics L SIL	Mimics H SIL	Mimics Cancer
Trichomonas, Candida, and most other inflammation	Herpes*	Repair
	IUD Atypia*	Reactive endocervical cells
	Atypia of atrophy*	Arias-Stella reaction
Atypia of maturity	Squamous metaplasia	(Also mimics of high-
Squamous metaplasia	Endometrial cells*	grade SIL)
Vitamin deficiency	Follicular cervicitis*	
Radiation	Histiocytes*	
Histiocytes	Decidual cells	
Decidual cells	Reserve cell hyperplasia*	

*May see hyperchromatic crowded groups

Histo-Cyto Correlation

In real life, there is not a perfect, one-to-one correspondence between the cytologic interpretation and the histologic diagnosis [Konikov 1969, Swinker 1994, Tabbara 1992, E Walker 1986]. Lack of correlation between histology and cytology does not necessarily mean that the Pap test was misinterpreted. Both colposcopy and biopsy are tests, which like other tests, are subject to variations in sampling and interpretation. Furthermore, there are no sharp demarcations between the various grades of dysplasia, eg, a "high-grade" mild dysplasia (L SIL) is essentially identical to a "low-grade" moderate dysplasia (H SIL). This is a concern in using the Bethesda System's squamous intraepithelial lesion terminology: there is no gray zone between L SIL and H SIL, and the distinction can be arbitrary [McGrath 2000, Selvaggi 1999b, Woodhouse 1999].

Cytology can offer certain advantages over histology in assessment of dysplasia. Cytology provides exquisite nuclear detail, making subtle nuclear abnormalities easier to appreciate. Also, because intact, rather than sectioned, cells are examined, direct one-to-one comparison makes subtle differences more apparent in cytology. And, importantly, a wider area—theoretically the entire ectocervix and endocervix—is sampled by cytologic methods.

For a screening test, a false-negative result (substantially undercalling or missing a lesion entirely) is, of course, the most serious problem, because the goal is to identify as many cases of disease as is reasonably possible. To enhance sensitivity, some test specificity may have to be sacrificed (it's like a teeter-totter—if sensitivity goes up, specificity goes down). Owing to interpretive difficulties, it is usually better to err on side of overinterpretation, because the consequences of undertreating may be substantially greater than those of overtreating. Of course, there are undesirable consequences of overtreatment, eg, infertility in women who want to have children—but consider the consequences of undertreatment: dead women don't have babies.

Atypical Squamous Cells

"Atypical" is a mystical cloud of unknowing. The problem of atypical cells is not new. Papanicolaou mentioned atypical cells in his 1943 atlas, *Diagnosis of Uterine Cancer by the Vaginal Smear,* and wondered if these borderline cases were incipient malignant changes [Papanicolaou 1943]. In the 1950s, the Papanicolaou classification system included a category for atypical cells (Class II). Then came a flood of "atypias," such as inflammatory atypia, benign atypia, and reactive atypia. "Nondiagnostic" squamous atypias were recognized as risk factors for underlying squamous lesions (dysplasia) [Melamed 1976]. In the 1970s, Patten gave formal cytologic criteria for atypical lesions that he designated "noninflammatory squamous atypia" and "atypical squamous metaplasia" [Patten 1978]. In 1988, the Bethesda System defined "atypical squamous cells of undetermined significance" (ASCUS) as squamous abnormalities that were more marked than reactive changes, but fell short of being diagnostic of a squamous intraepithelial lesion. Ironically, specific criteria, closely following those of Patten, were proposed for this nonspecific ASCUS category [Wilbur 1997a]. In the Bethesda System (TBS) 1991, ASCUS could be further

---

Atypical Squamous Cells

  ASC-US

    Squamous atypia + FLCs*

    (exclude L SIL)

  ASC-H

    Atypical squamous metapasia + FLCs*

    (exclude H SIL)

  Theory: Defines high risk woman

  Practice: Many have SIL, often high grade

  *FLCs=funny looking cells

---

subclassified as "favor reactive" or "favor SIL." In practice, ASCUS was usually used unqualified, and in TBS 2001, the "favor reactive" and "favor SIL" subcategories were dropped. However, a new category, atypical squamous cells-cannot exclude a high-grade SIL (ASC-H), was created, and in a breathtaking advance, a hyphen was added to ASCUS, becoming ASC-US. (Note: Although ASCUS and ASC-US are similar, they are not identical, since cells suspicious for H SIL could be included in the old ASCUS category, but would now be reported as ASC-H, not ASC-US. Many studies were done on ASCUS, not ASC-US, and the appropriate acronym has been retained in this text.)

In practice, there are two broad categories of atypical squamous cells [Wilbur 1996a, 1997a,b]. The first is characterized by relatively well-defined changes that Patten described as squamous atypia and atypical squamous metaplasia. Rather than being of "undetermined significance," these two interpretations have relatively well-defined significance, which can be conceptualized as "minimal dysplasia." The second group is, unfortunately, a vague wastebasket category for funny looking cells (FLCs) that are difficult to classify ("don't ask us!"). This group is one of irreproducible results that not only includes apples and oranges, but also zebras, black holes, and road kill, among other things.

The TBS 2001 category, ASC-US, more or less corresponds to Patten's squamous atypia *plus* funny looking cells that could be dysplastic, but are not thought to be H SIL. One could conceptualize this category as "atypical squamous cells-L SIL not excluded," or ASC-L, as long as it is clearly understood that there will be certain proportion of H SILs on biopsy. (Note well that ASC-L is *not* in the Bethesda System lexicon.) ASC-H more or less corresponds to Patten's atypical squamous metaplasia *plus* funny looking cells that could be H SIL, including those found in hyperchromatic crowded groups. Importantly, *either* of these cytologic interpretations (ASC-US or ASC-H) could be associated with a histologic diagnosis of H SIL, but H SIL is more likely in the ASC-H category. The following discussion will first consider minimally dysplastic lesions, as defined by Patten, and then atypical squamous cells, as defined by the Bethesda System.

Minimal Dysplasia: Squamous Atypia & Atypical Squamous Metaplasia

Minimal dysplasia can be thought of as "CIN $^1/_2$" or as a precursor to dysplasia (the first bubbles in boiling water). In theory, there are two basic forms of minimal, or very mild, dysplasia. The first occurs in mature squamous cells and is known as noninflammatory squamous atypia or, simply, squamous atypia. Squamous atypia resembles intermediate or superficial squamous cells with minimally abnormal nuclei. The second type of minimal dysplasia occurs in immature metaplastic cells and is also known as atypical squamous metaplasia. It resembles squamous metaplastic cells with minimally abnormal nuclei. Squamous atypia accounts for up to 80% of cases of minimal dysplasia [Stoler 1999]. The number of atypical cells is variable, but they are usually not numerous [Hoerl 2002].

Squamous Atypia

Minimal dysplasia of mature squamous cells is known as squamous atypia [11.59]. This lesion is characterized by intermediate or superficial cells with a "sick" nucleus ("dyskaryosis" to use Papanicolaou's term). Nuclear abnormalities are similar to those seen in low-grade dysplasia, but are less marked. The nuclei are enlarged, averaging about 100 μm² (range, 75 μm²- 120 μm²), which is about two to three times the area of an intermediate cell nucleus (35 μm²) [Patten 1978, Sheils 1997]. This compares with dysplasia in which the nuclei average 165 μm² (range from 120 μm²-210 μm²), ie, more than three times normal size [Patten 1978]. The nuclear

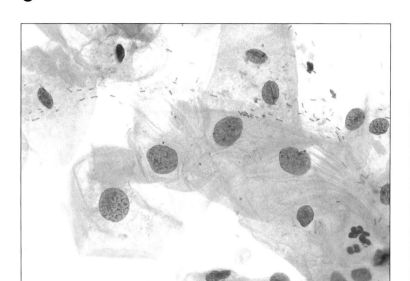

II.59
Squamous atypia (ASC-US) [C]

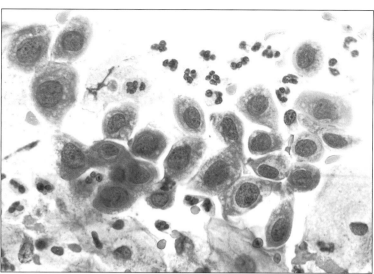

II.60
Atypical squamous metaplasia (ASC-H) [C]

membranes are usually smooth or only slightly irregular. The chromatin is fine, and tends to be slightly hyperchromatic, although sometimes it can be quite dark, but not coarse. Chromocenter formation is usually inconspicuous in both squamous atypia and mild dysplasia.

In squamous atypia the cytoplasm is thin, delicate, and transparent, very like the cytoplasm of a mature intermediate or superficial cell. The cytoplasm can stain blue or pink, or sometimes orange. In contrast, in mild dysplasia, not only is the nuclear abnormality more obvious, but also the dysplastic cytoplasm usually appears slightly thick and dense (ie, slightly immature), compared with normal mature cells or cells of squamous atypia. (In high-grade dysplasia, the cytoplasm appears still more immature, reminiscent of metaplasia, or is abnormally keratinized.)

Using the Bethesda System, squamous atypia is commonly interpreted as "atypical squamous cells-undetermined significance" (ASC-US). The main differential is between mild dysplasia and marked reactive changes.

Atypical Squamous Metaplasia

Minimal dysplasia of metaplastic squamous cells is known as atypical squamous metaplasia [II.60]. This lesion is characterized by nuclear abnormalities (size, outline, and chromatin) that are less marked than those of established dysplasia occurring in metaplastic cells. Compared with the normal metaplastic nucleus (50 μm^2), the nuclei of atypical squamous metaplasia are enlarged ~1.5 to 2 times normal (range, 65 μm^2-100 μm^2), which is about 2 to 3 times the size of an intermediate cell nucleus (35 μm^2) [Sheils 1997]. The nuclei are generally similar to those in squamous atypia. Nuclear membranes are smooth to slightly irregular. Chromocenters or small nucleoli may be present. The cytoplasm is diminished and dense, with rounded, sharply defined cell borders, and high N/C ratios, like ordinary squamous metaplasia. Very immature forms of atypical squamous metaplasia have smaller nuclei (35 μm^2-70 μm^2),

---

ASC-US: Squamous Atypia

Cells: Mature intermediate or superficial

Nuclear enlargement (< dysplasia)

   2–3 X (vs 4–6 X) intermediate nucleus

Smooth or minimally irregular membranes

Chromatin: ~ Normal to dark

In essence: Cytoplasm normal,

   Nucleus sick ("dyskaryosis")

Inflammatory change vs L SIL

---

markedly elevated N/C ratios, and variable cytoplasm that ranges from dense to frothy, the latter mimicking histiocytes [Wilbur 1997b].

Atypical squamous metaplasia is an extremely difficult cytologic interpretation [Hatem 1995, DE Jones 1987, Montes 1999]. In theory, atypical squamous metaplasia is simply intermediate in appearance between benign squamous metaplasia and metaplastic dysplasia. However, in practice, these distinctions can be exquisitely fine. The nuclear changes can be very subtle, and in contrast with squamous atypia, the cytoplasmic features are not helpful, since all metaplastic cells, whether benign or neoplastic, have immature cytoplasm by definition. Note in particular that the N/C ratio is completely useless in this differential (because both benign immature metaplastic cells and high-grade dysplastic cells have high N/C ratios). Moreover, these tiny little cells can be easy to miss altogether in screening [Frable 1994, Hatem 1995, Sherman 1992b, Wilbur 1997b].

Using the Bethesda System, questionable metaplastic lesions can be interpreted as "atypical squamous cells, cannot exclude high-grade squamous intraepithelial lesion" (ASC-H). The differential includes benign metaplasia, atypical squamous metaplasia, and metaplastic dysplasia. When little metaplastic cells with high N/C ratios are discovered, smooth nuclear membranes, fine, even chromatin, and nucleoli favor benign metaplasia, while irregular nuclear membranes and speckled chromatin

---

ASC-H: Atypical Squamous Metaplasia

Cells: Immature metaplasia, parabasal

Nuclei: Like those of squamous atypia

High N/C ratio (metaplastic cells)

Benign metaplasia vs H SIL

   Can be extremely difficult!

---

favor SIL. There is also a morphologic spectrum of atypical metaplastic cells: the more immature the cells, the higher the risk of H SIL on follow-up biopsy [D Gupta 2001a,b, Sheils 1997, Wilbur 1997b].

Significance of Minimal Dysplasia

Minimally dysplastic cells in the Pap test indicate that the full thickness of the epithelium is abnormal, at least focally. By the time cytologic abnormalities are visible in the light microscope, profound changes have occurred in the nucleus at the ultrastructural, and even molecular level [Rubio 1981a]. Women with these "minimal" lesions are often HPV-DNA positive, with high-risk viral types identified in many or most cases [H Bauer 1991, Borst 1991, Goff 1993, J Rader 1991, Stewart 1993a, Wagner 1984]. Further,

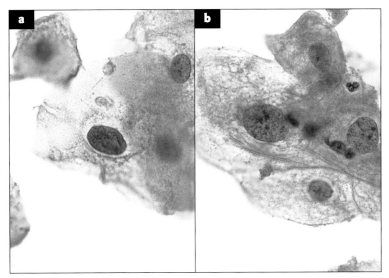

11.61
a, ASC-US HPV+ [C]; **b**, ASC-US HPV– [C]

11.62
a, "Candy" ASC-US HPV– [C]; **b**, "Trich" ASC-US [L]

these "minimal" abnormalities can be associated with aneuploidy [Bollman 2003b, Watts 1987]. What's more, significant squamous lesions are often found on follow-up biopsies. These "minimal" cellular changes, then, may not be so minimal after all.

In theory, when one of these minimally dysplastic lesions is identified in a Pap test, it is predicted that the biopsy results would be "negative," because the subtle cytologic abnormalities, by definition, fall short of being diagnostic of a squamous intraepithelial lesion. However, in practice, many women have SIL on biopsy, often enough H SIL, and a few even have cancer (discussed in more detail below) [Augor 1997, August 1991, Crabtree 2002, Dressel 1992b, Gatscha 2001, Kaufman 1996, Lindheim 1990, Massad 2001, Soutter 1986]). Therefore, these women are at high risk of having significant squamous lesions.

Atypical Squamous Cells: Undetermined Significance & Cannot Exclude H SIL

In TBS 1991, ASCUS could be qualified as "favor reactive" or "favor SIL," but these subcategories were dropped in TBS 2001. However, two new subcategories were defined: ASC-undetermined significance (ASC-US) and ASC-cannot exclude high-grade squamous intraepithelial lesion (ASC-H).

"Atypical squamous cells" (ASC) is a controversial and problematic cytologic interpretation ("can't live with it, can't live without it"). The ASCUS category is popular with cytologists because it formally recognizes the limitations of cytologic interpretation and provides "wiggle room" for diagnostic uncertainty. However, most clinicians despised it because of the confusion it caused as to its meaning, and therefore, management of women with this interpretation was unclear [R Nayar 2003]. Some authorities advocated eliminating the ASC category because: it is subjective, irreproducible, and overused; it has become a diagnostic wastebasket; it creates anxiety for women and management problems for clinicians; and it costs the health care system billions of dollars annually [Bonfiglio 2002, Cahill 2000, Frable 1999b, H Jones 1995, Kurman 1994, Raab 1998b, 1999c, Solomon 2001, Stoler 1999, 2001b]. However, the ASC category was maintained in TBS 2001 because: experience with eliminating it was limited to only a few cytology laboratories; there might be an increase in reporting of L SIL with a decrease in reporting of H SIL; and there is a risk of missing an underlying H SIL. In short, although eliminating ASC could increase specificity, it could also reduce sensitivity of the Pap test—not a desirable outcome for a screening procedure [R Nayar 2003, Pitman 2002, Raab

2000, Renshaw 2001b, Sodhani 2004]. Because follow-up recommendations for ASC are now more clearly defined [T Wright 2002a], much of the clinician's angst about this interpretation has been eliminated. It is possible that ASC-US rates will soar because of the financial incentive of reflex HPV-DNA testing (there's gold in them thar SILs). On the other hand, it could be argued that it is a *disservice* to women not to use the ASC-US interpretation liberally, because reflex HPV-DNA testing provides a "safety net" against false-negative cytologic results [Austin 2003b]. Women with false-negative results will not get early follow-up and referral for diagnostic testing.

Atypical Squamous Cells–Undetermined Significance (ASC-US)

Atypical Squamous Cells-Undetermined Significance (ASC-US) is defined as "cellular abnormalities that are more marked than those attributable to reactive changes, but that quantitatively or qualitatively fall short of a definitive diagnosis of a squamous intraepithelial lesion." ASC-US is used to designate cellular alterations that are neither definitely dysplastic nor definitely inflammatory. In other words, this is a negative definition, saying what the cells *are not,* rather than what they *are* [McGrath 2002]. (What is an orange? Well, it's not an apple [although it's a fruit] and it's not a baseball [although it's about the same size and shape].)

ASC-US refers to cytologic changes suggestive of SIL, but lack sufficient criteria for a specific interpretation [11.61a,b]. This terminology can also be used for other squamous cell changes that are less than diagnostic or of uncertain nature, in each case qualifying as best as possible the nature of the change, to aid in clinical management. An interpretation of ASC-US carries a significant risk of an underlying H SIL, but if there is a definite concern about H SIL, the interpretation should be ASC-H or H SIL, rather than ASC-US.

In ASC-US, the cells are mature superficial or intermediate squamous cells. The nuclei are enlarged from two to three times the area of a normal intermediate cell nucleus, they are round to oval, with minimal membrane irregularities, and are normochromatic or slightly hyperchromatic. The cytoplasm is polygonal in outline; abundant, thin, and transparent; and stains cyanophilic or eosinophilic. This definition corresponds almost exactly to Patten's noninflammatory squamous atypia [R Nayar 2003, Patten 1978, Sidawy 1997, Solomon 1998, 2002]. Inflammatory conditions, such as *Candida* infection ("candy ASC-US") [11.62a] and *Trichomonas* infection ("Trich ASC-US") [11.62b], can also cause mild nuclear enlargement and hyperchromasia, leading to ASC-US interpretations [Miguel 1997]. The differential is usually between a benign reactive process and L SIL. Minimal nuclear enlargement (<2 X intermediate nucleus), smooth nuclear membranes, fine even chromatin, and prominent nucleoli, favor a reactive process [T1.18].

T1.18 Comparative Features of Reactive Change, ASC-US, and L SIL

	Reactive	ASC-US[‡]	L SIL
Cells	Mature	Mature	Mature
Nuclei			
Area*	1-2 ×	2-3 ×	>3 ×
Stain	Pale or slt dark	Variably dark	Dark
Chromatin	Very fine or degenerated	Fine	Fine to coarse
Membrane	Smooth	Smooth/slightly irregular	Irregular
Nucleoli	Present	None or indistinct	None or indistinct
Cytoplasm			
N/C Ratio	Low	Low	Low
Quality	Degenerative change common ± small halos	Thin, delicate ± indistinct halos	Thick, dense ± koilocyte halos

[‡]*Similar to Patten's Squamous Atypia*
Compared with intermediate cell nucleus

In liquid-based cytology, the findings are similar, consisting of mild nuclear enlargement (2-3 times normal intermediate nucleus), occasional binucleation, and fine even chromatin in mature squamous cells. Perinuclear halos suggestive of koilocytes may be seen in either specimen type [I1.63a,b].

ASC-Cannot Exclude High-Grade Squamous Intraepithelial Lesion (ASC-H)

ASC-cannot exclude high-grade squamous intraepithelial lesion (ASC-H) will include true H SIL and its mimics owing to the interpretive uncertainty of this category [I1.64a,b]. In ASC-H the cells resemble immature parabasal or basal squamous cells. The nuclei are slightly enlarged, frequently hyperchromatic, and have irregular outlines. This definition corresponds well to Patten's atypical squamous metaplasia. The differential is usually between benign, reactive metaplasia and H SIL. Key features favoring SIL are irregular nuclear membranes and chromatin abnormalities (coarse, dark); favoring reactive changes are smooth nuclear membranes and nucleoli [T1.19] [Alli 2003, Sherman 1999]. Degeneration can cause hyperchromasia and nuclear irregularities; however, in degeneration, the chromatin often appears smudgy and the nuclei appear diffusely wrinkled or crenated. The differential also includes atypical repair, atypical parakeratosis, and atypia of atrophy [K Lee 1995, R Nayar 2003, Sherman 2001]. Reactive endocervical cells and histiocytes can also mimic dysplastic squamous cells in both conventional Pap smears and liquid-based cytology [Sherman2001].

Thick tissue fragments (ie, hyperchromatic crowded groups, HCGs) can be difficult to evaluate and can represent H SIL [I1.65] [DeMay 2000, Ramsamooj 2002, Selvaggi 2003]. Therefore, HCGs can placed in the ASC-H category when the cytologic findings are suspicious, but not definitive, for H SIL [R Nayar 2003, Sherman 1999]. However, in practice, such HCGs are probably more often interpreted as atypical glandular cells, helping explain the fact that women with atypical glandular cells on Pap test often have squamous lesions on biopsy. The differential includes squamous carcinoma in situ, endocervical glandular neoplasia, and benign aggre-

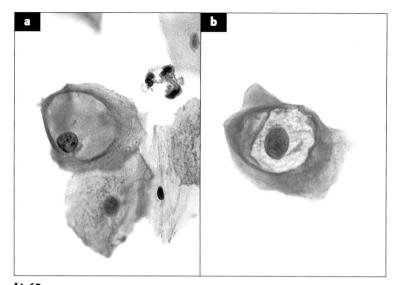

I1.63
a, ASC-US, halo HPV+ [L]; **b**, ASC-US, halo [L]

gates such as basaloid cells in atrophy, clusters of endometrial cells, and reactive endocervical cells [K Lee 1995, Sherman 2001].

In liquid-based cytology the findings are similar [Louro 2003, R Nayar 2003, Quddus 2001]. These can be summarized as immature squamous cells, with slight nuclear enlargement, slightly irregular nuclear membranes, variation in size and shape, and high N/C ratios. Hyperchromatic crowded groups can be just as difficult to interpret in LBC, if not more so, because it is more difficult to examine cells at the edge of the rounded up clusters.

Included in ASC

Cells suggestive of a squamous intraepithelial lesion, but their scarcity or degeneration preclude a definitive interpretation of SIL, can be placed in the ASC category. Atypical parakeratosis, atypical repair, and atypia of atrophy (all discussed below), and minimally dysplastic lesions (squamous atypia, atypical squamous metaplasia) can be included in ASC [Solomon 1998]. Cells suggestive of, but not definitive for, koilocytes can be interpreted as ASC (see minor cytologic criteria for

T1.19 Comparative Features of Squamous Metaplasia, ASC-H, and H SIL

	Metaplasia	ASC-H[‡]	H SIL
Cells	Immature	Immature	Immature
Nuclei			
Area*	1-2 ×	2-3 ×	>3 ×
Stain	Pale	Slightly dark	Variably dark
Chromatin	Fine	Speckled	Speckled to coarse
Membrane	Smooth	Slightly irregular	Irregular
Nucleoli	May be present	No or indistinct	No or indistinct
Cytoplasm			
N/C Ratio	High	High	High
Quality	Thick, dense	Thick, dense	Thick, dense

[‡]*Similar to Patten's Atypical Squamous Metaplasia*
Compared with intermediate cell nucleus

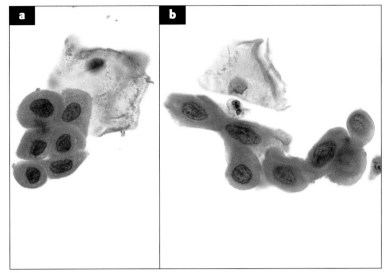

II.64
a, ASC-H HPV– [L]; **b**, ASC-H (H SIL) [L]

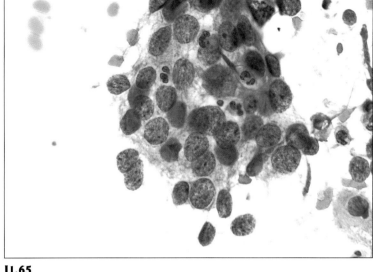

II.65
ASC-H, hyperchromatic crowded group [C]

condyloma, pg 50), but definitive koilocytes are placed in the L SIL category [R Nayar 1999, 2003]. Hyperchromatic crowded groups suspected of being neoplastic can also be included in ASC (in practice, ASC-H) [Solomon 1998]. In practice, ASC is often used as a wastebasket category that not only includes cells that are difficult to classify, but also atypical cells from compromised specimens that are difficult to visualize owing to poor preservation, obscuring material, etc [McGrath 2002, Mintzer 1999, Sebastião 2004, Solomon 1998]. Such compromised specimens may have poorly presented cells derived from significant abnormalities with SIL rates reported as high as 50% [Lindheim 1990, Noumoff 1987, Solomon 1998]. Use of liquid-based cytology (LBC) might be expected to decrease the number of ASC cases due to compromised specimens (air drying, obscuring inflammation, etc) [Anton 2001, Negri 2003, Solomon 1998]; however, a substantial number of ASC cases remain even when LBC is used [Emerson 2002].

Not Included in ASC

Cellular changes thought to be purely reactive in nature are not included in the category of ASC. Therefore, "reactive cellular changes" including Pap class II, reactive "atypia," inflammatory "atypia," and benign "atypia" are excluded from ASC. Hyperkeratosis and parakeratosis are excluded, although atypical parakeratosis or dyskeratocytes may be interpreted as ASC or squamous intraepithelial lesions, depending on the degree of nuclear abnormality [NCI 1993a,b]. Of course, mimickers of SIL, eg, inflammatory changes, Trich halos, glycogenated cells, benign metaplasia, atrophy, etc, are not included in ASC when they are recognized as imitators. However, it is not always obvious that these changes are only reactive in nature. In practice, reactive squamous "atypia," inflammatory changes, keratinization, and atrophy, as well as air-drying, degeneration, and other artifacts, are common explanations for ASC [Pinto 2002b].

ASC: An Irreproducible Result of Undetermined Significance?

"Atypical squamous cells" is not a distinct biological entity. It is a gray zone cytologic interpretation that will *never* find an exact histologic correlate because, if for no other reason, the term is not used in histopathology. (A

corollary is that there is no right or wrong ASC interpretation; some women have lesions and the others don't—that's what "undetermined significance" means!) Yet, "atypical squamous cells" is, by far, the most common cytologic abnormality reported in Pap tests [E Becker 2001]. At least 2 to 3 million American women receive this result every year [Raab 1998b, 1999c, Solomon 2001]. There is no "correct" rate for ASC interpretations [Solomon 1998]. An ASC rate of about 4% to 6% and an ASCUS/SIL ratio of 2 to 3 for an average population of women were suggested as targets (based on little or no data) [Kurman 1994].

According to a College of American Pathologists (CAP) survey of 759 laboratories conducted after implementation of the Bethesda System 2001 [T1.20], mean and median ASC (ASC-US + ASC-H) rates were 5.08% and 4.1%, respectively, and more than 25% of labs report ASC rates of >6% [Davey 2004]. A significant number (more than 10%) of the laboratories had ASC rates greater than 9%. The mean ASC/SIL+ rate was 1.55, although ASCUS/SIL ratios over 15 have been reported [Wachtel 2003]. Mean ASC and SIL rates are higher in LBC (5.31 and 3.76, respectively) than conventional Pap smears (4.29, 2.76), but the ASC/SIL+ ratio is lower in LBC (1.41 vs 1.55). The 5th and 95th percentiles for ASC/SIL+ ratios in the survey were 0.49 and 3.73, respectively, for conventional Pap smears, and 0.40 and 3.11 for LBC [Davey 2004].

T1.20 Mean Values in 2003 CAP Survey (% total cases)

	CPS+LBC	CPS	LBC
ASC (-US + -H)	5.08	4.29	5.31
SIL	3.27	2.76	3.76*
ASC/SIL+	1.55	1.55	1.41
ASC/SIL+ 5th, 95th percentile	0.50, 3.44	0.49, 3.73	0.40, 3.11

*Most of the increased SIL detection in LBC was L SIL.
[Davey 2004]

ASC rates are highly variable among observers [Kaufman 1996], and do not necessarily correlate with their education or years of experience [Gatscha 2001, Juskevicius 2001]. In high-risk populations, with a high prevalence of squamous intraepithelial lesions, there may be a correspondingly higher prevalence of ASC [Hudock 1995, Kurman 1994, Solomon 1998, Wachtel 2003]. High ASC rates and ASC /SIL ratios may also reflect increased medicolegal concerns together with widespread acceptance of the ASC terminology [Davey 1994, R Nayar 2003, Schoolland 1998, Stoler 1999].

There is some concern that clinicians may underestimate the risk of an underlying serious lesion for women with interpretations of "only" atypical squamous cells [Raab 2001b]. HPV-DNA testing is the method of choice in managing women with ASC-US (see pg 200) [J Kim 2002, Manos 1999, Solomon 2001, T Wright 2002a]. Anywhere from 15% to 90% of women with ASC-US are found to be HPV-DNA positive (the wide range reflects variable interpretive criteria) [Bruner 2004, Ferenczy 1995, I Hong 2002, Levi 2003, Lörincz 1986, Lu 2003, Manos 1999, Pirog 2004, Rowe 2004, Sarode 2003, D Scott 2002, Sherman 1994, 2001, 2002, Solomon 2001, T Wright 2002a]. For comparison, 10% to 40% of American women with normal Pap tests, and 60% to 90⁺% of those with SIL on Pap test, are positive for HPV [T1.21] [Pirog 2004, Scott 2002]. The prevalence of HPV positivity in women with ASC-US varies with age (more common before 30 years), clinical risk factors, pregnancy, and prior history of cytologic abnormality. HPV-positive ASC-US is essentially equivalent to an interpretation of L SIL and managed accordingly. Women with ASC-H should be referred to colposcopy [T Wright 2002a].

T1.21 Cervical Cytology and HPV-DNA

Pap Test Result	Total HPV +	High Risk HPV +
Normal	~10%*	2%-5%
ASCUS	20%-40%**	20%-30%***
L SIL	60%-85%	50%-80%
H SIL	80%-90%	80%-90%
Cancer	99%	>95%

*up to 40% in some series. **up to 90% in some series. ***75-85% of ASC-H cases
[S Anderson 2001 , Pirog 2004, Sherman 2001]

Age may have an important bearing on risk of cervical neoplasia. Younger women (<35 years) with ASCUS on Pap test have H SIL on biopsy more often than older women [Brotzman 1996, Kaminski 1989a,b, Kobelin 1998, Lousuebsakul 2000, 2001, A Rader 1999]. A prior history of an abnormal Pap test or treatment for cervical dysplasia also increases the risk of H SIL [H Jones 2000]. HPV-DNA positivity, particularly for high-risk viral types, increases the risk of dysplasia. Conversely, HPV-DNA negativity substantially reduces (indeed, practically eliminates) the risk of current cervical neoplasia.

Despite the morphologic criteria presented above, an interpretation of ASC is irreproducible even among (especially among?) top experts [Chhieng 2002, Cocchi 1997, Condel 2002, Confortini 2003, Crum 1999, Davey 1994, 1996, 2000, Ettler 1999, Gatscha 2001, Howell 1996, Quddus 2001, Renshaw 1997, Robb 1994, Sherman 1992c, 1994, Sidawy 1993, A Smith 2000, Solomon 1998, 2001, M Williams 1997, N Young 1994b]. Consensus among experts reviewing ASCUS results is rare. Interobserver reproducibility is poor, as measured by the kappa statistic, with κ scores of less than 0.40 (range 0.24 to 0.39) usually reported [Cocchi 1997, Crum 1999, Ismail 1989, Prasad 1994, Raab 1998a, D Stanley 1999, Tamiolakis 2001, M Williams 1997]. In one study, five experts reviewed 200 cases originally interpreted as atypical: not one single slide was interpreted as ASCUS by all five reviewers [Sherman 1994]. In the ASCUS-L SIL Triage Study (ALTS), only about half (55%) of cases submitted with a diagnosis of ASCUS were confirmed on review by the pathology quality control panel [Stoler 2001b]. In most cases in which a result is changed on review, the ASCUS interpretation is downgraded to negative (but of course, reviewers don't have to worry about lawsuits for false negatives!) [Al-Nafussi 2000, A Smith 2000, Sherman 1994]. Surprisingly, educational activities, such as review of the Bethesda Atlas, do *not* seem to improve reproducibility or accuracy (can't teach an old dog new tricks?) [A Smith 2000]. Of course, high levels of agreement do not necessarily translate into high levels of accuracy, sensitivity, or specificity (for centuries experts agreed that the sun revolved around the earth: they would have a high kappa statistic, but low accuracy) [Renshaw 1997].

Unfortunately, in reaction to the current onerous medicolegal climate, an interpretation of ASC is probably sometimes used as a defensive action against false negative reports because of the threat of litigation—a legitimate concern about loss of professional reputation and ability to earn a living ("cover your ASC-US") [Abu-Jawdeh 1994, Bonfiglio 2002, Briselli 1995, Frable 1994, Pitman 2002, Robb 1994, Scheiden 2003, Selvaggi 2001, Solomon 1998, D Stanley 1999, Stoler 1999, 2002, Wilbur 1997b, Workman 2000]. The constant threat of malpractice litigation has lowered the threshold for reporting cellular abnormalities in many cytology laboratories [Solomon 1998]. Laboratories that use the ASC interpretation liberally may actually be perceived as performing better than those that use the ASC interpretation more conservatively in external evaluations based on false-negative proportions [Frable 1999b, McGrath 2002, D Stanley 1999].

Statistically (it's tempting to say, sadistically) with ASC, the choices are between the devil and the deep blue sea. Decreasing the ASC rate increases specificity at the expense of sensitivity [Kaufman 1996]. Increased specificity is desirable, but the loss of sensitivity can lead to significant lesions being missed, which can not only cause harm, but can also lead to litigation. On the other hand, increasing the ASC rate increases sensitivity at the expense of specificity. Increased sensitivity is desirable for a screening test, but the loss of specificity can lead to investigation, and possibly therapy, of nonexistent lesions, which is not only expensive, but can also cause harm [A Goodman 2003, Solomon 1998, Wilbur 1996a]. Of course, the bottom line is that the Pap test is intended to prevent cancer.

Even though ASC is an irreproducible result, it nevertheless has important clinical implications [Al-Nafussi 2000, Cox 1999, 2001]. Roughly 25% (range 10% [Davey 1994] to 70⁺% [Dvorak 1999]) of women with ASC-US by cytology have SIL on biopsy; ~10% (range <3% [Suh-Burgmann 1998] to >20%) have H SIL; and rarely, invasive cancer (1 to 2 in 1000) [Abu-Jawdeh 1994, Alanen 1998, Anton 2001, Auger 1997, L Collins 1996, Davey 1994, 2000, Emerson 2002, Ferris 1998, Gatscha 2001, Ghoussoub 1997, A Goodman 2003, Lonky 1999, Manos 1999, Massad 2001, Morin 2000, Nygard 2003, Raab 1999c, Selvaggi 1995b, Sheils 1997, Sherman 1999, Sidawy 1993, Solomon 1998, 2001, Stastny 1997, Wilbur 1993, M Williams 1997, T Wright 1998, M Yang 1997]. (As a rule of thumb for women with ASC-US: 1 in 4 has SIL; 1 in 10 has H SIL; 1 in 1000 has cancer.) Atypical squamous cells may be the only cytologically detectable abnormality preceding a histologic diagnosis of H SIL [Sherman 1992b]. In fact, because it is so frequently used, ASC-US is the most common Pap test result preceding a histologic diagnosis of H SIL (33% to 45% of cases) [T1.22] [Cox 1999, Kinney 1998b, T Wright 2002a]. (ASC-US is the shotgun approach to hunting for a diagnosis: take a blunderbuss [ASC-US] and fire it two or three million times in the general direction of some ducks [dysplasia], and you are bound to hit a few.) Further, as many as ~75% of biopsy-proven high-grade lesions are preceded by negative, atypical, or low-grade SIL Pap test results [Howell 2004b, Kinney 1998b, Lonky 1999, Lyall 1995]. Morphologic predictors of significant squamous lesions include: immature metaplastic cytoplasm, irregular nuclear membranes, coarse chromatin, and hyperchromasia (ie, nuclear atypia) [Abu-Jawdeh 1994, Dvorak 1999, Ettler 1999, D Gupta 2001a,b, Morin 2000, Montes 1999, Sheils 1997, Wilbur 1997b]. Unfortunately, these cells can sometimes be difficult to find and difficult to interpret ("no-see-ums," litigation or jail cells) [Frable 1994, Hatem 1995, Montes 1999, Sherman 1992b, Wilbur 1997b].

T1.22 Pap Test Results Preceding Histologic Diagnosis of High-Grade SIL

ASCUS	39%
L SIL	20%
H SIL	31%
AGC	10%
Total	100%

Ref: Kinney 1998b

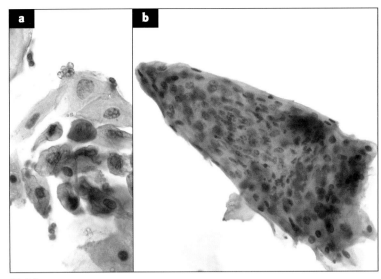

I1.66
a, Atypical parakeratosis [C]; **b**, Atypical PK, asperite [L]

In TBS 1991, an ASCUS interpretation could be subdivided into "favor reactive" and "favor SIL" categories. As expected, the "favor reactive" category was less commonly associated with SIL than the "favor SIL" category on follow-up biopsies [*Carozzi 2003, L Collins 1996, Eltabbakh 2000a, Ettler 1999, M Kline 1996, Lachman 1998, Solomon 1998, Vlahos 2000*]. Unfortunately, however, SIL rates ranging from <10% to >50% were reported in the "favor reactive" category, although this rate was still generally lower than for "favor SIL" [*Anton 2001, Genest 1998, González 1996, Guerrini 2001, M Kline 1996, Malik 1999, Raab 2001a*]. Even so, no prediction could be made for an individual woman [*Wilbur 1996a*]. Because both categories frequently correlated with SIL on biopsy, these qualifiers were dropped in TBS 2001 [*H Jones 2000*].

ASC-H was added to the Bethesda System in 2001. Although ASC-H is also irreproducible [*Quddus 2001, Sherman 1999, 2001*], it has significant predictive value for H SIL (CIN 2 or 3) on biopsy, intermediate between interpretations of ASC-US and H SIL [*Solomon 2002*]. ASC-H is associated with H SIL, very roughly, in about 50% of cases (range ~10% to 95%) [*Alli 2003, Ferris 1998, Genest 1998, Louro 2003, Malik 1999, Quddus 2001, Schoolland 1998, Selvaggi 2003, Sheils 1997, Sherman 1999, 2001, Solomon 2001*]. (In comparison, L SIL on Pap test is associated with H SIL on biopsy in at least 15% to 25% of cases, while H SIL on Pap test predicts H SIL on biopsy in about 60% to 75% of cases [*Cox 2003b, B Jones 1996, Sherman 2001*]. [T1.23]) The ASC-H category contains a mixture of true H SIL and its mimickers, such as inflamed/degenerated squamous metaplasia. The degree of maturity inversely correlates with the risk of SIL and, in particular, H SIL on biopsy. In other words, mature lesions (like squamous atypia) are less likely, and immature lesions (like atypical squamous metaplasia) are more likely, to predict SIL or H SIL on biopsy. Oncogenic HPV-DNA is detected in up to 70%-85% of ASC-H cases [*Pirog 2004, Sherman 2001*]. Because ASC-H is an equivocal, but potentially serious, interpretation, when no lesion is identified after colposcopy, review of the cytology, colposcopy, and histology results is recommended, if possible.

T1.23 Cyto-Histo Correlations

Cytology Result	H SIL on Biopsy
ASC-US	10% (5%-20%)
ASC-H	50% (10%-95%)
L SIL	15%-25+%
H SIL	60%-75%

In summary, there is no histologic equivalent of "atypical squamous cells" and even expert cytopathologists cannot agree on this interpretation [*Bonfiglio 2002, Pitman 2002*]. Furthermore, the "gold standard" biopsy diagnosis is only moderately-to-poorly reproducible [*Stoler 2001b*], and reproducibility is lower when the Pap test interpretation is ASCUS compared with biopsies taken for cytologic interpretations of SIL [*Grenko 2000*]. This makes meaningful intradepartmental and interdepartmental correlations difficult or impossible [*McGrath 2002*].

Ancillary techniques, HPV-testing, DNA ploidy, and cytogenetic analysis can help sort out real lesions from imitators [*Bollmann 2003b, Crabtree 2002, Duggan 2000, Emerson 2002, Khanna 2001, Nuovo 1998, Prasad 1994, D Scott 2002*]. Low-grade SIL and HPV-positive ASC-US are clinically equivalent; the risk of H SIL on biopsy for either is approximately 25% according to the ASCUS-L SIL Triage Study (ALTS) [*Cox 2003b*]. Review of "atypical" cases with knowledge of HPV status can be educational and serves as a quality improvement tool; however, the Pap test interpretation should not be altered based on the HPV results [*Davey 2003a*]. Management of women with ASC is discussed on pg 200. Briefly, reflex HPV DNA testing is recommended for ASC-US and colposcopy for ASC-H. Vaginal antibiotic therapy (to treat inflammatory changes mimicking SIL) is not recommended in management of women with ASC [*Connor 2002, Ferrante 2002*].

Some Other Atypical Squamous Cells

Atypical Squamous Cells
ASC-US (~Squamous Atypia)
ASC-H (~Atypical Squamous Metaplasia)
Atypical Parakeratosis
Atypical Repair
Atypia of Atrophy
Atypia of Maturity

In addition to mature and immature forms of atypical squamous cells (ASC-US and ASC-H; squamous atypia and atypical squamous metaplasia, respectively), there are other cell patterns that can be interpreted as atypical. These include atypical parakeratosis, atypical repair, and atypia of atrophy and maturity.

Atypical Parakeratosis

Atypical parakeratosis, also known as pleomorphic parakeratosis, is not specifically included in the Bethesda System lexicon, but is probably best considered a form of atypical squamous cells of undetermined significance (ASC-US) [*Solomon 1998*]. Atypical parakeratosis is composed of pleomorphic, miniature superficial cells; the nuclei and cytoplasm vary in size and shape, but the cells remain small [**I1.66a**] [*Voytek 1996*]. Caudate or elongate forms as well as nuclear enlargement or hyperchromasia can be present [*R Nayar 2003*]. Atypical parakeratosis resembles keratinizing dysplasia, but on a

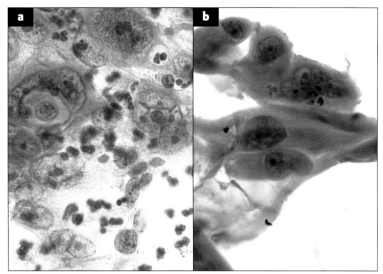

I1.67
a, Atypical repair [C]; **b**, Atypical repair [L]

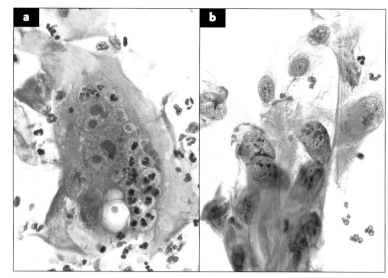

I1.68
a, Atypical repair [C]; **b**, Atypical repair [L]

miniature scale [Wilbur 1997a]. Atypical parakeratosis is also similar or identical to small dyskeratocytes discussed on pg 50.

Atypical Parakeratosis

PK-sized cells, any or all:
- *Pleomorphism*
- *Nuclear enlargement*
- *Hyperchromasia*

Single or clusters

~Miniature keratinizing dysplasia

In liquid-based cytology, the findings are similar. However, spike-like aggregates, corresponding to "asperites" of spike condyloma, may be more conspicuous than in conventional Pap smears [I1.66b].

Atypical parakeratosis is important not only because it can mask an underlying lesion, like ordinary parakeratosis, but it is also more commonly associated with a significant lesion (condyloma, dysplasia, or even squamous cell carcinoma [I1.18e]) [Abramovich 2003, Abu-Jawdeh 1994, Frable 1994, Vela Velasquez 1997, Voytek 1996]. Atypical parakeratosis is a marker for dysplasia that warrants further investigation [Voytek 1996]. If a more significant lesion cannot be identified, atypical parakeratosis can be reported as ASC-US.

Atypical Repair

Reparative cells that have cytologic abnormalities exceeding those of typical repair characterize atypical repair. Atypical repair is a form of atypical squamous (or glandular) cells associated with a wide spectrum of conditions, ranging from reactive to neoplastic. Atypical repair can mimic neoplasia, can co-exist with neoplasia, and may even be a form of neoplasia in some cases. Although "atypical repair" is not a Bethesda System interpretation, these changes can be categorized using Bethesda System terminology as "atypical squamous cells" or "atypical glandular cells."

Atypical Repair

Nuclear atypia, exceeding typical repair
- *Crowding, pleomorphism*
- *Irregular nuclear membranes*
- *Dark or irregular chromatin*
- *Nucleolar pleomorphism*

Single cells present, not numerous

No tumor diathesis, ± inflammatory background

High risk squamous (or glandular) lesions

"Repair in dysplasia"

Atypical repair presents as tissue fragments of immature squamous or glandular cells, resembling ordinary repair but having significant cellular abnormalities, such as crowding and piling up, nuclear enlargement and pleomorphism, and irregularities of nuclear outline and chromatin that go beyond those of typical repair [I1.67a,b, I.68a,b]. Admixture with neutrophils is common. Single atypical cells may be present, but are rare. When present in conventional Pap smears, they are usually in proximity to the abnormal groups; however, in liquid-based cytology, they are randomly scattered. Mitotic figures may be present. Single cells, nuclear pleomorphism, irregular nuclear membranes, prominent or irregular nucleoli, and mitotic activity are all features shared with malignancy [W-K Ng 2003c, Valente 1996]. Tumor diathesis and irregular, coarse dark chromatin are not present in atypical repair, and there tend to be fewer abnormal cells than in cancer.

The cells of atypical repair, having cytologic features of both repair and dysplasia, may be difficult to distinguish from true neoplasia. Some forms of atypical repair probably represent a reparative process occurring in a dysplastic epithelium. Many women are HPV-DNA positive [W-K Ng 2003c]. The risk of SIL in women with atypical repair is generally within the range reported for ordinary ASC-US (ie, ~25% SIL; ~10% H SIL) [Rimm 1996]. Even more ominously, some cases seeming to be atypical repair can actually represent invasive carcinomas that are difficult to recognize [J-H Chung 2000, W-K Ng 2002a, 2003c, Nunez 1985]. *If dysplasia or cancer cannot be excluded, refer to colposcopy.* Women with atypical repair are at high-risk!

Atypia of Atrophy and Maturity

Pap test abnormalities are common in postmenopausal women [Duffy 1976, Mandelblatt 1986, Siegler 1969, Soost 1982, Tambouret 2003]. However, the vast majority (up to 90%) of women with bona fide squamous intraepithelial lesions (dysplasia, condyloma) are younger than 35-40 years of age and SILs are uncommon in later life [Binder 1985, Carson 1993, Keating 2001c, R Reid 1986, Symmans 1992]. Therefore, Pap test screening may be less efficient in older women than younger ones (owing to more "false alarms") [Colgan 2002, Gustafsson 1995]. The corollary is that there is some truth to the adage, "Dysplasia is not a disease of old women." Keeping this in mind can be helpful when interpreting atrophic cytologic

FI.16 Relative Proportions of Dysplasia vs Carcinoma In Situ/Cancer by Age

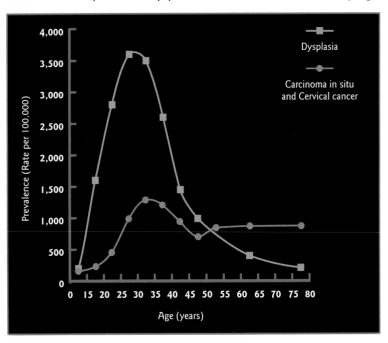

[Reid 1986]

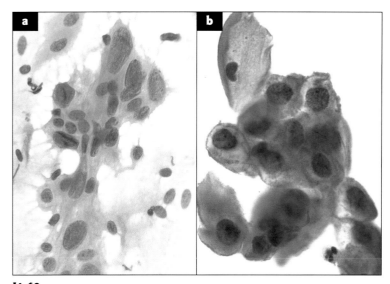

II.69
a, Atypia of atrophy [C]; **b**, Atypia of atrophy HPV– [L]

samples. Furthermore, squamous dysplasia usually occurs in a background of increased maturation, not atrophy [Fraser 1967, Patten 1978, Rubio 1973]. Note well, however, carcinoma (in situ or invasive) can occur in an atrophic background and the incidence of carcinoma generally increases with age. Before age 30, dysplasia is two to three times more common than in situ or invasive carcinoma, whereas after age 60, in situ or invasive carcinoma is two to three times more common than dysplasia [FI.16] [Binder 1985, Carson 1993, L Johnson 1968, R Reid 1986, Siegler 1969, E Stern 1963].

Most studies (but not all [Herrero 2000, E Smith 1997, 2004]) find that the prevalence of human papillomavirus diminishes substantially in older women [de Villiers 1992, Ferenczy 1997, Ley 1991, Melkert 1993, Nuovo 1989, Sellors 2002a, Tambouret 2003]. HPV-DNA triage is particularly helpful in older women [Schiffman 2000a, Sherman 2002]. HPV-DNA positive women are at increased risk of having bona fide neoplastic lesions and conversely, HPV-DNA negative women are at low risk [C-T Lin 2000, Mandelblatt 1992a]. Low-grade SIL is uncommon or rare in older women, because these women have usually cleared their HPV infections. However, high-grade lesions can occur in older women, possibly related in part to a decrease in immune response.

Because the transformation zone recedes with age and lesions mature distally, a squamous abnormality that appears low-grade in a Pap test may only be the "tip of the iceberg" of a more significant lesion occurring higher up in the endocervical canal in older women, particularly those who are postmenopausal. Also, exfoliation of cells may be reduced after menopause [A Roberts 1985]. These factors can lead to false-negative, or "undercall," cytologic results. Furthermore, histologic sampling and interpretive difficulties in elderly patients can lead to false negative biopsy diagnoses [G Acs 2000, Voytek 1996]. Therefore, all squamous abnormalities should be considered clinically significant and properly investigated [G Acs 2000, Kaminski 1989a,b]. Women with persistent abnormalities not explained by colposcopy/biopsy should be assessed for vaginal or vulvar lesions [Saminathan 1994]. Note also that neither "atypia of atrophy" nor "atypia of maturity" is recognized specifically in the Bethesda System. For these atypical cellular

changes, the interpretation of "atypical squamous cells" can be used, if warranted.

Atypia of Atrophy

Alarming microscopic findings can occur in benign atrophy and interpreting these atypical cells can be challenging ("challenging" is the politically correct word meaning "hard as heck," "heck" being the PC word meaning...) [G Acs 2000, Jovanovic 1995, Saminathan 1994, Symmans 1992]. Atrophic (basal/parabasal) cells normally have high nuclear/cytoplasmic ratios, and can sometimes show nuclear enlargement, pleomorphism, membrane irregularities, and hyperchromasia; these features can be difficult to distinguish from dysplasia or even cancer. Such benign change occurring in atrophy is known as "atypia of atrophy." The cytologic findings are probably related to inflammation, air-drying, estrogen deficiency, and other

Atypia of Atrophy

Parabasal cells, any or all:
  ·Big (>3 X), dark nuclei
  ·High N/C ratios
  ·Irregular nuclear outline
  ·Chromatin abnormalities
  ·Bizarre shape (tadpole, spindle)
Mimics H SIL or cancer
"Dysplasia not a disease of older women"
  Occurs in estrogenic environment
Note: CIS/CA in older women or atrophy
Estrogen test or Colposcopy
If HPV-DNA negative ⇒ low risk

metabolic changes occurring with age [G Acs 2000, Kaminski 1989a,b, A Rader 1999]. Most revert to normal cytology after a course of estrogen therapy (see estrogen test, below) [Batrinos 1975b, Kaminski 1989b].

The atypical cells are basal/parabasal sized, indicating atrophy. They occur singly, in sheets, in syncytial-like aggregates, or hyperchromatic crowded groups [II.69a,b]. The cells are often poorly preserved and degenerated, particularly in conventional Pap smears. The nuclei can be pleomorphic, hyperchromatic, and enlarged into the range seen in dysplasia (> 3 times an intermediate cell nucleus), with high N/C ratios that can mimic a high-grade lesion. The chromatin, however, remains uniformly distributed. Naked nuclei may be seen; these can cluster and mimic endometrial cells. The cytoplasm is usually blue-gray, sometimes pink, but occasional cells may be orangeophilic due to degeneration (ie, pseudokeratinized). Bizarre cells (tadpole, spindle) can occur. Syncytial-like aggregates of atypical basal/parabasal cells (hyperchromatic crowded groups) can be difficult to distinguish from carcinoma in situ or even invasive cancer [DeMay 2000]. More ominously, malignant tissue fragments can be mistaken for benign atrophy [Koike 1994]. A "dirty" background, composed of degenerated cells, debris, granular precipitate, fresh/old blood, and inflammatory cells, including neutrophils, histiocytes, and multinucleated giant cells, is common in severe atrophy ("atrophy with inflammation") [Van Peenen 1983]. This granular, dirty background resembles a tumor diathesis [Selvaggi 2002b].

In liquid-based cytology, nuclear enlargement is less pronounced and naked nuclei are fewer [11.69b]. The granular background material is less abundant and may adhere, or cling, to the cells, resulting in a cleaner background. Blue blobs and pseudoparakeratotic cells, discussed below, are rare or absent in LBC.

Nuclear enlargement and increased N/C ratios are nonspecific findings in atrophy; they must be coupled with nuclear membrane irregularities and chromatin abnormalities to be indicative of a dysplastic lesion [Abati 1998, G Acs 2000, Medley 1998, Teaff 1990]. In dysplasia, the chromatin is not only dark, but the texture is also *crisp*, ie, the chromatin particles are usually well preserved and almost seem to "sparkle" in the light of the microscope. In cancer, the chromatin particles tend to be coarser, irregularly arranged, and vary from cell to cell. In contrast, in atypia of atrophy, the chromatin is often poorly preserved and appears *smudgy*. When well preserved, the chromatin in atrophy is fine and even, and although it can be dark, it is not coarse, crisp, or irregular [Jovanovic 1995]. Compare the chromatin of the cell in question with that of a normal cell: similar chromatin favors benign atrophy, whereas coarser, darker chromatin favors neoplasia.

Hyperchromatic crowded groups (HCGs) commonly occur in the setting of benign atrophy, but may indicate a high-grade squamous lesion or cancer [DeMay 2000]. Here are some clues to correct interpretation. First, mitotic activity strongly suggests neoplasia, if a reactive/reparative process can be excluded, because mitotic figures are not expected in atrophic epithelium [C Buckley 1994]. Be aware, however, that neoplastic lesions in older women may have a paucity of mitotic figures; therefore, the absence of mitoses does not exclude neoplasia. Second, abnormal arrangement of the cells (chaotic architecture) favors a neoplastic process. Abnormal architecture (and hyperchromasia) can be easily appreciated at low power in the microscope. Third, the presence of an accompanying squamous dysplasia lends strong support to an interpretation of carcinoma in situ or cancer. Another warning, however, carcinoma in situ more commonly occurs as a pure lesion in older women, without an associated squamous dysplasia; thus, this valuable interpretive clue may be absent. Finally, marked pleomorphism in the form of tadpole or spindle cells, or atypical parakeratosis, suggests a true squamous abnormality [Abati 1998, R Nayar 2003, Solomon 1998].

Basophilic bodies, often called "blue blobs" because of their strong affinity for hematoxylin stain, are sometimes present in atrophy [Milligan 1959]. They can be alarming because they look rather like naked nuclei from some horrible malignancy [11.70] [Abdulla 2000, Milligan 1959, Naylor 1977, Ziabkowski 1976]. Blue

Atrophy ± Inflammation

Nuclear enlargement, slight hyperchromasia

Nuclear membranes, chromatin: Uniform

Naked nuclei (mimic endometrial cells)

"Blue blobs" (mummified cells)

Pseudokeratinization

Inflammation

Granular debris (benign diathesis)

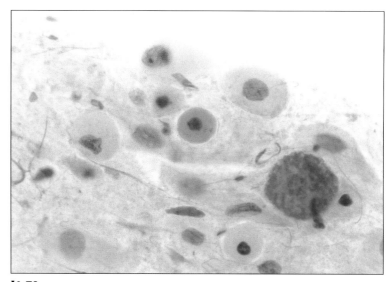

11.70
Atrophy, blue blob, pseudokeratosis [C]

blobs vividly reinforce the principle: never render an unequivocal malignant interpretation based only on naked nuclei. Blue blobs are the size and shape of parabasal cells. They are often coarsely granular and may seem to contain a large nucleolus, but on close inspection, blue blobs do not have the texture of chromatin and the "nucleolus" is really a nucleus. Blue blobs have been variously thought to be inspissated mucin or dystrophic calcification, but special stains are negative for both mucin and calcium [Abdulla 2000, Carson 1990]. Immunocytochemically, they are positive for cytokeratin, epithelial membrane antigen, and carcinoembryonic antigen, but negative for vimentin and muscle-specific actin [Abdulla 2000]. Ultrastructurally, there are cellular skeletons and degenerated nuclei [Abdulla 2000]. Thus, blue blobs apparently result from unusual precipitation of hematoxylin on mummified atrophic squamous cells. They do not indicate a neoplastic cellular abnormality.

Atrophic cells may also undergo coagulative necrosis. The cytoplasm becomes orangeophilic and the nuclei become small, dark, and pyknotic (pseudokeratosis) [11.70] [C Buckley 1994]. These small, orange, atrophic cells resemble parakeratosis or atypical parakeratosis, except that the cell outlines are rounded rather than polygonal and the cells are scattered randomly throughout the sample [G Acs 2000, Saminathan 1994, Weintraub 1987]. Note well, however, that bona fide atypical parakeratotic or dyskeratotic cells are markers for squamous intraepithelial lesions or cancer.

In theory, a trial of estrogen will cause atypical atrophic cells to mature, revealing their benign nature, while neoplastic cells will remain abnormal (although they too may mature somewhat), thereby contrasting sharply with the benign cells; this is the *estrogen test* [11.71a,b] [Kashimura 1987, Keebler 1974, Sheils 1997]. Koilocytes may appear following estrogen administration [Luzzatto 2000]. Note that if the lesion is already mature, eg, koilocytes, keratinizing dysplasia, or keratinizing squamous cell carcinoma, no additional information will be gained by performing an estrogen test. Also, the estrogen test does not help identify adenocarcinomas, or other kinds of neoplasms, such as sarcomas. Proliferation markers, such as MIB-1 (Ki-67), may help discriminate atrophy (low proliferative activity index) from H SIL (high proliferative activity index) [Bulten 2000a,b, Ejersbo 1999, Mittal 1999b, Smedts 2001], but may not be practical for a screening test. Management is discussed on pg 200.

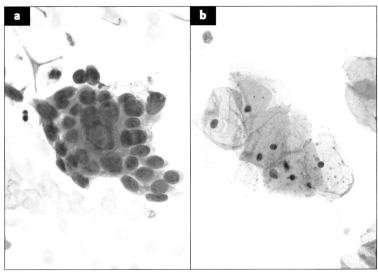

II.71
a, Atypia present, pre-estrogen [C]; **b**, Atypia absent, post-estrogen [C]

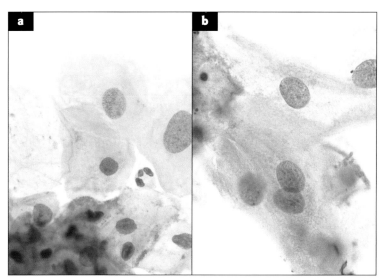

II.72
a, Atypia of maturity [C]; **b**, Atypia of maturity [L]

Atypia of Maturity

"Atypia of maturity" refers to mild nuclear abnormality occurring in mature (intermediate or superficial) cells in mature (older) women. The cells look like squamous atypia or ASC-US and they are commonly present in Pap tests from menopausal and post-menopausal women, particularly those on hormone replacement therapy [Ferenczy 1997, Menezes 2001, A Rader 1999, Sheils 19907, Symmans 1992]. Recall, however, that the rate of abnormal biopsy findings (SILs) decreases with age, with the vast majority of abnormalities occurring by 35-40 years of age [Kaminski 1989b, Nuovo 1990a]. Also, the ASCUS to SIL ratio tends to be higher in older, than younger, women [Keating 2001c, A Rader 1999]. Minimal cytologic abnormalities have lower predictive value for dysplasia in older women, partly because the prevalence of disease is lower than in younger women. In other words, false-positive (or false atypical) Pap test results are common in older women [A Rader 1999, Sheils 1997, Weintraub 1987].

The nuclear changes of atypia of maturity consist of nuclear enlargement into the range of squamous atypia (ASC-US) in mature cells; however, the nuclei are usually normochromatic and have smooth nuclear membranes [II.72a,b]. To qualify as a genuine squamous intraepithelial lesion, the nuclei should not only be enlarged, but also have significant hyperchromasia, irregular nuclear membranes, and abnormal chromatin texture. Marked pleomorphism, including bizarre (tadpole, spindle) shapes, also qualifies cells as indicative of a genuine abnormality [Abati 1998].

The vast majority (80%-90+%) of older women with minimal cytologic abnormalities (ASC-US-like changes) have negative colposcopy or biopsy findings, as well as negative HPV-DNA studies. Of those with underlying dysplasia, most have low-grade squamous intraepithelial lesions [Abati 1998, Bruner 2004, Cunnane 1993, Flynn 2001, Kaminski 1989a, Menezes 2001, A Rader 1999, Saminathan 1994,

---

Atypia of Maturity

Intermediate or superficial cells

· *Mild nuclear enlargement*

· *Mild hyperchromasia*

Mimics ASC-US or L SIL

Clue: No significant hyperchromasia,

irregular nuclear membranes,

abnormal chromatin texture,

pleomorphism

If HPV-DNA negative ⇒ low risk

Sheils 1997, Symmans 1992], although a few women have more significant squamous lesions [Cunnane 1993, A Rader 1999, Saminathan 1994].

The nuclear alterations in "atypia of maturity" seem to result from an accumulation of benign changes occurring with age. This may be related to defective DNA metabolism, perhaps akin to folate deficiency [Patten 1978], although many will respond to estrogen therapy [Kaminski 1989a,b]. In summary, "atypia of maturity," ie, mild nuclear enlargement without hyperchromasia in intermediate or superficial cells of older women, carries minimal risk of a significant underlying abnormality [Crum 2000, Jovanovic 1995, Keating 2001c].

Epidemiology of Cervical Neoplasia

Epidemiology is study of the spread of disease. Although Hippocrates wrote on this subject in ancient times (*On Airs, Waters, and Places*), epidemiology only developed as a formal science in the 19th century, out of the search for causes of human disease, especially of epidemics (the word, epidemiology, derives from the Greek: *epi* meaning upon, *demos* meaning people, and *logos* meaning study). One of the prime objectives of epidemiology is the identification of populations at high risk for a given disease, so that the cause can be identified and preventive measures undertaken. The primary investigational tool of epidemiology is statistics.

In 1713, the Italian physician, Bernardino Ramazzini, noted the relatively high incidence of breast cancer in nuns and wondered whether this was in some way related to their celibate lifestyle. This launched the field of cancer epidemiology and was the first indication that how people lived might affect their risk of cancer. In 1842, Domenico Antonio Rigoni-Stern, another Italian, analyzed 80 years of mortality records from the city of Verona [Rigoni–Stern 1842]. He reported that uterine cancer (*later* interpreted as mostly cervical cancer [Griffiths 1991]) was more common among married than unmarried women, and that it was rare in nuns (and also noted, as Ramazzini before him, that breast cancer was far more common in nuns than married women) [Kessler 1987, Scotto 1969, Stavola 1987]. A century later, Fabien Gagnon reported on the rarity of cervical cancer among nuns in Canada [Gagnon 1950]. Cervical cancer was considered to be rare in virgins and common in sex workers [Keighley 1968, Robboy 1978, 1984]. (It should be noted, however, that [with apologies to Chaucer] this "Nun's Tale" may not be as well proven as generally assumed [J Gardner 1974, Griffiths 1991, Skrabanek 1988, Towne 1955].) Furthermore, priority for the notion that cervical cancer is a venereal disease should probably be given to Jean Astruc, an 18th century French physician, who claimed that uterine cancer was caused by "injection of semen tainted with syphilis" in 1743 [Skrabanek 1988].

Risk Factors for Cervical Cancer

By the mid-20th century, epidemiologic evidence suggested that cervical cancer was related to early marriage and low socioeconomic status of the woman, with an additional component (thought possibly to be semen or smegma) related to the man [Aitken-Swan 1966, M Coppleson 1968, E Jones 1958, Stocks 1955, Terris 1980, C Walsh 1995]. Factors related to sexual behavior are now believed to be central to these epidemiologic findings [Brinton 1986c, 1992, Holly 1996, Kjær 1992, 1998, Murthy 2000, C Walsh 1995].

Risk Factors for Cervical Cancer

Coitus: early onset, multiple partners

High-risk male

Oral contraceptives

Cigarette smoking

Multiparity

Sexually transmitted diseases

[No Pap tests]

The Pap test made it possible to investigate the epidemiology of cervical cancer at an early stage of the disease, so that factors could be more directly related to etiology and onset [E Stern 1973]. Epidemiologic studies helped establish HPV as the cause of cervical cancer [Schiffman 1995a].

Coitus

Coitus is generally accepted as necessary for the development of cervical cancer and its precursors [Brinton 1987a, R Harris 1980, Kiviat 1989, LaVecchia 1986b, Reeves 1985, Rotkin 1967a, Singer 1975]. Next to coitus itself, the strongest epidemiologic associations are with *early age at first coitus* (before 18 years of age) [Aitken-Swan 1966, Biswas 1997, Boyd 1964, Brinton 1987a, Cuzick 1996, Kessler 1974a, Koutsky 1992a, C Martin 1967, Muñoz 1994, Pridan 1971, Rotkin 1962, 1967a, Wynder 1954] and history of *multiple sexual partners* (more than two) [Barron 1971, Brinton 1987a, Brinton 93, de Vet 1993, 1994, Edebiri 1990, Kessler 1974b, C Martin 1967, Pridan 1971, Rotkin 1973, Terris 1980]. Some increased risk also accrues to women initiating coitus before 21 years of age [Rotkin 1967a] or who have had more than one sexual partner [Brinton 1993, de Vet 1993, Kessler 1974b, Robboy 1984, Rotkin 1967a].

Male Factors

As long suspected, there is a male factor, not to say malefactor, in cervical carcinogenesis. Coitus with a "high risk male" increases the risk of a woman developing cervical neoplasia [R Burk 1996a, Singer 1976, Skegg 1982, Zunzunegui 1986], even if, by chance, this is her only lifetime sexual partner [SS Agarwal 1993, J Buckley 1981, Kjær 1991, D Thomas 1996b]. (Life is like a box of chocolates...) "High-risk males" have numerous sexual partners, penile condylomas, or previous partners with cervical neoplasia.

The epidemiologic evidence for a male role in cervical neoplasia is compelling. Populations with high rates of carcinoma of the cervix and penis, cluster geographically [J-Y Li 1982]. Wives of men who: have had numerous sexual partners [F Bosch 1996, Brinton 1989b, J Buckley 1981, Slattery 1989b, Zunzunegui 1986]; were

formerly married to women with cervical cancer [Kessler 1977]; or have penile condylomas or cancer [Boon 1988, S Graham 1979a, Kjær 1991, Martínez 1969, PG Smith 1980] are at increased risk of cervical cancer. The presence of HPV-DNA in the male's penis increases the female partner's risk of cervical cancer [F Bosch 1996].

Male partners of women with genital HPV infections have a high prevalence (up to 90%) of penile condylomas (which, like the cervical counterpart, may be invisible to the naked eye) [Boon 1988, Campion 1985, Kokelj 1993, Sand 1986, A Schneider 1988a, Sedlacek 1986, Wosnitzer 1988], and the virus detected is frequently the same viral type as the woman's HPV [Barrasso 1987, Kyo 1994, A Schneider 1987d]. Men who are regular sexual partners of women with CIN 3 have a high prevalence of penile HPV infection [Campion 1988]. Men with penile carcinomas have a high incidence of HPV [Boon 1989b, Varma 1991, Villa 1986] (although the association with HPV is not as strong as for cervical cancer, suggesting two pathways, as in vulvar cancer [Cubilla 2000, Garland 2002, Gross 2004]). Thus, the penis is a common host to HPV, which can infect the female genital tract (and, vice versa, like ping pong).

Historically, circumcision of men was believed to reduce the risk of cervical cancer in women [Adami 2002]. Later, circumcision was dismissed as a risk factor [Rotkin 1973, E Stern 1962, Terris 1973], but more recent evidence suggests that male circumcision may reduce the risk of cervical cancer after all [Castellsagué 2002, Kjær 1991, Schiffman 2003a]. Penile hygiene may also be a factor in cervical cancer [Jayant 1987]. Smegma, while not considered carcinogenic, could be important in transmission of the carcinogenic agent [Jayant 1987]. HPV-DNA can be detected in semen [Kyo 1994, Rintala 2004], but whether semen per se is important in development of cervical cancer is unproven [Fish 1982, French 1987, B Reid 1978] (see pg 87).

Contraceptive Method

A link between oral contraceptives (birth control pills) and cervical neoplasia was first postulated by Melamed et al in 1969 [Melamed 1969]. The relationship between oral contraceptives and cervical cancer is complex. Variables such as sexual and social behavior as well as Pap test screening can lead to confounding observations. Studies have found that oral contraceptives **are** associated with an increased risk of CIN and cervical cancer [Anonymous 1993b, Beral 1988, Brinton 1986a, 1991, Delgado-Rodriguez 1992, Gram 1992c, R Harris 1980, CJ Jones 1990, Kjær 1993b, Ley 1991, Meisels 1977a, Parazzini 1990b, E Stern 1970, S Swan 1982, D Thomas 1996a, Vessey 1983, WHO 1985] or that they **are not** associated with an increased risk of CIN and cervical cancer [E Clarke 1985, Castle 2002a, Kjellberg 2000, R Peters 1986b, Schiffman 1995a, D Thomas 1972, 1991]; the data are conflicting [Dallenbach-Hellweg 1984, Irwin 1988, LaVecchia 1986c, Ursin 1994, Vessey 1989b, WHO 1993]. Unfortunately, many of these studies were biased because the HPV status was unknown [Kjellberg 2000]. HPV-negative women, for all practical purposes, do not develop cervical neoplasia. However, oral contraceptives and human papillomavirus may interact [Hildesheim 1990b, Brinton 1991] and, unlike barrier contraceptives, oral contraceptives offer no protection from acquiring HPV infection. The current consensus seems to be that long-term use of oral contraceptives, by HPV-positive women, increases the risk of squamous neoplasia of the cervix [Brinton 1991, Chaouki 1998, LaVecchia 2001, Moreno 2002, Ylitalo 1999, Xi 2002, Zondervan 1996]. There may be an even stronger effect for cervical adenocarcinomas [Brinton 1986a, 87b, Chilvers 1987, Dallenbach-Hellweg 1984, MW Jones 1989, Kjær 1993a, Lacey 1999, 2000, Madeleine 2001, R Peters 1986a, Schiffman 1995a, S Schwartz 1986, Ursin 1994, Valente 1986, WHO 1993, Yeh 1991, Zaino 2000].

Barrier contraceptive methods (condom, diaphragm) decrease the risk of developing cervical cancer [Boyce 1977, Boyd 1964, Fasal 1981, CJ Jones 1990, C Martin 1967, Melamed 1969, Rotkin 1973, Slattery 1989b, Terris 1960, D Thomas 1996b, Worth 1972, N Wright 1978, Zondervan 1996]. Although barrier contraceptives do not prevent HPV infection [Ho 1998a, Winer 2003], it is plausible that the diaphragm or condom protects the cervix from HPV infection [Schiffman 1995a]. (A remarkable, although unconfirmed, report claimed that condom use cured intraepithelial cancer, perhaps by preventing reinfection! [Richardson 1981])

Spermacides may reduce risk [Hildesheim 1990a]. Vaginal spermicides (eg, nonoxynol-9) are capable of inactivating many sexually transmitted pathogens by their detergent effect on bacterial cell membranes and viral envelopes; however, papillomaviruses are non-enveloped [Hermonat 1992, Poindexter 1996]. Douching, which alters the vaginal milieu, could be related to development of cervical cancer [J Gardner 1991, S Graham 1979b, Rotkin 1968, J Zhang 1997]. Intrauterine contraceptive devices (IUDs) do not increase the risk of cervical cancer, and there may even be a trend to a protective effect for copper-containing IUDs [Lassise 1991]. Tubal ligation may be associated with a small decrease in risk [H–q Li 2000b]. Vasectomy, too, may reduce the risk of cervical cancer [S Swan 1979], although data are conflicting [R Harris 1979].

Cigarette Smoking

Cigarette smoking, as first proposed by Winkelstein in 1977, correlates epidemiologically with an increased risk of developing cervical cancer [Boardman 2002, Brinton 1986b, Brock 1989, E Clarke 1982, 1985, Greenberg 1985, R Harris 1980, Hellberg 1983, CJ Jones 1990, Kjær 1996a, LaVecchia 1986a, Licciardone 1989, D Luesley 1994, Lyon 1983, R Peters 1986b, Slattery 1989a, Szarewski 1998, Trevathan 1983, P Ward 1990, Winkelstein 1977, 1984, 1990]. Unexpectedly, the increased risk seems to be restricted to squamous cell carcinoma, not adenocarcinoma [Brinton 1986b, 1987b]. The risk is dose dependent [Brinton 1986, Brisson 1994, Brock 1989, E Clarke 1982, Coker 1992, Daling 1992, Daly 1998, Gram 1992a, Licciardone 1989] and quiting smoking reduces risk [Licciardone 1989, Slattery 1989a, Szarewski 1996]. Smoking by the male partner may also be a risk factor [M Clark 2000, Zunzunegui 1986].

Smoking also correlates with sexual behavior and socioeconomic status [Bornstein 1995, Hildesheim 1993]. Therefore, it is possible that when controlled for HPV infection and other risk factors, smoking could be found to be a confounding variable. Such studies have found conflicting results. Some have found that when HPV infection and sexual behavior are taken into account, the association of cervical cancer with cigarette smoking practically disappears [F Bosch 1992, Eluf–Neto 1994, Herrero 1989, Hildesheim 1994, Ho 1998b, Reeves 1987]. Others have found that cigarette smoking is one of the most important environmental risk factors for cervical cancer, even after controlling for HPV infection and sexual behavior [Acladious 2002, Castle 2002a, Kjellberg 2000, Moscicki 2001, Roteli–Martins 1998, Szarewski 1998, Ylitalo 1999]. It seems likely that the increased risk of cigarette smokers for cervical neoplasia may be partly, but not wholly, explained by confounding factors. In other words, cigarette smoking probably is a risk factor for cervical cancer [Doll 1996, A Phillips 1993]. (Several mechanisms have been proposed, see, pg 87.)

Other Possible Risk Factors

Although other factors, such as early age at first pregnancy, short time between pregnancies, abortions, early age of first marriage, poor genital hygiene, and venereal disease [Brinton 1987a, Levin 1942], may be risk factors, they are more likely to be confounding variables of sexual activity [Richart 1973]. Many other things have also been considered, eg, age of menarche [Brinton 1987a, E Jones 1958, Rotkin 1967a], menstrual patterns, use of tampons or vaginal deodorants [Brinton 1987a], masturbation, even coital positions [Rotkin 1967b], but these are not currently thought to be risk factors. After accounting for the number of sexual partners, studies fail to show any effect of lifetime frequency of intercourse [Boyd 1964, Brinton 1987a, E Jones 1958, C Martin 1967, Rotkin

1967a, Terris 1980]; this is consistent with the assumption that HPV is relatively easily transmitted during vaginal intercourse [Schiffman 1995a].

Parity was previously dismissed as an independent risk factor for cervical cancer [Boyd 1964, Rotkin 1967a, Wynder 1954]. However, after controlling for sexual behavior and HPV infection, multiparity may in fact be an independent risk factor for cervical cancer [T Becker 1994a, Brinton 1987a, 1989a, Muñoz 2002, Parazzini 1989, Schiffman 1993]. Possible explanations include: altered immune status, hormonal effects, cervical trauma, and nutrition; also, childbirth tends to maintain the transformation zone on the ectocervix, where it may be more vulnerable to carcinogenic agents for longer periods of time [Autier 1996, Schiffman 1995a]. A general decline in parity could partly explain a reduction in cervical cancer observed in most countries (ie, fewer children, fewer cancers) [Muñoz 2002].

Although cervical cancer rates vary by race, nationality, and religion, for the most part, these variables are not regarded as independent risk factors [Benard 2001, Ezra 2000, J Gardner 1995, Parham 1998]. However, the question of differences in biologic behavior of cervical neoplasia among races remains open [Baquet 1987, Harlan 1991, Mandelblatt 1993]. Recognized risk factors, such as age at first intercourse, number of sexual partners, or cigarette smoking, may reflect cultural, religious, and philosophical beliefs. Low socioeconomic status women are statistically at increased risk of HPV infection and cervical cancer [Hildesheim 1993, Schiffman 1995a]. Other correlates of low socioeconomic status, including poor nutrition, multiparity, and concurrent genital infections could be involved in carcinogenesis [Schiffman 1995a]. Women of lower socioeconomic status may also be poorly informed or lack access to health care [Chavez 1995, Rodney 2002]. Alcoholism is a possible risk factor [Weiderpass 2001]. Older women may be at increased risk of acquiring sexually transmitted diseases because of physiologic changes that naturally accompany the aging process. Also, because pregnancy is no longer an issue, use of barrier contraceptives, which can protect from infection, is less likely [D Patel 2003].

Several biologic cofactors are probably important in cervical carcinogenesis. These include immunocompetency, HIV infection, hormones, dietary, nutritional, and genetic factors. These co-factors are discussed in more detail later (see pg 85). Naturally, there is some overlap with the epidemiologic risk factors discussed above. For completeness, failure to obtain regular Pap tests is usually considered a significant risk factor for cervical cancer. However, lack of Pap tests does not cause cancer (think about it).

Summary

In summary, cervical cancer behaves, epidemiologically, like a venereal disease [Affandi 1993, Beral 1974, Kessler 1976, 1981, 1987, Kjær 1997, Slattery 1989b]. Sexual intercourse is a necessary prerequisite for the development of cervical cancer (and so, it is true, *everything* causes cancer!). The explanation is that a carcinogenic agent is passed from the male to the female at coitus [van Diest 2002]. The number of sexual partners and the age of first coitus are rough measures of likelihood of exposure to a carcinogenic agent and duration of exposure. The most likely vector is an infected ("high-risk") male. The data also suggest that a woman is more susceptible at a young age and with long-continued exposure [Herrero 1990]. The nature of the agent has been the subject of intense investigation. Naturally, infectious agents have long been suspected. Virtually every organism ever found in the female genital tract, including *Trichomonas*, *Treponema*, gonococcus, *Candida*, *Chlamydia*, cytomegalovirus, herpes simplex virus, and most recently human papillomavirus (HPV), has had its 15 minutes of fame as the possible cause of cervical cancer [Guijon 1985, M Morris 1996]. Except for HPV, these agents are now generally thought to be dependent variables of sexual behavior [T Becker 1994b, Kjellberg 1999].

Incidence and Prevalence

Before the Pap test, cervical cancer was a leading cause of cancer death in women [Janicek 2001]. Today, in the United States, less than 2% of cancer deaths in women, and less than 0.5% of all (female) deaths are attributable to cervical cancer [Jemal 2005]. Unfortunately, in developing countries where Pap test screening is not widely available, cervical cancer remains the second most common cancer, after breast cancer, and most common cause of cancer-related death, in women [Parkin 1999a,b, Pisani 1999, 2002, Robles 1996].

The incidence of squamous cell carcinoma of the cervix in 1940s, before the era of the Pap test, was about 33-44 per 100,000 women and is now about 5-8 per 100,000 in the United States. 10,370 cases of cervical cancer were expected in 2005 [Jemal 2005]. These figures indicate an overall reduction in incidence of cervical cancer of 75% to 90% since Pap test screening began [D Cramer 1974a,b, Devesa 1989, Nold 1998, Pretorius 1991, Stoller 2000c]. Mortality has also shown a similar remarkable decrease (current prevalence about 2.5/100,000), with a reduction of 70% to 80% in the same time frame [F1.17] [Boring 1991, D Fink 1988, Hartmann 2001]. 3,710 deaths were expected in 2005 [Jemal 2005]. Although the incidence and mortality have generally declined over the years, there was a distressing spike in incidence, followed by a small bump in mortality, beginning in the late 1980s, before resuming a downward trend in the 1990s. Incidence and mortality vary by race and ethnicity, but these variations are thought mostly to reflect cultural, social, and economic disparities, although biologic differences are possible [Baquet 1987, CDC 1990, Harlan 1991, Mandelblatt 1993]. Note that these figures include all women, *even those who have never had a Pap test*. It stands to reason that cervical cancer incidence and mortality has fallen still more among *regularly screened* women!

The overall 5-year survival is about 67%, ranging from about 90% for stage I cancers to <15% for late stage cancers [M Morris 1996]. Despite advances in medicine, the survival rate of women with cervical cancer has changed very little, stage for stage, since the 1950s [Kessler 1987, Pontén 1995]. Therefore, it is believed that the lower incidence and mortality rates for cervical carcinoma represent a triumph of the Pap test in achieving early cancer detection [Koss 1989a]. Lesions are now being detected earlier, while they are still in a more curable, often preinvasive, state. Before the Pap test was introduced into clinical practice, two of every three cervical cancers were invasive at the time of diagnosis. After Pap tests came into widespread use, at least three of four women were diagnosed while their cancers were still intraepithelial (ie, carcinoma in situ) [Kessler 1987]. Invasive cervical cancers detected by the Pap test are usually (80% to 90%) stage I, compared with those presenting for reasons other than abnormal Pap tests, of which one-third are stage II and one-quarter stage III or IV [J Carmichael 1984, Pretorius 1991].

While the number of invasive cancers has declined, *there has been a massive increase in precursor lesions* [Bibbo 1971a, Blohmer 1999, J Carmichael 1984, Kessler 1987, Sadeghi 1988, E Stern 1964, 1969, Wolfendale 1983]. The prevalence of SILs, including CIN 3, soared as much as 10 fold from the 1950s to the 1980s [SG Bernstein 1985, Bibbo 1971a, Blohmer 1999, CDC 1983, S Evans 1990, Kessler 1987, Mazur 1984a, Meisels 1977b, Richart 1987, Sadeghi 1988, E Stern 1969, Wolfendale 1983]. In a Q-probe study, about 2% of all Pap tests were reported as L SIL and an additional 0.5% were reported as H SIL, but much higher rates occur in some clinical settings [B Jones 2000]. Some estimate that up to 10% (or more) of Pap tests are interpreted as abnormal [Kurman 1994, McCance 1998] and, according to the Centers for Disease Control, approximately 20% of Pap test results in women under age 30 are abnormal [CDC 1994]. Very approximately 2.5 million SILs, including >300,000 H SILs, and 10,000 cervical cancers are detected annually in the United States [Davey 2000, Jemal 2005, Stoler 2003b, Wingo 1995].

Age

As the prevalence of preinvasive disease has been rising, *the average age at diagnosis has been falling* [G Anderson 1988, J Carmichael 1984, Cecchini 1982, G Cook 1984, Crowther 1995, Davies 1971]. The prevalence of SIL peaks in the third decade, and then decreases with age [Koutsky 1997, Lawson 1998, Meisels 1992, Mount 1999, Sadeghi 1988, Schiffman 1992]. Squamous intraepithelial lesions are *common* in teenagers and also occur in preteens [Economos 1994, Edelman 1999, M Feldman 1976, Hein 1977, Kahn 1999, Mount 1999, Sadeghi 1984, Simsir 2002, Snyder 1976]. Although the full range of dysplasia, including carcinoma in situ, can be seen in teenagers [Creasman 1972, J Ferguson 1961, Kaufman 1970, Sadeghi 1988, Wallace 1973], most of their lesions are low-grade SILs or ASC-US [Edelman 1999, Kahn 2001, Mount 1999, A Rader 1997, Sankar 1998, Silva 2002, Simsir 2002]. Although dysplasia is common, invasive cervical carcinoma is extremely rare in teenagers (the incidence is about 2/1,000,000) [Perkins 1996, Sankar 1998, Simsir 2002]. Most cervical cancers in teenagers are adenocarcinomas, including DES-associated clear cell carcinomas (now disappearing), but squamous cell carcinoma has been reported in teenagers, as young as 15 years old, although this is extremely rare [Bibbo 1971a, H Chung 1982, Crowther 1995, Dekel 1982, Hepler 1952, Kling 1973, Pollack 1947, Sankar 1998, Silva 2002]. (Seven *months* is apparently the earliest age at which cervical carcinoma, an adenocarcinoma, has been reported preceding the DES era [E Waters 1940].)

These alarming increases in cervical abnormalities are ascribed to changes in sexual behavior ("the sexual revolution") since the 1960s, when oral contraceptives ("the pill") became available. Earlier age of first coitus and multiple sexual partners are recurrent themes [Crowther 1995, Sadeghi 1984, Ylinen 1985]. In 1970, less than 30% (28.6%) of all adolescents were experienced sexually; by 1988, slightly more than half were (51.5%) [CDC 1991]. But, the times may be a-changing. The proportion of sexually active teenagers may have peaked in the late 1980s, and fallen, somewhat, since then, while condom use has increased—possibly as a response to the AIDS epidemic with an emphasis on abstinence and a trend toward "safer sex" [Anonymous 2002, Besharov 1997, Grunbaum 2002, S Seidman 1994].

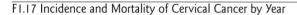

F1.17 Incidence and Mortality of Cervical Cancer by Year

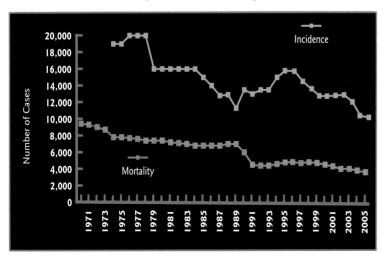

The median age of mortality from cervical cancer is 62 years [Brooks 1996]. The mean and peak (mode) ages for condyloma, degrees of dysplasia, and carcinoma in situ are estimated in [T1.24]. Average age increases more or less in direct proportion to the severity of the squamous abnormality, but there has been an overall shift to younger age groups [M Johnston 1988, Robboy 2002]. Since the curves are skewed, the peak (mode) age gives a better idea than mean age of the "average" woman actually seen in daily practice [Carson 1993].

T1.24 Mean and Peak Ages for Occurrence of Intraepithelial Lesions

Disease	Mean Age, y	Peak Age, y
Condyloma	28.2	19
Mild dysplasia	29.0	22
Moderate dysplasia	28.3	22
Severe dysplasia	30.3	23
Carcinoma in situ	36.0	30
Squamous cell carcinoma	52.8	39

[Carson 1993, Meisels 1977b]

As many as 90% of all squamous intraepithelial lesions occur before 35-40 years of age [Binder 1985, Carson 1993, Herbert 1999, Kinney 1998b, Meisels 1992, V Wright 1984] [F1.18]. The prevalence of squamous intraepithelial lesions rises, and then falls, with age. The prevalence of condyloma peaks between the ages of 16 and 25 years [Meisels 1981a, Oriel 1971, Schiffman 1995a], and diminishes greatly in women in their fifth and sixth decades of life [Melkert 1993]. However, there may be secondary peaks of HPV infection as well as H SIL after menopause [Herrero 2000]. Although dysplasia is relatively rare in women older than 40 years, cervical cancer becomes relatively more common [Bibbo 1971a, Carson 1993] [F1.19].

F1.18 Age Distribution of Dysplasia, Carcinoma In Situ, and Squamous Cell Carcinoma

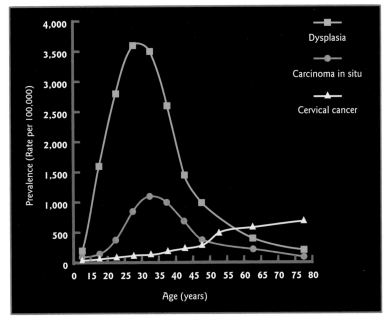

[Reid 1986]

Is Cervical Carcinoma Different in Young Women?

Both the incidence and mortality of cervical cancer appear to be increasing in women under 35 years of age [Anello 1979, Armstrong 1981, 1983, Beral 1986, Bourne 1983, Crowther 1995, Devesa 1989, Draper 1983, G Green 1978, 1979, N Larson 1994, Macgregor 1978b, Maddux 1990, M Morris 1996, Schiffman 1995a, Walton 1982, L Weiss 1994, Yule 1978], although not all agree [Berkowitz 1979, J Carmichael 1986, J Chu 1987, Devesa 1989, Kyriakos 1971, LaVecchia 1984a, Lowry 1989, Meanwell 1988, H Mitchell 1990b, Spanos 1989]. Although the mean age at diagnosis of cervical cancer is ~50 years, nearly half of cases are diagnosed before the age of 35 [Waggoner 2003]. The overall incidence of cervical carcinoma has decreased, while the incidence has increased in young women [Free 1991].

Some characteristics of cervical cancer seem to have changed since the 1960s [Crowther 1995]. Adenocarcinomas are increasing in incidence, particularly in younger women (<35 years of age, see pg 124). CIN is not only more common, but may also be progressing more rapidly than in the past, particularly in young women [Adcock 1982, Bain 1983, A Benoit 1984, Berkeley 1980, Berkowitz 1979, T Johnson 1994, Laskey 1979, LiVolsi 1984, Macgregor 1982, M Paterson 1984, Pedersen 1971, Prendiville 1980, P Schwartz 1988, Yule 1978]. The combination of increased incidence and more rapid progression of precursor lesions could result in more cancers [Beral 1974, Devesa 1987, A Levine 1993]. Rapid tumor growth, rather than delay in diagnosis, could account for poor outcome [P Symonds 2000]. The marked decline in the mortality rate for all age groups could conceal an increased mortality among younger women [G Anderson 1988, Parkin 1985]. Some authors suggest that the cancers of young women may also be more anaplastic [Prempree 1983] and aggressive [Elliott 1989, Prempree 1983, BG Ward 1985], with earlier recurrences [Prempree 1983] and poorer prognosis [Chapman 1988, Maddux 1990, Prempree 1983, Stanhope 1980]. Young women with cervical cancer are more likely to have had recently normal Pap tests, suggesting more rapid progression of tumors [Bain 1983, Bamford 1983, Berkeley 1980, Berkowitz 1979, Crowther 1995, H Mitchell 1990b]. However, large population-based studies have not confirmed a worse prognosis for younger women [Lowry 1989, Meanwell 1988, Russell 1987]. In fact, if anything, younger women are more likely to be diagnosed with earlier, more curable disease [Junor 1989, Meanwell 1988, Russell 1987]. (Younger women also have better performance factors than older women that allow them to tolerate aggressive therapy.) Nevertheless, more cancers could translate into more deaths.

F1.19 Cervical Squamous and Adenocarcinomas by Age

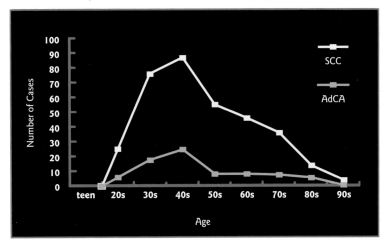

Age distribution for 416 invasive cervical cancers [University of Chicago] (note total absence of cervical cancer in teenagers)

Natural History of Squamous Intraepithelial Lesions

Optimal clinical management depends upon knowledge of the natural history of the disease. Squamous intraepithelial lesions can progress, regress, persist, or recur, but studies have found widely divergent rates. Meaningful data are notoriously difficult to obtain [Nyirjesy 1999]. The fundamental problem is that to observe the entire natural history, prospectively, would require allowing women to develop invasive cancer without any therapeutic intervention [Paul 1988], yet therapy interrupts the natural history of the lesions, making it impossible to determine what would have happened if left untreated [Holowaty 1999]. The very methods used to study a lesion, eg, biopsy, may substantially affect its natural history. Small lesions may be excised completely on biopsy. Lesions that are not completely excised may still be destroyed, or at least significantly affected, by the process of wound healing and the associated inflammatory reaction [Chenoy 1996, Koss 1963, Richart 1966b]. In other words, the biopsy can be therapeutic. This amounts to a Heisenberg Uncertainty Principle for SILs: "Study of the natural history of a lesion...by conventional means is further bedevilled by what amounts almost to a biological uncertainty principle analogous to that in nuclear physics. The act of observation, of making the diagnosis, may interfere significantly with the thing to be observed, in this case the natural history" [D Ashley 1966a]. (From the "nothing new under the sun" file, the unpredictability of atomic motion is an idea that had been around since at least Lucretius [in the 1st century BCE], who used this as an argument for free will and human freedom.) Numerous other difficulties include: studies employ different entry criteria, different diagnostic criteria, different study designs, including length of follow-up and follow-up procedures, and different statistical methodologies which makes comparisons among studies difficult [Kiviat 1996]. Cytologic or histologic follow-up can be misleading owing to variation in sampling and interpretation. Furthermore, dysplasia often recurs after biopsy, frequently in a different location [Koss 1963].

Though the natural history of these lesions is controversial, and still incompletely understood, the following are traditional teachings:

Squamous cell carcinoma is usually preceded by a dysplastic squamous lesion
New dysplastic lesions usually arise as mild dysplasia (CIN 1, L SIL)
Any grade of dysplasia can progress to carcinoma in situ
Most dysplastic lesions do not progress (corollary: more cases of L SIL than H SIL)
Many cases of carcinoma in situ will progress to cancer if left untreated
Invasive carcinoma can arise without first developing classic carcinoma in situ,
 but this is the exception

The longer a lesion persists, the more likely it is to progress. The more it progresses, the more likely it is to continue to progress, the more rapidly it progresses, and the less likely it is to regress. Though only a small minority of all dysplasias progress, those that do seem to "pick up steam" on their way to carcinoma in situ, where they may be held in check for some time before invading. Invasion usually occurs from the most advanced lesions (according to one careful study, >90% of squamous cell carcinomas arise from classic carcinoma in situ [A Ng 1969]), and then usually only after several years (5-10, or more) [MC Anderson 1985, Barron 1978, J Dunn 1967, Fidler 1968, S Jordan 1981, Richart 1969b, van Oortmarssen 1991]. However, invasive cancer can occasionally arise from any grade of dysplasia, even mild dysplasia [Burghardt 1976, J Nelson 1989], as well as from apparently normal epithelium (though this is very rare [perhaps transformed reserve cells can invade directly]) [A Ng 1969], without first developing classic carcinoma in situ [Koss 1978].

Progression of Disease

Only a tiny fraction of all dysplasias, left untreated, would progress to invasive cancer, but the risk increases with increasing grade of the lesion. In meta-analyses of many published studies, less than 10% of ASCUS progressed, 20% of L SILs progress, and 25% of H SILs progress in grade of CIN (dysplasia) within two years [Duggan 1998a, Melnikow 1998]. Well less than 1% of ASCUS or L SILs progress to cancer within two years, and only about 1.5% of H SILs progress to cancer within two years [Campion 1986, Duggan 1998b, Falls 1999, Greenberg 1999, Heinzl 1982, Kataja 1992, K Nasiell 1986, J Robertson 1988, Saw 2001].

It is believed that somewhere in the ballpark of 1% to 5% of L SILs will progress (or, up to 99% will *not* progress) all the way to invasive cancer *if left untreated* [Elkas 1998, Holowaty 1999, M Mitchell 1996, Östör 1993a]. High-grade lesions have a greater tendency to progress: the higher the grade, the greater the tendency to progress [S Jordan 1980]. Although long-term prospective studies find that anywhere from 0 to more than 80% of cases of classic carcinoma in situ progress to invasive carcinoma if left untreated [Albert 1981, A Chang 1990, Fidler 1968, Gad 1976, G Green 1970, M Jordan 1956, 1964, Kinlen 1978, Koss 1963, Kottmeier 1961, McIndoe 1984, BJ Morrison 1996, Östör 1993a, Petersen 1956, Richart 1973, Sörensen 1964, Spriggs 1971a, Te Linde 1973], the conventional wisdom is that about 20% to 35% of untreated carcinomas in situ (CIN 3) will ultimately develop into invasive carcinoma [V Schneider 2003b].

Regression and Recurrence

It is generally agreed that some—probably, most—dysplastic lesions can regress. The overall rate of spontaneous regression for cytologically detected dysplasia varies widely, ranging from less than 10% to greater than 95% [Campion 1986, D Eddy 1990, C Fox 1967, Macgregor 1978a, Melnikow 1998, Richart 1969b, J Robertson 1988, van Oortmarssen 1991]. The lower the grade of the lesion, the more likely it is to regress (conversely, the higher the grade, the less likely to regress) [C Fox 1967, J Hall 1968]. A meta-analysis found that about two-thirds of ASCUS regress, one-half of L SILs regress, and one-third of H SILs regress to normal within 2 years [Melnikow 1998]. Lesions tend to regress more often in younger women, than older ones [Moscicki 2004, Szarewski 2004, van Oortmarssen 1991].

It is not always obvious why some lesions regress spontaneously. Host immune status is probably an important factor not only in regression, but also in the development of the disease in the first place. Dysplastic epithelium may be fragile owing to decreased intercellular cohesion (a characteristic feature of neoplastic cells probably related to abnormal expression of cohesion molecules) [Felix 2003]. Therefore, minimal trauma, such as from coitus, tampon use, or even from obtaining a Pap test, could dislodge the lesion from the basement membrane [Berner 1980, Hellberg 1994]. There is a very high regression rate of dysplasia after childbirth, up to 50% to 75% [Kiguchi 1981], which could be related to trauma or a change in immune status [JL Benedet 1987, Hellberg 1987]. Biopsy has already been mentioned as a possible cure of some dysplastic lesions. It has even been hypothesized that the minor trauma from the very act of taking a Pap test could trigger an immune response to HPV, thereby reducing the risk of cervical cancer [Shapiro 2003]. Drugs, such as antibiotics and vitamins, might also influence the course of the disease [Koss 1978]. Local application of certain drugs, eg, tetracycline, can cause extensive shedding of abnormal epithelium [Koss 1963].

Lesions can also recur. Recurrences can be related to incomplete therapy, reinfection, or a reservoir of latent virus. Once a woman has been found to have a SIL, even if it subsequently regresses, she is still at risk for recurrence [McIndoe 1969]. A negative Pap test in the interim may give false reassurance that the lesion has gone away, never to return. Close surveillance of this high-risk population is important. Cytologic diagnosis after treatment is strongly related to the presence of HPV-DNA. Most women with negative cytology following therapy are HPV-DNA negative, while those with abnormal cytology following therapy are usually HPV-DNA positive [Bollen 1996]. Women with negative HPV tests are at low risk for recurrent disease [Bollen 1999].

Duration of Disease

It is estimated to take, on average, more than 10 years, and possibly as long as 20 years, for an invasive cancer to develop from a dysplastic lesion [Hartmann 2001, van Oortmarssen 1995]. The incidence of SILs peak in the 2nd and 3rd decades; cancer peaks in 5th and 6th decades. The time course is very variable, and probably follows something like a bell-shaped curve, with both rapidly and slowly developing cancers occurring over a range from a few months to several decades [Silcocks 1988].

The transit rates presented above are averages and, unfortunately, the data are dirty. For example, older data may have been skewed to shorter transit times by outmoded definitions of low-grade dysplasia, which included lesions that would now be recognized as carcinoma in situ (ie, lesions that have already progressed) [McKay 1959, Okagaki 1962, Richart 1969b]. On the other hand, the data can also be skewed in the opposite direction, to longer transit times, by low-grade squamous intraepithelial lesions caused by low-risk viral types, which may never progress. Shorter than average transit times are expected for those squamous intraepithelial lesions that are capable of progressing [Meisels 1981a, K Syrjänen 1981]. The bottom line is that an accurate prediction of the rate of progression cannot be made for an individual woman.

Rapidly progressing cancers, developing in less than a year or two, have been reported [Adcock 1982, Albert 1981, D Ashley 1966a,b, Bain 1983, Bamford 1983, A Benoit 1984, Berkeley 1980, Bolla 2000, J Dunn 1967, 1981, Fetherston 1983, Fidler 1968, Figge 1970, C Fox 1968, Hadjimichael 1989, E Hammond 1968, M Jordan 1964, Koutsky 1992a, Laskey 1979, W Liu 1967a, LiVolsi 1984, Macgregor 1982, P Martin 1972, H Mitchell 1990b, M Paterson 1984, Pedersen 1971, R Peters 1988, Prendiville 1980, Sandmire 1976, P Schwartz 1988, 1996, P Symonds 2000]. The women are frequently younger than 40 years. Their tumors tend to be poorly-differentiated, rapidly advancing, and widely disseminated, and respond poorly to therapy, with more frequent recurrences [Bolla 2000, Hadjimichael 1989, P Schwartz 1988, J Walker 1989]. They are frequently associated with HPV 18 and adenocarcinomas are overrepresented [Bolla 2000, Hildesheim 1999, Nakagawa 1996, P Schwartz 1996]. Mutations of cellular oncogenes, such as *ras*, may be an early predictive marker of rapid progression [Alonio 2003]. Women infected with human immunodeficiency virus may also have rapidly progressive cervical cancers [Branca 2000, Calore 1998, 2001, Duerr 2001, Ellerbrock 2000, Gallagher 2001, Ho 1994, Holcomb 1998, JC Johnson 1992, Y-C Lee 2000, Maiman 1990, 1991, 1998, Mayans 1999, Moodley 2001, Moscicki 2000, Robinson 2000, Rojansky 1996, X-W Sun 1997, Vermund 1991, ter Meulen 1992, AB Williams 1994, Womack 2000, T Wright 1994a,c] (see pg 87). Women with rapidly progressing cancers typically have had recently normal Pap tests [Berkeley 1980, Bolla 2000, R Peters 1988, Rylander 1977]. However, many so-called rapidly progressive cancers, particularly those with very brief transit times (weeks or a few months), may be related to sampling or interpretation variance of previous Pap tests, ie, false-negative results (unfortunately, Pap test interpretation is not an exact science) [Kenter 1996, Montes 1999, Rylander 1977, P Schwartz 1996].

Site

Cervical intraepithelial neoplasia usually occurs in the transition zone of the squamocolumnar junction, abutting the endocervical glandular epithelium. Like the Mid-East, this little area, only a few millimeters wide, is the site of a lot of turmoil. The anterior lip of the cervix is affected by cervical neoplasia twice as often as the posterior lip, while the lateral margins usually are spared [Richart 1965a]. This distribution of dysplasia corresponds to the location of the metaplastic epithelium on the cervix [Richart 1973].

Cervical intraepithelial neoplasia can grow by expansion to encompass the entire transitional zone [Richart 1973]. The anterior lip is in a position more exposed to trauma, eg, during intercourse (which could be important in the inoculation of a carcinogenic agent) or childbirth. However, condylomas are not necessarily confined to the transformation zone [Meisels 1977b].

Beginning at the squamocolumnar junction, cervical intraepithelial neoplasia spreads out distally on the cervix, like a ripple in a pond of squamous metaplasia, usually stopping abruptly at the shore of the native epithelium. However, the disease can occasionally grow proximally up the endocervical canal as far as the endometrium [Ferenczy 1971] or even the fallopian tube [Kanbour 1978]. There is a gradient of differentiation of the CIN lesion, with the proximal or endocervical portion being less differentiated (higher grade), and the distal portion being more differentiated (lower grade) [Richart 1973]. The maturity of the process has a distribution reminiscent of the metaplastic reactions: the more immature the lesion, the higher up in the endocervical canal the change is likely to be found.

Morphology

Mature metaplastic dysplasia is the most common form of dysplasia but, as might be expected from its high degree of differentiation, it is usually low-grade. High-grade dysplasia usually has a (immature) metaplastic morphology. Keratinizing dysplasias are difficult to grade, and may be undercalled or over-called by cytology [Faquin 2001, Hudock 1995, Navarro 1997]. Keratinizing dysplasia can also be difficult to distinguish from keratinizing squamous cell carcinoma. Unfortunately, it is impossible to predict morphologically which dysplasias will progress in an individual woman.

Pathogenesis

Carcinogenesis is a multistep process [Barron 1968]. Historically, there were two basic theories regarding the pathogenesis of cervical dysplasia [Richart 1973]. One held that the disease arises in a field of abnormal cells and progresses by transformation of other cells from normal to neoplastic [Burghardt 1983, M Coppleson 1970, Reagan 1969]. The other theory held that the disease is of unicellular origin, in which a clone of abnormal cells takes over. Supporting this single bullet (aka "Eve" or first cell) theory is colposcopic [Richart 1965a, 1966a], microscopic [Richart 1973], chromosomal [Spriggs 1971b], and biochemical (X-linked enzyme [JW Smith 1971]) evidence that the disease represents a clone of cells deriving from a single cell or a very small group of cells. The abnormal clone of cells then proliferates relatively rapidly and seems to plow the normal epithelium out of the way [Richart 1963a]. Resistance to chalones, which inhibit cell division, was suspected of playing a role in carcinogenesis [Richart 1969a].

These theories were developed before the concept that there are biologic differences between low-grade and high-grade lesions. Human papillomavirus (HPV) is now known to be critically important in the malignant transformation of the cells [Lehn 1985]. High-grade lesions are usually associated with a single HPV type, are frequently aneuploid, and contain integrated HPV-DNA. High-grade squamous intraepithelial lesions, thought to be the true precursor lesions, probably arise from a single cell within a low-grade lesion, and gradually expand as a clonal proliferation. It might be predicted that low-grade lesions are multicellular in origin, developing in a field of latently infected cells and associated with multiple HPV types. However, it has turned out that only those low-grade lesions associated with low-risk virus are polyclonal. Squamous intraepithelial lesions, whether low-grade or high-grade, associated with high-risk virus are usually monoclonal [El Hamidi 2003, T Park 1996]. This suggests that lesions associated with low-risk vs high-risk virus are different from their inception (discussed in more detail below, see pg 81). It is possible that clonality could predict which lesions are more likely to progress [El Hamidi 2003].

The traditional view of carcinogenesis is that lesions arise as low-grade dysplasia, progress through grades of dysplasia to carcinoma in situ, and then to invasive carcinoma. However, there is an alternative view: high-grade lesions develop de novo as a small focus within a low-grade lesion (or even normal tissue), and then expand in size. This gives the impression the lesion is progressing in grade, but according to this theory, it actually starts out high-grade [Tidbury 1992]. It has been postulated that cervical cancer arises from this aggressive CIN 3 lesion—widely present on the cervix and established years before invasion—rather than as a progression from a low-grade lesion [Kiviat 1992a, 1996, J Robertson 1994]. In support of this theory, some H SILs (possibly 5% to 10%, but mostly CIN 2, rather than CIN 3) have been reported to arise de novo in the absence of cytologically detectable L SIL, challenging the traditional view that L SIL is a precursor to H SIL [Koutsky 1992a, Nobbenhuis 1999, Schiffman 1995b, 2003a]. These two theories are not necessarily mutually exclusive; the traditional pathway could be the major pathway and the alternate pathway a minor one, for example. Or, there could be rapidly progressing CIN 1 lesions that advance quickly in grade. It is also quite possible that the de novo pathway, like some apparently rapidly developing carcinomas, could be an artifact of sampling or interpretation variations (ie, false-negative results) of prior cytologies or biopsies. (There is evidence that CIN 1 and CIN 2 are practically the same thing [M Mitchell 1996, Syrjänen 1992] and that the important biologic difference is between squamous dysplasia, any grade, and classic carcinoma in situ [A Ng 1969]. But, because differentiating severe dysplasia from CIS can be difficult in practice, this would put the critical division between CIN 2 and CIN 3, as the Europeans have it, not between CIN 1 and CIN 2, as the Bethesda System does [V Schneider 2003a].)

Squamous metaplasia is at its peak in young women, especially on the anterior lip of the cervix. HPV preferentially involves the immature (ie, metaplastic or reserve) epithelium of the cervix. The actual cell affected is also a matter of controversy, but is probably a primitive basal/reserve cell in the transformation zone [L Johnson 1969]. Because the vast majority (~90%) of dysplasias arise in the transformation zone, it is generally believed that a primitive cell at this site is involved. HPV appears to infect the basal or reserve cells [R Reid 1989], which are still capable of dividing, and may stimulate their proliferation. These facts may explain the importance of young age in cervical carcinogenesis and suggest a reason for its most common location, the transformation zone. Other, non-HPV, venereal diseases might help provide the soil for carcinogenesis to begin by inducing inflammatory reparative proliferation or metaplasia.

Viruses have the ability to usurp the host's DNA (cell cycle control) machinery in order to replicate. If a virus were to infect a cell and somehow throw a monkey wrench into the host's DNA machinery while the process of proliferation is already revved up, proliferation might get out of control, become neoplastic, and eventually malignant. The host cells could begin proliferating in a disorderly way, mimicking the benign proliferative reactions, and so on, down the dysplasia/CIS pathway to invasive cancer (see pg 83).

Human Papillomavirus

Introduction

It is no longer a mystery what causes cervical cancer: it's the lowly wart virus [Koutsky 1992a, Muñoz 1996, Schiffman 1993, K Syrjänen 1986a, zur Hausen 1974, 1981]. Human papillomavirus is now accepted as a necessary cause of virtually all cases of cervical cancer [Walboomers 1999]. As Thomas Kuhn, author of the classic book, *Structure of Scientific Revolutions*, might observe, there has been a transforming paradigm shift in our understanding of cervical cancer to include HPV infection as the cause.

Historical Context

Papillomaviruses co-evolved with humans over a span of millions of years [Bernard 1994, Ong 1993]. Lesions in animals, now known to be due to papillomaviruses, have been recognized for more than a millennium [Wick 2000]. The Roman physician, Celsus (25 BCE-50 CE), documented skin warts in the first century CE. Genital warts, or condylomas (Greek: knob, knuckle), were also described by ancient Greek and Roman writers [Burns 1992, Lutzner 1983, Oriel 1971]. These ancient authors associated condyloma with sexual contact [Sedláček 1999].

The etiology of warts began to be elucidated in 1898, when M'Fadyan and Hobday transmitted dog warts using cell-free extracts [zur Hausen 1999]. Ciuffo used the same method to produce human warts (papillomas or verruca vulgaris) by self-inoculation as early as 1907 [Ciuffo 1907]. In 1933, Richard Shope described the first papillomavirus, in the cottontailed rabbits he hunted in Iowa. The Shope papillomavirus was soon shown to be capable of causing cancer [Rous 1934, Rous 1935]. Peyton Rous, in 1911, had already established that infectious agents could cause cancer (proving that one animal could "catch" cancer from another, a notion considered ridiculous at the time). He described a sarcoma in chickens caused by what later became known as the Rous Sarcoma Virus [Rous 1911]. (More than half a century later, Rous was finally awarded the Nobel Prize, in 1965, for his discovery of tumor-inducing viruses. The committee had been "burned" once already, in 1926, by awarding the prize to Febinger, who claimed that worms caused cancer. This embarrassment may also have been a factor in Papanicolaou's failure to receive the prize [Koprowska 1985]. James Ewing severely criticized Rous for his suggestion that viruses caused cancer [van Helvoort 1999].) By mid century, circa 1947-1952, a rare hereditary condition, epidermodysplasia verruciformis, was found to be caused by papillomavirus infection; after a latency of about 20 years, squamous cell carcinomas of the skin develop in sun exposed verrucous plaques [zur Hausen 1999].

Barrett established venereal transmission of genital warts in 1954, finding they occurred in the wives of soldiers who had sexual relations with native Asian women during the Korean War [T Barrett 1954]. J. E. Ayre first described the distinctive halo cell, now known as the koilocyte, characteristic of condyloma in 1949 [Ayre 1949]. Papanicolaou described and illustrated these cells, without naming them, in his 1954 *Atlas* (plate A IV, numbers 8 & 9) [Papanicolaou

1954]. The term, koilocyte (Greek for "hollow cell"), was derived from Koss and Durfee's 1956 description of koilocytotic atypia in tissue sections [Koss 1956]. Prophetically, Fred Stewart often used the term, "warty atypia," for cervical biopsies demonstrating this abnormality [Frable 1995]. In 1960, Ayre speculated that the koilocyte, which he called the "halo cell," was a viral change in premalignancy. He wrote:

"a viral nucleic acid might enter a host cell and be incorporated into the genetic structure of the cell....The viral nucleic acid...would be subject to...carcinogenic agents—which could cause it to...greatly increase its rate of replication, and thus to act as an independent functional unit. The result would be production of a mutant, perhaps cancerous, cell.... The significant feature of the [koilocyte] would seem to be that it represents a steppingstone between normal cells and malignant or premalignant cells.... The thought is, then, that [koilocytes] represent the earliest manifestation of malignancy in human cells, that they are caused by some nucleic acid-viral infectious activity in an estrogenic environment which produces derangement of cell metabolism and orderly replication of cells, and that they are probably a mutant deviation towards malignant cell growth" [Ayre 1960].

This was the first time that the koilocyte was attributed to the effect of a virus and, prophetically, it summarizes what we now think about cervical carcinogenesis [Meisels 1983]. Yet, in spite of this early progress, the wart virus was not suspected of having a significant role in cervical carcinogenesis, largely because dysplasias typically were not wart-like, but flat. Koilocytes were dismissed as being important in cervical carcinogenesis [Sagiroglu 1963]: "It is unlikely that the koilocytotic lesion is a part of the natural history of more than a fraction of cervix cancers" [Koss 1956]. Efforts to link HPV to cervical neoplasia were hampered by insensitive detection techniques. For a long time, before the development of highly sensitive recombinant DNA technology, herpes simplex virus was thought to be the culprit in cervical carcinogenesis [Aurelian 1974, Bornstein 1995, R Burk 1999, Fish 1982, Galloway 1983, S Graham 1982, Kessler 1974a, Kremar 1986, McLachlin 2000, A Ng 1970a, Pacsa 1975, Rawls 1969, Vonka 1984, zur Hausen 1983].

Virus particles were first identified ultrastructurally in skin warts in 1949 [M Strauss 1949] and in venereal warts in the 1960s [A Dunn 1968, Melczer 1965]. In 1976, Meisels and Fortin proved that koilocytosis is due to HPV infection [Meisels 1976b, 1983]. The next year, Purola and Savia from Finland, and Meisels and Fortin from Canada, independently described the flat condyloma, identified the koilocyte as being the cytopathic effect of HPV, and suggested that most "dysplasia" was really viral infection [Meisels 1977b, Purola 1977]. Prior to that time it was thought that condylomas (ie, visible genital warts) were rare on the cervix [Marsh 1952, Woodruff 1958]; this discovery (of flat lesions) indicated that condylomas were common.

In the mid-1970s researchers began to postulate that HPV might play a role in cervical cancer [Josey 1976, zur Hausen 1976, 1977]. In 1974, zur Hausen, et al, published the first, albeit unsuccessful, experiments searching for papillomavirus DNA in cervical cancer [zur Hausen 1974]. In 1978, Laverty, et al, first described finding viral particles by electron microscopy in flat condylomas [Laverty 1978]. In 1980 Gissman first reported partial characterization of an HPV from genital warts, which was designated HPV 6 [Gissmann 1980]. HPV 16 and HPV 18 were first isolated from cervical cancer in 1983 and 1984, respectively [Boshart 1984, Dürst 1983]. In 1985, Dürst, et al, isolated specific types of HPV-DNA in the majority of squamous cell carcinomas and precursor lesions [Dürst 1985]. Modern techniques, such as PCR, have confirmed an extremely strong relationship between HPV and cervical cancer, 10 to 20 *times* stronger than

the relationship between cigarette smoking and lung cancer, for example [F Bosch 2002a, Meijer 1992, Pisani 1997, Unger 2001, T Wright 2003b].

Beginning in the 1980s, scientific investigation began unraveling the molecular biology of human papillomavirus and the actual cellular mechanisms of cervical infection and carcinogenesis [zur Hausen 2002]. The expression of early viral genes, E6 and E7, and demonstration of deletions of part of the viral genome after integration in cervical cancer was reported in 1985 [Schwarz 1985]. Transforming properties of E6 and E7 were described in 1989 [Münger 1989a,b]. In 1992, it was shown that E6 and E7 viral genes are necessary factors for the malignant phenotype of HPV-positive cervical cancer cells [von Knebel Doeberitz 1992]. The first epidemiologic study of HPV infection was published by de Villiers et al in 1987 [de Villiers 1987]. This was followed by large-scale epidemiologic studies that provided solid evidence that HPV is the primary risk factor for cervical cancer [Muñoz 1992, 1996, 2000]. In 1995, the World Health Organization officially recognized certain human papillomaviruses (specifically, HPV types 16 and 18) as human carcinogens [IARC 1995]. HPV has now been found guilty of causing cervical cancer beyond any reasonable doubt [F Bosch 2002a,b, Richart 1998]. However, while HPV may be the ring-leader, it is not sufficient by itself to cause cancer, and its suspected accomplices (cofactors) remain at large.

Epidemiology of HPV Infection

Human papillomavirus infection is thought to be the single most common venereal infection [Kiviat 1992b, Koutsky 1997]. Clinically detected lesions are, relatively speaking, rare (~1% of all infections), and represent only the tip of the iceberg compared with the total number of infections [McGlennen 2000]. Most infections are asymptomatic [C Mao 2003]. Microscopy is not very sensitive in detecting HPV infection [de Villiers 1992, Sherman 1994]. Older laboratory detection techniques were also relatively insensitive and underesti-

Human Papilloma Virus

Most common STD

Millions of cases per annum

50%-90% sexually active women

20-50 million currently infected

2.5 million SILs/year

10,000 cervical cancers/year

Persistent infection major risk factor

Most women clear HPV in 1-2 years

mated the number of cases. Using modern tools, such as PCR, the prevalence of HPV infection has been found to be very high [Anonymous 1987, H Bauer 1991, Bevan 1989, Borg 1995, de Villiers 1992, M Johnson 1990, Koss 1993a, Pasetto 1992, Schiffman 1991, A Schneider 1992a, Tidy 1989a, L Young 1989]. More than 5 million American women and men become infected annually, with an estimated 20 million to 50 million currently infected [L Alexander 1998]. By comparison, there are, very approximately 2.5 million SILs, including >300,000 H SILs, and 10,000 cervical cancers detected annually in the United States [Davey 2000, Jemal 2005, Stoler 2003b, Wingo 1995]. Somewhere between 50% and 90% of sexually active women will acquire anogenital HPV infection at some point in their lives. Genital HPV infections are probably about equally common between the sexes, but are more difficult to detect in men [Fife 2003, Schiffman 1995a]. The overall prevalence of HPV infection in adults is thought to be, very approximately, 20%, but prevalence changes with age [R Nayar 2003, Stoler 2001a]. Several studies indicate that 35% to 50% of American and Western European women in their 20s are infected, falling to less than 20% of women in their 30s, and to 5%-10% after 50 [Baay 2004, R Burk 1996b, Ferenczy 1997, Jacobs 2000, Schiffman 1992, 1995a, 2003a, Stoler 2000a]. (Note: not all studies show this decline in prevalence with age [Herrero 2000, E Smith 1997, 2004].) Adolescents may be biologically more susceptible to HPV infection than adults [Kahn 2001, Moscicki 1998, Shew 1994], possibly owing to large ectopy with exposure of vulnerable metaplastic cells, inadequate cervical mucus production, less resistance to minor trauma during intercourse, cervical cell membrane differences that enhance interaction with virus, and lack of protective immunity due to not having had prior exposure to HPV [Ducan 1990, Jacobson 2000a, Moscicki 1999, Moss 1991].

The risk of infection is directly related to the number of sexual partners, particularly recent sexual partners [H Bauer 1991, Burkett 1992, Kjær 1990, Moscicki 2001]. Genital HPV infection is highly contagious, with infection rates ranging from 50% to 85% of sexual partners [Ferenczy 1983, Gomousa–Michael 1997, Winer 2003]. It is possible to acquire oral HPV infection from oral sex [L Gilbert 2003, Kashima 1992, Winer 2003]. HPV, including high-risk anogenital types, can be detected in women with apparently normal oral mucosa [J Carr 2000]. The same HPV types associated with cervical cancer, predominantly HPV 16 and 18, also seem to be responsible for some head & neck cancers (although most cases are associated with cigarette smoking and alcohol abuse) [J Carr 2000, Gillison 2000, 2001, Premoli–De–Perceco 1998, S Schartz 1998]. Common hand or plantar warts are caused by viral types that generally do not infect the genital tract. HPV infection is usually silent (latent infection); in other words, most of those infected are unaware of it, because they do not have symptoms, genital warts, abnormal Pap tests, or other clinical manifestations of HPV [C Mao 2003, Trofatter 1997]. However, they can still transmit the virus to a sex partner. Rarely, pregnant women can pass HPV to their baby during vaginal delivery (vertical transmission). HPV-DNA can be detected in the oral cavity and foreskin of babies born to infected mothers, and these infants can also develop laryngeal condylomas (papillomas) or other HPV infections [Mounts 1984, Rice 1999, Roman 1986, Sedlacek 1989]. It has been suggested that HPV causes some spontaneous abortions [Hermonat 1997].

For two uninfected individuals, who have never had any other sexual partners besides each other, there is no risk of acquiring genital HPV infection during sex, even if they are swinging from the chandeliers (or whatever) [Azocar 1990, J Carr 2000]. Condoms do not effectively prevent HPV infection [Ho 1998a, Winer 2003], although they may decrease the risk of H SIL and cancer [Manhart 2002]. Abstinence is the surest way to prevent HPV infection, but were this approach to be entirely successful, we could kiss the human race goodbye. However, vaccination against HPV 16 and 18, prior to onset of sexual activity, has the potential to be highly effective in preventing many cervical cancers.

It may be possible to transmit the virus on fomites (objects that spread infectious agents) contaminated with exfoliated HPV infected squames, such as shared underwear or swimsuits [Bergeron 1990, T Wright 1990], or even instruments used in caring for women with HPV infections, such as surgical gloves, towels, speculums, and possibly fumes from lasers [Bergeron 1990, Ferenczy 1989, McCance 1986, Roden 1997]. Believe it or not, toilet seats have been investigated, and yes, they can be contaminated with HPV infected cells [S Strauss 2002]. HPV is resistant to desiccation, heat, and some disinfectants, including 90% ethanol and Savlon (chlorhexidine and cetrimide) [J Carr 2000, Roden 1997].

The epidemiology of HPV infection mirrors, in many ways, the epidemiology of cervical cancer [Munk 1997, Tortolero–Luna 1999]. Studies have found that virgins are usually HPV negative, while young, sexually active women are frequently HPV positive [Andersson–Ellström 1996, H Bauer 1991, R Burk 1996a,b, Fairley 1992, Kjær 2001, Ley 1991, Pao 1992, Rylander 1994, Schiffman 2003a]. The number of male vaginal sexual partners is the major risk factor for acquiring HPV infection [Andersson–Ellström 1996, Azocar 1990, R Burk 1996a, Giuliano 2002, Ho 1998a, Karlsson 1995, Kjær 2001]. Although virgins can acquire HPV of the vulva from nonpenetrative sexual contact [Winer 2003], the cervix is usually negative [Andersson–Ellström 1996, Blackledge

1998, Carter 1996, Ley 1991], and they do not have cervical cytologic abnormalities [A Peters 1994].

Most HPV infections are transient, particularly in young women (<30 years), with a median duration of about a year; by two years, the vast majority of HPV infections become nondetectable by sensitive HPV DNA tests, except those that lead to precancer [Elfgren 2000, Evander 1997, Ho 1998a, Moscicki 1998, MH Schiffman 1995a, 2003a, CB Woodman 2001]. Because most HPV infections resolve spontaneously, the prevalence decreases with age [R Burk 1996b, de Villiers 1992, Jacobs 2000, Ley 1991, Melkert 1993, Sherman 2002]. However, reinfections by different HPV types (serial infections) are common in sexually active women. Infection with multiple viral types occurs in 20% to 50% of infected women [H Bauer 1993, Cuschieri 2004, Kalantari 1997, Kiviat 1992b, Moscicki 1998, Rousseau 2003]. Cytologic abnormalities, mostly ASC-US, develop in 17% to 36% of women within 5 years of testing positive for HPV [Castle 2002b, Ho 1998a, CB Woodman 2001].

The peak incidence of HPV infection is between 16 and 25 years, which coincides with the usual age of onset of sexual activity [Sellors 2000a]. By age 35-40 years, the large majority (>90%) of women have apparently cleared their infections and tests for HPV-DNA are negative [Schiffman 1992, 1995a]. The number of recent (<5 years) sexual partners is a better predictor of current HPV infection than total number of partners, probably because of the transient nature of the infection [R Burk 1996a,b, Fairley 1994, JP Figueroa 1995, Hildesheim 1993]. The factors responsible for controlling infection are not entirely clear, but immunologic response and viral type, combined with less exposure to new HPV types owing to fewer new sexual partners, seem to be important [Schiffman 1995a]. However, a few women remain HPV positive (persistent infection) [Melkert 1993]. Infections in older women are more likely to persist [Schiffman 1992].

Persistent HPV infection is a major risk factor for developing cervical cancer [Chua 1996, K Cooper 1997, Ellerbrock 2000, Harnsel 1999, Ho 1995, Hopman 2000, Josefsson 2000, Nobbenhuis 1999, Remmink 1995, Schlecht 2001, X–W Sun 1997, Wallin 1999, Ylitalo 2000a]. Persistent infection can be defined as the same *specific* type of HPV-DNA detected consecutively at least twice over a period of one or more years [R Burk 1999]. This definition requires a detection system capable of identifying specific viral types. Merely finding a woman to be "high-risk" virus positive more than once does not necessarily mean the HPV infection is persistent (could be a new infection with another high-risk viral type; such multiple, serial infections are common). The longer a lesion persists, the more likely it is to progress [IARC 1995, Schiffman 1995b]. The higher the grade of the lesion, the less likely it is to regress [Nobbenhuis 2001]. The corollary is that women who clear their infections are at low-risk of cervical cancer [T Wright 2003b]. However, persistent infection is not a prerequisite for development of H SIL; some high-grade lesions develop rapidly [Koutsky 1992a, CB Woodman 2001]. Thus, it is possible that persistent HPV infection might be necessary to maintain a SIL [CB Woodman 2001]. (Chicken and egg problem: Does H SIL develop because HPV persists or does HPV persist because H SIL develops?)

Persistent infections are more common with high-risk viral types [Giuliano 2002, X–W Sun 1997]. Smoking, multiparity, long-term use of oral contraceptives, and possibly other sexually transmitted infections, eg, *Chlamydia,* chronic inflammation, and nutritional factors, increase the risk of persistent infection [Schiffman 2003a]. High viral load may be predictive of persistent cervical abnormalities and the development of significant precursor lesions [K Cooper 1997, C Johnston 2000, Josefsson 2000, D Swan 1999, Ylitalo 2000b]. However, viral load seems to wax and wane during the course of HPV infection [C Wheeler 1996, CB Woodman 2001], and not all investigators have found high viral load to be predictive of H SIL [Lörincz 2002]. Women who are HPV negative after therapy for SILs are at low risk of recurrence

(<5%); those who are HPV positive after therapy are at high risk (~33%) of recurrence [Milde–Langosch 2000, Paraskevaidis 2001]. Women treated for H SIL who have recurrent lesions are almost always HPV positive [Chua 1996]. Recurrences can be due either to activation of endogenous virus [Ferenczy 1985, Krebs 1990, 1991] or reinfection with a different viral type [Crum 1995, Nuovo 1990b]. Immunity undoubtedly plays an important role in preventing recurrences [Nuovo 1991a, Richart 1980b, Rosenfeld 1992].

HPV-DNA can be detected in urine samples in women with cervical infections [Jacobson 2000b]. Vaginal HPV types correlate well with cervical HPVs [Finan 2001]. HPV-DNA can be detected using self-collected samples [D Harper 1999, Sellors 2000b, Tong 2003, T Wright 2000a]. Interestingly, HPV-DNA can be detected in the blood of some women with cervical cancer [Pornthanakasem 2001].

Finally, it should be noted that although it is often assumed that a negative HPV-DNA test means the virus has been completely cleared from the body, it could be that the viral load has merely diminished to the point of being nondetectable by currently available diagnostic methods. At least some infections become latent for long periods of time and can be reactivated, possibly related to change in immune status [Schiffman 2003a]. This is important because if the virus has been truly cleared, then a new sexual contact would be required to place the woman at risk for cervical cancer. However, if the virus is merely latent, then the woman would remain at risk for cervical cancer.

Microbiology of HPV

Papillomaviruses were formerly classified with the Papovavirus family (*papillomavirus*, *polyomavirus*, simian *vacuolating* virus). Papovaviruses comprised a heterogeneous group of double-stranded DNA tumor viruses, although they have similar action in cells, eg, they replicate in the nucleus. However, papillomavirus is physically larger, has a larger genome, no sequence relatedness, and has a different gene transcription process, than the other members of the Papovavirus family. Accordingly, *Papovaviridae* has now been divided into two families, the *Polyomaviridae* and the *Papillomaviridae*, while the Papovavirus family has been eliminated [de Villiers 2001, Garland 2002]. Papilloma is an ex-Papova. Papovavirus is no more! It has ceased to be!

Papillomaviruses are ubiquitous, and infect a broad range of animal hosts, including all vertebrates, often producing warts or other epithelial proliferations. Papillomaviruses are species specific, eg, some infect only cows, others only humans. Papillomaviruses are also tissue specific; like homing pigeons they roost in specific epithelial or mucosal sites. Certain HPVs infect skin, eg, HPV-1 causes plantar warts, while HPV-2 and HPV-4 cause common warts, whereas other HPVs infect mucosal sites, eg, HPV-6 and HPV-11 cause anogenital condylomas. Some HPVs, eg, HPV-16 and HPV-18, are associated with anogenital cancers and may be a significant factor in some oropharyngeal cancers.

Human papillomavirus looks something like a golf ball under the scanning electron microscope. It measures about 55nm in diameter, and consists of an icosahedral capsule enclosing a circular DNA genome. The virus is non-lipid-containing (naked, ie, nonenveloped). There are 72 capsomeres. The DNA is double-stranded, circular, and composed of about 7,900 base pairs [Alani 1998, Beutner 1997b, J Carr 2000, Prasad 1995]. The viral genome is supercoiled and bound to histones.

Through the 1960s, it was thought that there was only one type of HPV, because all papillomaviruses were alike based on studies with investigational tools, such as electron microscopy, available at the time. However, beginning in the 1970s, with the advent of molecular techniques that revolutionized biology, more than 200 HPV genotypes are now suspected, of which more than 40 can infect the female (and male) genital tract, and about 20 can cause cervical cancer [Garland 2002, Monk 2004, Wick 2000, Wolf 2003]. Each HPV type is a separate genetic species and each should be considered a separate infection when identified [Schiffman 2003a].

Formerly, HPV was classified according to its nucleotide sequence homology by hybridization and then numbered in order of discovery. Those HPVs having less than 50% homology with known HPV viruses were considered new types; those with greater than 50% homology were considered variants or subtypes. However, this assay overestimated sequence differences. Classification is currently based on DNA sequencing. To be considered a new HPV type, the HPV genome must differ by more than 10% from known types. HPV subtypes have between 2% and 10% sequence divergence; variants have <2% divergence [Garland 2002]. DNA sequence assay is easier, can be computerized, and allows formation of a central database. Many HPVs have now been fully cloned.

Methods of Detection of HPV Infection

The life cycle of human papillomavirus (HPV) is usually tightly linked to squamous differentiation. Complete HPV replication only occurs in mature, terminally differentiated squamous cells. Therefore, replicating the virus in culture is problematic. Permissive infection refers to those lesions that permit full viral DNA replication and capsule formation, with complete infectious viral particle formation, eg, well-differentiated flat or warty condyloma (low-grade squamous intraepithelial lesions). Glandular cells, atypical immature metaplasia, latent infections, high-grade dysplasia/carcinoma in situ, and cancer do not permit full viral expression with formation of viral capsule and complete virions; hence, they are considered nonpermissive infections (see pg 82 for further discussion).

The Pap Test

The Pap test can detect koilocytes, which are pathognomonic of condyloma and HPV infection [Boras 1989, Koss 1987b, 2000b, Meisels 1981a, 1982, 1983, Naib 1961b]. Koilocytes are present, histologically, in at least 80% of permissive HPV infections [11.51a] [S Sato 1986]. Koilocytes form predominantly in the intermediate to superficial cell layers, but the surface of the lesion is often covered with dyskeratotic cells. Therefore, the Pap test is not very sensitive in the detection of HPV infection by koilocytosis, because it samples the epithelial surface. Koilocytes are identified, cytologically, in only about 20% to 33% of women with condylomas diagnosed histologically [11.51b,1.52a,b] [Mayelo 1994, Okagaki 1992, V Schneider 1989]. Further, koilocyte formation diminishes with increasing

Human Papilloma Virus
- *Species specific, tissue specific*
- *Cause epithelial proliferations*
  - *Warts to cancer*
- *>200 known HPV types*
- *~40 infect anogenital tract*
  - *67%: 6, 11, 16, 18*
- *~20 potentially oncogenic*
  - *80%: 16, 18, 31, 45*
- *HPV causes >99% cervical cancer*

Human Papilloma Virus
- *Non-encapsulated, non-enveloped*
- *Icosahedral, 55 nm diameter*
- *HPV Genome: Circular, double stranded DNA*
  - *7900 base pairs*
- *Coding region: 8 early, 2 late*
- *Noncoding, transcription, replication*

grade of cervical intraepithelial neoplasia. In summary, koilocytes are usually present, histologically at least, in L SILs (permissive infection), but they are usually absent in both in situ and invasive carcinoma (nonpermissive lesions) as well as in latent infections [A *Schneider* 1989a]. (Koilocytes are discussed in more detail on pg 49.)

Electron Microscopy

Electron microscopy can only detect viral particles (requires permissive infection), although the virions need not be completely mature [II.73a] [*Coleman* 1977, Hills 1979, S *Sato* 1986, J *Smith* 1983]. Since the tissue concentration of virions is low, electron microscopy is not very sensitive for diagnosis, unless preselected areas are examined (which amounts to an ultrastructural confirmation of a light microscopic diagnosis).

Immunocytochemistry

Immunocytochemical staining can detect viral capsular antigens (in permissive infections) [II.73b]. However, viral capsule formation is a late and focal event. Immunocytochemistry is positive in only 50% to 80% cases of classic condyloma and mild dysplasia (ie, low-grade squamous intraepithelial lesions). Because viral production diminishes, the detection rate declines as the dysplasia becomes more advanced and may be zero in carcinoma in situ [*Kurman* 1983, S *Sato* 1986]. In other words, the more advanced the dysplasia, the *less* likely that HPV will be demonstrated by immunocytochemistry [S *Sato* 1986]. In practice, koilocytosis (ie, routine histologic diagnosis) is more sensitive than immunostaining in detection of HPV infection.

DNA Hybridization

DNA hybridization techniques detect HPV-DNA or RNA and are more sensitive and specific methods of diagnosing HPV infection than light microscopy, electron microscopy, or immunocytochemical staining, and, unlike those techniques, hybridization can detect nonpermissive viral infections in which the viral DNA is integrated into the host genome (important for cancer development). Hybridization techniques can also usually determine the specific type of HPV.

Three types of nucleic acid hybridization technologies include: direct nucleic acid probes (eg, Southern blot and in situ hybridization), hybridization signal amplification (eg, Digene Hybrid Capture® System), and target amplification (eg, polymerase chain reaction) methods [*Qureshi* 2003, S *Syrjänen* 1990, *Trofatter* 1997, *Unger* 2000, 2001, *Wick* 2000].

HPV-DNA is detected by the extent of homology ("hybridization") with a labeled probe (purified HPV-DNA or RNA labeled with a radionucleotide or biotin, etc). Filter hybridization uses denatured, single stranded DNA on a filter support, which binds the DNA. Hybridization depends on the extent of nucleic acid homology as well as the conditions under which the test is performed: the higher the degree of base pair similarity, the stronger the hybridization.

Southern Blot

Southern blot, the old reliable, but still useful test, was named for the scientist who first introduced this technique that revolutionized molecular biology [E *Southern* 1975]. Southern blot is still considered the "gold standard" technique for HPV diagnosis [*Hubbard* 2003, *Koutsky* 1988]. It is a modification of the filter hybridization technique that measures HPV without amplification. Its sensitivity is 10-40 virions per cell. The DNA is

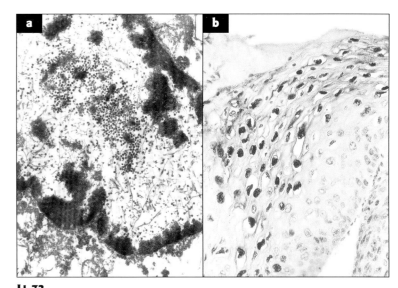

II.73
a, Ultrastructure HPV; **b**, Immunochemistry HPV [*Meisels* 1997]

extracted from cells and digested with restriction enzymes to cut the DNA at specific sites. The procedure separates the DNA fragments (using electrophoresis), which are then transferred to a filter support and hybridized with labeled probes [T *Wright* 1990]. This dual characterization, by migration pattern and hybridization, is highly specific. In addition, it can assess the physical state of the virus (episomal vs integrated). Unfortunately, Southern blot technique cannot localize the individual infected cells, requires fresh or frozen tissue and relatively large amounts of DNA, is relatively insensitive, and laborious to perform.

In Situ Hybridization

In situ hybridization (ISH) is another method of HPV detection in which a labeled probe is applied directly to an ordinary tissue section or cytologic specimen. Its sensitivity is about 10-100 virions per cell. The method requires DNA or RNA probes of known viral types. The probes can be labeled with radioactive substances (such as tritium or sulfur 35) or nonradioactive substances (such as biotin). Biotin labeled probes can be detected by immunocytochemistry. Tests using nonradioactive probes, though less sensitive, are faster and easier to perform than those using radioactive probes. In contrast with filter techniques, in situ hybridization can be applied to fixed tissue and allows localization of infected cells. This allows their morphology to be studied, and archived specimens can be examined. However, it is not as sensitive as filter hybridization, cannot detect latent infections, and is not well suited for typing HPV-DNA.

DNA Hybrid Capture

DNA hybrid capture (Digene Hybrid Capture® System) is a new-generation hybridization assay that can detect nucleic acid targets directly. It is a signal amplification assay using antibody capture and chemiluminescent signal detection. An alkaline solution is added to the specimen, which disrupts the virus (the method can also be applied to bacteria), releasing the target DNA. The target DNA combines with specific RNA probes, forming RNA-DNA "hybrids." (Currently, the high-risk probe include: HPV 16, 18, 31, 33, 35, 39, 45, 51, 52, 56, 58, 59, and 68; the low-risk probe include: 6,

I i, 42, 43, and 44.) Multiple RNA-DNA hybrids are "captured" on a solid phase (tube or microtiter plate) with universal capture antibodies specific for RNA-DNA hybrids. Captured RNA-DNA hybrids are labeled for detection using multiple antibodies conjugated to alkaline phosphatase. The resulting signal can be amplified at least 3000 times. The bound alkaline phosphatase is detected with a chemiluminescent dioxetane substrate, which when cleaved by alkaline phosphatase, produces light that is measured with a luminometer in relative light units (RLUs). The amount of light emitted is proportional to the amount of target nucleic acid in the specimen. The results are nearly as specific as Southern blot and nearly as sensitive as PCR [S Anderson 2001, Clavel 1998]. The FDA-approved cut-off value is I pg HPV-DNA/mL, which corresponds to about 5,000 viral copies. This cut-off has a high sensitivity for detecting H SIL and cancer. However, women with fewer than 5,000 viral copies will test negative for HPV. Also, women with viral types not included in the probes will test negative.

Polymerase Chain Reaction

Believe it or not, some HPV genotypes are patented. (What were the bureaucrats at the Patent Office thinking? But it raises an interesting question: If someone "owns" an HPV strain, are they responsible for any injuries or death it may cause? If your dog bites, you're responsible! PS: I hereby formally claim a share of all resulting legal compensation!) The law prohibits commercial use of these proprietary sequences unless the patent holder grants a license. Unfortunately for women, a business enterprise holds exclusive rights to many high-risk HPV sequences; this has limited commercialization of HPV tests intended for in vitro diagnostic use. However, in 2002, in what one hopes will become a trend, HPV intellectual property was transferred to the owners of polymerase chain reaction (PCR) technology. PCR holds great promise for HPV testing [Hubbard 2003].

Polymerase chain reaction, which uses enzymatic DNA amplification, is currently the most sensitive method of HPV detection. This technology can also be used for viral load quantitation, DNA sequencing, and mutation analysis [Hubbard 2003]. The method is a target amplification system, based on the identification of a region of DNA to be amplified. The exact nucleotide sequence must be known. However, the most widely used PCR methods use "consensus" (generic) primers that amplify the L1 HPV gene; this gene is almost identical among HPV types and therefore, this method can identify almost all anogenital HPV infections with a single test. The amplified DNA can then be further analyzed, using gel electrophoresis or hybridization methods, to determine the specific type(s) of HPV.

In performing PCR, heat is used to denature the DNA into two chains. Automated successive cycles amplify the target DNA. This is followed by hybridization with primers to the selected DNA. Each cycle includes primer extension, denaturation, and reannealing, using a heat stable DNA polymerase. The cycles can be repeated multiple times, producing enough DNA for Southern blot analysis. By selecting specific primers, new types of HPV can be identified; by selecting common primers, the presence of HPV can be documented without specific identification. PCR is simple, rapid, and extremely sensitive. In theory, PCR is capable of detecting a single viral particle in 1,000,000 (10^6) cells [Anonymous 1989a, A Schneider 1989a]. In practice, however, the sensitivity is 10-100 virions per sample. Unfortunately, the extreme sensitivity of the method makes it prone to false-positive diagnoses due to contamination, which diminishes specificity, if proper precautions are not taken [Tidy 1998a].

Summary

Standard methods of detection of HPV infection fail to find viral DNA in 5%-10% of invasive cancers [F Bosch 1995, Lombard 1998, zur Hausen 2002], 10%-15% of H SILs, and 20%-30% of L SILs [Bergeron 1992, Lörincz 1992, Lombard 1998]. However, false-negative results can occur owing to methodological problems or presence of viral types not yet identified [Crum 1998, deVilliers 2001, Walboomers 1997]. Using more powerful research tools, such as PCR, HPV is detected in almost, but not quite, 100% of cervical cancers [Walboomers 1999], including rare types [Matthews–Greer 2004]. Most women who test positive for HPV-DNA have no cytologic or histologic abnormalities [F Bosch 1995, Burrows 1990, Lombard 1998, Rozendaal 1996, Walboomers 1997]. Although some of these may represent false-positive results, most are true-positive interpretations in women with latent infections.

Low-Risk and High-Risk HPV

HPVs that infect anogenital cells are divided into low-risk and high-risk types. "Low-risk" and "high-risk" were defined *retrospectively*, ie, certain viral types are more commonly found in cancer, ergo, "high risk," and some are rarely if ever found in cancer, ergo, "low risk." Prospectively, *all* HPV types are low-risk because very few infections (<1%) develop into cancer; thus, from a clinical perspective, "high-risk" is a misnomer [Richart 1998]. (Everything's relative.)

Practically all (90%-99⁺%) neoplastic lesions of the cervix, from L SIL to cancer, are associated with HPV [de Roda Husman 1994, A Schneider 1987c, Walboomers 1999]. All anogenital HPVs can induce low-grade lesions (which correlate with productive infection), because this is necessary for viral replication; these low-grade lesions are common. However, only a few "high-risk" types of HPV are associated with H SILs and cancers; these lesions are relatively rare.

"Low-risk" viral types, eg, HPV 6 and 11, are unlikely to integrate into the host genome or be associated with cancer. Less than 1% (0.15%) of cervical cancers have only "low-risk" virus [F Bosch 1995, Ngelangel 1998, Walboomers 1999, T Wright 2002b]. "High-risk" viral types, eg, HPV 16 and 18, are more likely to integrate and be associated with high-grade dysplasia and cancer [J Nelson 1989, zur Hausen 1987] (although virus is not integrated in every cancer). It is now known that only the E6 and E7 genes of high-risk, or oncogenic, virotypes are able to immortalize cells and cause neoplastic changes [zur Hausen 2002]. Although any of the HPVs that infect the female genital tract, including both low-risk and high-risk types, can cause low-grade SILs [Ambros 1990], it has turned out that most (>80% of cases) L SILs are actually caused by "high-risk" viruses [Adam 1998, 2000, Anonymous 2000, Bergeron 1992, Franquemont 1989, Nuovo 2000, Stoler 2000b, G Willett 1989]. Moreover, high-risk HPV is frequently present in the genital tract of apparently healthy women with normal Pap tests [Meanwell 1987, Murdoch 1988, Tidy 1989a, L Young 1989]. However, women with high-risk viruses are more likely than women with low-risk viruses to have abnormal Pap tests [Nuovo 1991b].

About 30% of CIN I lesions (L SIL) contain more than one type of virus. CIN 2 is a gray area [Schiffman 1995b]. Although high-risk virus is present in most CIN 2 lesions, some contain viral types not found in cancer (low-risk virus) [F Bosch 1995, Lörincz 1992]. However, practically all CIN 3 lesions and cervical cancers contain high-risk viral types. In cancer, multiple HPVs, including mixtures of both high- and low-risk types, have been found within a single neoplasm [Griffin 1990], and rarely, invasive carcinomas are associated with only low-risk HPV types.

The prognosis for invasive cancers of the uterine cervix correlates with the oncogenic potential of the associated HPV type. Women with HPV

16, and particularly 18, have significantly poorer prognosis than those with HPV 31, 33, 35, and others [*L–W Huang 2003, Lombard 1998, Nakagawa 1996, Zuna 2004*]. However, viral type is not by itself completely predictive of biologic behavior. (Note: HPV testing is not recommended for triage of women with SIL on Pap test, although viral type can facilitate management of women with ASC-US, see pg 200 [*Anonymous 2000*].)

HPV 6 and 11 are prototypical low-risk viruses that primarily cause anogenital warts and L SILs, but are rarely found in H SIL or cancer. Other low risk viral types include 40, 42, 43, 44, 54, 61, 70, 72, 81, and CP6108.

Human Papilloma Virus

Low risk: Rarely found in cancer

    6, 11; also 40, 42, 43, 44,

    54, 61, 70, 72, 81, CP6108.

High risk: Commonly found in cancer

    16, 18; also 31, 33, 35, 39, 45,

    51, 52, 56, 58, 59, 68, 73, 82

Prospectively: all low–risk

HPV 16 and 18 are prototypical high-risk viruses that are commonly found in cancer; other high-risk viral types include: 31, 33, 35, 39, 45, 51, 52, 56, 58, 59, 68, 73, and 82 [*Muñoz 2003, Wolf 2003*]. Types 26, 53, and 66 are probably carcinogenic. Together, four HPV types (6, 11, 16, 18) account for about two-thirds of all anogenital squamous lesions.

HPV 16 is the most common viral type to infect the cervix, and is associated with a whole spectrum of lesions, ranging from genital warts to L SIL to H SIL to invasive carcinomas, including squamous and, less commonly, glandular cancers. HPV 16 accounts for most (>50%) cervical cancers, followed by HPV 18 (~15%), HPV 45 (~10%), and HPV 31 (~5%) (thus, these four viral types, HPV 16, 18, 45, and 31, account for four-out-of-five cervical cancers) [*F Bosch 1995, Hernandez–Avila 1997, Herrero 1999, Lörincz 1992, Shah 1997, Schiffman 2003a*]. Keratinizing SCC is usually associated with HPV 16; nonkeratinizing SCC is associated with multiple high-risk viral types [*Zehbe 1997*].

HPV 18 is more commonly associated with nonsquamous cancers (particularly cervical adenocarcinoma) and aggressive biologic behavior [*R Burger 1996, Crum 1995, Tase 1988, Nakagawa 1996, Wilczynski 1988a, b*]. In squamous lesions, HPV 18 seems to "short circuit" the sequence of progression: HPV 18 associated lesions may invade directly from low-grade SILs (ie, mild dysplasia) [*Arends 1993, 1998, Beaudenon 1986, Bergeron 1987, Brescia 1986, Fuchs 1988, Gissmann 1983, Kadish 1992, Koutsky 1988, Kurman 1988, Lörincz 1987a, b, 1992, Lutzner 1983, JS Park 1991, R Reid 1987, Wilczynski 1988a, G Willett 1989, CB Woodman 2003, T Wright 1990*]. HPV 18 is relatively commonly identified in L SIL, but is uncommonly found in H SIL [*Kadish 1992, McLachlin 1994, 1997*]. Although HPV 18 may occur in squamous cell carcinoma, it is the most common HPV type in adenocarcinomas and small cell neuroendocrine carcinomas [*Crum 1995, Nakagawa 1996, Stoler 1991*]. In HPV 18-associated cancers, the viral genome is invariably integrated (vs episomal) [*Cullen 1991, Crum 1995*]. Rapidly progressive cervical cancers probably occur, and these more aggressive cancers are often associated with HPV 18 [*Barnes 1988, 1990, Nakagawa 1996*]. HPV 18 positivity is a risk factor for recurrence of cervical cancer after therapy [*Rose 1995*]. Women with HPV-18 positive cervical cancers are more likely than others to have recently negative Pap tests [*Bjersing 1991, J Walker 1989, CB Woodman 2003*].

HPV has now been found in all major types of cervical cancer, including not only squamous cell carcinoma, but also adenocarcinoma (in situ, invasive, and metastatic) [*Smotkin 1986, Tase 1989a, Walboomers 1987, Wilczynski 1988a, b*], adenosquamous carcinoma, including glassy cell carcinoma [*Smotkin 1986*], small cell neuroendocrine carcinoma [*Stoler 1991*], and metastases [*Lancaster 1986, Nagai 2001*] and recurrences [*Holloway 1991*] of cervical cancer.

Molecular Biology of HPV

The physical state of the virus in the cell (ie, episomal or integrated) is important in the clinical outcome. When the viral DNA is free in the nucleus (extrachromosomal or episomal), full viral expression and productive infection can occur: ie, complete virions are produced in association with koilocyte formation (condyloma). The morphology (flat, warty) depends on the degree of maturation of the infected epithelium; koilocytosis and complete virus production require mature cells—the lesions are well-differentiated. These low-grade lesions usually regress without therapy, but some persist or progress. When the viral DNA is integrated into the host genome (into the "immortal" basal/reserve cell), the viral DNA is not fully expressed, although it remains present, perhaps for the life of the woman (latent infection). In advanced dysplasia, with little squamous maturation, koilocytes are not formed, and complete virions are not produced (nonproductive infection)—the lesions are poorly-differentiated. High-grade lesions are more likely to persist or progress than low-grade lesions.

The Viral Genome

The viral genome consists of circular, doubled-stranded DNA, of about 7,900 base pairs. This modest amount of DNA contains the information necessary to code for all viral gene products, including proteins that transiently control host cell proliferation and differentiation, as well as for structural proteins that make up the viral capsid. The viral genome is divided into three regions: a noncoding region, and a coding region, with early and late genes. Early and late refer to the time in the viral life cycle when the genes are expressed.

The *noncoding region* (NCR) is also known as the long control region (LCR) or upstream regulatory region (URR) [*F Chang 1990*]. The noncoding region is short (~1,000 base pairs). It contains DNA sequences for the major promoter of viral transcription (p97 in HPV 16) and is important in regulating viral replication. This region may be involved in tissue tropism, through interaction with transcription factors found in specific tissue types.

The *coding region* contains six early and two late open reading frames (ORFs) without stop codons. RNA polymerase reads the ORFs as specific units, analogous to genes, during transcription. The early region is about 4,500 base pairs, with up to eight genes encoding non-structural regulatory gene products (E1-E8). However, E3 and E8 are present in only a minority of papillomaviruses and their functions are currently unknown [*Sandemente 2002*]. The late region is about 2,500 base pairs, with two genes encoding two structural capsid proteins (L1, L2) [*Richart 1998, Wolf 2001*].

The early genes are involved in viral replication and oncogenesis. Early gene products are probably transcribed before DNA replication. E1 codes for proteins involved in maintenance and replication of the viral genome. E2 codes for two DNA binding proteins that interact with the upstream region and regulate viral transcription. E4 encodes proteins that bind and disrupt cytokeratin, producing classic koilocytes [*Sandemente 2002*]. E4 is most highly expressed in well-differentiated cells [*Stoler 2000a*]. E5 could be involved in malignant transformation; it stimulates cell cycle progression by upregulating

---

Early Viral Genes

    Viral replication, oncogenesis

    E1: Maintenance, replication viral genome

    E2: DNA binding proteins that

        regulate viral transcription

    E4: Viral function?; Binds, disrupts host–

        Cytokeratin → koilocytes

        Cell membrane → viral particles escape

    E5: Transformation, lost with integration

---

epidermal growth factor receptor, which is essential to progress through the G1 phase of the cell cycle [McCance 1998]. However, E5 is often lost when the virus in integrated, so its actual role in carcinogenesis is uncertain [Stoler 2000a].

E6 and E7, as discussed below, are essential in carcinogenesis. They are involved in regulating viral gene expression and regulation, and can recruit the host enzymatic machinery. They also encode proteins that control host cell mitosis and differentiation [McGlennen 2000]. E6 and E7 of oncogenic HPVs code for proteins that can transform and immortalize cells, properties necessary for malignant transformation [McGlennen 2000, Münger 1993]. E6 and E7 are the only genes that are found in all HPV-associated diseases, from condylomas to SILs to cancer. Taken together, these proteins, E6, E7, and possibly E5, can stimulate cells into S-phase of the cell cycle [McCance 1998]. Viral protein can also interfere with the mitotic spindle apparatus, and particularly with high-risk viral types, lead to abnormal mitotic figures.

E6 & E7 Viral Genes

  Key in carcinogenesis:

  ·*Involved in gene expression, regulation*

  ·*Recruit host enzyme machinery*

  ·*Can disrupt cell cycle*

  ·*Interact with p53, RB, respectively*

  Only genes found in all HPV disease

The late genes, L1 and L2, code for the major and minor viral capsid proteins, respectively, that form the protein coat of the virus. These structural proteins are required for viral infection. L1 major capsid protein is highly immunogenic; this protein is similar in all papillomaviruses [Crum 1998]. The L1 antigen is frequently used for HPV typing and encodes the common papillomavirus antigen that is the target of many monoclonal antibody detection systems [Jacobs 1997]. L2 minor capsid protein appears to be involved in assembly of the virion, but may also play a role in cell surface receptor specificity. L2 protein varies greatly among viral types, largely accounting for differences in antigenicity. Because they are expressed late, L1 and L2 probably do not play a role in malignant transformation of infected cells.

Late Viral Genes

  L1: Codes for major capsid protein

  L2: Codes for minor capsid protein

   Proteins required for infection

  L1 highly antigenic, ~identical all types

  L2 viral assembly, varies greatly

  Late genes not involved carcinogenesis

Viral gene expression is usually tightly linked to host cell differentiation. Early genes are expressed in the basal cell layers and late genes are expressed in differentiated intermediate to superficial cell layers. Consequently, in well-differentiated squamous lesions, such as condyloma and mild dysplasia (L SIL), many late (capsid) proteins are present. In poorly-differentiated squamous lesions, such as severe dysplasia/carcinoma in situ (advanced forms of H SIL), there is little or no capsid protein and few whole virions. Note, however, that L SILs and H SILs can co-exist in the cervix.

Life Cycle of HPV

The life cycle of the papillomavirus is unique. It differs from all other known viruses in that infection requires epithelial cells still capable of cell division [zur Hausen 2002]. In the cervix, HPV infects the basal/reserve cell of immature metaplastic epithelium in the transformation zone, with α6β4 integrin (a cell surface protein) possibly acting as a receptor [Alani 1998, Evander 1997]. It is believed that microtrauma during intercourse enhances the chances of HPV gaining access to these cells [Ferenczy 1996b, A Schneider 1992b]. HPV can remain in the basal/reserve cell as low copy number episomal viral genomes (50-100 episomes per cell), replicated only once per cell cycle [McMurray 2001]. These infected cells can provide a reservoir of virus in morphologically *normal* looking cells. Episomal replication is tightly linked to epithelial differentiation, and only occurs in concert with host cell DNA replication. Limited expression of specific early genes, such as E5, E6, and E7, results in enhanced proliferation of the infected cells and their lateral expansion. Complete virions are not formed, but HPV-DNA can be detected using molecular techniques [T Wright 1990]. The virus is usually cleared in a year or two, but can persist in this stable episomal state for extended periods of time. This is nonproductive, or latent, infection.

For reasons currently unknown, but possibly related to the host immune response, a latent infection can change into a productive infection, in which viral DNA replication occurs independently of host DNA replication and complete virions are produced. In productive infection, as the basal cell starts to differentiate and enters the parabasal cell layer, late genes begin to be expressed. The viral genome is replicated and structural proteins form. In the upper layers of the epithelium, abundant complete infectious viral particles are assembled. Also, a specific cytopathic effect, koilocyte formation, occurs in the intermediate to superficial cell layers. Infectious cells are sloughed from the surface.

HPV can also infect glandular epithelium [Farnsworth 1989, Higgins 1992, Tase 1988], neuroendocrine cells, or possibly a multipotential stem cell [Crum 2000]. The following discussion applies primary to squamous cell carcinoma. Adenocarcinomas and neuroendocrine carcinomas are considered separately.

HPV in Cervical Carcinogenesis

Oncogenic human papillomaviruses cause cervical cancer and may be associated with other cancers (including some carcinomas, lymphomas, melanomas), particularly carcinomas of the head & neck, and possibly some lung cancers [Y Chen 2004, Herrero 2003, Lazo 1999]. Cervical cancer is undoubtedly one of the most intensively studied and best understood human malignancies.

Two host proteins are particularly important in regulating normal cell division: retinoblastoma (Rb) protein and p53 [Wolf 2003]. Two viral gene products, E6 and E7, bind and inactivate these two regulatory proteins, causing the cell to reproduce without restraint. The cell literally grows wild, and as it does, it accumulates more damaged DNA that cannot be repaired. The accumulated genetic mutations eventually turn the abnormally proliferating cell into a cancer cell.

Cervical intraepithelial neoplasia is a common and early manifestation of HPV infection (average, 4 to 24 months) and invasive cervical cancer is a rare and late manifestation of HPV (average, 10 to 20, or even 30 years) [CB Woodman 2001, Xi 2002]. HPV, like many other DNA viruses, replicates by interfering with the normal cell cycle control mechanisms [Crum 2000]. Damage to the DNA of a cell ordinarily induces cell cycle arrest, DNA repair or apoptosis (programmed cell death). Two viral proteins, E6 and E7, are essential to the oncogenic effects of high-risk HPVs [von Knebel Doeberitz 1988]. E6 and E7 oncoproteins can disrupt the cell cycle by interacting with host regulatory genes and their proteins, such as the retinoblastoma gene and *p53*, respectively, that normally suppress cell growth. This impairs the ability of the cell to repair DNA damage, resulting in genetic instability and accumulation of genetic defects. The molecular mechanisms that ultimately result in malignant transformation of the cell are being elucidated and have been extensively reviewed [Alani 1998, Arends 1998, Beutner 1997b, Campo 1998, G Dell 2001, Garland 2002, Jin 2001, Kaufman 2000, Lazo 1999, McGlennen 2000, McLachlin 2000, Milde–Langosch 2000, Sedlacek 1999, S Southern 1998, MA Stanley 2001, Vernon 1998, Villa 1997, Wolf 2001, zur Hausen 2000].

Integration of viral genetic material into the host genome is a critical event in carcinogenesis [K Cooper 1997, Ho 1995, TW Park 1995]. Viral integration appears to induce aneuploidy [*Waggoner 1990*]. Integration is accompanied by a morphologic change from low-grade to high-grade cervical intraepithelial neoplasia with increasing cytologic atypia, disorganization, and abnormal mitotic figures [*Richart 1990*]. Integration of HPV genome occurs in different human chromosomes, but usually into regions that contain highly transcribed genes important for cell viability [*Klimov 2002*]. The entire HPV genome need not be integrated; however, integration of the E6 and E7 genes is critical in carcinogenesis. Cells that contain integrated viral genome have a selective growth advantage over cells containing non-integrated HPV-DNA, leading to further proliferation and dedifferentiation of cells with integrated HPV-DNA [*G Dell 2001, Milde–Langosch 2000*]. This growth advantage is thought to be due to overexpression of E6 and E7 oncoproteins.

Viral DNA is usually not integrated into the host genome in low-grade squamous intraepithelial lesions [*Lehn 1988*]. In contrast, in high-grade lesions and squamous cell carcinoma (and adenocarcinomas [*K Cooper 1992*]), the viral DNA is usually [*Lehn 1988*], but not always [*Dürst 1985*], integrated. Up to 25% of HPV 16 associated carcinomas contain only nonintegrated extrachromosomal (episomal) viral DNA [*Cullen 1991, Matsukuma 1989*], whereas the virus is usually integrated in HPV 18, 31, and 35 associated carcinomas [*W Hall 1997, Lombard 1998, Pirami 1997*]. Integration of HPV-DNA into the host chromosome makes the infection irreversible. A significant number of H SILs progress to cancer if left untreated, although this may require several years or even decades [*Schiffman 1995a*]. HPV oncoproteins can disrupt the cell cycle in ways analogous to functions already known for SV40 and adenovirus [*S Southern 1998*].

Integration consistently disrupts the viral genome at the E1-E2 region [*Tidy 1989b*]. This interrupts the life cycle of the virus, and thus complete virions are not formed (nonproductive infection). So, for the virus, integration is a biologic dead end, although it guarantees perpetual expression of viral oncogenes [*Crum 2000*]. Viral integration inactivates the E2 gene. The E2 protein suppresses E6 and E7 oncogenes that control viral growth; therefore, inactivation of E2 results in uncontrolled expression of E6 and E7 genes [*Tidy 1989b*]. Loss of E2, with overexpression of E6 and E7, is the first stage in transformation.

E6 and E7, key factors in cervical carcinogenesis, are consistently expressed in malignant cells, and inhibiting their expression blocks the malignant phenotype [*zur Hausen 2002*]. E6 and E7 code for proteins that bind, respectively, the gene products of p53 [*Werness 1990*] and retinoblastoma (Rb) genes [*Dyson 1989, Münger 1989a,b*], which are important tumor suppressors. The E6 and E7 proteins of various HPV types have varying efficiency in transformation: those of HPV 16 and HPV 18 are highly potent in oncogenic transformation, whereas those from HPV 6 and HPV 11 are incapable of binding or inactivating p53 or Rb [*Crook 1991a, Heck 1992*].

E6 binding of p53 targets this tumor suppressor for rapid degradation via an ubiquitin-dependent pathway. This mimics the biological effect of p53 genetic mutation [*Inman 1993*]. (There may be some very rare cervical cancers in which actual p53 mutation occurs [*Crook 1991b, 1992, Tsuda 2003*].) Loss of p53 prevents p21 inhibition of cyclin dependent kinases and also prevents p53-dependent apoptosis. Loss of p53-mediated apoptosis is an important event in tumor progression. With loss of p53, popularly known as the "guardian of the genome," genetic lesions accumulate [*D Lane 1992*]. Protein p53 monitors cells as they progress through the cell cycle (G1) and if there is a problem, such as DNA damage that is likely to disrupt a normal cell cycle, it will stop cells in G1 until the problem is resolved. Thus, loss of p53 may allow genetically damaged cells to reproduce with gradual accumulation of mutated genes [*McCance 1998*]. Low-risk and high-risk viral types have different effects on p53 and p21 expression [*Giannoudis 2000*].

E7 binds and inactivates the retinoblastoma (Rb) protein, which frees E2F, a potent transcription factor, to bind to DNA and induce cell proliferation and growth. E2F apparently can override the inhibitory function of the Rb protein and stimulate the host replication machinery [*McCance 1998*]. This leads to accelerated cell cycle progression and proliferation. E6 and E7 cooperate in inducing tumor formation [*S Song 2000*].

You ain't heard nuthin' yet…

The picture is still more complicated and new details are being learned all the time [*Alani 1998, Milde–Langosch 2000, S Syrjänen 1999*]. E6 oncoprotein binds to p53 protein via another cellular protein (p100) and targets it for degradation via an ubiquitin-dependent pathway. E6 also interacts with the pro-apoptotic protein, Bax, which results in resistance to apoptosis (programmed cell death) and increased chromosomal instability [*S Jackson 2000, Kokawa 1999*]. In addition, the E6 oncoprotein activates telomerase, resulting in immortalization of infected cells [*Gorham 1997, Kawai 1998, Klingelhutz 1996, Nowak 2000, S Riethdorf 2001, Veldman 2001, P–S Zheng 2000*], and may inhibit degradation of SRC-family kinases, which contributes to the HPV-transformed phenotype [*Oda 1999*]. (SRC stands for sarcoma; src protein was the first tyrosine kinase to be discovered.) The cyclin dependent kinase inhibitor, p16 (also known as INK4a, or p16^{INK4a}), seems to counteract these functions and decelerate the cell cycle [*Sano 1998, zur Hausen 2002*].

E7 oncoprotein prevents the retinoblastoma protein from binding to the host transcription factor, E2F. E2F is then free to bind host cell promoters, thereby activating transcription of genes, like c-myc, whose proteins cause the cell to divide. High E2F activity may also lead to apoptosis in E7 expressing cells. E7 oncoprotein stimulates the cyclin A and cyclin E, S-phase genes that are important regulators of cell cycle progression [*Schulze 1998, Vogt 1999, Zerfass 1995*]. It also seems to inhibit the function of cyclin–dependent kinase inhibitors, p21/WAF1 and p27/KIP1, blocking their binding to cyclins, disrupting cell cycle control [*Funk 1997, DL Jones 1997, Zerfass–Thome 1996*]. By inducing centriole amplification, which leads to abnormal mitoses, E7 also induces aneuploidy of E7-expressing cells, which contributes to tumorigenesis [*Duensing 2001*]. E7 oncoprotein also upregulates INK4a (p16) [*Dyson 1989, Kiyono 1998*].

E6 and E7 are cell-transforming genes that target tumor suppressor genes, p53 and RB, thereby escaping cellular growth regulation. E6 and E7 can immoralize cells independently [*Band 1990, Halbert 1991*], but work synergistically with increased efficiency. But nowhere is it written in the Bible that E6 seems to be impaired by INK4a, whereas E7 bypasses this inhibition and directly activates cyclins A and E. E6, in turn, prevents E7-induced apoptosis by degrading the apoptosis-inducing proteins, p53 and BAX [*M Thomas 1998, Zerfass 1995*]. Progesterone and glucocorticoids may also facilitate transcription of E6 and E7 [*W Chan 1989, Villa 1997*].

A common polymorphism of the p53 amino-acid sequence results in the presence of either a proline or an arginine at position 72. The arginine form of p53 is significantly more susceptible than the proline form to E6 mediated degradation. It has been reported that cervical cancers, including adenocarcinomas, are more common in women who are homozygous for arginine-72 p53 compared with heterozygotes [*Storey 1998, Y–C Yang 2001*]. Note, however, these findings have been questioned [*Inserra 2003, Klaes 1999*].

High-risk HPV infection results in substantial upregulation of p16 (INK4A), which although functionally inactive (because E7 induces cyclin A and E, bypassing its interference in the cell cyle), can be readily detected in cells and tissues using immunocytochemistry. Because p16 (INK4A) overexpression is a specific marker for dysplastic and neoplastic cells, and can be demonstrated using immunocytochemical techniques, this could provide a new approach to screening for high-risk HPV infections and cervical cancer, including adenocarcinoma [Bibbo 2002, 2003, Keating 2001a,b, Klaes 2001, McCluggage 2002, N Murphy 2003, Pientong 2003, 2004, Sahebali 2003, Saqi 2002, Trunk 2004]. Note that p16 is diffusely expressed in endometrium and focally in tubo-endometrial metaplasia [L Riethdorf 2002].

In a significant minority of cervical cancers (possibly 25%), the HPV 16 virus is not integrated, but present as an episome [Pirami 1997]. In cancers with episomal HPV, mutations of ying yang 1 [I'm not making this up] (YY1) silencer elements within the regulatory region are frequent. YY1 elements are binding sites for the transcription factor YY1, which regulates a large number of genes. Mutations of YY1 elements that abolish its binding can greatly enhance E6/E7 oncogene expression [May 1994, Milde-Langosch 2000].)

Viral Carcinogenesis

Key event: viral integration

Disrupts, inactivates E2 gene

→ overexpression E6, E7

E6 & E7 inactivate tumor suppressors

p53 & Rb, respectively

→ accelerated cell cycle progression, and

cellular proliferation

Finally, it has never been clear why L SILs are common, H SILs are unusual, and cancers are rare, but mutations of *ras* oncogenes may be involved [Alonio 2003, Rincón-Arano 2003, Soh 2002, Stenzel 2001].

To summarize briefly: viral integration is a key event in carcinogenesis. With integration, the HPV gene, E2, is disrupted and inactivated. This leads to overexpression of E6 and E7. E6 and E7 bind and inactivate tumor suppressors, p53 and Rb, respectively, which results in accelerated cell cycle progression and cellular proliferation.

Molecular Model of Cervical Carcinogenesis

A possible molecular model of HPV-mediated cervical carcinogenesis has been proposed [F1.20] [Stoler 1996, 2000a, 2003a]. HPV infects germinal basal/reserve cells in the transformation zone. In most cases, the virus is maintained at low levels (latent infection) and then is eradicated, but in some cases, lesions develop.

Germinal cells are the only cells normally capable of division; differentiated cells cannot divide. These germinal cells are also pluripotential and capable of differentiating along squamous, glandular, or neuroendocrine lines. The following model is for squamous carcinogenesis, but it is possible that something similar happens in adenocarcinomas and neuroendocrine carcinomas [M Parker 1997].

Low-Grade Squamous Intraepithelial Lesion

Productive HPV gene expression is tightly linked to cell differentiation, and is only permitted in differentiated cells that do not divide. The result of the host-virus interaction in differentiated cells is L SIL, the only source of infectious virions (productive infection). Koilocytotic changes often occur, but are not obligatory [Milde-Langosch 2000]. These well-differentiated lesions usually regress within a year or two, but can persist for a long time.

The cytomorphology of L SIL is characterized by mature (differentiated) cells, with nuclear atypia consisting of enlargement and hyperchromasia, and koilocyte formation. At the molecular level, the nuclear atypia is probably caused by E6, E7-driven host DNA synthesis. Viral DNA alone is inadequate to account for the relatively marked nuclear changes. Koilocyte formation may be related to the E4 protein, some forms of which can bind and disrupt the keratin apparatus forming cytoplasmic vacuoles [Stoler 2000a].

High-Grade Squamous Intraepithelial Lesion

High-grade SILs probably develop within low-grade SILs by clonal expansion of atypical cells with increasingly undifferentiated phenotype and high

F1.20 Molecular Model of Cervical Carcinogenesis

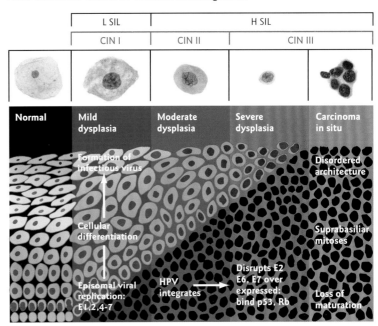

L SIL: The virus infects the basal/reserve cell. There is episomal viral replication with expression of early genes. As the infected cells differentiate, and enter the parabasal cell layers, late genes begin to be expressed, with eventual formation of infectious virions released at the mucosal surface. Koilocytes, the characteristic cytopathic effect, may be seen in the intermediate to superficial cell layers.

H SIL: Viral integration is a key event in carcinogenesis. This consistently disrupts E2, resulting in overexpression of E6/E7, which bind and inactivate p53 and Rb. With these tumor suppressors inactivated, there is loss of maturation, increased proliferation with suprabasalar mitoses, and disordered architecture, the morphologic expression of H SIL.

proliferative potential [Milde-Langosch 2000]. H SILs are monoclonal lesions that harbor high-risk HPV types in almost all (>90%) cases. The main molecular difference from L SIL is the high expression of E6 and E7 in H SIL [Milde-Langosch 2000].

The cytomorphology of H SIL is characterized by immature cells and evidence of increased proliferation. With progression to H SIL, the linkage between cellular differentiation and early viral gene expression is lost, resulting in cellular proliferation of basaloid cells. Viral integration disrupts E2, allowing uncontrolled expression of E6 and E7 oncogenes in cells that can still divide. E6/E7 can also prevent cellular differentiation. Inhibited cellular differentiation and increased proliferation results in morphologic progression to H SIL. Interestingly, these changes only become apparent after several generations, mimicking the long natural history of CIN [Stoler 2000a].

And On to Cancer

Cervical cancer cells are usually characterized by viral integration, high E6/E7 gene expression, disruption of cellular control mechanisms, and accumulation of additional genetic defects, leading to aneuploidy [Bollmann 2003a, Milde-Langosch 2000]. Aneuploidy correlates with malignant potential [Bibbo 1989b, Böcking 1986, Bollmann 2003a, JR Davis 1989, Fu 1981, 1983, 1989, Hanselaar 1988, 2001, Hering 2000, Kurtycz 1996, Mourits 1992, R Reid 1984a,b, Watts 1987, Wilbanks 1967, G Willett 1989]. L SIL is rarely aneuploid (<5% of cases), while H SIL is usually aneuploid (~80% of cases) [Bollmann 2001]. Aneuploidy puts a woman at high risk, even if the lesion appears to be L SIL [Boone 1992, Fu 1981, Lungu 1992]. Abnormal mitotic figures, probably caused by disordered mitosis [Richart 1973], are excellent markers of aneuploidy [Bergeron 1987, Fu 1988, Hering 2000, Winkler 1984]. Oncogenic HPV types are associated with abnormal mitoses [Crum 1984b].

Proliferating cells, such as those of H SILs, are at increased risk of acquiring further genetic errors, perhaps related to cigarette smoking , host factors, oral contraceptives, parity, other sexually transmitted diseases, nutrition, etc [Franco 2001, Herrington 1995a,b, Popescu 1990a,b]. This could account for the importance of other risk factors in cervical carcinogenesis. Another possible viral factor is naturally occurring sequence variation within viral types that alters its biological properties [Etherington 1999, Giannoudis 2001, Hildesheim 2001, Lizano 1997, Xi 1997, 2002, Zehbe 1998]. As with HPV types, HPV variants may differ in incidence and outcome of infection.

Chromosomal abnormalities, such as 3q amplification [Heselmeyer 1996] and 3p deletions [J Rader 1996] may be important in the transition from in situ to invasive carcinoma [Shah 1997, Silverberg 1999, Wolf 2001]. Loss of heterozygosity at chromosome 3p (specifically 3p14-25), has been found in as many as 70% of cervical cancers and about 30% to 60% of precursor lesions, suggesting this may be an early event in carcinogenesis [T Chu 1998, Huettner 1998, A Larson 1997a, Montgomery 1995, J Rader 1998, Wistuba 1997, Wolf 2001]. The tumor suppressor gene, a fragile histidine triad or FHIT, is located in this area of chromosome 3 (3p14.2) and may be disrupted [Hendricks 1997, A Larson 1997b, Vecchione 2001]. Microsatellites (repeating DNA sequences) may play a role in DNA repair; abnormalities could cause genetic instability [Kersemaekers 1998, Wistuba 1997, Wolf 2001]. Microsatellite instability has also been found in many cervical cancers [Ou 1999, Rha 2001]. Genital HPVs are unique among DNA viruses in requiring steroid hormones for their expression in infected tissue [McGlennen 2000]. It has long been known that dysplasia usually occurs in an estrogenic environment [Fraser 1967, Patten 1978, Rubio 1973].

Escape from immune surveillance is undoubtedly an important factor in progression to frankly invasive carcinoma [M Stanley 2001a,b]. Most women who develop lesions mount an effective cell mediated immune response, clear the virus, and the lesions regress. Localized delayed hypersensitivity, CD4+ lymphocytes, cytokines, including interleukin-12, cytotoxic T cells, NK cells, and Langerhans cells are probably all involved [Caorsi 1986, Connor 1999, McArdle 1986, H Morris 1983a,b, Sonnex 1998, Tay 1987a, Viac 1990]. Failure of the cell-mediated response could result in persistent infection. Humoral immunity can protect against subsequent viral challenge. Finally, Folkman reported that growth of solid tumors and their metastasis is dependent upon angiogenesis [Folkman 1971]; vascular endothelial growth factor in cervical cancer correlates well with local tumor progression and metastasis [W-F Cheng 1999].

HPV-Negative H SILs and Cancers?

The International Biological Study on Cervical Cancer reported detection of HPV in 99.7% of cervical cancers [Walboomers 1999]. Thus, HPV-negative cervical cancers and high-grade CINs are possible, though they would be very rare [Herrington 1999, Mittal 1995, Walboomers 1997, CB Woodman 2001]. It has been suggested that HPV-negative high-grade CIN, if it exists, has little malignant potential [Herrington 1999]. However, the risk of progression of high-grade CIN has not been shown to be different when HPV cannot be detected [Shah 1996]. There is additional support for the notion of HPV-negative H SILs and cancers. There appear to be some differences in risk factors for HPV-positive vs HPV-negative CIN [M Burger 1996, Krüger- Kjær 1999, Tabrizi 1999]. HPV-negative cancers may have a worse prognosis [Higgins 1991, Riou 1990]. Genetic mutation, eg, of the p53 oncogene, could account for HPV-negative tumors. Overexpression of cyclin D has been implicated in carcinomas [G Nichols 1996].

The PRAD 1 or bcl 1 oncogene, on chromosome 11q13, is activated by translocation, and is identical to cyclin D1 [S Southern 1998]. E7 protein has cyclin D-like activity, which overexpression of cyclin D could mimic.

Summary

The old concepts were that practically everyone was currently infected with anogenital HPVs and that low risk virus caused low-grade lesions, while high-risk virus caused high-grade lesions. The new concepts are that most sexually active women become infected at some point in their lives, but they usually clear their infections in 1 to 2 years, and by their mid-30s, most women are HPV negative (at least by currently available tests). It is not infection, per se, but rather,

> **HPV Summary**
> *Infects most sexually active women*
> *But usually clear 1-2 years*
> *By mid-30s, most negative*
> *HPV causes ~all cervical cancer*
> *Risk: Not infection, but persistence*
> *Most SILs due to high-risk virus*
> *Few SILs develop into cancer*
> *Cofactors probably important*

persistent infection, that is risky (owing to increased risk of viral integration) [Ellerbrock 2000, Hopman 2000]. The large majority of L SILs and practically all H SILs are associated with "high-risk" viral types, but relatively few SILs develop into cancer.

It is now accepted that HPV is a necessary cause of nearly all cases of cervical cancer [Chichareon 1998, Franco 1999, Stoler 2000a]. The evidence for this statement is compelling. As a transmissible agent, HPV fits the epidemiologic data that implicate multiple sexual partners and early onset of coitus in the development of the disease [Kjær 1996b, Schiffman 1993, K Syrjänen 1984]. HPV-DNA has been found in >90% of invasive cervical cancers worldwide [F Bosch 1995, Chichareon 1998, Ngelangel 1998], and using extremely sensitive techniques, in >99% of cases [Walboomers 1999]. On the other hand, HPV infection is very common, and cancers relatively rare, so there must be more to the story. In other words, there must be some other important co-factors in cervical carcinogenesis.

Possible Cofactors in Cervical Carcinogenesis

Human papillomavirus is a necessary, but not sufficient condition, for the development of cervical cancer [Bornstein 1995, Campo 1998, Franco 1999, Kadish 2001, R Reid 1989]. Why a cell progresses from latent infection to a clinically apparent lesion to invasive cancer is not known, but probably involves interaction with some cofactor(s) [Chichareon 1998, Kessler 1987, Ngelangel 1998]. The cofactors might, for example, cause an increase in the rate of integration of the HPV into the host genome or failure of the immune system.

> **Cofactors in Cervical Carcinogenesis**
> *Genetic susceptibility*
> *Host factors, eg, HLA type*
> *Immunosuppression*
> *Chromosomes*
> *Trauma*
> *Pregnancy*
> *Steroids*
> *Venereal disease*
> *Male factors*
> *Cigarette smoking*
> *Diet, including vitamins*

Genetic Susceptibility

The rare autosomal recessive disease, epidermodysplasia verruciformis, is associated with a defect in epithelial maturation and cellular immunity. In this disease, specific types of HPV produce multiple wart-like lesions on sun-exposed skin, that progress, in about one third of cases, to invasive cancers, after many years. This pattern (HPV infection, precursor lesion, cofactor[s], and time) is similar to the multistep development of cervical cancer, providing not only a model of the disease, but also suggesting that genetic predisposition may be a cofactor in its development [T Wright 1990]. Cervical cancer and its precursors can show significant familial clustering [Bender 1976, Brinton 1987b, Furgyik 1986, Magnusson 1999, 2000]. Genetic predisposition probably plays a role in susceptibility to HPV infection as well as persistence of infections [Lynch 1998]. Epidemiologic data indicate that genetic host factors contribute significantly to cancer risk [Magnusson 1999].

Host Factors

The human leukocyte antigen (HLA) system is critical in presenting peptides to antigen-specific T cell receptors. Certain HLA types, particularly the D locus, may be associated with susceptibility to cervical neoplasia [Apple 1994, 1995, Gostout 2003, Hilders 1994, Hildesheim 1998, Krul 1999, Madeleine 2002, Raju 1994, Torres 1993]. There is a significant association between HLA DQw3 and cervical neoplasia, possibly because these women are less able to mount an effective immunoresponse to HPV infection [David 1992, Mehal 1994, Wank 1991]. Permissiveness of the individual host cell may be a factor. Infection with various types of HPV is site specific (epitheliotropic). For example, HPV 11 proliferates better in foreskin and cervix than in other epithelia [Kreider 1987].

Immunologic Factors

Altered immune status is known to be important in some cases of cervical neoplasia [Hachisuga 2001, Laverty 1978]. Immune deficiency could theoretically facilitate infection in the first place, and also allow for escape of abnormal cells from immune surveillance. Cell-mediated and humoral immunity play important roles in human papillomavirus induced cervical neoplasia [M Stanley 2001a,b]. Langerhans cells are depleted in women with persistent cervical dysplasia [Fukuda 1993]. Cervical mucus immunoglobulin levels fluctuate during the menstrual cycle and in response to exogenous hormones [Franklin 1999]. Immunosuppressive drugs may themselves be carcinogenic.

Immunosuppressed women (eg, those with organ transplants [Alloub 1989, Busnach 1993, Ghazizadeh 2001, Halpert 1986, Kay 1970, Ozsaran 1999, Porreco 1975, V Schneider 1983], malignant lymphoma [R Katz 1987], systemic lupus erythematosis [Bateman 2000, Dhar 2001], or other immunosuppressive diseases or therapies [Shokri-Tabibzadeh 1981]) are at increased risk of HPV infections, which are also refractory to therapy [Krebs 1986]. Immunosuppressed women are also at increased risk of cervical neoplasia [Cerilli 1974, Porreco 1975, Sasadeusz 2001, V Schneider 1983] (as well as other malignancies) [A Evans 1990, Matas 1975].

Human immunodeficiency virus (HIV) infection is an independent risk factor for development of HPV-related cervical neoplasia [Adachi 1993, K Chin 1998, Heard 2000, MJ Henry 1989, Henry–Stanley 1993b, Kobayashi 2002, Kuhn 1999, Maiman 1990, 1991, Mandelblatt 1992b, Palefsky 1991, Petry 1994, Provencher 1988, Robinson 1996]. HIV infection is not only associated with a higher prevalence of cervical neoplasia, but the lesions also persist longer, progresses more rapidly, and are more refractory to therapy, than in women not infected with HIV [Branca 2000, Calore 1998, 2001, Duerr 2001, Ellerbrock 2000, Gallagher 2001, Ho 1994, Holcomb 1998, JC Johnson 1992, Y–C Lee 2000, Maiman 1990, 1991, 1998, Mayans 1999, Moodley 2001, Moscicki 2000, Robinson 2000, Rojansky 1996, X–W Sun 1997, Vermund 1991, ter Meulen 1992, AB Williams 1994, Womack 2000, T Wright 1994a,c]. Women with concurrent HIV and HPV infection have a mani-

fold increase risk of developing invasive cervical cancer [A Feingold 1990]. Factors besides depressed cellular immunity may be involved. HIV also alters the natural history of HPV infection, mirrored in a different molecular pathway, marked by microsatellite instability caused by interaction via viral proteins [B Clarke 2002]. In 1993, the Centers for Disease Control, added cervical cancer to the list of AIDS-defining illnesses in women with HIV infection [CDC 1993]. Pap tests may be less reliable in HIV seropositive women, underestimating the grade of lesions or missing them altogether [M Fink 1994, Fruchter 1994, Tweddel 1994, T Wright 1994a]; although, of course, false-negatives occur in both HIV-positive and HIV-negative populations [Adachi 1993, Korn 1994, Robinson 1997, Spinillo 1998, T Wright 1994a,c]. However, discrepancies have also been reported in non-HIV infected women who are immunosuppressed [Alloub 1989]. For these women, HPV-DNA testing may have a role in screening [Petry 1999]. This population should be screened carefully and managed aggressively [J Cohn 2001, Jay 2000, C Johnston 1996, Korn 2001, Robinson 1996, T Wright 1996].

Cervical carcinoma cells are known to be antigenic, expressing tumor-associated antigens [McCoy 1981]. In women with SILs, there is depletion of intraepithelial Langerhans (antigen presenting) cells, which may be the first line of host defense [Barton 1989a, Koutsky 1988, H Morris 1983a,b]. There are also fewer CD4+ helper lymphocytes and more CD8+ suppressor cells, resulting in a lower CD4+/CD8+ ratio [M Cardillo 2001, Koutsky 1988, Tay 1987b]. In addition, there is increased macrophage [Tay 1987d] and natural killer cell [Tay 1987c] infiltration in women with HPV infection and cervical intraepithelial neoplasia.

Chromosomes

Chromosomal abnormalities, particularly of chromosomes 1 and 11, can be induced by HPV-DNA and EJ-ras in human fibroblasts [Matlashewski 1988]. These two chromosomes, as well as chromosomes 3 and 17, are commonly abnormal in cervical tumors [Teyssier 1989]. Integration of HPV-DNA causes aneuploidy, which might lead to activation of oncogenes or inactivation of anti-oncogenes, such as p53 [Dürst 1987a,b, Pirisi 1987, 1988]. Tetraploidy in atypical cervical cells may be a risk factor for developing more advanced lesions [Olaharski 2004].

Trauma

Condyloma, dysplasia, and cancer all commonly arise in the anterior cervix, a site exposed to trauma during childbirth and during intercourse. Trauma could cause mucosal defects and facilitate inoculation of a virus.

Pregnancy

Pregnancy is associated with an altered immune status and change in lymphoid cell function necessary for fetal allograph survival [Petrucco 1976]. As first noted by Woodruff and Peterson, in 1958, condylomas are more common in pregnancy, and the majority regress post-partum [Woodruff 1958]. Subsequent studies confirmed that condylomas and cervical intraepithelial neoplasia are more frequent during pregnancy [Oriel 1971, A Schneider 1987a] and may progress more rapidly during pregnancy, but have a high postpartum regression rate [JL Benedet 1987, Hellberg 1987, Kiguchi 1981]. HPV-DNA is detected more often in pregnant women [A Schneider 1987a]. An increase in risk of cervical cancer, in direct proportion to the number of pregnancies, has been reported, possibly related to trauma, hormones, or immunodeficiency [Brinton 1989a].

Steroid Hormones

Epidemiologic studies indicate that long-term use of oral contraceptives probably increases the risk of both glandular and squamous cervical neoplasia (see pg 70). Oral contraception is associated with cervical ectopy, which could increase the exposure of the transitional zone to infection [*Critchlow 1995*]. An increased occurrence of dysplasia and cervical cancer has been reported in women exposed to diethylstilbestrol in utero ("DES daughters") [*Ben Baruch 1991, Fowler 1981, Hatch 2000, 2001, Piver 1988, Robboy 1984, Stafl 1974, Verloop 2000, Vessey 1989a*]. It has been known for many years that dysplasia usually occurs in an estrogenic environment [*Fraser 1967, Patten 1978, Rubio 1973*]. In the 1960s, it was shown that steroid hormones promote the development of cervical cancer in animals [*T Dunn 1969, Kaminetzky 1966*]. Genital HPVs are unique among DNA viruses in requiring steroid hormones for their expression in infected tissue [*McGlennen 2000*]. Estrogen can alter HPV gene expression [*Arbeit 1996*]. The estrogen metabolite, 16 α-hydro-oxyestrone, causes DNA damage [*Telang 1992*], which could result in accumulation of genetic mutations [*Auborn 1991, Newfield 1998*]. High prevalence of HPV DNA correlates with high serum progesterone levels [*Kedzia 2000*]. Progesterone, or closely related derivatives, has been associated with oncogenic transformation of cells by HPV [*A Pater 1990*]. At the molecular level, the HPV genome contains multiple steroid responsive elements, which are inducible by steroid hormones. When these response elements are bound by activated hormone receptor, viral gene transcription is enhanced [*McGlennen 2000*]. Steroid hormones, including estrogen, can increase HPV transcription and possibly oncogenic transformation [*Auborn 1991, Gloss 1987, Mitrani-Rosenbaum 1989, Monsonego 1991, A Pater 1990, M Pater 1988*]. Thus, oral contraceptives may promote the activity of HPV once infection has occurred [*Schiffman 1995a*].

Venereal Infections

Inflammation could be a risk factor for cervical neoplasia [*Castle 2001, Cuzick 2001*]. Venereal infections may increase the risk of acquiring HPV by causing inflammation, ulceration, or squamous metaplasia [*Koutsky 1988, 1992a*]. Herpes simplex, although it probably does not play a central role in cervical carcinogenesis, may be an important cofactor in some women [*Brinton 1992, Di Luca 1987, 1989, Fenoglio 1982, Galloway 1983, S Graham 1982, Hildesheim 1991, Iwasaka 1988, Kremar 1986, Rawls 1986, Vonka 1984, zur Hausen 1982*]. Herpetic lesions could facilitate infection with HPV [*Moscicki 2001*]. Herpes virus increases HPV transcription [*Gius 1989*] and may lead to oncogenic transformation [*Iwasaka 1988*]. Cytomegalovirus infection may also be associated in some way with development of cervical intraepithelial neoplasia [*Koutsky 1992a*]. The cervix frequently harbors Epstein-Barr virus; however, its role, if any, in cervical carcinogenesis remains to be elucidated [*Blackett 1994, T Sasagawa 2000, S Taylor 1994, Y Taylor 1994*]. *Chlamydia* has also been suspected of being a possible cofactor in cervical cancer [*Allerding 1985, Anttila 2001, Cevenini 1981, E Claas 1992, de Sanjosé 1994, M Hare 1982, Jha 1993, Kjær 1997, Koutsky 1992a, M Lehmann 1999, J Schachter 1982, K Syrjänen 1986b, Wallin 2002, Zenilman 2001*]. Multiple infections may [*Schmauz 1989*] or may not [*de Sanjosé 1994*] play a role in cervical carcinogenesis [*Boyle 1999*]. HIV was discussed under Immunologic Factors, above.

Male Factors

The male is the most likely vector for an infectious agent. Other possible male factors in cervical neoplasia could include semen or smegma. Semen is alkaline and rich in protein; these can inhibit the normal vaginal flora, possibly facilitating infection, including HPV infection. Semen also contains immunodepressants that inhibit lymphocyte function [*N Alexander 1987*]. These immunodepressants may not only facilitate impregnation, but also HPV infection. HPV DNA can be detected in semen [*Kyo 1994, Rintala 2004*].

Cigarette Smoking

There are at least three possible mechanisms to account for the association between cigarette smoke and cervical cancer: direct carcinogenic effect, co-carcinogenic effect, and local immunosuppression [*M Morris 1996*]. Products of cigarette smoke, including carcinogens, are concentrated in the cervical mucus of women who smoke (as well as those merely exposed to cigarette smoke, or passive smokers) [*Hellberg 1988, McCann 1992, Prokopczyk 1997, Sasson 1985, Szarewski 1998, Tay 2004*], resulting in "mutagenic mucus" [*Holly 1986*]. Smoke products can also be identified in cervical cells [*Mancini 1999, Simons 1996*]. Micronuclei, formed from chromosomes or their fragments that fail to be included in the nucleus during cell division, are more common in Pap tests from cigarette smokers. Smoking leads to increased modification and damage to DNA in cervical epithelium, providing biochemical evidence for smoking as a cause of cervical cancer [*Cerqueira 1998, Simons 1993, 1994, 1996*]. Smoking has also been reported to affect immunocompetent cells, both locally in the cervix [*Barton 1988*] and systemically [*L Miller 1982, B Phillips 1985*]. Smoking reduces the number of cervical Langerhans cells, which could diminish viral antigen presentation, and allow viral persistence [*Barton 1989a, Poppe 1995, Szarewski 1998*]. Smoking can alter CD4+/CD8+ lymphocytes ratios, causing an effect similar to HIV-related immunodeficiency discussed above [*Poppe 1995*]. The prevalence of oncogenic HPV infection increases with the number of cigarettes smoked [*M Burger 1993*]. There may be a synergistic relationship between cigarette smoke and HPV infection, and the development of cervical cancer [*X Yang 1996*]. In summary, although HPV is necessary for cervical carcinogenesis, cigarette smoking may promote its development [*Ho 1998b*].

Diet

There is growing evidence of a relationship between diet and cancer [*Block 1992, Giuliano 2000, Potischman 1996, Rock 2000, W Willett 1984a,b*]. Diet may be important not only for cancer prevention [*Correa 1992, Schiffman 1995a*], but also in cancer survival [*J Brown 2001*]. For example, fruits and vegetables may be protective against cervical cancer [*Steinmetz 1991a,b*]. Deficiencies of micronutrients, such as vitamins [*T Liu 1993, Potischman 1993, A Schneider 1989b, VanEenwyk 1992*] and minerals (eg, magnesium [*S Johnson 2001*], selenium [*Thompson 2002*]), may be related to development of cancer, including cervical cancer [*Giuliano 1998, 2003, M Mitchell 1995, Ziegler 1990*]. However, dietary factors in cervical cancer prevention may diminish when infection with HPV is taken into account [*Wideroff 1998*].

Vitamin A

Retinoids, which include vitamin A, are necessary for growth and development of epithelial cells [*A Bernstein 1984, DeLuca 1972*]. Dietary deficiencies of vitamin A may increase the risk of SILs in the cervix, and conversely, women with high dietary levels of vitamin A have a reduced risk [*Cuzick 1990*]. Retinoids apparently suppress expression of HPV E6 and E7 proteins, perhaps by secreting transforming growth factor, TGF-β. Carotenoids and retinoids may help prevent the development of squamous cell carcinomas not only in the genital tract, but also in the head & neck and other sites [*Giuliano 1998, 2000, LaVecchia 1984b, Romney 1981*]. Beta-carotene is the most common and active dietary carotenoid. When converted to vitamin A, it helps regulate epithelial differentiation and also functions as a free radical scavenger, which may explain its cancer-protective effects [Steinmetz 1991a,b].

Vitamin B

Folate (folic acid, a B vitamin) is involved in DNA synthesis, repair, and methylation, which are necessary for normal cell growth and differentiation. Folate deficiency can cause megaloblastosis in red blood cells and chromosomal damage [Yunis 1984]. Folic acid deficiency may lead to reversible cytologic changes similar to those induced by radiation, eg, formation of macrocytes [van Niekerk 1966]. Low folate levels may enhance susceptibility to HPV infection [Butterworth 1992a,b]. Oral contraceptive use is associated with (reversible) folate deficiency, which is more marked in women with dysplasia [Butterworth 1982, J Harper 1994]. Folate deficiency may have a crucial role in early in cervical carcinogenesis [Butterworth 1992c].

Vitamin C

There is a strong association of hypovitaminosis C with cervical dysplasia and carcinoma in situ [Romney 1985, Wassertheil-Smoller 1981]. Its role in preventing colds remains open.

Normal Flora, Inflammatory Change, Infections

While the detection of premalignant and malignant lesions of the cervix is the main focus of the Pap test, inflammatory conditions are important, not only in-and-of themselves, but also because they can mimic dysplasia (and vice versa). Pap test interpretation is not simply a matter of separating normal cells from neoplastic ones, like separating white marbles from black ones. Unfortunately, it is much more complex. There are many epithelial changes, informally referred to as "atypias," that can sometimes mimic dysplasia almost perfectly. So, the Pap test is not a simple test with only "true or false" (black or white) answers, but rather more like a multiple-choice test with numerous difficult distractors and sometimes more than one correct answer (shades of gray).

Most nondysplastic epithelial changes, or "atypias," are due to chemical factors (eg, douching, intravaginal medications), mechanical factors (eg, local trauma, diaphragms, pessaries, and surgical procedures such as biopsy), or biological factors (eg, response to infectious agents other than HPV, such as *Chlamydia*, trichomonas, etc). "Atypia" can also be present with repair/regeneration, vitamin deficiencies, atrophy, and radiation/chemotherapy. Remember, the key to interpretation is the nucleus: the nucleus reveals the health of a cell. Before considering these epithelial changes, normal flora and cytolysis will be discussed.

Normal Flora and Cytolysis

The normal vaginal flora is a complex, dynamic ecosystem. Its composition varies with the woman's age, hormonal status, sexual activity, and general state of health, including immune competence, as well as presence of vaginal blood, foreign bodies, medications, etc [K Gupta 2000, Keane 1997, Larsen 1982a, Mårdh 1991, Newton 2001]. What constitutes "normal" vaginal flora is difficult to define for all women at all times. However, some organisms are commonly encountered in asymptomatic women, while others are usually associated with symptoms. Those organisms occurring in asymptomatic women can be considered nonpathogenic ("normal"); organisms occurring in symptomatic women can be considered pathogenic ("disease"). When the normal biologic balance is disturbed, pathogenic organisms may gain a foothold, and cause vaginitis.

The predominant normal bacteria, originally described by Albert Döderlein in the late 19th century [Döderlein 1894], belong to the genus, *Lactobacillus*, and are known, colloquially, as *Bacillus vaginalis* or *Döderlein bacilli* [Donders 1999, Eschenbach 2000, Giacomini 1989, C Morris 1967]. Lactobacilli are relatively large, gram-positive rods. Lactobacilli are ubiquitous in the environment and colonize plants and animals. In humans, they colonize the mouth, intestines, and vagina [Ahrné 1998, Pavlova 2002]. Several species of lactobacilli can be isolated from the vagina, and historically, *Lactobacillus acidophilus* was thought to be most common. However, using molecular genetic techniques, *L crispatus* and *L jensenii*, followed by *L iners*, and *L gasseri*, have been found to be the most common species, and *L acidophilus* is actually rare [Antonio 1999, Burton 2003, Giorgio 1987, Pavlova 2002, Tarnberg 2002, Vallor 2002, Vásquez 2002]. Other vaginal species include *L fermentum, L vaginalis, L ruminis, L oris,* and *L reuteri,* among others [Y-L Song 1999, Vásquez 2002]. Furthermore, so-called *Lactobacillus acidophilus* is actually a complex of six distinct species that cannot be distinguished by classic biochemical techniques [E Du Plessis 1995, Lauer 1980, Vásquez 2002].

In addition to Lactobacilli, the normal vaginal flora consists of a wide variety of genera and species, including anaerobes (such as peptococci, *Prevotella* [formerly, *Bacteroides*], peptostreptococci, and Eubacteria) and aerobes (such as *Staphylococcus epidermidis*, corynebacteria) [Bartlett 1977, 1978, 1984, Giacomini 1989, Gorbach 1973, Larsen 1980, J Lindner 1978, Masfari 1986, Redondo-Lopez 1990]. Usually, only two to five bacteria colonize the vagina at any one time, including one *Lactobacillus* species [Antonio 1999, Redondo-Lopez 1990]. Although lactobacilli usually predominate, the presence of "mixed bacteria" (cocci and bacilli) in the Pap test is normal for some women [Keane 1997]. Culture is necessary to identify the specific organisms.

Lactobacilli are amazing little critters! They play a key role in preventing illness, including bacterial vaginosis, yeast infections, sexually transmitted diseases, urinary tract infections, and possibly even cancer [G Reid 2002]. The mechanisms by which lactobacilli control disease include: preventing pathogens from attaching to vaginal cells by blocking adhesion receptors; competing with pathogens for nutrients; and producing substances that inhibit pathogens such as organic acids, hydrogen peroxide, bacteriocins, and possibly biosurfactants [Boris 2000, Osset 2001]. Lactobacilli may help prevent cancer by interacting with reactive oxygen species, such as superoxide anion, hydroxyl radicals, and hypochlorous acid [G Bauer 2001].

On the other hand, some forms of lactobacilli are potentially pathogenic (causing "lactobacillosis") [Eschenbach 1989, Harty 1994]. In some cases of lactobacillosis, long filamentous forms of lactobacilli are observed (see Leptothrix, pg 102) [B Horowitz 1994]. In addition, excessive lactobacterial cytolysis can be associated with vaginosis-like symptoms ("cytolytic vaginosis") [Demirezen 2003a]. This is a little known, but common cause, of vulvovaginal complaints, including itching, burning, and discharge, in women of reproductive age that is frequently misdiagnosed as *Candida* infection [Cibley 1991, B Horowitz 1994, Hutti 2000, Paavonen 1995, Secor 1992, Wathne 1994].

Vaginal glycogen is transformed into glucose, which lactobacilli metabolize into lactic acid, the principal acid of the vagina [Boskey 2001, Wylie 1969]. Vaginal epithelial cells also contribute to vaginal acidity by producing organic acids, including lactic acid [Boris 2000, Preti 1975]. The vaginal pH is normally about 4 ± 0.5 [Andersch 1986, L Cohen 1969, J Paavonen 1983, Tevi-Bénissan 1997]. The normal glycogen-rich, acidic environment of the vagina is the perfect medium for lactobacilli to proliferate, while acidity inhibits most other organisms, including pathogenic ones. In addition, most vaginal strains of lactobacilli, including 95% of *L crispatus* and *L jensenii*, produce hydrogen peroxide, which inhibits many microorganisms, encompassing bacteria and viruses, including human immunodeficiency virus [Hawes 1996, Hillier 1998, H Martin 1999, Martius 1988, Vallor 2001]. Peroxidase and halide ions (eg, chloride) are present in the vagina, and when combined with hydrogen peroxide, produce acids such as hypochlorous acid that greatly promote this inhibitory system [Boris 2000, Klebanoff 1991]. Lactobacilli may also produce bacteriocins, proteins that have broad-spectrum bactericidal activity [Aroutcheva 2001, Valore 2002]. Vaginal pH is critical in all this: as the pH rises, bacteriocins lose their effectiveness, hydrogen peroxide is degraded, and lactobacilli cannot compete against other bacteria [Aroutcheva 2001].

Lactobacilli are particularly prominent during: the second half of the menstrual cycle; pregnancy; use of progestational drugs, including oral contraceptives; and sometimes menopause, particularly in diabetic women. Lactobacilli cannot thrive when the vaginal pH is alkaline. Menstrual flow increases the pH of ("alkalinizes") the vagina, peaking near pH 7 on days 2 and 3, but there follows a rapid return to the normal, mildly acidic pH that persists until day 21, when the pH begins steadily to increase [Redondo–Lopez 1990]. Semen increases the pH of the vagina, allowing an opportunity for fertilization [Redondo–Lopez 1990, Tevi–Bénissan 1997], since sperm are quickly inactivated at pH 4 [Olmsted 2000]. Lactobacilli return the vaginal pH to normal within several hours after intercourse [Boskey 2001, Eschenbach 2001]. After menopause, lactobacilli diminish, unless the woman is on hormone replacement therapy [Larsen 1982b]. Premenarchic girls usually have skin commensals and fecal organisms, rather than lactobacilli, owing to the alkaline vaginal pH [Hammerschlag 1978, Keane 1997]. Antimicrobial agents can disturb the ecological balance of the vaginal flora [Sullivan 2001].

Lactobacilli are gram-positive, rod shaped bacteria, about 3 to 6 μm long, that are pale blue in the Pap stain. They are able to lyse glycogen-rich intermediate cells, a process known as cytolysis. Cytolysis is characterized by normal-appearing intermediate cell nuclei floating in cytoplasmic debris, with numerous lactobacilli in an otherwise clean (noninflammatory) background [II.74]. Abundant cytolysis (>50% of cells) may be mentioned as a quality indicator in the Bethesda System, but the specimen should not be regarded as "Unsatisfactory" unless nearly all of the cells are damaged.

In liquid-based cytology, lactobacilli may look similar, but typically are attached to squamous cells or trapped in mucus, and not dispersed in the background. However, cytolysis can cause a noninflammatory "dirty" background.

Cytolysis is common in the second half of the menstrual cycle, during pregnancy, and in diabetes mellitus, but can also occur in premenarche and with steroid hormone therapy (including estrogen, progesterone, and androgens). Cytolysis is essentially limited to glycogen-containing intermediate cells and rarely affects other cells. Superficial cells are resistant to cytolysis and samples containing primarily parabasal cells (ie, atrophy) are usually free of lactobacilli [Wied 1955b]. Dysplastic cells are unaffected because of their low glycogen content (the basis of the Schiller iodine test). Cytolysis is also uncommon in inflammatory conditions and infections. Infectious agents inhibit growth of the normal lactobacilli responsible for cytolysis. Inflammation can cause nonhormonal maturation to superficial cells, which do not contain significant glycogen, and rarely undergo lactobacterial-induced cytolysis. However, enzymes released from inflammatory cells can damage epithelial cells leading to destruction of both the nucleus and the cytoplasm (inflammatory cytolysis or catalysis). The differential of cytolysis also includes

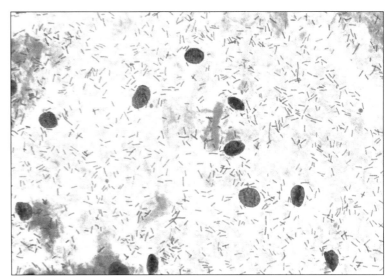

II.74
Lactobacilli, cytolysis [C]

endocervical mucus, in which naked (endocervical) nuclei float in pools of mucus, rather than cytoplasmic fragments.

Inflammation and Inflammatory Change

Vaginitis is the most commonly diagnosed gynecologic abnormality [M Egan 2000]. Pruritus and leukorrhea (itching and abnormal discharge) are among the most common symptoms for which a woman seeks medical advice from her gynecologist. Although a small amount of discharge is normal, leukorrhea usually indicates an infection, and occasionally a neoplasm. Most infections are due to bacterial vaginosis, *Candida*, or *Trichomonas*. The Pap test can be useful in identifying specific infectious agents, but it should not be used in lieu of more effective tests [Roongpisuthipong 1987].

Infectious agents can gain access to the vagina, but are normally controlled by several interrelated factors, including physical barriers such as the squamous mucosa; chemical barriers, such as normal vaginal acidity; and biologic barriers, such as presence of other microbiological agents, and general immune competence [Enhörning 1970]. The delicate endocervical glandular epithelium affords little protection from infection; therefore, women with ectropion, common in adolescents, young adults, or during pregnancy, are at increased risk of nonspecific inflammation as well as specific infections [Critchlow 1995, Singh 1999].

Causes of Inflammatory Change
Infection: Viral, bacterial, fungal, protozoal
Physical: IUD, tampon, diaphragm, pessary, polyps, trauma, including childbirth, etc
Hormonal: Oral contraceptives, atrophy, lactation
Chemical: Douches, gels, foams
Cancer and cancer therapy (radiation, chemotherapy)
Nonspecific, idiopathic

Oral contraceptives, which also can cause ectopy, are associated with inflammatory changes in Pap tests [Bertolino 1992, Brunham 1984, Eckert 1995, Kiviat 1985a, J Wilson 1990]. Women with atrophic vaginal mucosa are at increased risk of inflammation and infections. The endometrium is protected by regular shedding during the reproductive years.

Inflammation is a common finding in Pap tests, reported in 5% to 25% of cases, with even higher rates in some clinical settings [Bertolino 1992, B Kelly 1990, Lawley 1990, Malik 2001]. Inflammation is not synonymous with infection: *most women with inflammation do not have an infection* [Bertolino 1992, Malik 2001, Marshall 1997, W Parsons 1993]. Besides infection, other causes of inflammation of the female genital tract include physical, hormonal, chemical, neoplastic (and therapeutic) as well as nonspecific or idiopathic causes, alone or in combination. In addition, inflammatory cells easily traverse the endocervical epithelium and a few white blood cells are normally present in Pap tests. In women who have had a hysterectomy, the background of inflammatory cells often clears, even though they may be subjected to the same physical, chemical, or microbiologic assaults as before surgery.

The Cells of Inflammation

The general features of inflammation include leukocytosis, epithelial cell changes, and cell debris. Sometimes, pathogens are identified.

Erythrocytes

Erythrocytes, or red blood cells (RBCs), are biconcave discs, with pale staining centers, that measure about 6-8 µm in diameter. Intact or lysed RBCs are a common finding in Pap tests, particularly in relationship to menses, or minor bleeding associated with obtaining the sample. However, blood can be an abnormal finding that may indicate inflammation or tissue damage, and hence, can be a warning sign of cancer [Boon 2002, 2003]. In some cases, blood obscures or dilutes the epithelial cells; when extensive, these cases may be unsatisfactory for evaluation. Hemosiderin-laden macrophages indicate chronic ("old") bleeding.

Neutrophils

Polymorphonuclear leukocytes, or neutrophils (PMNs), have three to five nuclear lobes; "drumsticks" representing sex chromatin (Barr bodies) may be identifiable. Neutrophils average about 8 µm-12 µm, slightly larger than RBCs. *Neutrophils do not necessarily indicate acute inflammation.* Neutrophils in low numbers are a common, physiologic accompaniment of the premenstrual and menstrual phases of the normal menstrual cycle. However, numerous neutrophils do indicate inflammation or infection. Neutrophils adherent to squamous cells are sometimes referred to as "cannonballs" or "pusballs" [11.96d]. Cannonballs are associated with *Trichomonas* infection, but are not specific for it. Abundant neutrophils sometimes obscure the epithelial cells, possibly including abnormal cells. A specimen with excess exudate may be unsatisfactory for evaluation, and repeating the Pap test after therapy may be indicated for proper cancer surveillance.

Eosinophils

Eosinophils usually have two nuclear lobes, the cytoplasmic granules are visible individually, and are dull orange (rusty) in Pap stain [11.75a]. Eosinophils may have a physiologic role in cervical ripening after onset of labor during childbirth [Knudsen 1997]. Increased numbers of eosinophils may mean that the woman has an allergic reaction to microorganisms (eg, *Candida*), chemicals, medications, powders, or even semen or sperm (a possible cause of infertility) [B Levine 1973, Moraes 2000, Swerdloff 1988, Witkin 1989]. Charcot-Leyden crystals are rare findings in Pap tests [Kaur 1999]. Allergic vaginitis is frequently unrecognized or misdiagnosed clinically, resulting in

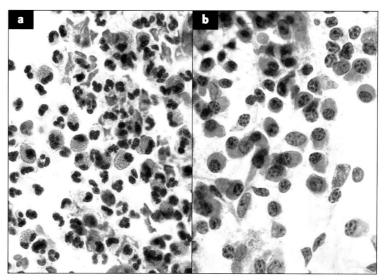

11.75
a, Eosinophils [C]; **b**, Plasma cells [C]

inappropriate therapy. Therefore, it may be worthwhile to report the presence of eosinophils in a Pap test, although this is not routine practice. Eosinophils are also associated with invasive squamous carcinoma [Papanicolaou 1941, G Spiegel 2002, van Driel 1999]. Some other cancers, too, may be associated with eosinophils (eg, glassy cell adenosquamous carcinoma).

Lymphocytes and Plasma Cells

Lymphocytes and plasma cells are characteristic of chronic inflammation. Lymphocytes have single, round nuclei with coarse chromatin, no visible nucleoli, and scant cytoplasm. They measure about 8 µm-10 µm in diameter. Plasma cells have eccentric, round nuclei, with very coarse ("clockface") chromatin, and a perinuclear pale zone ("hof"), which corresponds to the Golgi apparatus. Plasma cells are slightly larger than lymphocytes and occasionally are binucleated [11.75b]. Mild chronic cervicitis is so common—in histology—that it is considered essentially normal. However, lymphocytes and plasma cells are seldom found in normal Pap tests; their presence usually indicates significant inflammation (see also, follicular cervicitis). Plasma cells are classically associated with syphilis, but are not specific for this disease. Plasma cell cervicitis, which can produce a tumorous mass, can be mistaken for malignancy [Doherty 1993, Qizilbash 1974a]. Also, a lymphoplasmacytic infiltrate is a common response to invasive carcinoma. (See also lymphoma pg 179.)

Histiocytes (Macrophages)

Histiocytes originate from bone marrow-derived monocytes. Monocytes are transformed into macrophages in the peripheral tissues. Like vacuum cleaners, macrophages ingest various materials, such as bacteria and cell debris. Histiocytes, like neutrophils, can

Histiocytes
Common, especially during exodus (days 6-10)
Also: Postpartum; postmenopause*
(*Minor risk factor for Endometrial CA)
Multinucleated giant cell histiocytes:
Postmenopausal women†
(†Not risk factor for Endometrial CA)
Post-therapy: Radiation or surgery

be present either physiologically or pathologically [11.76a,b,c]. They are a normal component of the Pap test just before and after menses. Histiocytes

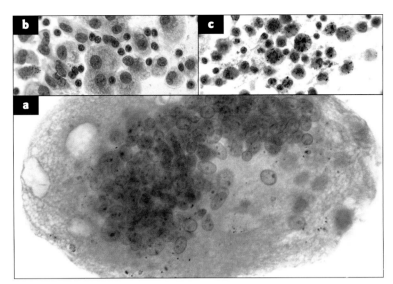

II.76
a, Giant cell histiocyte [C]; **b**, Histiocytes [C]; **c**, Siderophages [C]

In liquid-based cytology, histiocytes may form fairly dense clusters. The cytoplasm also tends to appear dense because the cells round up in fluid.

Large histiocytes often have phagocytosed material in their cytoplasm (including debris, bacteria, white blood cells, red blood cells, etc). If the cytoplasm contains lipid or hemosiderin particularly after menopause, there is an increased risk of endometrial hyperplasia/neoplasia, because these histiocytes may indicate tissue destruction (lipophages) or old bleeding (siderophages [II.76c]).

Multinucleated giant cell histiocytes are common postpartum and in postmenopausal women; they also occur after radiation therapy or surgery [c Evans 1984, Murad 1985, Tweeddale 1968]. [II.76a]. Characteristically, the nuclei closely resemble each other, like sisters ("sister image nuclei"). Differential possibilities include "syncytial" parabasal cells that may be present in long-standing atrophy (with squamous cytoplasm) and syncytiotrophoblastic cells (central, degenerated nuclei, dense cytoplasm with tails, see pg 168). Multinucleated tumor giant cells usually have obvious malignant features. The characteristic nuclear chromatin and foamy/granular cytoplasm identifies a cell as histiocytic. Multinucleated giant cell histiocytes have no significance in detection of endometrial hyperplasia or neoplasia.

(along with glandular endometrial cells) may be present in large numbers between days 6 and 10 of the menstrual cycle. This part of the cycle was designated "exodus" (Greek, the road [*hodus*] out [*ex*], ie, exit) by Papanicolaou [Papanicolaou 1953]. Morphologically similar cells originate from the superficial endometrial stroma and are recognized by their tendency to form loose aggregates ("sticky histiocytes") (see "Endometrial Stromal Cells" pg 116).

Histiocytes may be present in the Pap test in early or late pregnancy, postpartum or following abortion. Numerous histiocytes after menopause or in the second half of the menstrual cycle, may be associated with endometrial hyperplasia or neoplasia, but the association is weak (see pg 118). Histiocytes are also associated with foreign bodies, eg, sutures, IUDs, and tampons; chronic inflammation, including that associated with infections (eg, tuberculosis, fungus, parasites) and ulcers; as well as radiation, biopsy, or cryotherapy [Bardales 1995, Safäll 1966]. Histiocytes can also be present in rare diseases ranging from malakoplakia to Langerhans cell histiocytosis [Axiotis 1991, Issa 1980, Steppeler 2003].

Histiocytes are classified as being small, large (often associated with phagocytosis), or giant (multinucleated) [II.76a,b]. Histiocytes may be present singly or in loose aggregates, but do not form tightly cohesive or molded groups. The histiocyte nucleus varies in size and is eccentrically located. While the histiocyte nucleus is most characteristically bean-shaped, it usually appears round to oval. The chromatin is usually fine and pale, or it may have a characteristic "salt-and-pepper" pattern. One or more small nucleoli may be present. Mitotic figures may be seen.

The cytoplasm of a histiocyte usually has a foamy (delicate, vacuolated) or granular texture, although sometimes, the cytoplasm is dense, like that of a squamous cell, particularly in liquid-based cytology. However, it lacks the waxy or glassy appearance of squamous cytoplasm (as well as keratin rings).

Histiocytes are great impersonators ("Judy, Judy, Judy..."). They can mimic many other cell types, including squamous, endocervical, endometrial, reserve cells at one end of the spectrum and dysplastic or malignant cells at the other. A good clue to the true identity of a histiocyte is its characteristic "salt-and-pepper" chromatin texture. Also, the histiocyte nucleus is typically eccentrically located in the cytoplasm, secretory vacuoles are absent, and there is no perinuclear halo.

Inflammatory Change ("Inflammatory Atypia")

Distinguishing inflammatory change from dysplasia is a common, everyday problem in Pap test interpretation. This can lead to both false-positive results (overinterpreting inflammatory changes as dysplasia), and false-negative results (underinterpreting dysplasia as inflammatory change) [Renshaw 2004b,d]. Rather than completely destroying cells, inflammation more commonly merely changes them [Kiviat 1985a]. "Inflammatory changes" have many features in common with dysplasia, including nuclear enlargement, nuclear membrane irregularities, chromatin abnormalities, and cytoplasmic alterations [II.77a,b][Coach 2001]. And, therein lies the problem: separating inflammatory change from dysplasia. As a general rule, the difference between inflammatory change and dysplasia is a matter of degree: the nuclei of dysplasia are more enlarged, more pleomorphic, more irregular, with more extensive chromatin abnormalities, more prominent cytoplasmic halos (ie, koilocytic vs inflammatory halos), and the cell arrangements are more disorderly. Inflammatory change can mimic either low-grade dysplasia or high-grade dysplasia. Note well, however, that *inflammatory change and dysplasia can, and frequently do, coexist* [Reagan 1956a]. As a rule of thumb: if a cell looks dysplastic, it probably is dysplastic. A word of warning—do not underestimate the difficulty of these interpretive problems!

Inflammatory Change

Nuclei: Minimal enlargement (< 2 X)
  Bi- or multi-nucleation
  Smooth to wrinkled membranes
  Fine chromatin, pale to mildly dark
  Degeneration (clumped, lysed)
Cytoplasm: Polychromasia, vacuolization,
  pseudokeratinization, raggedy,
  perinuclear halos (not koilocytes)
Background: "Dirty," inflammatory
  Can mimic tumor diathesis

Inflammatory Change vs Dysplasia

Common, everyday interpretive problem
Matter of degree, dysplasia has:
  •More pleomorphic, larger nuclei
  •More irregular nuclear outline
  •More abnormal chromatin
  •More prominent halos
  •More cellular disorder
...than inflammatory change

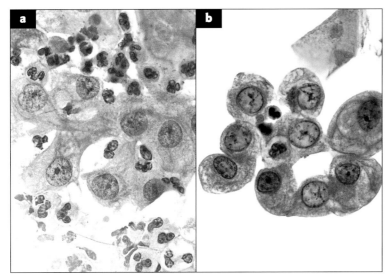

II.77
a, Inflammatory change [C]; **b**, Inflammatory change [L]

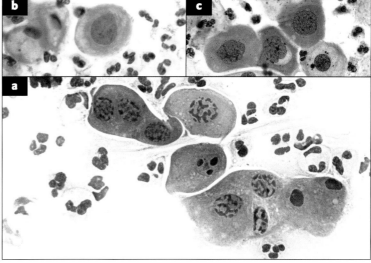

II.78
a, Karyorrhexis [C]; **b**, Red chromatin, inflammation [C];
c, Blue chromatin, dysplasia [C]

Nuclear Features

Nuclear alterations in inflammation include changes in size, staining, and number as well as presence of nucleoli and nuclear vacuolization. Nuclear condensation (pyknosis), disintegration (karyorrhexis), and dissolution (karyolysis) are common degenerative changes associated with inflammation. Occasional binucleation or multinucleation may be observed.

Nuclear features are the key to distinguishing inflammatory and degenerative changes from dysplasia. In inflammation, the nuclei are frequently big, but not dark (in fact, pale) compared with a normal intermediate cell nucleus. In degeneration, the nuclei are frequently dark, but not big, compared with normal. However, in some cases, inflammatory nuclear enlargement and hyperchromasia occurs that can mimic the "big, dark" nuclei of dysplasia, but the inflamed nuclei are usually not *too* big and not *too* dark. In contrast, in dysplasia, the nuclei are usually distinctively both bigger *and* darker than normal [T1.25].

Inflammatory Change vs Dysplasia

Nuclear features: Key to interpretation

Dysplasia:

 "If it's big & it's dark, it's dysplasia"

 Dark blue nuclei, indistinct/no nucleoli

Inflammation:

 Big, but not dark; Dark, but not big

 Red nuclei, prominent nucleoli

Cytoplasm: "Trich" vs koilocyte halos

T1.25 Nuclear Size & Staining with Likely Interpretation

	Not Big	Big
Not Dark	Normal	Inflamed
Dark	Degenerated	Dysplasia

Hydropic degeneration (the cells imbibe too much water) is common in inflammation. Fluid absorption leads to nuclear (and cytoplasmic) enlargement and decreased nuclear staining intensity, or chromatolysis. Thus, inflamed nuclei are usually less than about twice the area of an intermediate cell nucleus (<75 μm², ie,

not too big), and they usually have fine and pale (not dark) chromatin. The changes vary from cell to cell, and this causes apparent nuclear pleomorphism (actually, anisonucleosis or variation in nuclear size).

Occasionally, inflamed nuclei are not only enlarged, but also hyperchromatic, mimicking dysplasia. This is particularly common in *Trichomonas* infection, but not specific for it. Dysplastic nuclei are characterized by still greater nuclear enlargement (>120 μm², >3× an intermediate nucleus) and pleomorphism, with darker, coarser chromatin, and frequently, higher N/C ratios.

Bland, hypochromatic nuclei are unlikely to be mistaken for dysplasia. However, there is a form of dysplasia with pale-staining nuclei ("pale dyskaryosis" or dysplastic "pale bland cells," PBCs) that can easily be mistaken for inflammatory change. In "pale dyskaryosis" the dysplastic nuclei may be enlarged, but are hypochromatic (big and pale). This can occur as a fixation artifact, particularly in liquid-based cytology, or may possibly represent a hypodiploid chromosome complement in some cases [Dudding 1996a, PA Smith 1997]. Interpretive clues to dysplastic pale bland cells include nuclear pleomorphism, irregular nuclear membranes, and chromatin variations, such as speckling (see pg 57).

The nuclear borders are usually round and uniform in inflammation, but may be wrinkled. The nuclear membrane often appears "thickened" due to margination of chromatin, with clearing of the center of the nucleus. This "empty look" of inflammation contrasts with dysplasia, in which the nuclear membranes are often deeply folded and the chromatin is diffusely coarse throughout the nucleus.

The chromatin typically appears smudgy and indistinct in inflammation, rather than crisp and distinct as in dysplasia. Although the chromatin of inflamed cells may clump, it is a degenerative, rather than neoplastic change. Inflammatory nuclear degeneration commonly results in karyopyknosis, karyorrhexis [II.78a], or karyolysis. Pyknotic nuclei stain intensely, but are small (ie, dark, but not big). The clumped chromatin particles of degenerated nuclei tend to be rounded, like beads of mercury, while those in dysplasia tend to be angular, like shards of pottery. In short, the nuclei of inflammatory change "do not have the chromatin of dysplasia."

Redness (rubor) is classically associated with inflammation. Interestingly, inflamed nuclei have a tendency to "shine red," ie, the chromatin may have a peculiar red quality in some cells in conventional Pap smears [II.78b]. This contrasts with dysplastic nuclei that have granular, dark blue chromatin [II.78c].

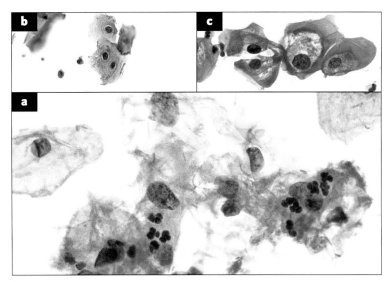

II.79

a, Inflammatory change, raggedy cytoplasm [C]; **b**, Inflammatory halos, pseudokeratinization [L]; **c**, Koilocyte halos [L]

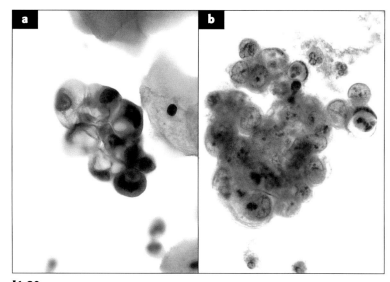

II.80

a, Vacuolated metaplastic cells [C]; **b**, Adenocarcinoma [L]

Nucleoli *strongly* favor a reactive process over a dysplastic one, particularly in conventional Pap smears [Patten 1978]. Nevertheless (there being no hard and fast rules in cytology), indistinct or micronucleoli can occur in dysplasia [Meisels 1976b], particularly in liquid-based cytology. Dysplastic cells are probably not immune to inflammation and can show secondary inflammatory alterations (see also, atypical repair, pg 66). Dysplastic cells having unexpectedly vesicular chromatin with nucleoli, instead of the expected hyperchromatic, granular chromatin pattern without nucleoli, are particularly difficult to distinguish from reactive cellular changes [Sherman 1999].

Nuclear vacuolization is common in inflammation. Binucleation or multinucleation are also common. However, neither vacuolization nor hypernucleation is specific for inflammation.

Cytoplasmic Features

Cytoplasmic reactions to inflammation include staining alterations, perinuclear halos, cytoplasmic vacuolization, and cytolysis. Polychromasia ("two-tone" pink and blue staining) may occur, or the cytoplasm may stain less intensely as a result of inflammation [II.79a]. Commonly, however, especially in *Trichomonas* infection, the cytoplasm becomes eosinophilic or orangeophilic [Papanicolaou 1943]. "Pseudokeratinized" cytoplasm plus enlarged, dark nuclei (also common with *Trichomonas* infection) can mimic low-grade keratinizing dysplasia [II.79b].

A perinuclear halo is a small, clear space around the nucleus of inflamed squamous cells. It forms when an edematous, swollen nucleus shrinks due to fixation, leaving a gap, or halo, around the nucleus. Perinuclear halos are common in inflammation, particularly in *Trichomonas* infection, where they are known as "trich halos" (they can trick the unwary into an interpretation of condyloma by mimicking koilocytes) [II.79b,c]. As a rule, the width of an inflammatory halo (ie, the space between nucleus and cytoplasm) is less than the diameter of an intermediate cell nucleus and the outline of the halo is poorly defined. Inflammatory perinuclear halos usually do not occur in dysplastic cells. However, koilocytes are common in dysplasia (see pg 50); their halos are usually much larger and more sharply defined, and their nuclei appear "dysplastic" (big and dark).

Cytoplasmic vacuolization is a common inflammatory change. Vacuolar cytoplasmic degeneration is particularly prevalent in metaplastic cells, sometimes giving them a soap bubble appearance. The cytoplasmic vacuoles often contain ingested neutrophils. The combination of vacuolated cytoplasm and atypical (reactive) nuclei may suggest glandular cancer. In practice, highly vacuolated cells are more likely to be benign metaplasia [II.80a] than adenocarcinoma [II.80b], particularly in the presence of inflammation (see also, "IUD Effect" pg 163). The cell borders often appear frayed or raggedy in inflammation. Eventually, the cytoplasm dissolves completely: this is inflammatory cytolysis.

Background Features

Severe inflammation is frequently associated with a protein-rich exudate, manifested as a finely granular protein precipitate and fibrin strands. In addition, mucus, bacteria, inflammatory cells, and lysed cells add to the "dirty background" characteristic of inflammation. This inflammatory background can mimic a tumor diathesis [II.81a,b]. In liquid-based preparations, the inflammatory material often has a "ratty" appearance (dirty, tattered) and clings to reactive/degenerated epithelial cells.

Summary

Inflammatory change is frequently characterized by enlarged, but pale nuclei with nucleoli, or small, dark, degenerated nuclei, plus cytoplasmic polychromasia, pseudokeratinization, vacuolization, and frayed cell outlines. The background is typically "dirty," characterized by inflammation, granular debris, and sometimes, microbiologic agents. (See also discussion of reactive endocervical cells, pg 112).

The findings are similar in liquid-based cytology. In brief, reactive changes are characterized by slight nuclear enlargement (usually < 2 times an

Causes of Repair/Regeneration

Severe inflammation, eg, Trichomonas

Cautery, cryotherapy, or laser therapy

Biopsy, surgery

Childbirth

Radiation

Spontaneous, idiopathic

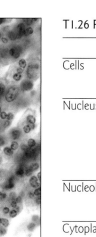

I1.81
a, Inflammatory background [C]; **b**, Inflammatory background [L]

T1.26 Repair vs Cancer

	Repair	Cancer
Cells	More cohesive	Less cohesive
	Few single cells	More single cells
Nucleus	Hypochromatic, pale	Hyperchromatic, dark
	Smooth membranes	Irregular membranes
	Fine, even chromatin	Coarse, dark chromatin
	Mitoses possible	Abnormal mitoses
Nucleoli	Prominent, all cells	Variable among cells
	± Irregular shape	± Irregular shape
Cytoplasm	Adequate	Decreased
	N/C ratio WNL	N/C ratio high
	Not keratinized	May be keratinized
	Polychromasia	Monochrome
	Ingested PMNs common	Ingested PMNs uncommon
Background	Inflammatory	Tumor diathesis
Summary	Order, cohesion	Disorder, dyshesion
	Fine chromatin	Coarse, dark chromatin
	Smooth membranes	Irregular membranes

intermediate cell nucleus), smooth nuclear membranes, fine chromatin, nucleoli, and frequently, degenerated or vacuolated cytoplasm. Inflammatory nuclear halos also occur (differential: koilocyte halos). The background inflammatory material often has a "ratty" appearance (dirty, tattered looking material) that clumps or "clings" to reactive/degenerated epithelial cells.

Repair/Regeneration

When the mucosa is denuded, damaged, or destroyed, the epithelial cells at the periphery proliferate to repair the defect. The cytologic changes reflect cellular regeneration, ie, the rapid growth and protein synthesis necessary for repair. The nuclei become enlarged, pleomorphic, and develop prominent nucleoli; mitotic figures may be present. These changes can mimic neoplasia. Distinguishing repair/regeneration from dysplasia/carcinoma, and vice versa, can be tricky. In fact, repair/regeneration is a difficult and irreproducible category, one of the most common sources of error in Pap test interpretation [Colgan 2001b, Renshaw 2003, 2004d, Yelverton 1996].

Although repair is most common in younger women, no age is spared. For example, repair occurs in young women after childbirth and also in older women after radiation therapy. Repair/regeneration results from an extremely heterogeneous group of injuries, ranging from the common, eg, severe inflammation or mechanical injury (such as biopsy) to the exotic, eg, Behçet disease (named after Hulusi Behçet [pronounced "beh-chet"], a Turkish doctor, and characterized by a triad of aphthous stomatitis, genital ulcers, and uveitis) [Wilbur 1993]. Some cases are seemingly idiopathic (Gr: same root as in idiot), with no obvious cause. Women with repair are at increased risk of having or developing SILs [Bibbo 1971b, JH Chang 1996, Patten 1978, Soofer 1997].

Repair/Regeneration
Flat cohesive, well-ordered sheets
Single cells absent/rare
Nuclei line up ("nuclear streaming")
± Macronucleoli
Chromatin: Fine, pale
± Mitotic figures, not abnormal
Inflammatory background

Reparative cells can resemble squamous, glandular, or metaplastic epithelium [T1.26]. Benign reparative cells usually exfoliate in cohesive sheets, and may have a swirling tissue culture-like appearance. Nuclear "atypia" ranges from mild to severe, and may suggest malignancy (see also, atypical repair, pg 65).

There are a few key points regarding regeneration/repair [Bibbo 1971b, Colgan 2001b, Epstein 1972, Geirsson 1977, González–Merlo 1973, Sugimori 1982, Ueki 1992]. Because it is a benign process, repair maintains a high degree of orderliness. The cells tend to form fairly orderly ranks and files. The nuclei line up in rows ("nuclear streaming" that looks like a school of fish) and have little or no overlap or crowding [I1.82a,b,c,d,e].

Sheets of reparative cells tend to be very cohesive and single cells are usually absent or sparse. In contrast, single cells are usually prominent in cancer. When single cells are present in repair, they are usually in proximity to a group in conventional Pap smears, but are randomly distributed in LBC. Unfortunately, single reparative cells are more common in the most atypical reparative processes—cases that are cytologically more difficult to distinguish from cancer.

Nuclear enlargement (usually < 2-3 times), pleomorphism, and multinucleation are common in repair, but the chromatin pattern is usually fine and pale, although in some cases it may be slightly coarse and hyperchromatic. Cancer is associated with abnormal chromatin that usually is distinctly coarse and hyperchromatic. Each cell has adequate cytoplasm; therefore, the N/C ratio is relatively normal or only somewhat increased in repair, while in cancer, the N/C ratio is typically high. Perhaps surprisingly, nucleoli can sometimes be *more* prominent in repair than cancer. Nucleoli with irregular contours may also be present in benign repair. Normal mitotic figures can occur in either repair or cancer, but abnormal mitotic figures point to cancer. In sum, mitotic figures (unless clearly abnormal), macronucleoli, or irregular nucleoli are *not* necessarily indicative of malignancy [Sugimori 1982].

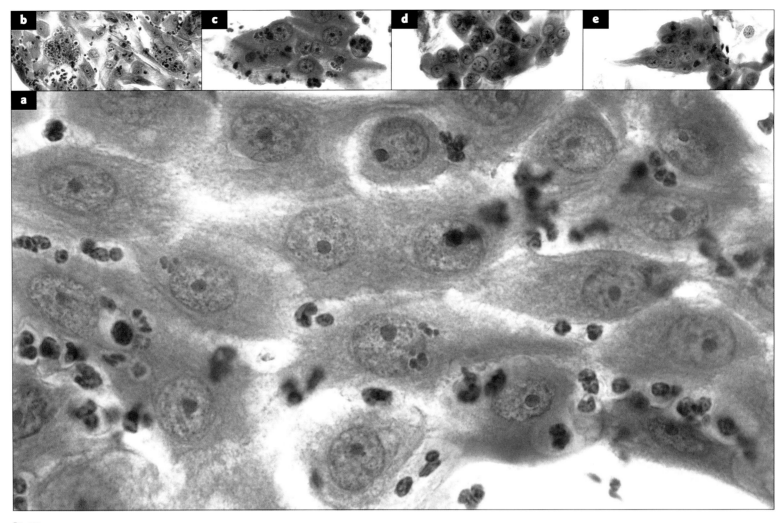

11.82
a, Repair/regeneration [C]; **b**, Repair/regeneration [C]; **c**, Repair/regeneration [C]; **d**, Repair/regeneration [L]; **e**, Repair/regeneration [L]

The cytoplasm of repair is relatively abundant, usually stains blue, sometimes pink, or commonly, both (polychromatic), but does not stain bright orange (ie, does not keratinize). Cell boundaries range from well-defined to poorly-defined ("syncytial"). The cytoplasmic edges are frequently irregular or ragged. Cytoplasmic vacuolization may be present. Acute inflammatory cells mixed within the sheets of epithelial cells with an inflammatory background are common [Rimm 1996]. Repair is often accompanied by inflammation or pathogenic organisms.

The cytology of repair is similar in liquid-based cytology (cohesive, orderly sheets, smooth nuclear membranes, fine chromatin, occasional mitoses), except that the groups appear more rounded or folded, with greater depth of focus, and the characteristic "streaming" pattern may be less apparent because the cells are not spread, or "smeared," on the slide [W-K Ng 2003c]. Nucleoli may be more prominent.

Benign repair can sometimes be quite alarming in appearance, and the distinction from cancer is not always straightforward. Benign proliferating cells have a high degree of orderliness not characteristic of cancer, which usually appears chaotic (crowded, loss of polarity, etc). Benign cells also have cell-to-cell similarities, such as similar number of chromocenters and nucleoli, similar chromatin distribution, etc. Cancer, on the other hand, tends to have marked vari-

ability of these features from cell-to-cell. Single cells are rare in repair, but common in cancer. Repair forms flat sheets of cells; cancer cells pile up. Repair has fine, pale, evenly distributed chromatin; cancer usually has coarse, dark, irregular chromatin. Reparative cells are cohesive, cancer cells dyshesive. Neutrophils in the cytoplasm favors repair, keratinized cytoplasm favors cancer. Cancer is associated with a tumor diathesis, while repair has a clean or inflammatory background, in which inflammatory cells are commonly present. However, occasionally it can be difficult to distinguish a "dirty" background of inflammation from a tumor diathesis, and cancers can be associated with inflammation.

Repair vs Carcinoma

Favors carcinoma:
- *Poorly cohesive, disorderly cells*
- *Many single cells*
- *Irregular nuclear membrane*
- *Chromatin: Coarse, dark, irregular*
- *Cytoplasm: If keratinized*
- *Cell-to-cell variation*
- *Tumor diathesis*

Favors repair:
- *Cohesion, order, fine pale chromatin*
- *Smooth nuclear membrane*

Not too helpful:
- *Nucleoli, unless very variable*
- *Mitoses, unless abnormal*

In summary, in repair there is a disparity between the abnormal appearing, pleomorphic nuclei with prominent nucleoli versus the orderliness of

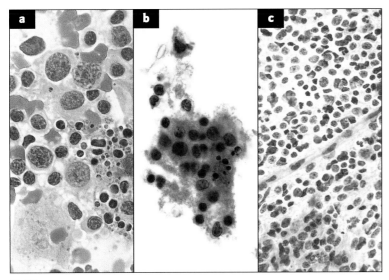

II.83
a, Follicular cervicitis [C]; **b**, Follicular cervicitis [L];
c, Follicular cervicitis, capillary [C]

membranes, no visible nucleoli, and very little cytoplasm. The immature lymphocytes (follicular center cells) vary in size, but are larger than mature lymphocytes. Immature lymphocytes have more open chromatin and somewhat more cytoplasm, and may have irregular nuclear membranes or prominent nucleoli. Mitotic figures may be observed. Plasma cells, histiocytes, and neutrophils may also be present.

Tingible body macrophages contain cellular debris in their cytoplasm, which is visualized microscopically as tingible (ie, stainable) bodies. The debris is the result of cell turnover in the germinal center (ie, necrobiosis [the word kind of sends a chill up your spine, doesn't it?]). Tingible body macrophages suggest the diagnosis of follicular cervicitis, but can be seen in other conditions, including high-grade lymphomas and invasive carcinomas. Capillaries, the smallest blood vessels, are tubular structures that typically contain erythrocytes.

In liquid-based cytology, the inflammatory cells may clump, forming dense, three-dimensional aggregates that can mimic endometrial cells, or other hyperchromatic crowded groups of cells. Look for tingible body macrophages to help identify follicular cervicitis.

Pleomorphic (lymphoid) cells with coarse chromatin and nucleoli can appear quite alarming and could be mistaken for carcinoma in situ, small cell carcinoma, endometrial carcinoma, or malignant lymphoma. In contrast with epithelial neoplasia, there is little or no molding, nor are there true epithelial groupings, such as clusters, sheets, or glands, in conventional Pap smears (although as mentioned, in liquid-based cytology, marked clumping of the cells can occur, which can make evaluation difficult [Halford 2002]). Although women with follicular cervicitis are in the high-risk group for developing cervical dysplasia, dysplasia does not necessarily accompany follicular cervicitis. In contrast, dysplasia usually accompanies carcinoma in situ.

The differential of follicular cervicitis also includes malignant lymphoma. Primary lymphoma of the cervix is very rare and is associated with a mass or barrel-shaped cervix. Follicular cervicitis is common by comparison and does not produce a grossly abnormal cervix. Follicular cervicitis presents a polytypic lymphoid population ("range of maturation") and tingible body macrophages, indicative of follicular center formation and a benign reactive lymphoid process. Malignant lymphoma, on the other hand, is characterized by a block in maturation of the lymphoid cells. The classic cytologic appearance of lymphoma is a monotypic population of cells, often lacking tingible body macrophages (except when high-grade). (See pg 179 for further discussion of lymphoma.)

Granulomatous Cervicitis
Causes of granulomatous cervicitis include infections, foreign body reactions, and cancer [II.84a]. Tuberculous cervicitis, which is rare, can mimic squamous cell carcinoma of the cervix grossly (see pg 104). Other organisms, including *Chlamydia* (lymphogranuloma venereum), *Calymmatobacterium granulomatis* (Donovanosis, granuloma inguinale), schistosomes, and amoeba, can also cause granulomatous inflammation of the cervix [Christie 1980]. Foreign body granulomatous reactions are commonly observed after radiation therapy (reaction to squamous cells or altered ground

the cells with bland chromatin. In cancer, all of the abnormal cellular features point to malignancy. This disparity of cytologic features is an important warning to be cautious in reporting cancer. The key features of repair are: high degree of orderliness and cohesion of the cells, fine chromatin pattern, and smooth nuclear membranes. In practice, there is a spectrum of reactive/reparative changes, including atypical forms, and repair is a common source of error, including both false-positive and false-negative results [Colgan 2001b, Davey 1993, Koss 1993b, Moriarty 2003b]. Atypical repair is covered on pg 66.

Follicular Cervicitis
Lymphoid follicles, complete with follicular (germinal) center formation, occur occasionally in the cervix (or vagina). This condition is known as follicular cervicitis (or vaginitis or cervicovaginitis). It is frequently (50% to 75% of cases) associated with *Chlamydia* infection [P Gupta 1979, M Hare 1981, 1982, Paavonen 1982, Winkler 1987]. Follicular cervicitis can occur at any age, but is both more common and more likely to be detected in Pap tests in postmenopausal women, who have a thin, atrophic overlying epithelium, than in younger women with a thick, mature overlying epithelium [T Roberts 1975].

The cytologic appearance of follicular cervicitis looks like a "touch-prep" of a reactive lymph node [II.83a,b,c] [Eisenstein 1965]. The two main cytologic features are: range of maturation of the lymphoid cells ("mature" and "immature" lymphocytes in varying stages of differentiation) and presence of tingible body macrophages. Capillaries may also be present.

Lymphoid cells lie singly, have high N/C ratios, do not form tight groups, and lack significant nuclear molding. Most of the lymphoid cells are small, mature lymphocytes with coarse, dark chromatin, smooth nuclear

Follicular Cervicitis
Any age; associated with Chlamydia
~ Imprint Reactive Lymph Node
·Range of maturation
·Small lymphs predominate
·Follicular center cells
·Tingible body macrophages
Lymphoma → grossly abnormal cervix
Extremely rare at this site

Granulomatous Cervicitis
Infections: Tuberculosis, other
Foreign body (eg, suture)
Posttherapy reaction (radiation, surgery)
Reaction to squamous cell carcinoma
Misc: Wegener, Sarcoidosis, etc

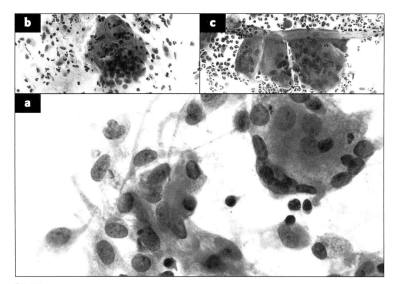

II.84
a, Granuloma [C]; **b**, Reaction to squames [C]; **c**, Suture granuloma [C]

extending from the main cytoplasmic mass. The nuclei are pleomorphic and active in appearance, with large, prominent nucleoli, but pale chromatin. Mitotic figures may be present. Radiated myofibroblasts and endothelial cells from the stroma in radiation-induced ulcers, can appear frankly bizarre, possibly suggesting a sarcoma (see pg 159). However, highly atypical cells are relatively sparse. The history of radiation must be provided by the clinician.

Specific Infections

Although the Pap test can provide valuable information about vaginal pathogens, it is not a substitute for formal microbiologic studies. Gonorrhea, syphilis, staphylococci, streptococci, and mycoplasma infections, among others, can all cause inflammation, but the changes in the Pap test are usually nonspecific [Donders 2002, W McCormack 1973]. On the other hand, some agents, such as viruses, can produce more or less characteristic cytologic changes [Coleman 1979]. Some organisms produce toxins that can cause disease (such as staphylococci and toxic shock syndrome) [Anonymous 1980]. Multiple infections are the rule, not the exception. Some infections, including viral infections, *Trichomonas,* syphilis, gonorrhea, *Chlamydia,* and *Candida,* have

Specific Organisms

Bacillus vaginalis: Normal flora, cytolysis

Herpes: 3Ms

(multinucleation, molding, margination)

→ ground glass chromatin (key) ± inclusions

Gardnerella: Normal vs bacterial vaginosis,

clue cells

Leptothrix: Long thin bacteria, + Trichomonas

Actinomyces: Filaments + other bacteria

"dust bunnies," associated with IUDs

Chlamydia: Pap test not reliable for detection

Candida: Pseudohyphae/spores; balloon

dogs; shish kabob

Trichomonas: Pear-shaped, must see nucleus

May see red granules; Flagellae (in LBC)

seasonal variation in prevalence [Smolensky 1981, Sodhani 1994]. Squamous intraepithelial lesions also may have some seasonal variation [Rietveld 1997].

substance) [II.84b] or after surgery (including suture granuloma) [II.84c] [Almoujahed 2002, Bardales 1995]. Granulomas may also be present as a response to infiltrating squamous cell carcinoma. Wegener granulomatosis and sarcoidosis are among the rare causes of granulomatous cervicitis [Almoujahed 2002, Malamou-Mitsi 2000].

Granulomatous cervicitis is a possible explanation for finding giant cells in the Pap test [Kuttch 1992]. Aggregates of epithelioid histiocytes and giant cells are characteristic of granulomas [II.84a] [Angrish 1981]. In exfoliative cytology, epithelioid histiocytes frequently have a tapered "carrot" shape and may even stain orange. In foreign body reactions, the giant cells tend to surround and ingest the foreign material.

Granulation Tissue

Granulation tissue forms in reaction to severe inflammation, including biopsy, cryotherapy, surgery, and radiation, and is sometimes sampled in the Pap test [Montanari 1968]. The lesion may be grossly visible as a nubbin of red tissue. Histologically, granulation tissue is composed of a network of proliferating capillaries, surrounded by histiocytes and other inflammatory cells, as well as proliferating myofibroblasts.

An inflammatory background, mononucleated and multinucleated histiocytes, repair, blood and blood vessels characterize the cytology of granulation tissue. The most characteristic finding is small blood vessels, capillaries or venules, surrounded by histiocytes. Blood vessels are small tubular structures, sometimes with red blood cells in the lumen. The endothelial lining cells may appear reactive or "atypical." When occurring singly, reactive endothelial cells resemble small endocervical cells or small histiocytes with eccentric nuclei. A longitudinal groove is typically present in the nuclear membrane. The chromatin is very fine, pale, and regularly distributed. A small, but distinct, nucleolus may also be present. The cytoplasm is very delicate, with indistinct cell boundaries. A pale zone may be present in the perinuclear cytoplasm.

In addition, reactive myofibroblasts may be sampled. Myofibroblasts produce collagen and have a role in scar contraction. They have spindle to stellate shapes. A characteristic feature of these cells is the presence of thin little "rootlets"

Viruses

Herpes Simplex Virus

Although herpetic (Greek, to creep, referring to serpentine) genital lesions were described over a century ago [Naib 1966b], herpes simplex virus was first isolated from the female genital tract in 1946 [Slavin 1946]. Genital herpes infections are common; it is estimated that nearly 50 million Americans have been infected. Herpes simplex virus (HSV)-1 is the cause of most nongenital tract herpes infections, but HSV-1 can also infect the genitals, eg, by orogenital contact. HSV-2 is typically associated with genital tract infections [Nahmias 1968]. The old rule of thumb was that HSV-1 caused infections "above the waist," and HSV-2 caused those "below the waist," but genital tract lesions caused by HSV-1 are now more common than those caused by HSV-2 in some populations [C Roberts 2003, Samra 2003].

Many people infected with herpes are not aware of their infection. In some people, however, signs and symptoms can be severe, particularly with the first (primary) infection [Corey 1983a,b, Wald 1998]. When anogenital lesions occur, they typically appear as blisters. The blisters break, leaving painful ulcers that may take two to four weeks to heal the first time they occur. Because antibodies are produced, subsequent episodes are usually less frequent and less severe. The virus can remain dormant in the body for long periods of time. "Reinfection," which is actually reactivation of latent virus, often coincides when another infection is

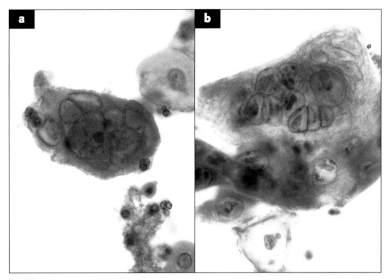

II.85
a, Herpes [L]; **b**, Herpes [L]

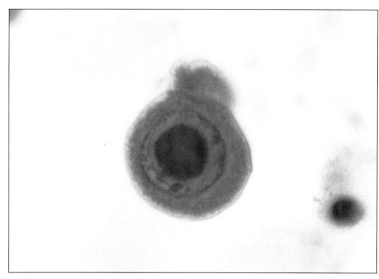

II.86
Cytomegalovirus [C]

contracted, such as *Trichomonas* or gonorrhea. Virions can be released from sores or from unbroken skin, during or between acute episodes.

Herpes simplex can cause herpes neonatorum, a rare, but potentially fatal infection in infants, if the mother is shedding virus at the time of vaginal delivery [Wald 1998]. If a pregnant woman has active genital herpes near delivery, a cesarean delivery is usually indicated. Although herpes is an important finding in pregnant women, *the Pap test is not reliable for detection of herpes infection.* There is a high false-negative rate, even in women with grossly visible lesions [R Ashley 1993, Corey 1982, Elnashar 2003, Koutsky 1992b, Maccato 1992, Morse 1974]. Herpes infection can make people more susceptible to HIV infection, and it can also make HIV-infected individuals more infectious. At one time suspected of causing cervical cancer, a primary role of HSV in cervical carcinogenesis is now doubtful. However, women with sexually transmitted diseases, including herpes infections, are in the high-risk group for cervical neoplasia.

There is no cure for herpes, but antiviral medications can shorten and prevent outbreaks. Although condoms decrease the risk of infection, when signs or symptoms are present, abstinence is safer.

Herpes is a double-stranded DNA virus. It has a capsid, produced by the virus, and a lipid envelope, derived from the host cell membrane. After penetrating the host, it is able to enter neurons and move up to the sensory sacral ganglia where it may remain latent for long periods. Recurrent infection represents reactivation of latent virus. The immune system of the host plays a key role in defense against reactivation [Maccato 1992].

The morphologic changes caused by Herpes simplex types 1 and 2 are indistinguishable [II.85a,b]. The most characteristic cells are multinucleated, with enlarged nuclei and nuclear molding (3Ms: multinucleation, molding, margination). The chromatin marginates, resulting in a homogeneous, ground glass appearance. Ground glass nuclei are key cytologic findings in herpes [Coleman 1982, Naib 1966b, Stowell 1994, Vesterinen 1977]. Ground glass nuclei contain viral particles. The nuclear membrane appears irregularly thickened due to condensed chromatin. Cowdry type A intranuclear inclusions are highly characteristic when present, but are found in less than half of cases [Stowell 1994]. These inclusions are said to be more typical of secondary infection [A Ng 1970b], but may simply be markers of cell death.

In liquid-based cytology, the usual features of herpes are seen, including multinucleation, molding, and margination of chromatin, leading to a ground glass appearance of the nucleus. Intranuclear inclusions, outlined by halos, may appear particularly prominent in LBC. Also, mononucleated infected cells may be more conspicuous.

The late changes, described above, are the most characteristic findings in herpes infection. Early cytologic changes in herpes infection include mononucleated cells, with high N/C ratios, and abnormal chromatin. Early changes can mimic CIN 3. However, CIN 3 has granular, clumped chromatin, irregular nuclear membranes, and is accompanied by lower-grade dysplasia, while herpes has ground-glass chromatin, smooth but thick nuclear membranes, and is accompanied by cells with classic herpetic changes. Necrotic herpetic lesions can mimic cervical cancer, clinically. Of course, cervical neoplasia and herpes infection share risk factors and can coexist [Rawls 1969].

Multinucleated endocervical cells can also mimic herpes infected cells, but nuclear molding is minimal or absent in endocervical cells and they also lack the highly characteristic ground glass chromatin and nuclear inclusions [Stowell 1994]. Other multinucleated cells that may be seen in a Pap test include: giant cell histiocytes, syncytiotrophoblasts, and malignant cells. A Pap test interpretation of herpes infection can be confirmed by other diagnostic tests [G Anderson 1985].

Other Viruses

Cytomegalovirus

Cytomegalovirus is a DNA virus that is a member of the herpes virus family. Although serologic evidence of prior CMV infection is very common (50%-80% of adults), morphologic evidence of CMV is rarely identified in Pap tests [Coleman 1982, Gideon 1991, Henry–Stanley 1993a, J Huang 1993, Morse 1974, Mulford 1991, Naib 1966a, Sickel 1991, Vesterinen 1975]. Glandular cells are usually involved, but squamous cells can be infected [JL Hunt 1998, Sekhon 2004]. Classic cytologic features of CMV include: cellular enlargement, nuclear enlargement, large nuclear inclusion surrounded by a halo ("owl's eye"), and small satellite nuclear or cytoplasmic inclusions [II.86] [Z Goodman 1979, Kasnic 1982]. Multinucleation can occur, but the nuclei do not mold significantly. Characteristic cells, if present at all, are usually sparse. If detected during pregnancy, there is a possibility of fetal infection. The cytologic findings are similar in LBC [Sekhon 2004].

Human Immunodeficiency Virus

Human immunodeficiency virus (HIV), although it can be transmitted sexually, does not have characteristic findings in Pap tests. The virus can be present in cervical secretions of infected women; therefore, vaginal fluid is potentially infectious. Sexually transmitted diseases appear to increase transmission of HIV; women with HIV are at increased risk of developing infections as well as cervical neoplasia. The CDC classifies cervical cancer as an AIDS defining illness in women with HIV infection [Anonymous 1993a] (see pg 87).

Human Papillomavirus

Human papillomavirus (HPV) is associated characteristic koilocytes, which have already been beaten to death in this manuscript (see pg 49), and so, will not be further discussed here. HPV is also important in cervical carcinogenesis; if this point somehow eluded you...go to jail, go directly to jail, do not pass Go, do not collect $200.

Other Viral Infections

Other viral infections, such as due to molluscum contagiosum, vaccinia, and adenoviruses, can be detected, rarely, in Pap tests. These viruses are associated with characteristic morphologic findings [S Brown 1981, Laverty 1977, Montone 1995]. Epstein-Barr virus and polyoma virus can cause genital ulcers, but the cytologic findings are nonspecific [S Taylor 1994, Y Taylor 1998].

Bacteria

In routine Pap tests, bacteria may be present, and their shape and arrangement can be noted, eg, cocci in clusters—staphylococci. However, it is not possible to determine whether the bacteria are gram-positive or gram-negative, let alone identify them specifically, in a routine Pap test. Culture is necessary for specific diagnosis. Normal flora was discussed previously (pg 88). This section discusses potentially pathogenic bacteria.

Bacterial Vaginosis

In 1955, Gardner and Dukes defined a clinical disease, nonspecific vaginitis, and reported that *Haemophilus vaginalis* was its cause [H Gardner 1955]. *H. vaginalis* was later renamed *Gardnerella vaginalis* (in honor of Herman Gardner) and the condition is now known as "bacterial vaginosis." "Bacterial" implies that bacteria, rather than fungi or parasites, cause the disease. "Vaginosis" (as opposed to vaginitis) is preferred because evidence of inflammation is typically absent [Eschenbach 1993, C Spiegel 1983, 1991].

Bacterial vaginosis (BV) is the most common cause of abnormal vaginal discharge in women of childbearing age [Sobel 1997]. It predominantly affects young, sexually active women, and although it can occur in nonsexually active women, it usually does not affect post-menopausal women unless they are on hormone replacement therapy [Sobel 2000]. Bacterial vaginosis can cause mild symptoms characterized by an abnormal vaginal discharge, with an unpleasant "fishy" or ammonia-like odor, especially pronounced after intercourse. The discharge is usually thin, homogeneous, and white or gray. Vaginal erythema and inflammation are absent and the cervix appears normal; if inflammation is present, it is caused by something else [Sobel 2000]. Many women with bacterial vaginosis are asymptomatic or consider their "symptoms" normal [Prey 1999].

Bacterial vaginosis is not caused by a single organism, but instead represents a polymicrobial syndrome. The normally predominant lactobacilli are replaced by the "BV organisms": *Gardnerella vaginalis*, *Prevotella* (formerly *Bacteroides*), *Mobiluncus*, peptostreptococci, and genital mycoplasmas *Mycoplasma hominis* and *Ureaplasma urealyticum* [JD Davis 1997, Eschenbach 1989, Giacomini 1992, Hawes 1996, Hill 1993, Hillier 1993b, DM Jones 1967, Mårdh 1971, Osborne 1982, Pybus 1999, Schwebke 1999, Thorsen 1998]. These organisms can be present in low numbers normally, but overgrow massively (100 to 1000 times normal) in bacterial vaginosis [Pybus 1999, Sobel 1997]. Thus, changes in vaginal flora can be thought of as a continuum, with the clinical syndrome of bacterial vaginosis being at one end of the spectrum [Schwebke 1999]. Women without evidence of vaginitis commonly have transient shifts in vaginal flora, eg, during menses [Bartlett 1977, Priestley 1997, Schwebke 1999]. In fact, only a minority of healthy women maintain "normal" vaginal flora consistently [Keane 1997, Schwebke 1999]. Factors associated with a shift in vaginal flora include multiple sexual partners, IUD use, douching, vaginal medications, spermicides, cunnilingus, prior pregnancy, and cigarette smoking [Amsel 1983, Avonts 1990, Barbone 1990, Hawes 1996, Hellberg 2000, Moi 1990, N Peters 1995, Schwebke 1999, Sobel 2000, Wolner-Hanssen 1990].

In bacterial vaginosis, the vaginal pH rises because of the lack of lactic acid-producing lactobacilli. Not only are the protective effects of lactobacilli lacking, but products from the BV organisms, such as sialidases and mucinases, can also facilitate more invasive infection [Soper 2002]. Overgrowth of vaginal anaerobes is associated with increased production of proteolytic enzymes, which break down peptides to amines (eg, putrescine, cadaverine, and trimethylamine); raise the vaginal pH; and increase vaginal transudation and cellular exfoliation, causing a malodorous discharge [Hillier 1993a, Wolrath 2002]. When the vaginal pH is increased above normal, *Gardnerella vaginalis* adheres more efficiently to squamous cells, causing "clue cell" formation, a characteristic finding in bacterial vaginosis [Sobel 2000]. *Gardnerella* is recovered in vaginal cultures in almost all (>90%) women with bacterial vaginosis, but it can also be cultured from roughly half (range 0 to 70%) of healthy, asymptomatic women [H Gardner 1955, Giacomini 1987, Mikamo 2000, Sobel 1997]. Therefore, a positive vaginal culture is not helpful in diagnosis of bacterial vaginosis, although a negative culture would practically exclude the diagnosis [Hillier 1993a, Mikamo 2000, Sobel 1997].

Complications of bacterial vaginosis are uncommon, but potentially serious, even in asymptomatic women [Giacomini 2000]. Bacterial vaginosis predisposes women to mucopurulent cervicitis, upper genital tract inflammation, and pelvic inflammatory disease. This can lead to other problems, including infertility, postoperative infections, premature labor, and premature or low-birth weight babies [JD Davis 1997, Demirezen 2003c, Hillier 1995, Mass 1999, C Spiegel 1991]. It may also increase a woman's susceptibility to other sexually transmitted diseases, such as *Chlamydia* and gonorrhea, and possibly HIV [CR Cohen 1995, Sewankambo 1997]. Bacterial vaginosis is common among women with CIN referred for colposcopy [Byrne 1991, Guijon 1992], and invasive cervical cancer is often associated with growth of anaerobic organisms [Mead 1978]. Nitrosamines, which are metabolic byproducts of anaerobic vaginal flora, may be potential chemical carcinogens [Harington 1975, Pavic 1984]. However, studies have reported conflicting results regarding whether bacterial vaginosis is associated with an increased risk of squamous intraepithelial lesions [N Peters 1995, Platz-Christensen 1994].

The clinical diagnosis of bacterial vaginosis can be made when three of the following four signs are present: thin, homogeneous discharge;

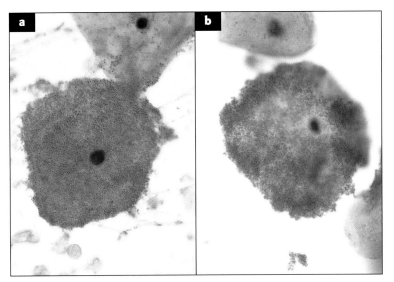

II.87
a, Clue cell, vaginosis [C]; **b**, Clue cell, vaginosis [L]

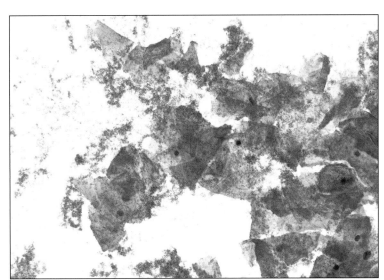

II.88
Desquamation and coccoid bacteria, bacterial vaginosis [C]

positive whiff test; vaginal pH > 4.5; and clue cells [Amsel 1983, Eschenbach 1988, Forsum 2002, Hellberg 2001, Nugent 1991]. The whiff test is performed by adding 10% potassium hydroxide (KOH) to the discharge; this releases amines and intensifies the fishy odor. The presence of clue cells is the single most reliable predictor of bacterial vaginosis [Eschenbach 1988, Hellberg 2001, Nugent 1991]. A shift from the normal *Lactobacillus* dominated vaginal flora to a predominance of coccobacilli in the Pap test provides supportive evidence of a clinical diagnosis of bacterial vaginosis [NCI 1993a, b]. Bacterial vaginosis is treatable with appropriate antimicrobial medicines [Soper 2002].

Pap Test in Bacterial Vaginosis

  "Shift in vaginal flora"

  Clue cells

  No lactobacilli

  No inflammation

Gardnerella vaginalis is a small, comma-shaped coccobacillus (gram negative/gram variable, facultative anaerobe) [Metzger 1998]. It is one of the major species associated with bacterial vaginosis. The bacteria tend to stick to squamous cells, forming "clue cells" [II.87a,b]. Clue cells are characterized by tiny bacteria that seem to be glued to squamous cells, forming a "velvety coat," and they also spread beyond the cell border, obscuring the cell margin, giving a "shaggy" appearance to the cell [Metzger 1998, Schnadig 1989]. Other bacteria, including lactobacilli, *staphylococci, streptococci,* and *Neisseria gonorrhoeae,* can adhere to cells [Bibel 1987, Ocana 2001]; therefore, to be considered a *true* clue cell, the bacteria must be tiny coccobacilli consistent with *Gardnerella* [Schnadig 1989]. Although the organisms must extend past the cell edges, the entire cell need not be covered with bacteria to be considered a clue cell.

Besides clues cells, the small coccobacilli also form a characteristic granular blue background in conventional smears, often described as filmy or sandy. This cytologic picture, historically known as "coccoid bacteria" or "cocci," is designated "shift in vaginal flora" in the Bethesda System [Ayre 1958]. Coccoid bacteria and clue cells are two manifestations of the same disorder [Giacomini 1987, 2000]. Coccoid bacteria, and sometimes clue cells, can be present in specific infections, such as those due to *Trichomonas* or yeast; this is not interpreted as bacterial vaginosis [Demirezen 2003c].

Mobiluncus organisms may be seen. They are small (1 μm-3 μm) curved (gram-negative, anaerobic) rods with tapered ends [C Spiegel 1983].

Lactobacilli are conspicuous by their absence (the dog that didn't bark in the night) [Schnadig 1989]. Inflammation is also notably absent, unless there is a coexisting infection [Prey 1999]. The absence of leukocytes in most women with bacterial vaginosis likely is due to lack of interleukin-8 induction [Cauci 2002]. Enhanced cellular desquamation with the presence of abundant anucleated squames is a common feature of bacterial vaginosis [II.88]. The squames are not hypermature (ie, this is not hyperkeratosis); desquamation is caused by the toxic nature of the amines [Amsel 1983, Giacomini 1998]. Slight parakeratosis is common.

In liquid-based cytology, the findings are generally similar (including clue cells), except that the background tends to be clean, in contrast to filmy background of small coccobacilli seen in conventional Pap smears.

In summary, the cytologic features of bacterial vaginosis are: presence of shift in vaginal flora ("coccoid bacteria") and clue cells, and absence of lactobacilli and inflammation. These findings in the Pap test are highly specific (~95%) for clinical bacterial vaginosis [JD Davis 1997, J Greene 2000, Tokyol 2004]. "Coccoid bacteria" (with or without clue cells) is frequently associated with clinical signs of bacterial vaginosis [Giacomini 1987, 1998]. Clue cells alone are highly predictive of bacterial vaginosis [Platz-Christensen 1994, 1995]. Although some authors have reported low sensitivity of cervical cytology for clinical bacterial vaginosis [JD Davis 1997, Greene 2000], sampling the vagina increases detection, probably because the vagina, rather than the cervix, is the primary site of disease [JD Davis 1997, Giacomini 1998, Greene 2000, Hillier 1993a]. A shift in vaginal flora is easily identified in the Pap test, and has the added advantage that several other conditions can be detected at the same time [U Bedrossian 1999, Giacomini 1998, Mass 1999].

In the Bethesda System, the findings described above are reported as "shift in vaginal flora suggestive of bacterial vaginosis." This interpretation is not considered definitive for bacterial vaginosis, but must be correlated clinically to arrive at a diagnosis. Many women with a shift in vaginal flora are asymptomatic.

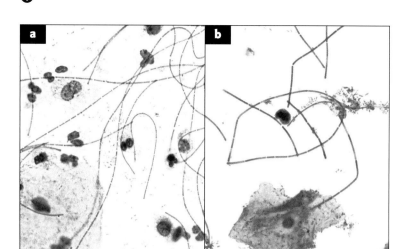

II.89
a, *Leptothrix* [C]; **b**, *Leptothrix* [L]

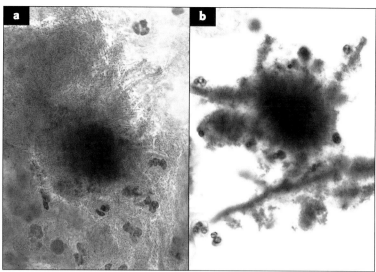

II.90
a, *Actinomyces* [C]; **b**, *Actinomyces* [L]

Leptothrix

Leptothrix is a commonly used, but outmoded term, for long filamentous bacteria, including mixed lactobacilli or *Actinomyces* [II.89a,b]. The organisms are long, thin (less than half as thick as *Candida*), and usually limp, like spaghetti. If *Leptothrix* is present, *Trichomonas* usually is also present ("spaghetti and meatballs"), but the reverse is not true, ie, *Trichomonas* is often present without *Leptothrix* [Bibbo 1972]. If you see spaghetti, look for the meatballs. In liquid-based cytology, *Leptothrix* has a tendency to form clumps that look a bit like balls of yarn.

Actinomyces

Actinomycosis of the female genital tract is rare. Most human cases are due to *Actinomyces israelii* and the vast majority are superficial colonizations, rather than invasive infections [Valicenti 1982]. Actinomycosis is predominantly associated with IUDs, occasionally, with other foreign objects (eg, pessaries, tampons), and rarely, occurs spontaneously [Bhagavan 1978, Brenner 1967, Christ 1978, deMoraes–Ruehsen 1980, Duguid 1980, DT Evans 1993, P Gupta 1976, 1982, Henderson 1973, Jarvis 1985, Luff 1978, Schmidt 1980, Spence 1978, Traynor 1981]. The organisms are part of the normal flora of the mouth and bowel, and can be introduced into the vagina from these sites [Merki–Feld 2000]. *Actinomyces* species can be grown in vaginal cultures from up to 25% of asymptomatic women [Lippes 1999], but organisms are identified microscopically in <10% (range 0% to 36%) of long-term IUD users [Fiorino 1996, Perlow 91] and in <1% of all Pap tests [Petitti 1983]. The risk increases with duration of IUD use [Chatwani 1994, Keebler 1983, Mali 1986, M Nayar 1985, Petitti 1983, Valicenti 1982] and possibly, composition of the IUD (more common with copper-containing than plastic-only IUDs) [Keebler 1983, Merki–Feld 2000, M Nayar 1985]. Although not considered a venereal disease, orogenital contact and multiple sexual partners increase risk [Fiorino 1996].

Most women with *Actinomyces* in their cytologic samples are asymptomatic, but some have a malodorous brownish discharge [P Gupta 1982]. Pain (pelvic, menstrual, dyspareunia) suggests invasive infection or pelvic inflammatory disease [Burkman 1982]. Disseminated infection, however, is rare [de la Monte 1982]. The presence of *Actinomyces* in the Pap

test should alert the clinician to the possibility of pelvic inflammatory disease.

Grossly visible sulfur granules, as described in sputum, are rarely observed in cervicovaginal actinomycosis. Microscopically, *Actinomyces* species are gram-positive, non-acid fast, branching, filamentous bacteria. In Pap tests, the organisms live symbiotically with colonies of bacteria, forming characteristic fuzzy dark-blue masses ("dust bunnies" or "Gupta bodies" [P Gupta 1976]) [II.90a,b, I.91a]. These have dense, granular blue bodies (bacteria) with delicate, red-tinged, spidery legs (*Actinomyces*). Coccoid bacteria usually replace the normal lactobacilli. There may be an associated acute inflammatory background. Possible clues to an invasive infection are: clubbing of the filaments at the periphery (Splendore-Hoeppli phenomenon, due to antigen-antibody reaction) [II.91b] and neutrophils adherent to the collections of organisms.

In liquid-based cytology, *Actinomyces* is seen as more three-dimensional "woolly" balls of tangled, branching filaments [II.90b]. Splendore-Hoeppli phenomenon (clubbing) may be present at the periphery of the filaments. The filaments are associated with colonies of nonfilamentous bacteria. Neutrophils are often present in the background.

The differential of filaments in the Pap smear includes other filamentous organisms, eg, *Candida*, *Leptothrix*, Eubacterium nodatum, botryomycosis, *Aspergillus*, *Nocardia*; fibers, eg, fibrin, cotton, synthetic fibers; mucin strands; and other foreign material [P Gupta 1982, Fiorino 1996, Hill 1992, MC Jones 1979, Merki–Feld 2000, Valicenti 1982]. Cockleburs (radiate crystalline arrays often associated with pregnancy, see pg 168) may be a particularly tempting misinterpretation if the clinical history is unknown. Clusters of other anaerobic bacteria can mimic actinomycotic granules. Culture is the most reliable method of diagnosis. After removal of the IUD, the organisms usually disappear from the Pap test [deMoraes–Ruehsen 1980, Valicenti 1982, Keebler 1983, K Mao 1984].

Therapy is controversial. For asymptomatic women, some recommend both IUD removal and antibiotic therapy; others recommend only one or the other [Bonacho 2001, Dybdahl 1991, DT Evans 1993, P Gupta 1982, Valicenti 1982]. For symptomatic women, antibiotics are usually indicated [Perlow 1991].

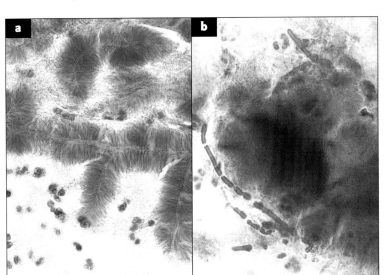

II.91
a, Variant *Actinomyces* [C]; **b**, Splendore-Hoeppli (arrows) [C]

Gonorrhea

Gonorrhea (gono-seed; rrhea-flow) is a common venereal disease. Each year approximately 650,000 American are infected with gonorrhea, and the incidence is increasing. In the United States, most cases occur in 15 to 29 years olds.

Gonorrhea is caused by *Neisseria gonorrhoeae*. It usually is spread through sexual contact (vaginal, oral, or anal), but can infect other parts of the body by contact with infective material. Symptoms are often mild and non-specific, but may include a painful or burning sensation when urinating and a vaginal discharge that is yellow or occasionally bloody. Untreated gonorrhea can ascend the female genital tract, and lead to pelvic inflammatory disease (PID). Women with gonorrhea should also be screened for other sexually transmitted diseases, including *Chlamydia*.

The organisms are bean-shaped cocci, slightly larger than coccoid bacteria, and occur in pairs as diplococci, often in mosaic arrangements [Heller 1974]. Intracytoplasmic diplococci (in neutrophils) are characteristic of gonorrhea, but not specific for it. The diplococci can also adhere to the surface of squamous cells. There is usually abundant purulent exudate. Although the organism can sometimes be detected in Pap tests [Arsenault 1976], this is tedious, time consuming, and has low sensitivity [Genvert 1980]; therefore, culture or other microbiologic testing must be performed to diagnose gonorrhea definitively.

Chlamydia Trachomatis

Chlamydia trachomatis is the most common sexually transmitted, bacterial infection in the United States. An estimated 3 million new *Chlamydia* infections occur each year [Holland–Hall 2004]. The cost of care for untreated chlamydial infections and their complications is estimated to exceed $2 billion annually [Peipert 2003].

Sexually active young women are especially susceptible to infection. Oral contraceptives and pregnancy may increase risk. By age 30, 50% of all sexually active women have had a Chlamydial infection. After age 30, the incidence drops off sharply. *Chlamydia* species can also cause other infections, including lymphogranuloma venereum, psittacosis, trachoma, and

conjunctivitis. *Chlamydia pneumoniae* has been associated with Alzheimer disease and cardiovascular disease [A Hudson 2001, Kalayoglu 2002].

Chlamydia can be transmitted by sexual intercourse and can also infect babies during vaginal childbirth. *Chlamydia* acquired during delivery is a leading cause of neonatal pneumonia and inclusion conjunctivitis (pinkeye). *Chlamydia* is known as a "silent" disease because the infection is usually (85% to 90% of cases) asymptomatic. However, about a third of women have local signs of infection on examination, particularly mucopurulent cervicitis and hypertrophic cervical ectopy [Peipert 2003]. Unfortunately, the disease is frequently not diagnosed until complications, such as pelvic inflammatory disease (PID) or infertility, develop [Turner 2002]. Barrier contraception reduces the risk of infection.

Chlamydia initially attacks the cervix and the urethra in women. Symptoms, when they occur, usually appear within 1 to 3 weeks of exposure, and may include an abnormal vaginal discharge or burning on urination. When the infection ascends from the cervix to the fallopian tubes, some women have lower abdominal pain or low back pain, nausea, fever, dyspareunia, or intermenstrual bleeding; but other women are asymptomatic. When the upper reproductive system is involved, it may lead to pelvic inflammatory disease with permanent damage.

Mucopurulent cervicitis (yellow exudate) is clinically characteristic. The presence of a neutrophilic infiltrate is a sensitive microscopic indicator of *Chlamydia* infection, but is not specific [Brunham 1984]. Screening tests for *Chlamydia* are available, which can be performed on the residual of liquid-based Pap tests (although the value of the Pap test itself for the detection of *Chlamydia* is limited, read on). When diagnosed early, *Chlamydia* can be easily treated and cured with appropriate antibiotics. All sex partners should be treated.

An association between *Chlamydia trachomatis* and the development of cervical neoplasia has been reported [Allerding 1985, Anttila 2001, Cevenini 1981, E Claas 1992, de Borges 1984, de Sanjosé 1994, M Hare 1982, Kjær 1997, Koutsky 1992a, M Lehmann 1999, Paavonen 1979, J Schächter 1975, 1982, K Syrjänen 1986b, Wallin 2002, Zenilman 2001]. *Chlamydia* infection has also been described in women who have received radiotherapy for cervical cancer [Maeda 1990]. However, the role of *Chlamydia*, if any, in cervical carcinogenesis seems to be minimal after controlling for sexual risk factors and HPV infection [E Claas 1992, Edelman 2000, L Lindner 1985]. Infection with *Chlamydia* may be a risk factor for ovarian cancer [Ness 2003].

There are four species of Chlamydia: C. trachomatis, C. pneumoniae, C. psittaci, and C. pecorum. C. trachomatis is subdivided into 15 serotypes. *Chlamydia* was not recognized as a sexually transmitted disease until recently. The name, *Chlamydia*, derives from the Greek, *chlamys*, a cloak draped over the shoulders, to describe intracytoplasmic inclusions draped over the nucleus [Taylor–Robinson 1980]. *Chlamydia* is generally considered a bacterium, but it also has viral properties. Like bacteria, *Chlamydia* contains both DNA and RNA, has cell walls, and is sensitive to antibiotics. Like viruses, *Chlamydia* is an obligate intracellular organism that multiplies by binary fission, forms cellular inclusions, and cannot synthesize its own adenosine triphosphate (ATP) that is necessary for cellular energy. The genome of *Chlamydia* is ~500-1000 kilobases and contains both RNA and DNA. C. trachomatis targets endocervical glandular cells and metaplastic cells.

Chlamydia trachomatis can cause several cytologic changes in cells, including granular cytoplasmic inclusions, discussed in more detail

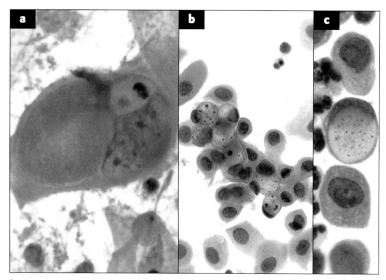

II.92
a, *Chlamydia* [C]; **b**, Nonspecific vacuoles [C]; **c**, Faux chlamydia [C]

In theory, detection of *Chlamydia* is based upon identification of these cytoplasmic inclusions that represent different stages of the life cycle [Weisenberg 2001]. Inclusions occur in endocervical cells or metaplastic squamous cells, but not mature squamous cells [R Phillips 1987]. Elementary bodies supposedly can be identified as numerous fine intracytoplasmic "coccoid" structures, surrounded by narrow clear zones [P Gupta 1979, 1988]. Reticulate bodies supposedly can be identified as fine vacuoles containing somewhat larger inclusions, giving the cell a "moth-eaten" appearance [P Gupta 1988]. With time, these merge to form dense, targetoid inclusions within larger vacuoles. Moth-eaten metaplastic cells are said to correlate with a high risk of infection [P Gupta 1988]. However, targetoid cytoplasmic inclusions are not definitive for Chlamydial infection [II.92b,c]. Many are actually mucin vacuoles, or contain bacteria, cell debris, or other artifacts [E Claas 92, R Clark 1985, P Gupta 1979, 1988, MR Henry 1993, Paavonen 1980, Purola 1982, Shafer 1985, Shiina 1985].

Nebular bodies may be more specific for *Chlamydia*, but are rarely identified [MR Henry 1993, S Waters 1991]. Shiina first described nebular bodies in 1985 [Shiina 1985, 1990]. Nebular bodies are variably-sized vacuoles, with thin walls and finely granular inclusions, that neither displace the nucleus nor distend the cytoplasm [Shiina 1985]. This contrasts with non-specific targetoid vacuoles, which have thick walls and coarsely granular inclusions, that may (or may not) displace the nucleus or distend the cytoplasm.

In practice, specific recognition of these various bodies is difficult and their significance is questionable. Cytoplasmic vacuolization is extremely common and the causes are legion [Crum 1984c, Vinette-Leduc 1997]. Trying to sort out all the different kinds of vacuoles is an exercise in futility. Conclusive diagnosis of Chlamydial infection requires confirmation by culture, immunologic techniques, or molecular diagnostic methods, such as polymerase chain reaction or ligase chain reaction [E Chan 2000, H Claas 1990, Crum 1984c, D Feldman 2001, Hori 1995, Kobayashi 1987, Kuo 1974, L Lindner 1985, 1986, 1988, Singh 2002, Tam 1984, Vela 1998, Vinette-Leduc 1997]. It is noteworthy that *Chlamydia* is not included as an interpretation/result in the Bethesda System lexicon.

Tuberculosis

Rare in the United States, tuberculous cervicitis and endometritis are more common in developing countries. The disease is usually secondary to tuberculosis elsewhere in the female genital tract, particularly the fallopian tube, which itself may follow primary pulmonary or intestinal tuberculosis. Advanced cervical tuberculosis can mimic invasive cancer on clinical examination. Histologically, the lesion is characterized by multiple granulomas ("tubercles") with central caseous necrosis, epithelioid histiocytes, and multinucleated Langhans giant cells, surrounded by a heavy lymphoplasmacytic infiltrate.

The cytology reflects the histology: epithelioid histiocytes, Langhans giant cell histiocytes (with peripheral nuclei), ordinary histiocytes, lymphocytes and plasma cells, and granular ("caseous" or cheesy) necrosis [Angrish 1981, Coleman 1969, Kobayashi-Kawata 1978, Meisels 1975, Misch 1976]. Epithelioid histiocytes have elongated, slender nuclei with irregular outlines (like footprints or bananas), very fine chromatin, tiny nucleoli, and ill-defined, fibrillar cytoplasm. In exfoliative cytology, they often have a carrot shape and may even stain orange. Acid-fast stain can be used to identify characteristic beaded, red mycobacteria ("red snappers"). Definitive diagnosis can be made by culture or polymerase chain reaction of cervicovaginal specimens [Ferrara 1999]. The differential includes foreign body granulomas, which are common after surgery or radiation (reaction to foreign material or necrotic tissue [C Evans

below [II.92a] [P Gupta 1979]. Nuclear changes include nuclear enlargement, increased N/C ratio, hyperchromasia, and multinucleation; nucleoli are rare or absent. These nuclear changes can mimic dysplasia, usually low-grade, but true dysplasia can coexist [Boon 1983]. *Chlamydia trachomatis* can also cause cellular enlargement (20 μm-100 μm).

Chlamydia trachomatis is strongly associated with follicular cervicitis [M Hare 1981, 1982, Kiviat 1985a,b, Paavonen 1982, Winkler 1987]. Transformed lymphocytes, plasma cells, or histiocytes are frequently increased in women with *Chlamydia* [Freund 1992, Kiviat 1985a,b], but these findings are nonspecific [L Lindner 1985]. Neutrophils are a common (sensitive, but nonspecific) finding in women with *Chlamydia* infection [Páler 2000]. *Chlamydia* may be suspected in young women with marked acute inflammation, particularly when another infectious agent, such as *Trichomonas*, cannot be identified [Dimian 1992, J Wilson 1990].

The value of the Pap test in specifically identifying *Chlamydia* has been hotly debated [Addiss 1990, Bernal 1989, R Clark 1985, Dorman 1983, Forster 1985, Geerling 1985, Ghirardini 1989, 1991, P Gupta 1988, Kiviat 1985a, L Lindner 1985, Naib 1970, Pandit 1993, T Quinn 1987, Roongpisuthipong 1987, Sekhri 1988, Shafer 1985, Spence 1986, Weisenberg 2001]. Cytoplasmic inclusions, said to be diagnostic, were first described in scrapings of conjunctival mucosa by K Stargardt in 1909, and shortly thereafter, in cells in cervical smears by L Halberstaedler and S von Prowazek [Naib 1970]. Reported sensitivities and specificities are all over the map: sensitivity ranges from <10% [Arroyo 1989b] to 100% [Pánuco 2000] and specificity from <5% [Caudill 1994] to 100% [Kiviat 1985b].

The life cycle of *C trachomatis* consists of two stages, elementary bodies and reticulate bodies [M Lehmann 1999, Swanson 1975, Taylor-Robinson 1980]. Elementary bodies, analogous to metabolically inactive spores, are the infectious particle. They enter the cell, by endocytosis, and are contained in small vacuoles derived from the cell membrane. Individual elementary bodies are about 0.2 μm to 0.4 μm in diameter [Hori 1995]. Elementary bodies then "germinate" into reticulate bodies, which are noninfectious, but metabolically active. They divide by binary fission, forming a cytoplasmic inclusion. Reticulate bodies condense to reform infectious elementary bodies; eventually, the vacuole contains 100 to 1000 elementary bodies, which are then released from the cell by exocytosis or cell lysis [Winkler 1987].

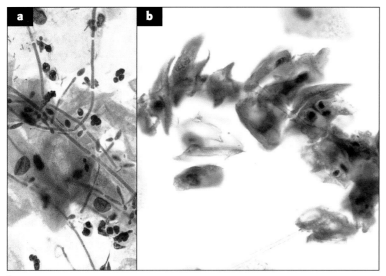

II.93
a, *Candida* [C]; **b**, *Candida* shish kebab [L]

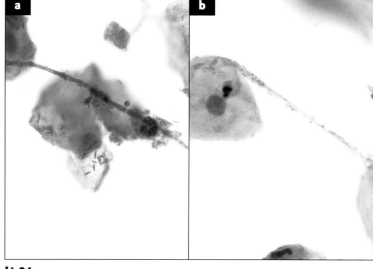

II.94
a, *Candida* [L]; **b**, Mucus strand [L]

1984]). Also, other infections, such as syphilis, schistosomiasis, granuloma inguinale [de Boer 1984], and lymphogranuloma venereum [M Chandra 1991, Leiman 1986]; foreign bodies, such as sutures, crystals, or cotton fibers; sarcoidosis; and squamous cell carcinoma can be associated with granulomatous inflammation.

Syphilis

Treponema pallidum, the spirochete that causes syphilis, cannot be identified in routine Pap tests, and requires special staining (eg, silver stains, immunofluorescence) to be visualized. The Pap test findings in syphilis are nonspecific, but may include granulomas, chronic inflammation with plasma cells, histiocytes, and debris [Gutmann 1995].

Fungi
Candida Species

Candida, formerly known as Monilia, accounts for the vast majority of mycotic vulvovaginal infections [Kearns 1963]. Vulvovaginal Candidiasis, or "yeast" infections, are extremely common in women during the reproductive years, particularly during pregnancy and the late luteal phase of the menstrual cycle [Kalo–Klein 1989]. It is estimated that up to 75% of all women have a *Candida* infection sometime in their lives and 5% have chronic, recurrent infections [Sobel 1997]. Candidiasis is not traditionally considered a sexually transmitted disease because it can occur in virgins and *Candida* can be part of the normal vaginal flora [Sobel 1997]. However, there is an increased incidence of Candidiasis in women following the onset of regular sexual activity.

The presence of *Candida* in Pap tests is associated with changes in vaginal glycogen, flora, or pH. Other predisposing factors include: immunosuppression, including HIV infection [Rhoads 1987] and diabetes mellitus; debilitating disease; steroids (oral contraceptives, corticoids); broad-spectrum antibiotics, chemotherapy; alkaline douches; and even soap, any of which can disrupt the normal vaginal flora and allow *Candida* to proliferate. Clinical findings include itching, with red inflamed mucous membranes, and discharge that is characteristically thick and

white, like cottage cheese, but not malodorous. Complications are rare [Valdivieso 1976].

Candidiasis is often self-diagnosed and self-treated. A concern is that several conditions can mimic Candidiasis, including allergic or chemical reactions and herpes. The Pap test is not a particularly good test for *Candida*; it is detected in many asymptomatic women and is not detected in many women who are symptomatic [Donders 1992, Shurbaji 1999].

> ### Pap Test in Candida Infection
> *Yeasts, pseudohyphae*
> *Mild nuclear enlargement,*
> *slight hyperchromasia*
> *Mimics squamous atypia ("Candy ASC-US")*
> *Slight hyperkeratosis, neutrophil lysis (clues)*

Obviously, the presence of *Candida* in the Pap test does not necessarily indicate a clinically significant infection. Microscopic examination, although less sensitive than fungal culture, correlates better with clinical symptoms than culture [Shurbaji 1999]. Ultimately, clinical signs and symptoms play a decisive role in determining whether therapy is necessary.

Both pseudohyphae (sticks) and yeast (stones) usually occur, and together look like "balloon dogs" [II.93a,b, I.94a]. Yeasts measure about 3 μm-7 μm, and may bud. Pseudohyphae usually stain pale pink or blue, and are surrounded by a small, clear halo. Pseudohyphae may appear to impale mature squamous cells, giving a "shish kebab" or "paper spindle" effect (who remembers "do not fold, *spindle*, or mutilate" in this day of yellow sticky notes?). The number of organisms is highly variable and does not correlate with symptoms [Shurbaji 1999].

In liquid-based cytology, the organisms are usually beautifully highlighted and easy to identify. The shish kebab effect tends to be particularly prominent in LBC [II.93b, 1.94a]. However, mucus strands, common in LBC, can closely mimic *Candida*; look for constrictions (budding) that make *Candida* resemble strings of sausages [II.94a,b].

Up to 90% of yeast infections are due to *Candida albicans* [Kearns 1963]. If only pseudohyphae are seen, consider *Geotrichum* (*Geotrichum candidum*); if only yeasts are seen, consider *Torulopsis* (*Candida glabrata*) [Boquet–Jiménez 1978]. However, *Candida* cannot be speciated based on

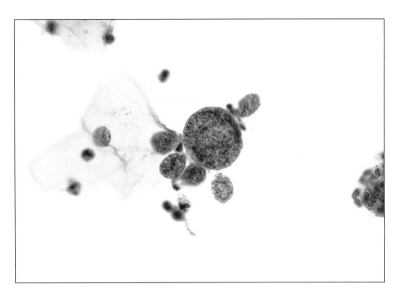

11.95
Cokeromyces [L]

morphology alone; culture is necessary, but probably not important because therapy is the same. Candidiasis is usually associated with an increase in neutrophils, but they vary considerably in number from case to case [Shurbaji 1999]. Other findings associated with *Candida* in the Pap test include: neutrophil lysis (free nuclear lobes that look like little blue BBs in the background), mild hyperkeratosis, and minimal nuclear abnormalities, mimicking squamous atypia (*Candida* atypia, aka "Candy ASC-US") [Heller 1971, Miguel 1997].

In summary, Pap test sensitivity for presence of *Candida* is approximately 80% [Siapco 1986]. However, *Candida* in the Pap test does not necessarily indicate symptomatic infection.

Other Fungi

Rarely, other fungi besides *Candida* are identified in Pap tests [Colino 1976]. These include *Blastomyces* [Dyer 1983, Sen 1997], *Paracoccidioides* [Sheyn 2001], *Fusarium* [S Gupta 2003a], and *Cokeromyces* [11.95] [Kemna 1994, McGough 1990, Munipalli 1996, Ribes 2000, Rippon 1979, 1980].

Protozoa

Trichomonas vaginalis

Alfred Donné (1801-1878) first discovered the parasite that he named *Trico-monas vaginalis*, in 1836, when he visualized motile microorganisms in the vaginal discharge of symptomatic women. This was apparently the first description of a living pathogenic organism in humans. In 1845, he published the first medical book using photomicrographs (*Cours de Microscopie*, also the first cytology text and atlas) as the basis for illustrations (an image of *Trichomonas* was included). Donné's "wet prep" technique is still the mainstay of diagnosis of *Trichomonas* infection [Campbell 2001, Fouts 1980, Hajdu 1998].

Trichomoniasis, caused by the protozoan, *Trichomonas vaginalis*, is one of the most common sexually transmitted diseases, mainly affecting 16-to-35-year old women, but can occur even in postmenopausal women. It is estimated that at least 2 million women in the US become infected each year. It can also infect men, causing urethritis or prostatitis, although symp-

toms are more common in women [W Gardner 1986, Kuberski 1980]. Having multiple sexual partners is the primary risk factor for infection [McLellan 1982, Z-F Zhang 1996]. Condoms decrease risk.

Trichomoniasis typically causes a frothy, yellow-green or gray-white vaginal discharge with a strong odor. Itching and irritation are common [Wolner-Hanssen 1989]. Infection can also cause discomfort during intercourse or urination. In rare cases, lower abdominal pain occurs. Symptoms usually appear within 5 to 28 days of exposure in women, but many women are asymptomatic [Burja 2001, McLellan 1982, Spence 1980]. Trichomoniasis in pregnant women can cause premature rupture of the membranes and preterm delivery [Herzberg 1996].

A possible link between *Trichomonas* infection and cervical neoplasia was first suggested in the 1950s [Bechtold 1952, Frost 1962, Koss 1959, Z-F Zhang 1994]. Earlier studies failed to account for HPV as a confounding factor [Sardana 1994, Yap 1995]. However, some risk remains after controlling for HPV [Gram 1992b]. Although no longer believed to be a primary cause, *Trichomonas* infection could promote cervical cancer, eg, by production of abnormal amines [Boyle 1999, Harington 1975].

On exam, the vaginal wall and cervix are typically congested and have pinhead-sized hemorrhages, resulting in the classic "strawberry" appearance [Koss 1959]. Detection of *Trichomonas* is traditionally made by wet mount or by Pap test. The Pap test sensitivity ranges from 35% to 85%; specificity ranges from 80% to 100% [Felman 1979, Fleury 1979, J Krieger 1981, 1988, Lara-Torre 2003, Lobo 2003, Lossick 1991, Spence 1980, Thomason 1988, Weinberger 1993, Wiese 2000, Wolner-Hanssen 1989]. A meta-analysis reported that the sensitivity of the Pap test was 57% and the specificity 97% [Wiese 2000]. However, confirmation of a Pap test interpretation of *Trichomonas* is recommended before treatment of asymptomatic women [Weinberger 1993, Wiese 2000]. Culture is the current "gold standard" for diagnosis, but it is not perfect, with sensitivity ranging from 86% to 97% [Burja 2001, Lawing 2000, Lossick 1988, Thomason 1988, Weinberger 1993]. Newer diagnostic techniques, such as polymerase chain reaction, are also available [Lawing 2000, Lobo 2003, Okuyama 1998, B Paterson 1998, Ryu 1999]. Trichomoniasis usually can be easily cured with appropriate antibiotics. All sexual partners should be treated to eliminate the parasite.

Trichomonas vaginalis is an oval or pear-shaped organism that ranges from 8 μm-30 μm (ie, from the size of an intermediate *nucleus* to parabasal *cell*) [Frost 1962, Papanicolaou 1955b] [11.96a,b,c]. An inverse relation between the size of the organism and the severity of the infection has been reported (smaller size, more severe) [Winston 1974]. The Trichomonad nucleus (thin, elliptical, pale, eccentrically located) *must* be seen to identify this organism specifically (the nucleus distinguishes the parasite from cytoplasmic fragments, other debris). Red granules are frequently present in cyanophilic to gray cytoplasm, and help to locate the organisms. Flagella (3-5 anterior, 1 posterior) are practically never seen in conventional Pap smears, but may be identified, occasionally, in liquid-based Pap tests [11.96c].

Pap Test in Trichomonas Infection
Protozoans, plus:
*Pseudokeratinization**
*Slight nuclear enlargement**
*Hyperchromasia**
*Perinuclear vacuoles**
Dirty background
Cannonballs
**Features can mimic L SIL*

Richard M DeMay

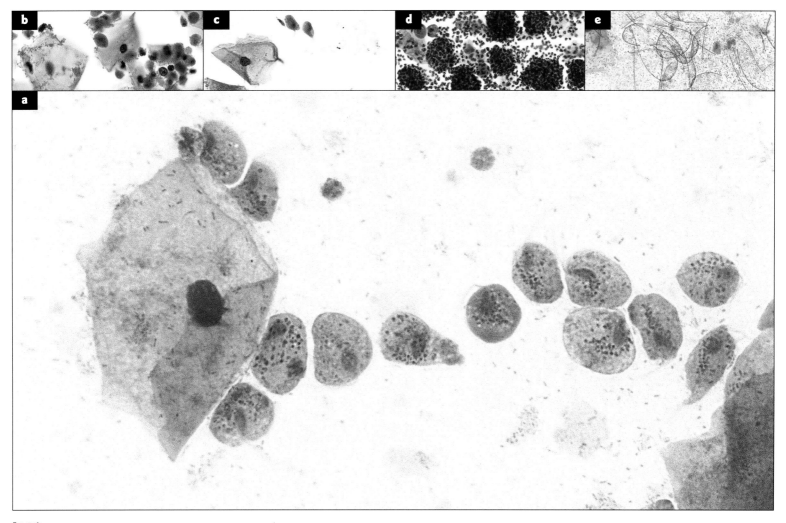

11.96
a, *Trichomonas* [C]; **b**, *Trichomonas* [L]; **c**, *Trichomonas*, flagella [L]; **d**, *Trichomonas*, cannonballs [C]; **e**, *Trichomonas*, *Leptothrix* [C]

In liquid-based cytology, Trichomonads appear smaller and as mentioned, flagella are sometimes identified. The organisms are usually oval to pear-shaped, as in conventional Pap smears, but sometimes are angular, and may look like little kites (particularly if flagella are identified). Also, the nuclei are smaller and the red granules may be less apparent in LBC.

Trichomonas infection commonly causes nonhormonal maturation, or "pseudomaturation," of the squamous epithelium [Frost 1962, Koss 1959, Papanicolaou 1955b]. Superficial cells, generalized eosinophilia, and pseudokeratinization characterize pseudomaturation. Slightly enlarged, dark nuclei and inflammatory perinuclear halos are common, mimicking low-grade dysplasia or condyloma (L SIL) [11.53a] [Bechtold 1952, Koss 1959, Papanicolaou 1955b]. Atypical parakeratosis can occur [Voytek 1996].

Marked inflammatory changes are common in *Trichomonas* infection. Numerous neutrophils, often agglomerated onto squamous cells forming characteristic "cannonballs" (or "pusballs") [11.96d], as well as lots of lymphocytes [Kiviat 1985a] and many mast cells [Kobayashi 1983b] may be observed. Marked reparative changes can mimic malignancy; on the other hand, malignancy may be misinterpreted as benign repair when a

distracting *Trichomonas* infection is present [Renshaw 2004d]. The background typically appears "dirty" owing to lysed cells, inflammation, and debris, and the normal flora is replaced by coccoid bacterial overgrowth [Papanicolaou 1955b]. Erythrophagocytosis can occur; RBCs provide nutrients, eg, iron and lipids, for the organism [Demirezen 2000b, 2001]. In some cases, long bacteria (so-called Leptothrix) are present **[11.96e]** [Papanicolaou 1955b]—when leptothrix is present, look for Trichomonads. However, the background can also be clean rather than inflammatory [Herzberg 1996]. Neither the number of organisms nor the degree of inflammation correlates well with clinical symptoms [Burja 2001].

The differential of *Trichomonas* organisms includes cell fragments, cytoplasmic debris, bare epithelial nuclei, small mucus aggregates, and even neutrophils [Herzberg 1996, Weinberger 1993]. Identification of the nucleus of the parasite helps avoid misinterpretation. *Trichomonas* infection can lead to both false-positive and false-negative results. The combination of a dirty background plus atypical cellular changes can be overinterpreted as squamous neoplasia (dysplasia, cancer); conversely, squamous neoplasia can be underinterpreted as benign changes resulting from *Trichomonas* infection [Neal 1999, Renshaw 2004d].

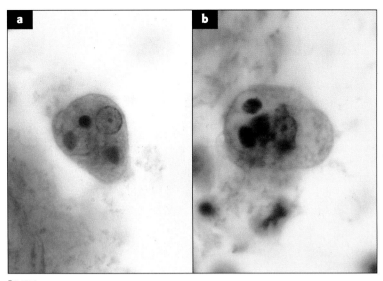

II.97
a, *Entamoeba histolytica*; **b**, *Entamoeba gingivalis*

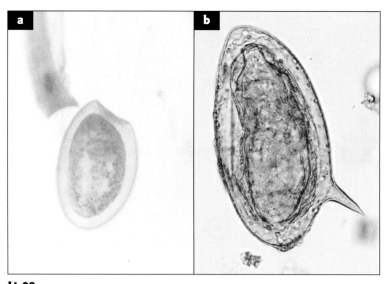

II.98
a, *Enterobius vermicularis*; **b**, *Schistosoma mansoni*

Other Organisms

Other organisms can infect the female genital tract and can *sometimes* be identified in Pap tests [De Torres 1973, Feldmeier 2001, S Gupta 2003a, Learmonth 1990, Sheyn 2001]. These include amoebae (*Entamoeba histolytica* [II.97a] [Arroyo 1989a, Bhambhani 2001, C Cohen 1973, De Torres 1973, R Gupta 2003, Kobayashi 1985, Munguia 1966] and *E gingivalis* [II.97b] [Arroyo 1989c, deMoraes-Ruehsen 1980, McNeill 1978] (see also IUD effect pg 163), and ova and parasites such as *Enterobius vermicularis* (pin worm) [II.98a] [Avram 1984, Bhambhani 1985, Das 2002, Garud 1980, Mali 1987, San Cristobal 1976], *Schistosoma hematobium* and *S mansoni* [II.98b] [Adeniran 2003, Berry 1966, 1976, DeMille 1995, el Tabbakh 1989, Feldmeier 2001, Mainguené 1998, Poggensee 2001, Rand 1998, Sharma 2001], *Strongyloides stercoralis* [Avram 1984, Daneshbod 2004, Murty 1994], *Trichuris trichuria* (thread worm), *Tenia solium* [Bhambhani 1985], *Vorticella* [P Kumar 2001], *Taenia* [Bhambhani 1985], *Loa loa* [Stelow 2003], echinococcus, *Ascaris lumbricoides* [Bhambhani 1984, 1985, Garud 1980, Mali 1987] and *filaria* [de Borges 1971, Mali 1987, Sharma 1971, Vaghese 1996], including *Wuchereria bancrofti* [K Chandra 1975, Mehrotra 1998].

Arthropods, such as body lice, *Pediculus humanus*, or the pubic louse, *Phthirus pubis*, "crabs," are identified, rarely, in Pap tests [II.99] [Suurmeijer 2002]. Various artifacts and contaminants also occur that could be misinterpreted as infectious agents (see pg 192) [Demirezen 2000a].

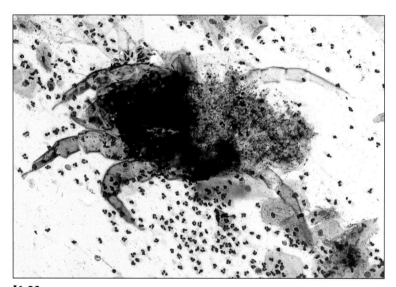

II.99
Phthirus pubis ("crab") [C]

II. Cytology of the Glandular Epithelium

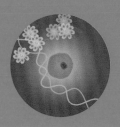

Glandular epithelium of the female genital tract includes the lining of the cervix (endocervix), uterus (endometrium), and fallopian tube (endosalpinx). These structures and their corresponding glandular cells are of Müllerian origin and their malignancies, adenocarcinomas, are by far the most common invasive cancers of the female genital tract. Adenocarcinoma of the cervix has been increasing in incidence, despite widespread screening, and currently accounts for up to a third of all invasive cervical cancers. Endometrial adenocarcinoma is even more common, but adenocarcinoma of the fallopian tube is rare. Although it is sometimes possible to detect adenocarcinomas and their precursor lesions by exfoliative cytology, to date, Pap test screening has had no significant effect in preventing adenocarcinomas.

Interpreting glandular cells and their lesions on Pap tests can be challenging. Even the basic distinction between glandular and squamous cells can be tricky: abnormalities thought to be *glandular* on Pap test often turn out to be *squamous* on biopsy! Interpretive problems can arise because the glandular cells are sparse or degenerated, particularly those of endometrial origin. On the other hand, even when the cells are abundant and well preserved, interpretive problems can still occur. For example, an endocervical brush can harvest large, densely cellular aggregates, which can have a host of morphological appearances that can be difficult to classify. Benign glandular cells may have reactive changes mimicking both glandular and squamous neoplasia [Chakrabarti 1994, Lickrish 1993]. Malignant glandular cells can be cytologically bland and look benign. Even normal endocervical cells have a spectrum of cytomorphologies that can lead to interpretive problems.

Endocervical Cytology

Knowledge of normal histology is helpful in interpretation of endocervical cytology. First of all, the endocervix does not really have "glands" in the usual sense of having a secretory unit, with secretory cells, connected to a surface by a duct, lined with ductal cells. Rather, the endocervix is a series of grooves or clefts, ie, deep infoldings of mucosa that may tunnel into the endocervical stroma forming crypts that, histologically, look like compound, racemose glands, but are not [Fluhmann 1957, E Stern 1973]. A single layer of endocervical columnar cells lines these mucosal folds, which are termed plicae palmatae [I2.1].

Location, location, location: glandular cells are a normal component of the endocervix and a key component of Pap tests that indicate that the transformation zone was sampled. However, endocervical cells occurring in the vagina (as opposed to the cervix) indicate vaginal adenosis (see pg 161). Collections of small endocervical "glands," known as tunnel clusters, could be histologically mistaken for well-differentiated adenocarcinoma [MA Jones 1996]. Moreover, the morphology of endocervical cells depends upon their location in the endocervix. The classic morphology of endocervical cells, as obtained by the Ayre spatula and derived from low in the endocervix, is described below. So-called "high endocervical cells," as obtained by an endocervical brush and derived from high in the endocervix, are also described.

Endocervical Cells

"Classic" endocervical cells are tall and columnar; most are secretory [I2.2a,b, 2.3a,b], some are ciliated [I2.4a,b]. They commonly range from 20 μm-30 μm in height and 8 μm-10 μm in width. "Pencil-thin" endocervical cells are elongated and slender, sometimes resembling smooth muscle cells [I2.5a,b]. These skinny cells can result from application of Lugol iodine solution (which is hypertonic) or acetic acid to the cervix, or from electrocautery (heat artifact) [Benda 1987, Cronjé 1997, Griffiths 1989, D Hammond 1980, Holmquist 1976]. Mitotic figures are rare in normal endocervical cells; their presence is a red flag warning to look carefully for evidence of neoplasia.

Secretory endocervical cells have generous cytoplasm that contains either multiple fine mucin vacuoles or one large one [I2.2a,b, 2.3a,b]. These cells can be particularly "plump and juicy" in the luteal phase of the menstrual cycle, in pregnancy, in response to some oral contraceptives or hormone therapies, and in endocervical polyps [Affandi 1985]. Endocervical cell mucin contains sulfated, sialic acid, mucopolysaccharides. Endocervical mucus is alkaline, which contrasts with the normal acid pH of the vagina. Estrogen promotes, and progesterone inhibits, mucus secretion [E Stern 1973].

Ciliated endocervical cells look like ciliated respiratory ("bronchial") cells [I2.4a,b]. They have denser cytoplasm than secretory endocervical cells and, most characteristically, terminal bars and cilia. The number of ciliated endocervical cells increases during the first half, or estrogenic phase, of the menstrual cycle. As in the lung, ciliated cells probably have a role in propelling mucus. Rarely, ciliated cells "blow their tops" and the little red wigs detach from the cells (see ciliocytophthoria, detached ciliary tufts pg 192). Ciliated cell malignancies are as rare as hen's teeth [Maksem 1997]. So, it pays to look carefully for cilia because ciliated cells are almost always benign, even when they look atypical (Cilia: When these you divine, that's a fine benign sign!).

Endocervical cells can be seen singly, in strips, or in sheets. Two-dimensional sheets, seen *en face*, appear as regular, orderly ranks and files of uniform cells [I2.3a,b]. Each cell lines up in a row and the cells all look alike—like a "print" with a repeating pattern (think of a checkerboard). Slight prominence of the cell membranes where the cells attach to one another results in a well-ordered "honeycomb" appearance—the classic finding in benign glandular cells in any site. There are normally no glandular structures (papillae, cell balls, microacini or rosettes, etc). Malignant cells are unruly little devils, and typically crowd and pile up, resulting in a disorderly appearance.

Strips of endocervical cells, viewed from the side, line up—like pickets in a fence—forming a palisade of uniform, orderly cells [I2.2a,b]. Single cells have a columnar configuration, with basal nuclei and apical cytoplasm ("basal" and "apical," of course, depend on the spatial orientation of the cells; "nucleocytoplasmic polarity" is more politically correct because it is not "spacist"). Nucleocytoplasmic polarity is characteristic of glandular differentiation. ("Honeycomb," "picket fence," and "palisade" are buzzwords that imply a benign process to those in the know.)

Endocervical nuclei usually are single, but occasionally binucleation or multinucleation occurs, particularly in reactive conditions. The nucleus of an endocervical cell looks like a normal intermediate cell nucleus, although it is slightly larger (~55 μm^2 vs 35 μm^2), or about the size of a parabasal cell nucleus (~50 μm^2) [Patten 1978]. It is round to oval and the nuclear membrane is usually smooth, but sometimes there is a protrusion, or "nipple" [Koizumi 1996, RS Taylor 1984]. Papanicolaou suggested that nuclear nipples are normal and noted an association with estrogen [Papanicolaou 1954], while others have observed an association with progesterone, eg,

---

Endocervical Cells

Columnar cells

Sheets, "honeycomb"

Strips, "palisades"

Single, N–C polarity

Secretory > ciliated

Presence ⇒ TZ sampled

Also: high endocervical cells

LBC: More rounded, more "reactive"

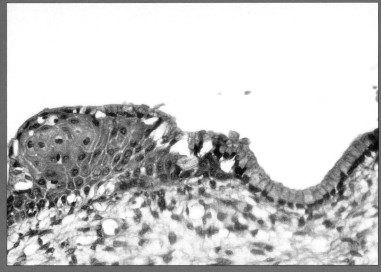

I2.1
Squamocolumnar junction

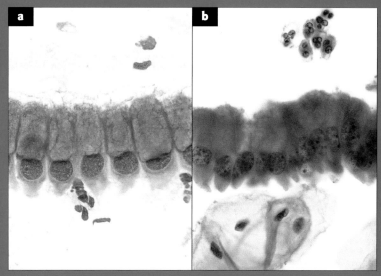

I2.2
a, Endocervical cells [C]; **b**, Endocervical cells [L]

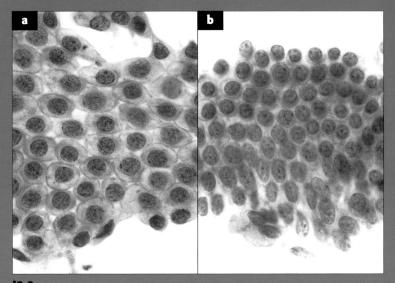

I2.3
a, Endocervical cells [C]; **b**, Endocervical cells [L]

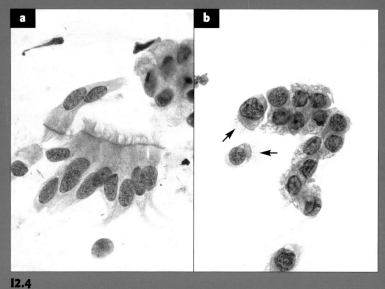

I2.4
a, Ciliated endocervical cells [C]; **b**, Ciliated endocervical cells (arrows) [L]

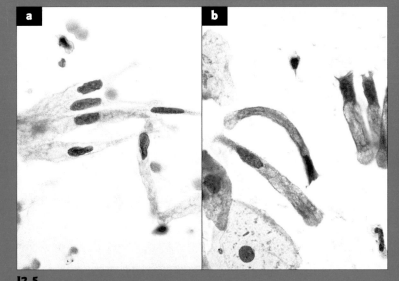

I2.5
a, Pencil thin endocervical cells [C]; **b**, Pencil thin endocervical cells [C]

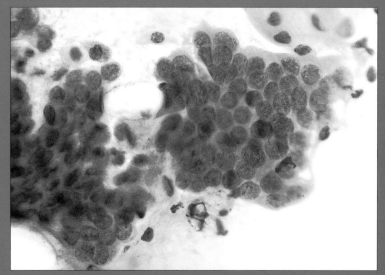

I2.6
High endocervical cells [C]

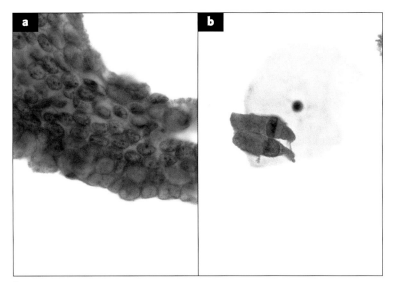

I2.7
a, Endocervical cells [L]; **b**, Endocervical cells [L]

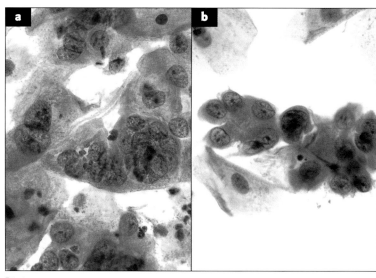

I2.8
a, Reactive endocervical cells [C]; **b**, Reactive endocervical cells [L]

in oral contraceptives [McCallum 1988]. Nipples are probably nonspecific findings [Koizumi 1996]. The N/C ratio averages about 30%. The chromatin is normally fine and evenly distributed. There may be one or more inconspicuous micronucleoli.

The cytoplasm of endocervical cells is delicate and often strips from the nucleus. When this occurs, naked endocervical nuclei lounge about in finely granular or wispy blue pools of degenerated cytoplasm and mucus, the so-called endocervical mucus. Endocervical mucus is *not* considered a good indicator of the adequacy of transformation zone sampling in a Pap test. Naked nuclei are common in other conditions ranging from cytolysis to squamous carcinoma in situ.

High endocervical cells, obtained with an endocervical brush from high in the endocervix, can exfoliate crowded groups of cells with hyperchromatic nuclei (HCGs), high N/C ratios, and scant cytoplasm [I2.6]. They do not look like the usual mucinous, columnar endocervical cells that are typically obtained with the Ayre spatula. Although these cells are normal for their location, they may suggest a neoplastic process [Raab 2000]. Reactive changes (nuclear pleomorphism, dark chromatin, crowding, palisading, feathering, and rosettes) may be present [Babkowski 1996, Soofer 2000]. In general, high endocervical cells are uniform, with round, bland nuclei that look like normal endocervical nuclei, and lack mitotic figures. In liquid-based cytology, high endocervical cells can have dense cytoplasm, mimicking immature squamous metaplasia.

In liquid-based cytology, endocervical cells occur in small or large groups, and large sheets [I2.2b, 2.3b, 2.7a,b]. Dissociation of endocervical cells is more prominent in LBC; single endocervical cells can be more difficult to identify while screening, particularly when trapped in mucus or clumps of leukocytes. Aggregates of endocervical cells tend to "round up" or fold, forming denser, more three-dimensional clusters, or hyperchromatic crowded groups, that are more difficult to distinguish from endometrial cells or other, more ominous entities, including glandular neoplasia. Normal endocervical nuclei often look more "reactive" than in conventional Pap smears, with small, but more conspicuous nucleoli.

Oxyphilic metaplasia can occur in endocervical (and endometrial) cells. Oxyphilic cells are large and polygonal, with abundant, finely granular, eosinophilic cytoplasm. Nuclear atypia can occur, including enlargement, irreg-

ularity, hyperchromasia, and multinucleation, which could lead to interpretive errors [Ghorab 2000, MA Jones 1997].

Neuroendocrine cells also occur in the endocervix. These are not specifically recognizable in Pap tests without special studies [Fetissof 1991].

Reactive Endocervical Cells

Reactive changes are common in endocervical cells [I2.8a,b, 2.9a,b]. Hormonally induced hyperplasia, endocervicitis, or endocervical polyps, among a 1001 other things, can cause these changes.

Reactive endocervical cells "lie flat" (ie, form two-

<table>
<tr><td>*Reactive Endocervical Cells*</td></tr>
<tr><td>*Common!*</td></tr>
<tr><td>*Minimal crowding: cells "lay flat"*</td></tr>
<tr><td>*Nuclear enlargement, hyperchromasia*</td></tr>
<tr><td>*Smooth nuclear membranes*</td></tr>
<tr><td>*Prominent nucleoli*</td></tr>
<tr><td>*N/C ratios maintained*</td></tr>
<tr><td>*Mitoses possible—but be careful!*</td></tr>
</table>

dimensional flat sheets) with minimal nuclear crowding or overlap, and have well-defined cell borders ("honeycombs"). The cells are usually columnar in shape, with nucleocytoplasmic polarity. The N/C ratios are within normal limits, or only modestly increased.

Nuclear enlargement, sometimes up to four or five times the normal area, hyperchromasia, and prominent or macronucleoli characterize reactive changes [Bose 1994, DiTomasso 1996, Ghorab 2000, Nasu 1993, Sidawy 1997]. Binucleation is common. Multinucleation, with slight nuclear molding, can also occur; this could be mistaken for herpes virus effect (but ground-glass chromatin and viral inclusions are lacking) [Stowell 1994]. Although mitotic figures can sometimes be present in benign, reactive endocervical cells, mitotically active glandular cells raise the specter of neoplasia.

The cytoplasm is well defined, pale, and cyanophilic, with occasional mucous vacuoles. Inflammatory cells are often present in the background [Bose 1994, DiTomasso 1996, Ghorab 2000].

Reactive endocervical cells are common causes of misinterpretations [Goff 1992, K Lee 1995, Sidawy 1997]. Big, dark nuclei, prominent nucleoli, and mitotic figures are features that reactive and neoplastic cells share. Neoplastic endocervical

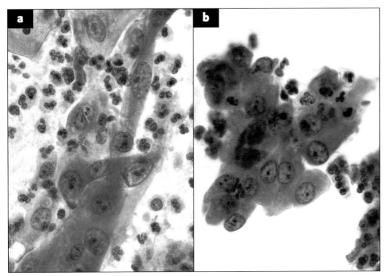

I2.9
a, Reactive endocervical cells [C]; **b**, Reactive endocervical cells [L]

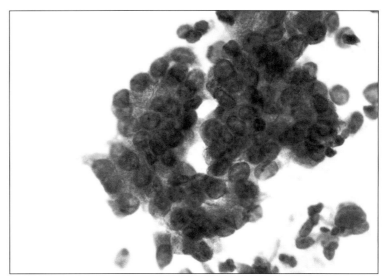

I2.10
Microglandular hyperplasia [C]

cells typically form markedly crowded, three-dimensional clusters, with feathery edges or microacinar structures (rosettes), indistinct cell borders, elongated (cigar shaped) or irregular nuclei, with coarse dark chromatin, high N/C ratios, mitosis, and apoptosis (see pg 140). Reactive cells are more orderly, with well-defined (honeycomb) cell borders, round to oval (not cigar shaped) nuclei, with smooth (or only slightly irregular) nuclear membranes, and fine chromatin. Although not regarded as a preneoplastic condition, reactive endocervical cells in a Pap test forecasts squamous intraepithelial lesions on biopsy in a significant number of women [*Ghorab 2000, Goff 1992, Nasu 1993*].

Microglandular Hyperplasia

Microglandular hyperplasia of the endocervix was first described by Taylor et al in 1967 [*H Taylor 1967*]. This is a benign, nonneoplastic proliferation of endocervical glands [I2.I0]. It is a common condition that usually occurs in women of reproductive age, but it can sometimes be present after menopause. Microglandular hyperplasia has been associated with oral contraceptives, particularly progestins, and pregnancy [*Chhieng 2001d, Chumas 1985, TS Kline 1970, Leslie 1984, Nucci 2002, R Young 1989b*]. However, it is not necessarily related to hormones, and in a large series of cases, no statistical association with progestins was found [*Greeley 1995*]. Human papillomavirus DNA is absent from these proliferations [*Okagaki 1989, Tase 1989b*]. Microglandular hyperplasia is not related to the development of adenocarcinoma, although the two conditions can coexist [*MW Jones 1989, K Lee 2000a*]. Also, microglandular hyperplasia, particularly atypical forms of microglandular hyperplasia, can mimic adenocarcinoma [*Mikami 1999, Valente 1994b, R Young 1989b*]. Conversely, adenocarcinoma can mimic microglandular hyperplasia [*Shidham 2000, R Young 1992*].

Histologically, microglandular hyperplasia has an interlacing pattern of orderly endocervical glands, with minimal stratification, and absent or rare mitotic figures. Occasional cases have atypical features, such as cells with enlarged, hyperchromatic nuclei, and increased mitotic activity, that could lead to false-positive interpretations of neoplasia [*R Young 1989b*].

Cytologically, the findings are usually within normal limits, or there are nonspecific reactive/reparative changes in glandular cells, precluding specific recognition of this entity in the Pap test [*Yahr 1991*]. Clusters of uniform glandular cells with microacini ("fenestrations") have been described as being a characteristic finding when present [*Alvarez–Santin 1999*]. Plasma cells or other inflammatory cells may accompany microglandular hyperplasia.

On the other hand, some examples of microglandular hyperplasia have striking cytologic atypia mimicking malignancy [*Selvaggi 2000*]. Hyperchromatic crowded groups (with nuclear crowding and loss of polarity), nuclear enlargement, hyperchromasia, coarse chromatin, prominent nucleoli, karyorrhexis, and mitotic figures may be present, which may suggest endocervical glandular neoplasia or a high-grade squamous intraepithelial lesion [*Chhieng 2001d, DeMay 2000, T Nichols 1971, Rizzo 1989, Selvaggi 1997, 2000, Shidham 2004, Valente 1994b, Yahr 1991*]. Atypical glandular cells, engulfing neutrophils, may suggest endometrial carcinoma [*Selvaggi 1999a*]. Fine chromatin, smooth nuclear membranes, lack of "feathery" edges, and presence of cilia or terminal bars point to a benign interpretation [*Valente 1994b, 1996*]. Extensive immature squamous metaplasia can occur, which could lead to interpretations of atypical squamous cells-high grade SIL not excluded (ASC-H) [*Shidham 2004*]. Carcinoembryonic antigen is usually negative in microglandular hyperplasia, but frequently positive in adenocarcinoma [*Nucci 2002, Speers 1983*]. Pseudoparakeratosis is a possible clue to microglandular hyperplasia.

Pseudoparakeratosis

Pseudoparakeratosis is characterized by masses of single, degenerated endocervical cells, often in linear arrays in conventional smears or dense clusters in liquid-based preparations. This is most commonly observed in the second half of the menstrual cycle in women taking oral contraceptives [I2.I1a,b,c]. The cells typically have pyknotic nuclei and orangeophilic cytoplasm, due to degeneration or coagulative necrosis. These small orange glandular cells with ink-dot nuclei mimic squamous parakeratosis and, therefore, are

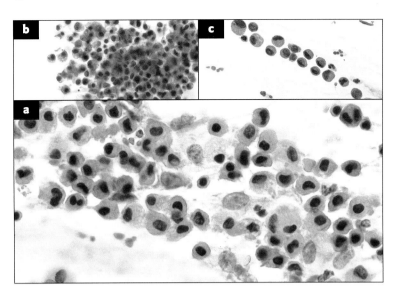

I2.II
a, Pseudoparakeratosis [C]; **b**, Pseudoparakeratosis [L];
c, Pseudoparakeratosis [C]

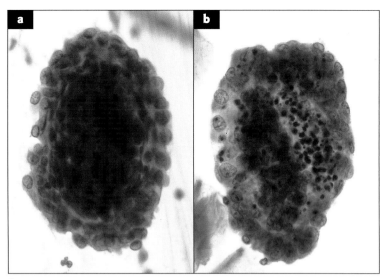

I2.12
a, Endometrial cells, double contour [C]; **b**, Endometrial cells, double contour [I]

known as pseudoparakeratosis [M Clarke 1993, Patten 1978, Valente 1994b]. Orangeophilia, however, is a staining artifact related to degeneration and is not always present. Recognizable endocervical cells are usually in the vicinity, which aids in identification. Also, the degenerated endocervical cells have a finely vacuolated or granular cytoplasm (vs waxy cytoplasm of true parakeratosis). The differential includes histiocytes, particularly during exodus (look for ciliocytophthoria) and high-grade dysplasia (which can also shed atypical small cells in strands of mucus—in conventional Pap tests).

Atypical Endocervical Cells and their differential are covered beginning on pg 144.

Endometrial Cytology

The lining of the uterine corpus, the endometrium, comprises endometrial "glands" (without ducts) surrounded by stroma. The histology varies with the day of the menstrual cycle and is also affected by factors such as age and hormones. During the proliferative phase, days 5-14, the glands proliferate, beginning with straight outlines that become curved. The cells change from cuboidal to columnar; mitoses are prominent, but secretions are minimal. During the secretory phase, days 14-28, the glands are tortuous (corkscrew) and secretion is active until day 21, when involution begins. During menses, day 1 to 5, the glands break down and endometrial glandular and stroma cells are shed. Regeneration begins from the residual glands and stroma to start the cycle over again.

The following discussion of endometrial cytology pertains primarily to *spontaneously* exfoliated cells, rather than to directly sampled endometrium (see pg 148). During menses, blood, inflammatory cells, and histiocytes typically accompany endometrial cells. During "exodus" (days 6-10), endometrial cell balls and stromal histiocytes are prominent in the Pap test [Papanicolaou 1953]. Exodus sees the elimination of debris at the end of menstrual bleeding. Endometrial cells shedding after day 10-14 or in menopause is considered abnormal. There are two major types of endometrial cells, glandular and stromal, although it is not always possible to distinguish the two in Pap tests, particularly in liquid-based cytology.

Endometrial Glandular Cells

Spontaneously shed endometrial cells usually exfoliate in crowded, three-dimensional groups, with or without central stroma. They rarely, if ever, form honeycomb sheets or palisades when exfoliated spontaneously. Single endometrial cells are difficult to identify specifically in Pap tests. Although cyclic variations in morphology occur, they are too subtle to be of consequence in interpretation of spontaneously exfoliated endometrial cells [Coscia-Porrazzi 1986].

Double-contour cell balls, or "wreaths," with darkly staining stroma inside and lighter staining epithelium wrapped around the outside, are the arrangements most characteristic of endometrial cells [Papanicolaou 1953, Wolfson 1983] [I2.12a,b]. Papanicolaou noted that endometrial wreaths are prominent from days 6 to 10 of the menstrual cycle, which he called "exodus" [Papanicolaou 1953]. Endometrial stromal histiocytes are commonly associated with the endometrial wreaths during exodus. Wreaths may also be present during menses as well as in women with benign polyps or endometrial hyperplasia.

Three-dimensional clusters of endometrial glandular cells, without central stroma, also occur. The cells are small and crowded, and the nuclei usually are degenerated and hyperchromatic, ie, they form hyperchromatic crowded groups (HCGs) that can mimic carcinoma in situ [DeMay 2000]

Endometrial Glandular Cells
Small clusters (HCGs); few single cells
Degenerated small cells
Nucleus: ~ Size intermediate nucleus
Round to irregular, single inconspicuous nucleoli
Cytoplasm: Scant, basophilic, ± vacuoles
Cilia ⇒ tubal metaplasia
LBC: Nuclei larger, more variable;
Chromatin, nucleoli more conspicuous

Double Contour Cell Balls
Highly characteristic of EMs
Outside:
Paler staining glandular cells
Inside:
Darker staining stromal cells
Associated with "Exodus" (days 6-10)

[I2.13a,b]. Time of the menstrual cycle and presence of nearby endometrial stromal histiocytes help to identify endometrial cells.

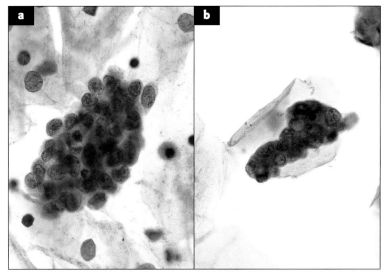

I2.13
a, Endometrial cells [C]; **b**, Endometrial cells [L]

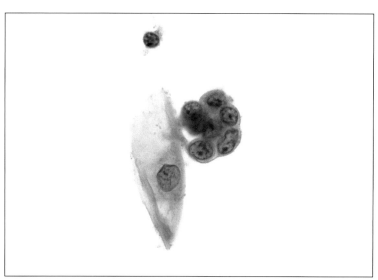

I2.14
Endometrial cells, nucleoli [L]

Normal endometrial cells are round to oval, and smaller than endo-cervical cells, averaging about 10 μm-15 μm in largest diameter. They resemble lymphocytes, but are usually degenerated owing to ischemia associated with menstrual shedding and time spent in the vaginal pool before collection.

The nuclei are round to oval and usually eccentrically located in the cell. In contrast with endocervical cells, binucleation or multinucleation of endometrial cells is rare. The mean nuclear area is 35 μm²-40 μm², essentially the same size as an intermediate cell nucleus (35 μm²). The nuclear contour varies in outline, as a degenerative change. The chromatin is fine and evenly dispersed when well preserved, but often is coarse to pyknotic due to degeneration. Small chromocenters may be present. Nucleoli are normally absent or indistinct in conventional Pap smears, but may be more conspicuous in LBC [I2.14]. Mitotic figures are not normally present in spontaneously shed endometrial cells. However, apoptosis, cell fragmentation, chromatin clumping, margination, or pyknosis can occur, particularly during the proliferative phase (or in conditions with breakdown and proliferative glands, but without intervening secretory phase, such as anovulatory bleeding or disordered proliferative endometrium). Lysed red blood cells may be seen in the background during menses.

The cytoplasm is variable in amount, but generally scant, with ill-defined cell borders. It usually stains basophilic or amphophilic, but may have an eosinophilic cast due to degeneration. The cytoplasm is finely vacuolar or granular. In contrast with endocervical or metaplastic cells, distinct vacuoles are infrequent and, if present, rarely contain neutrophils.

In liquid-based cytology, endometrial nuclei are slightly larger and more variable in size and shape, the chromatin details are accentuated, and nucleoli may be visible [I2.14]. These features, though normal in LBC, would be worrisome in conventional Pap smears, and could lead to unnecessary interpretations of atypical endometrial cells in LBC. The cytoplasm may appear more distinctly vacuolated in LBC. Also, apoptosis (single cell necrosis) may be more obvious. The background looks cleaner, especially in menstrual samples, compared with conventional Pap smears. Other endometrial cell features, such as double contour cell balls and small crowded groups, are similar in LBC, although the aggregates tend to focus above the plane of the squamous cells,

particularly in gradient-based methods such as SurePath™. (See also endometrial stromal histiocytes in LBC, below.)

Metaplastic changes can occur in endometrial cells. Fallopian tubal metaplasia is characterized by ciliated cells. Other metaplasias, including eosinophilic or oncocytic (oxyphilic), papillary syncytial, mucinous, and squamous metaplasia may involve the endometrium. These metaplasias can sometimes be associated with cytologic atypia that could conceivably cause interpretive problems. However, these endometrial metaplasias are more commonly encountered in directly sampled endometrium than in spontaneously exfoliated cells.

A common, everyday, and sometimes difficult problem in Pap test interpretation is distinguishing endometrial cells from endocervical cells [Simsir 2003] [T2.1]. This can be important, since shedding of endometrial cells is abnormal in the second half of the menstrual cycle (especially past 40 years of age) or any time in postmenopausal women. Abnormal shedding of endometrial cells may be associated with endometrial hyperplasia or neoplasia, and so is considered a risk factor for endometrial pathology.

Endocervical cells do not form the wreaths that are so characteristic of endometrial cells. Crowding (ie, the way endometrial cells are "packed together" forming berry-like clusters), degeneration, and smaller cell size point to endometrial origin. Honeycomb sheets, binucleation or multinucleation, more abundant

T2.1 Endocervical vs Endometrial Cells

Endocervical cells	Endometrial cells
Larger	Smaller
More variable	More uniform
Flat 2D sheets	Crowded, 3D balls
Honeycombs, palisades	Double contour cell balls
Nuclei vary size, not shape	Nuclei vary shape, not size
Multinucleation common	Multinucleation rare
Abundant cytoplasm	Scant cytoplasm
Better preservation	Degeneration

Clue: compare with similar glandular cells of known origin

cytoplasm, and distinct cytoplasmic vacuoles point to endocervical origin. Endocervical nuclei remain round, but can be variably sized; endometrial nuclei can be variably shaped, but remain small. In other words, endocervical nuclei vary in size, but not shape; endometrial nuclei vary in shape, but not size.

Clusters of naked nuclei may resemble aggregates of endometrial cells [II.4d, II.8b]. Naked nuclei can derive from syncytial-like aggregates of parabasal cells in atrophy, which is common post menopause. Shedding of endometrial cells is abnormal postmenopause, and raises the suspicion of endometrial pathology. Helpful clues are the total lack of cytoplasm and the similarity of the naked nuclei to those in the aggregates of atrophic cells. Clusters of naked nuclei can also be seen in association with hormone replacement therapy or Tamoxifen therapy; in these settings, the endometrial-like clusters of naked nuclei tend to stand out against a mature squamous background.

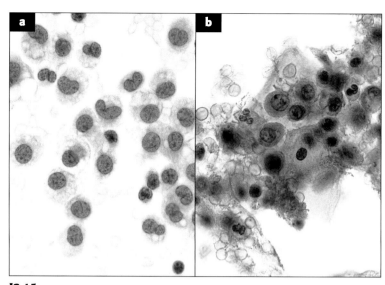

I2.15
a, Stromal histiocytes [C]; **b**, Stromal histiocytes [L]

Endometrial Stromal Cells

Endometrial stromal cells, like endometrial glandular cells, are normally present only during the first half of the menstrual cycle. By long tradition, two types of endometrial "stromal" cells have been recognized in Pap tests. These are superficial and deep stromal cells, supposedly originating from the stratum functionalis and stratum basale of the endometrium, respectively. However, so-called superficial stromal cells are probably bone marrow-derived histiocytes, not true mesenchymal stromal cells.

Endometrial Stromal Cells

  Superficial stromal cells
    "Sticky histiocytes"
  Deep stromal cells
    Round to spindle
    Small oval nuclei
    Scant cytoplasm

Deep Stromal Cells

Deep stromal cells are typically small, spindle or stellate cells, with scant cytoplasm, which usually stains cyanophilic or amphophilic [I2.16a,b]. The nuclei are oval to spindle-shaped, and frequently have a longitudinal groove in the nuclear membrane. The chromatin structure is similar to that of histiocytes. The findings are similar in liquid-based cytology. Deep stromal cells are rarely identified in Pap tests. Decidualized stromal cells (decidual cells) are discussed on pg I67.

Superficial Stromal Cells (Stromal Histiocytes)

Superficial stromal cells, or stromal histiocytes, are most prominent in Pap tests during exodus (days 6 to I0) and help eliminate endometrial debris toward the end of menstrual bleeding (vacuum cleaners). These cells are indistinguishable from ordinary small histiocytes, but tend to form loose aggregates ("sticky histiocytes") or, more problematically, strings of these cells that can be difficult to distinguish from CIN 3 [I2.15a,b]. The cells are small, only slightly larger than endometrial glandular cells. The nuclei are round to oval, or bean-shaped, and often eccentrically located in the cell. They have a moderate amount of delicate, finely vacuolated cytoplasm and ill-defined borders. In contrast, ordinary histiocytes can range from small to large, or even giant, tend to be single, and may have phagocytosed debris in their cytoplasm. In some cases, ciliocytophthoria in the vicinity provides an interpretive clue. As mentioned, these cells are probably histiocytes rather than actual stromal cells. They express CD68, a histiocytic marker, unlike true endometrial stromal cells [A Chang 2001].

In liquid-based cytology, stromal histiocytes commonly form dense, three dimensional aggregates that can be difficult to distinguish from clusters of endometrial glandular cells (this is true of conventional Pap smears, as well). In addition, the nuclei can be slightly pleomorphic, with nuclear membrane irregularities, and darker, granular chromatin. This could lead to unnecessary interpretations of atypical endometrial cells. Individual cells round up, have denser cytoplasm, enhanced nuclear details, and high N/C ratios; these findings can mimic H SIL. Granular/foamy vs dense squamoid cytoplasm and fine details of nuclear morphology are key features to evaluate in the differential. In contrast with conventional Pap smears, strings of cells are not seen in LBC.

Abnormal Shedding of "Normal" Endometrial Cells

Exfoliation of normal-appearing endometrial cell during the first part of the menstrual cycle (from day I to days I0-I4) is normal, physiologic shedding . Exfoliation of endometrial cells, whether glandular or stromal, at any other time of the menstrual cycle is abnormal, "out-of-phase" shedding. During the second half of the menstrual cycle, endometrial cells are present in only 2% of Pap tests; the percentage rises again in the premenstrual phase (after day 25) [W Liu 1963, Vooijs 1987b]. Postmenopausal shedding of endometrial cells is always abnormal. Although there are many possible benign causes (see below), abnormally shed endometrial cells raises the spectre of serious uterine pathology, including adenocarcinoma. The risk of malignancy is small, but increases with age [Cherkis 1988, Gondos 1977, Kempsack 1998, A Ng 1974b, Yancy 1990, Zucker 1985]. The Bethesda System 2001 recommends reporting the presence of normal-appearing endometrial cells in women 40 years of age or older, regardless of menstrual status (reported under the general category of "Other"). (Of course, abnormal-appearing endometrial cells are always abnormal, see below.)

Shedding of Normal Endometrial Cells
  ·Glandular, stromal, double-contour balls
  Normal: First half of menstrual cycle (only)
    Physiologic shedding
  Abnormal: 2nd half of cycle or
    postmenopause
  (> 40 yrs in TBS = "Other")
    Risk factor for endometrial pathology
  Shedding abnormal endometrial cells
    Always abnormal

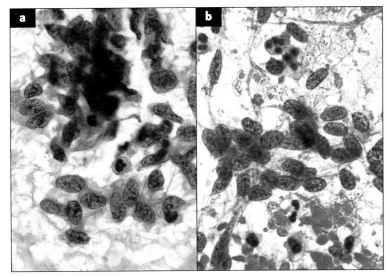

I2.16
a, Deep stromal cells [C]; **b**, Deep stromal cells [C]

F2.1 Abnormal Shedding of Normal-Appearing Endometrial Cells

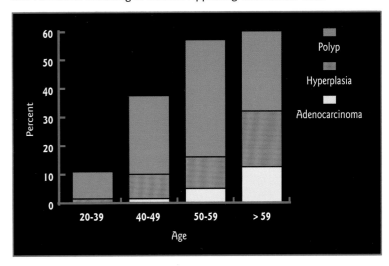

The risk of endometrial carcinoma increases with age, but is rare before 40 years.
[A Ng 1974a,b]

A vaginal pool sample, from the posterior vaginal fornix, is a good source of spontaneously exfoliated endometrial cells, and can significantly increase detection of occult endometrial carcinoma compared with a routine Pap test [Koss 1984]. Days 15 to 24 are theoretically the most opportune time to detect endometrial lesions in premenopausal women, although in practice, the Pap test is not a good screening test for these lesions. Cervical, as opposed to vaginal or endocervical, samples do not contribute significantly to detection of endometrial disease [Koss 1981]. Endometrial cells can be obtained, inadvertently, at any time with an endocervical brush; directly sampled endometrium is not considered abnormal shedding. Abnormally shed endometrial cells are often sparse and degenerated; directly sampled endometrial cells are usually numerous and well preserved (see pg 148).

The causes of abnormal shedding of endometrial cells run the gamut from benign to malignant, but fortunately, most causes are benign, including: anovulatory changes, atrophy, post-partum state, status post-abortion, recent instrumentation, intrauterine contraceptive devices, endometriosis, tuboendometrial metaplasia, endometritis, pyometra, submucous leiomyomas, and polyps. In many cases, no underlying abnormality can be identified. Hormone replacement therapy (HRT) is a recognized cause of post-menopausal shedding of endometrial cells; some regimens, particularly sequential combinations of estrogen and progesterone, induce menstrual-like endometrial shedding in some women [Akkad 1995, Archer 1994, 2000, Nand 1998, Spencer 1997, Symons 2000]. The incidence of endometrial cancer is increased with unopposed estrogen therapy, but not with combined estrogen and progestin use [H Nelson 2002]. Oral contraceptives (birth control pills, BCPs) may be associated with midcycle breakthrough bleeding and abnormal shedding of endometrial cells. Of course, the primary concern of abnormal shedding of endometrial cells is the possibility of underlying endometrial hyperplasia and particularly, endometrial carcinoma.

Causes of Abnormal Shedding

Endometriosis, Endometritis
Postpartum, Abortion, IUD
Instrumentation
Hormonal therapy: BCPs, HRT
Dysfunctional uterine bleeding
Submucosal myoma
Endometrial polyp
Endometrial hyperplasia
*Endometrial carcinoma**
**Risk increases after age 40*

Abnormal shedding of endometrial cells raises the possibility of endometrial cancer, even if the cells look normal [F2.1]. Before 40 years of age, the association ("risk") is low, but increases with age and postmenopausal status [D Anderson 1976, Cherkis 1988, Gondos 1977, Moriarty 2003a, A Ng 1974b]. Abnormally shed endometrial glandular cells (with or without stromal cells) are of most concern; however, a few cancers (~5%) shed endometrial stromal cells only, if they shed any endometrial cells at all [A Ng 1974b]. The risk of endometrial carcinoma in postmenopausal women shedding cytologically benign endometrial cells averages about 5% (range 0 to 20%), the risk of hyperplasia averages about 10%, and the combined risk of significant endometrial pathology averages between 15% and 20% [Ashfaq 2001, Brogi 2002, A Chang 2001, Cherkis 1988, Doornewaard 1993, Gomez-Fernández 2000, Gondos 1977, J-A Gray 1999, Karim 2002, Kerpsack 1998, Montz 2001, A Ng 1974b, Sarode 2001, A Schneider 1985, M Schneider 1986, van den Bosch 1998, Webster 2000, Wu 2001, Yancy 1990, Zucker 1985]. For women receiving hormone replacement therapy, the risk of malignancy is probably closer to 1%, but not zero [A Chang 2001, Feeley 2001, Montz 2001, Sarode 2001, Yancy 1990].

The Bethesda System does not *require* reporting the presence of endometrial cells in women younger than 40 years of age, because significant pathology is rarely discovered when otherwise asymptomatic women are investigated. However, some cytology laboratories *always* report endometrial cells in Pap tests, regardless of the woman's age or menstrual status, to document that the cells were identified and interpreted as benign. This is because neoplastic lesions can exfoliate hyperchromatic crowded groups (HCGs) that can be practically indistinguishable from benign endometrial cell aggregates [DeMay 2000]. Further, the "last menstrual period" is unreliable information: not only are the dates untrustworthy, but abnormal bleeding may also be reported as a menstrual period. And, of course, no one ever fibs about their age!

Atypical Endometrial Cells

Shedding *abnormal* appearing endometrial cells is always abnormal, regardless of age or menstrual status. However, the abnormalities range from benign to malignant, including endometrial polyps, chronic endometritis, IUD changes, tubal metaplasia, endometrial hyperplasia, and endometrial carcinoma. Some women shedding what seem to be atypical "endometrial" cells actually have high-grade *squamous* lesions or cancer [Chhieng 2001b, Soofer 2000, Zhou 1998b]. Criteria for separating atypical endometrial cells into "favor reactive" vs "favor neoplastic" are not well defined, and the category is not further subdivided in the Bethesda System [Solomon 1998].

Atypical endometrial cells are usually shed in small loose or tight clusters of small glandular cells [Solomon 1998]. Atypical or abnormal findings in endometrial glandular cells include: nuclear enlargement, hyperchromasia, irregular chromatin,

---

Atypical Endometrial Cells

Shedding is always abnormal

Two key atypical features:

· Nuclear enlargement

(> Intermediate nucleus)

· Prominent nucleoli

LBC: Chromatin, nucleoli more distinct

No criteria: reactive vs neoplastic "atypia"

Significant risk factor postmenopause

---

and nucleoli. Not all features need be present. The two best indicators of endometrial atypia are nuclear enlargement (greater than an intermediate cell nucleus) and prominent nucleoli [Salomao 2002]. Chromatin and nucleoli are normally more distinct in LBC.

Mild atypia includes nuclear enlargement and increased N/C ratio; moderate atypia adds hyperchromasia with abnormalities of the chromatin; and marked atypia adds presence of nucleoli. The cytoplasm is scant and cell borders ill defined. Endometrial cell abnormalities can be difficult to appreciate owing to cellular degeneration. On the other hand, normal endometrial cells, which are abundant during menses, can show reactive changes (slight nuclear enlargement and pleomorphism) or degenerative changes that could be misinterpreted as abnormal, particularly in LBC. Clinical history must be provided for accurate interpretation.

A substantial number (>50%) of postmenopausal women who shed atypical endometrial cells have significant endometrial pathology, including adenocarcinoma [Cherkis 1987, Chhieng 2001b, Doornewaard 1993, van den Bosch 1998]. The risk of malignancy increases with age and degree of cytologic atypia. Atypical endometrial cells are often found in a background of high maturation (>20% superficial cells). A tumor diathesis favors frank malignancy.

Other Cytologic Risk Factors for Endometrial Pathology

It has been known since the 1940s that uterine cancer cells can sometimes be detected in Pap tests [Papanicolaou 1943]; however, this is rare. In 1962, Koss and Durfee proposed additional criteria to enhance cytologic detection of endometrial carcinoma, including abnormal shedding of normal appearing endometrial cells, shedding of abnormal endometrial cells, increased histiocytic activity, excess blood, and high postmenopausal maturation index [Koss 1962]. Short of finding indubitable ("no doubt about") cancer cells, none of these is specific. Unfortunately, endometrial carcinoma may not shed any characteristic cells at all, or only intermittently, and when shed, the cells may be sparse and degenerated, making critical assessment difficult or impossible. Hence, even frankly malignant endometrial cells can be indistinguishable from normal endometrial cells in Pap tests.

Increased maturation of the squamous epithelium ("estrogen effect") in a postmenopausal woman is a possible risk factor because endometrial hyperplasia/neoplasia is associated with unopposed estrogen stimulation [Cassano 1986, Y

Chang 1963, Efstratiades 1982, Gronroos 1986, W Liu 1970, Ritchie 1965]. However, an atrophic background by no means excludes the possibility of endometrial cancer [Y Chang 1963, W Liu 1970]. For practical purposes, a specimen with >20% superficial cells in a postmenopausal woman can be considered increased maturation. Inflammation or infection can cause non-hormonal maturation ("pseudo-maturation") [T Lin 1972].

Histiocytes, in moderate or heavy numbers ("increased histiocytic activity"), in Pap tests from postmenopausal women have been

---

---

considered risk factors for endometrial carcinoma [Abadi 2000, Wen 2003]. This is because women with endometrial carcinoma often shed histiocytes [Blumenfeld 1985, Dressel 1992a, A Ng 1974b, TN Nguyen 1998]. However, women shedding histiocytes rarely have endometrial carcinoma [A Chang 2001, T Hall 1982, Tambouret 2001, Zucker 1985]. (Similarly, most women with endometrial carcinoma have abnormal uterine bleeding, but most women with abnormal bleeding do not have endometrial carcinoma [although the risk increases with age] [H Mitchell 1995c, Nassar 2003, Zucker 2001].) Histiocytes are commonly associated with benign endometrial diseases, such as endometritis, and even more commonly, derive from the cervix where they have nothing at all to do with endometrial disease [T Hall 1982]. Furthermore, women with endometrial carcinoma shedding histiocytes usually also have other abnormal signs or symptoms; histiocytes are rarely the only indication of malignant disease. To make a long story short, just remember: histiocytes are poor predictors of endometrial adenocarcinoma [Blumenfeld 1985, Nassar 2003, TN Nguyen 1998, Tambouret 2001, Wen 2003].

Histiocytes containing hemosiderin, lipid, neutrophils, or cell debris, on the other hand, are a little more worrisome [Karim 2002, TN Nguyen 1998]. Foam cells, which are large lipid-laden macrophages, are markers for endometrial malignancy, but can be present in benign conditions, such as adenomatous hyperplasia [Dawagne 1982, Fechner 1979]. Foam cells have abundant, finely vacuolated cytoplasm and small central nuclei. Multinucleated giant cell histiocytes are common findings in postmenopausal women, and are not important in the detection of endometrial carcinoma [Koss 1962].

Necrosis and old (ie, degenerated, not fresh) blood are also associated with increased risk of endometrial carcinoma in postmenopausal women. However, these, too, are nonspecific findings.

Some further considerations…

Clinical history, including age, day of cycle, or menopausal status, is critical in evaluation of endometrial cells. Other important information includes: clinical signs/symptoms, hormonal therapy, use of intrauterine contraceptive device, recent instrumentation, etc. The clinician must provide this information. Postmenopausal bleeding is a suspicious sign. Although postmenopausal bleeding can be caused by benign conditions [Choo 1985, Webster 2000], abnormal bleeding must always be investigated clinically, regardless of Pap test results.

More endometrial cancers could be detected from vaginal pool or cervical canal aspiration samples [Blumenfeld 1985, Creasman 1976, Koss 1962, McGowan 1974, Reagan 1980, Vuopala 1977]. There is evidence that liquid-based cytology may increase detection of endometrial carcinomas compared with conventional Pap smears, possibly by virtue of reducing obscuring blood and inflammation making it easier to detect a few abnormal cells [Guidos 2000, Schorge 2002]. Although endometrial aspiration could further increase the yield, the sample must be obtained under sterile conditions and the procedure is uncomfortable (few will submit to it more than once or twice). Endometrial aspiration cytology specimens are also difficult to interpret [Maksem 2000, Tajima 1998, Wu 2000]. Direct endometrial sampling in asymptomatic women has a high false-positive rate, resulting in unnecessary endometrial biopsies ("battered uterus syndrome") [Ferenczy 1984, Valente 2001]. Therefore, most pathologists prefer histologic processing of endometrial specimens. Screening asymptomatic women for endometrial carcinoma does not significantly reduce mortality and has not been recommended as a public health measure [Jobo 2003].

Although many women (range, ~20% to 70%) with endometrial carcinoma have endometrial cells in routine Pap tests (whether benign-, atypical-, or malignant-appearing) [Bibbo 1974, J Burk 1974, Christopherson 1971, DuBeshter 1991, Frick 1973, Fukuda 1999, H-S Kim 1991, Koss 1962, D Larson 1994, Lederer 1973, Lozowski 1986, McGowan 1974, H Mitchell 1993a, Nahhas 1971, A Ng 1974a, A Schachter 1980, M Schneider 1986, Sjolin 1970], the vast majority of these women also have symptoms, particularly abnormal uterine bleeding [Ashfaq 2001, Brogi 2002, Gomez-Fernández 1999, 2000, Gondos 1977, Karim 2002]. It is rare for the Pap test to be the only sign of endometrial cancer in otherwise asymptomatic women [Cherkis 1988, Koss 1962, A Ng 1974b, Wu 2001, Zucker 1985], although these women may have a better prognosis by virtue of early detection [Koss 1962]. The chance of finding atypical endometrial cells increases with the grade and stage of the tumor [Demirkiran 1995, DuBeshter 1991, 1999, 2003, G Eddy 1997c, Fukuda 1999, Gu 2001, D Larson 1994, Lozowski 1986, M Schneider 1986, Zuna 1996]. This can be helpful prognostically, ie, women shedding malignant cells are more likely to have advanced stage disease, including pelvic and para-aortic lymph node metastases [D Larson 1994]. Note, however, that false positive Pap test interpretations of endometrial carcinoma also occur [J-A Gray 1999, H Mitchell 1993a].

In summary, *the Pap test is not a reliable screening procedure for detection of endometrial disease* [J Burk 1974, Koss 1962, Pritchard 1989, Solomon 2002, Waddell 1997]. There is no reasonable expectation that Pap test screening can reduce the morbidity or mortality of endometrial carcinoma in the general population. Although some asymptomatic endometrial cancers can be detected by routine Pap tests, this is the exception. Most women with endometrial carcinoma have symptoms at the time of diagnosis, particularly, abnormal uterine bleeding. Women at risk of endometrial carcinoma must be carefully followed clinically; those with suspicious symptoms, such as abnormal bleeding, must always be investigated, regardless of the Pap test results. Endometrial biopsy or dilatation and curettage (D & C) is usually required for definitive diagnosis.

Endometrial Hyperplasia and Carcinoma

Endometrial adenocarcinoma is the most common invasive gynecologic malignancy. Most patients are perimenopausal or postmenopausal, and the disease rarely occurs before 40 years of age. 40,880 new cases of endometrial carcinoma, with 7,310 deaths, were expected in 2005 [Jemal 2005]. The incidence of endometrial adenocarcinoma peaked in the early 1970s, fell back to 1950s levels, reaching a nadir in the late 1980s, but has increased again since then [Gusberg 1989a, Robboy 1979a, N Weiss 1976, Jemal 2005]. The rise and fall of endometrial cancer paralleled the prescription of estrogen, supporting its role in endometrial carcinogenesis [Gusberg 1989b, Gwinn 1986, Sherman 2000]. Addition of progestin reduces risk. Oral contraceptives that include progesterone may reduce the risk of endometrial carcinoma.

Two Clinical Types of Endometrial Carcinoma

There are at least two clinical groups of women with endometrial carcinoma, one associated with endometrial hyperplasia (classical, type I) and the other apparently arising de novo (type II) [T2.2] [Bokhman 1983, Koss 1984, Silverberg 1980]. The archetypal morphology of type I cancer is endometrioid endometrial carcinoma; these tumors account for up to 80% of cases. Type II cancers are characterized by nonendometrioid (eg, serous, clear cell) morphology [Bokhman 1983, Sherman 2000]. This may well represent an oversimplification and other epidemiologic groups have been suggested (which are beyond the scope of the present discussion) [Sivridis 1998].

T2.2 Two Clinical Types of Endometrial Carcinoma

Type I (Classic)	Type II
More common	Less common
Classic risk factors	Lack classic risk factors
Obese, hypertensive, diabetic; nulliparous	Thin, multiparous
Younger, perimenopause	Older, postmenopause
Arises in hyperplasia	Atrophy, true CIS
Low grade	High grade
Microsatellite instability; *ras* & PTEN mutations	p53 mutations
Responds to hormones	Aggressive
Favorable prognosis	Unfavorable prognosis

Type I Endometrial Carcinoma

Type I endometrial adenocarcinoma is the end product of abnormal proliferation, a sequence of endometrial hyperplasia, atypical hyperplasia, and finally carcinoma [F2.2]. It takes about a decade for endometrial hyperplasia to develop into endometrial carcinoma, and only a minority runs the full course [Kurman 1985]. Prolonged estrogen excess is important in pathogenesis of type I cancers. Estrogen induces endometrial hyperplasia and acts as a promoter of endometrial cancer. Because adipose tissue is a major source of aromatase, an enzyme that converts (adrenal and ovarian) androgens to estrogens, obesity is a risk factor for endometrial carcinoma [Sherman 2000]. Prolonged, excessive, and unopposed estrogen production can also be due to ovarian lesions, including granulosa cell tumor, thecoma, polycystic ovary disease, and hyperthecosis. Exogenous sources of estrogen include estrogen hormonal therapy. Tamoxifen, a nonsteroidal estrogen antagonist, can also have weakly estrogenic properties, and increases the risk of endometrial carcinoma [Sherman 2000].

F2.2 Evolution of Type I (Classic) Endometrial Carcinomas

Proliferation	Adenomatous hyperplasia	Atypical hyperplasia	Adeno-carcinoma

The classic risk factors for type I endometrial carcinoma, include diabetes mellitus (or abnormal glucose tolerance), obesity, hypertension,

Classic Clinical Risk Factors
for Endometrial Carcinoma
Diabetes mellitus
Obesity
Hypertension
Hyperestrinism
Nulliparity
Late menopause

signs of hyperestrinism, nulliparity, and late menopause [S Feldman 1995, MacMahon 1974, Sherman 1997]. The women are typically perimenopausal with a median age of about 60 years. These cancers are usually low to intermediate grade, endometrioid morphology, associated with endometrial hyperplasia, respond to hormones, and have a favorable prognosis. The endometrial hyperplasia-carcinoma pathway is associated with microsatellite instability and *ras* and PTEN mutations [Sherman 2000].

Type II Endometrial Carcinoma

Type II endometrial carcinoma tends occur in women who lack the risk factors classically associated with endometrial cancer, described above [Sherman 1997, 2000]. These women are typically older, multiparous, postmenopausal, and may be thin. These cancers arise spontaneously from endometrial carcinoma in situ (endometrial intraepithelial carcinoma), characterized by markedly atypical glandular cells, without associated endometrial hyperplasia [Sherman 1992a, 2000, G Spiegel 1995]. These cancers are typically high-grade, often serous morphology, arise in atrophic endometrium, and are aggressive. These tumors are associated with p53 mutations [Sherman 2000]. Although type II cancers represent a minority of all endometrial carcinomas, they account for a disproportionate number of recurrences and deaths [Hendrickson 1982].

Histology of Endometrial Hyperplasia and Carcinoma

Type I, or classic type endometrial adenocarcinoma evolves through a spectrum of abnormal proliferation to invasive carcinoma [I2.17a,b,c]. The commonly used histologic classification recognizes simple and complex hyperplasia, with or without cytologic atypia [Kurman 1985]. Classification of spontaneously exfoliated endometrial cells according to this histologic system is well beyond the scope of a routine Pap test. A simplified histologic classification is presented here, although ability to transmogrify even this simple system into a specific cytologic interpretation is beyond the ken of most mortal cytologists. The precursor lesion for type II carcinoma, endometrial adenocarcinoma in situ (or endometrial intraepithelial lesion), is distinguished by high-grade cells that could be detected fortuitously in a Pap test [D Wheeler 2000], although the lesion itself is clinically silent. Endometrial biopsy or dilatation and curettage (D&C) is required for definitive diagnosis of endometrial abnormalities.

Adenomatous Hyperplasia

Adenomatous hyperplasia is characterized by glandular and stromal proliferation. The glands are crowded, and have increased cellular stratification and mitotic activity. Cytologic atypia is negligible. Hyperplasia without cytologic atypia rarely progresses to cancer.

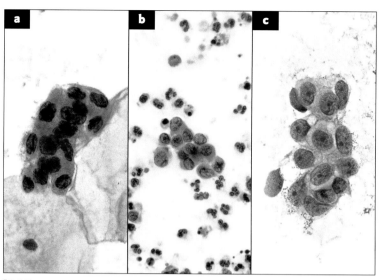

I2.17
a, Endometrial hyperplasia [C]; **b**, Low-grade adenocarcinoma [C]; **c**, High-grade adenocarcinoma [C]

Atypical Hyperplasia

Atypical hyperplasia features marked crowding and irregular gland outlines, in which fanciful shapes, such as puppy dogs or sailing ships, may be imagined (like looking at clouds). Cytologic atypia (eg, nuclear enlargement, irregular membranes, coarse chromatin, prominent nucleoli) is variable. Hyperplasia with atypia more commonly progresses to cancer.

Endometrial Adenocarcinoma

Endometrial adenocarcinoma is characterized, histologically, by invasive "back to back" glands and definite cytologic atypia. Invasion into myometrium or lymphatics, or metastasis, are also malignant characteristics.

Cytology of Endometrial Hyperplasia and Carcinoma

In theory, there are cytologic differences among hyperplasia, atypical hyperplasia, and adenocarcinoma, but the differences can be subtle even in well-preserved samples obtained by endocervical or endometrial aspiration. The more or less theoretical cytologic features are summarized below and in [T2.3].

T2.3 Endometrial Hyperplasia, Atypical Hyperplasia, & Adenocarcinoma

	Hyperplasia	Atypical Hyperplasia	Well-Differentiated Adenocarcinoma
	# Cells and cell & nuclear size progressively increase		
Average # groups	5	10	20
Average # cells	150	250	350
Nuclear area	45 μm²	55 μm²	60 μm²
Hyperchromasia	++	++	+
Irregular chromatin	5%	30%	80%
Nucleoli	5%	25%	75%
Diathesis	0	0	90%

[A Ng 1973a]

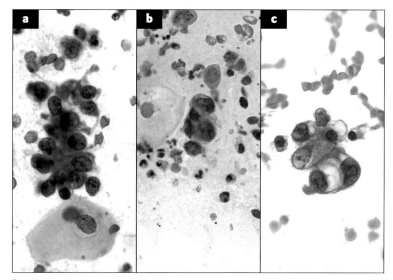

I2.18
a, Low-grade endometrial carcinoma [C]; **b**, Low-grade endometrial
carcinoma [C]; **c**, High-grade endometrial carcinoma [C]

Although the average nuclear area increases from normal to hyperplasia to
cancer, there is significant overlap, and nuclear size alone is insufficient to
separate these categories [Skaarland 1985]. Therefore other features, such as
nuclear hyperchromasia, chromatin granularity, nucleolar size, cytoplasmic
vacuolization, and background are also evaluated [Arrighi 1958, Bibbo 1970,
Boschann 1958, DeBrux 1958, Ferreira 1958, Y Ishii 1997, Kashimura 1988, A Ng 1973a, Skaarland
1985]. In practice, exfoliation of endometrial cells is inconsistent and the
cells are frequently poorly preserved, usually precluding any specific interpretation. In many cases of endometrial pathology, the endometrial cells—
if present at all—appear normal, in other cases, they appear nonspecifically
abnormal, ie, as "atypical endometrial cells" or "atypical glandular cells." Of
course, sometimes, the cells appear frankly malignant.

Endometrial Hyperplasia

Endometrial hyperplasia usually sheds few endometrial cells and
they usually appear normal. Either glandular or stromal cells can be exfoliated, but glandular cells usually predominate; rarely are stromal cells the
only indication of endometrial hyperplasia. The cells form small, loose, flat
groups or sometimes, glandular structures. Single cells can also occur;
however, tight three-dimensional cell balls are usually not present. The
nuclei are only slightly enlarged (~45 µm²), with uniform fine chromatin,
and rare micronucleoli, but no prominent nucleoli. There may be cytoplasmic vacuoles, with or without neutrophils. The background is clean and
an estrogen effect may be evident [A Ng 1973a].

Atypical Hyperplasia

Atypical endometrial hyperplasia features more cells, often
comprising a mixture of normal, hyperplastic, and atypical cells. Most of the
cells are glandular, and occur in groups of 5-25 cells. Aggregates are similar
to those in hyperplasia; however, the cells are more variable in size and
there may be loss of polarity. Single cells, but usually not tight groupings or
cell balls, may also be present. The nuclei are more obviously enlarged
(~55 µm²), slightly hyperchromatic, and have fine chromatin with two or
three chromocenters. Some nuclei have irregular chromatin distribution.

Single micronucleoli are present in up to 25% of cells, but prominent
nucleoli are rare [A Ng 1973a]. As in hyperplasia, the background is clean and
an estrogen effect is common.

Endometrial Adenocarcinoma

The morphology of endometrial adenocarcinoma depends on
the grade of the tumor as well as its subtype [I2.18a,b,c]. The cells usually
exfoliate as loose or tight aggregates (including "hyperchromatic crowded
groups" [DeMay 2000]), distorted glandular structures, cell balls, papillae, or
sheets. Single cells may also be present, but are difficult to recognize as
malignant in well-differentiated tumors. Degenerated single cells are easily
confused with histiocytes [AV Berry 1969]. Well-formed rosette-like structures,
peripheral palisading, pseudostratified strips, or feathering—all common in
cervical adenocarcinoma—are rare in endometrial adenocarcinoma.

Malignant endometrial cells tend to be relatively uniform, round-
to-oval, or cuboidal, with a mean cell area of ~150 µm² (range 100 µm²-
200 µm²), roughly 10 µm-15 µm in diameter. Columnar cells are unusual
and bizarre cells are rare.

The nuclei are irregularly arranged, crowded, and round-to-irreg-
ular, with a mean area of 70 µm² (range 50 µm²-90 µm²). Loss of nuclear
polarity is an important, but not specific, malignant feature. Marked hyperchromasia is unusual in endometrioid endometrial carcinoma; in fact, the
nuclei usually stain *less* intensely than normal. The chromatin is finely granular, but irregularly distributed, with areas of clearing that vary from cell to
cell. Nucleoli, usually small, are present in most tumor cells; the size and
number increase with grade of the tumor [M Long 1958]. Mitoses can be
present, but are unusual.

The cytoplasm is usually scanty, cyanophilic, and finely vacuolated. However, large degenerative vacuoles, often containing neutrophils,
are common and characteristic, but not pathognomonic, of endometrial
carcinoma [I2.19a,b] [Berg 1958].

The background may reflect the characteristic clinical sign of a
watery vaginal discharge. This appears in the Pap test as a finely granular,
basophilic diathesis, known as a watery diathesis, particularly in low-grade
tumors [AV Berry 1969] [I2.18b]. Watery diathesis may be subtle and difficult
to detect, especially in LBC. The diathesis may also contain fresh and old
blood, fibrin, cellular debris, and necrosis, particularly in high-grade tumors,
similar to that seen in invasive cervical cancers. Large numbers of histiocytes may be present, particularly in well-differentiated tumors [Reagan 1973].
Rarely, psammoma bodies are present; however, these are usually associated with the serous subtype [Karpas 1963, R Weaver 1967].

The number, size, and degree of atypia of the malignant cells
tend to increase with tumor grade, although the total number of abnormal
cells is usually far less than in primary cervical cancers (unless the cervix
is involved [Morimura 2002]). Adenocarcinoma exfoliates single cells and
clusters of cells that range from tightly packed aggregates, like those in
menses, to loose agregates to papillary groups. If the tumor invades the
cervix, large sheets of malignant cells may be sampled. As the grade
increases, the nuclei enlarge, the nuclear membranes become irregular and
thickened, and the nucleoli become larger, more numerous, and irregular.
The chromatin becomes more abnormal (coarse and irregular). The tumor
diathesis becomes more conspicuous with increasing grade; in high-
grade tumors, hemorrhage and necrosis may dilute or obscure the tumor
cells. An estrogen effect is common in low-grade (type I) tumors, while

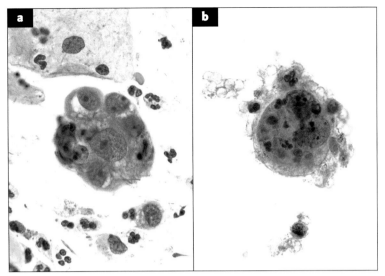

I2.19
a, Endometrial carcinoma, neutrophils [C];
b, Endometrial carcinoma, neutrophils [L]

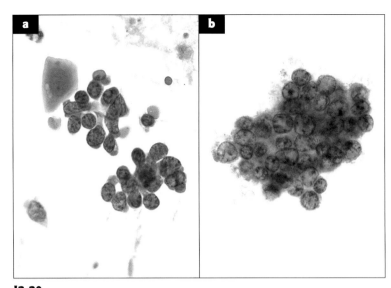

I2.20
a, Low-grade endometrial carcinoma [C]; **b**, Low-grade endometrial carcinoma [L]

high-grade (type II) tumors are more likely to occur in an atrophic background [Reagan 1973].

Well-Differentiated Endometrial Adenocarcinoma

Well-differentiated endometrial adenocarcinomas tend to occur in younger women in a background of endometrial hyperplasia (ie, type I cancers) [I2.17b, 2.18a, 2.20a,b]. The malignant cells resemble normal or hyperplastic endometrial cells, but the nuclei are larger. The mean nuclear area of grade I adenocarcinoma is approximately 60 μm² (vs 40 μm² for normal endometrial nuclei and 35 μm² for intermediate squamous cell nuclei) [F2.3] [Reagan 1973]). The chromatin is abnormal and tends to aggregate irregularly, resulting in areas of chromatin clearing. In low-grade endometrial adenocarcinoma, the nuclei may stain *less* intensely than either normal or hyperplastic endometrial cell nuclei. Micronucleoli are seen in most (70%) tumor cells, macronucleoli are unusual. The amount of cytoplasm is slightly more generous than normal. A watery tumor diathesis is typical of low-grade endometrial carcinomas. A high maturation index ("estrogen effect") is common. Foamy histiocytes are frequently seen [Reagan 1973]. Sparse, cytologically bland or minimally atypical endometrial cells in a background of high maturation characterize well-differentiated endometrial adenocarcinoma in LBC.

Endometrial Carcinoma

Increase with grade:

· *Nuclear size*

· *Hyperchromasia*

· *Chromatin granularity*

· *Nucleolar size*

Cytoplasm: Scant or vacuolated

Background: Watery diathesis

Poorly-Differentiated Endometrial Adenocarcinoma

Poorly-differentiated endometrial adenocarcinomas tend to occur in older women without a history of endometrial hyperplasia (ie, type II cancers) [I2.17c, 2.18c, 2.21a,b]. These poorly-differentiated tumors usually have serous/clear cell morphology. The cells tend to form three-dimensional clusters or loose aggregates [Akin 1999]. The tumor cells have obvious malignant features, as described above. The mean cell area is 190 μm², and the mean nuclear area is ~90 μm². Many tumors cells have nucleoli, which are often prominent and multiple. Bizarre tumor cells may

be present. A tumor diathesis, with marked inflammation and necrosis similar to invasive cervical carcinoma, may be present. An atrophic maturation pattern is typical [Reagan 1973]. Increased cellularity, more cytologic atypia (nuclear enlargement, irregular membranes, chromatin abnormalities, nucleoli), and a background of atrophy characterize poorly-differentiated endometrial adenocarcinoma in LBC.

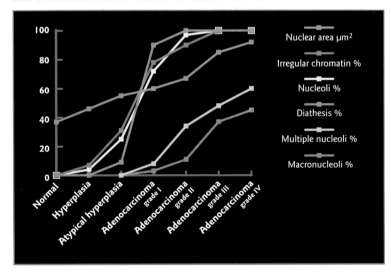

F2.3 Differential Nuclear Features of Endometrial Cells

Nuclear area μm²
Irregular chromatin %
Nucleoli %
Diathesis %
Multiple nucleoli %
Macronucleoli %

[A Ng 1973,1974a]

Descending from the Olympian heights to the real world of daily practice, an attempt is made to classify endometrial cells in a Pap test into three groups: normal [I2.22a], atypical [I2.22b], or malignant appearing [I2.22c]. Endometrial cells are often found in a background of high maturation ("estrogen effect"). In general, as the severity of the lesion progresses, there is an increase in: the size and number of endometrial cells; number of single cells; nuclear size; chromatin abnormalities; and nucleolar prominence. A diathesis favors a malignant interpretation. Remember, however, that even invasive endometrial carcinoma can shed cells that appear to be normal cytologically, or it may shed no cells at all.

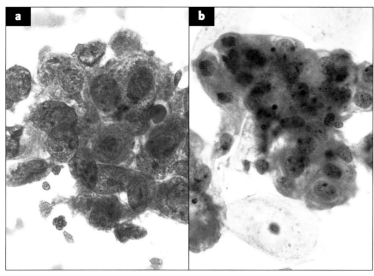

I2.21
a, High-grade endometrial carcinoma [C]; **b**, High-grade endometrial
carcinoma [L]

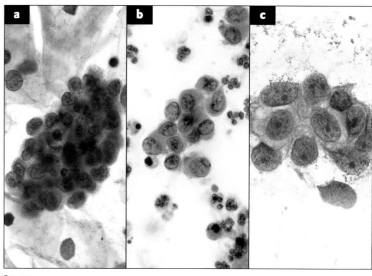

I2.22
a, Normal endometrial cells [C]; **b**, Atypical endometrial cells [C];
c, Malignant endometrial cells [C]

The differential of endometrial vs endocervical carcinoma is discussed on
pg 129. The differential of endometrial carcinoma also includes: menstrual phase
endometrium, endometritis, endometriosis, endometrial hyperplasia, endometrial
polyps, postpartum changes, Arias-Stella reaction, trophoblasts, IUD effect, atrophy,
clusters of naked nuclei, reserve cell hyperplasia, immature squamous metaplasia, repair, radiation effect, reactive endocervical cells, micro-glandular hyperplasia, and tubal

---

EC vs EM Carcinoma

Favors endometrial origin:
Fewer, smaller, rounder cells
Smaller nuclei, less cytoplasm

---

metaplasia [Babkowski 1996, J Benoit 1996, Chhieng 2000b, de Peralta–Venturino 1995, Ducatman 1993,
Ehrmann 1975, Frank 1991, J–A Gray 1999, P Gupta 1978, Hanau 1997, Heaton 1996, H–S Kim 1991, Kobayashi
1983a, Mulvany 1994, 1999, Murad 1981, Shidham 2000, Shrago 1977, Tajima 1998, von Ludinghausen 1984].
Any of these can be associated with Pap test misinterpretations, including both false-
positive and false-negative results.

Benign conditions can shed atypical glandular/endometrial cells (AGC),
consisting of crowded groups of cells with nuclear enlargement, prominent nucleoli,
and cytoplasmic neutrophils suggesting adenocarcinoma. Benign cells are typically
cohesive and have uniform nuclei, with smooth nuclear membranes, and regular chromatin. Endometritis, endometrial polyps, endometrial hyperplasia, and intrauterine
contraceptive devices can all be associated with abnormal shedding of atypical
endometrial cells. (The differential of atypical glandular cells is discussed on pg 146.)
On the other hand, well-differentiated endometrial adenocarcinoma may shed cytologically benign appearing cells, if it sheds any cells at all. Poorly-differentiated adenocarcinoma may shed sheets of tumor cells, which can resemble nonkeratinizing
squamous cell carcinoma. Squamous cell carcinoma tends to have more cells, with
denser cytoplasm, well-defined cell borders, coarser, darker chromatin, and less prominent nucleoli. Note, also, that adenocarcinoma with squamous differentiation is relatively common in the endometrium, so mixtures are possible (see below) [Berg 1958].
The differential also includes metastatic adenocarcinomas, which are uncommon.

Variants of Endometrial Carcinoma

There are several variants of endometrial carcinoma. These are discussed
below.

Adenocarcinoma With Squamous Differentiation

Some adenocarcinomas have a squamous component; these tumors
are designated adenocarcinoma with squamous differentiation [I2.23a]. The
squamous element is usually, but not always, nonkeratinizing and can have a
bland, benign appearance ("adenoacanthoma") or can be clearly malignant
("adenosquamous carcinoma"). Benign-appearing squamous elements closely
resemble squamous metaplasia. Squamous morules, pearls, or keratin bodies can
sometimes be seen, but are not specific [S Becker 1976, Blandamura 2002, Buschmann
1974]. Malignant squamous elements can be keratinizing or nonkeratinizing, or
have a spindle cell appearance [I2.23b]. The glandular component usually
predominates; the glandular and squamous components may be found together
or separately; and the squamous element is not always apparent in the Pap test
[A Ng 1973b]. Squamous differentiation apparently has no effect on prognosis when
the glandular component is
compared grade for grade and
stage for stage with pure adenocarcinoma [Zaino 1991].

Serous Adenocarcinoma

Serous adenocarci-
noma is a high-grade malignancy,

Endometrial Carcinoma Variants
Adenocarcinoma with squamous differentiation
Serous adenocarcinoma
Clear cell carcinoma
Mucinous adenocarcinoma
Secretory adenocarcinoma
Other

---

by definition [Sherman 2000]. Histologically, in serous carcinoma, high-grade nuclear
features are often associated with well-differentiated architectural features (glands
or papillae). In contrast, in endometrioid carcinoma, nuclear and architectural
abnormalities are usually concordant [Sherman 2000]. Cytologically, serous adenocarcinoma typically has numerous papillary clusters, coarse to smudgy dark chromatin, prominent nucleoli, and dense bulky cytoplasm [I2.24a,b]. Bizarre tumor
giant cells are characteristic. Psammoma bodies are most common in this variant
[Kuebler 1989, C Wright 1999]. It is identical to its homolog, high-grade serous carcinoma
of the ovary.

Clear Cell Adenocarcinoma

Clear cell adenocarcinoma is a poorly-differentiated tumor with abundant, delicate cytoplasm, highly abnormal nuclei, prominent, irregular nucleoli, many

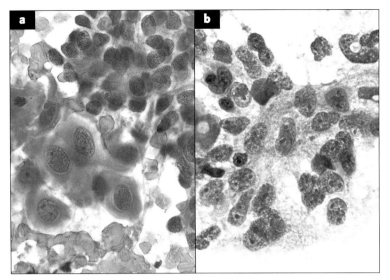

I2.23
a, AdCA, squamous differentiation [C]; **b**, AdCA, spindle cells [C]

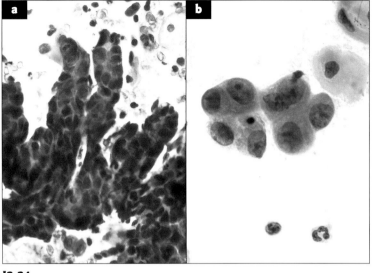

I2.24
a, Papillary serous carcinoma [C]; **b**, Papillary serous carcinoma [C]

naked nuclei, and a tumor diathesis [*Ohwada 1998, Wolinska 1980*] [I2.25a,b,c]. Glycogen explains the cytoplasmic clarity. (See Clear cell cervical carcinoma pg 133.)

Mucinous Adenocarcinoma

Mucinous carcinoma is an uncommon tumor of the endometrium that resembles the more common endocervical tumor. It is usually a low-grade, mucin-positive adenocarcinoma, occasionally with signet ring cells, and mucus in the background. Neutrophils may be present in the cytoplasm. The differential includes not only endocervical adenocarcinoma, but also secretory carcinoma, clear cell carcinoma, endometrial carcinoma, and secondary gastrointestinal carcinoma, as well as benign mucinous metaplasia of the endometrium and tubal metaplasia [*Galera-Davidson 1989*].

F2.4 Squamous Cell and Adenocarcinoma of the Cervix

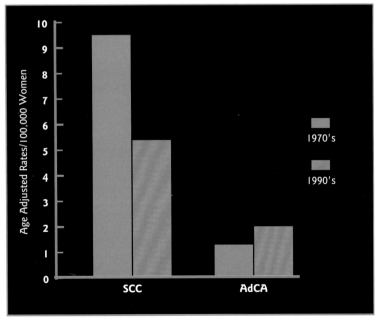

[*H. Smith 2000*]

Secretory Adenocarcinoma

Secretory adenocarcinoma is a rare, well-differentiated adenocarcinoma. It tends to shed large clusters of bland cells, with minimal cytologic atypia, moderate amounts of delicate, glycogen-positive cytoplasm, and round nuclei with fine chromatin [I2.26] [*Kusuyama 1989*]. The differential includes histiocytes and reactive endocervical cells as well as clear cell carcinoma.

Other Rare Variants

Other rare variants of endometrial carcinoma include: endometrial carcinoma with argyrophilic cells [*Prade 1982*], small cell neuroendocrine carcinoma [*Proca 1998*], minimal deviation endometrioid adenocarcinoma [*Rahilly 1992*], villoglandular adenocarcinoma (see cervical counterpart, pg 131), primary squamous cell carcinoma [*Houissa-Vuong 2002, Simon 1988, White 1973*], transitional cell (urothelial) carcinoma, and ciliated cell carcinoma [*Maksem 1997*].

Cervical Adenocarcinoma

Introduction

Over the past several decades, since the Pap test was introduced, the incidence of invasive squamous cell carcinoma has fallen remarkably. In striking contrast, the incidence of adenocarcinoma of the cervix has *increased* since the 1970s [*Alfsen 2000, Devesa 1989, Franco 2003, Gallup 1977, Kjær 1993a, Kudo 1992, R Peters 1986a, S Schwartz 1986, Stockton 1997, Vesterinen 1989, Vizcaino 1998, Zaino 2000, 2002, T Zheng 1996*]. Most of the increase has occurred in women born since 1935 [R Peters 1986a, T Zheng 1996]. These are women who became sexually active since the "sexual revolution" and the widespread use of oral contraceptives. In the 1950s, squamous cell carcinoma accounted for 95% of cervical cancers [*Fu 1987, Gallup 1977, Hepler 1952, Shingleton 1981*]. Today, cervical adenocarcinoma accounts for

Endocervical Adenocarcinoma
Increasing in frequency
Despite widespread screening
Pap test not proven effective in prevention
Cause: HPV, esp type 18

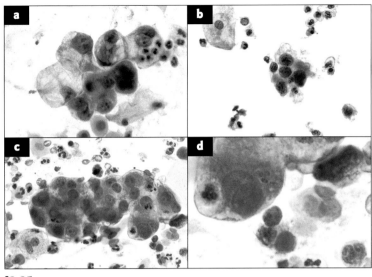

I2.25
a, Clear cell carcinoma [C]; **b**, Clear cell carcinoma [L];
c, Clear cell carcinoma [C]; **d**, Clear cell CA, glycogen [C]

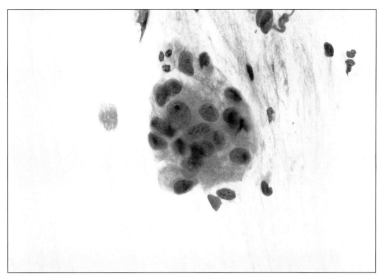

I2.26
Secretory carcinoma [C]

one-fifth to one-third of all invasive cervical cancers [Berek 1985, Brand 1988, JR Davis 1975, Franco 2003, H Goodman 1989, Greer 1989, I Horowitz 1988, Mayer 1976, B Miller 1993, R Peters 1986a, S Schwartz 1986 Shingleton 1981, Shorrock 1990, H Smith 2000, Tamimi 1982, Tasker 1974, Vesterinen 1989, R Weiss 1986]. At the University of Chicago, adenocarcinomas (including adenosquamous carcinomas) accounted for one-third (32.6%; 140/430) of all invasive cervical cancers diagnosed histologically over a recent period. In addition, 42 cases of adenocarcinoma in situ were diagnosed, histologically, in the same time period. These numbers reflect both a relative and an absolute increase in incidence of cervical adenocarcinoma [F2.4].

The mean age at diagnosis has fallen as the incidence of invasive cervical adenocarcinoma has risen [B Miller 1993]. The average age is now in the 40s and 50s. Most women are older than 30 years; a few women are in their 20s, and very rarely, are even younger [Pollack 1947, Saigo 1985] (see F1.18 pg 73). The ages are similar to, or slightly older than, those with invasive squamous cell carcinoma, which also is occurring in younger women than before.

The cell of origin is thought to be the reserve cell, probably the same primitive, pluripotential cell implicated in squamous dysplasia and carcinoma [Alva 1975, Boon 1981a,b, Brinton 1993, L Brown 1986, Burghardt 1970, Christopherson 1979, Colgan 1990, Cullimore 1989a, Duggan 1995, Glücksmann 1956, Hitchcock 1993, L Johnson 1964, Kashimura 1990, Kjær 1993a, Kudo 1991, Kurian 1999, Lauchlan 1967, Laverty 1988, G-K Nguyen 1984b, Noda 1983, Parazzini 1990a, Rollason 1989, Smedts 1992, Teshima 1985, van Aspert-van Erp 2004b, Yamakawa 1994]. In fact, endocervical glandular neoplasia is frequently associated with squamous intraepithelial lesions and adenosquamous carcinomas are also relatively common [Alva 1975, Maier 1980]. Roughly 50% (range 25% to 75%) of glandular lesions have coexisting squamous lesions; however, only about 5% of squamous lesions have coexisting glandular lesions [E Andersen 1989, Bose 1994, L Brown 1986, Colgan 1990, Denehy 1997, Fu 1987, Gloor 1982, Goff 1992, Kohan 1985, Maier 1980, Nasu 1993, Qizilbash 1975].

Human papillomavirus is the cause of most cases of cervical adenocarcinoma. HPV-DNA can be detected in most cervical adenocarcinomas, including endocervical, endometrioid, and adenosquamous types as well as other rare variants, which account for the vast majority (>90%) of all cervical adenocarcinomas [A Ferguson 1998, Pirog 2000]. Some rare variants of cervical adenocarcinoma, including clear cell, serous, and mesonephric subtypes, and minimal deviation adenocarcinoma ("adenoma malignum"), may be unrelated to human papillomavirus, at least in

some cases [A Ferguson 1998, Milde-Langosch 1993, Pirog 2000, Toki 1999]. HPV 16 and 18 are the most frequently detected viral types (also, 45, 52, and 35), but in contrast with squamous cancers, HPV 18 is more common than HPV 16 [Altekruse 2003, Bjersing 1991, F Bosch 1995, K Cooper 1992, Duggan 1993, Iwasawa 1996, Leminen 1991, Lizano 1997, Nakagawa 1996, Okagaki 1989, Smotkin 1986, Tase 1988, 1989a, Tenti 1996, Yokoyama 1994]. HPV cannot replicate in glandular cells (nonproductive infection); consequently, only high-risk viral types are identified, whereas low-risk viral types (HPV 6, 11, 42, 43, 33, etc) rarely if ever occur in glandular lesions. When squamous and glandular lesions coexist, they often share the same viral type [Jaworski 1990].

Epidemiologically, cervical adenocarcinoma shares many of the risk factors associated with squamous carcinoma that implicate sexual transmission, eg, early age of first intercourse and multiple sexual partners. In contrast, cigarette smoking may not be related to adenocarcinoma, and the women tend to be of higher socioeconomic status than those with squamous cell carcinoma [Brand 1988, Brinton 1987b, 1993, I Horowitz 1988, Parazzini 1988, 1990a, Ursin 1996, Zaino 2000]. Long-term use of oral contraceptives is more strongly associated with cervical adenocarcinoma than squamous cell carcinoma [Brinton 1986a, 1987b, Chilvers 1987, Dallenbach-Hellweg 1984, MW Jones 1989, Kjær 1993a, Lacey 1999, 2000, Madeleine 2001, R Peters 1986b, Schiffman 1995a, S Schwartz 1986, D Thomas 1996a, Ursin 1994, Valente 1986, WHO 1993, Ydh 1991, Zaino 2000]. However, the increased risk diminishes after accounting for HPV infection, and the overall risk is low and may diminish further in the future owing to lower hormone doses in modern contraceptive pills. Endocervical glandular neoplasia may also share some risk factors classically associated with endometrial cancer, particularly nulliparity and obesity (possibly also hypertension and diabetes mellitus) [Altekruse 2003, Brinton 1987b, Kjær 1993a, M Korhonen 1980, Lacey 2003, Parazzini 1988, 1990a, Ursin 1996, Valente 1996, Ydh 1991].

Clinically, the majority (~75%) of women with invasive cervical adenocarcinoma present with abnormal bleeding, although some present with vaginal discharge or pelvic pain [Hurt 1977]. Unfortunately, symptoms usually indicate advanced disease [Ydh 1991]. About 10% to 20% are asymptomatic [Brand 1988, Leminen 1990, Saigo 1985]. The tumor may present as an ulcer, as a nodular or polypoid mass, or as a barrel-shaped cervix. About one third have a grossly normal appearing cervix.

Adenocarcinoma arises in or near the squamocolumnar junction/transformation zone [Jaworski 1988, Teshima 1985]. (The endometrioid variant may arise, rarely, from ectopic endometrial glands or endometriosis [Noda 1983].) Invasive cervical adenocarcinomas are often large, grow endophytically, have a propensity for early dissemination, and may have poor prognosis relative to squamous cell carcinoma [Bertrand 1987, Cullimore 1992, S Liu 2001]. Although the data do not show a clear-cut prognostic difference, clinicians tend to believe adenocarcinomas are more aggressive than squamous cell carcinomas, and therefore, treat early glandular lesions more aggressively [Fu 1982, Hopkins 1991a, Shingleton 1981, 1995].

Colposcopy, and colposcopically directed biopsy, are generally viewed as unreliable in detecting endocervical neoplasia because of lack of well-defined diagnostic criteria and the location of most of the lesions high in the endocervix or deep in the glands [Ayer 1987, Jaworski 1988, Lickrish 1993, Teshima 1985, Yeh 1991]. Also, because the transformation zone recedes into the endocervical canal over time, early detection becomes more difficult with age [Fu 1987]. Consequently, the colposcopic examination may be falsely interpreted as benign in 20% to 30% of cases of invasive adenocarcinoma (with higher false negative rates for adenocarcinoma in situ, see pg 136) [M Korhonen 1978].

Pap tests cannot detect all adenocarcinomas; sensitivity ranges from <50% to >90% [G Anderson 1992, Angel 1992, Boddington 1976, Boon 1987, M Costa 1991b, Hayes 1997, Hurt 1977, H S Kim 1991, M Korhonen 1978, Krane 2001, Kristensen 1991, B Miller 1993, M Mitchell 1996, Saigo 1985, Sasieni 2001, Schoolland 2002a, van Aspert-van Erp 2004, Yeh 1991]. Difficulties include problems with sampling, screening, and interpretation [Boon 1987, K Lee 1997b, Raab 2000]. Although women with invasive cervical adenocarcinoma often have cytologic abnormalities, the abnormalities are not necessarily specific [Angel 1992, Leminen 1990, Saigo 1985, 1986b]. Negative cytology does not exclude the possibility of malignancy [Peete 1965, Schoolland 2002a]. The false-negative rate is as high as 50%, even in women with grossly identifiable lesions, and as high as 80% if there is no gross lesion [Hurt 1977]. The rate of cytologic detection of adenocarcinoma increases with stage and grade of the tumor [M Korhonen 1978]. Of course, not all adenocarcinomas detected in the Pap test originate in the cervix; some arise in the endometrium, fallopian tubes, ovaries, or distant sites [Pretorius 1996, M Sasagawa 2003]. It is also worth noting again that the incidence of cervical adenocarcinoma has increased despite widespread Pap test screening (see Early Glandular Neoplasia, pg 135, for further discussion.)

Classification of Cervical Adenocarcinomas

I. Pure Adenocarcinomas
  A. Typical Endocervical Type
    Variant: Villoglandular Adenocarcinoma
  B. Mucinous Adenocarcinoma
    Variants:
      1. Adenoma Malignum
      2. Intestinal-type
        a. Signet Ring Cell Adenocarcinoma
        b. Colloid Adenocarcinoma
  C. Endometrioid Adenocarcinoma
    Variant: Minimal Deviation Adenocarcinoma
  D. Clear Cell Adenocarcinoma
  E. Serous Adenocarcinoma
  F. Mesonephric Adenocarcinoma
II. Mixed Adenocarcinomas
  A. Adenosquamous Carcinoma
  B. Glassy Cell Carcinoma
  C. Adenoid Cystic Carcinoma
  D. Adenoid Basal Carcinoma
  E. Adenocarcinoma with neuroendocrine
    differentiation

Histology of Cervical Adenocarcinoma

The major morphologic types of cervical adenocarcinoma are: endocervical (the usual type, accounting for at least 80% of cases); mucinous types (adenoma malignum and intestinal types [including signet ring cell and colloid carcinoma]); and endometrioid, as well as clear cell, serous, and mesonephric. There are also adenocarcinomas with a non-glandular component, including adenosquamous carcinoma, glassy cell carcinoma, adenoid basal carcinoma, adenoid cystic carcinoma, and adenocarcinoma with neuroendocrine

differentiation [R Young 2002]. Villoglandular adenocarcinoma is a variant of typical endocervical adenocarcinoma.

Although endocervical adenocarcinomas are sometimes described as "mucinous," the typical type usually has little or no mucin, although there are mucinous forms such as adenoma malignum. Nevertheless, mucin stains can help detect glandular differentiation in tumors thought to be purely squamous. On the other hand, immunochemistry contributes little to diagnosis of these tumors. A histologic diagnosis of invasion is made when neoplastic glands extend beyond the normal crypt depth, although this determination can be difficult in practice. Lymphatic and vascular invasion beyond 3 mm-5 mm, or confluence of early invasive glands, indicates frankly invasive adenocarcinoma. A chronic inflammatory or desmoplastic stromal response is characteristic of invasive carcinoma, but not always present. Precursor lesions of frankly invasive cervical adenocarcinoma, including endocervical glandular dysplasia, adenocarcinoma in situ, and microinvasive adenocarcinoma, are discussed separately. There are also benign mimickers of adenocarcinoma. The presence of an obvious mass typical of carcinoma speaks for a malignant diagnosis, although even deeply invasive tumors can be deceptive grossly [R Young 2002].

Cytology of Cervical Adenocarcinoma

The first cytologic clue to invasive cervical adenocarcinoma is finding an *abundance* of (atypical) endocervical cells in the Pap test—assuming the lesion was adequately sampled. Acinar formation, columnar cells, and cytoplasm vacuolization indicate glandular differentiation. The malignant cells are usually larger than normal endo-

Endocervical Glandular Neoplasia

1st clue: Abundance of endocervical cells
Abnormalities of:
  ·Architecture
  ·Nuclei
SILs often present

cervical cells, with big nuclei, and increased N/C ratios. Well-differentiated adenocarcinoma is characterized by tall columnar cells, with elongated (cigar-shaped) nuclei, and coarse, dark chromatin; this can be difficult to distinguish from adenocarcinoma in situ [Boon 1981b]. As the grade of the tumor increases, things become more "loosey-goosey." The cells tend to become more loosely arranged; they lose their well-formed columnar shape and their well-defined cell borders (loss of "honeycomb"). With increasing grade, there is more pleomorphism, larger nuclei, *finer* chromatin, and more prominent nucleoli. Endometrioid endocervical adenocarcinoma may have densely packed, *smaller* cells, with nuclear molding and scant mucin production.

Architectural and *nuclear abnormalities* are important in cytologic recognition of cervical adenocarcinoma [12.27]. Not as much emphasis is placed on evaluation of single cells as on the groups, although the conspicuous presence of single cells suggests invasion [12.28a,b]. However, it may be easier to appreciate subtle glandular features, such as nucleocytoplasmic polarity, prominent nucleoli, and delicate vacuolated cytoplasm, in single cells than in groups of cells.

Architectural abnormalities include abnormal glandular arrangements such as rosette-like structures [12.29a] and secondary gland openings in sheets of endocervical cells [12.29b] [Krumins 1977]. With no true glands in the endo-

Architectural Abnormalities

Marked cellular crowding
HCGs with feathery edges
Abnormal gland arrangements
  Microacini, rosettes
Indistinct cell borders

cervix, sheets of endocervical cells with well-formed glandular lumens, or crypt openings, are the equivalent of the "gland-in-gland" pattern characteristic of

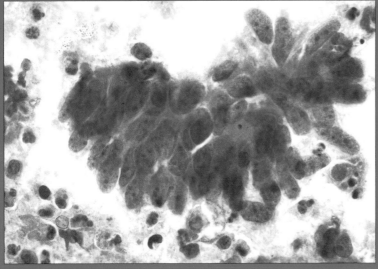

I2.27
Endocervical carcinoma [C]

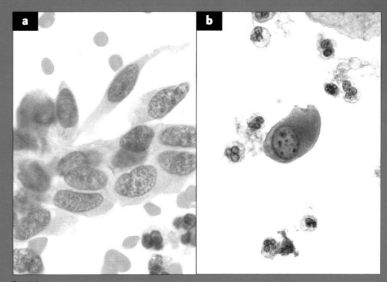

I2.28
a, Endocervical carcinoma [C]; **b**, Endocervical carcinoma [L]

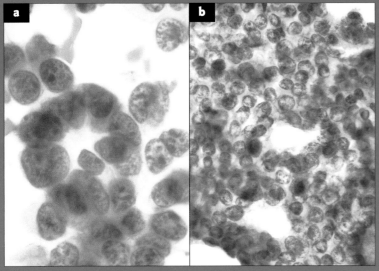

I2.29
a, Endocervical carcinoma, rosette [C]; **b**, Secondary gland openings [C]

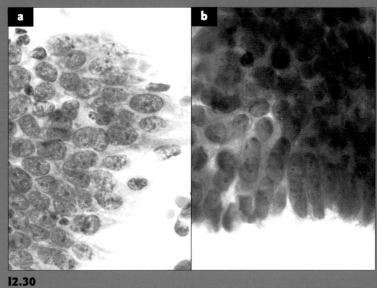

I2.30
a, Hyperchromatic crowded group [C]; **b**, Hyperchromatic crowded group [L]

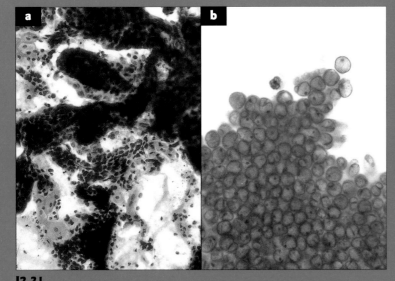

I2.31
a, Endocervical carcinoma, papillae [C]; **b**, Supercrowding [C]

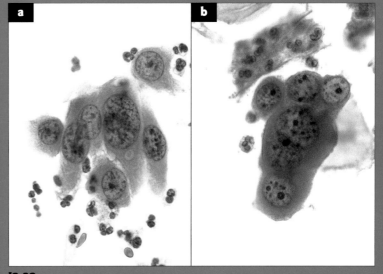

I2.32
a, Endocervical CA, high grade [C]; **b**, Endocervical CA, high grade [L]

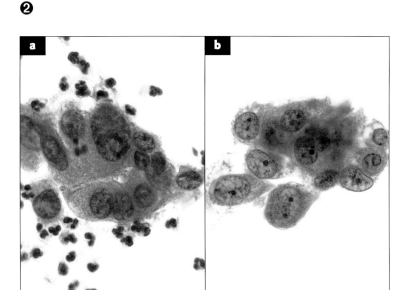

I2.33
a, Endocervical CA, high grade [C]; **b**, Endocervical CA, high grade [L]

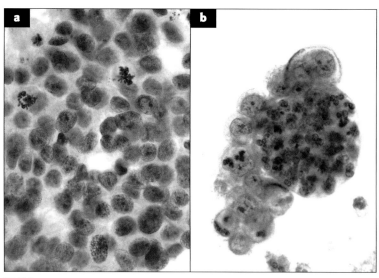

I2.34
a, Endocervical CA, mitoses [C]; **b**, Endocervical CA, neutrophils [L]

adenocarcinomas. Occasionally, however, sheets of malignant endocervical cells can be unexpectedly orderly, even in high-grade adenocarcinoma, and rarely, rosettes and secondary glandular openings can be present in benign endocervical cells.

Syncytial-like aggregates (hyperchromatic crowded groups, HCGs) are sometimes present, in which glandular differentiation may not be obvious [I2.30a,b]. These aggregates can be difficult to distinguish from squamous carcinoma in situ or other HCGs [DeMay 2000]. In adenocarcinoma, the hyperchromatic crowded groups typically have "feathery" edges, particularly in well-differentiated tumors and adenocarcinomas in situ [Ayer 1987, 1991, Bose 1994, Bousfield 1980]. Feathering refers to the protrusion of nearly naked nuclei from the edges of crowded cell clusters, resulting in an irregular, raggedy, or frayed outline. Well-developed feathery edges rarely occur with benign glandular cells [K Lee 1991].

Loose, disorderly two-dimensional sheets and palisades are more common than three-dimensional cell balls in the cytology of invasive adenocarcinoma. Although papillae can occur in ordinary cervical adenocarcinoma [R Young 2002], they suggest villoglandular adenocarcinoma, when the component cells are well-differentiated, and serous carcinoma, when the cells are poorly-differentiated [I2.31a].

Nuclear abnormalities include crowding, which is often marked ("supercrowded"), particularly in well-differentiated and in situ adenocarcinomas [I2.31b].

Nuclear Abnormalities

Nuclear enlargement

Elongated or irregular outlines

High N/C ratios

Coarse, dark chromatin

Small or indistinct nucleoli

Mitotic figures highly suspicious!

Strips of irregularly stratified cells with hyperchromatic nuclei recapitulate the histologic appearance of adenocarcinoma. Sheets of cells also have marked nuclear crowding and irregular overlapping. Poorly-differentiated cervical adenocarcinomas, however, usually do not have the marked nuclear crowding characteristic of well-differentiated tumors.

Nuclear size generally increases with the grade of the tumor, ranging from 73 µm^2 to 165 µm^2 [Reagan 1973]. The mean nuclear area is 86 ± 17 mm^2, compared with 55 µm^2 for the normal endocervical nucleus [Reagan 1961b]. (Occasionally, cervical adenocarcinomas have *smaller* nuclei than normal, see endometrioid type, below.) The N/C ratios are elevated. In well-differentiated tumors, the chromatin is coarse and dark [I2.27, 2.30b], but becomes paler, finer, and more irregularly distributed in high-grade cancer [I2.32a,b, 2.33a,b]. As the grade of the tumor increases, nucleoli tend to become larger and more numerous. Mitotic figures, including abnormal forms, as well as apoptotic bodies, may be present [I2.34a].

The cytoplasm stains variably, but is typically basophilic, with granular texture and decreased mucin content. Multiple fine vacuoles can also be present, especially in low-grade adenocarcinoma. With increasing grade, granularity of the cytoplasm becomes more apparent, and vacuolization diminishes. Leukophagocytosis can occur [I2.34b], but is less common than in endometrial adenocarcinoma.

A background of tumor diathesis indicates invasion [I 2.27] [I2.35a,b]; however, it is not always present [Bose 1994, DiTomasso 1996, Keyhani-Rofagha 1995, K Lee 1991, Schoolland 2002a]. Heavy blood staining is a common finding in invasive adenocarcinoma; this could be mistaken for a menstrual smear containing endometrial cells [Schoolland 2002a]. An increase in single abnormal cells, with more chromatin abnormalities (irregular distribution), and more prominent nucleoli are also features of invasion. It is important to emphasize that cytology can suspect, but not exclude, invasion.

Suggest Invasion

More single cells

Irregular chromatin

Prominent nucleoli*

Tumor diathesis*

*Key features

Cannot exclude invasion by cytology!

Accompanying squamous intraepithelial lesions or invasive squamous carcinomas are present in a significant number of women [Keyhani-Rofagha 1995, G-K Nguyen 1993]. This could result in the glandular lesion being misinterpreted as purely squamous in a Pap test.

In liquid-based cytology, the chromatin is more open and vesicular, and nucleoli are more prominent [I2.32b, 2.33b]. Three dimensional clusters, single cells, and irregular nuclear membranes are similar to conventional Pap smears, although "feathering" is less prominent in LBC [I2.30b, 2.34b]. The cytoplasm is finely vacuolated and N/C ratios are elevated. The tumor diathesis may be less conspicuous and tends to cling to cells [I2.35b]. It looks a bit like tissue paper, which is different from the granular, necrotic diathesis seen in conventional Pap smears [JE Johnson 1999]. Dense, three dimensional clusters of

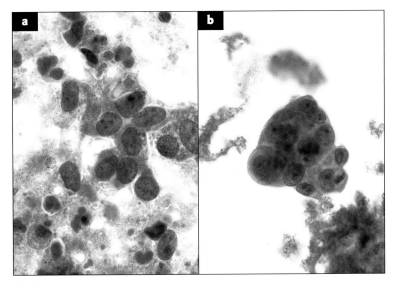

I2.35
a, Tumor diathesis [C]; **b**, Tumor diathesis [L]

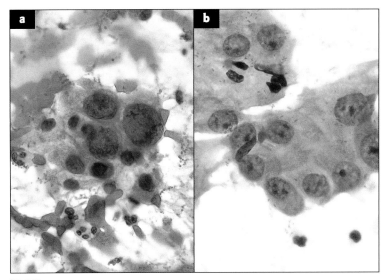

I2.36
a, Benign endocervical cells (brush artifact) [C]; **b**,Reactive endocervical cells [C]

malignant endocervical cells, more common in LBC, may be difficult to distinguish from endometrial adenocarcinoma.

Well-differentiated cervical adenocarcinoma is cytologically similar to adenocarcinoma in situ [I2.27, 2.30b]. Features that favor invasive carcinoma over in situ carcinoma include: numerous single atypical cells, irregular chromatin distribution, prominent nucleoli, and tumor diathesis. Prominent nucleoli and a tumor diathesis are probably the two most helpful features that suggest invasion.

Poorly-differentiated cervical adenocarcinoma is characterized by irregularly arranged sheets of abnormal cells with marked nuclear atypia, including large size, irregular nuclear membranes, pale or slightly dark chromatin, and prominent, multiple, or irregular nucleoli [I2.32a,b]. The cytoplasm has a granular texture and vacuolization is minimal. Leukophagocytosis is more common in poorly-differentiated tumors (and still more common in endometrial carcinoma). The differential includes endocervical repair and nonkeratinizing squamous cell carcinoma [Saigo 1985]. Searching for areas of better-differentiated tumor may provide a helpful clue.

Cytologic atypia, such as nuclear enlargement, anisonucleosis, hyperchromasia, prominent nucleoli, and (normal) mitotic figures, may be present in benign endocervical cells [I2.36a,b]. Such "atypical" changes are common in reactive/reparative conditions, cervical polyps, microglandular hyperplasia, tubal metaplasia, and radiation (see Atypical Glandular Cells, pg 144) [DiTomasso 1996]. If the atypical endocervical cells form two-dimensional sheets (ie, "lie flat"), without significant crowding or overlapping, have well-defined cell borders (ie, maintain "honeycomb"), round nuclei, smooth nuclear membranes, and fine chromatin, they are probably benign. Significant nuclear crowding, overlapping, feathering, high N/C ratios, elongated nuclei, irregular nuclear membranes, distinctively coarse chromatin, abnormal mitotic figures, and apoptosis point to a malignant interpretation. However, some cervical adenocarcinomas shed small cells or cytologically bland cells [Bousfield 1980]. This can cause false-negative interpretations [Krane 2001]. Very well-differentiated adenocarcinomas, such as minimal deviation adenocarcinoma ("adenoma malignum") and villoglandular carcinoma, are also potential sources of false-negative results. When adenocarcinoma is suspected on Pap test, colposcopy and biopsy are the next steps in clinical management.

Differential: Endocervical vs Endometrial Adenocarcinoma

A common problem is differentiating endocervical from endometrial adenocarcinoma [I2.37a,b] [T2.4]. Many of the observed differences between the two result from the way in which the cells are collected. Cells from cervical adenocarcinoma may be sampled directly, while those of endometrial carcinoma are usually exfoliated spontaneously. Therefore, cervical adenocarcinoma is characterized by the presence of an abundance of well-preserved cells, while endometrial carcinoma typically has fewer, more

T2.4 Differential Features of Endocervical and Endometrial Carcinomas

	Favors Endocervical CA	Favors Endometrial CA
Cellularity	Abundant	Sparse
Cells	Larger	Smaller
	Tall columnar	Rounder
	Preserved	Degenerated
Groups	Crowded groups, rosettes	Balls
	Feathering	Molded groups
Nuclei		
Shape	Elongated	Round
Size	Larger (75-165 μm^2)	Smaller (60-90 μm^2)
	~2-5× intermediate	<3× intermediate
Multinucleation	Common	Rare
Chromatin	Coarser, darker	Finer, paler
Nucleoli	Multiple, larger	Single, smaller
Cytoplasm		
Texture	Granular	Vacuolar
Stain	More acidophilic	More basophilic
PMNs	Uncommon	More common
Associations	SILs	Clinical risk factors
Diathesis	Coarse	Watery
Immunochemistry	CEA	Vimentin
Hormone receptors	(−)	(+)
HPV	(+)	(−)

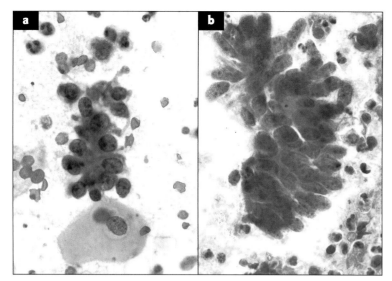

I2.37
a, Endometrial carcinoma [C]; **b**, Endocervical carcinoma [C]

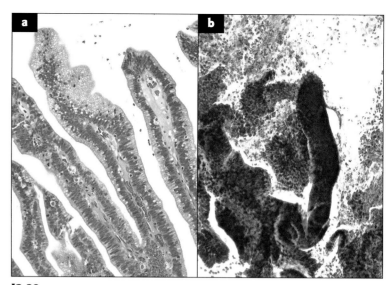

I2.38
a, Villoglandular carcinoma; **b**, Villoglandular carcinoma [C]

degenerated cells, unless the tumor has invaded the endocervix. Grade for grade, malignant endocervical cells are larger, have bigger nuclei, more hyperchromasia, coarser chromatin, and more and bigger nucleoli than malignant endometrial cells.

Cervical adenocarcinoma typically exfoliates two-dimensional rosettes or clusters with feathery edges, while endometrial carcinoma tends to exfoliate rounded, three-dimensional cell balls. As the grade of tumor increases, cellular aggregates may become tighter in endometrial carcinoma, while they tend to become looser in endocervical carcinoma. Malignant endocervical cells tend to maintain their columnar shape, while malignant endometrial cells tend to round up [Nasu 1993]. Multinucleation is common in cervical adenocarcinoma, but not in endometrial carcinoma [Reagan 1973]. The nuclei of cervical adenocarcinoma usually are elongated and dark, and may have prominent, multiple nucleoli.

Endometrial carcinoma, on the other hand, typically sheds cells that are rounded, with smaller, rounder nuclei, finer chromatin, and a conspicuous central nucleolus. The cytoplasm is usually vacuolated in endometrial carcinoma, and is usually more granular in cervical adenocarcinoma. Cytoplasmic basophilia or cyanophilia favors endometrial carcinoma, while cytoplasmic acidophilia favors cervical origin (depending on the individual stain). Neutrophils are more commonly present in the cytoplasm of malignant endometrial cells, but do not exclude cervical adenocarcinoma.

Cervical adenocarcinomas are frequently associated with squamous intraepithelial lesions. Endometrial carcinomas are frequently associated with classic clinical risk factors. Cervical adenocarcinoma is usually associated with HPV DNA, while endometrial carcinoma is not [McCluggage 2002, A Nielsen 1990]. Carcinoembryonic antigen (CEA) is not expressed in normal endocervical cells, but is frequently (~60% to 100%) expressed in cervical adenocarcinoma, while only a few endometrial carcinomas also express this antigen [Wells 2002]. Some benign lesions, such as florid microglandular hyperplasia, can also have focal cytoplasmic CEA positivity [Cina 1997]. In sum, CEA expression suggests malignancy in endocervical cells, and favors endocervical over endometrial carcinoma, but it is neither highly sensitive nor specific [S Agarwal 1990, C Cohen 1982, P Cooper 1987, Dabbs 1986, Wahlström

1979, Wells 2002]. Estrogen and progesterone receptors are identified in only a minority cervical adenocarcinomas, but are present in the majority of endometrial adenocarcinomas [Staebler 2002]. Both tumors are usually CK7 positive and CK 20 negative. Expression of vimentin or bcl2 favors endometrial origin [Dabbs 1986, Marjoniemi 2004].

Endometrioid variant of cervical adenocarcinoma is morphologically identical to primary endometrial adenocarcinoma, but arises in the cervix (discussed below). Endometrial carcinoma extends into the endocervix in about 10% of cases, making cytologic distinction difficult or impossible [Morimura 2002, Reagan 1973]. The bottom line is that it is not always possible to separate cervical adenocarcinoma from endometrial adenocarcinoma by cytology alone, and even in tissue studies, this distinction can sometimes be difficult [M Costa 1991b, Valente 1996].

Variants of Cervical Adenocarcinoma

Other forms of cervical adenocarcinoma include villoglandular adenocarcinoma (a well-differentiated variant of typical endocervical adenocarcinoma), adenoma malignum, intestinal type adenocarcinoma (including signet ring and colloid carcinomas), and endometrioid types. There are also other types, including clear cell, serous, mesonephric, etc. Mixed adenocarcinoma and neuroendocrine carcinoma is discussed with neuroendocrine tumors (see pg 173). Although cytologic criteria

Endocervical Carcinoma Variants

Villoglandular: Papillae, low-grade cells
Adenoma malignum: Repair-like cells
Intestinal-type: Goblet-like cells
Endometrioid: Small cells
Clear cell: guess what?
Serous: Papillae, high-grade cells
Mesonephric: Nonclear cells
Adenosquamous: Squamoid cells
Glassy cell: Ground glass cells
Adenoid cystic: Basaloid cells, globules
Adenoid basal: Basaloid cells, acini

for these variants have been described, they may be difficult to implement in routine practice [Ayer 1988, Hayes 1997, Tobón 1988].

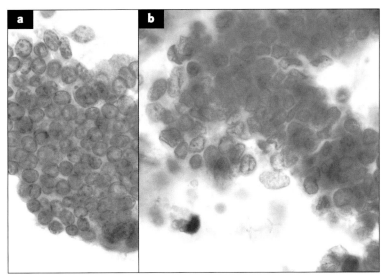

I2.39
a, Villoglandular carcinoma [C]; **b**, Villoglandular carcinoma [L]

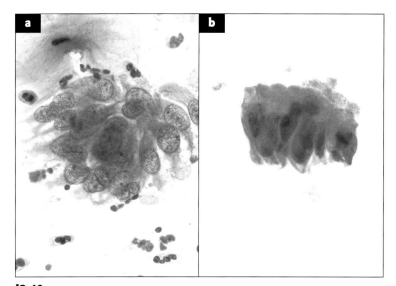

I2.40
a, Villoglandular carcinoma [C]; **b**, Villoglandular carcinoma [L]

Villoglandular Adenocarcinoma

Villoglandular adenocarcinoma, first described by Young and Scully in 1989 [R Young 1989a], is a distinct variant of cervical adenocarcinoma that tends to occur in younger women (<40 years of age), is usually only minimally invasive, and has an excellent prognosis [Collinet 1999, MW Jones 1993, Zaino 2000]. The tumor is well-differentiated (grade I) by definition, with papillary fronds comprised of fibrovascular cores lined by mildly atypical glandular cells (with endocervical, endometrioid, or intestinal features), morphologically similar to villous adenomas of the gastrointestinal tract. The papillae are usually tall and thin [I2.38a], but can occasionally be short and broad [R Young 2002]. These tumors have been associated with oral contraceptive use and high-risk HPV types [MH Jones 1992, MW Jones 2000].

Abundant endocervical cells are, as usual, clues to the presence of a neoplastic glandular lesion of the cervix, including villoglandular adenocarcinoma [Ballo 1996]. Typically, there are large, crowded sheets of uniform tumor cells, with minimal cytologic abnormalities and partial loss of prominent cell borders (honeycomb). Villous fronds, true papillae with fibrovascular cores, and little cytologic atypia suggest this lesion [I2.38b] [Ajit 2004, Ballo 1996, W Chang 1999, Khunamornpong 2002, Novotny 1997]. Sheets, rosettes, and strips of crowded cells may be present [I2.39a,b], but feathery edges are minimal or absent, unless the tumor is mixed with ordinary cervical adenocarcinoma. Single, intact atypical cells are sparse, but naked nuclei may be numerous [Ajit 2004].

Individual cell atypia is minimal by definition [R Young 2002]. The nuclei are uniform, round to oval (not cigar shaped), have increased N/C ratios, and mild to moderate, but not marked, atypia [I2.40a,b]. The chromatin is moderately hyperchromatic, granular, and evenly distributed. Nucleoli are inconspicuous or absent. Mitotic figures are an important clue to a neoplastic process. Psammoma bodies are present only rarely [R Young 1989a]. Because the tumor is usually minimally invasive, a tumor diathesis is usually minimal. HPV has been reported in this tumor, with type 18 predominating over type 16, as in other cervical adenocarcinomas [MW Jones 2000, Yamazawa 2000].

Villoglandular adenocarcinoma is often misinterpreted in Pap tests [W Chang 1999]. Many cases are reported as atypical glandular cells, or more ominously, reactive endocervical cells, as may be present in endocervical

polyps, for example. Villoglandular carcinoma could also be misinterpreted as squamous carcinoma in situ and ordinary glandular neoplasia, in situ or invasive, and these lesions can also coexist [MW Jones 1993]. Clues to villoglandular adenocarcinoma include: true papillary fragments, nuclear crowding, subtle cytologic atypia, and mitotic figures. Three dimensional tumor clusters may suggest endometrial adenocarcinoma; however, the groups are usually more numerous and the cells larger in villoglandular adenocarcinoma. Papillary architecture can occur in other cervical adenocarcinomas; however, these other papillary carcinomas are usually serous or clear cell carcinomas characterized by high-grade, rather than low-grade, tumor cells.

Minimal Deviation Adenocarcinoma ("Adenoma Malignum")

Adenoma malignum was first reported in 1870 by Gusserow [Gusserow 1870], and McKelvey and Goodlin [McKelvey 1953] rediscovered it in 1953 [K Ishii 1998]. Silverberg and Hurt apparently first applied the term "minimal deviation adenocarcinoma" to this tumor in 1975 [Silverberg 1975]. By any name, this is a rare malignancy. It is composed predominantly of highly differentiated, mucin-rich glandular cells, although there may be a small (<10%) component of ordinary adenocarcinoma [Hart 2002]. Because the tumor is so well-differentiated, it is easily misinterpreted as benign, both histologically and cytologically [Kaku 1983, H Michael 1984, R Young 1990, 1993].

The age ranges from about 25 to 75 years (average ~42 years) [Hart 2002]. Profuse, mucinous vaginal discharge is a characteristic symptom of adenoma malignum, but can also occur in women with fallopian tube carcinoma [Hirai 1998]. There is an association with Peutz-Jegher syndrome (rare, autosomal dominant disorder characterized by circumoral pigmentation and intestinal polyposis, with increased risk of cancers of pancreas, breast, lung, ovary, and uterus) [R Young 1982, Szyfelbein 1984, Valente 1996, Zaino 2000].

The hallmarks of adenoma malignum include a gross lesion present in the hysterectomy specimen; the cervix is often very hard and the mucosal surface may be hemorrhagic, friable, or mucoid [R Young 2002]. Histologically, the glands are oddly shaped, sometimes cystically dilated, and lined by innocuous looking, uniform, mucinous columnar cells. However, there is usually at least focal moderate to severe atypia that is a helpful diagnostic clue. Occasional mitotic

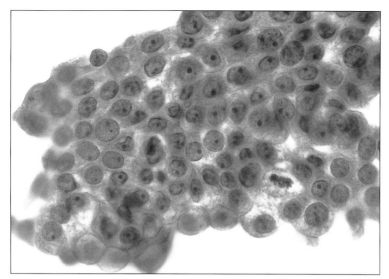

I2.4I
Adenoma malignum, note mitosis [C]

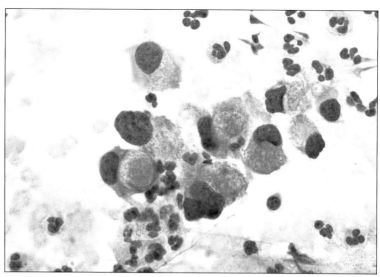

I2.42
Intestinal-type adenocarcinoma [C]

figures and apoptosis are further clues [Kaku 1983, H Michael 1984, R Young 1993]. (This disease is one reason why mitotic figures in endocervical cells, although not diagnostic of malignancy, should be viewed with suspicion.) There is often a desmoplastic stromal response to invasive tumor. The presence of obviously malignant glands and vascular or perineural invasion establishes a malignant diagnosis.

Cytologically, the tumor cells are deceptively bland, resembling benign endocervical cells, which can make cytologic recognition of this tumor difficult or impossible [I2.4I]. The cytologic picture resembles endocervical repair in some cases. Subtle architectural and nuclear abnormalities may be the only cytologic clues to this disease [Valente 1996]. Characteristically, there are numerous large sheets of cells with abundant, clear, mucinous cytoplasm, and fairly innocuous looking nuclei [Fukazawa 1992, Granter 1996, G-K Nguyen 1993, Vogelsang 1995]. The tumor may exfoliate cells in multilayered or slightly crowded groups, including honeycomb arrangements and palisades, as well as single cells. Very large sheets of glandular cells provide an interpretive clue. The nuclei may be somewhat more irregular in size, shape, and outline than normal. The chromatin ranges from fine to granular, and tends to be slightly hyperchromatic. Macronucleoli may be present in some cases providing another interpretive clue [Kudo 1987, Vogelsang 1995]. Mitotic figures are rare, but helpful when present [Szyfelbein 1984]. Abundant mucus in the background is another possible clue to this tumor [Granter 1996, K Ishii 1999].

Adenoma malignum has been reported to express gastric cell phenotypes, including gastric-type mucin secretion [Ishii 1998, 1999, S Sato 2000, Toki 1997]. Golden-yellow staining of cytoplasmic mucin (vs normal pale pink or pale blue mucin) is another potential clue to adenoma malignum. Although not present in normal endocervical cells, gastric-type mucin can occur in benign lesions, eg, pyloric metaplasia and "lobular endocervical glandular hyperplasia" [Hata 2002, K Ishii 1999, McCluggage 2002, Mikami 2000, 2001]. Ultimately, the diagnosis of malignancy should be based on histopathology, not mucin stains.

Adenoma malignum is treacherous because it is so difficult to recognize, even in histopathology [Gilks 1989]. The difficulties are related to several factors, including: rarity of the tumor, extremely well-differentiated

tumor cells, and absence of a specific tumor marker [Ishii 1999]. The malignant cells are often indistinguishable from benign reactive/reparative endocervical cells in the Pap test [Granter 1996]. Nevertheless, the Pap test can sometimes aid in its detection, eg, by finding atypical glandular cells [Granter 1996, Hart 2002, Hirai 1998, Silverberg 1975]. A less differentiated component may be present that indicates malignancy. Owing to its deceptively benign appearance, the disease is often left untreated until the clinical signs and symptoms of malignancy are so overwhelming that the diagnosis is finally made.

Carcinoembryonic antigen may be helpful in interpretation; it is usually expressed in the cytoplasm, in at least some of the malignant cells [Hart 2002, Steeper 1986]. Some, but not all, cases have been associated with HPV [A Ferguson 1998, Fukushima 1990, Hart 2002, Pirog 2000, Wilczynski 1988b].

Minimal deviation endometrioid carcinomas and clear cell carcinomas also occur. These, too, could be misinterpreted as benign lesions [R Young 1993].

Intestinal-type Adenocarcinoma

Intestinal-type adenocarcinoma is a rare variant of cervical adenocarcinoma that resembles colorectal adenocarcinoma [H Fox 1988, R Young 2002]. The cells are arranged in three-dimensional clusters and disorganized honeycomb sheets. Goblet-like cells, with irregular nuclei, coarse chromatin, large nucleoli, and generous cytoplasmic mucin vacuoles, are characteristic [I2.42]. "Terminal bar-like" apical cytoplasmic densities are typical of intestinal-type cells. Occasional Paneth cells and argentaffin cells may be demonstrable with special studies [Azzopardi 1965, K Lee 1990]. Extracellular mucin is usually conspicuous. The differential includes reactive endocervical cells and metastatic gastrointestinal carcinoma. Keratin immunostaining can be helpful in the latter differential. Metastatic intestinal carcinoma is usually CK 7 negative and CK 20 positive, while the reverse is usually true of cervical carcinoma, although these findings are not specific [Raspollini 2003].

Rare signet ring and still rarer, *colloid*, variants have also been recognized [Ebrahim 2001, Konishi 1990, R Young 2002]. These can occur either in pure form or as a component of typical cervical or intestinal-type adenocarcinoma [Haswani 1998].

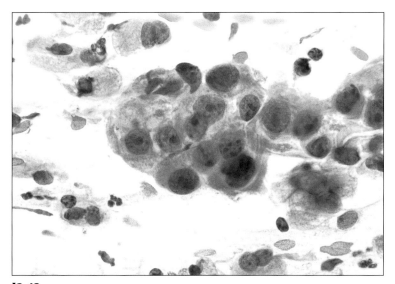

I2.43
Clear cell carcinoma [C]

Endometrioid Cervical Adenocarcinoma

Endometrioid adenocarcinoma is an uncommon variant of cervical adenocarcinoma that is morphologically indistinguishable from endometrial adenocarcinoma [Alfsen 2000]. Women with this cervical tumor are at increased risk of endometrioid ovarian carcinomas [Kaminski 1984]. The endometrioid variant usually arises at the squamocolumnar junction, but rarely arises in cervical endometriosis [S Chang 1971]. The tumor sheds loose clusters of relatively small cells (syncytial balls), with eccentric, round nuclei, fine-to-coarse chromatin, small nucleoli, and scant cytoplasm, without peripheral palisading or feathering of nuclei. Squamous differentiation can occur (see adenosquamous carcinoma, below). Distinguishing endometrial adenocarcinoma and endometrioid cervical adenocarcinoma on biopsy or cytology is a common problem that may require evaluation of a hysterectomy specimen to resolve. The endometrioid variant can also be mistaken for benign glandular cells on cytology, leading to false negative interpretations [Krane 2001]. There is also a deceptively benign appearing minimal deviation endometrioid adenocarcinoma [Rahilly 1992, R Young 1993]. Also, rarely, ciliated cells can occur in well-differentiated endometrioid carcinomas [R Young 2002]. Vimentin is expressed in the majority (80%) of endometrioid endometrial adenocarcinomas, but only a minority (<15%) of endometrioid cervical adenocarcinomas [Dabbs 1996].

Clear Cell Carcinoma

Clear cell carcinoma of the cervix or vagina is a rare tumor of Müllerian origin [Baird 1977, A Clark 1986b, Gompel 1976, Hasumi 1978, Herbst 1970a,b, Mawad 1974, Silverberg 1972]. Although it can occur sporadically, it occurred more commonly in daughters of women who took diethylstilbestrol (DES) during pregnancy [Hanselaar 1991, Herbst 1971, 1974, 1975, Wingfield 1991]. (DES has not been prescribed during pregnancy since the early 1970s, see pg 161.) The age peak for clear cell carcinoma in DES daughters was between 14 to 22 years [Herbst 1990b]. Non DES-associated clear cell carcinoma generally occurs in an older age group, although there is a wide age range (13-80+ years), and more often in nulliparous women [Kaminski 1983]. The prognosis may be slightly worse than for ordinary cervical adenocarcinoma [Herbst 1979b, Reich

2000]. The tumors are morphologically identical whether or not associated with DES. Because clear cell carcinomas can recur decades after first diagnosis, prolonged follow-up is required [Burks 1990, Herbst 1979a,b, 1990b].

In histology, the tumor has three basic growth patterns: tubulocystic, solid, and papillary [R Young 2002]. The cells have apical "hobnail" nuclei, prominent nucleoli, and clear cytoplasm [A Clark 1986b, Dickersin 1980].

In cytology, the cells are present singly or in sheets, clusters, or occasionally, papillae. Abundant, delicate, finely vacuolated to finely granular, glycogen-rich cytoplasm is characteristic [I2.43]. Rarely, the cells have abundant oxyphilic cytoplasm. Intracytoplasmic mucin can be present in occasional cells, sometimes resulting in a signet ring appearance. Nuclei are large, pale, round to irregular, with prominent nucleoli. Naked nuclei are common owing to the delicate nature of the cytoplasm [Hanselaar 1999, G-K Nguyen 1993, Suzuki 2002, Taft 1974, Y Watanabe 2002, Q Young 1978]. Tigroid (striped) background, similar to that described in dysgerminomas, and basement membrane-like material may be present [Hirokawa 2000]. The majority (>60%) of clear cell carcinomas are HPV-DNA negative; however HPV-DNA has been detected in both DES and non-DES associated tumors [Duggan 1995, Milde-Langosch 1993, Pirog 2000, Stoler 1994, Tenti 1996, Waggoner 1994]. The differential includes clear cell squamous carcinoma and clear cell adenosquamous carcinoma, tumors that are strongly associated with human papillomavirus [Fujiwara 1995].

Serous Adenocarcinoma

Serous adenocarcinoma of the cervix is rare [Gilks 1992]. It is morphologically similar to the more common ovarian or endometrial tumor of the same cell type (which must be excluded before accepting cervical origin of this tumor) [R Young 2002]. Cervical serous carcinoma has a bimodal age distribution, with one peak occurring before age 40 and another after age 65, coinciding with the peak incidences of uterine serous carcinoma [Zhou 1998a]. The tumor has high-grade malignant cells and grows in a complex papillary or budding pattern. The nuclei are large, pleomorphic to bizarre, and have macronucleoli. Endometrial gland-like cells and squamoid cells with abundant, dense cytoplasm, may be encountered. The background is bloody and necrotic, and neutrophils may be numerous. Psammoma bodies are uncommon in the cytologic specimens [G-K Nguyen 1997, Zhou 1997]. Tumors associated with germline BRCA-1 mutation are HPV negative; others may be HPV positive [Pirog 2000]. The tumor is aggressive and has a poor prognosis. Villoglandular adenocarcinoma also has papillae, but the cells are well-differentiated. Morphologically similar or identical tumors can arise in other sites in the female genital tract and metastasize to the cervix.

Mesonephric Adenocarcinoma

Mesonephric adenocarcinoma is an extremely rare tumor that arises from the mesonephric (Gartner or Wolffian) ducts located deep in the lateral cervical stroma [Buttenberg 1960, Clement 1995, Lang 1990]. The age ranges from about 35 to 75 years (average, 52 years) [Hart 2002]. It is glycogen-negative, mucin-negative, non-clear cell tumor, distinct from the relatively more common glycogen-positive clear cell carcinoma of Müllerian origin. Gland lumens typically contain PAS positive hyaline-like secretions [I2.44] [R Young 1990, 2002]. The tumor can grow in a ductal, tubular, retiform, solid, or sex cord-like pattern; some cases have a sarcomatoid (spindle cell) component [Hart 2002, R Young 2002]. Endocrine differentiation can occur [Stewart 1993b].

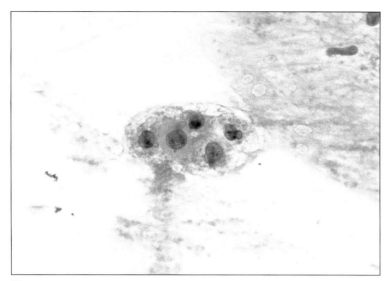

I2.44
Mesonephric carcinoma (putative)[C]

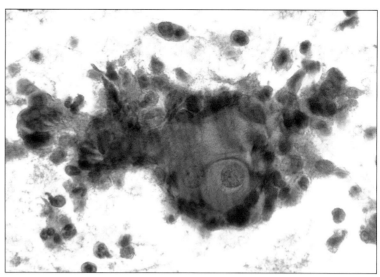

I2.45
Adenosquamous carcinoma [C]

Epithelial markers are universally positive; interestingly, most tumors also express calretinin, a mesothelial marker [Hart 2002]. One example tested negative for HPV-DNA [Pirog 2000]. Although the cytology of mesonephric carcinoma has been described [Hausdorfer 1985, Rosati 1973], many older cases would probably be reclassified as clear cell carcinoma of Müllerian type [Hart 2002, R Young 2002]. Benign mesonephric remnants can also occur and cause abnormal Pap tests [Ferry 1990a, MA Jones 1993, Lang 1990, J Seidman 1995, Welsh 2003].

Adenosquamous Carcinoma

On careful analysis, about one-third of cervical adenocarcinomas are mixed adenosquamous carcinomas [Benda 1985, G-K Nguyen 1993, R Young 1990]. This combined differentiation probably reflects the dual potential of the reserve cell. The adenocarcinomatous component is usually typical endocervical type, but can be mucinous, endometrioid, or clear cell type [R Young 2002]. Malignant appearing squamous elements can be keratinizing, nonkeratinizing, or poorly-differentiated squamous cell carcinoma [I2.45]. Cervical adenocarcinomas with cytologically bland squamous metaplasia are classified as adenocarcinomas with squamous differentiation. Eosinophils may be prominent. Some well-differentiated forms of adenosquamous carcinoma resemble mucoepidermoid carcinoma of salivary gland [R Young 2002]. A papillary variant has been described [W-K Ng 2003e]. Cervical adenosquamous carcinoma may have a worse prognosis than pure adenocarcinoma or squamous carcinoma [Benda 1994, Fu 1987]. Adenosquamous cervical carcinomas are usually HPV DNA positive [Anciaux 1997, Duggan 1995, Matthews-Greer 2004, Pirog 2000, Stoler 1994, van Muyden 1999, Yamakawa 1994]. The differential diagnosis includes "collision tumors" in which two separate primary neoplasms occur, one glandular, the other squamous.

Glassy Cell Carcinoma

Glassy cell carcinoma was first described by Glücksmann and Cherry in 1956 [Glücksmann 1956]. Glassy cell carcinoma is a rare form of malignancy of the female genital tract that usually involves the cervix. A poorly-differentiated variant of adenosquamous carcinoma, it ultrastructurally has evidence of both glandular and squamous differentiation [L Richard 1981, Ulbright

1983]. Distinct cell borders, ground glass cytoplasm, large nuclei, prominent nucleoli, and eosinophils characterize this tumor histologically [H Gray 2002, Mhawech 2001]. Those affected are often relatively young (most < 35 years of age). The tumor is aggressive, as would be expected for a poorly-differentiated malignancy [Talerman 1991]. Some authorities do not regard glassy cell carcinoma as a bona fide pathologic entity, preferring to designate it simply as poorly-differentiated adenosquamous carcinoma.

Glassy cell carcinoma features large tumor cells, with abundant, finely granular ("ground glass") cytoplasm, large, pleomorphic nuclei, coarse, irregular chromatin, and prominent nucleoli [I2.46] [Littman 1976, Mhawech 2001, W-K Ng 2004, G-K Nguyen 1993, Nunez 1985, Pak 1983, Reis-Filho 2001, JH Smith 2000, R Young 1990, Zaino 1982]. The cells occur mostly in sheets, clusters, or syncytia; single cells are less conspicuous [J-H Chung 2000]. Occasional bizarre and atypical multinucleated cells tumor may be present. Mitoses, including atypical forms, can be numerous. Cytoplasmic vacuoles may occur. The cytoplasm may contain glycogen, which can be demonstrated with the PAS stain. Eosinophils, lymphoplasmacytic infiltrate, and tumor diathesis are also typical findings. Occasionally, keratin pearls, abortive glands, signet ring cells, or mucin are present. HPV-DNA has been detected in this tumor [Kenny 1992, Matthews-Greer 2004, Pirog 2000, Stoler 1994]. The differential encompasses other large cell lesions, including: poorly-differentiated nonkeratinizing squamous cell carcinoma, lymphoepithelioma-like carcinoma, metastatic carcinoma, melanoma, and an atypical reparative process [J-A Gray 2002, W-K Ng 2002a, 2003c].

Adenoid Cystic Carcinoma

Adenoid cystic adenocarcinoma is a very rare lesion of the cervix, first described at this site by Paalman and Counsellor in 1949 [Paalman 1949]. This tumor resembles the salivary gland tumor of the same name, although in the cervix, it more commonly has high nuclear grade, increased mitotic activity, and necrosis [Grafton 1976, Yeh 1991]. There is a stromal reaction to the infiltrating tumor. The cancer tends to occur in elderly, postmenopausal women, although younger women can be affected. Although slow growing, it is aggressive [Ferry 1988, Ramzy 1975].

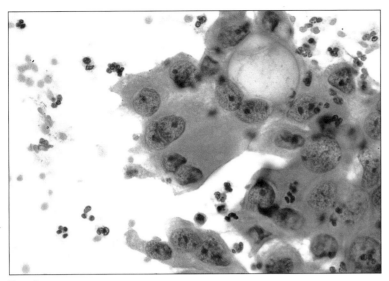

I2.46
Glassy cell carcinoma [C]

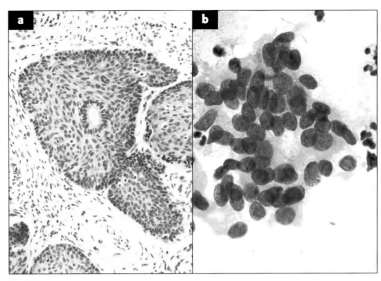

I2.47
a, Adenoid basal carcinoma; **b**, Adenoid basal carcinoma acinus [C]

The cells are typically small and round ("basaloid"), but have dark nuclei, occasional small nucleoli, and scant cytoplasm without mucin [Dayton 1990, Ravinsky 1996, Vuong 1996]. They often form cell balls, which may contain hyaline globules (basement membrane-like material) [Mazur 1982]. Necrosis, mitosis, and nuclear pleomorphism are more common than in the salivary gland tumor. This malignancy is frequently mixed with ordinary adenocarcinoma or squamous neoplasia; mucinous ovarian tumors may also occur [Ramzy 1975, Vuong 1996]. High-risk HPV types, particularly HPV 16, have been reported [Grayson 1996, 1999, Pirog 2000].

The tumor cells are easily confused with benign endocervical or, especially, endometrial cells. The differential includes ordinary cervical adenocarcinoma, endometrial adenocarcinoma, and small cell (neuroendocrine) carcinoma as well as poorly-differentiated squamous carcinoma, squamous carcinoma in situ, and basaloid carcinoma [Daroca 1980].

Adenoid Basal Cell Carcinoma

Adenoid basal cell carcinoma was first distinguished from adenoid cystic carcinoma by Baggish and Woodruff in 1966 [Baggish 1966]. However, the tumors probably share a common ancestor (the pluripotent reserve cell) and may actually form a biologic spectrum of basaloid cervical cancers [Grayson 1999].

Adenoid basal carcinoma is a rare invasive, but indolent, tumor that tends to occur in older postmenopausal women, but has a wide age range (~30 to 90 years). It seems to affect nonwhite women disproportionately [Brainard 1998, Hart 2002].

Histologically, adenoid basal carcinoma is composed of small, infiltrating nests of basaloid cells with peripheral palisading and no stromal reaction [I2.47a]. Lumens may form in the centers of the nests, which can become cystically dilated. These spaces can be lined with mucinous cells, clear cells, basaloid cells, or squamous or transitional-like cells. The cells have bland nuclei and mitotic figures are sparse. The tumor is usually associated with a high-grade squamous intraepithelial lesion that may lead to cytologic abnormalities [Langlois 1995, Peterson 1995, Powers 1996, R Young 1990, 2002].

Cytologically, the tumor forms hyperchromatic crowded groups (HCGs) that may have peripheral nuclear palisading and a tendency to acinar formation [I2.47b]. Nests and cords of small basaloid cells, foci of squamous differentiation or gland-like or cystic spaces filled with necrotic debris, can also be present. The tumor cells are small, bland, and uniform, with few mitotic figures [Langlois 1995, Peterson 1995, Powers 1996]. There is a strong association with HPV 16 [Crum 2000, Grayson 1999, MA Jones 1997, Matthews–Greer 2004, Pirog 2000].

Adenoid basal carcinoma differs from squamous carcinoma in situ chiefly by the presence of columnar cells and small gland openings. Adenoid basal carcinoma has smaller, more uniform cells, lacks microcystic spaces containing hyaline material, and has a better prognosis than adenoid cystic carcinoma. The differential also includes reactive endocervical cells and adenocarcinomas (cervical, endometrial). Owing to its rarity and resemblance to other more common lesions, it is unlikely that this tumor would be recognized specifically in Pap tests, except in retrospect. Moreover, because the lesion may be covered by an intact epithelium, no tumor cells may be sampled, although an associated H SIL may bring the lesion to attention.

Early Endocervical Glandular Neoplasia

Endocervical glandular dysplasia, adenocarcinoma in situ, and microinvasive adenocarcinoma are thought to be intermediate steps down the path to frankly invasive cervical adenocarcinoma [Alva 1975]. However, early glandular neoplasia, particularly dysplasia and microinvasive adenocarcinoma, are not as well defined as the squamous counterparts. Histologic confirmation of a Pap test interpretation of endocervical glandular neoplasia is required.

Cervical Adenocarcinoma In Situ

Noninvasive endocervical glandular malignancy was described as early as 1894 by G. Hauser [Hauser 1894]. By the mid 20th century, in 1952, TK Hepler and colleagues described highly atypical cells lining endocervical glands

adjacent to invasive cervical adenocarcinoma [Hepler 1952]. (Hepler's name is frequently misspelled "Helper" in the medical literature, suggesting that his work is cited more often than read.) The next year, Friedell and McKay introduced the term "adenocarcinoma in situ" (AIS) of the endocervix to describe histologic lesions believed to be precursors of invasive cervical adenocarcinoma [Friedell 1953]. In the early 1970s, the first cytologic illustrations of AIS were published [R Barter 1970, Weisbrot 1972]. Cytologic criteria for interpretation of adenocarcinoma in situ soon followed [R Barter 1970, Christopherson 1979, Krumins 1977, Qizilbash 1975].

Evidence supports the notion that adenocarcinoma in situ is a true precursor lesion. First of all, the cells of in situ and invasive adenocarcinoma are morphologically similar [Qizilbash 1975]. Adenocarcinoma in situ is frequently associated with invasive adenocarcinoma [Abell 1962, Hepler 1952, LiVolsi 1983, JC Parker 1977]. Cases of AIS progressing to adenocarcinoma have been reported [Hocking 1996, Hopkins 1988, Kashimura 1990, Krivak 2000]. As would be expected of a precursor lesion, women with AIS range from 5 to 20 years younger than those with invasive adenocarcinoma [Ayer 1987, Boon 1981a, L Brown 1986, Christopherson 1979, Colgan 1990, Denehy 1997, Gloor 1982, Hopkins 1988, Im 1995, Kaspar 1993, Kurian 1999, K Lee 1991, 2000a, Östör 1997, Plaxe 1999, Poynor 1995, Qizilbash 1975, Shingleton 1981, Teshima 1985, Van Aspert-van Erp 2004a, Wolf 1996]. Note that if the preinvasive phase is closer to the lower end of this range, as suggested by a meta-analysis that showed women with AIS were only ~5 years younger than those with early invasive adenocarcinoma (38 years vs 43 years) [K Lee 2000a], then there is only a small "window of opportunity" to detect preinvasive glandular lesions. Retrospective review of cervical cytologies or biopsies sometimes discloses atypical glandular cells preceding invasive cancer by several years [Boddington 1976, Boon 1981a, Bousfield 1980, Jaworski 1988, Kashimura 1990, Krumins 1977, Qizilbash 1975, Zaino 2002], supporting the existence of precursor lesions—and also underlining the difficulty of identifying these lesions prospectively [Cox 1997a, Richart 2000].

Although widely accepted as a precursor lesion, the natural history of adenocarcinoma in situ is not known [Syrjänen 2004]. In sharp contrast with high-grade squamous precursor lesions, which far outnumber invasive squamous carcinomas, adenocarcinoma in situ is less common (or at least, less commonly recognized) than invasive adenocarcinoma [Plaxe 1999, SS Wang 2004]. The ratio of AIS to invasive adenocarcinoma is as low as 1 to 10, whereas ratios as high as 10 to 1 occur with squamous CIS to invasive squamous cell carcinoma [E Andersen 1989, Azodi 1999, Betsill 1986, Kurian 1999, SS Wang 2004]. The risk of women with AIS developing cancer is unknown.

The typical woman with cervical adenocarcinoma in situ is young, white, and asymptomatic [Betsill 1986]. Those women with symptoms may complain of abnormal vaginal bleeding (postcoital, postmenopausal, or intermenstrual) or rarely, an abnormal vaginal discharge. The colposcopic, histologic, and cytologic recognition of AIS is difficult. AIS lacks specific colposcopic features and most cases (up to 95%) of AIS look benign in the colposcope, eg, normal ectopy, microglandular hyperplasia, or immature metaplasia [Ayer 1987, E Andersen 1989, Etherington 2001, Ferris 1996, Lickrish 1993, Zaino 2002]. Therefore, colposcopically directed biopsy is not reliable for establishing the diagnosis, extent of disease, or presence of invasion. A few cases are diagnosed fortuitously in endocervical curettage or biopsies performed for other reasons. The histologic diagnosis of AIS is also problematic. Many cases may be simply overlooked [Boon 1981a, Christopherson 1979, van Roon 1983]. Reactive/reparative changes, microglandular hyperplasia, tubal metaplasia, and endometriosis can all present problems in diagnosis of AIS.

Unfortunately, Pap testing is unreliable in detecting AIS [Renshaw 2004d]. The sensitivity of the Pap test may be no better than 50% owing to problems with sampling and interpretation [E Andersen 1989, Denehy 1997, J Roberts 1999, Ruba 2004, Schoolland 2002b, Shin 2002, Shipman 2001, H Smith 2002, Solomon 1998, van Aspert-van Erp 2004a]. First of all, glandular lesions are rare. High-grade squamous lesions (CIN 3) are 25 to 250 *times* more common than AIS [Boon 1981b, Christopherson 1979, H Mitchell 2004], although the incidence of AIS is apparently increasing (from 0.02/100,000 in 1973 to 0.61/100,000 in 1995, an annual increase of 12.25% [Plaxe 1999]). When the prevalence of disease is low, so is the predictive value of the test (independent of sensitivity and specificity of the test). Sampling glandular lesions can be problematic owing to their size and location. Lesions high in the endocervical canal or deep in the glands are difficult to sample [Boon 1987, Teshima 1985, Ursin 1994, Wells 1986]. Endocervical sampling devices, such as the endocervical brush, may facilitate obtaining a suitable cytologic specimen [Boon 1986, K Lee 1997b]. However, endocervical brushes have been in widespread use for many years, yet adenocarcinomas have increased in incidence. Interpretation of atypical glandular cells remains problematic. As in histology, many cases are simply overlooked, even when the cells are plentiful and well preserved [K Lee 1997b]. Interpretive criteria can be difficult to apply in practice [B Jones 1995], in part due to problems with the criteria themselves and the presence of many mimickers of AIS. Recognizing AIS and distinguishing it from non-neoplastic changes, such as reactive endocervical cells, endometrial cells, tubal metaplasia, etc, can be difficult [Gero 1996, K Lee 1997b, Shin 2002]. The recognition of AIS is particularly difficult in the presence of a coexisting squamous lesion [Gloor 1986, Kurian 1999, Lauchlan 1967, Luesley 1987, Raab 2000, van Aspert-van Erp 2004b]. Reproducibility of an interpretation of AIS is poor [Renshaw 2004c]. Specificity is also poor, as low as 17% [K Lee 1995, Novotny 1992, Waddell 1997]. An interpretation of "atypical glandular cells" is even less specific for AIS (see Atypical Glandular Cells, pg 144).

In theory, if AIS could be detected, adenocarcinoma could be prevented [Boddington 1976, Laverty 1988, K Lee 2000a, Syrjänen 2004, Valente 1996]. In practice, even though cytologic criteria for recognition of preinvasive glandular lesions have been available since the 1970s [R Barter 1970, Krumins 1977, Qizilbash 1975]; "atypical glandular cells" has been in the Bethesda System lexicon since the 1980s; and "adenocarcinoma in situ" was added to the Bethesda System in the 1990s; to date, Pap testing has had little or no effect on reducing the incidence of adenocarcinoma [Andersson 2003, Austin 2003b,c, A Benoit 1984, Bergström 1999, Bjersing 1991, Boddington 1976, Boon 1987, Brinton 1987b, J Burk 1974, Canavan 2000, Christopherson 1979, Colgan 2001a, Crum 2002, Erzen 2002, Etherington 2001, Franco 2003, Fry 1969, Fu 1987, Hayes 1997, Herbert 2001, Herrero 1992, Janerich 1995, Jaworski 1990, Keyhani-Rofagha 1995, H-S Kim 1991, Kinney 2003, Krane 2002, K Lee 1997b, 1998, 1999, 2002, S Liu 2001, Makino 1995, A Miller 1995, H Mitchell 1988, 1990c, 1993a, 1995a, Mody 1999, Moriarty 2003a, G-K Nguyen 1993, Nieminen 1995, Ollayos 1997, Parkin 1985, R Peters 1986a, Renshaw 2004c, Ruba 2004, Sasieni 2001, Schoolland 2002a,b, H Smith 2000, Stockton 1997, Vizcaino 1998, SS Wang 2004, Zappa 2004, T Zheng 1996]. In addition to these problems, it is possible that the biologic behavior of glandular lesions is different from their squamous counterparts, making detection and prevention more difficult. The very fact that cervical adenocarcinomas have been increasing in frequency despite widespread screening would seem to be prima facie proof that the Pap test cannot prevent adenocarcinoma. Still, there is hope that with improved sampling of the transformation zone and further dissemination of criteria for pre-invasive glandular lesions, the Pap test may begin to have some effect on preventing cervical adenocarcinomas [Herbert 2001, Kinney 2003, H Mitchell 2003, Ruba 2004, Sasieni 2001, H Smith 2000, 2002]. Nevertheless, the bottom line is that *the Pap test has never been proven effective in preventing adenocarcinoma.*

Topographically, AIS seems to begin in the transformation zone/squamocolumnar junction in most or all cases [Zaino 2002]. The disease usually involves the superficial canal epithelium with extension into deep crypts; the deep glands tend to be more involved than the surface [E Andersen 1989]. Rarely,

deep disease occurs without superficial disease. The actual surface, however, may be covered by squamous epithelium, which may be normal, metaplastic, or dysplastic, precluding sampling of the glandular lesion by the Pap test. AIS can be focal or extensive, and frequently involves multiple quadrants, but true "skip" lesions are unusual [Bertrand 1987, Colgan 1990, Friedell 1953, Gloor 1982, Jaworski 1988, 1990, Östör 1984, Shipman 2001, Qizilbash 1975, Zaino 2002].

Biologically, AIS is strongly associated with human papilloma virus, predominantly HPV 18, less commonly HPV 16 (or other high-risk types) [Duggan 1994, Leary 1991, Okagaki 1989]. AIS is associated with squamous intraepithelial lesions or invasive squamous cell carcinoma in at least 50% of cases [Bertrand 1984, G Casper 1997, Colgan 1990, Jaworski 1988, Luesley 1987, Laverty 1988, Mulvany 1997, Östör 1984, Qizilbash 1975, Zaino 2002]. This suggests common origin from the reserve cell with its capacity for divergent differentiation [Alva 1975, Boon 1981a,b, Brinton 1993, L Brown 1986, Burghardt 1970, Christopherson 1979, Colgan 1990, Cullimore 1989a, Duggan 1995, Glücksmann 1956, Hitchcock 1993, L Johnson 1964, Kashimura 1990, Kjær 1993a, Kudo 1991, Kurian 1999, Lauchlan 1967, Laverty 1988, G-K Nguyen 1984b, Noda 1983, Parazzini 1990a, Rollason 1989, Smedts 1992, Teshima 1985, van Aspert-van Erp 2004b, Yamakawa 1994].

Cone biopsy is usually the next procedure following a histologic diagnosis of AIS, to determine extent of disease and exclude invasion. The prognosis is generally excellent for AIS lesions that are completely excised, although there is a slight risk of recurrence even with negative conization margins [E Andersen 1989, Azodi 1999, Bertrand 1987, Denehy 1997, Etherington 2001, Goldstein 1998b, Hopkins 1988, Houghton 1997, Im 1995, Jaworski 1988, DM Luesley 1987, Muntz 1992, Narayansingh 2001, Nicklin 1991, Östör 1984, 2000b, Poynor 1995, Shin 2000, Shipman 2001, Qizilbash 1975, Widrich 1996, Wolf 1996]. Another consideration in management of AIS is that many women in the reproductive age group may desire to maintain fertility [Azodi 1999].

Histology of Adenocarcinoma In Situ

Adenocarcinoma in situ is characterized by endocervical glands lined by atypical columnar cells that cytologically resemble those of invasive adenocarcinoma, but lack invasion [12.48a]. There is often an abrupt transition between normal and abnormal glandular cells. The glands have numerous outpouchings and complex papillary infoldings, and may grow in a cribriform pattern, focally. The cells are crowded and pseudostratified. They have elongated cigar-shaped nuclei, high N/C ratios, coarse, dark chromatin, and diminished mucin secretion. Mitotic figures, including atypical forms, and apoptotic bodies are frequent [Biscotti 1998, Moritani 2002]. Subtypes, such as endocervical (most common), endometrioid, and intestinal, are recognized (see below).

Cytology of Adenocarcinoma In Situ

Adenocarcinoma in situ is a rare cytologic finding, reported in well less than 1% of all Pap tests (range 0.0002% to 0.025%) [Bousfield 1980, Goff 1992, Laverty 1988, Nasu 1993, Östör 1984]. Cytologic mimickers of AIS, including reactive endocervical cells, tubal metaplasia, etc, as well as squamous neoplasia, are far more common. Adenocarcinoma in situ is not reliably detected by cytology, even though interpretive criteria have been available since the 1970s [R Barter 1970, Krumins 1977, Qizilbash 1975] and widely disseminated since the 1980s [Boon 1981a,b, Keyhani-Rofagha 1995, Laverty 1988, DM Luesley 1987, G-K Nguyen 1993, Poynor 1995, Qizilbash 1975, Valente 1996, Weisbrot 1972]. Unfortunately, application of these criteria is difficult, even with experience, and there are numerous pitfalls that lead to both false positive and false negative results [Renshaw 2004c, Ruba 2004, Sidawy 1992, Valente 1996, van Aspert-van Erp 2004a,b].

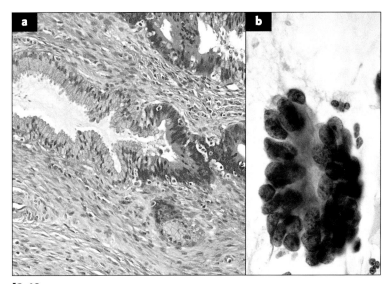

12.48
a, Adenocarcinoma in situ; **b**, Adenocarcinoma in situ [C]

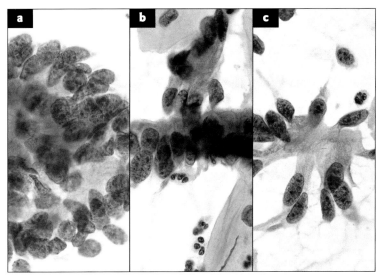

12.49
a, AIS, hyperchromatic crowded group [C]; **b**, AIS, crowded strip [C];
c, AIS, rosette [C]

A simple definition of AIS is noninvasive malignant glands. The cytology recapitulates the histology [12.48a,b]. In theory, cytologic interpretation is relatively straightforward. It consists of both architectural and nuclear abnormalities. Architectural abnormalities include: hyperchromatic crowded groups, crowded strips, and rosettes [12.49a,b,c]. The aggregates characteristically have nuclei protruding from the margins, giving the clusters a frayed look, referred to as "feathery edges," a concept introduced by Bousfield [12.50a,b] [Bousfield 1980]. Nuclear abnormalities

Adenocarcinoma In Situ
Features similar to adenocarcinoma
Abnormalities of:
  •Architecture
  •Nuclei
Cannot exclude invasion!

include: nuclear enlargement, elongation, inconspicuous or micronucleoli, distinctively coarse, dark chromatin, and mitotic figures/apoptotic bodies [I2.51a,b]. There is no tumor diathesis [Ayer 1987, 1988, Betsill 1986, Biscotti 1997, Boon 1981b, Bousfield 1980, A Clark 1986a, DiTomasso 1996, Ehrmann 1996, Jaworski 1988, 1990, Keyhani-Rofagha 1995, Krumins 1977, Lickrish 1993, Nasu 1993, G-K Nguyen 1993, Östör 1984, Solomon 1998, Tobón 1988, Wilbur 1995].

There usually are moderate numbers of neoplastic endocervical cells associated with normal or reactive endocervical cells. The cells are usually relatively normal size in size, but the nuclei are large and have high N/C ratios. Small cell variants (see endometrioid type, below) can be sources of false negative results [Krane 2001]. Architectural abnormalities and nuclear hyperchromasia can usually be appreciated at low, scanning power in the microscope [Biscotti 1997, Bousfield 1980, Solomon 1998]. Then, nuclear detail can be evaluated at high power.

Architectural abnormalities are characterized by disorderly arrangements ("chaotic architecture," "loss of nuclear polarity") and marked crowding ("supercrowding") of the cells [I2.52a,b] [Biscotti 1997, DeMay 2000, K Lee 1991]. The normal honeycomb pattern (including prominent cell borders) is usually lost. Abnormal groups take three forms: rosettes [I2.48b, 2.49c], pseudostratified strips [I2.49b], and three-dimensional, syncytial-like aggregates (hyperchromatic crowded groups) with feathery edges [I2.50a,b, 2.51a]. Single abnormal cells may be present, but are usually inconspicuous in noninvasive lesions. A rosette refers to a group of cells, arranged in a circle, with centrally oriented cytoplasm and peripheral nuclei. Pseudostratification refers to nuclei at different levels compared with their neighbors, but the cells are not truly stratified, with more than one cell layer (as in a stratified squamous epithelium). Feathering is a characteristic feature of AIS (and well-differentiated cervical adenocarcinoma) [Biscotti 1997, Bousfield 1980, DiTomasso 1996, K Lee 1991]. Secondary gland (or crypt) openings can also be present in sheets of neoplastic endocervical cells [I2.53a].

Nuclear abnormalities are characterized by elongation ("cigar shape") or irregularity; less commonly, the nuclei are round, which makes interpretation more difficult. The nuclear area averages about 75 μm² (vs 55 μm² for normal endocervical nuclei). Cells with high N/C ratios are usually present [Biscotti 1997, K Lee 1991, Nasu 1993]. In rare cases, nuclei are of normal or small size; this also makes interpretation more difficult (see endometrioid subtype, below) [K Lee 1998, 1999, Ruba 2004]. The chromatin pattern of AIS is distinctive: although generally similar to that of squamous carcinoma in situ, it is characteristically coarser and darker, particularly in conventional Pap smears [I2.49c, 2.50a] [Biscotti 1997, Bousfield 1980, A Clark 1986a, K Lee 1991, Nasu 1993]. However, some cases have unexpectedly bland chromatin, which can lead to false-negative interpretations. Nucleoli are present in about half of cases [Renshaw 2004c], but they are usually inconspicuous, and seen in only a minority of cells [Ayer 1987]. Macronucleoli are usually rare or absent in noninvasive glandular lesions; prominent nucleoli suggest invasion. (Nucleoli are more conspicuous in LBC, see below.) Mitotic figures vary in number, and may be rare or absent in cytologic specimens, but their presence is an important clue to a neoplastic glandular lesion [I2.50b, 2.51a] [Ayer 1987, Biscotti 1997, DiTomasso 1996, Jaworski 1988, K Lee 1991]. Mitotic figures are rare in normal endocervical cells, although reactive/reparative endocervical cells may be mitotically active.

The cytoplasm is typically delicate to finely granular, and amphophilic to basophilic, with poorly defined cell borders. Mucin production is usually markedly diminished. These findings contrast with the mucinous cytoplasm and prominent cell borders (honeycomb) of normal or reactive endocervical cells. Apoptotic bodies are usually present in AIS [I2.51b] and are at least as important as mitotic figures, if not more so, in identifying malignant endocervical cells [Biscotti 1997, 1998, Jaworski 1988, Moritani 2002].

A tumor diathesis is characteristically lacking in AIS [Tobón 1988]. However, an inflammatory background is common. Adenocarcinoma in situ is frequently associated with squamous dysplasia or carcinoma in situ.

To summarize: look for HCGs with big, dark nuclei, which suggest a high-grade lesion; stratified strips, rosettes, and feathery edges suggest glandular differentiation. These features are usually present in AIS, and relatively easy to see when they occur [Ruba 2004].

In liquid-based cytology, the architectural and nuclear abnormalities of AIS are similar to those in conventional Pap smears. Typical features, such as numerous, variably-sized disorderly hyperchromatic crowded groups, crowded sheets, stratification, rosette formation, high N/C ratios, nuclear elongation, nuclear membrane irregularities, and mitotic figures can all be seen in LBC [I2.50b, 2.52a,b, 2.53b]. However, there can be some important variations resulting from differences in cytopreparation. Architectural abnormalities, such as crowding, rosettes, and feathery edges may be less apparent in liquid-based Pap tests [2.54a]. The cell clusters tend to be more rounded and very three-dimensional, although large sheets of crowded cells can still be appreciated. Feathering is less conspicuous or may even be absent in LBC. The cytoplasm is finely vacuolated and cell border are usually indistinct; however, remnants of honeycomb structures may sometimes be present [I2.53b]. Nuclear abnormalities are generally similar to those in conventional Pap smears, including hyperchromasia, crowding, and mitotic figures, but dissimilarities may occur in LBC, including: the nuclei appear more rounded (although membrane irregularities may be more obvious), the chromatin more open, and nucleoli more prominent [I2.50b, 2.54a,b]. Note in particular that the distinctively coarse, dark chromatin of AIS may be lost altogether in LBC, replaced in some cases with pale, vesicular nuclei (and conspicuous nucleoli). On the other hand, nuclear detail, mitotic figures, and apoptotic bodies may be easier to appreciate in LBC [JE Johnson 1999, Ozkan 2004, Selvaggi 2002a]. Single cells are more conspicuous in liquid-based cytology because the specimens are agitated during processing. The background remains clean or inflammatory without a tumor diathesis [Burja 1999, JE Johnson 1999, Siziopikou 1997].

Carcinoembryonic antigen (CEA) is frequently (67%) expressed in the cytoplasm, whereas CEA is absent or has only luminal expression in normal endocervical glands [Hurlimann 1984]. Most cases of AIS also express cytoplasmic CA-125. HPV DNA is usually present, as previously discussed.

Variants of Adenocarcinoma In Situ

Subtypes of AIS have been recognized histologically [Gloor 1982, Hasumi 1978, Jaworski 1988, 1990, Kudo 1992, K Lee 1998, Nasu 1993, Noda 1983, Tobón 1988, Zaino 2002]. In addition to the classic or endocervical type, there are also endometrioid, intestinal, adenosquamous, clear cell, and others, including poorly-differentiated, variants. Although the cytology of subtypes has been described, subclassification is difficult in practice, and mixtures of cell types can coexist. Fortunately, subclassification has little clinical significance other than the possibility of mistaking these variants of AIS for benign conditions.

Endometrioid Variant of AIS

The endometrioid variant of AIS is characterized by markedly crowded aggregates of small cuboidal cells with little cytoplasm that resemble well-differentiated endometrial adenocarcinoma [2.55a,b]. Thick chunky strips, rosettes, pseudostratified strips, feathering, coarse, dark chromatin, and mitoses are typically present [Ayer 1987, K Lee 1998, G-K Nguyen 1993]. The nuclei are small and dense, and the scant cytoplasm lacks mucin. This variant can be difficult to

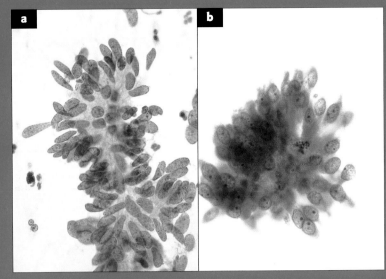

I2.50
a, AIS, feathering [C]; **b**, Feathering, nucleoli [L]

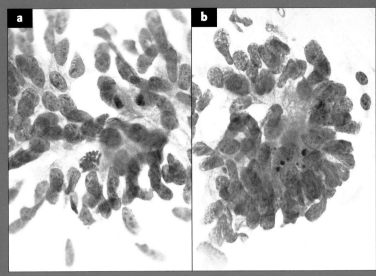

I2.51
a, AIS, mitosis [C]; **b**, AIS, apoptosis [C]

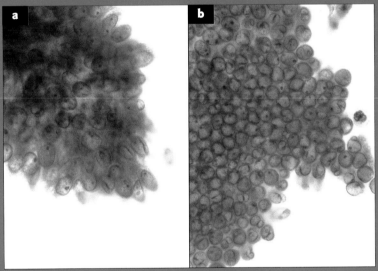

I2.52
a, AIS, chaotic architecture [L]; **b**, AIS, supercrowding [L]

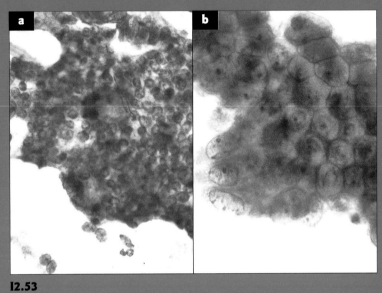

I2.53
a, AIS, secondary gland [C]; **b**, Remnants of honeycomb [L]

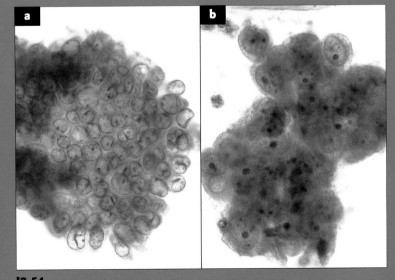

I2.54
a, AIS, well differentiated [L]; **b**, AIS, poorly differentiated [L]

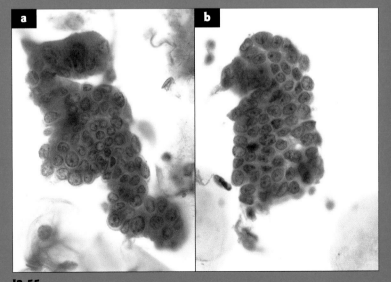

I2.55
a, AIS, endometrioid [L]; **b**, AIS, endometrioid [L]

distinguish from directly sampled benign endometrium, lower uterine segment, or tubal metaplasia, leading to false-negative interpretations [K Lee 1997b, 1999]. In contrast with endometrium, AIS lacks endometrial stroma, tubular glands, and uniform flat sheets of cells; however, high N/C ratios, hyperchromasia, and mitotic figures can be present in either AIS or benign endometrium [K Lee 1998].

Intestinal Variant of AIS

The intestinal variant of AIS is characterized by papillae and sheets of cells, including goblet cells. Goblet cells have more abundant cytoplasm, with large secretory vacuoles containing mucin (sialomucin). The nuclei are larger, rounder, and more pleomorphic, with more prominent nucleoli, than the usual type of AIS [Ayer 1987, G-K Nguyen 1993].

Adenosquamous Variant of AIS

The adenosquamous variant of AIS is composed of either a mixture of squamous and glandular type cells or formed of a uniform population of cells with characteristics intermediate between squamous and glandular cells. The cells are polyhedral to columnar and have moderate to abundant cytoplasm [Christopherson 1979].

Poorly-Differentiated Variant of AIS

The poorly-differentiated variant of AIS has more cytoplasm and larger, rounder nuclei, vesicular chromatin, and prominent nucleoli or macronucleoli [12.54b] [Ayer 1987, 1988, Kudo 1991, Sidawy 1992]. These cytologic features can also be present in invasive adenocarcinoma [Kudo 1991, K Lee 1991]. Some consider this the serous variant of AIS. The differential includes benign repair.

Ciliated Variant of AIS

The ciliated variant of AIS is composed of atypical fallopian tube-type cells, including cells with cilia [Schlesinger 1999]. Although this rare lesion flouts the rule that ciliated cells are always benign, it is still true that ciliated cells, even when cytologically atypical, are *almost* always benign and HPV-DNA negative [K Lee 2000a].

Differential of Adenocarcinoma In Situ

The differential of adenocarcinoma in situ includes reactive endocervical cells, squamous carcinoma in situ (H SIL), tubal metaplasia, and endometrial cells, particularly when directly sampled or in cases of cervical endometriosis. Distinguishing between AIS and reactive endocervical cells is probably the most common problem. Reactive change in endocervical cells is common; AIS is rare.

Endocervical "No No's"

Crowding, piling up, feathering

Elongated or irregular nuclei

Coarse, dark chromatin

Mitosis, apoptosis

Reactive endocervical cells usually exfoliate in sheets, with minimal nuclear crowding or overlap, and no feathering, but maintain the honeycomb pattern. Reactive endocervical nuclei can be "big and dark," and vary in size, but usually are round, with smooth membranes, fine chromatin, and, frequently, prominent nucleoli. Although mitotic figures can be present in benign reactive/reparative endocervical cells, they are worrisome findings in endocervical cells. Apoptotic bodies are even more worrisome in endocervical cells.

The differential also includes other conditions that exfoliate hyperchromatic crowded groups, including squamous carcinoma in situ (CIS) and tubal metaplasia [DeMay 2000]. Squamous CIS tends to have rounder nuclei and

finer chromatin than AIS; AIS usually has feathering and pseudostratification. Rosette-like structures can be present in either squamous or glandular carcinoma in situ, but are usually better developed in AIS. Tubal metaplasia can mimic AIS almost to perfection in some cases, even including feathering and mitotic figures. Cilia and terminal bars, when present, are "benign signs" that argue strongly against malignancy (look for cilia, it won't kill ya). Although a ciliated-variant of AIS has been described [Schlesinger 1999], atypical ciliated cells are usually benign and negative for HPV [K Lee 2000a]. Directly sampled endometrium, cone biopsy artifact, and cervical endometriosis, can also be difficult to distinguish from AIS and vice versa. Spontaneously exfoliated endometrial cells are usually smaller, rounder, and may be associated with endometrial stromal cells, but lack feathering.

The cytologic features suggestive of invasive adenocarcinoma include: marked cellularity and more single cells; increased nuclear size and pleomorphism; irregular chromatin distribution; numerous macronucleoli (a key feature); more generous cytoplasm; and a tumor diathesis (another key feature) or heavy bloodstaining in the background [DiTomasso 1996, Keyhani-Rofagha 1995, Schoolland 2002a,b, Sidawy 1997]. A substantial minority of cases thought to be adenocarcinoma in situ by cytology, turn out to be invasive adenocarcinoma by histology [Laverty 1988, K Lee 1991, 1995, Nasu 1993, G-K Nguyen 1993]. Therefore, adenocarcinoma in situ is ultimately a histologic, not a cytologic, diagnosis—despite the inclusion of AIS in the Bethesda System lexicon. *Invasion cannot be excluded by cytology!*

Endocervical Glandular Dysplasia

Squamous carcinoma is preceded by a spectrum of premalignant change (dysplasia/CIS; CIN; SIL). Therefore, it is reasonable to suggest that invasive adenocarcinoma, like its squamous counterpart, also has a pre-invasive phase. And, in fact, cervical adenocarcinoma in situ (AIS) is widely accepted as a precursor of invasive adenocarcinoma [Ayer 1987, Boon 1981a, Bousfield 1980, G Casper 1997, Cullimore 1992, Jaworski 1990, Laverty 1988, K Lee 2000a,b, DM Luesley 1987, Mohammed 2000, G-K Nguyen 1993, Östör 1984, Qizilbash 1975, Teshima 1985, Valente 1996]. But, whether there is a *spectrum* of premalignant change preceding adenocarcinoma, ie, "endocervical glandular dysplasia," analogous to grades of squamous dysplasia, is the subject of vigorous debate [Ioffe 2003, K Lee 2003]!

There are basically two schools of thought regarding endocervical glandular dysplasia (aka cervical glandular intraepithelial neoplasia [CGIN] or atypical glandular hyperplasia). Some believe that there is no precursor lesion less severe than AIS: the cell goes directly from normal to full-blown AIS without an intervening dysplastic stage [Goldstein 1998a]. Others believe in the existence of endocervical glandular dysplasia, ie, that there is a spectrum of glandular atypia preceding adenocarcinoma in situ. In support, glandular dysplasia is recognized in other body sites, such as Barrett esophagus [Geisinger 1992, Hamilton 1987, Hughes 1998]. There is also a middle ground in which endocervical glandular dysplasia is believed to exist, but all grades have similar significance, a concept comparable to that of cervical intraepithelial neoplasia (CIN). This would diminish the importance of grading of endocervical glandular dysplasia [Wells 1986]. The following discussion presents evidence for the existence of endocervical glandular dysplasia and possible criteria for its recognition.

A possible definition of endocervical glandular dysplasia (EGD) is that it has features similar to, but less advanced than, AIS or, alternatively, EGD has some, but not all, features of AIS (and it is not associated with inflammation, ie, it is a non-inflammatory lesion) [Ioffe 2003, Yeh 1991, Zaino 2000, 2002]. The first reference to "glandular dysplasia" was made in 1970, by Barter, who also used the term "columnar cell dysplasia" [R Barter 1970]. A decade later, in 1980, Bousfield provided the first direct study of EGD [Bousfield 1980]. The first attempt to grade EGD was reported by van Roon in 1983 [van Roon 1983].

There are several lines of evidence that endocervical glandular dysplasia exists [Zaino 2002]. For example, there is a spectrum of atypical glandular morphology leading up to full-blown adenocarcinoma in situ (seeing is believing). EGD is frequently associated with adenocarcinoma and AIS (guilt by association) [L Brown 1986, Deligdisch 1984, Gloor 1986, Higgins 1992, Jaworski 1988, Kurian 1999, Leary 1991, Tase 1989b]. These observations imply that EGD is a precursor to AIS.

EGD occurs at a slightly younger average age than AIS, as would be expected for a lesion preceding AIS. The mean ages are summarized: EGD–31.5 to 40 years; AIS–35.2 to 46 years; microinvasive adenocarcinoma–43-44 years; adenocarcinoma–43.1 to 57 years [Bousfield 1980, L Brown 1986, G Casper 1997, Kurian 1999, DM Luesley 1987, Wells 1986]. One study showed a mean age progression from low-grade EGD to high-grade EGD/AIS to invasive adenocarcinoma of 39, 43, and 48 years, respectively [Kurian 1999]. So, there also seems to be a mean age progression, as would be expected for a precursor lesion [Boon 1981a, Higgins 1992, Qizilbash 1975]. EGD is more common than AIS, suggesting that like other precursor lesions, only a proportion progress to more advanced disease [L Brown 1986, Wells 1986].

Like AIS, EGD is frequently associated with squamous dysplasia suggesting a common etiology [Anciaux 1997, L Brown 1986, Lawrence 1991, DM Luesley 1987]. HPV can be detected in many EGD cases and is frequently associated with high-risk viral types [Higgins 1992, K Lee 2000b, A Nielsen 1990]. In various studies, HPV was detected in 0 to 46% of cases of EGD, 15% to 83% of invasive adenocarcinomas, and 42% to 89% of cases of AIS. Normal epithelium is negative for HPV [Anciaux 1997, Farnsworth 1989, Jaworski 1990, Leary 1991, K Lee 1993b, Okagaki 1989, Samaratunga 1993, Tase 1989b, Wilbur 1995]. The range of HPV positivity in EGD is intermediate between normal and AIS. The relatively wide ranges are partly explained because different methods of HPV detection, with varying sensitivities, were used in these studies. Also, in actual practice, the category of "EGD" probably includes benign (nonneoplastic) conditions. Using highly sensitive techniques, HPV is found in up to 95% of cases of endocervical glandular dysplasia [Zaino 2002].

Nuclear areas increase along a line from normal (37.8 μm^2) to EGD (45.0μm^2) to AIS (57.4μm^2) and adenocarcinoma (55.6 μm^2) [Goldstein 1998a, Rosenthal 1982, van Roon 1983]. Nuclear size in EGD, intermediate between normal and AIS, also suggests a spectrum. Endocervical glandular dysplasia can have aneuploid DNA patterns similar to squamous dysplasia [Alva 1975].

Epithelial glycoprotein secretion has been measured in normal cells, adenocarcinoma, and EGD. In normal cells, sulfomucin predominates. In adenocarcinoma, sialomucin predominates. EGD expresses both sialomucin & sulfomucin, ie, an intermediate reaction [Gloor 1986, Kase 1999]. Lectin binding has also been studied. Lectins are proteins that bind cell surface glycoproteins, similar to antigen-antibody reactions. Differences in lectin binding have been shown among normal, dysplastic, and malignant cells [Gloor 1986]. Human milk fat globule-1 antibody reactivity is a marker of altered growth or neoplastic change. Normal cells have predominantly cuticular luminal reactivity (26 of 28 cases), while cervical adenocarcinoma has mixed cytoplasmic reactivity and cuticular reactivity (13 of 14 cases). EGD reactivity is similar to AIS and adenocarcinoma in being predominantly mixed (13 of 15 cases), indicating a relationship of EGD to glandular carcinoma [L Brown 1987]. Epithelial-Specific Antigen expression has also been studied. Normal cells

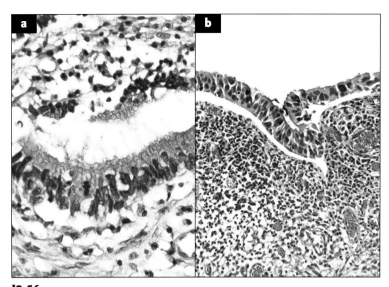

I2.56
a, EGD, low grade; **b**, EGD, high grade

have basolateral staining only (10/10); AIS and adenocarcinoma have diffuse cytoplasmic membrane staining only (20/20). EGD shows an intermediate pattern of diffuse staining (6/11) [Umezaki 1997]. Amylase was expressed in 39/40 cases of invasive adenocarcinoma, 6/7 cases of AIS, 6/6 cases of high-grade EGD, and 12/14 cases of low-grade EGD, but only 2/18 normal endocervices [Griffin 1989]. Novel expression of complex carbohydrates is found in 90% of adenocarcinomas, 92% of high-grade glandular intraepithelial neoplasia, and 63% of low-grade intraepithelial neoplasia, in contrast with normal glands [Griffin 1994].

Silver binding nucleolar organizing regions, AgNORs, have been evaluated in glandular neoplasia and normal cells. The number of AgNORs increases from normal to AIS to invasive carcinoma [Darne 1990]. In one study, the number of AgNORs in "transitional" areas was the same as normal, which might be viewed as evidence against EGD. However, "transitional" was defined in that study as "*apparently normal* bordering areas" [emphasis added] and so does not detract from an argument for the existence of EGD [Cullimore1989b].

Finally, some studies have shown various interpretive criteria for EGD reach statistical significance. These include criteria to recognize EGD, to separate it from reactive changes on the one hand and adenocarcinoma on the other, and to divide EGD into low and high-grades [DiTomasso 1996, Ioffe 2003, van Aspert-van Erp 1995a,b, 1996a, 1996b, 1997]. These findings imply that EGD not only exists, but can also be graded.

Morphologic Criteria for Endocervical Glandular Dysplasia

The morphologic features of EGD that have been described include: crowding and stratification present, but less marked than AIS; nuclei larger and more oval/elongated than normal, but less than AIS; nuclear pleomorphism and irregularity may be *more* marked than in AIS; increased N/C ratio, but less than AIS; chromatin abnormal, but less dense, more uniform, and finer than AIS; nucleoli less conspicuous; mitoses/apoptosis less than AIS; cytoplasm slightly more abundant; paradoxically, EGD may have *more* cellular variation within clusters than AIS (broader spectrum of differentiation?); mucin depletion increases with increasing grade **[I2.56a,b]**

T2.5 Endocervical Glandular Dysplasia (EGD) vs Adenocarcinoma In Situ (AIS)

Nuclear feature	EGD	AIS
Enlargement	Less	More
Pleomorphism	More	Less
Chromatin	Fine-moderate coarse	Coarse
Nucleoli	Inconspicuous	Indistinct or small
Shape	Oval	Elongate to irregular
Stratification	Mild	Marked
Mitosis	Occasional	Frequent
Apoptosis	Less	More

[Modified from Jaworski 1990]

[T2.5] [Bose 1994, Bousfield 1980, G Casper 1997, Gloor 1986, Jaworski 1990, Kudo 1992, Samaratunga 1993, Valente 1996, Wells 1986, Wilbur 1995, Yeh 1991]. The lower the grade of EGD, the more difficult it is both to sample (less extensive) and to interpret (mimics reactive changes) [Hayes 1997].

Some authors have attempted to grade endocervical glandular dysplasia. A three or four grade system, such as has been applied to squamous abnormalities, is probably unrealistic for glandular abnormalities. Differences would be very subtle and irreproducible. A two grade system, low-grade and high-grade glandular intraepithelial lesions ("dysplasia"), analogous to the Bethesda System's squamous intraepithelial lesions, has been proposed [I2.57a,b], although even a two-grade system has significant problems in practical application [T2.6].

Normally, endocervical cells have small, round nuclei and abundant, mucinous cytoplasm. As the cells become abnormal ("dysplastic"), the most obvious changes begin in the nuclei, which become more oval than round, distinctly hyperchromatic, and somewhat crowded and piled up, with loss of polarity. The cytoplasm becomes less abundant and mucin content diminishes. Cell borders may not be as conspicuous as normal (losing honeycomb). Rare mitotic figures may occur, but few are abnormal. Mitotic figures are abnormal in

T2.6 Reactive Changes, Low-Grade & High-Grade Endocervical Dysplasia

Feature	Reactive	LG EGD	HG EGD/AIS
Cell			
Size	WNL/slt ↑	WNL/slt ↑	Slt/mod ↑
Borders	Well-defined	Well-defined	Ill-defined
Nuclei			
Shape	Round/oval	Oval, irregular	Elongate, irregular
Size	Increased	Increased	Increased
Pleomorphism	Can be marked	Little	More
Crowding	Minimal	Mild	Marked
Chromatin	Fine	Moderate	Coarse
Hyperchromasia	Variable	Mild/moderate	Marked
Nucleoli	Prominent	Rare, small	Indistinct, small
N/C ratio	WNL to increased	Slight increase	Marked increase
Mitosis/apoptosis	None	Rare	Few
Cytoplasm	Abundant	Decreased	Scant
Background	Clean/Inflammatory	Clean/Inflammatory	No diathesis

[Modified from Jaworski 1990, Nasu 1993]

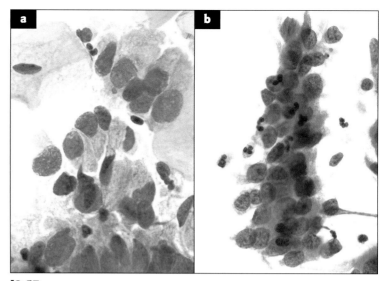

I2.57
a, EGD, low grade [C]; **b**, EGD, high grade [C]

endocervical epithelium; their presence suggests a neoplastic lesion (or repair/regeneration).

With increasing abnormality (advancing dysplasia), the nuclei become more elongated (cigar shaped) or irregular; more crowded; and more disorganized (may form hyperchromatic crowded groups) with feathering. Mitotic figures become more frequent and some are abnormal. Apoptosis mirrors mitosis. The amount of cytoplasm and mucin diminishes further. Cell borders become inconspicuous (honeycomb lost).

Low-Grade Endocervical Glandular Dysplasia

Low-grade endocervical glandular dysplasia (LG EGD) is morphologically similar to reactive changes, preserving honeycombs and distinct cell borders, but has greater nuclear crowding and irregularity [I2.56a, 2.57a]. LG EGD also has features similar to AIS, including: nuclear enlargement, hyperchromasia, and elongation (compared with normal endocervical nuclei), but compared with AIS, LG EGD has less stratification, rare/no mitoses, fewer vesicular nuclei; the chromatin is finer, but mildly to moderately hyperchromatic. The mildest form of EGD has: minimal crowding, stratification; minor variations in nuclear size, shape, staining; minimal hyperchromasia; minimal nuclear irregularities; and rare or absent mitosis/apoptosis. The differential encompasses: reactive changes, including repair, and hormonal effects [L Brown 1986, DiTomasso 1996, Drijkonigen 1996, Gloor 1986, Nasu 1993, van Aspert-van Erp 1995a].

High-Grade Endocervical Glandular Dysplasia

High-grade endocervical glandular dysplasia (HG EGD) has abnormalities only slightly less marked than those of AIS [I2.56b, 2.57b]. The nuclei are crowded, stratified, enlarged, pleomorphic, and elongated (cigar-shaped), with increased N/C ratios. The chromatin is coarse and dark. Nucleoli range from absent to inconspicuous to prominent. Mitoses are present, but rare [L Brown 1986]. There may be a vague honeycomb pattern, but cell borders are poorly defined. The differential includes: AIS and invasive adenocarcinoma [L Brown 1986, DiTomasso 1996, Gloor 1986, Nasu 1993, van Aspert-van Erp 1995a].

There are very real problems not only in recognizing EGD, but particularly, with grading it [K Lee 2003]. The interpretation is highly subjective, being

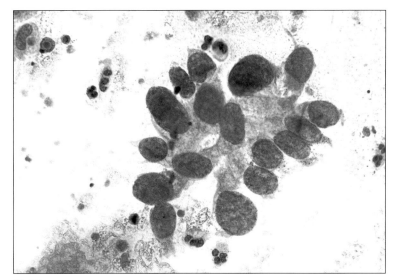

I2.58
Microinvasive adenocarcinoma [C]

based on AIS, which itself is not well-defined and reproducible. Because of interpretive problems, some cases thought to be EGD are really AIS, or reactive changes [*Valente 1996*]. Presently, EGD is of unknown biologic significance: if it is accepted that AIS and EGD form a spectrum, then no sharp division is possible. EGD does not lend itself to grading the way squamous dysplasia does. Squamous dysplasia is graded by degree of replacement of the epithelium with undifferentiated cells. Glands are normally only one cell thick. Therefore, progressive architectural alteration is not present; the degree of replacement is not applicable to diagnosis and interpretation rests more on individual cell morphology, even in histology.

Because there are no uniform diagnostic criteria for AIS, EGD also lacks uniform diagnostic criteria. Observers are more likely to agree at the far end of the spectrum of glandular precursor lesions, ie, indisputably malignant, but noninvasive, cells. The other end of the spectrum is more problematic, ie, what is minimum degree of atypia required for EGD: Where does reactive change end and EGD begin? Similarly, where does EGD end and AIS begin? Moreover, pathologists are reluctant to diagnose EGD in the first place. At the University of Chicago, only one histopathologist, and no cytopathologists, currently uses EGD as a diagnosis. The IAC Task Force discourages use of low-grade or mild glandular dysplasia [*Solomon 1998*]. Obviously, these factors make the histologic/cytologic correlation difficult or impossible [*Jaworski 1990, Solomon 1998, Wilbur 1995*].

In summary, there is evidence for the existence of a precursor of adenocarcinoma, less advanced than AIS, known as endocervical glandular dysplasia, and for a spectrum of abnormality (low to high-grade) analogous to squamous precursor lesions. However, although EGD may well exist, and can possibly even be graded in theory—practice is another matter. Adenocarcinoma in situ (or even invasive adenocarcinoma!) probably cannot be recognized reliably and reproducibly in Pap tests. The ability to interpret EGD accurately is almost certainly lower than the ability to interpret AIS accurately. The practical importance of EGD is that, first, it probably does exist, and second, it may be the explanation for finding atypical glandular cells in a Pap test. The bottom line is that *a reliable/reproducible cytologic interpretation of endocervical glandular dysplasia is currently not possible* (and forgeddabout grading EGD!).

Microinvasive Cervical Adenocarcinoma

Microinvasive cervical adenocarcinoma is very rare (and non-existent for those who believe *any* invasion indicates frank adenocarcinoma) [*Ayer 1988, Betsill 1986, Jaworski 1990, Kurian 1999, Mulvany 1997, G-K Nguyen 1984a, Nicklin 1999, Östör 1997, 2000a, Qizilbash 1975, Schorge 1999, Webb 2001a, Zaino 2002*]. Even in the most experienced hands, cytology is unreliable in the differential of microinvasive adenocarcinoma vs both adenocarcinoma in situ and frankly invasive adenocarcinoma [*Ayer 1988, Laverty 1988, Mulvany 1997*]. Microinvasive adenocarcinoma is not well defined either microscopically or by its clinical behavior. Like its squamous counterpart, microinvasive adenocarcinoma requires thorough histologic evaluation before the diagnosis is accepted. This is particularly important because microinvasive adenocarcinoma is more often multifocal than microinvasive squamous cell carcinoma [*Buscema 1984, Nicklin 1999, Östör 1997*]. Although the prognosis is generally favorable when adequately treated, microinvasive adenocarcinoma has a risk of lymph node metastasis and recurrence [*Balega 2004, Berek 1985, Buscema 1984, Fu 1987, Kaku 1997, Östör 2000a, Schorge 1999, Webb 2001a*].

The histologic definition of microinvasive adenocarcinoma is generally similar to that used for microinvasive squamous cell carcinoma, and includes controversies regarding acceptable depth of invasion (range 1 mm-5 mm) [*Shipman 2001*]. Some question the very existence of microinvasive adenocarcinomas. The earliest histologic sign of stromal invasion is when AIS shows an abrupt glandular change, the cell becoming enlarged, with abundant eosinophilic squamoid cytoplasm [*Kurian 1999, Mulvany 1997, Östör 1997, Rollason 1989*]. The histologic criteria for microinvasive carcinoma generally include: invasion to 5 mm or less; complete obliteration of normal endocervical crypts; extension beyond normal glandular field; and a stromal response characteristic of invasive carcinoma [*Östör 2000a*]. Not all criteria are always present, however.

In theory, the cytologic features of microinvasive adenocarcinoma are intermediate between in situ and fully invasive adenocarcinoma [I2.58]. In practice, it is probably not possible to recognize microinvasive adenocarcinoma specifically in Pap tests, although criteria have been suggested [*Ayer 1988, Mulvany 1997, G-K Nguyen 1984b*].

Possible interpretive criteria include the usual findings in adenocarcinoma in situ (eg, cellular samples, crowded clusters, rosettes, pseudostratified strips, feathering, high N/C ratios, enlarged nuclei, and coarse, dark chromatin) plus significant numbers of single atypical cells [*Ayer 1988*]. The tumor cells in microinvasive adenocarcinoma and adenocarcinoma in situ are cytologically similar [*Betsill 1986, G-K Nguyen 1984b*]. However, the nuclei of microinvasive adenocarcinoma are said to be more round (than oval), with irregular chromatin clumping, contain prominent nucleoli, including macronucleoli, and have more abundant cytoplasm [*Kudo 1991, K Lee 2000a, Mulvany 1997*]. Dense squamoid cytoplasm is a common finding and there is frequently an associated squamous lesion, probably reflecting the common origin from reserve cells [*Colgan 1990, Kudo 1991, K Lee 2000a, Mulvany 1997*]. This can make differential with squamous lesions difficult. A tumor diathesis usually indicates invasion, but is present in only a minority of cases of microinvasive disease [*Ayer 1988, Mulvany 1997*]. Variants, such as endometrioid or intestinal subtypes, can also occur [*K Lee 2000a*].

Bottom line: microinvasive cervical adenocarcinoma is a histologic, not a cytologic, diagnosis. Even in histology, the diagnosis is difficult and controversial.

Differential of Early Endocervical Glandular Neoplasia

Reactive endocervical cells, repair, tubal metaplasia, squamous carcinoma in situ, brush artifact, and invasive cervical adenocarcinoma all factor into

T2.7 Reactive Endocervical Cells, Adenocarcinoma In Situ, & Adenocarcinoma

	Reactive	AIS	Adenocarcinoma
Crowding	±	+++	++
Feathering	0	+++	++
Rosettes	±	+++	++
Cilia	±	0	0
Mitoses	±	++	++
Nuclear irregularity	±	+	+++
Chromatin irregularity	0	±	+++
High N/C ratio	±	+++	++
Nucleoli	Variable	Small, indistinct	Prominent
Normal endocx cells	+++	++	+
Diathesis	0	0	++

the differential of early glandular neoplasia [T2.7]. Benign/reactive conditions can be mistaken for neoplastic/malignant ones, or more ominously, neoplastic/malignant conditions can be mistaken for benign/reactive ones.

The major cytologic features of cervical adenocarcinoma in situ are similar to those of well-differentiated invasive cervical adenocarcinoma, consisting of tightly crowded aggregates of columnar cells with hyperchromatic, oval-to-elongated nuclei, and high N/C ratios (ie, hyperchromatic crowded groups) [Boon 1991, K Lee 1991]. Rosettes, secondary gland (crypt) openings, and feathery edges are also features shared with invasive cervical adenocarcinoma [Ayer 1987]. However, invasive adenocarcinoma characteristically has more atypical cells, more single cells, more pleomorphism, more abnormal chromatin patterns, more frequent and larger nucleoli, and a tumor diathesis. Compared with adenocarcinoma in situ, the cell groups tend to be looser, syncytial-like clusters less common, and the N/C ratios lower in invasive adenocarcinoma. Two of the most important cytologic features of invasive adenocarcinoma are prominent nucleoli and a tumor diathesis. However, the presence of nucleoli does not necessarily indicate invasion, nor does the absence of a diathesis exclude invasion [K Lee 1991]. A key point to remember is that invasion can be suspected, but not excluded, by the Pap test.

A common, everyday problem in Pap test interpretation is to differentiate the wide range of reactive cellular changes that can be present in benign endocervical glandular cells from cellular changes present in malignancy [Nasu 1993]. Reactive endocervical cells can be *more* pleomorphic than malignant endocervical cells. Reactive nuclei can be markedly enlarged (up to 5 times normal area) and hyperchromatic (ie, "big and dark"), but tend to remain round, have smooth nuclear membranes, and prominent nucleoli. In contrast, the nuclei of in situ, or low-grade invasive, adenocarcinoma tend to be elongated (cigar shaped), with distinctively coarse dark chromatin and inconspicuous nucleoli (particularly in conventional Pap smears). Marked crowding is present in malignancy, while benign cells tend to "lay flat" and maintain their prominent cell borders ("honeycombs"). Ciliated cells are (almost) always benign. Most reported cases of ciliated cell adenocarcinoma in situ [Betsill 1986, K Lee 1991] probably represent misinterpretation of tubal metaplasia [Jaworski 1988, Pacey 1988], although ciliated adenocarcinomas have been described [Schlesinger 1999, R Young 2002]. Note that ciliated benign cells do not exclude the possibility of co-existing neoplasia.

In brief, when endocervical cells crowd, stratify, "feather," form rosettes or gland openings, and have cigar shaped nuclei with high N/C ratios, consider

an interpretation of endocervical glandular neoplasia [Bose 1994, K Lee 1991, Siziopikou 1997]. Multinucleation, pleomorphism, nuclear enlargement, prominent nucleoli, can be present in reactive conditions, but benign cells tend to lay flat and maintain their honeycomb arrangements. Macronucleoli in every cell suggest endocervical repair or high-grade adenocarcinoma. Reactive changes in endocervical cells are common, while cervical adenocarcinoma in situ is rare.

It also can be difficult to distinguish endocervical *glandular* neoplasia from *squamous* neoplasia (in situ or invasive carcinoma). Both can shed hyperchromatic crowded groups (HCGs) and both can have features suggesting glandular differentiation, including palisading, columnar cells, microacinar or rosette-like structures, and even some feathering [W Andersen 1988, DeMay 2000, Drijkoningen 1996, K Lee 1995, P Levine 2002, Mattosinho 2003, Nasu 1993, Raab 2000, Selvaggi 1994, Siziopikou 1997, Solomon 1998, Valente 2001, van Hoeven 1996b, Wilbur 1995]. Features favoring a glandular lesion include: well-defined feathery edges, columnar cell shape, nuclear-cytoplasmic polarity, elongated nuclei, distinctively coarse chromatin, and granular amphophilic cytoplasm. Favoring a squamous lesion: more single cells, scanty, undifferentiated cytoplasm, rounder nuclei, finer chromatin, occasional dyskeratotic cells, and an associated squamous dysplasia. Flattening at the edge of groups and whorling in the center favor squamous origin of hyperchromatic crowded groups [Sidawy 1997].

Endocervical glandular neoplasia coexists with squamous dysplasia or carcinoma in situ in 25% to 75% of cases [E Andersen 1989, Bose 1994, L Brown 1986, Colgan 1990, Denehy 1997, Fu 1987, Gloor 1982, Goff 1992, Kohan 1985, Nasu 1993, Qizilbash 1975]. However, there is more to the story. Given a glandular lesion, a squamous lesion is commonly also present, but given a squamous lesion, a glandular lesion only rarely co-exists (< 5% of cases). Therefore, as a practical matter, finding good evidence of a squamous lesion makes a glandular lesion unlikely.

Atypical Glandular Cells

Atypical cells, apparently glandular in origin, that are not readily classifiable as either reactive or neoplastic in nature, are commonly encountered in Pap tests. These cells are known as "atypical glandular cells" (AGCs) in the Bethesda System 2001 (formerly, atypical glandular cells of uncertain significance, AGUS). AGCs can be further subcategorized as "favor endocervical" or "favor endometrial," as well as "favor neoplastic," "adenocarcinoma in situ," and "not otherwise specified." However, a "favor reactive" subcategory was eliminated in the Bethesda System 2001. The recommended follow-up for all AGC categories is similar (ie, colposcopy), except for atypical endometrial cells (recommend endometrial sampling, see pg 201).

In many cases, it is not even possible to distinguish glandular from squamous lesions by cytology. This distinction can sometimes be difficult in histology as well. Many studies report that when atypical glandular cells (AGC) are identified on Pap tests, the majority of lesions found on biopsy are squamous. What's more, many studies of "atypical glandular cells" find that in a substantial number of cases, significant lesions are not present at all [Bose 1994, Currie 1994, Goff 1992, T Kim 1999, K Lee 1995, Pisharodi 1995, Ronnett 1999, Wilbur 1994, 1995]. When encountering atypical hyperchromatic crowded groups, and it is not certain whether the cells are squamous or glandular, a convenient Pap test interpretation is: "Atypical glandular cells, high-grade squamous intraepithelial lesion not excluded"; follow with colposcopy.

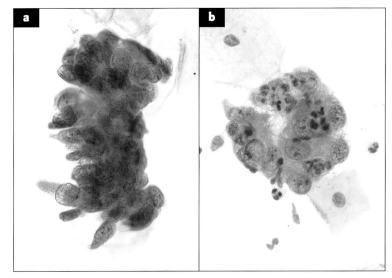

I2.59
a, AGC (benign, mimics AIS) [C]; **b**, AGC (malignant, mimics reactive) [C]

T2.8 Benign/Reactive vs Atypical Endocervical Cells

	Reactive Endocervical Cells	Atypical Endocervical Cells
Architecture	Cells lie flat, minimal crowding/overlap	HCGs, rosettes; Feathering
Cell borders	Well defined	Indistinct
Cytoplasm	Adequate, mucinous	Scant, mucin depleted
N/C ratio	WNL or slightly increased	High
Nuclei	Round, can be large	Oval/elongated to irregular
Chromatin	Usually fine, can be dark	Usually coarse & dark
Nucleoli	Often prominent	Absent or small (in situ)
Background	Clean/inflammatory	Diathesis ⇒ invasion
Other	Cilia	Mitoses/apoptosis

Note: Both reactive and atypical endocervical cells can have big, dark nuclei

Criteria for atypical endometrial cells in TBS are: small groups, slight nuclear enlargement, slight hyperchromasia, no or small nucleoli, ill-defined cell borders, and scant cytoplasm [NCI 1993a,b]. Nuclear enlargement and prominent nucleoli are two key features of atypical endometrial cells (see pg 117 for more discussion).

Criteria for atypical endocervical cells are: disorderly sheets or crowded groups, diminished cytoplasm, increased N/C ratios, round to oval nuclei, smooth to slightly irregular nuclear membranes, granular chromatin, conspicuous nucleoli [I2.59a,b] [T2.8]. Three dimensional crowding, rosette or microacinar formation, and mitoses/apoptosis are three key features of atypical endocervical cells. Not all features need be present for an interpretation of atypical glandular cells. The findings are similar in both conventional Pap smears and liquid-based cytology, although nuclear detail and nucleoli tend to be more prominent in LBC. Although TBS recommends specifying the cell of origin (endocervical vs endometrial), even this basic distinction can sometimes be impossible in practice (poor interobserver reproducibility) [Simsir 2003].

The goal of the Pap test is to identify women with significant cervical lesions (sensitivity), without including those who do not have lesions (specificity). By this definition, the Pap test performs poorly for glandular lesions. Therefore, the category of Atypical Glandular Cells was added to increase sensitivity of the Pap test to glandular neoplasia [Moriarty 2003a]. Unfortunately, the category pretty much stinks—it does a poor job of identifying women with significant glandular lesions (low sensitivity) and it also includes many women who do not have any significant lesions at all (low specificity) [Gornall 2000]. It has turned out that "atypical glandular cells" are not always glandular, nor even abnormal [Bose 1994]. On the other hand, enough women have serious underlying abnormalities that the "AGC" interpretation requires careful clinical follow-up.

The incidence of AGC interpretations on Pap tests ranges from about ~0.1% to 2.5% [Bose 1994, R Cheng 1999, Chhieng 2000a, 2001c, 2003, A Chin 2000, Cox 1998b, Davey 2000, DiTomasso 1996, Duska 1998, G Eddy 1997b, Eltabbakh 2000b, Goff 1992, Hammoud 2002, Kennedy 1996, Koonings 2001, Korn 1998, K Lee 1995, Manetta 1999, Mulligan 1998, Nasu 1993, Nasuti 2002, Parellada 2002, Raab 1995, 1997, 1999b, 2000, J Roberts 2000, Soofer 2000, RR Taylor 1993, Veljovich 1998, Zweizig 1997]. This translates into roughly *one million* AGC results in the United

States every year [Raab 1995, 1998a]. And, the annual number of AGC interpretations may be increasing [Cangiarella 2003, Chhieng 2001c, G Eddy 1997b].

AGC raises the old philosophical question, "is the glass is half full or half empty?" From the "half empty" perspective, the sensitivity of an interpretation of AGC for adenocarcinoma (in situ or invasive) is only about 50%, the specificity is < 20%, and the predictive value is a miserable 5% to 10% (range, 0 to 34%). Most of the significant lesions detected (average ~75%, range ~25% to 100%) are squamous, not glandular, and what's more, most women (average, ~60%; range ~15% to 80%) do not have significant lesions at all. From the "half full" perspective, however, AGC is a high-risk result that predicts adenocarcinoma in 5% to 10% of cases and clinically significant abnormalities in up to 80% of cases. However, most of the invasive cancers detected are endometrial, not endocervical, adenocarcinomas. As usual, there is a trade-off between sensitivity and specificity: those studies reporting higher sensitivity generally have lower specificity and vice versa [G Acs 2000, E Andersen 1989, Bose 1994, Burja 1999, Burnett 2000, Cangiarella 2003, R Cheng 1999, Chhieng 2000a, 2001a, 2001c, 2003, A Chin 2000, Cox 1998b, 2001, Cullimore 1992, Currie 1994, Davey 2000, DiTomasso 1996, Duska 1998, G Eddy 1997a, Eltabbakh 2000b, Geier 2001, Goff 1992, Gornall 2000, Hammoud 2002, Hecht 2002, SR Jackson 1996, Kennedy 1996, T Kim 1999, Korn 1998, K Lee 1995, 1997b, Leeson 1997, L Levine 2003, Manetta 1999, Mathers 2002, Meath 2002, H Mitchell 1994b, Mount 1999, Mulligan 1998, Nasu 1993, H Nguyen 1999, Nyirjesy 1998, Ollayos 1997, Parellada 2002, Raab 1995, 1997, 1998a, 1999b, 2000, Reuss 2001, J Roberts 1999, 2000, Ronnett 1999, Schindler 1998, Selvaggi 1999a, Simsir 2003, Solomon 1998, Soofer 2000, RR Taylor 1993, Valente 2001, van Aspert–van Erp 1995a, Veljovich 1998, Wilbur 1994, 1995, Zweizig 1997].

In sum, although AGC is an interpretive quagmire, it is generally a riskier category than ASC-US. Unfortunately, surveys suggest that AGC is not managed as comprehensively as has been recommended by professional organizations, such as the American College for Obstetricians and Gynecologists (ACOG) or the American Society for Colposcopy and Cervical Pathology (ASCCP) [ACOG 1993, Cox 1997a, 2001, 2003a, Partridge 1999, Smith-McCune 2001] (see pg 244ff for management guidelines). Long-term follow-up is indicated for women with atypical glandular cells despite initial negative findings [Chhieng 2004]. HPV-DNA, MiB-1, and p16[INKa] may provide additional information relevant to management of women with AGC [Boon 2004, Krane 2004, Nieh 2004, Oliveira 2004].

For women with Pap test interpretations of AGC, squamous intraepithelial lesions are more common in younger women and in those with a prior history of cervical abnormality; glandular lesions and invasive cancers are more common in older women and those with a history of abnormal bleeding [Chhieng

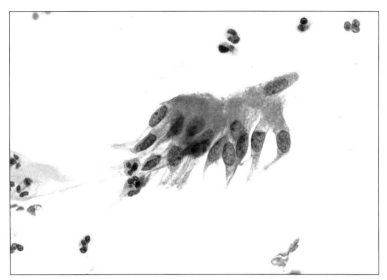

I2.60
Benign feathering [C]

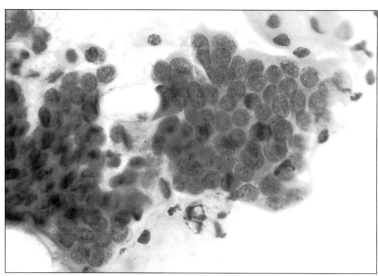

I2.61
High endocervical cells [C]

2000a, 2001a, A Chin 2000, Duska 1998, G Eddy 1997a, Geier 2001, A Hare 2003, Koonings 2001, Leeson 1997, Nasuti 2002, Obenson 2000, Raab 1999b, Veljovich 1998, Zweizig 1997]. In some cases, atypical glandular cells may indicate an occult or metastatic malignancy [Manetta 1999, Patsner 2002, Zweizig 1997]. Also, remember that squamous and glandular lesions commonly coexist.

It is thought that better endocervical sampling could increase yield. Unfortunately, "improved" endocervical sampling devices, such as the endocervical brush, are two-edged swords: they probably have increased the number of precursor lesions detected (true-positives), but at the expense of a large number of "atypical," but nonneoplastic, cases (false-positives) owing to high cellularity, cell clumping, cell distortion, toothpick or brush artifacts, and interpretive problems related to sampling of high endocervix/lower uterine segment, tubal metaplasia, microglandular hyperplasia, etc [Babkowski 1996, Boon 1991, Chakrabarti 1994, Cox 1998b, de Peralta–Venturino 1995, Heaton 1996, SR Jackson 1996, Krane 2001, Raab 2000]. Other sources of interpretive problems related to "atypical" glandular cells include: reactive endocervical cells, endometriosis, radiation effect, cone biopsy artifact, pregnancy associated changes, and endosalpingiosis [Soofer 2000].

A finding of "atypical glandular cells" is an irreproducible result, even among experts [Simsir 2003]. In one study, 133 conventional Pap smears and 131 liquid-based Pap tests originally diagnosed as atypical glandular cells were reviewed by 5 pathologists. The original atypical glandular cells interpretation was not retained by *any* reviewer in ~20% of conventional smears and nearly half (48.1%) of liquid-based cytologies, and was almost never (<5% of cases) retained by *all five* reviewers [K Lee 2002]! The overall interobserver agreement, including all subcategories, was poor [K Lee 2002]. In another study, 100 Pap smears, originally classified as atypical glandular cells, were reviewed by four expert cytopathologists. In *no* case did all four agree with the original atypical glandular cells interpretation. The kappa (κ) statistic for pairwise comparison ranged from 0.16 to 0.27, which, according to the author, indicated "terrible agreement" (good agreement is κ > 0.6) [Raab 1998a, 2000]. About one-in-seven cases of "atypical" glandular cells was downgraded to benign on review; however, adenocarcinomas and high-grade dysplasias were eventually found in some of these downgraded cases!

It is no great wonder that glandular lesions are difficult to interpret. First, the abnormal cells often exfoliate as "hyperchromatic crowded groups,"

which can present difficult differential interpretations. Further, the cytologic criteria for glandular lesions are not well defined and consistent. For example, "feathering" is often considered a classical feature of AIS, but has been reported in a range from nearly 90% of cases [Biscotti 1997] to less than 5% of cases [Siziopikou 1997], and occasionally is observed in benign Pap tests [I2.60]. The cells of AIS are usually larger than normal endocervical cells, but in some cases, they are small [K Lee 1997b]. Nucleoli are not considered a usual feature of AIS in conventional Pap smears, and yet can be seen ~25% to 75% of cases [Chhieng 2003]. Typical cytologic features, when present, may be diffuse, or focal. Finally, interpretive criteria for glandular lesions, such as they are, can be difficult to apply in actual practice [Raab 1999b, 2000]. Although education improves performance, not all cases can be interpreted accurately even after instruction: some benign cases are still misclassified as neoplastic and more ominously, some neoplastic cases are still misclassified as benign [K Lee 1999, Raab 1997]. When expert academic (ivory tower) cytologists cannot achieve perfection, even after review of specific criteria, perfection certainly cannot be expected from those practicing in the real world [Mody 1999]!

In summary, a possible definition of Atypical Glandular Cells is that they have some, but not all, features of adenocarcinoma. (Note the similarity of this definition to that of endocervical glandular dysplasia—the very existence of which is debated—a fact that may help explain why these lesions are so difficult to interpret.) Atypical findings in endocervical cells include: exfoliation of hyperchromatic crowded groups, rosette formation, loss of honeycomb pattern, nuclear elongation (cigar shape) or irregularity, coarse dark chromatin, high N/C ratios, mitotic figures or apoptotic bodies, and focal feathering. The "atypical" nuclei tend to be intermediate in size between normal and definitively neoplastic ones (average ~136.6 μm^2) and exhibit variability in size and shape [Cenci 2000a,b]. The differential includes both glandular and squamous lesions [Betsill 1986, Chhieng 2003, Fiorella 1994, Gloor 1982, Jaworski 1988, K Lee 1988, Pacey 1988].

Differential of Atypical Glandular Cells

"Atypical" glandular cells are more common in cytologic samples obtained with specialized endocervical sampling devices (brush, broom, etc) compared with glandular cells obtained with a spatula [L Levine 2003]. Highly

Richard M DeMay

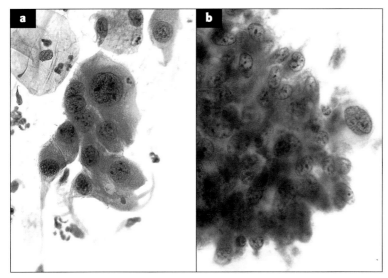

12.62
a, Reactive endocervical cells [C]; **b**, Reactive endocervical cells [L]

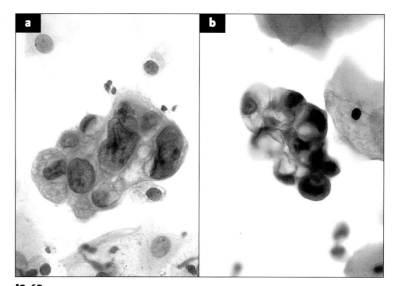

12.63
a, Chemotherapy effect [C]; **b**, Vacuolated metaplastic cells [C]

cellular specimens, containing abundant, dense clusters of endocervical cells, are commonly encountered when using these sampling devices. In some cases, the nuclei are enlarged, pleomorphic, and hyperchromatic, possibly reflecting polyploidy ("brush atypia"). Also, endocervical cells derived from high in the endocervical canal, or even endometrial cells, may be sampled using an endocervical brush. These glandular cells are normally more crowded and have higher N/C ratios, than those obtained with an ordinary spatula [Babkowski 1996, K Lee 1993a]. They may form hyperchromatic crowded groups (HCGs) mimicking neoplasia, which can lead to false-positive (or "false atypical") interpretations [Babkowski 1996, DeMay 2000, Hoffman 1993]. Reactive changes can be superimposed on these cells making them seem even more atypical. There are many other explanations for "atypical" glandular cells, ranging from tubal metaplasia to Arias-Stella reaction to endocervical glandular neoplasia. Squamous lesions (especially carcinoma in situ) can also exfoliate HCGs mimicking glandular lesions.

The following discusses the differential of atypical glandular cells. Remember, the AGC category is a gray-zone. When the cells are thought to be benign or reactive, such as reactive endocervical cells or tubal metaplasia, or indicative of a specific neoplastic lesion, such as adenocarcinoma, do not use the interpretation "atypical glandular cells." AGC is for those times when you can't tell for sure what's going on, but you're worried about what you see. Recall the dilemma with ASC (the devil vs the deep blue sea, pg 64)? On the

Atypical Endocervical Cells
- *High endocervical cells*
- *Reactive endocervical cells*
- *Endocervical brush artifact*
- *Endocervical repair*
- *Endocervical polyps*
- *Directly sampled endometrium*
- *Lower uterine segment*
- *Cone biopsy artifact*
- *Endometriosis*
- *Tubal metaplasia*
- *Microglandular hyperplasia*
- *IUD effect*
- *Postpartum atypia*
- *Arias-Stella reaction*
- *Squamous carcinoma: in situ, invasive*
- *Endocervical glandular neoplasia*
- *Metastatic adenocarcinoma*

one hand, interpretations of AGC will unnecessarily subject some women to time-consuming, expensive, and unpleasant follow-up procedures such as colposcopy and biopsy. On the other hand, an AGC result sometimes correlates with very serious abnormalities, including cancer. Keep in mind that most of the entities described below can exfoliate hyperchromatic crowded groups or HCGs (see pg 182).

High Endocervical Cells

High endocervical cells, obtained with an endocervical brush from high in the endocervix, can exfoliate hyperchromatic crowded groups (HCGs) of cells, with high N/C ratios, and scant cytoplasm [12.61]. Although these cells are normal for their location, they may suggest a neoplastic process [Raab 2000]. They do not look like the usual mucinous, columnar endocervical cells that are typically obtained with the Ayre spatula. In some cases, nuclear pleomorphism, abnormal chromatin patterns, and abnormal architectural arrangements, such as nuclear crowding, palisading, feathering, and rosettes may be present (see also, brush artifact, below) [Babkowski 1996, Soofer 2000]. In general, high endocervical cells are uniform, with round, bland nuclei that look like normal endocervical nuclei, and lack mitotic figures. In liquid-based cytology, these cells can resemble immature squamous metaplasia.

Reactive Endocervical Cells

Reactive endocervical cells may be somewhat crowded, with nuclear enlargement, hyperchromasia, and prominent nucleoli (see pg 112) [12.62a,b]. Mitotic figures may be present, but should be regarded suspicious findings [K Lee 1995]. Reactive endocervical cells may be seen in numerous circumstances, including endocervicitis, polyps, oral contraceptives, intrauterine contraceptive devices, postpartum, and following radiation or chemotherapy [12.63a] [Doss 1995, Frierson 1990, K Lee 1991]. Reactive endocervical cells may be difficult to distinguish from squamous dysplasia or carcinoma in situ, in some cases, because reactive endocervical cells can have big, dark nuclei occurring in unexpectedly dense cytoplasm or undifferentiated cytoplasm, respectively [Goff 1992, K Lee 1995]. The differential also includes benign metaplastic cells [12.63b] and adenocarcinoma.

Endocervical Brush Artifact

Endocervical brush artifact includes an increased number of endocervical cells, with increased thickness and crowding of groups (sheets, strips) [Fiorella 1994]. Also, large, dark nuclei (possibly due to polyploid DNA) may be present. In some cases, nuclear crowding, enlargement, and hyperchromasia may be worrisome, leading to a false impression of a serious lesion, such as carcinoma in situ or invasive carcinoma [12.64] [Covell 1992, Valente 1996]. Maintenance of honeycomb pattern, flat sheets, and round nuclei are clues to a benign process.

Endocervical Repair

Endocervical repair features macronucleoli in every cell, with pale chromatin, plenty of cytoplasm, and orderly, cohesive cell groups. Marked crowding and hyperchromasia [12.65a,b] favor neoplasia (see pg 95 for more discussion).

Endocervical Polyps

Endocervical polyps are usually accompanied by non-specific cytologic findings, such as reactive endocervical cells. However, atypical reactive/reparative changes, including mitotic activity, can lead to false-positive interpretations [12.66a,b] [Valente 2001]. Rarely, intact micropolyps are present; these tissue fragments have smooth borders outlined with columnar cells, pale intermediate zones, and dark inner cores made up of numerous small, dark stromal cells.

Adenomyomatous polyps and polyps of lower uterine segment also occur. They can exfoliate atypical glandular cells, including sheets or aggregates, with nuclear crowding, elongation, and hyperchromasia, rosettes, and focal feathering [Baschinsky 1999, Chhieng 2000b, Kimura 2003, Ngadiman 1995].

Directly Sampled Endometrium

Endometrium (directly sampled) features hyperchromatic crowded groups of endometrial cells [DeMay 2000]. Endometrial cells may be obtained at any time during the menstrual cycle: using an endocervical brush (endometrial cells directly sampled from the lower uterine segment or even the endometrial cavity itself); in the presence of cervical endometriosis; or in women who have undergone cone biopsy (in whom the endocervical canal is shortened, see "cone biopsy artifact" below) [K Lee 1993a]. The endometrial tissue is hormonally responsive. Plasma cells indicate chronic endometritis [Namiq 2004]. Mitotic figures may be present, and can be numerous during the proliferative phase of the menstrual cycle. These benign endometrial cells can mimic endocervical neoplasia. A clue: although the endometrial cells are tightly packed, they are usually well-organized and uniform. Biphasic glandular-stromal complexes [12.67a], with capillaries in the stroma [12.67b], help identify directly sampled endometrium (see lower uterine segment, below). Of important note is that only spontaneously exfoliated, not directly sampled, endometrial cells are reported in the Bethesda System in women 40 years of age and older.

Endometriosis

Endometriosis refers to ectopic endometrial glands and stroma. Endometriotic implants commonly involve the ovaries, uterosacral ligaments, rectovaginal septum, and peritoneum, but diverse sites can be involved, rarely. Apparently first described by the German physician, Daniel Shroen, in 1690 [Knapp 1999], endometriosis is estimated to affect about 5% to 10% of reproductive age women, and can cause problems ranging from chronic pelvic pain to infertility [Eskenazi 1997, Giudice 1998].

Cervical endometriosis was first reported by Erich Fels in 1928 [Fels 1928], and occurs more commonly following trauma, such as biopsy or possibly delivery [HL Gardner 1966]. Areas of cervical endometriosis appear as one or more, small, blue or red nodules. Contact bleeding may occur. Endometriosis can be the source of (very) atypical glandular cells identified in Pap tests [Hanau 1997, Mulvany 1999, D Symonds 1997]. Rarely, adenocarcinoma arises in endometriosis [McCluggage 2001b, S Chang 1971].

The classic interpretive triad for endometriosis is: endometrial glandular cells, endometrial stromal cells, and hemosiderin, but the full triad is not always present, particularly in cytologic specimens [12.68a,b]. The cytologic findings are nonspecific; therefore, specific recognition of cervical endometriosis is usually not possible in Pap tests, unless the woman has had a hysterectomy. The importance of cervical endometriosis is that it can simulate malignancy, both clinically and microscopically.

The endometrial glandular cells exfoliate in strips, sheets, and hyperchromatic crowded groups of endometrial cells. The cells are usually more numerous and better preserved than when spontaneously exfoliated. Nuclear crowding, pseudostratification, focal "feathering," and rare rosettes can occur in glandular clusters. Endometrial cells have high N/C ratios and dark coarse chromatin; nucleoli are variable. Because the tissue is hormonally responsive, mitotic figures, apoptotic bodies, and varying degrees of nuclear atypia may be present. The background of the sample is frequently bloody. These "atypical glandular cells" could easily be misinterpreted as H SIL (carcinoma in situ), adenocarcinoma in situ, or adenocarcinoma [Hanau 1997, Jaworski 1990, T Johnson 1996, K Lee 1991, Lundeen 2002, Mulvany 1999, G–K Nguyen 1993, Novotny 1992, Pacey 1988, Symonds 1997, Szyfelbein 2004, Valente 1996]. Helpful clues: *presence* of overall monotonous appearance of the glandular cells, endometrial stromal cells, and ciliated cells; and *absence* of frankly malignant appearing cells, prominent feathering, rosettes, single atypical cells, and tumor diathesis.

Lower Uterine Segment

The lower uterine segment can be sampled, inadvertently, using an endocervical brush or broom, and endometrial-like cells can then be present without any relationship to the menstrual cycle. The lower uterine segment consists of fragments and sheets of glandular cells, with or without stromal cells [12.69a,b,c]. Entire tubular glands, straight or branching, may be present. The glandular cells are crowded, but retain some degree of order or honeycombing. Neither stratification nor feathery edges occur, but mitotic figures may be present. Stromal cells are uniform, plump to spindle shaped, with bland nuclei and delicate cytoplasm. Stromal aggregates can form hyperchromatic crowded groups, leading to interpretive problems. Capillaries often traverse the tissue fragments, sometimes yielding a "lollipop" appearance. Capillaries, which occur in the stroma, are never seen in the epithelium of dysplasia or carcinoma in situ.

In liquid-based cytology, the findings are similar. Tissue fragments, often large, may show characteristic biphasic glandular epithelial cells and spindle-shaped stromal cells. The glandular cells have round, uniform nuclei and indistinct cytoplasm. The epithelium can suggest atypical glandular cells. The stroma can form hyperchromatic crowded groups. Capillaries, if present, are a clue to interpretation.

Cells from the lower uterine segment can be mistaken for endometriosis, glandular atypia, and in situ or invasive carcinomas, including squamous, endocervical, and endometrial types [de Peralta–Venturino 1995, Heaton 1996, K Lee 1991, 1995, Sidawy 1997]. In fact, hyperchromatic crowded groups of glandular cells from high in the endocervix or lower uterine segment are among the most common sources of

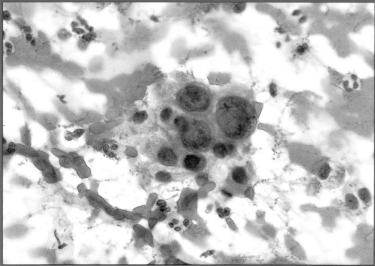

I2.64
Brush artifact [C]

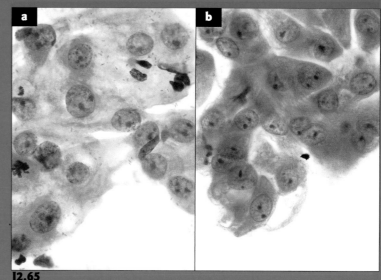

I2.65
a, Endocervical repair [C]; **b**, Endocervical repair [L]

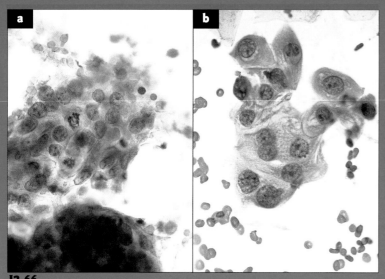

I2.66
a, Endocervical polyp [C]; **b**, Endocervical polyp [C]

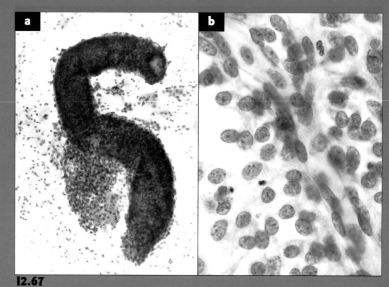

I2.67
a, Endometrium, biphasic [C]; **b**, Endometrium, stromal capillary [C]

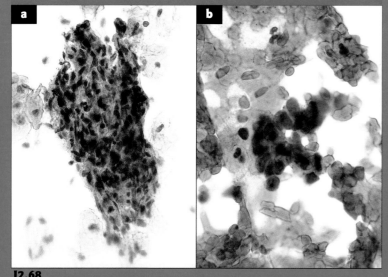

I2.68
a, Endometriosis [C]; **b**, Endometriosis [C]

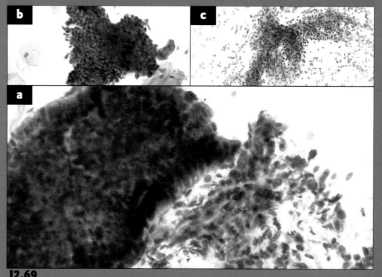

I2.69
a, Lower uterine segment, biphasic [L]; **b**, Lower uterine segment, glands [L];
c, Lower uterine segment, stroma [C]

false-positive interpretations in Pap tests [Fiorella 1994, K Lee 1991, 1995]. To complicate matters, adenocarcinomas can arise in the lower uterine segment [Masuda 1999]. Tubular glands, glandular-stromal complexes, and presence of capillaries are three clues to endometrium/lower uterine segment [Solomon 1998].

Cone Biopsy Artifact

Cone biopsy artifact refers to direct sampling of the lower uterine segment and endometrial cells following cervical conization biopsy [12.70]. These cells can be readily obtained because of mechanical shortening of the endocervical canal. Tubal metaplasia can also occur. Cone biopsy artifact can lead to exfoliation of hyperchromatic crowded groups (HCGs) of atypical glandular cells, with high N/C ratios, coarse, dark chromatin, rosettes, focal feathering, and mitotic figures, mimicking malignancy [DeMay 2000, Frauchiger 1998, Heaton 1996, S Hong 2001, Ismail 1991, K Lee 1988, 1991, 1993a, Pacey 1988]. In cone biopsy artifact, there are usually fewer abnormal cells and they are less crowded than in neoplasia. They typically form a morphologic spectrum that includes clearly benign cells of endometrial or endocervical origin. Nuclei are usually smaller and more uniform, with rounder, smoother outlines, and finer chromatin than in neoplasia. Ciliated cells or endometrial stroma associated with glandular cells are generally indicative of a benign process. Mitotic figures are suspicious findings in HCGs, but they can be present in benign glandular cells, particularly proliferative endometrium. The clinician must provide the history of a prior cervical cone biopsy for correct interpretation [G-K Nguyen 1993].

Tubal Metaplasia

Tubal metaplasia is benign, nonneoplastic replacement of the normal endocervical (or endometrial) epithelium with cells characteristic of the fallopian tube [12.71a,b]. It is very common, particularly after age 35, and can be identified, histologically, in 30% to 90% of cervices [Al-Nafussi 1993, Babkowski 1996, Jonasson 1992]. Although there may be an association with estrogen, tubal metaplasia does not appear to be related to the phase of the menstrual cycle, inflammation, or dysplasia [Jonasson 1992]. Tubal metaplasia usually occurs high in the endocervical canal, a site not commonly sampled in the past. However,

---

Tubal Metaplasia

Now common (endocervical brush)

Cells: HCGs, stratified strips, rosettes

   Pleomorphism, hyperchromasia

Nuclei: Dark, but fine even chromatin

Cytoplasm: Terminal bars and cilia (!)

   Also, tiny bubbles

---

owing to widespread use of the endocervical brush, tubal metaplasia has become a fairly common finding in Pap tests that can cause perplexing interpretive problems. Tubal metaplasia is clinically insignificant, but can be mistaken for glandular neoplasia, particularly adenocarcinoma in situ (AIS), in histology or cytology, prompting unnecessary work-up. More ominously, glandular neoplasia may be mistaken for benign tubal metaplasia in the Pap test and the woman may be lost to follow-up [Bose 1994, Ducatman 1993, Hirschowitz 1994, Jaworski 1988, Jonasson 1992, K Lee 1991, 1995, Novotny 1992, Pacey 1988, Sidawy 1997, Suh 1990, Van Le 1991].

Tubal metaplasia comprises ciliated, secretory, and intercalated (peg) cells, although rarely are all three cell types recognized specifically in Pap tests. The number of cells varies greatly. Secretory cells have round, basal nuclei and pale vacuolated cytoplasm. Intercalated cells are small and tend to be triangular, with high N/C ratios and scant, dark, granular cytoplasm [Ducatman 1993]. The morphologic findings, described below, are similar in both conventional Pap smears and liquid-based cytology .

Ciliated cells are most helpful in recognizing tubal metaplasia [12.72a,b], although they are not pathognomonic, because a few cells with cilia are normally present in the endocervix. The cells typically form crowded sheets or three-dimensional clusters, or may occur singly. The cells are usually smaller than ordinary endocervical cells, but can have larger nuclei. The nuclei are round to oval, with finely granular, but dark chromatin. Nucleoli are usually inconspicuous or absent. Mitosis can be present, but apoptosis is rare (see below) [Solomon 1998]. The cytoplasm is usually uniform, dense, cyanophilic, and may have tiny discrete vacuoles (tiny bubbles) [12.71b]. Secretory cells, similar to goblet cells, may also be present. This two-cell pattern of ciliated and secretory cells can help identify tubal metaplasia. The background is usually clean.

Recognition of ordinary tubal metaplasia, as described above, is usually fairly straightforward. However, atypical tubal metaplasia can mimic endocervical glandular neoplasia almost perfectly in some cases [Novotny 1992, Solomon 1998]. Both tubal metaplasia and glandular neoplasia can feature hyperchromatic crowded groups of columnar cells, with enlarged, pleomorphic nuclei, high N/C ratios, and conspicuous hyperchromasia [12.73a]. Increased single cells, occasional rosettes, focal feathering, and even occasional mitotic figures or rare apoptotic bodies—all features of glandular neoplasia—can sometimes be present in benign tubal metaplasia [12.73b]. Although the differential with AIS can be difficult in some cases, it is rare for the full spectrum of architectural and nuclear abnormalities of AIS to be present in tubal metaplasia

---

Tubal Metaplasia vs EGN

Favors Endocervical Glandular Neoplasia

   Marked crowding, feathery edges, mitoses

   Nuclear elongation, coarse dark

      chromatin

Cilia ⇒ Benign, but can degenerate

[Chhieng 2003, DeMay 2000, Hirschowitz 1994, K Lee 1991, Novotny 1992, Pacey 1988, Wilbur 1995]. On the other hand, a mixture of cell types, when present in an aggregate, is a clue to tubal metaplasia (vs a more serious lesion such as AIS). Similarly, AIS usually shows monotonous hyperchromasia, while in tubal metaplasia nuclear staining may be more variable.

Two helpful clues to tubal metaplasia are the presence of tiny, discrete, clear cytoplasmic vacuoles, and of course, terminal bars and cilia. Terminal bars and cilia *strongly* favor a benign interpretation [Ducatman 1993, Hirschowitz 1994, Novotny 1992, Van Le 1991], but unfortunately, these structures degenerate readily [Novotny 1992]. It has also been suggested that atypical tubal metaplasia can sometimes be a neoplastic precursor lesion [Schlesinger 1999]. However, most examples, by far, of atypical ciliated cells are benign and HPV-DNA negative [K Lee 2000a].

In addition, the cell groups tend to be more orderly in tubal metaplasia than in AIS. The nuclear outline is usually more round-to-oval and more uniform in tubal metaplasia, whereas it more elongated or irregular in AIS. On average the nuclei of tubal metaplasia are smaller than those in AIS; however, occasionally, huge (benign) nuclei pop out of the background of tubal metaplasia (like the Martian Popping Thing™ squeeze toy [McPhee 2003]) [12.73a]. Also, tubal metaplastic cell nuclei usually lack the distinctively coarse, dark chromatin pattern of AIS. Nucleoli are usually inconspicuous in both tubal metaplasia and AIS, but prominent in invasive adenocarcinoma. Numerous mitotic figures, and particularly, atypical mitoses, favor a neoplasia. The background is clean in tubal metaplasia and AIS, but a tumor diathesis is typical of invasive cancer. Carcinoembryonic antigen is not helpful in distinguishing tubal metaplasia from cervical adenocarcinoma [Marques 1996].

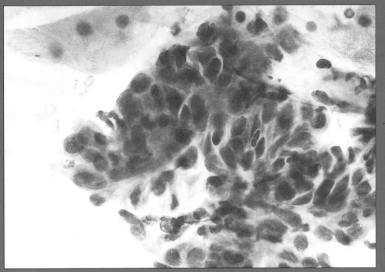

12.70
Cone biopsy artifact [C]

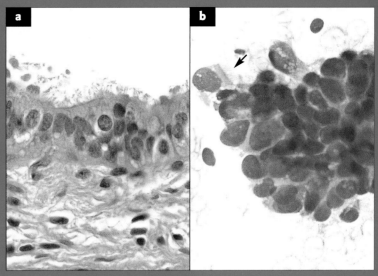

12.71
a, Tubal metaplasia; **b**, TM, bubbles, cilia (arrow) [C]

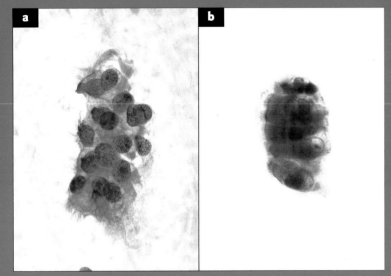

12.72
a, Tubal metaplasia [C]; **b**, Tubal metaplasia [L]

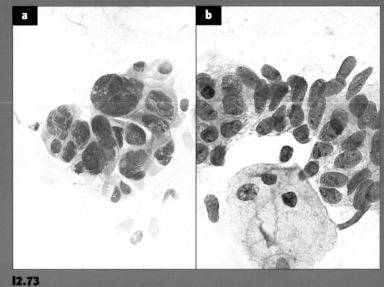

12.73
a, TM, cytologic atypia [C]; **b**, TM, mimics AIS [C]

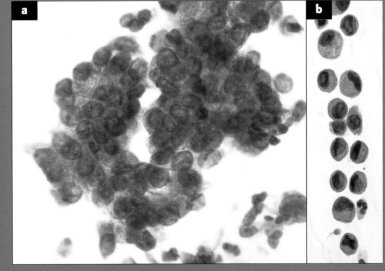

12.74
a, Microglandular hyperplasia [C]; **b**, Pseudoparakeratosis

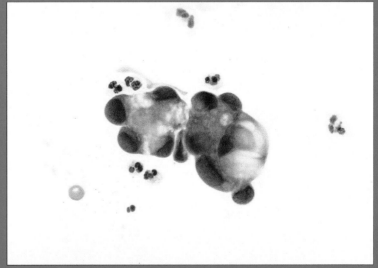

12.75
IUD effect, mimics adenocarcinoma [C]

Other forms of metaplasia, including endometrial metaplasia, tuboendometrioid metaplasia [*Hirschowitz 1994*], gastric or intestinal metaplasia [*Azzopardi 1965, Mikami 1999, Trowell 1985*], and rarely sebaceous or epidermoid metaplasia [*Ionescu 2004*], can also occur in the cervix. Transitional cell (urothelial) metaplasia is described on page 48. Of course, the mere presence of any of these benign metaplasias does not exclude the possibility of a coexisting neoplastic lesion [*Solomon 1998*]. Unfortunately, however, these benign findings may confound interpretation. Say, for example, there are several hyperchromatic crowded groups (HCGs) in the specimen. On careful search, *some* have cilia: t'would be easy to conclude they are all benign, but it ain't necessarily so.

Microglandular Endocervical Hyperplasia

Microglandular hyperplasia usually sheds endocervical cells that may show nonspecific reactive changes [12.74a]. However, some cases display cytologic atypia that can mimic malignancy [*Selvaggi 2000*]. Hyperchromatic crowded groups, with nuclear enlargement, hyperchromasia, nucleoli, and mitotic figures may suggest endocervical or endometrial neoplasia, or high-grade squamous intraepithelial lesions [*Chhieng 2001d, DeMay 2000, T Nichols 1971, Rizzo 1989, Selvaggi 1997, 1999a, 2000, Shidham 2004, Valente 1994b, Yahr 1991*]. Absence of coarse chromatin, irregular nuclear membranes, and "feathery" edges, or presence of cells with cilia or terminal bars point to a benign interpretation [*Valente 1994b, 1996*]. Pseudoparakeratosis is a possible clue to microglandular hyperplasia (see pg 113) [12.74b]. Extensive immature squamous metaplasia can also occur, which could lead to interpretations of atypical squamous cells-high grade SIL not excluded (ASC-H) [*Shidham 2004*].

Intrauterine Contraceptive Device Effect

Intrauterine contraceptive device (IUD) effect displays clusters of reactive glandular cells of either endocervical or endometrial origin, and clusters of vacuolated metaplastic cells, which can mimic adenocarcinoma [12.75]. Also, single endometrial cells can be present, which can mimic squamous CIN 3. *Actinomyces*, if present, supports the interpretation. The clinician must provide the history of IUD use (see pg 163 for more discussion of IUD effect).

Postpartum Atypia

Postpartum atypia is common in the obstetrical population. Highly atypical reactive/degenerative epithelial and stromal cells may occur [12.76]. The cytologic differential includes: reactive/reparative changes, microglandular hyperplasia, and Arias-Stella reaction vs bona fide squamous or glandular neoplastic lesions [*Chhieng 2001d, C Michael 1997*]. (Pregnancy and postpartum change are discussed in more detail in section IV.)

Arias-Stella Reaction

Arias-Stella reaction is characterized by marked nuclear atypia (enlargement, pleomorphism, hyperchromasia, and prominent nucleoli) and abundant cytoplasm that could easily be mistaken for adenocarcinoma, particularly clear cell carcinoma [*Jaworski 1990, G-K Nguyen 1993, Shrago 1977*]. No stratification or crowding occurs, and mitotic figures are absent or rare [12.77]. Similar cells can be present in cases of chemotherapy effect [12.63a] [*Doss 1995*] (see pg 166, for more details).

Squamous Carcinoma In Situ

Squamous carcinoma (particularly carcinoma in situ involving endocervical glands) can be indistinguishable from adenocarcinoma. Both squamous

and glandular carcinomas in situ can be associated with hyperchromatic crowded groups. Both lesions can have similar nuclei (coarse, dark chromatin) and cytoplasm (delicate, nonkeratinizing). Furthermore, squamous carcinoma in situ *commonly* has rudimentary glandular features (such as nuclear palisading, columnar cells, microacinar or rosette-like structures, feathering) that can mimic endocervical glandular neoplasia [12.78] [*W Andersen 1988, Cangiarella 2003, DeMay 2000, Drijkoningen 1996, K Lee 1995, P Levine 2002, Mattosinho 2003, Nasu 1993, Raab 2000, Renshaw 2004c, Selvaggi 1994, Siziopikou 1997, Solomon 1998, Valente 2001, van Hoeven 1996b, Wilbur 1995*]. Presence of *well-formed* glandular structures and mucin, of course, points to glandular origin. Glandular lesions tend to have more elongated nuclei (vs rounder), distinctively coarse, dark chromatin, and more prominent feathering than squamous lesions. Look at the edges of the HCGs: feathering favors glandular origin, while flattening favors squamous origin. Within the HCGs, well-formed rosettes favor glandular origin, while whirling or spindling favors squamous origin. In the background, squamous dysplasia favors squamous carcinoma in situ. In some cases, this dilemma may have to be resolved by tissue biopsy, and even then the differential can sometimes be difficult. Finally, it is not uncommon for squamous and glandular lesions to coexist; these lesions are more difficult to interpret accurately [*Gloor 1986, Kurian 1999, Lauchlan 1967, Luesley 1987, Raab 2000, van Aspert-van Erp 2004b*].

Invasive Squamous Cell Carcinoma

Invasive squamous cell carcinoma can sometimes mimic atypical glandular cells, particularly in liquid-based cytology where aggregates of cells tend to round up [12.79a,b,c]. The cells of squamous carcinoma generally have denser cytoplasm and more central nuclei than adenocarcinoma. Keratinization or dysplastic squamous cells, of course, strongly favors squamous origin, but does not exclude the possibility of a coexisting glandular lesion or adenosquamous carcinoma. Irregular or raggedy outlines of the HCGs favors invasive carcinoma over carcinoma in situ. The differential of poorly-differentiated neoplasms is difficult, since their features are "poorly-differentiated" by definition.

Neoplastic Endocervical Cells

Neoplastic endocervical cells (in brief review) typically have marked crowding, rosettes, feathery edges; tall columnar cells; enlarged, oval to elongated nuclei, with distinctively coarse, dark chromatin; and mitoses/apoptosis [12.80a]. Irregular chromatin, prominent or macronucleoli, and tumor diathesis are classically associated with invasion. Variants of endocervical carcinoma as well as endometrial carcinoma also enter into the differential of atypical glandular cells. Even benign glandular cells can sometimes pose interpretive problems [12.80b].

Metastatic Adenocarcinoma

Metastatic adenocarcinoma exfoliates clusters of malignant-appearing cells, most characteristically lacking a tumor diathesis. There is almost always a known history of cancer and there is usually evidence of metastasis at other sites, although rarely, the Pap test is the first indication of occult malignancy [*Patsner 2002*] (see pg 181) [12.81].

Other Conundrums

Several other conditions, including herpes, pemphigus vulgaris, repair/regeneration, radiation effect, severe atrophy, vaginal adenosis, gland cells post-hysterectomy, small cell carcinoma, can from time to time mimic atypical glandular cells or shed hyperchromatic crowded groups.

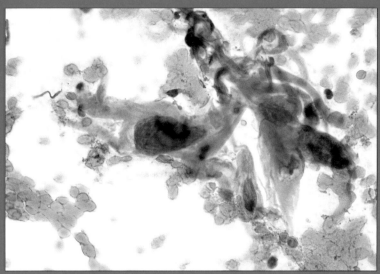

I2.76
Postpartum atypia [C]

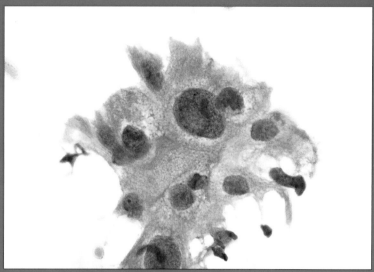

I2.77
Arias-Stella reaction [C]

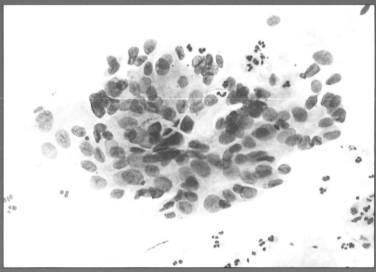

I2.78
Squamous CIS with "glands" [C]

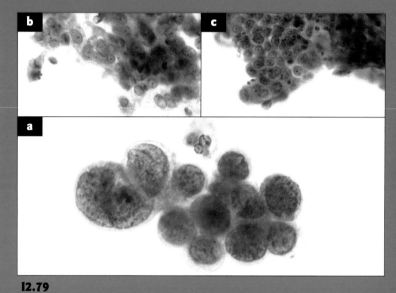

I2.79
a, SCC, gland-like clusters [L]; **b**, SCC, gland-like clusters [L]; **c**, SCC, gland-like clusters [L]

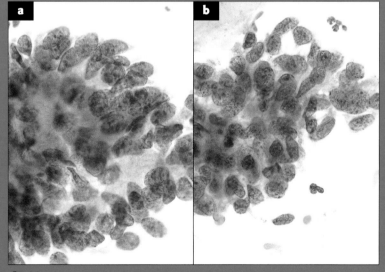

I2.80
a, AIS vs endometrium (= AIS) [C]; **b**, AIS vs endometrium (= EMs) [C]

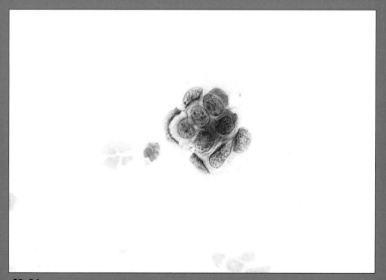

I2.81
Metastatic carcinoma, breast [C]

III. Cytology of Iatrogenic Conditions

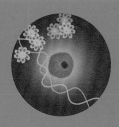

Jatrogenic (Greek: *iatros,* physician; *-genic,* produced) conditions can be induced unintentionally by medical treatment or investigational procedures, including Pap tests. An extreme example is a woman who required open-heart surgery to replace a cardiac valve that became infected following a routine Pap test [Mong 1997]. Less extreme, but still serious, iatrogenic conditions range from the possibility of transmitting HPV infections via vaginal specula to overtreatment of nonexistent lesions, with attendant risks and complications of surgical procedures [Bourgain 2004, J McCormack 1989].

Artifactual changes related to improper collection, fixation, or preparation of the specimen could be considered iatrogenic, and can lead to misinterpretation of the cells. These changes may include cellular or nuclear enlargement and pleomorphism, cytoplasmic vacuolization and eosinophilia, hyperchromasia or hypochromasia, other chromatin alterations, such as irregular clumping or clearing, and nuclear vacuolization. Liquid-based cytology may help reduce the number of artifactual changes [J Wright 2003].

Effects of radiation, chemotherapy, immunosuppressive drugs, surgical procedures, hormonal therapy, and contraceptive devices in Pap tests are discussed in this section. The clinician must supply an accurate history for proper cytologic interpretation [Frable 1973].

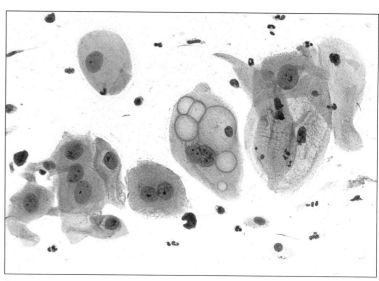

I3.I
Radiation, cytomegaly and vacuoles [C]

Radiation Cytology

Not long after Roentgen discovered x-rays, in 1895, and the Curies isolated radium, in 1898, Cleaves first described the use of radioactive radium to treat cervical cancer in 1903 [Cleaves 1903, Shield 1992]. Radiation therapy is now widely used for cancer of the female genital tract, particularly squamous cell carcinoma of the cervix. Radiation can be quite effective in destroying cancer cells (To paraphrase Cato the elder: *Cancer delenda est! Cancer must be destroyed!*), which are generally more sensitive to radiation than benign cells, but it can affect native cells, causing cytologic changes that may be transitory (acute) or may persist (chronic), sometimes for life [Abitbol 1974, Koss 1961, R Graham 1947a,b]. Radiation can affect the genetic code of germinative cells, possibly causing permanent damage to subsequent generations [Shield 1995, Zimmer 1959].

Cytology is a simple, accurate, and cost-effective method to detect residual cancer in women who have been treated for cervical carcinoma [Friedell 1961, H Kraus 1979, McKenzie 1996, Shield 1992]. Although many women with residual disease have abnormal signs or symptoms [McKenzie 1996, Muram 1982], cytology can be the first clinical indicator of recurrent or persistent carcinoma [Muram 1982]. However, interpreting the postradiation sample can be difficult, because radiation can produce striking cellular alterations of both benign and malignant cells. Benign radiation changes can be misinterpreted as malignant (false-positive result) and conversely, residual carcinoma can be misinterpreted as benign radiation effect (false-negative result). False-negative results can also occur owing to problems with sampling, eg, deep pelvic recurrences, poor cellularity, subsurface tumor, etc [Muram 1982]. False-negative results are reported to be in the range of ~50% to 75% [Muram 1982, Shield 1991, J Wright 2003]. Cytology can also detect postradiation dysplasia, which may portend a poor prognosis [Murad 1985, Wentz 1970].

A variety of radiation sensitivity tests have been proposed to try to predict which women will respond well to radiation therapy. None is currently thought to be clinically useful. The most important clinical predictors of radiation effectiveness are the histologic type of the tumor and its extent (stage). The qualitative effects of radiation are independent of type of radiation and method of administration. However, the quantitative effects are dependent on several variables such as dosage and duration of radiation.

The cause of this effect, or rather say, the cause of this defect, for this effect defective comes by cause, is that radiation can disrupt the cell and the cell cycle by damaging the cell's DNA, proteins, lipids, and even its water (with free radical formation) [Little 1968]. The cumulative effect can be the demise of the cell [E Hall 1985]. Sensitivity of cells to radiation varies with cell type, mitotic activity, and oxygen content (hypoxic cells are radioresistant) [Murad 1985, Thar 1982]. Cells are most sensitive to radiation during the mitotic, or M, phase, and premitotic, or G2, phase of the cell cycle. Cells are most resistant to radiation during DNA synthesis, S phase, and are moderately resistant after DNA synthesis is complete.

Cells with a high rate of turnover, such as those of small cell carcinoma, are the most sensitive to radiation since they spend relatively more time in the vulnerable phases. However, while small cell carcinoma is among the most radiosensitive of the cervical cancers, it is one of the least radiocurable (it melts away, but then comes back with a vengeance) [Wentz 1965].

Histologically, acute radiation changes are characterized by tissue degeneration and necrosis; vascular damage and inflammatory changes resulting in erythema and edema; and desquamation and sloughing of tissue. Chronic radiation changes are characterized by regeneration and persistent changes such as sclerosis in vessels and connective tissue, and epithelial atrophy [Shield 1995]. In most women, acute changes subside within a few months after treatment, but in some cases, enlarged or bizarre cells persist for years [Abitbol 1974, Koss 1961, Shield 1995].

Radiation Effect

Radiation can effect cytologic changes, sometimes marked, that affect epithelial and mesenchymal cells, and can mimic condyloma, dysplasia, carcinoma, or even sarcoma. However, criteria for defining radiation

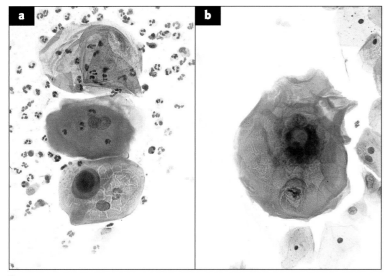

I3.2
a, Radiation, macrocytes [C]; **b**, Macrocyte, polychromasia [C]

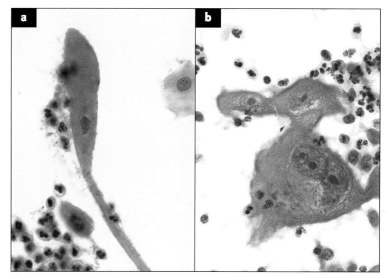

I3.3
a, Radiation, bizarre cell [L]; **b**, Radiation, nuclear abnormalities [C]

changes have not been standardized [J Wright 2003]. Consequently, radiation changes have been reported to occur in ~30% to 90% of those treated and affect 5% to 70% of the cells. The changes are usually most marked immediately following therapy and usually resolve within a year or two, but can persist [S Gupta 1982, Masubuchi 1969, Rintala 1997, Shield 1992]. An individual woman's response is unpredictable: some show marked radiation changes following a low dose of radiation; others may have no discernable effect after high dosage.

Radiation Effect

Macrocytes → Cytomegaly

Cells: Enlarged, some bizarre

Nuclei: Enlarged/multiple, pale/dark

Cytoplasm: Polychromatic, vacuolated

N/C ratios relatively unchanged

Repair/regeneration common

May regress or persist for life

Similar changes in chemotherapy

Cytoplasmic vacuolization is the earliest effect of radiation, but is non-specific [I3.1] [R Graham 1955]. Polychromasia, and particularly, cytomegaly are characteristic features of radiation change [I3.2a,b]. Bizarre cells may be present [I3.3a]. Atrophy is common after treatment [Ceelen 1966, Shield 1995]. The cytologic effects are divided into acute and chronic radiation changes, which are similar morphologically [Murad 1985].

Acute Radiation Change

When first administered, radiation induces a severe inflammatory reaction, with a "diathesis" consisting of white blood cells, histiocytes (including giant cells), debris, and necrosis, plus evidence of epithelial regeneration and repair. In this milieu, dead and dying, as well as viable appearing, tumor cells are expected for up to 8 weeks following therapy. During this acute phase, cytologic samples are unsatisfactory for evaluation of the presence of residual carcinoma. Then, tumor cells usually clear relatively rapidly and the maturation pattern often becomes atrophic (if the ovaries were sterilized) [S Gupta 1987]. After a grace period of 6 to 8 weeks following therapy, a baseline Pap test can be assessed for tumor cells and a radiation reaction. The presence of tumor cells or the absence of a good radiation reaction after the grace period are poor prognostic signs.

Squamous Cells

Cytomegaly (ie, the formation of macrocytes) [I3.2a,b] is the single most characteristic radiation-induced change in squamous cells [Ceelen 1966, R Graham 1955, McLennan 1975a, K Masubuchi 1969, Murad 1985, Powers 1995, Rintala 1997, S Whitaker 1990]. The cells are enlarged by at least one-third, but can grow to enormous size, sometimes > 200 μm in diameter (several times the area of a normal mature cell). The nuclei and the cytoplasm usually enlarge in concert, so that the N/C ratio remains relatively normal or only modestly increased. Radiation-induced nuclear and cytoplasmic abnormalities can cause benign cells to appear bizarre (snakes, tadpoles, etc); this finding can be difficult to distinguish from malignancy [Powers 1995]. Although bizarre cells tend to command attention, they are numerically rare (no more than 1% of cells) [R Graham 1955].

Nuclear changes typically include enlargement of both nuclei and nucleoli [I3.3b] [R Graham 1955, Powers 1995]. Multinucleation is common and the nuclei can be of unequal size. Nuclear membrane irregularity ("wrinkling") can occur in radiated benign cells, which may suggest neoplastic changes, but the nuclear membrane does not appear thickened. The chromatin, when well preserved, is typically finely granular and bland. However, radiation can cause chromatin clumping and hyperchromasia; in this case, the chromatin usually looks smudgy and degenerated, not crisp and distinct as in cancer. Nuclear vacuolization can further distort the chromatin, mimicking malignant chromatin irregularities. Other signs of nuclear degeneration, such as chromatolysis, karyolysis, karyorrhexis, or pyknosis, are also common as the radiated cells die [Powers 1995]. Nucleoli can be prominent and sometimes pleomorphic.

Cytoplasmic changes typically include enlargement and polychromasia: the generous cytoplasm tends to stain both pink and blue (polychromatic or "two-tone" staining), but usually not orange [I3.3b]. Dense orangeophilia (heavy keratinization) suggests malignancy. Cytoplasmic vacuolization is both early and common, and is particularly characteristic of acute radiation change. The vacuoles range from fine to coarse, and may contain ingested neutrophils, other cells, or debris. Extremely large vacuoles can follow radiation; these can form signet ring cells or mimic koilocytotic vacuoles. As mentioned, the shape of the cell can be irregular or abnormal, or sometimes even bizarre. Cell shape is not a reliable malignant criterion in this setting.

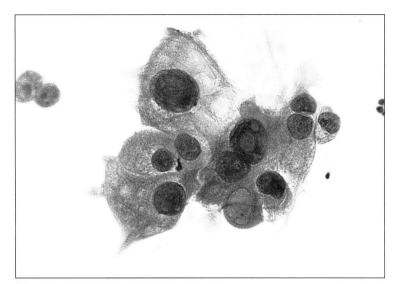

I3.4
Radiation, glandular cells [C]

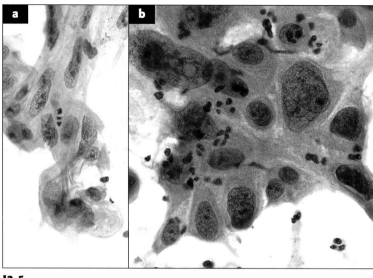

I3.5
a, Radiated repair [C]; **b**, Radiated repair [C]

Background findings include evidence of inflammation and necrosis. An acute inflammatory exudate, with a marked histiocytic reaction, cell debris, and blood, is a common, early observation that usually indicates a good radiation response. Histiocytes may appear unusually active, with prominent nucleoli and phagocytosis of red blood cells, hemosiderin, and debris. Multinucleated giant cell histiocytes and lymphocytes appear later. Large sheets of atrophic (parabasal) squamous cells or reparative cells may be present, particularly in the acute phase. Naked nuclei, sometimes sticking together in small clusters, derive from atrophic epithelium. These may suggest poorly-differentiated carcinoma, especially small cell type.

Glandular Cells

Glandular cells undergo changes similar to those that have been described for squamous cells, including cellular enlargement and vacuolization [Shield 1995] [I3.4]. The cytologic picture may be one of atypical repair in glandular cells. The cells are present singly or in clusters, but clusters may lack the typical honeycomb appearance [Frierson 1990]. Radiated glandular cells can show macrocytosis, vacuolization, large or multiple nuclei, hyperchromasia, prominent nucleoli, irregular cell shapes, and mucinous cytoplasm. The nuclei tend to be round to oval with minimal membrane irregularities, although intranuclear cytoplasmic invaginations may occur. The cytologic changes can be mistaken for malignancy [Tabatabai 2003]. As with radiated squamous cells, the N/C ratio usually remains within normal limits [Doss 1995, Frierson 1990, Lesack 1996]. Since similar changes can occur in reactive, nonradiated glandular cells, radiation changes are better assessed in squamous cells.

Radiated Repair

Radiated repair is one of the most strikingly abnormal, yet benign, changes that can be present in a Pap test. The cells can look wild, with the atypia of radiation superimposed upon the atypia of repair [I3.5a,b]. Ordinary repair is common after radiation and usually readily recognized as such, but repair with radiation changes can lead to interpretive problems [Shield 1995]. Radiated repair retains the usual features of benign repair (eg, cohesive groups, relatively orderly arrangements) but also has superimposed radiation change

(eg, bountiful and colorful cytoplasm together with enlarged, often multiple, nuclei and prominent nucleoli). Clinical history is paramount in interpretation.

Stromal Cells

Stromal cells, including fibroblasts and endothelial cells, can exhibit striking cytologic atypia following radiation [I3.6a,b]. Cellular enlargement, with big, dark nuclei, and peculiar cytoplasmic extensions (legs) may give rise to weird octopus-like cells or la cucarachas. These cells, when present in a Pap test, usually indicate the presence of an ulcer (because they live in the stroma). Histologically, the stroma is fibrotic to hyalinized, with thick walled blood vessels. The differential includes sarcoma, which although rare, can occur as a late (≥10 years) complication of radiation therapy [Shield 1995]. Most carcinomas recur within three years of therapy [van Nagell 1979], although late recurrences are possible [McLennan 1975a].

Chronic Radiation Change

Chronic radiation change is arbitrarily defined as lasting at least 6 months to a year. Upon entering the chronic phase, inflammation fades and repair resolves. Other morphologic features of chronic radiation change are similar to those of acute radiation change, in particular, the persistence of macrocytes [Ceelen 1966]. Pleomorphic cell shapes and polychromasia are also characteristic of chronic radiation change. The squamous epithelium usually remains atrophic, unless the ovaries are functional or hormone replacement therapy is prescribed [McLennan 1975a]. Foreign body giant cell histiocytes, as well as ordinary histiocytes, are commonly present [Shield 1995]. The background is usually clean, or may be inflammatory ("atrophy with inflammation"). Many specimens are unsatisfactory for evaluation owing to inadequate numbers of squamous cells or lack of an endocervical/transformation zone component [Shield 1995].

Residual Carcinoma

Pap tests following radiation therapy can be classified as showing a good radiation response (rapid clearing of cancer cells), delayed response, or poor response. In most (>80%) cases, there is a good response to therapy, and cancer cells

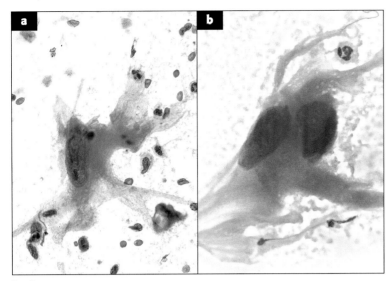

13.6
a, Radiated stromal cell [C]; **b**, Radiated stromal cell [C]

are "cleared" by 6-8 weeks. However, some cancer cells may persist with acute radiation changes for up to 8 weeks after therapy. These tumor cells are biologically inactive, and have no effect on survival.

Cancer After Radiation

  Allow 8 week grace period

  Tumor (vs radiation effect):

    ↑ *N/C ratios, crisp chromatin*

  Persistent tumor

    Tumor with radiation effect

    Mitoses ⇒ viability

  Recurrent tumor

    Tumor without radiation effect

    Viable ± mitoses

Persistence of cancer cells beyond the grace period is a poor prognostic sign [S Gupta 1982, 1987, McLennan 1975a], although curative therapy is still possible for early, localized recurrences [Muram 1982, S Whitaker 1990].

After a 6-8 week grace period, the Pap test can be used to evaluate the presence of residual viable malignant cells and to distinguish them from radiated benign cells. The interpretive criteria for residual malignancy are similar to those used for the initial diagnosis of malignancy. Cervicovaginal cytology cannot detect all residual tumors, because many occur deep in the pelvis or in metastatic sites, [Powers 1995, Rayburn 1980, van Nagell 1979]. Even neoplasms located in the cervix or vagina fail to exfoliate cells unless the lesion involves the mucosal surface [Muram 1982]. Furthermore, sampling can be difficult owing to radiation-induced vaginal stenosis, atrophy, or adhesions [Muram 1982].

The effects of radiation on malignant cells are similar to those seen in benign cells, but in addition, residual tumor cells have typical malignant features [Koss 1961]. Residual tumor cells usually more or less resemble the original tumor cells. Therefore, it can be helpful to compare with pretreatment biopsy or cytology specimens [Powers 1995]. Cells with bizarre, irregular configurations, particularly if numerous or keratinized, suggest cancer. Nuclear enlargement occurs in both radiated benign cells and malignant cells; however, the *N/C ratio* is one of the most helpful features in differentiating malignant cells (high N/C ratio) from benign radiated cells (low N/C ratio). Nuclear membrane irregularity can be present in either benign or malignant radiated cells, but in malignant cells, the membrane often appears thickened. Similarly, nuclear hyperchromasia may occur in either cell type, but the *chromatin quality* is helpful in the differential: it usually appears smudgy and degenerated in benign radiation effect vs

crisp and distinct in cancer. Enlarged or irregular nucleoli are not necessarily indicative of cancer, because they can also be present in benign repair. Mitotic figures can be present in both benign repair and malignant cells; however, their presence indicates the cells were viable (at the time of sampling). Abnormal mitotic figures are indicative of malignancy.

Other conditions that may be confused with radiation effect include atrophy caused by hormonal therapy and inflammatory changes not induced by radiation. Also, cytotoxic drugs, vitamin deficiencies (folate, B_{12}), and condyloma can cause cytomegaly, nuclear enlargement, multinucleation, and other nuclear abnormalities similar to those seen in radiation effect [van Niekerk 1966].

Persistent vs Recurrent Carcinoma

Cytologic samples that contain malignant cells after radiation therapy can be divided into two general groups: those in which the disease was never actually controlled (persistent disease), and those in which the disease was clinically controlled, ie, a complete response, but came back after therapy (recurrent disease). The cytology of these two groups is, theoretically, quite different, although tumor cells are usually numerous in both. *Persistent disease* often has small cell ("undifferentiated") morphology, because women with aggressive small cell tumors are more likely to fail radiation therapy [R Graham 1964]. *Recurrent disease* often has more differentiated cells, although small cell morphology can also be present [H Kraus 1979]. Look carefully for small tumor cells, particularly in women lacking a good radiation reaction in the benign cells. Even in women with a good radiation reaction, small malignant cells can be difficult to find in a "busy" background. The differential includes small, atrophic (basal/parabasal) squamous cells and clusters of naked nuclei, which could be mistaken for small tumor cells [H Kraus 1979].

Positive cytology may be the first indication that the malignancy has not been controlled. If malignant tumor cells *with* radiation effect are found after the 6-8 week grace period, this suggests that they were present when the radiation was completed and, therefore, is consistent with *persistent* tumor. While these radiated tumor cells may not be biologically active (viable), they are a worrisome finding. Mitoses prove viability. On the other hand, if malignant tumor cells *without* radiation effect are present after the grace period, this suggests that the tumor came back after cessation of radiotherapy. This is consistent with *recurrent* cancer. (Note, however, that proof of tumor recurrence, as opposed to persistence, requires clinical or biopsy evidence of a disease-free interval.)

In summary, the Pap test is not very sensitive in detection of tumor persistence or recurrence, but it is highly specific [Shield 1991, S Whitaker 1990]. False-negative results are often due to sampling problems; false-positive results can occur due to presence of atypical repair and bizarre cells in an inflammatory/necrotic background occurring in benign radiation effect. Finding tumor cells in the Pap test after therapy (beyond the 6-8 week grace period) is a poor prognostic sign—proof that the cancer has not been cured. Further therapy is indicated without waiting for clinical symptoms of relapse. Negative cytology at the end of treatment does not guarantee cure, but most tumors that recur, do so in less than 3 years, although late recurrences are possible [McLennan 1975a]. Recurrence has a poor prognosis [van Nagell 1979]. The clinical stage is particularly important in women who have negative cytology findings; their likelihood of death correlates with the stage of the disease at presentation [Campos 1970].

Postradiation Dysplasia

Unfortunately, some women treated with radiation, usually for squamous cell carcinoma of the cervix—who had apparently been cured—develop a new lesion, postradiation dysplasia, from 6 months to many years (or even decades) after therapy [Davey 1992a, Friedell 1961, Koss 1961, Patten 1963, Wentz 1970, J Wright 2003]. Older studies reported rates of approximately 20% of treated patients [S Gupta 1982, McLennan 1975a, Patten 1963, Wentz 1970]. Studies also indicated that postradiation dysplasia had a poor prognosis, particularly if it occurred within 3 years of radiation [Muram 1982, Patten 1978, Wentz 1970]. However, since November 1999, the standard of care for advanced stage cervical cancer has changed; many patients now receive cisplatin therapy, a radiation sensitizer. There is evidence that the rate of postradiation dysplasia and its association with recurrence is much lower than in the past [J Wright 2003]. Although postradiation dysplasia could be related to ionizing radiation, HPV can be detected in exfoliated cells following radiation [Filho 1997], and recurrent carcinomas are usually HPV positive [Ikenberg 1994]. Rarely, postradiation sarcomas develop following therapy (see pg 175 for discussion of sarcomas) [Fehr 1974, Norris 1965].

Postradiation dysplasia is a risk factor for residual carcinoma. Recurrence is usually not in continuity with the dysplasia, but instead occurs at a distant site, eg, deep in the pelvis (parametria) or lymph node metastases [Patten 1963]. The risk of recurrence does not correlate well with the grade of dysplasia, although aneuploidy may increase the risk of clinical recurrence [Davey 1998, Okagaki 1974].

Cytologically, postradiation dysplasia usually looks like ordinary dysplasia, often keratinizing type, occurring in a background of radiation effect [Koss 1961, Patten 1963, Powers 1995, Shield 1992]. Common dysplastic changes include enlarged, hyperchromatic ("big and dark") nuclei, with coarse distinct chromatin, increased N/C ratios, and polygonal to irregular cell outline [RH Kaufman 1961, Patten 1963, Wentz 1970, Zimmer 1959]. The dysplastic cells are present singly or in sheets. Like ordinary dysplasia, postradiation dysplasia usually occurs in a mature (nonatrophic) epithelium. In contrast, benign radiation change is characterized by macrocytes with relatively normal N/C ratios, polychromasia, cytoplasmic vacuolization, phagocytosis, fine or smudgy chromatin, and occasionally, macronucleoli. In practice, however, it is difficult to distinguish mild postradiation dysplasia (L SIL) from benign radiation effect.

A small cell type of postradiation dysplasia, reminiscent of CIN 3, also occurs, often in an atrophic background [Patten 1963]. The small cells have high N/C ratios and hyperchromatic, distinct chromatin. The large (mature) cell type of postradiation dysplasia is more common in younger women, while the small cell (CIN 3) type is more common in an older age group [Patten 1963].

The persistence of maturation after radiotherapy ("estrogen effect") indicates that the milieu is right for postradiation dysplasia or residual cancer to occur [Rubio 1966]. In practice, maturation means the formation of superficial cells (>20% of cells). Close cytologic follow-up of all postradiation patients,

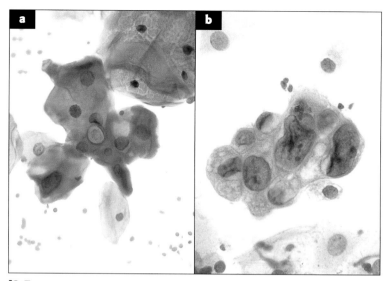

I3.7
a, ChemoRx, macrocyte [C]; **b**, ChemoRx, glandular cells [C]

particularly those with increased maturation, is indicated, looking for evidence of postradiation dysplasia or persistent/recurrent carcinoma [S Gupta 1982].

In summary, postradiation dysplasia is a possible risk factor for recurrent carcinoma, particularly when occurring within 3 years of therapy. Women with postradiation dysplasia should undergo colposcopy. A careful pelvic examination and appropriate diagnostic tests, possibly including pelvic FNA biopsy, should be conducted in an effort to detect residual carcinoma. Postradiation dysplasia developing after 3 years does not guarantee the woman is completely safe from recurrence, but the risk is reduced.

Finally, it can be very difficult to distinguish among benign radiation changes, repair, postradiation dysplasia, and residual carcinoma in some cases [McLennan 1975a]. DNA analysis may be helpful; aneuploidy is rarely, if ever, present in benign radiation changes [Davey 1992a].

Chemotherapy Cytology

Although not as well defined as cytologic changes due to radiation, chemotherapy can also cause morphologic alterations in cells. Some forms of systemic chemotherapy cause effects similar to radiation change; other drugs, such as busulfan, cause changes that can be difficult to distinguish from neoplasia [Doss 1995, M Feingold 1969, P Gupta 1969, Gureli 1963, Koss 1965, H Kraus 1977, A Schachter 1983, Schramm 1970]. However, in most cases, a normal cellular pattern is observed in women receiving chemotherapy [K Liu 1999]. Also note that prolonged chemotherapy can cause cancer [Takamizawa 1973] and immunosuppressed women are at increased risk of cervical neoplasia.

Macrocytes can be present in radiation and chemotherapy (as well as condyloma, and vitamin deficiency [folate or B_{12}]) [I3.7a] [van Niekerk 1966]. Multinucleation of nonneoplastic cells is common following chemotherapy. Atypical epithelial cells with large, irregular nuclei, but smudgy chromatin, suggest therapeutic effect. Chemotherapy can also induce a reversible atrophic maturation pattern. Arias-Stella-like reaction in nonneoplastic glandular cells can be induced by chemotherapy [I3.7b] [Doss 1995].

Immunosuppressive Drugs

Immunosuppressive drugs probably have no specific effects on Pap tests. However, women who are immunosuppressed, including those with AIDS, transplant recipients, and others, are particularly susceptible to human papillomavirus infections and are at increased risk of cervical carcinoma. Close clinical follow-up is indicated to detect precursor lesions.

Surgery, Electrodiathermy, Laser, and Cryotherapy

Surgical procedures, including biopsies, electrodiathermy (eg, LEEP [loop electrocautery excision procedure]), laser, or cryotherapy, are commonly used to treat epithelial lesions; these procedures can cause cytologic alterations detected in Pap tests [*Bellina 1980, Buckovsky 1985, Frauchiger 1998, Gondos 1970, Hasegawa 1975, Holmquist 1976, Ioffe 1999, Sharp 1984, P Thomas 1996*]. A cytologic sample taken within a few days will often have degenerative changes, such as nuclear pyknosis and karyolysis, and cytoplasmic vacuolization, with an inflammatory or necrotic background. Regenerative changes of nuclear enlargement and hyperchromasia could be confused with cells derived from squamous intraepithelial lesions. As the wound heals, repair/regeneration will be in evidence. Thermal changes in cells ("heat artifact"), consisting primarily of formation of spindle cells with elongated nuclei and cytoplasmic tails, are associated with laser or LEEP therapy. The affected nuclei appear degenerated, with smudgy chromatin and the cytoplasm is coagulated. "Pencil-thin" endocervical cells can also be present as a thermal artifact [13.8] [*Holmquist 1976*]. Follow-up Pap tests should not be obtained until after the treatment site has had an opportunity to heal. Long-term consequences of cone biopsy may include tubal metaplasia and "cone biopsy artifact," as previously discussed (see pg 150). Massive exfoliation of endometrial cells, probably due to ischemia, has been reported following uterine artery embolization therapy [*Kobayashi 2001*].

Hormone Therapy-Related Cytology

Diethylstilbestrol

Diethylstilbestrol (DES), a synthetic estrogen, was marketed as a "miracle drug" that could prevent miscarriage and enable women to deliver stronger, healthier babies. Although its effectiveness began to be questioned as early as 1953, aggressive marketing of DES ultimately resulted in this drug being prescribed to 5 million women between 1938 and 1971 [*Dieckmann 1999*]. Then, in 1970, Herbst, et al, implicated DES, and related drugs, in the development of a rare form of vaginal cancer, clear cell adenocarcinoma, in daughters of treated women [*Herbst 1970a,b, 1971*]. Consequently, in 1971, the Food and Drug Administration (FDA) advised physicians to stop prescribing DES during pregnancy. Nevertheless, DES continues to affect daughters (and possibly sons [a role in ductal-type prostate cancer?]) of women who took DES while pregnant. The DES-related injuries do not become apparent for many years, or even decades, because the "birth defects" are internal, including cervical ectropion and vaginal adenosis [*McDonnell 1984*]. Moreover, many women are unaware that their mothers took DES. It was sold under many brand names, and that was many years ago. Because DES has not been prescribed during pregnancy

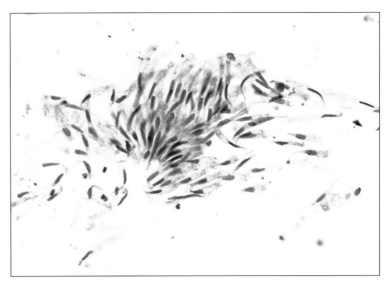

13.8
Thermal artifact, pencils [C]

since 1971, its associated diseases have diminished in incidence, but there are still many DES daughters being followed. It is possible that there will be a second wave of malignancies in these women as they age, but it is unlikely that the daughters of DES daughters will be affected [*Kaufman 2002*].

Vaginal Adenosis

Vaginal adenosis, defined as persistence of Müllerian glandular epithelium in the vagina after birth, was first described in 1877 by von Preuschen [*Antonioli 1975, Sandberg 1968, von Preuschen 1877*]. Vaginal adenosis is characterized cytologically by endocervical-like glandular cells, or metaplastic squamous cells, or both, in a vaginal specimen [*Bibbo 1975, Hart 1976a,b, A Ng 1975, 1977, Robboy 1976*]. Endometrioid columnar-like cells can also occur. For a time, most cases were associated with DES, but today vaginal adenosis usually occurs in women exposed to other hormones, drugs, trauma, inflammation, laser, radiation, or chemotherapy (eg, 5-fluorouracil), as well as idiopathically [*Chattopadhyay 2001, Kurman 1974, Robboy 1986, Sedlacek 1990, Vooijs 1973*]. During the DES era, an autopsy study of postpubertal women, who had no history of gynecologic abnormality, reported vaginal adenosis in 41% of cases [*Sandberg 1968*]. Although nowadays the prevalence of vaginal adenosis may be closer to 10%, this still represents a substantial number of women [*Chattopadhyay 2001, Kranl 1998, Kurman 1974*]

The p63 gene product determines whether Müllerian duct epithelium becomes uterine or vaginal cells. DES causes irregularities in p63 expression leading to vaginal adenosis [*Kurita 2001*]. These women are at risk of neoplasia, including the rare clear cell adenocarcinoma [*Antonioli 1979, Herbst 1971, Robboy 1977*], and the common squamous dysplasia or cancer [*Ben Baruch 1991, Fowler 1981, Hatch 2000, 2001, McDonnell 1984, Orr 1981, Piver 1988, Robboy 1979b, 1981, 1984, Stafl 1974, Verloop 2000, Vessey 1989a*]. Glandular dysplasia has also been described in vaginal adenosis [*Robboy 1976, Scurry 1991*]. Hyperkeratosis, characterized by anucleate squames, is common in women exposed to DES *in utero*. The development of these lesions depends upon the dose of DES and the time of pregnancy. Oncogenic HPVs may be involved in the development of clear-cell adenocarcinoma of the vagina or cervix, though this association is less than that reported for squamous or non-clear-cell adenocarcinomas [*Waggoner 1990*].

Hormone Replacement Therapy

Steroid sex hormones, including oral contraceptives and hormone replacement therapy, can affect both the squamous and the glandular epithelium. The effects depend upon the balance of estrogens and progesterone. Hormone replacement therapy (HRT) in postmenopausal women causes increased maturation of the squamous epithelium. HRT is also a common cause of benign abnormal shedding of endometrial cells in postmenopausal women; however, women receiving HRT (unopposed estrogen therapy) are at increased risk of endometrial carcinoma [H Nelson 2002]. Oral contraceptives and HRT have both been associated with microglandular endocervical hyperplasia (see pg 113). Atypical glandular cells, including reactive, degenerative, and Arias-Stella changes, can also occur, Arias-Stella changes being particularly associated with progesterone.

Oral Contraceptives

Oral contraceptives (birth control pills, or simply, "the pill"), which initiated the "sexual revolution" of the 1960s, are associated with numerous things that can affect the Pap test. Oral contraceptive pills can disrupt the normal vaginal flora and allow *Candida* to proliferate. Oral contraceptives may also increase the risk of *Chlamydia* and other infections. Nippling of endocervical nuclei has sometimes been associated with progesterone, which is present in oral contraceptives [McCallum 1988]. Reactive endocervical cells and Arias-Stella-like changes can occur

Oral Contraceptive Effects

Reactive endocervical cells

Microglandular hyperplasia

Abnormally shed endometrial cells

Decidual cells, Arias–Stella reaction

Candida infections

Cockleburs

Psammoma bodies

↑ risk SILs, SCC, Adenocarcinoma

in women taking oral contraceptives [Affandi 1985, K Lee 1991]. Microglandular hyperplasia has also been associated with oral contraceptives, particularly those that contain progestins [Chumas 1985, TS Kline 1970, Leslie 1984, Nucci 2002, R Young 1989b]. This can lead to exfoliation of pseudoparakeratotic cells, which are degenerated endocervical cells. Breakthrough bleeding at midcycle can lead to abnormal shedding of endometrial cells. However, oral contraceptives containing progesterone may reduce the risk of endometrial carcinoma. Cockleburs (radiate crystalline arrays) [Minassian 1993], psammoma bodies [Valicenti 1977], and decidual cells [V Schneider 1981b] can also be present in Pap tests of women taking oral contraceptives.

Abnormal cytology, ranging from atypia to frank cancer, has long been associated with use of oral contraceptives [W Liu 1967b]. Long-term use of oral contraceptives, by HPV positive women, increases the risk of squamous neoplasia of the cervix [Brinton 1991, Chaouki 1998, LaVecchia 2001, Moreno 2002, Ylitalo 1999, Xi 2002, Zondervan 1996]. There may be an even stronger effect for cervical adenocarcinomas [Brinton 1986a, 1987b, Chilvers 1987, Dallenbach–Hellweg 1984, MW Jones 1989, Kjaer 1993a, Lacey 1999, 2000, Madeleine 2001, R Peters 1986a, Schiffman 1995a, S Schwartz 1986, D Thomas 1996a, Ursin 1994, Valente 1986, WHO 1993, Yeh 1991, Zaino 2000]. Oral contraceptives can cause cervical ectopy, which is associated with inflammation on Pap tests [Bertolino 1992, Brunham 1984, Eckert 1995, Kiviat 1985a,b, J Wilson 1990].

Ectopy could also increase the exposure of the transition zone to HPV infection [Critchlow 1995]. Unlike barrier contraceptives, oral contraceptives offer no protection from acquiring cervical HPV infections. Furthermore, oral contraceptives may promote the activity of HPV once infection has occurred [Auborn 1991, Brinton 1991, Gloss 1987, Hildesheim 1990b, Mitrani–Rosenbaum 1989, Monsonego 1991, A Pater 1990, M Pater 1988, Schiffman 1995a]. Oral contraceptives may induce

folate deficiency, which can not only cause epithelial changes mimicking dysplasia, but may also be a cofactor in carcinogenesis [Butterworth 1982, J Harper 1994, Kitay 1969, Whitehead 1973]. Oral contraceptives possibly can produce cytologic changes mimicking squamous or glandular lesions, which could lead to interpretations of atypical squamous or glandular cells, ASC-US or AGC [Chretien 1998, Kjaer 1996, K Lee 1991, C Morrison 2003].

Long-Acting Hormonal Contraception

Oral contraceptives usually allow normal maturation of the squamous mucosa [Reyniak 1969]. However, long-acting progestin-only contraceptives (eg, depomedroxyprogesterone acetate, Depo-Provera® and levonorgestrel, Norplant®) inhibit pituitary gonadotropin and ovarian hormone synthesis, which inhibits ovulation, thickens the cervical mucous barrier to sperm, and causes loss of endometrial glycogen needed to support implantation [Mishell 1996]. Amenorrhea is a common side effect of long-acting hormonal contraceptives. Serum estradiol (E2) levels are markedly reduced; this can cause decreased bone density and high-density lipoprotein levels [Jeppsson 1977, Mishell 1996]. An early effect of administration of progestins is glycogenation of intermediate cells, similar to navicular cell changes present in pregnancy [Volk 2000]. In long-term users, the hypoestrogenic state can lead to thinning of the vaginal mucosa (atrophy) with a left shift (to intermediate and parabasal cells) in the maturation index [Bahamondes 2000, Bonte 1977, Heber 1975, Kaptain 2002, Mauck 1999, Mishell 1968, Tambouret 2003, Valente 1998]. This, and diminished lactobacilli [Kaptain 2002, L Miller 2000], could compromise the vaginal barrier to infection, including HIV infection [H Martin 1998]. Additionally, changes similar to those occurring in postmenopausal women, described as "atypia of atrophy," may occur and be difficult to differentiate from H SIL [Valente 1998]. However, there is no proven increased risk of dysplasia [Anonymous 1994a,b, Mascarenhas 1998, Misra 1995, 2003].

Megace®

Megace® (megestrol acetate) has a chemical structure similar to the endogenous hormone progesterone. It is used as a treatment for certain cancers, such as those of breast and endometrium. It also has been approved as an appetite stimulant in certain settings. In the Pap test there is an intermediate predominant maturation pattern. Atypical glandular cells, including Arias-Stella-like reactions and decidualization, may be associated with progesterone therapy [13.9].

Tamoxifen®

Tamoxifen® (as well as other anti-estrogen therapy) is commonly used to treat carcinoma of the breast, and more recently, to prevent breast cancer. Tamoxifen is in fact the most important and successful hormonal drug therapy for breast cancer available, and one of the most widely prescribed drugs in the world today [Vrscaj 2001]. Breast cancer cells often have hormone receptors with a strong affinity for estrogen. When estrogen binds to receptor-bearing tumor cells, they are stimulated to grow and divide. Tamoxifen is a nonsteroidal anti-estrogen that blocks estrogen stimulation by binding to estrogen receptors. However, Tamoxifen has paradoxical estrogen-like activity in some tissues.

In addition to its antiestrogen effect, Tamoxifen is known to have certain positive side effects, including increasing bone density (reducing osteoporosis) and reducing the risk of cardiovascular disease. However, Tamoxifen also has negative side effects. In premenopausal women, Tamoxifen disrupts the menstrual cycle and causes ovarian cysts, while in postmenopausal women, it induces ovarian cystic

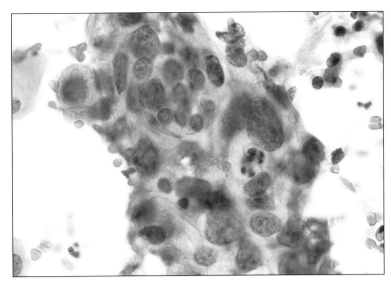

I3.9
AGC, Megace® effect [C]

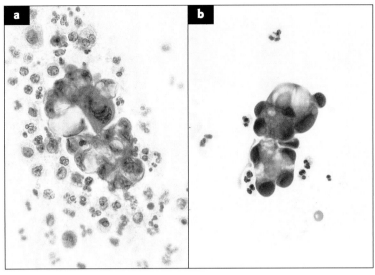

I3.10
a, IUD, mimics adenocarcinoma, note stromal histiocytes [C];
b, IUD, mimics adenocarcinoma [C]

tumors and endometriosis [*Varras 2003*]. Tamoxifen has a toxic effect on endometrium, leading to atrophy, polyps, and uterine fibroids, as well as increased climacteric symptoms, including "hot flashes" and postmenopausal bleeding [*Neven 1993, Vrscaj 2001*]. Further, the International Agency for Research on Cancer (IARC) lists Tamoxifen as a human carcinogen [*IARC 1996*]. There is an increased risk of endometrial carcinoma [*Fornander 1989, Neven 1998, J Seidman 1999, Sherman 2000, Stearns 1998, Suh–Burgmann 1999*], first noted by Killackey et al in 1985 [*Killackey 1985*] and, possibly, other cancers [*Ganesan 1999*].

In premenopausal women, Tamoxifen can cause atrophy of the vaginal mucosa [*Athanassiadou 1992*]. However, in postmenopausal women, Tamoxifen can cause an estrogen-like effect on squamous maturation in Pap tests [*Abadi 2000, Athanassiadou 1992, Bertolissi 1998, Boccardo 1981, Eells 1990, Ferrazzi 1977, Gu 1997, K Liu 1999, Love 2000, Rayter 1994, YJ Yang 2001*]. Vaginal adenosis has been reported in women taking Tamoxifen [*Ganesan 1999, J Johnson 1999*]. Women on Tamoxifen therapy who are shedding endometrial cells may be at increased risk of endometrial carcinoma [*Abati 2000*]. ASCUS-like changes (nuclear enlargement, hyperchromasia, perinuclear halos) have been reported [*B Gill 1998*].

Tamoxifen has also been associated with shedding of clusters of naked nuclei (small, dark, round to oval, with bland chromatin, inconspicuous nucleoli, and slight molding). These nuclei, probably of squamous origin, are similar to those seen in atrophy, but tend to stand out in background of mature squamous cells induced by Tamoxifen therapy [*Opjorden 2001, YJ Yang 2001*]. The differential includes: high-grade squamous lesions, endometrial cells, endometrial carcinoma, and metastatic breast carcinoma as well as rare small blue cell tumors. In cases of doubt, women should receive appropriate follow-up, to exclude a more serious underlying abnormality [*Suh–Burgmann 1999*].

Intrauterine Contraceptive Device (IUD) Changes

Intrauterine contraceptive devices (IUDs) can be associated cellular alterations ("atypia"), which though benign, can be disturbing [*Fornari 1974, P Gupta 1982*]. Because IUDs can cause cytologic changes mimicking glandular or squamous

neoplasia, the clinician must provide history of IUD use. Whether these women are at increased risk of actual squamous intraepithelial lesions, and if so, why, are unresolved questions [*Engineer 1981, B Kaplan 1998, Misra 1989, 1991, Risse 1981*]. Certain infections, such as *Actinomyces*, are more common in women using IUDs.

Reactive endometrial cells and increased numbers of neutrophils and histiocytes are exfoliated soon after insertion of the IUD. Foreign body giant cells and histiocytes containing sperm may be present [*Sagiroglu 1970, 1971*]. Atypical glandular cells, including Arias-Stella-like changes, may occur (discussed below) [*Kobayashi 1997*]. IUD changes can persist for months after removing the device.

Endometrial cells can be shed at any time during the menstrual cycle in women using an IUD. Furthermore, the endometrial cells may appear atypical. Endometrial cells shed singly (see below) or in clusters. The clusters usually are composed of cells with uniform nuclei and scant cytoplasm. However, reactive/degenerative changes are common, including nuclear abnormalities and cytoplasmic vacuolization. There may be evidence of inflammation ("endometritis"). Endometrial stroma, if present nearby, is a good clue to an endometrial origin of the glandular cells [I3.10a]. The differential with adenocarcinoma may be difficult. Features favoring adenocarcinoma include: nuclear enlargement, pleomorphism, abnormal chromatin, prominent nucleoli, and a watery tumor diathesis.

Endocervical cells and metaplastic squamous cells can shed in clusters or papillary aggregates in women using IUDs. These reactive cells are often distended by large, clear cytoplasmic vacuoles, which may contain neutrophils [I3.10b]. The nuclei can be enlarged, hyperchromatic, vary moderately in size, have prominent nucleoli, and be mitotically active. Psammoma bodies occur rarely [*J Barter 1987, Boon 1981c, P Gupta 1978, 1982, Highman 1971*]. Leukophagocytosis may suggest

> ### IUD Changes
> *Endometrial cells, any time of cycle*
> *Reactive glandular or metaplastic cells*
>   *Prominent nucleoli*
>   *Hypervacuolated*
>   *Clean background*
>   *Mimics metastatic adenocarcinoma*
> *Single endometrial cells*
>   *Few, small, high N/C ratios*
>   *Mimics CIN 3*
> *Actinomyces; Ameba; Psammoma bodies*

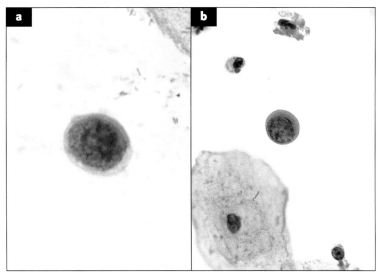

I3.II
a, IUD cell, mimics CIN 3 [C, oil]; **b**, IUD cell, mimics CIN 3 [L]

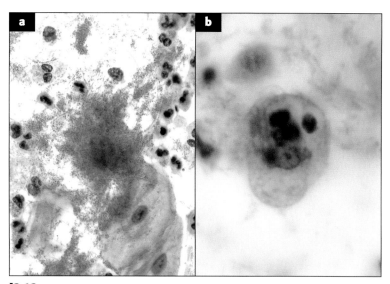

I3.I2
a, IUD, *Actinomyces* [C]; **b**, IUD, amoeba

endometrial adenocarcinoma. Papillary aggregates or clusters of atypical cells, possibly associated with psammoma bodies, in a clean background, can be practically indistinguishable from metastatic adenocarcinoma, particularly of ovarian origin, in a Pap test. *Be cautious reporting adenocarcinoma in a woman using an IUD!*

"IUD cells," which are single, atypical endometrial cells, can also be exfoliated. "IUD cells" resemble single cells of CIN 3 [P Gupta 1978] [I3.IIa,b]. These small cells have high N/C ratios, hyperchromatic nuclei, and finely undulating nuclear membranes. Prominent nucleoli and multinucleation are not seen. The nuclei of CIN 3 usually have chromatin abnormalities and deeply folded ("raisinoid") membranes. "IUD cells" are rare and single, do not form syncytia (hyperchromatic crowded groups), and are not accompanied by a spectrum of squamous dysplasia.

In liquid-based cytology, the findings are similar. Clusters of glandular cells with high N/C ratios, prominent nucleoli, and cytoplasmic vacuolization, sometimes forming signet ring cells, can mimic adenocarcinoma. Single cells with high nuclear/cytoplasmic ratios can mimic H SIL. Although nucleoli can be seen in these single cells, this does not exclude H SIL in liquid-based cytology.

Actinomyces may be discovered in Pap tests of some women using an IUD for long periods of time [I3.I2a] [Arroyo 1989c, Duguid 1980, P Gupta 1976, Schmidt 1982]. In this setting, *Actinomyces* usually indicates only an infestation or superficial infection, rather than deeply invasive disease. Treatment of *Actinomyces* associated with IUD use is controversial (see pg 102).

Amoebae that resemble *Entamoeba gingivalis* are present, rarely, in Pap tests of women using IUDs [I3.I2b] [Arroyo 1989c, deMoraes–Ruehsen 1980, McNeill 1978]. In contrast with *Entamoeba histolytica*, they do not contain red blood cells. *Actinomyces* or Amoebae, if present, supports an interpretation of IUD effect.

IV. Cytology of Pregnancy

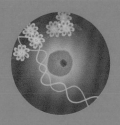

During pregnancy, the glands and stroma of the cervix undergo changes similar to those occurring in the endometrium. The cervical glands become hyperplastic and hypersecretory, producing a mucous plug that seals the uterus like a cork. The cervical stroma becomes decidualized, and softens by action of collagenases, accompanied by accumulation of gel-like mucopolysaccharides and fluid. The cervix enlarges and pushes out into the vagina with eversion of cervical glands (ectopy). Extensive squamous metaplasia follows. The Pap test reflects these physiologic changes [C Michael 1997].

Cytology of Pregnancy

Pap test cannot determine pregnancy!

Intermediate predominant MI (0:100:0)

Navicular cells

Arias-Stella reaction

Decidual cells

Trophoblastic cells

Cockleburs

SILs, cancer can occur!

In the past, cytologists attempted to use the Pap test to predict the time of delivery, fetal maturation, fetal sex, or inevitable abortion, but without much success [Kobayashi 2000]. The Pap test cannot even reliably determine if a woman is pregnant [Meisels 1966b, von Haam 1961]. There are, however, characteristic cellular alterations, and some interpretive traps, that accompany pregnancy [Danos 1968, Fiorella 1993a, Klaus 1971, Kobayashi 1980, Murad 1981, Papanicolaou 1925, Soloway 1969, van Niekerk 1966]. Pregnancy is also a good opportunity to screen for neoplastic cervical lesions as well as for potentially serious infections, including some that could compromise the pregnancy [C Michael 1999, Wied 1963]. In addition, the cytologic method can be useful in evaluation of a wide variety of complications of pregnancy (including amniotic fluid cytology and amniotic fluid embolism) that are beyond the scope of this discussion [M Cohen 1987, Ramzy 1978].

Hormonal Cytology of Pregnancy

During pregnancy, as the corpus luteum (and later the placenta) gear up to manufacture progesterone, the maturation index of the cervical epithelium shifts to intermediate predominance pattern ("shift to the middle" of the maturation index) [Bercovici 1973, Meisels 1966b, 1968, Ortner 1977, Sen 1972]. The intermediate cells are characteristically heavily glycogenated, causing many of the cells to assume an elongated, angular shape, like little boats, known as navicular cells (navicular is the diminutive form of *navis*, which is Latin for ship, the same root as in navy) [Papanicolaou 1933, 1948]. The glycogen stains golden yellow [14.1]. Cytolysis may be extensive.

The placenta uses fetal adrenal hormones as building blocks to manufacture pregnancy-associated hormones, including progesterone. Therefore, a truly atrophic pattern occurring during pregnancy could indicate intrauterine fetal demise. However, parabasal cells of atrophy can be similar to those of immature squamous metaplasia, which is common and can be extensive during pregnancy, mimicking atrophy. At the other extreme of the maturation index, a superficial predominant pattern occurring after the first trimester may suggest intrauterine fetal distress. With decreased fetal adrenal function, decreased progesterone production could result in relative excess of maternal estrogen. However, far more commonly, inflammation/infection causes pseudomaturation.

During the postpartum period, with the fall in hormone levels, the cervicovaginal mucosa atrophies to varying degrees. Atrophy occurs in about one

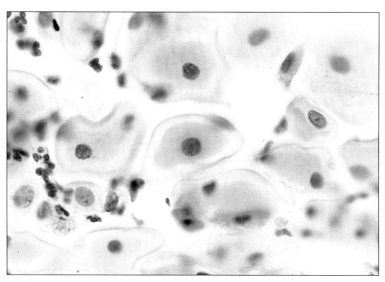

14.1
Navicular cells [C]

third of nonlactating and two thirds of lactating mothers (parabasal predominant maturation pattern). The mucosa matures again within a few weeks, unless the woman is breast-feeding, in which case the mucosa may remain atrophic for the duration of lactation. If the maturation does not return to normal by 1 year, there may be a serious endocrine problem.

The Cells of Pregnancy

Glycogenated intermediate cells (navicular cells), as mentioned, are characteristic of pregnancy [Papanicolaou 1933, 1948]. Increased numbers of histiocytes are also typical, especially early and late in pregnancy. In addition, during pregnancy, endocervical cells tend to be present on the ectocervix (ectropion), where they can be more easily sampled. The endocervical cells often appear reactive ("plump and juicy") during pregnancy, and remain so postpartum, possibly resulting in a cytologic interpretation of atypical glandular cells. Furthermore, noninfectious reactive/reparative changes are common postpartum. This "postpartum atypia" can take up to 8 weeks to regress after delivery [Rarick 1994].

In addition to these cells, there are three types of cells more or less specifically associated with pregnancy. They derive from Arias-Stella reaction, decidua, and trophoblast. These atypical-appearing pregnancy-associated cells can be a source of interpretive errors [Danos 1967, 1968, Frank 1991, Hilrich 1955, Kobayashi 1980, 2000, Murad 1981, Naib 1961a, Soloway 1969, Youseff 1963].

Arias-Stella Reaction

Javier Arias-Stella first called attention to a distinctive, hypersecretory glandular change associated with hyperprogestational states, particularly pregnancy, in 1954 [Arias-Stella 1954]. The changes can begin within days of fertilization [Holmes 1973, V Schneider 1981a]. Arias-Stella reaction can also be caused by oral contraceptives, ovulation-inducing drugs, or other hormonal therapies, particularly those containing progestins. Similar cells can be present in chemotherapy effect [Doss 1995] and in association with intrauterine contraceptive devices (IUDs) [Kobayashi 1997].

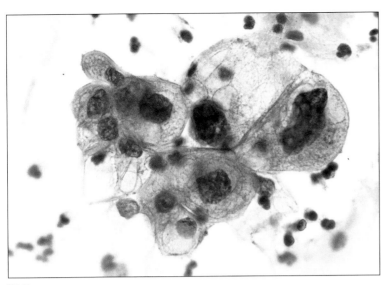

I4.2
Arias-Stella reaction [C]

I4.3
a, Decidual cells [C]; **b**, Decidual cells [C]

Arias-Stella reaction most commonly affects endometrial glands, but can also involve other glands including those of the fallopian tube and endocervix [*Cove 1979, Rhatigan 1992, Silverberg 1972*]. Rarely, Arias-Stella reaction is encountered in Pap tests, where it can lead to interpretive problems, including false-positive results for adenocarcinoma or viral effect [*Albukerk 1974, 1977, J Benoit 1996, Cariani 1966, Chhieng 2001d, Hilrich 1955, V Schneider 1981a*].

Arias-Stella Reaction

Hypersecretory with polyploidy

Nuclei: Big, dark, pleomorphic

Cytoplasm: Abundant, secretory

Differential: Adenocarcinoma (clear cell)

Arias-Stella cells occur singly or in small, loose groups, in a clean background [*Pisharodi 1995*] [I2.77, I4.2]. The cells are large and pleomorphic, with atypical nuclei and voluminous pale ("clear") cytoplasm. The nuclei are big and eccentric (which refers to its location in the cytoplasm, not eccentric like your nutty uncle). The chromatin is hyperchromatic, and ranges from fine to granular to ground glass or smudgy [*J Benoit 1996, Kobayashi 1997*]. Nucleoli are variable, but can be prominent and occasionally multiple [*Shrago 1977*]. Intranuclear cytoplasmic invaginations may be present [*J Benoit 1996, Mulvany 1994, V Schneider 1981a, Yates 1997*]. The nuclei are polyploid (but not aneuploid) [*Kobayashi 1983a*]. Mitotic figures are absent or very rare (be careful if mitoses are present) [*Albukerk 1977, Nucci 2002, R Young 2002*]. Naked nuclei are often present. The abundant cytoplasm is fine to coarsely vacuolated with ill-defined cell borders [*Albukerk 1974, 1977, Kobayashi 1980, 1983a, 1997*]. Occasional bizarre epithelial cells with irregular, giant nuclei may be present [*Mulvany 1994*].

The large, atypical glandular cells of Arias-Stella reaction can be very similar to adenocarcinoma, particularly clear cell type [*Yates 1997*]. Carcinoma produces a mass lesion and is mitotically active; clear cell carcinoma is rare in young women in the post-DES era. *Be cautious reporting clear cell carcinoma during pregnancy or postpartum!* Arias-Stella cells could also be mistaken for herpes viral effect, an important finding in a pregnant woman.

Decidual Cells

Decidual cells are altered stromal cells that contain abundant glycogen and glycoproteins. Decidual cells are present, rarely, in Pap tests of preg-

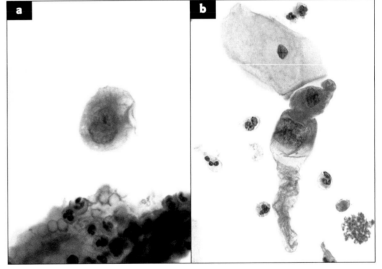

I4.4
a, Decidual cells [L]; **b**, Decidual cells [L]

nant or postpartum women, as well as some women taking oral contraceptives or other hormonal therapies, particularly those containing progestins, such as Megace [*Danos 1967, 1968, Fiorella 1993a, Gladwell 1974, Kobayashi 1980, C Michael 1997, Murad 1981, Pisharodi 1995, V Schneider 1981b, Soloway 1969*]. Their presence in a Pap test usually indicates that the cervical stroma has been decidualized, which is more common in late pregnancy.

Decidual Cells

Parabasal-sized cells

Large nuclei (~ dysplasia)

Chromatin: Bland to reactive

Nucleoli present

Differential: Repair, HSIL, cancer

Decidual cells can be present singly or in small, loose clusters [I4.3a,b, 4.4a,b]. The cells are usually about the size of parabasal to intermediate cells, occasionally larger. They have more or less polygonal outlines, but may have cytoplasmic extensions [C Michaels 1997]. The cytoplasm is finely vacuolated or fibrillar. Decidual cells are usually mononuclear, sometimes have two or three nuclei, but rarely more [Kobayashi 2000, Murad 1981]. The nuclei are large, on average 3 to 4 times the area of an intermediate cell nucleus, but occasionally, they are much larger [V Schneider 1981b]. When well preserved, they have bland, finely granular chromatin. However, degenerative/regenerative changes are common in Pap tests, and can cause nuclear atypia, including condensed, dark chromatin, and prominent nucleoli, mimicking neoplasia. Decidual cells can be mistaken for H SIL (particularly moderate dysplasia in mature metaplastic cells) [C Michaels 1997]. Dysplasia has coarse chromatin, increased N/C ratios, but nucleoli are absent or indistinct. The differential also includes repair, carcinoma, and sarcoma [Danos 1967]. Repair has cohesive sheets, few single cells, and may have mitotic figures. Carcinoma has crowded groups, abnormal chromatin, and may have mucin secretion in adenocarcinoma. Sarcoma has a predominance of single cells, often spindle or pleomorphic shapes, and abnormal chromatin.

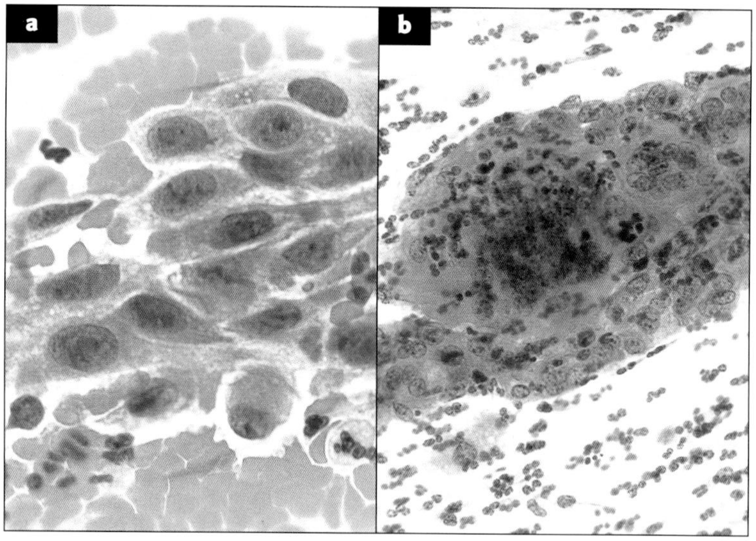

I4.5
a, Cytotrophoblasts [C]; **b**, Trophoblasts [C]

Trophoblasts

Cytotrophoblasts and syncytiotropoblasts derive from the placenta. Trophoblastic cells are rarely present in Pap tests, but they sometimes occur in late pregnancy or following delivery, and exceptionally, can be detected in Pap tests for up to one year following delivery [Fiorella 1993a, Frank 1991]. Although they have been described in the setting of threatened abortion [Holmquist 1967a, Kobayashi 1980, Naib 1961a, Wagner 1968], their presence is not a reliable indicator of an adverse pregnancy outcome [Fiorella 1993a]. If trophoblastic cells are numerous, or abnormal appearing, suspect trophoblastic disease (see pg 178) [Ishi 1998b]. Trophoblastic cells can be mistaken for a neoplastic process [Frank 1991, Naib 1961a, Tambouret 2003].

Trophoblastic Cells
- *Cytotrophoblasts*
  - *Mononucleated*
- *Syncytiotrophoblasts*
  - *Giant cells ~ pomegranates*

Cytotrophoblasts

Cytotrophoblasts occur singly or in small sheets or cohesive clusters [I4.5a,b]. They are small, round to polyhedral cells, with moderately high N/C ratios. The nucleus, usually single, is enlarged, irregular, and hyperchromatic, with a conspicuous nucleolus [Kobayashi 1980]. The cytoplasm is moderate in amount, dense, and may be vacuolated. These cells are rarely present, and difficult to identify specifically, but may suggest a high-grade squamous intraepithelial lesion or poorly-differentiated carcinoma [Frank 1991, Naib 1961a].

Syncytiotrophoblasts

Syncytiotrophoblasts are multinucleated giant cells, with up to 50 or more nuclei [I4.5b, 4.6a,b]. They characteristically have a cytoplasmic extension, or tail, where they detached from the placenta. Syncytiotrophoblasts resemble multinucleated histiocytes—which are far more common in Pap tests—except that trophoblastic nuclei are typically concentrated in the center of the cell. When well preserved, the nuclei have finely granular chromatin, and basophilic or eosinophilic cytoplasm with granular texture [Fiorella 1993a]. With degeneration, which is common, the cytoplasm characteristically stains red-orange and the nuclei stain dark. Hence, syncytiotrophoblasts often look like pomegranates, owing to the central mass of dark nuclei in red-orange cytoplasm. After an abortion, syncytiotrophoblasts can be atypical-to-bizarre appearing, perhaps suggesting choriocarcinoma, a rare malignancy. Weird trophoblastic giant cells can lead to false-positive results for malignancy [Frank 1991, Naib 1961a, Pisharodi 1995]. The differential of multinucleated giant cells in pregnancy includes not only syncytiotrophoblasts and multinucleated giant cell histiocytes, but also herpes infection (an important consideration in pregnancy; look for molding, ground glass chromatin, and inclusions), tumor giant cells (malignant cytologic features), and macrocytes in dysplasia/condyloma (big, dark nuclei in squamous cytoplasm).

Giant Cells in Pregnancy
- *Syncytiotrophoblasts*
- *Giant cell histiocytes*
- *Herpes infection (!)*
- *Dysplasia/Condyloma*
- *Tumor giant cells*

Cockleburs: Pseudoactinomycotic Radiate Granules

Pseudoactinomycotic radiate granules are better known as "cockleburs" (cockleburs!? ...in a Pap test??). These cockleburs are not stickers from weeds, rather they are radiating arrays of golden, refractile material [Bhagavan 1982] [I4.7]. Cockleburs typically measure about 50 μm-100 μm in diameter, are composed of thick, club-shaped spokes, and are usually surrounded by histiocytes. As a general rule (>80% of cases), cockleburs are detected during pregnancy, particularly the second half [Capaldo 1983, Hollander 1974a, Zaharopoulos 1985a,b]. However, less than 5% of pregnant women have cockleburs in their Pap tests [Capaldo 1983]. Their presence apparently has no effect on maternal or fetal prognosis [Capaldo 1983, Minassian 1993].

Cockleburs
- *Pregnancy associated, not specific*
- *Radiate crystalline arrays*
- *Not hematoidin or actinomyces*
- *Up to 100 μm in diameter*
- *Club-shaped spokes*
- *Reddish to golden brown*
- *Histiocytes surround*
- *No affect maternal/fetal prognosis*

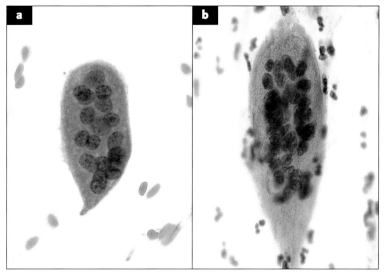

I4.6
a, Syncytiotrophoblast [C]; **b**, Syncytiotrophoblast [C]

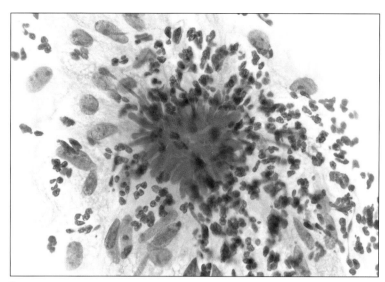

I4.7
"Cocklebur" [C]

Cockleburs can also occur in nonpregnant women, usually in association with use of oral contraceptives or IUDs [Minassian 1993]. Sometimes no obvious cause can be identified. Similar crystalline bodies, related to the Splendore-Hoeppli phenomenon, can be found in nongenital sites, where they are most commonly associated with microorganisms, particularly *Actinomyces*, or foreign bodies. However, Splendore-Hoeppli phenomenon is thought to be an antigen-antibody reaction, and contains immunoglobulin. Cockleburs contain neither *Actinomyces* nor immunoglobulins.

Cockleburs in the female genital tract apparently form in stagnating secretions from products of degenerating cells, which surround microorganisms or biologically inert substances [Zaharopoulos 1985a,b]. Cockleburs are composed of nonimmune glycoprotein, lipid, and calcium and do not contain immunoglobulin, glycogen, or mucin [Bhagavan 1982]. In contrast with actinomycotic granules, genital cockleburs do not have visible central filaments in the radiating spokes.

The cockleburs discussed here are *not* hematoidin radiate crystals, which are also sometimes known as "cockleburs" or "chestnut burs." Hematoidin is an iron-free, bile-like pigment formed in hypoxic tissue from hemoglobin and usually indicates old bleeding. Hematoidin crystals are far less common in Pap tests than the cockleburs under discussion. Hematoidin crystals are present not only as radiate forms, but also as spherules, rhomboids, or irregular shapes. Hematoidin crystals are usually much smaller than genital cockleburs and the crystalline rays of hematoidin burs are much finer [Zaharopoulos 1985a,b].

Cervical Neoplasia During Pregnancy

Pregnancy is an ideal opportunity for Pap test screening, since women usually seek health care at this time [Creasman 2001, Fry 1969, C Michael 1999]. Women in their reproductive years are also the primary age group at risk for squamous intraepithelial lesions [Boutselis 1972, DePetrillo 1975, Kashimura 1991, M Smith 1968]. HPV infection and dysplasia are at least as common in pregnant as in non-pregnant women [K Kaplan 2004, Lu 2003, Oriel 1971, A Schneider 1987a]. Moreover, cervical cancer (and breast cancer) are the most common malignancies diagnosed during pregnancy, but fortunately, still rare [Bokhman 1989, Creasman 2001, Haas 1984, Hannigan 1990, K Kaplan 2004, W Jones 1996, Pavlidis 2002, R Ward 2002]. The cytobrush has been found safe to use during pregnancy, although minimal traumatic bleeding may occur [Orr 1992].

There are no significant differences in the cytologic features of dysplasia (or cancer) between pregnant and nonpregnant women: dysplasia is dysplasia. Cytologic interpretation is reasonably accurate during pregnancy [Bertini–Oliveira 1982, Fowler 1980, Kashimura 1991, LaPolla 1988, Reagan 1961a, Richart 1963b, Rutledge 1962, Yoonessi 1982]. However, inflammatory changes and increased activity of various cell types can mimic dysplasia, sometimes resulting in a difficult differential. The endocervix is shorter and slightly dilated, so the squamocolumnar transformation zone may be more accessible, theoretically making it easier to obtain abnormal cells. On the other hand, in practice, clinicians may be concerned about taking a vigorous endocervical sample during pregnancy. Postpartum atypia can also present interpretive challenges [I4.8].

Cervical Neoplasia in Pregnancy
L SIL to Cancer
Usual criteria for interpretation
Pregnancy ideal time to screen
High regression rate postpartum,
but lesions may recur

Many dysplasias, particularly low-grade lesions, regress postpartum, perhaps related to trauma during delivery or change in immune status after delivery [Ahdoot 1998, JL Benedet 1987, Hellberg 1987, A Kaplan 1967, K Kaplan 2004, Kiguchi 1981, Siddiqui 2001, Yoonessi 1982]. A meta-analysis of 8 published series showed that about 15% of SILs progressed, 35% persisted, and 50% regressed during pregnancy [K Kaplan 2004]. In addition, many SILs, particularly H SILs, recur within 5 years [Hellberg 1987, K Kaplan 2004].

While the morphology of dysplasia does not change in pregnancy, the management may be very different. *The primary goal is to rule out invasive cancer.* If a noninvasive lesion is detected cytologically, it should be followed by careful, repeated colposcopy, cytology, and possibly directed biopsies [Creasman 2001, Economos 1993, Hellberg 1987, Kirkup 1980, Kohan 1980, LaPolla 1988, Lundvall 1989, McDonnell 1981, Yoonessi 1982]. Cone biopsy and cryotherapy should be avoided if at all possible. If microinvasive squamous cell carcinoma is suspected, the abnormal area should be excised to exclude frankly invasive cancer. If microinvasive disease is

Cytology of Pregnancy

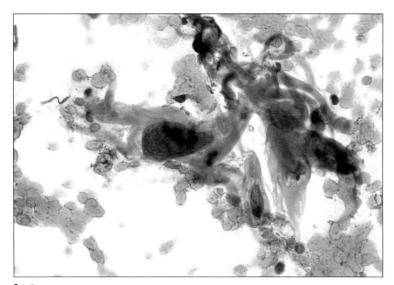

I4.8
Postpartum atypia [C]

Miscellaneous Pregnancy Findings

Puerperal Endometritis

Puerperal endometritis, due to bacterial infection, can occur following abortion or delivery. Before the age of antibiotics, this was a dreaded complication of pregnancy, but fortunately is now rare. Retained products of conception can be a source of bleeding. A Pap test might contain reactive trophoblastic elements (irregularly distributed chromatin, molding, prominent nucleoli), fresh and old blood, neutrophils, histiocytes, fragmentation of nucleus and cytoplasm, or foreign body-type giant cells.

Vitamin Deficiency in Pregnancy

Folate deficiency, when it occurs, usually does so in postmenopausal women. However, it may occur during pregnancy, preeclampsia, and dietary deficiency [Kitay 1969]. The cytologic effects are exactly the same as in folate deficiency in nonpregnant women, and is manifested mostly by macrocytes (see pg 172).

Cells of Fetal Origin

Fetal Squamous Cells

Anucleate squamous cells may indicate rupture of the amnion. In theory, squamous cells of fetal origin can be distinguished from maternal anucleate squames by the presence of intracytoplasmic lipid that stains with Nile blue [Kittrich 1963]. In practice, after the 36th week, a dry, unfixed smear (best obtained by pipette from the internal cervical os) is stained; fetal cells stain pink and are diagnostic of rupture of membranes [Fry 1969].

Fetal Erythrocytes

Fetal erythrocytes can sometimes be found in Pap tests associated with abortion [Kobayashi 2000]. They have orangeophilic cytoplasm with a central India ink dot-like nucleus.

confirmed, definitive therapy can be delayed until after delivery [Giuntoli 1991, Sivanesaratnam 1993]. However, if frankly invasive cancer is found or strongly suspected, it must be treated definitively, which usually means terminating the pregnancy (abortion or early delivery [cesarean section preferred]). A short delay in cancer therapy, particularly for stage I disease, may be carefully considered if the fetus is near viability and the woman is willing to take the risk [Canavan 2000, Creasman 2001]. Note that the detection of trophoblastic disease and choriocarcinoma by the Pap test is unreliable. These diseases occur at some distance from the cervix and the cells do not shed consistently.

V. Cytology of the Rare and Sundry

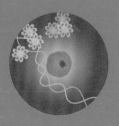

Most of the clinically important lesions that can be detected in Pap tests are the common squamous and glandular lesions described in mind numbing detail above. Believe it or not, there are still many more, often rare, conditions that can affect the cervix; some of these are discussed below. Not only can it be important to recognize these conditions specifically, but some of them could also be mistaken for other lesions. Pemphigus vulgaris is a good example of a rare benign disease that can easily be misinterpreted as malignant in a Pap test. Rare variants of squamous cell carcinoma, such as verrucous carcinoma, and rare variants of adenocarcinoma, such as adenoid cystic carcinoma, were discussed previously. Now get out your toothpicks and prop your eyes open to read the following...

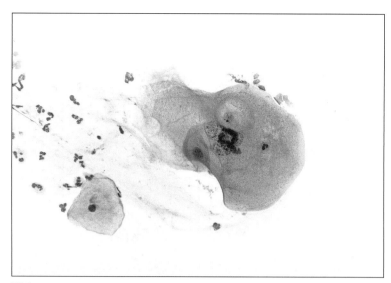

15.1
Macrocyte [C]

Non-Neoplastic Conditions

Vitamin Deficiency Cytology

In the face of either folate or B_{12} vitamin deficiency, cellular changes can occur that are similar to those present secondary to radiotherapy (in essence, polychromatic macrocytes) [van Niekerk 1966]. Folate and vitamin B_{12} are coenzymes in DNA synthesis. B_{12}-methyl deficiency leads to thymine deficiency, which mimics radiation DNA injury. Folate deficiency is relatively common in late pregnancy, postmenopause, and with use of some oral contraceptives [Kitay 1969, Whitehead 1973]. Epithelial cell changes can antedate megaloblastic changes in the bone marrow by several weeks.

The characteristic cytologic changes are primarily nuclear and cytoplasmic enlargement with the formation of macrocytes. Macrocytes can also be present in radiation or chemotherapy (particularly folate antagonists, eg, methotrexate and cyclophosphamide) and in condyloma [15.1]. Similar cells can rarely be present in other viral infections such as measles [Heimann 1992]. Abnormalities of an enzyme (polymorphism of methylenetetrahydrafolate reductase) involved in folate metabolism and DNA synthesis may increase the risk of cervical intraepithelial neoplasia [M Goodman 2001, Lambropoulos 2003, Piyathilake 2000].

Cells with enlarged nuclei may be essentially indistinguishable from dysplasia, usually of mild degree (low-grade squamous intraepithelial lesion) [Kitay 1969], which is probably far more common than cytologic manifestations of vitamin deficiency. Although a course of vitamin therapy, followed by the disappearance of the changes on repeated Pap test supports the notion of vitamin effect, women with persistent epithelial changes should be considered for colposcopy. Here's a hot tip: if you suspect vitamin deficiency, count lobes of neutrophils (<5 lobes is normal; more than a few neutrophils with 5 lobes, or any with ≥6 lobes, indicates megaloblastic anemia).

Pemphigus Vulgaris

Pemphigus vulgaris is a rare autoimmune, blistering disease in which autoantibodies against one of the cadherins, desmoglein3, are formed. This leads to lysis of the intercellular connections (desmosomes) of the epithelial cells, resulting in acantholysis of skin and mucous membranes that results in separation of the cells of the spinous cell layer with consequent formation of vesicles and bullae (blisters). The junction between epithelium and connective tissue is not affected. When the blisters rupture they leave a raw, ulcerated surface.

The mouth is almost always affected. In women with generalized disease, the cervix is commonly involved [RH Kaufman 1969, Lonsdale 1998, G Mikhail 1967]. The cervix can be affected by pemphigus in the absence of other manifestations of the disease; in these cases, the Pap test is more likely to be misinterpreted as positive for malignancy [D Friedman 1971, RH Kaufman 1969, Krain 1973, Libcke 1970]. Owing to the autoimmune destruction of desmosomes, a blister forms, leaving a zone of basal/parabasal cells, known as Tzanck (acantholytic) cells, attached to the basement membrane. The Nikolsky sign may be positive (the blister extends laterally with pressure) [Sagher 1974, C Wright 2000]. The denuded area can be mistaken, clinically, for cervical ectopy ("erosion") [D Friedman 1971].

Tzanck cells are parabasal-sized, present singly and in loose clusters. They are characterized by round nuclei, with smooth, thin nuclear membranes, fine pale chromatin, and prominent, irregular nucleoli (classically, bullet shaped) [15.2] [E Chan 1998, S Gupta 2003c, Krain 1973, Libcke 1970, Valente 1984, C Wright 2000]. In cytologic samples, these cells mimic repair, except for the striking predominance of single cells (because of the damage to the intercellular junctions). Single cells, with high N/C ratios, prominent nucleoli, and mitotic figures may erroneously suggest malignancy. Clues to a benign process include, first and foremost, clinical history of the disease (which must be provided by the clinician); uniform nuclear size; smooth, thin nuclear membranes; fine pale chromatin; and often, a characteristic perinuclear acidophilia (red staining cytoplasm around the nucleus). Irregular nuclei, coarse dark chromatin, and a necrotic background favor a neoplastic process [E Chan 1998, Dvoretsky 1985]. Without being provided with the history of pemphigus, Tzanck cells could be misinterpreted as malignant [RH Kaufman 1969, Krain 1973, Libcke 1970, C Wright 2000]. Note, however, it is possible for both genital tract neoplasia and pemphigus to occur in the same patient (in a blue moon) [Krain 1973, Dvoretsky 1985].

Malakoplakia

Malakoplakia was first described by Michaelis and Gutmann in 1902 [Michaelis 1902], followed by von Hansemann in 1903 [von Hansemann 1903]. It is a rare, chronic inflammatory disease usually associated with *Escherichia coli*, but also other with organisms such as *Klebsiella*, *Mycobacterium*, *Staphylococcus aureus*, and even fungi. Although the exact pathogenesis is still uncertain, it is probably

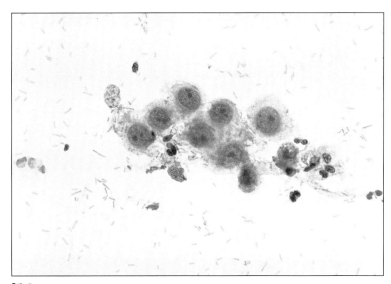

I5.2
Pemphigus, cervix [C]

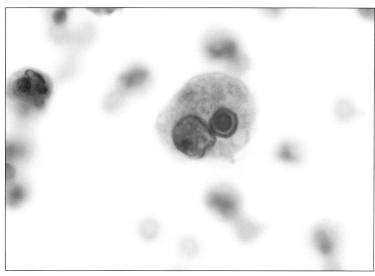

I5.3
Malakoplakia, bladder [C]

related to the inability of macrophages to digest phagocytozed bacteria completely, owing to an enzymatic defect in lysosomes. Immunodeficiency, such as in transplant recipients, autoimmune disease, or AIDS, is also associated with the development of malakoplakia.

The term "malakoplakia" is derived from the Greek *malakos* and *plakos* meaning "soft plaque," which describes the characteristic lesions. Malakoplakia most commonly affects the urinary tract, especially the bladder and kidney, but rarely, many other bodily organs can be involved, including the female genital tract [K Chen 1985, Pfeifer 1999, Saad 1993]. Women with genital tract involvement are usually elderly and present with postmenopausal bleeding. Friable lesions can clinically look malignant.

Cervical malakoplakia has been identified in Pap tests [Falcón-Escobedo 1986, Kapila 1989, Stewart 1991, Wahl 1982]. Microscopically, the lesion consists of a xanthogranulomatous proliferation dominated by sheets of histiocytes with granular cytoplasm (von Hansemann histiocytes). Scattered plasma cells and lymphocytes also occur. Pathognomonic Michaelis-Gutmann (MG) bodies are present in some of the histiocytes [I5.3]. MG bodies are ~4 μm-10 μm, basophilic, laminated ("targetoid"), intracytoplasmic inclusions. They are composed of mucopolysaccharides and lipids similar to those in bacterial cell walls, especially of *E. coli*, supporting bacterial origin of the inclusions. These organic elements constitute the matrix for the deposition of calcium and other inorganic salts, thereby forming the distinctive targetoid inclusions. MG bodies can be highlighted with von Kossa (calcium) stain, Perl (iron) stain, or periodic acid-Schiff (PAS) stain.

Treatment of malakoplakia involves surgical excision, or incision and drainage, in conjunction with antibiotic therapy, and discontinuation of any immune suppressing drugs, if feasible. The mortality for those treated is ~15%, but is greater than 80% in the untreated [Van der Voort 1996].

Neoplastic Conditions

Neuroendocrine Carcinomas

Neuroendocrine carcinomas of the cervix, first described in 1976 by Albores-Saavedra et alia [Albores-Saavedra 1976], are rare neoplasms that run the gamut from well-differentiated carcinoid tumors to poorly-differentiated small cell carcinomas. Large cell neuroendocrine carcinomas and mixed large cell/small cell neuroendocrine carcinomas can also occur. Because these tumors are morphologically similar to their pulmonary counterparts, a similar classification system has been adopted (typical carcinoid tumor, atypical carcinoid tumor, small cell neuroendocrine carcinoma, large cell neuroendocrine carcinoma,and combined tumors) [Albores-Saavedra 1997]. These tumors can be difficult to recognize specifically in Pap tests. The use of special studies, formerly, silver stains [Albores-Saavedra 1976, Mullins 1981] or electron microscopy [Groben 1985, Mackay 1979, Ueda 1989, A Watanabe 2000], but nowadays, immunocytochemistry [R Barrett 1987, van Nagell 1988], can facilitate interpretation, but are impractical for a screening test.

Small Cell Neuroendocrine Carcinoma

Small cell neuroendocrine cervical carcinoma is uncommon, accounting for 1% to 5% of cervical malignancies, although it is the most common neuroendocrine carcinoma of the uterine cervix [Abeler 1994, Conner 2002, van Nagell 1988]. The age peak is in the late 30s to early 40s, younger than the average woman with squamous cell carcinoma, but there is a wide age range (~18-90 years) [J Chan 1989, Conner 2002, Mannion 1998, Reich 1996, Viswanathan 2004]. The clinical presentation is similar to ordinary cervical carcinoma, but rarely some women have clinical or biochemical evidence of hormone production, including Cushing syndrome, carcinoid syndrome, hypoglycemia, or syndrome of inappropriate antidiuretic hormone secretion (SIADH) [Hashi 1996, Ishibashi-Ueda 1996, A Watanabe 2000]. The tumor is associated with squamous or glandular carcinomas, in situ or invasive, in about one-half of cases [Eichhorn 2001].

Unfortunately, the Pap test cannot prevent small cell carcinoma [Abeler 1994, Gersell 1988, Hoerl 2000, P-H Wang 1998, A Walker 1988, Zhou 1998b]. There is no known precursor lesion for the Pap test to detect and tumor can develop rapidly in the interval between screenings. However, the frequent association with H SIL may lead to fortuitous early detection in some cases. This malignancy is aggressive and has a poor prognosis [Connor 2002, Hoskins 1995, Viswanathan 2004, Weed 2003]. A further note: the poor prognosis attributed to small cell squamous carcinoma may have been unduly influenced by inadvertent inclusion of small cell neuroendocrine carcinomas.

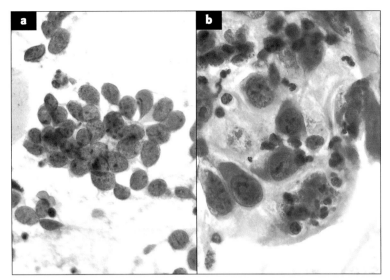

I5.4
a, Small cell carcinoma [C]; **b**, Non-small cell component [C]

Small cell neuroendocrine carcinoma of the female genital tract histologically and cytologically closely resembles its pulmonary counterpart [Albores-Saavedra 1997, Bing 2004, Ciesla 2001, J Chan 1989, Fujii 1986, Gersell 1988, Groben 1985, Hoerl 2000, R Joseph 1992, Kamiya 1993, Y Kim 2002, Mannion 1998, W-K Ng 2003a, Proca 1998, Reich 1996, Zhou 1998b] [I5.4a]. Cytologically, the tumor usually shows moderate to high cellularity [Y Kim 2002]. The malignant cells lie singly or in small clusters. They are small, round-to-oval or irregular in outline, and have prominent nuclear molding, very high N/C ratios, fine, dark chromatin, inconspicuous or absent nucleoli, and very scant delicate cytoplasm. Mitoses and apoptosis may be present. Hyperchromatic crowded groups may suggest squamous or glandular neoplasia. Rosettes and focal feathering may suggest glandular differentiation [Ciesla 2001, Zhou 1998b]. Crush artifact may be prominent in conventional Pap smears. The background is necrotic [A Watanabe 2000]. The common association with squamous or glandular neoplasia is probably related to their shared viral etiology. Finally, as with the pulmonary counterpart, some small cell carcinomas have a large cell component (mixed small cell/large cell carcinoma) or may be combined with squamous or adenocarcinoma [I5.4b] [Conner 2002].

In liquid-based cytology, the cytologic findings are similar, except that crush artifact is absent and molding is less prominent. However, nucleoli may be slightly more conspicuous in LBC [Ciesla 2001, Hoerl 2000, W-K Ng 2003a].

Small cell neuroendocrine carcinoma of the cervix is strongly associated with human papillomavirus, particularly type 18 [Abeler 1994, Ambros 1991, W-K Ng 2003a, Stoler 1991, Wistuba 1999], while lung cancer is only rarely HPV positive [Clavel 2000b]. Thyroid transcription factor-1 (TTF-1) is characteristically associated with pulmonary small cell carcinoma, but is also expressed in about one-third of small cell neuroendocrine carcinomas of the female genital tract [Agoff 2000, Bing 2004, Cheuk 2001, W-K Ng 2003a, Ordonez 2000].

Epithelial and neuroendocrine immunomarkers are characteristically expressed. Neuroendocrine immunomarkers include neuron-specific enolase, chromogranin, and synaptophysin; epithelial immunomarkers include epithelial membrane antigen and cytokeratins [Ambros 1991, R Joseph 1992, Kamiya 1993, A Watanabe 2000]. A confounding factor, however, is that some squamous cell carcinomas and adenocarcinomas may undergo focal neuroendocrine differentiation, but this is usually limited to isolated cells [Ambros 1991, R Barrett 1987, S Lee 1994, Savargaonkar 1996],

while up to one-half of cervical small cell neuroendocrine carcinomas fail to express neuroendocrine markers [Ambros 1991, Conner 2002, Gersell 1988]. Thus, the bottom line is that the recognition of small cell neuroendocrine carcinoma of the cervix remains a morphologic interpretation, not an immunocytochemical one [Conner 2002].

Malignancies with small tumor cells are a "mixed bag" of neoplasms that includes not only small cell neuroendocrine carcinoma and carcinoid tumor, but also poorly-differentiated squamous cell carcinoma, poorly-differentiated adenocarcinoma, adenoid cystic carcinoma, and adenoid basal cell carcinoma [Albores-Saavedra 1976]. In addition, lymphomas, sarcomas, and melanoma can be composed of "small blue cells." Small cell neuroendocrine carcinomas can also be difficult to distinguish from normal or atypical endometrial cells, well-differentiated endometrial carcinoma, metastatic carcinoma (eg, breast), inflammatory exudate, and follicular cervicitis, particularly when the cells are poorly preserved [Ciesla 2001]. Clusters of naked nuclei, such as in atrophy, can also mimic small cell carcinoma. Of course, metastatic small cell carcinoma from another site, usually lung, must be excluded before accepting a primary tumor in the cervix. Because of the aggressive nature of small cell neuroendocrine carcinoma and possible therapeutic differences, it is important to try to separate it from other, more common tumors such as poorly-differentiated (small cell) squamous cell carcinoma [Conner 2002].

Small cell squamous carcinoma has somewhat more and denser cytoplasm, better-defined cell borders, and less crush artifact than small cell neuroendocrine carcinoma. Coarse chromatin with parachromatin clearing, more conspicuous nucleoli, and less nuclear molding also favor squamous origin. Abnormal keratinized cells favor squamous carcinoma, but do not completely exclude neuroendocrine carcinoma since it can be associated with a squamous lesion. Either tumor type can have spindle cells.

Endometrial adenocarcinoma is more pleomorphic, with coarser chromatin, and more prominent nucleoli than small cell carcinoma. Rosettes in neuroendocrine tumors may be difficult to distinguish from rudimentary gland lumens in adenocarcinoma, but columnar cell shape or mucin points to adenocarcinoma.

Other Neuroendocrine Tumors

Neuroendocrine tumors include carcinoid tumor (well-differentiated neuroendocrine carcinoma) and atypical carcinoid tumor (moderately-differentiated neuroendocrine carcinoma). These tumors form a spectrum with small cell (poorly-differentiated) neuroendocrine carcinoma. Large cell neuroendocrine carcinoma is an aggressive, rare tumor in the cervix.

Carcinoid Tumors

Carcinoid tumors (well-differentiated neuroendocrine carcinomas) of the uterine cervix are very rare. However, they are morphologically similar to carcinoids occurring at other body sites, although clinical syndromes are less common and classic carcinoid syndrome is rare [Albores-Saavedra 1979, 1997, H Fox 1964, Koch 1999, Mannion 1998, Scully 1984, Stockdale 1986, Tateishi 1975]. Also, some cases may represent adenocarcinoids, as seen in the gastrointestinal tract (and recall that scattered neuroendocrine cells can often be found in ordinary cervical cancers on diligent search using special stains).

The cytology of carcinoid tumor is characterized by small, round, uniform cells, with scant cytoplasm and high N/C ratios, that are present singly or in small aggregates [Hirahatake 1990, Miles 1985]. The cells resemble small lymphocytes or plasma cells (lymphoplasmacytoid cells) or, uncommonly, small spindle cells. "Salt and pepper" chromatin and cytoplasmic neurosecretory granules are characteristic features. Mitotic figures are absent or rare. Papillary structures, psammoma bodies, and amyloid have been reported in neuroendocrine carcinoma [Albores–Saavedra 1997, Russin 1987]. The background is clean without necrosis. Carcinoid tumors often co-exist with squamous or glandular lesions, including carcinomas [Mullins 1981, Stahl 1981, Warner 1978].

Atypical carcinoid tumor (moderately-differentiated neuroendocrine carcinoma) also occurs, very rarely, in the cervix. These tumors are intermediate in morphology and behavior between typical carcinoid and small cell carcinoma. There is mild to moderate nuclear atypia, some mitotic activity, and focal necrosis [Eichhorn 2001].

Large Cell Neuroendocrine Carcinoma

Large cell neuroendocrine carcinoma is an aggressive poorly-differentiated tumor. Although rare, it may be more common than generally appreciated because it cannot be recognized specifically without the use of special studies, such as immunocytochemistry [Eichhorn 2001]. Morphologically, it can be mistaken for squamous or adenocarcinoma. The patients average 34 years of age (range, ~20 to >60 years) [Gilks 1997]. The prognosis is poor. Histologically, the tumor grows in trabeculae or solid sheets and may form glands (or gland-like spaces) [Krivak 2001, Y Sato 2003].

Cytologically, the tumor may exfoliate hyperchromatic crowded groups. The tumor cells are large and have moderately abundant cytoplasm. The nuclei are about 3 to 5 times the size of an intermediate cell nucleus and have irregular outlines, but pleomorphism is not usually marked. The chromatin is coarse; there are 2 or more prominent nucleoli, and mitotic figures are present. There is often extensive necrosis in the background [Albores–Saavedra 1997, WY Lee 2002, Rhentula 2001]. Neuroendocrine and epithelial markers are positive. Like small cell neuroendocrine carcinoma, this tumor can be associated with squamous or glandular lesions [Gilks 1997, Yun 1999]. HPV has been reported, suggesting common origin [Cui 2001, Yun 1999].

Large cell neuroendocrine carcinoma differs from atypical carcinoid in being more pleomorphic, more mitotically active, and having more extensive necrosis. It differs from small cell neuroendocrine carcinoma by larger cell size, larger nuclei, coarser chromatin, more prominent nucleoli, and more abundant cytoplasm, and lacks nuclear molding and crush artifact. The differential with nonkeratinizing squamous carcinoma may be difficult or impossible, in some cases, without the use of special studies. However, squamous cell carcinoma tends to have more marked nuclear pleomorphism and denser cytoplasm [WY Lee 2002].

Mesenchymal Tumors

Both benign and malignant mesenchymal tumors can involve the cervix or vagina. Leiomyomas are, by far, the most common benign "soft tissue tumors" of these sites. Other benign mesenchymal tumors that can be encountered include: hemangiomas, nerve sheath tumors, granular cell tumors, and lipomas, among other rare tumors [G Nielsen 2001]. None of these is likely to be shed cells in Pap tests unless the cervix is involved and the overlying epithelium is denuded; even then, exfoliation of tumors cells is uncertain [Oda 2004].

Sarcomas, ie, malignant neoplasms of mesenchyme, are rare [Bonfiglio 1976, Ito 2004]. They account for less than 10% of uterine (corpus) cancers and only about 1% of cervical cancers, as well as a small number of malignancies of fallopian tube, ovary, vagina, and vulva. Stromal sarcomas and leiomyosarcomas comprise ~90% of uterine sarcomas, not counting carcinosarcomas (malignant mixed Müllerian tumors) which are actually metaplastic epithelial malignancies. Morphologically, sarcomas can be pure mesenchymal tumors (eg, leiomyosarcoma, endometrial stromal sarcoma, rhabdomyosarcoma, fibrosarcoma, neuroectodermal tumors) or mixed with epithelial elements, which can be either benign-appearing or malignant (see mixed Müllerian tumors, pg 177) [G Nielsen 2001].

Pap tests usually cannot detect sarcomas of the female genital tract because characteristic cells rarely exfoliate. Exfoliation is affected by several factors, including the location of the tumor, ulceration, necrosis, and inflammation. When numerous, well-preserved tumor cells are present in the specimen, sarcomas can often be recognized as malignant, but they may be difficult to classify specifically, by cytology alone. Sarcomas shedding few, small, or cytologically bland cells are difficult to detect [Ito 2004].

General Cytologic Features of Sarcomas

Sarcomas, characteristically, shed predominantly as single cells. True tissue aggregates and cellular or nuclear molding are less common in sarcomas than carcinoma. The tumor cells frequently look very "ugly," with obvious malignant features, although the chromatin tends to be fine in well preserved cells. Multinucleated giant tumor cells or nonkeratinized spindle tumor cells suggest sarcoma [Ces-Blanco 1977]. The cytoplasm often has a fibrillar, granular, or glassy quality, unlike that seen in carcinomas, and tends to stain cyanophilic or orange. Cell borders are usually poorly defined. In many cases, the tumor cells are small and degenerated [R Graham 1958a]. Small sarcoma cells may be confused with isolated cells originating from virtually any small cell type of lesion [Patten 1978]. Because these tumors arise in stroma, they usually must be ulcerated to exfoliate cells; therefore, a tumor diathesis is common in Pap tests of sarcomas [X Wang 2002]. Immunomarkers can support mesenchymal origin and specify differentiation, eg, smooth muscle, but are too costly for screening.

Sarcoma
  Usually easy to recognize as malignant
  ...but can be difficult to classify
  Most are spindle cell sarcomas
    Cells: Mostly single, "ugly"
    Nuclei: Very abnormal
    Cytoplasm: Glassy or fibrillar

Sarcomas
  Leiomyosarcoma
    Spindle or epithelioid cells
    Low or high grade
  Stromal sarcoma
    ~ Endometrial stroma cells
  Rhabdomyosarcoma
    Cross-striations
  Primitive neuroectodermal tumor
    Small blue cells
  Immunomarkers helpful

Leiomyoma and Leiomyosarcoma

Smooth muscle tumors are the most common soft tissue tumors of the uterus. They can be benign or malignant, ie, leiomyomas or leiomyosarcomas. It is not necessarily easy to distinguish these cytologically: benign smooth muscle tumors can show marked cytologic atypia, while malignant ones can be cytologically bland. The final diagnosis depends upon histologic analysis of cellularity, nuclear atypia, and mitotic count.

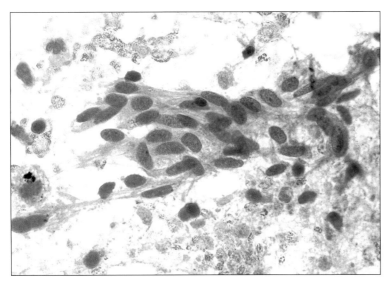

I5.5
Leiomyoma [C]

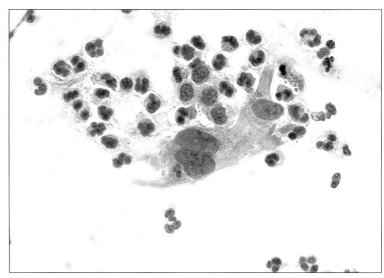

I5.6
Leiomyosarcoma [C]

Leiomyoma

Leiomyomas are hormonally dependent, benign tumors of smooth muscle cells. Leiomyomas are the most common tumors of the uterus, although the cervix is less commonly affected than the corpus. They arise in the myometrium and cannot be identified in Pap tests, unless they involve the cervix and the overlying epithelium ulcerates. The smooth muscle cells usually are spindle shaped cells, with cigar-shaped nuclei, fine chromatin, small nucleoli, and fibrillar cytoplasm [I5.5]. Degeneration may cause nuclear hyperchromasia, suggesting malignancy, but the degenerated chromatin appears smudgy. Ulceration with necrosis mimics a tumor diathesis. Nonneoplastic smooth muscle cells can sometimes be found in Pap tests, eg, following uterine trauma [Kobayashi 2000].

Leiomyosarcoma

Leiomyosarcoma accounts for about half of sarcomas of the uterine corpus, but cervical or vaginal origin is rare [Curtin 1995]. It predominantly affects women older than 40 years. It can arise de novo or as malignant change occurring in a benign leiomyoma (which is rare). Leiomyosarcomas are divided into low-grade and high-grade neoplasms, which has important prognostic implications. Mitotic activity and nuclear anaplasia are important prognostic features. Low-grade tumor cells often resemble benign smooth muscle; high-grade tumor cells can be difficult to classify specifically.

Leiomyosarcoma does not exfoliate cells readily [X Wang 2002]. When tumor cells are present, they are found singly or in small loose clusters with indistinct cell borders. The tumor cells are usually spindle-shaped but occasionally are plump and epithelioid [Ito 2004, Massoni 1984]. Cells vary (from case to case) from uniform and small to pleomorphic and giant [I5.6]. Cytoplasm is ill defined, transparent, or fibrillar. Nuclei of low-grade tumor cells are usually oval to cigar-shaped, with finely granular, irregular chromatin. High-grade tumor cells exhibit marked nuclear pleomorphism, irregular nuclear membranes, coarse, dark chromatin, and prominent or irregular nucleoli. A myxoid background occurs in some cases (myxoid leiomyosarcoma). Epithelioid tumor cells are oval to polygonal, instead of spindle or pleomorphic, have large nuclei, containing prominent nucleoli, and the cells may form three-dimensional clus-

ters. Epithelioid leiomyosarcoma could be misinterpreted as carcinoma, although the cytoplasm tends to be pale and fibrillar in sarcoma. The differential also includes atypical repair, decidual cells, and metastatic tumors, such as melanoma. Benign leiomyomas can show cytologic atypia and necrotic background mimicking leiomyosarcoma.

Endometrial Stromal Sarcoma

Endometrial stromal tumors scale the range from benign stromal nodules to high-grade stromal sarcomas. Endometrial stromal sarcoma accounts for about 40% of uterine sarcomas. The average age is the fifth decade. Abnormal uterine bleeding is the most common symptom. In theory, abnormal shedding of endometrial stromal cells could be a potential clue to this entity. However, in practice, endometrial stromal sarcoma would be an extremely unusual explanation for this finding in a Pap test.

Endometrial stromal sarcomas have traditionally been divided into low-grade and high-grade types, although diagnostic criteria are variable. Most are low-grade tumors and resemble benign stromal cells; high-grade tumors may be confused with other pleomorphic tumors, but must bear at least some resemblance to stromal cells, by definition. Some authorities do not recognize a high-grade stromal sarcoma, preferring to classify these tumors as undifferentiated sarcoma. Grade correlates with prognosis. Mitotic rate helps separate grades, but there is overlap in mitotic counts between grades. Low-grade tumors usually have less than 3 mitotic figures per 10 high power field in histologic sections, while the mitotic rate in high-grade tumors is usually greater than 10 per 10 high power fields. Invasion is a characteristic feature of malignancy. A benign stromal tumor, known as a stromal nodule, is noninvasive and the mitotic rate is usually low, and often zero, but can be higher.

Low-grade stromal sarcoma exfoliates cells that resemble benign endometrial stroma, which can make the tumor cells difficult to distinguish from benign stromal cells [I5.7a,b,c]. A clue is the presence of "too many (stromal) cells" with mild cytologic atypia in the Pap test. The tumor cells occur singly or in small groups. They are uniform, small, and plump, or sometimes, spindle or comet shaped with cytoplasmic tails. The nucleus is somewhat larger than normal, with

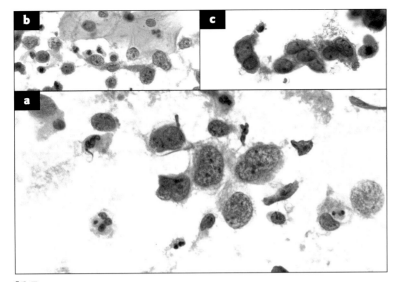

15.7
a, Stromal sarcoma [C]; **b**, Stromal sarcoma [C]; **c**, Stromal sarcoma [L]

granular, hyperchromatic chromatin and micronucleoli. The cytoplasm is scant with high N/C ratios and ill-defined cell borders [S Becker 1981, Hsiu 1979, Ito 2004, Massoni 1984, Morimoto 1982].

High-grade stromal sarcoma exfoliates small to medium sized, oval to elongated cells, with enlarged, hyperchromatic nuclei, coarse, irregular chromatin, and prominent nucleoli. The cytoplasm is scant, but has a delicate, fibrillar appearance, stains basophilic, and has ill-defined cell borders. Necrosis and tumor diathesis are common.

The differential includes other types of sarcomas, squamous cell carcinoma, follicular cervicitis, and lymphomas. Carcinosarcoma (malignant mixed Müllerian tumor) may include an element of stromal sarcoma (see below) [Izumi 1985].

Rhabdomyosarcoma

Rhabdomyosarcoma is a rare malignant tumor with striated muscle differentiation. It is the most common vaginal neoplasm of infants and children; 90% occur before age 5 years, but adults can be affected. In infants, the tumor frequently forms multiple grape-like vesicles known as botryoid sarcoma (Gr: *botryo* = grape). The prognosis of classic botryoid sarcoma is excellent, with 10 year survival >90% [Leuschner 2001].

Rhabdomyosarcoma is a classic example of a "small blue cell tumor" of childhood, but in the female genital tract, it characteristically comprises spindle and strap cells (ie, rhabdomyoblasts) in a myxoid background [Howdon 1964]. The nuclei are oval to elongated, with irregular membranes, granular chromatin, and conspicuous nucleoli. Cytoplasmic "cross-striations" are pathognomonic of skeletal muscle differentiation, but observed only rarely [Ito 2004]. Bizarre tumor cells may occur [Matsuura 1999]. Skeletal muscle markers, such as desmin, are typically expressed by tumor cells.

Primitive Neuroectodermal Tumor

Primitive neuroectodermal tumor (PNET) is a rare "small blue cell tumor" derived from fetal neuroectodermal cells. PNETs can occur, rarely, in the female genital tract; most patients are postmenopausal, but there is a wide age

range. Cytologically, the tumor is composed of small to medium sized cells, with round to oval, hyperchromatic nuclei, granular chromatin, distinct nucleoli, and scant cytoplasm [BS Ward 2000]. Neuroendocrine and epithelial markers are expressed. The differential includes: neuroblastoma, small cell neuroendocrine carcinoma, rhabdomyosarcoma, cervical stromal sarcoma, lymphoma, poorly-differentiated squamous or adenocarcinomas, as well as benign entities, such as follicular cervicitis and endometrial cells.

Other Sarcomas

Other sarcomas have also been reported in which malignant cells were identified in Pap tests [Bonfiglio 1976, Massoni 1984]. Rhabdoid cells, containing dense paranuclear inclusions, occur in rhabdoid tumors [Niemann 1994]. Alveolar soft part sarcoma may have characteristic PAS-positive cytoplasmic crystals [Zaleski 1986]. In a Pap test from a woman with a sarcoma, you're lucky if you can detect the lesion at all, let alone determine the exact type.

Mixed Müllerian Tumors

Mixed Müllerian tumors are rare neoplasms of the female genital tract composed of both epithelial and mesenchymal elements. The most common site of origin is the endometrium, but the tumors can arise in the cervix, fallopian tubes, or rarely, the ovary. This category includes carcinosarcoma (both elements malignant); adenofibroma (both elements benign); adenosarcoma (benign-appearing epithelial, but malignant mesenchymal elements); and carcinofibroma (malignant epithelial, but benign-appearing mesenchymal elements).

Carcinosarcoma (Malignant Mixed Müllerian Tumor)

Carcinosarcoma (malignant mixed Müllerian, or mesodermal, tumor; MMMT) is an uncommon, but highly aggressive, mixed epithelial and "mesenchymal" malignancy that usually occurs in postmenopausal women. It more commonly involves the uterine corpus than the cervix [Clement 1998], presenting as a fungating uterine mass, which may protrude from the cervical os. Some cases are associated with prior radiation, eg, for squamous cell carcinoma of the cervix [Abdl 1973]. The prognosis is generally poor, but depends on the type of carcinoma [Barwick 1979].

> *Carcinosarcoma (MMMT)*
> *Malignant Mixed Müllerian Tumor*
> *Adenocarcinoma + Sarcoma*
> *Sarcomatous elements*
> *·Homologous:*
> *eg, Stromal, Leiomyosarcoma*
> *·Heterologous:*
> *eg, Rhabdomyo-, Chondro-sarcoma*
> *Derive from epithelium by metaplasia*
> *⇒ MMMT better than carcinosarcoma*

Epithelial elements usually include endometrial adenocarcinoma, which can range from well-differentiated to anaplastic, but high-grade adenocarcinoma usually predominates. In more than 50% of cases, the carcinomatous component is uterine serous carcinoma. Other types of carcinoma, such as squamous (usually nonkeratinizing), papillary, clear cell or undifferentiated carcinomas, can also occur.

Stromal elements can be composed of cells that are either native or foreign to the uterus. Native cells (homologous elements) include smooth muscle or endometrial stroma (leiomyosarcoma or stromal sarcoma, respectively). Fibrosarcoma and unclassified sarcoma are more common, and considered homologous elements. Foreign cells (heterologous elements) include striated muscle,

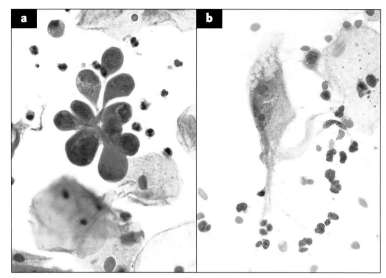

I5.8
a, MMMT, carcinoma [L]; **b**, MMMT, sarcoma [C]

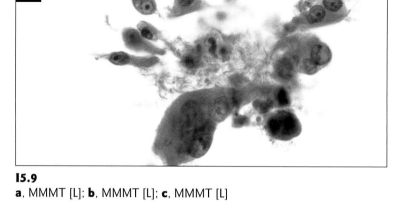

I5.9
a, MMMT [L]; **b**, MMMT [L]; **c**, MMMT [L]

cartilage, or bone (rhabdomyosarcoma, chondrosarcoma, or osteosarcoma). The morphologic appearance of the sarcomatous element does not appear to affect prognosis [Silverberg 1990]. In fact, *all* "sarcomatous" elements are probably of epithelial (metaplastic) origin, ie, metaplastic carcinoma [Bitterman 1990, Guarino 1998, Silverberg 1990] (so the old designation, MMMT, is better than the new one, carcinosarcoma).

The cytology often is bloody and necrotic, and therefore, the cells may be sparse and degenerated. Tumors that do not involve the cervix may not shed any characteristic cells at all. Owing to these problems, false-negative results are common [Barwick 1979, Casey 2003, M Costa 1992]. When tumor cells are exfoliated, the adenocarcinomatous component is more likely than the sarcomatous component to shed characteristic cells [I5.8a, 5.9a,b] [An-Foraker 1985, Casey 2003, M Costa 1992, Holmquist 1962, Massoni 1984, JE Parker 1964]. Therefore, the cytology may be interpreted simply as adenocarcinoma, often high-grade. The adenocarcinomatous component has the usual malignant features, including pleomorphism, high N/C ratios, abnormal chromatin, and conspicuous nucleoli. Look for atypical spindle cells or bizarre tumor cells (ie, a sarcomatous component), in addition to adenocarcinoma, to suggest the specific interpretation of MMMT [I5.8b, 5.9c]. Other neoplastic cell types, including clear cells, endocervical-like cells, and squamous cells, as well as malignant stromal cells, smooth or striated muscle cells, cartilage, or osteoid, may be identified rarely [Boram 1972, Howdon 1964, Izumi 1985]. The differential includes other tumors with a biphasic pattern, such as adenosquamous carcinoma and leiomyosarcoma (with spindle and epithelioid cells).

Adenosarcoma

Adenosarcoma is rare; it usually arises in the endometrium in postmenopausal women. It is less aggressive than carcinosarcoma. Adenosarcoma consists of a (probably metaplastic) sarcomatous element plus benign-appearing endometrial glandular cells. Psammoma bodies have been reported [Hidvegi 1982, Takeshima 2001].

Carcinofibroma

Carcinofibroma is composed of malignant epithelial cells (adenocarcinoma) and benign-appearing mesenchymal elements, which can be homologous

(eg, fibrous or smooth muscle tissue) or heterologous (eg, adipose or chondroid tissue). The mesenchymal component usually consists of benign-appearing spindle cells with minimal nuclear atypia and no mitotic activity [Imai 1999].

Gestational Trophoblastic Disease

Gestational trophoblastic disease is a spectrum of lesions characterized by proliferation of trophoblastic tissues associated with pregnancy. The lesions encompass hydatidiform mole (partial/complete), invasive mole, choriocarcinoma, and placental site trophoblastic tumor.

Hydatidiform Mole

Hydatidiform mole is characterized by cystic swelling of chorionic villi accompanied by varying degrees of trophoblastic proliferation. In complete moles, all of the villi are edematous and there is diffuse hyperplasia with cytologic atypia. In partial moles, only some of the villi are edematous and there is only focal trophoblastic proliferation without cytologic atypia. Rarely, complete moles are precursors to choriocarcinoma; partial moles hardly ever are. Invasive moles invade myometrium and blood vessels and can metastasize to extrauterine sites.

The cytology of various forms of hydatidiform moles is similar, except for cytologic atypia. Two cell types, cytotrophoblasts and syncytiotrophoblasts, are characteristic. Cytotrophoblasts have single nuclei and relatively abundant cytoplasm. Syncytiotrophoblasts are multinucleated giant cells. Cytologic atypia is associated with complete or invasive moles; it can be difficult to separate moles with atypia from choriocarcinoma. (These cells are described in more detail in the section on pregnancy cytology, see pg 168.)

Choriocarcinoma

Choriocarcinoma is not a single entity with a single cytogenesis. Some are trophoblastic in origin; these are practically limited to reproductive age women. Others are of germ cell origin and can occur in males as well as

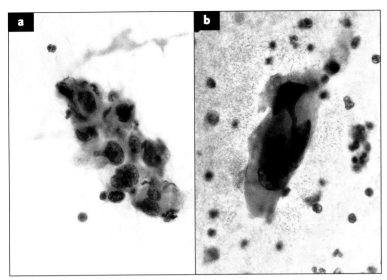

I5.10
a, ChorioCA, cytotrophoblast [C]; **b**, ChorioCA, syncytiotrophoblast [C]

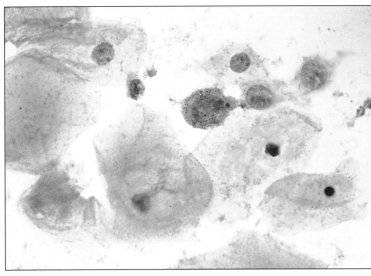

I5.11
Melanoma [C]

females. Some probably represent "dedifferentiation" of another malignant neoplasm.

Choriocarcinoma consists of a biphasic proliferation of mononucleated cytotrophoblast and multinucleate syncytiotrophoblast [I5.10a,b]. The cytotrophoblast is the malignant element, whereas the syncytiotrophoblast is nonmalignant, differentiated cytotrophoblast. Choriocarcinoma invades the uterus; hemorrhage and necrosis are typical. Formerly uniformly fatal, the tumor is highly responsive to modern chemotherapy.

The syncytiotrophoblastic cells are large, pleomorphic cells, with dense cytoplasm, and 3 to 6 central nuclei, dark, irregular coarse chromatin, and prominent nucleoli. Malignant cytotrophoblastic cells are pleomorphic, parabasal sized, with delicate cytoplasm, large nuclei, granular chromatin and prominent nucleoli. The background is bloody. Marked increased concentration of serum β-human chorionic gonadotropin (β-HCG) is characteristic.

Placental Site Trophoblastic Tumor

Placental site trophoblastic tumor is a rare lesion characterized by proliferating trophoblastic tissue invading deep into the myometrium. Serum β-HCG is low. The tumor is composed of intermediate trophoblasts, without cytotrophoblast. Intermediate trophoblasts are large, but mononucleated cells, with more abundant cytoplasm and more irregular, darker nuclei, than typical cytotrophoblasts [Ishi 1998b]. The tumor is locally aggressive, but widespread metastases are rare.

Germ Cell Tumors

Yolk sac tumor (endodermal sinus tumor) of cervicovaginal origin is extremely rare, and most cases are diagnosed in girls younger than 4 years old. Clinically, serum α-feto-protein (AFP) is usually elevated. Cytologically, the tumor cells form aggregates or are single, have malignant appearing nuclei, and high N/C ratios. Cytoplasmic hyaline globules, often containing AFP, are characteristic. Schiller-Duval bodies, also characteristic, are unlikely to be observed in exfoliative cytology specimens [Ishi 1998a].

Melanoma

Of malignant melanomas in females, 5% to 10% arise in the genital tract (vulva, vagina) [DasGupta 1964], although primary melanoma of the cervix is a *rara avis* in the annals of gynecologic oncology [Morrow 1976, Santoso 1990]. Metastatic melanoma is relatively more common in the female genital tract, but many cases are diagnosed only at autopsy [J Patel 1978]. Few cases are detected by cytology; misinterpretations are common [Deshpande 2001, D Hall 1980, H Jones 1971, Krishnamoorthy 1986, Mudge 1981, Pajtler 2003, Podczaski 1990, Visvalingam 2000]. It helps if the clinician mentions the funny, pigmented lesion seen during pelvic examination [Pajtler 2003]!

The cytology of melanoma can be quite variable from case to case [I5.11] [Deshpande 2001, Ehrmann 1962, Feichter 1995, Fleming 1994, Garcia-Valdecasas 1974, S Gupta 2003b, Hajdu 1974, D Hall 1980, Holmquist 1988, H Jones 1971, Krishnamoorthy 1986, S Masubuchi 1975, Mudge 1981, Pajtler 2003, Podczaski 1990, Sagebiel 1978, Schlosshauer 1998, Takeda 1978, Takehara 1999, Yamada 1972, Yu 1987]. The cells are usually dissociated, and range from small to large, oval, spindle, pleomorphic, or frankly bizarre. The nuclei can be pale or dark, and may have irregular membranes, prominent nucleoli, and intranuclear cytoplasmic invaginations. The cytoplasm ranges from delicate to dense. Of course the most characteristic feature is melanin pigment, but this is not always identifiable. The tumor cells usually express S100 protein and HMB-45 as well as other melanoma markers, but not cytokeratins (which helps separate this tumor from carcinoma), using immunochemistry [Takehara 2000]. The differential is wide and varied, including benign and malignant conditions. The tumor cells could be mistaken for squamous carcinoma, adenocarcinoma, or sarcoma. Melanin pigment could be mistaken for hemosiderin [Mudge 1981]. Benign nevi can also occur on the cervix and can be mistaken for melanomas [Goldman 1967, Jiji 1971].

Lymphoma and Leukemia

Lymphoreticular malignancies involving the female genital tract, including Hodgkin and non-Hodgkin lymphomas, leukemias, and myelomas, are rare. Most cases represent disseminated disease; less than 1% of primary extranodal lymphomas originate in the female genital tract (including ovary,

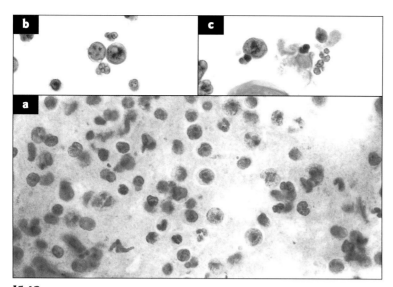

I5.I2
a, Myeloid tumor [C]; **b**, Lymphoma [L]; **c**, Lymphoma [L]

uterus, and cervix) and only a very tiny fraction of primary cervical malignancies are malignant lymphomas [Chorlton 1974, Ferry 1990b, H Fox 1965, Freeman 1972, N Harris 1984, Komaki 1984, Ohwada 2000, Perren 1992, D Whitaker 1976].

To be considered a primary lymphoma of the cervix, the tumor must be confined to the cervix and there should be no evidence of lymphoma elsewhere for at least several months [Renno 2002, P-H Wang 1999a]. Women with primary uterine lymphomas range from 20 to 80 years of age, with a median in the early 40s [N Harris 1984]. Most patients present with abnormal uterine bleeding, which can be severe, and most have a mass lesion or "barrel-shaped cervix" [Ferry 1990b]. Large B cell non-Hodgkin lymphoma is the most common type, but other types also occur [N Harris 1984, Vang 2000]. When the disease is localized, cure is possible with appropriate therapy, which may include surgery [Muntz 1991].

Lymphomas and leukemias, though rare, can mimic carcinoma of the cervix clinically [I5.I2a,b,c]. Unfortunately, the value of the Pap test in lymphoreticular malignancy is limited [Al-Talib 1996, Cahill 1997, MR Cardillo 1987, Ferry 1990b, Grace 1999]. In most cases (60% to 90%), the cytology is negative [SJ Andrews 1988, Grace 1999, N Harris 1984, C Johnson 1957, King 1997, Komaki 1984, Stransky 1973, Tunca 1979]. In other cases, the cytology is reported as abnormal [Cahill 1997, Delgado 1976, King 1997, Komaki 1984, Mann 1987] or malignant [Matsuyama 1989, JW Welch 1963, CJ Wright 1973], but the nature of the lesion is not correctly identified, eg, reported as endometrial carcinoma [Matsuyama 1989] or squamous cell carcinoma [Katayama 1973]. Neoplastic cells will not be sampled unless the lesion is ulcerated, and even then exfoliation may be limited by sclerosis, which is common in cervical/vaginal lymphomas, and interpretation may be limited by cellular degeneration [N Harris 1984]. The differential with inflammation, including follicular cervicitis, or with other small cell tumors can be difficult [SJ Andrews 1988, Dhimes 1996, King 1997, D Whitaker 1976]. Specifically typing lymphomas based only on exfoliative cytology is also difficult or impossible. Nevertheless, the Pap test can sometimes at least suggest this general class of disease, and facilitate appropriate clinical evaluation [Katayama 1973, Krumerman 1978, Taki 1985, D Whitaker 1976].

The cytology varies according to the specific type of tumor. In general, lymphomas are characterized by shedding single cells, without true tissue aggregates [I5.I2b,c]. However, pseudoaggregates (formed by artifactual cellular grouping or clustering of naked nuclei) can be seen. The tumor cells are relatively small (even so-called large cell lymphomas usually have fairly small cells) and have high N/C ratios.

From case to case, the nuclear membranes range from smooth to irregular; chromatin fine to coarse; and nucleoli invisible to prominent. Nuclear "nipples" can occur in lymphomas. The cytoplasm is usually scant and lacy, with indistinct cell borders. A dirty inflammatory/hemorrhagic background is typical [Al-Talib 1996, Cahill 1997, MR Cardillo 1987, Dhimes 1996, Ferry 1990b, JM Figueroa 1978, Katayama 1973, Krumerman 1978, Matsuyama 1989, M Mikhail 1989, Taki 1985, D Whitaker 1976].

Hodgkin Lymphoma

Hodgkin lymphoma is even more rare than non-Hodgkin lymphoma of the cervix. The Pap test may have large Reed-Sternberg cells or Hodgkin cells in a reactive inflammatory background [M Nasiell 1964, Uyeda 1969]. The differential includes many other malignancies with large tumor cells.

Extramedullary Myeloid Tumor

Extramedullary myeloid tumor, also known as granulocytic sarcoma and chloroma, is associated with myelogenous leukemia [I5.I2a]. It can involve the female genital tract [H Friedman 1992]. Reasonably well-differentiated tumors have eosinophilic myelocytes that can be recognized cytologically. Eosinophilic myelocytes are mononuclear myeloid cells with distinct eosinophilic granulations in the cytoplasm. Poorly-differentiated tumors mimic malignant lymphoma. Biopsy with special studies is required for definitive diagnosis [Ceelen 1962, Delaflor-Weiss 1999, Spahr 1982, Vang 2000].

Plasmacytoma

Plasmacytoma arising in the female genital tract is extremely rare and secondary involvement is not common. This lesion is composed of diffuse collections of neoplastic cells, ranging from mature-appearing plasma cells to anaplastic tumor cells with marked cytologic atypia [Fischer 2003]. Anaplastic forms may be difficult to recognize as plasmacytic. Well-differentiated plasma cell neoplasms could be mistaken for chronic inflammation, or conversely, chronic plasma cell cervicitis could be mistaken for plasmacytoma [Doherty 1993, JM Figueroa 1978, Fischer 2003, Qizilbash 1974a].

Differential

The major differential of lymphoreticular malignancy is follicular cervicitis, which is far more common. Lymphoma, in contrast with follicular cervicitis, deforms the cervix by producing a tumor mass that is detectable clinically. *Be extremely wary of making an interpretation of malignant lymphoma in the absence of a mass lesion!* Also, most women with evidence of lymphoma or leukemia in their Pap tests will have a well-documented history of the disease, which the clinician must provide. Inflammatory conditions are characterized by polymorphous lymphoid infiltrates, plasma cells, tingible body macrophages, and plasma cells [Al-Talib 1996, Matsuyama 1989, T Roberts 1975]. (See follicular cervicitis pg 97.)

Poorly-differentiated carcinomas, including squamous, neuroendocrine, and adenocarcinomas, may shed small cells, but carcinomas usually form true tissue aggregates and the cells may have conspicuous nuclear molding, unlike lymphoma/leukemia. The differential also includes other small cell lesions, such as high-grade dysplasia (CIN 3), endometrial stromal sarcoma, small round cell components of carcinosarcomas, small cell variant of melanoma, and "small blue cell tumors" such as Ewing/primitive neuroectodermal tumor [Vang 2000]. Biopsy and appropriate use of immunochemical markers or other special studies are indicated.

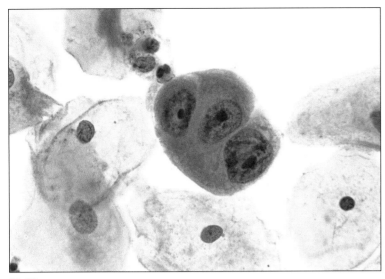

I5.13
Metastatic carcinoma, note clean background [L]

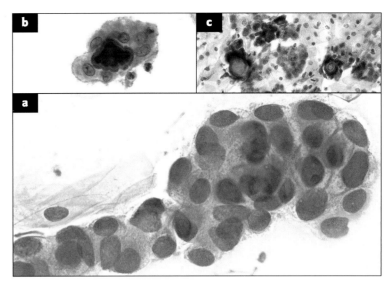

I5.14
a, Papillary group [C]; **b**, Psammoma body [L]; **c**, Psammoma bodies [C]

Metastases

Metastases to the cervix are rare, accounting for less than1% of cases in autopsy series [Abrams 1950]. Frech, in 1949, was apparently the first to report metastatic carcinoma in a Pap test [Frech 1949]. Most patients have a known history of cancer; it is particularly rare for the Pap test to be the first indication of an extrauterine malignancy, although this can occur [McGill 1990, Patsner 2002]. Extrauterine cancer can also masquerade as a primary uterine neoplasm [M Benoit 2004, N Kumar 1982]. Women may present with abnormal uterine bleeding. A history of ascites is common [Daw 1972]. The tumor cells are often obviously malignant-appearing and typically occur in a clean background [Dance 1970].

Pap Test in Metastatic Malignancy

Most have known primary tumor
Pap test rarely first indication
Sites: Ovary most common; GI, breast, lung
 Also: Melanoma
Cells usually clearly malignant
 Adenocarcinoma most common
Background: Clean (no diathesis)
Looks like "floater"

Virtually any malignancy can metastasize to the cervix, where it can exfoliate cells if the overlying epithelium is breached [Chong 1994, Hoda 2004, Olsen 2000]. However, ovary, followed by breast (often lobular type) and gastrointestinal tract (including colon/rectum, stomach, and pancreas) are the most common sources of metastatic cervical malignancies; lung, pancreas, melanoma, and others, have been reported, but are rare [Bhagavan 1969, Chagpar 2001, De Alvarez 1956, R Graham 1962, D Gupta 1999, Huijssoon 2001, Jiménez-Ayala 1996, N Kumar 1982, Lammens 2002, Lemoine 1986, Mazur 1984b, L Parsons 1953, Pomerance 1962, Scharpe 2003, Queiroz 1999, D Rubin 1963, Stemmermann 1961, Way 1980]. Tumors can also involve the cervix by direct extension, eg, endometrium, GI tract, bladder, and mesothelioma [Way 1980]. Malignant cells from the lower genital tract, including extramammary Paget disease, can sometimes be present in Pap tests [Costello 1988, Hendsch 2002]. Also, tumor cells, particularly in women with malignant ascites, can migrate down the fallopian tubes, without actual metastasis to the uterus or cervix [Maher 1996, P-H Wang 1999b].

Adenocarcinoma, often poorly-differentiated, is by far the most common morphology of metastatic malignancy [A Ng 1974c]. Metastatic squamous cell carcinomas, urothelial carcinomas, sarcomas, lymphomas, or melanomas can also occur [Bokun 1985, S Chong 1994, Epstein 1976, D Gupta 1999, Hájdu 1969, A Ng 1974c, YS Song 1957, Takeshina 1988b].

Metastatic malignancies usually exfoliate fewer abnormal cells than primary tumors. Large nuclei, hyperchromasia, prominent nucleoli, and cytoplasmic vacuolization are common in extrauterine cancers [D Gupta 1999, Kashimura 1983]. Metastatic carcinoma usually (up to 80% of cases) lacks a tumor diathesis [A Ng 1974c, Takashina 1988b], unless the metastasis becomes locally invasive. Classically, metastatic tumor looks like a contaminant "floater," ie, it looks foreign to the sample [I5.13] [A Ng 1974c, W-K Ng 2002a]. Tumors that invade the cervix or vagina directly, such as colorectal carcinomas, are usually associated with a marked tumor diathesis. Consider a metastasis when the cytomorphology is unusual for a primary cervical or uterine tumor, eg, signet ring cells or small "neuroendocrine" cells.

Although the cytomorphology may not allow definitive determination of the primary site, some clues may be helpful in suggesting possible origin of a tumor [Garret 1959, D Gupta 1999] [T5.1]. Papillary groups or psammoma bodies suggest ovarian origin, but neither finding is specific [I5.14a,b,c] [D Gupta 1999, A Ng 1974c,

T5.1 Clues to Primary Site of Metastasis

Clue	Possible Site
Papillary groups	Ovary, other, eg, renal cell carcinoma
Psammoma bodies	Ovary, other including benign conditions
Single file cell chains	Breast, Stomach
Intracytoplasmic lumens	Breast
Clear cells	Renal (exclude Müllerian tumor)
Signet ring cells	Stomach, breast
Pollywogs ("cercariform" cells)	Urothelial carcinoma
Small "neuroendocrine" cells	Lung (cervical primary possible)
Tall cells, cigar nuclei, "terminal bars," goblet cells, dirty necrosis	Colorectal carcinoma

Consider metastatic malignancy when adenocarcinoma occurs in a "clean" background or the cytomorphology is unusual for a primary cervical or uterine tumor.

Takashina 1988b, JM Welch 2000]. Papillary groups can be present in renal cell carcinoma, urothelial carcinoma, pancreatic carcinoma, and mesothelioma, for example [D Gupta 1999]. Psammoma bodies can be present in a wide variety of benign and malignant conditions (see pg 190.) Single file chains of cells suggest breast or gastric cancer [15.15]. Intracytoplasmic lumens (ICLs, targetoid mucin vacuoles) strongly suggest breast cancer [15.15] [D Gupta 1999, Mallow 1997, Pambuccian 2000, Rau 2003, Vadmal 1997]. Clear cells are consistent with renal cell carcinoma; however, a primary tumor of Müllerian origin must be excluded [15.16a] [Queiroz 1999]. A signet ring pattern not only suggests a metastasis, but also suggests origin from stomach or breast [15.16b,c] [Fiorella 1993b, Franchi 2000, D Gupta 1999, Kashimura 1983, Mallow 1997, Matsuura 1997, Pambuccian 2000, Taxy 1994, Vadmal 1997]. So called "cercariform" cells, which is a fancy term for tadpole or pollywog forms, are associated with urothelial carcinoma [15.17a]. A small cell "neuroendocrine" pattern suggests origin in lung, although a primary tumor is possible [15.17b] (see pg 173). Tall columnar cells, stratified cigar-shaped nuclei, terminal bar-like edges, scattered goblet cells, and "dirty" necrosis suggest colonic cancer [15.18].

Metastatic malignancies can mimic primary tumors of the uterus or cervix [Matsuura 1997, Pomerance 1962]. Also consider the possibility of IUD effect, which can shed papillary aggregates of atypical cells, complete with psammoma bodies in some cases [15.19]. Many cases of metastatic carcinoma may simply be interpreted as "atypical glandular cells" (see pg 146 for differential of atypical glandular cells). Estrogen and progesterone receptors and HPV-DNA status may be helpful in the differential in selected cases [Vinette-Leduc 1999]. Immunocytochemistry can also be helpful, in some cases, by highlighting cellular markers [Malle 2001, Mallow 1997]. For example, colon cancer is usually CK20 positive, while breast cancer is usually CK7 positive.

Odds & Ends

Hyperchromatic Crowded Groups (HCGs)

An important problem in interpretation of Pap tests is the evaluation of "hyperchromatic crowded groups" or "HCGs," also known as tissue fragments or microbiopsies [DeMay 2000]. This problem has been addressed throughout the text, but summarized here. HCGs are among the most common sources of interpretive (as opposed to screening) errors in Pap test evaluation. (The problem is not finding them, they're easy to see; the problem is figuring out what they are.) HCGs are defined as: three-dimensional aggregates, of crowded cells, with hyperchromatic nuclei.

HCGs usually represent benign entities, such as clusters of endometrial cells, aggregates of basaloid cells in severe atrophy, or fragments of endocervical tissue, the latter occurring with increased frequency due to the widespread use of the endocervical brush. Tubal metaplasia is another common, benign, source of HCGs. However, occasionally, HCGs represent serious lesions, such as carcinoma in situ, invasive squamous cell carcinoma, and glandular neoplasia, either in situ or invasive. Unfortunately, it is not always easy to distinguish between the common, benign HCGs and the relatively rare, neoplastic HCGs.

Hyperchromatic Crowded Groups
  Aka tissue fragments, microbiopsies
   •3D aggregates
   •Crowded cells
   •Hyperchromatic nuclei

There are several interpretive problems pertaining to HCGs. First, as mentioned, HCGs usually represent benign entities: probably 99% of the time they are benign, including normal or reactive conditions. Therefore, since they are encountered every day in screening, one becomes inured to them and blithely pass them by as "nothing," which in fact, they usually are. Due to the nature of Pap test screening, if something is considered benign or insignificant, like endometrial cells in young women, they fade into the unnamed background of things that are simply passed by in the search for significant findings. Only in retrospect are these entities named [15.20]

Hyperchromatic Crowded Groups
  Usually benign
   Endometrial cells
   Severe atrophy
   Tubal metaplasia
  Occasionally neoplastic
   Carcinoma in situ
   Squamous cell carcinoma
   Glandular neoplasia

Unfortunately, when HCGs are bad, they are really bad: the least bad thing they are likely to represent is carcinoma in situ. If a low-grade lesion is missed, in a certain way, the woman may actually have been done a favor [Sawaya 2000]. Current follow-up recommendations call for colposcopy and biopsy for every squamous intraepithelial lesion, even low-grade. This is expensive and unpleasant, and can lead to still more expensive and unpleasant procedures, such as cone biopsy, and even hysterectomy, with their attendant risks, including infertility. Yet, most low-grade lesions will disappear on their own, even without therapy. (Get out your pens and write this down, it is very important: I am *not* advocating intentionally overlooking dysplasia in screening, only pointing out risks vs benefits.)

On the other hand, if an HCG is interpreted as benign when it isn't, the lesion is probably at least carcinoma in situ, and it may even be invasive cancer. In other words, HCGs, when they are neoplastic, will *never* represent a low-grade lesion; they will probably *not* go away on their own; and if they are misinterpreted as "nothing" this is a potentially serious error, that could have important patient consequences and could lead to malpractice litigation. In fact, most Pap test litigation revolves around misinterpretation of HCGs (particularly failure to detect squamous carcinoma in situ or adenocarcinomas) [Austin 2003b].

An unfortunate problem is that benign HCGs can be morphologically very similar to neoplastic ones. But, simply being aware of the problem will go a long way toward solving it. Stop and look carefully at HCGs. When carefully evaluated, HCGs can usually be correctly interpreted; however, there is an important subset of cases that are extremely difficult, or impossible, to classify accurately. Not surprisingly, these cases may be passed off as benign, since there may be no reliable criteria by which to recognize them as neoplastic. For example, some cases of carcinoma in situ occurring in older women shed aggregates of extremely bland cells, that are not mitotic active, and closely mimic syncytial-like aggregates of benign basal cells in severe atrophy.

HCGs: Interpretive clues
  Low power
   Chaotic architecture
   Hyperchromasia
  High power
   Coarse dark chromatin
   Mitotic figures
  More clues
   CIS + squamous dysplasia
    spectrum of abnormality
  Glandular neoplasia:
   Feathery edges
   Well-formed microacini
   Elongated nuclei, coarse, dark chromatin

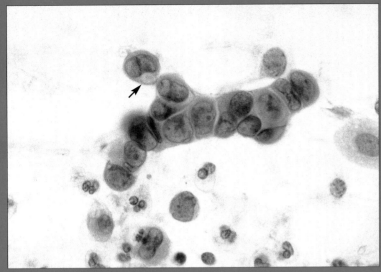

I5.15
Single file, note ICL (arrow) [C]

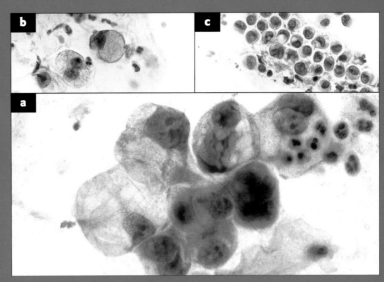

I5.16
a, Clear cell carcinoma [C]; **b**, Signet ring cells [C]; **c**, Signet ring cells [C]

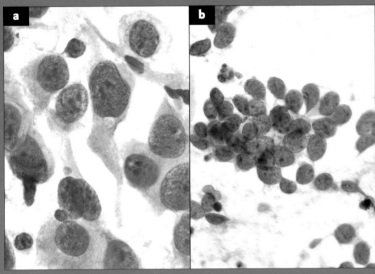

I5.17
a, Urothelial CA, pollywog [C]; **b**, Small cell carcinoma, primary [C]

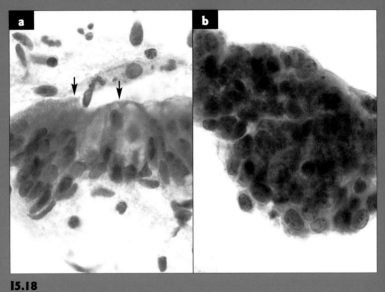

I5.18
a, Colon CA, note "terminal bar" (arrows) [C]; **b**, Colonic carcinoma [L]

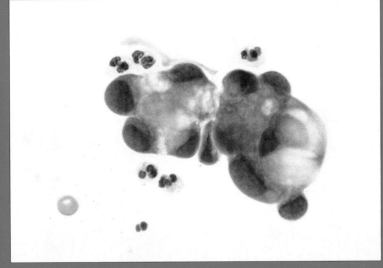

I5.19
IUD effect, mimics metastasis [C]

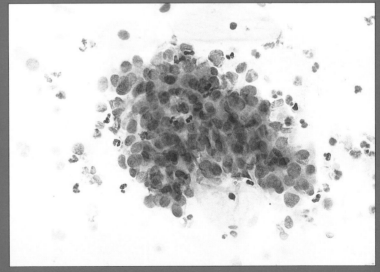

I5.20
HCG, benign vs malignant? [C] (villoglandular adenocarcinoma)

(Conversely, basal cells in atrophy can form similar aggregates of small, closely packed cells with dark nuclei and scant cytoplasm, ie, hyperchromatic crowded groups, mimicking CIS.)

When evaluating HCGs, there are several important cytologic clues to the presence of a serious abnormality. First, at low power, look for disorderly cellular arrangements, referred to as "loss of nuclear polarity" or "chaotic architecture" [15.21]. Then, at high power, look at cytologic details, such as irregular nuclear membranes, coarse, dark chromatin, and mitotic figures, which strongly favor a significant lesion, such as carcinoma in situ [15.22]. Architectural abnormalities and hyperchromasia are often more apparent at low power, than high power, microscopy.

There are often other clues to the recognition of neoplastic HCGs. For example, squamous carcinoma in situ is usually accompanied by squamous dysplasia, representing a spectrum of abnormality (ie, mild, moderate, severe dysplasia plus CIS). On the other hand, HCGs in glandular neoplasia typically show feathery edges, well-defined microacini, and elongated nuclei

---

Carcinoma In Situ (Classique)

Syncytial aggregates
  Tightly bunched cells
High N/C ratios
  Scant cytoplasm
Abnormal nuclei
  Irregular membranes
  Coarse chromatin
  Mitoses

---

with distinctly coarse, dark chromatin (the nuclei in squamous CIS tend to be rounder with somewhat finer chromatin).

The usual textbook description of carcinoma in situ is: syncytial-like aggregates of tightly bunched cells, with high N/C ratios, scant cytoplasm, and abnormal nuclei with irregular membranes, coarse chromatin, and mitotic figures: this CIS classique.

However, it is important to broaden the conception of what CIS actually looks like: this is CIS nouveau. For example, rudimentary microacini or rosettes, ie, gland-like structures, are *common* in HCGs from CIS [15.23].

Carcinoma In Situ (Nouveau)

Microacini common! (reserve cell)
  Mimics reactive/neoplastic endocervical cells
Low nuclear/cytoplasmic ratios
Nuclei: bland, smooth membranes,
  fine chromatin, few/no mitoses
Nuclei: mistake for reactive changes
No accompanying dysplasia (lose clue)

Although it has been suggested that this indicates glandular extension, it could also represent the dual potential of the reserve cell to differentiate into either a squamous or a glandular cell. (Furthermore, high-grade lesions are generally extensive lesions; therefore, CIS is likely to extend into glands regardless of its subtle cytologic features [Abdul Karim 1982]. Also, glandular extension, by definition, occurs deep in the tissue, whereas the surface is sampled in a Pap test. Of course, glandular and squamous lesions can also co-exist; these are difficult to interpret accurately [Gloor 1986, Kurian 1999, Lauchlan 1967, Luesley 1987, Raab 2000, van Aspert–van Erp 2004b].) Less ominously, CIS with "glands" could lead to erroneous interpretations of endocervical glandular neoplasia, but the woman should still be referred for appropriate follow-up (colposcopy). More ominously, these "acinic" HCGs of CIS could be misinterpreted as benign/reactive endocervical cells, and the woman could be lost to follow up.

In some cases, CIS has lower N/C ratios than usually expected that could lead to cytologic misinterpretations [15.24]. This is particularly true of the large cell type of CIS, which can have fairly abundant cytoplasm. Moreover, it is not rare for cells of CIS to be unexpectedly bland, with smooth

nuclear membranes, fine chromatin, and little or no mitotic activity, particularly in postmenopausal women [15.25]. Nucleoli are not a traditional feature of CIS, and yet they can be present in CIS [15.26]. This is not a particularly rare event, and it can be misleading. On the one hand, nucleoli suggest the possibility of an invasive process, which could lead to overinterpretation of CIS as squamous cell carcinoma. However, these women will likely receive appropriate follow-up and so the misinterpretation is not a serious one. On the other hand, nucleoli also suggest a benign, reactive/reparative process, which could lead to false-negative results; these women will probably not receive appropriate follow-up.

As a rule, squamous carcinoma in situ is accompanied by squamous dysplasia, ranging from mild to severe, representing a spectrum of abnormality. The accompanying dysplasia provides an important clue that the HCGs in question represent carcinoma in situ and not benign mimickers. In fact, when a high-grade squamous dysplasia is reported, the patient will likely receive appropriate follow-up, even if the true nature of the HCGs was not specifically recognized as carcinoma in situ. Unfortunately, in some cases of CIS the accompanying squamous dysplasia is sparse or absent. In these cases, an extremely valuable interpretive clue may not be apparent, compounding the difficulty of accurately classifying HCGs. Pure CIS lesions are more common in older women. A similar problem is that invasive squamous cell carcinoma can also shed HCGs in which differentiated squamous cells may be sparse or absent. Look for marked nuclear abnormalities, particularly irregular chromatin distribution, to indicate frank malignancy [15.27]

As can be seen, these neoplastic HCGs do not always "follow the rules" in terms of their expected morphology. Therefore, they may be difficult to recognize as being a significant abnormality. HCGs lacking standard interpretive criteria may be passed off as benign, even by reasonable, competent cytologists. An easy solution would be to refer every patient with HCGs to colposcopy. Unfortunately, however, because benign HCGs are so common, and neoplastic HCGs so rare, the Pap test would lose its value as a screening if this were done.

As if the differential outlined above were not problematic enough, there are several other potential sources of HCGs in Pap tests. These, too, can cause serious problems in interpretation.

Atypia of atrophy can be associated with syncytial aggregates of pleomorphic cells, with enlarged, hyperchromatic nuclei, and high N/C ratios, ie, HCGs mimicking carcinoma in situ or even invasive cancer [15.28, 5.29]. Conversely, malignant tissue fragments may be difficult to distinguish from

---

More Hyperchromatic Crowded Groups

Atypia of atrophy
Atypical endocervical cells
Brush artifact
High endocervical cells
Endometrial cells
Cone biopsy artifact
Tubal metaplasia
Microglandular hyperplasia
Endocervical glandular neoplasia

---

benign atrophy. In severe atrophy there is frequently a dirty background, with degenerated cells, debris, granular precipitate, fresh/old blood, and inflammatory cells, including neutrophils and histiocytes ("atrophy with inflammation"). This granular background can resemble a tumor diathesis. Crisp and distinct chromatin texture favors a neoplastic process, while smudgy, degenerated chromatin favors a benign process. The presence of mitotic figures suggests neoplasia, if a reactive/reparative process can be excluded, but the absence of mitotic activity does not exclude a serious

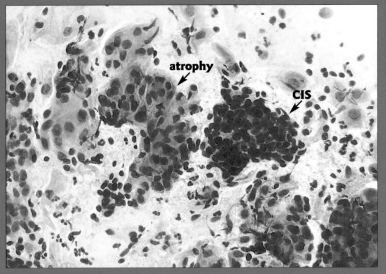

I5.21
Low power: architecture, hyperchromasia (CIS in atrophy) [C]

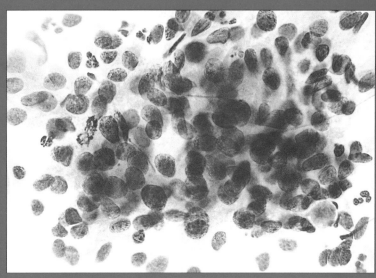

I5.22
High power: cytologic detail, note mitosis (CIS) [C]

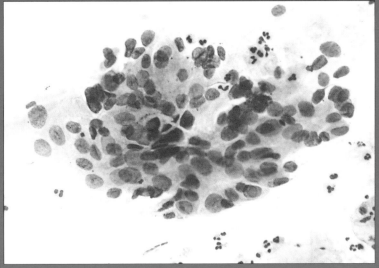

I5.23
HCG CIS with "glands" [C]

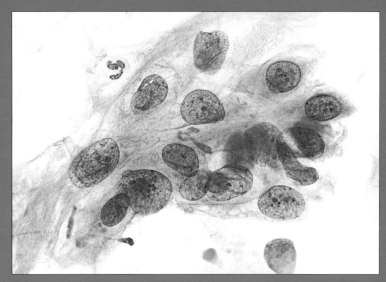

I5.24
HCG CIS, low N/C ratios [C]

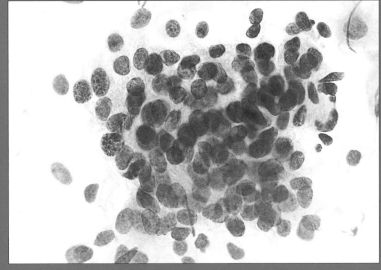

I5.25
HCG CIS, bland cells [C]

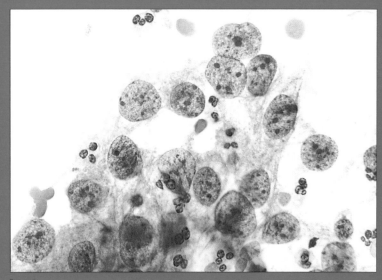

I5.26
HCG CIS, nucleoli [C]

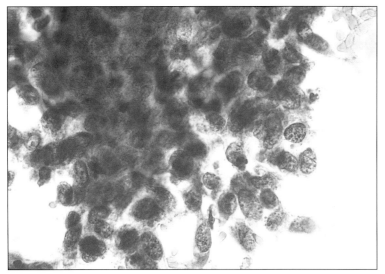

I5.27
HCG SCC, irregular chromatin [C]

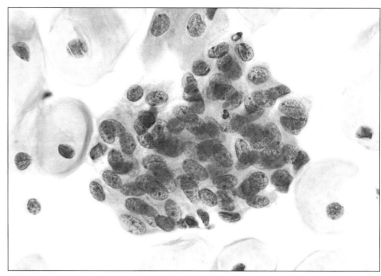

I5.28
HCG Atrophy [C]

abnormality [I5.30]. Abnormal arrangements of the cells (chaotic architecture) favors a neoplastic process. An accompanying bona fide squamous dysplasia supports a diagnosis of carcinoma in situ or cancer; however, particularly in older women, carcinoma in situ may occur as a pure lesion, without an associated dysplasia, and the cells may be cytologically bland with a paucity of mitotic figures.

Atypical endocervical cells are commonly seen in samples obtained with the endocervical brush. In some cases, the nuclei are enlarged, pleomorphic, and hyperchromatic, possibly reflecting polyploidy ("brush atypia") [I5.31a]. Also, endocervical cells obtained high in the endocervical canal, which may be sampled using an endocervical brush, are normally more crowded, with higher N/C ratios, than those obtained with an ordinary spatula [I5.31b]. These "high endocervical cells" can form hyperchromatic crowded groups mimicking neoplasia. However, the nuclei are bland and round, and resemble other endocervical nuclei. No mitotic figures are present.

Endometrial cells (spontaneously shed) can form three-dimensional clusters of hyperchromatic glandular cells, without central stroma [I5.32a,b]. The cells are small and crowded, and the nuclei are usually degenerated and hyperchromatic, ie, they form hyperchromatic crowded groups that can mimic carcinoma in situ, and vice versa. Possible clues to endometrial origin include the time of the menstrual cycle and presence of nearby endometrial stroma. Mitotic figures are not present in spontaneously exfoliated endometrial cells, but can be numerous in directly sampled endometrium. Apoptotic bodies can occur in benign endometrium.

Endometrium (directly sampled) and endometriosis both feature hyperchromatic crowded groups of endometrial cells with high N/C ratios, possibly secondary gland openings, and mitotic figures [I5.33a]. Such cells can mimic endocervical neoplasia [I5.33b]. Some possible clues to interpretation: the endometrial glandular cells usually have a uniform, benign appearance and may be intimately associated with endometrial stromal cells (yielding a characteristic biphasic pattern). Endometrial cells may be obtained, at any time during the cycle, with: an endocervical brush (which can obtain cells directly from the lower uterine segment or even the endometrial cavity itself); in patients with cervical endometriosis (classic triad: glands, stroma, hemosiderin);

or in patients who have undergone cone biopsy (in whom the endocervical canal is shortened).

Cone biopsy artifact may be associated with hyperchromatic crowded groups of atypical glandular cells [I5.34a]. Cone biopsy alters the anatomy and shortens the endocervical canal, allowing direct sampling of lower uterine segment and endometrium. These endometrial cells may show reactive/regenerative changes and exfoliate hyperchromatic crowded groups mimicking neoplasia; however, there tend to be fewer abnormal cells, and they are less crowded and more orderly than in neoplasia. They are part of a morphologic spectrum that includes clearly benign cells, which may appear of endometrial or endocervical origin. Nuclei tend to be uniform with fine chromatin, but mitotic figurs can occur. Ciliated cells imply a benign process, but may not be present.

Microglandular hyperplasia can shed hyperchromatic crowded groups (nuclear overlap, crowding, and loss of polarity) showing cytologic atypia, including nuclear enlargement, hyperchromasia, nucleoli, and mitotic figures, which may suggest endocervical glandular neoplasia or high-grade squamous intraepithelial lesions [I5.34b]. Absence of coarse chromatin and "feathery" edges, and presence of cells with cilia or terminal bars point to a benign diagnosis. Pseudoparakeratosis is a potential interpretive clue [I5.34c].

Tubal metaplasia features crowded columnar cells, which can have enlarged, somewhat pleomorphic nuclei, elevated N/C ratios, and moderate hyperchromasia that may suggest endocervical glandular neoplasia, particularly adenocarcinoma in situ [I5.35a,b]. Small, discrete, clear cytoplasmic vacuoles are common, and terminal bars and cilia are characteristic. For practical purposes, the presence of cilia excludes malignancy. Unfortunately, the cilia may degenerate or be difficult to visualize.

Endocervical glandular neoplasia characteristically sheds cells in hyperchromatic crowded groups that can cause interpretive difficulties [I5.31c] [Renshaw 2004c, Ruba 2004]. The aggregates typically have "feathery" edges. Secondary gland openings can also be seen in sheets of neoplastic endocervical cells. The nuclei are characteristically oval to elongated or irregular. The cells have high N/C ratios. The chromatin is markedly hyperchromatic and moderately coarse, similar to squamous carcinoma in situ. As mentioned above, HCGs of squamous CIS can share features with those of endocervical glandular neoplasia. To help distinguish them, look at the edges of the HCGs: feathering favors glandular origin, while

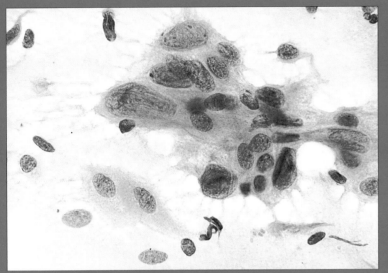

I5.29
HCG Atypia of atrophy [C]

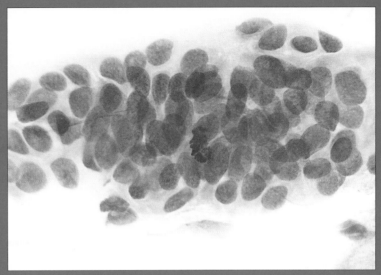

I5.30
HCG Bland CIS, note rare mitosis [C]

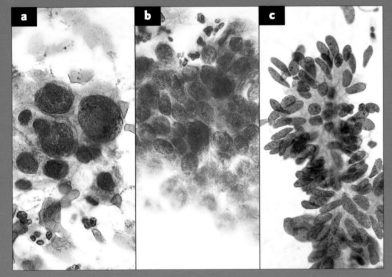

I5.31
a, HCG Endocervical brush artifact [C]; **b**, HCG High endocervical cells [C];
c, HCG Adenocarcinoma in situ [C]

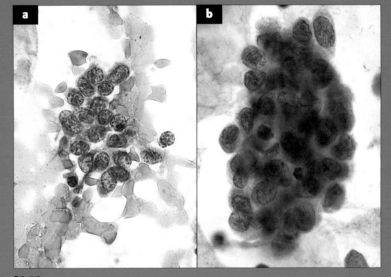

I5.32
a, HCG Endometrial cells [C]; **b**, HCG Endometrial cells [C]

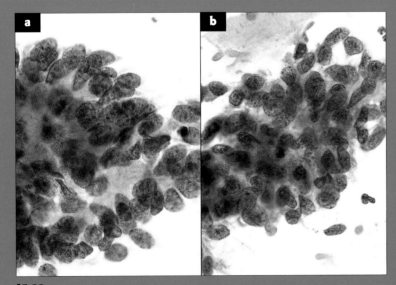

I5.33
a, HCG Endometrium vs AIS (EMs) [C]; **b**, HCG Endometrium vs AIS (AIS) [C]

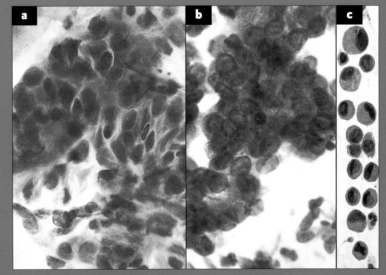

I5.34
a, HCG Cone biopsy artifact [C]; **b**, HCG Microglandular hyperplasia [C];
c, Pseudoparakeratosis [C]

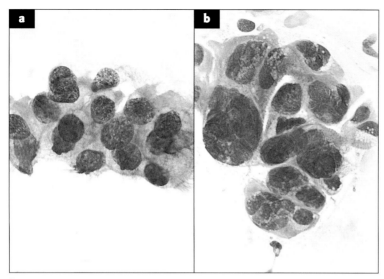

I5.35
a, HCG Tubal metaplasia [C]; **b**, HCG Tubal metaplasia [C]

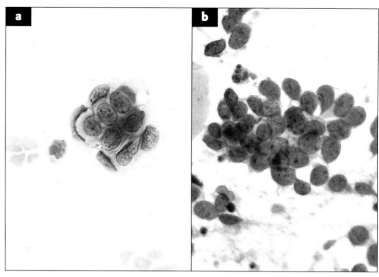

I5.36
a, HCG Metastatic carcinoma [C]; **b**, HCG Small cell carcinoma [C]

flattening favors squamous origin. Within the HCGs, well-formed rosettes favor glandular origin, while whirling favors squamous origin. Macronucleoli suggest an invasive process, but can occur in the poorly-differentiated variant form of in situ adenocarcinoma. In fact, invasive adenocarcinoma may be indistinguishable from in situ adenocarcinoma, and vice versa. However, in general, invasive adenocarcinomas usually show more cytologic atypia, single cells, and a tumor diathesis. Invasion can be suspected, but not excluded, by cytology.

Metastatic carcinoma is another potential source of HCGs [I5.36a]. The Pap test is rarely the first place that a nongenital malignant neoplasm is detected; patients with metastatic tumors usually have a known history of malignancy. The typical cytology of a metastasis shows tumor aggregates in a clean background. A "floater" may be considered in the differential. Small cell carcinoma, primary or metastatic, also exfoliates HCGs [I5.36b].

In summary, HCGs are important sources of error in Pap test interpretation. HCGs are seen everyday in screening and it is easy to become so used them that we may fail to recognize that occasionally they represent serious abnormalities. The first step in preventing an error is to be aware of the problem. Then, the next step is to classify the HCGs accurately. On careful evaluation, one can usually—*but not always*—correctly identify their true nature. One final thought: HPV-DNA testing may be very helpful in evaluating women with equivocal HCGs [Austin 2003b].

Fallopian Tube Cells

Cells from the fallopian tube, or oviduct, are rarely present in the Pap test. More commonly, ciliated fallopian tube-like cells indicate tubal metaplasia of the endometrium or endocervix. The cells can be cytologically atypical—cilia provide a benign clue. Fallopian tube cells can also appear similar to normal or reactive ciliated endocervical cells. The cytology of fallopian tube cells is discussed in more detail under tubal metaplasia, pg 150.

Carcinoma of the Fallopian Tube

Carcinoma of the fallopian tube was first described by Renaud in 1847 [O Jones 1965]. Fallopian tube carcinoma is rare and still more rarely sheds cells

detected in a Pap test [Backelandt 2000, P Benson 1974, Besserer 1953, Boutselis 1971, Brewer 1956, Case 1951, Deden 1955, Fidler 1954, C Fox 1978, A Frankel 1956, T Green 1962, Hirai 1987, Hopfel-Kreiner 1978, Hu 1950, Israel 1954, Isbell 1947, Kernodle 1948, E Larsson 1956, Papanicolaou 1954, Patsner 2002, Podobnik 1993, Rahimpanah 2000, Safret 2004, M Sasagawa 2003, Sedlis 1961, YS Song 1955, Takeshima 1997, Warshal 1999, Yoonessi 1979]. In 1948, Dr. J. Ernest Ayre may have become the first person in history to suggest the diagnosis of fallopian tube carcinoma, preoperatively, from a Pap test [Fidler 1954]. Most patients are postmenopausal (although the disease has been reported even in teenagers [Yoonessi 1979]); many are nulliparous [C Schneider 2000]. Abnormal vaginal discharge or bleeding is common, but the classic syndrome, "hydrops tubae profluens" (colicky pain relieved by profuse watery vaginal discharge), is rare [Backelandt 2000].

The cells typically exfoliate in papillary or glandular clusters in a clean background [I5.37] [Minato 1998, Wachtel 1961]. The malignant cells usually (80% of cases) have serous adenocarcinoma morphology [C Schneider 2000]. The cells are medium sized, with high N/C ratios; dark, irregular nuclei; abnormal chromatin; prominent nucleoli; and dense, but often vacuolated, cytoplasm. Psammoma bodies may be present [Luzzatto 1996, Parkash 2002, Zreik 2001]. In women whose Pap tests indicate adenocarcinoma or adenosquamous carcinoma, but who have (1) negative cone biopsy findings (to exclude cervical adenocarcinoma), (2) negative dilatation and curettage findings (to exclude endometrial adenocarcinoma), and (3) no known primary tumor, consider fallopian tube adenocarcinoma (or primary peritoneal carcinoma) [P Benson 1974, Hirai 1987, Olsen 2000, Takashina 1985, P-H Wang 1999b, J Wright 2002]. Other tumors of the fallopian tube, such as lymphomas, carcinosarcomas, and sarcomas, are vanishingly rare [Wachtel 1961].

Benign Glandular Cells Posthysterectomy

Finding benign-appearing glandular cells in a Pap test from a woman who has had a hysterectomy is not especially rare, occurring in anywhere from 1% or 2%, up to 13%, of posthysterectomy cytology specimens [Eren 2004, Ramirez 2000, Tambouret 1998] [I5.38]. This now has a place in the Bethesda System lexicon, which may increase the frequency of reporting this finding [Eren 2004]. It may be explained by any of the following:

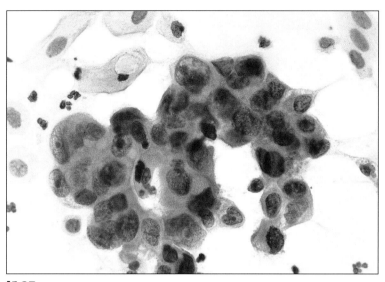

I5.37
Fallopian tube carcinoma [C]

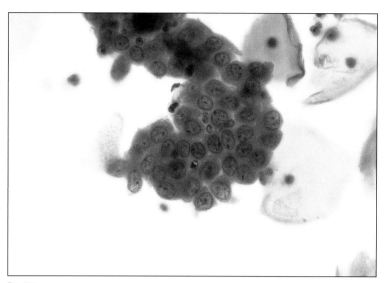

I5.38
Benign gland cells, post-hysterectomy [L]

The history is wrong [Frable 1973]. For example, either no hysterectomy, or a subtotal hysterectomy (leaving the cervix), was performed. Radiation shrinks the cervix, making it difficult to visualize clinically, giving the misleading impression that a hysterectomy was performed.

Vaginal adenosis is probably more common than generally appreciated. During the DES era, the number of women affected may have been as high as ~40% [Sandberg 1968], but nowadays may be closer to 10%, still a substantial number of women [Chattopadhyay 2001, Kranl 1998, Kurman 1974].

Glandular Cells Posthysterectomy

Not rare, possible explanations:

Wrong history

No hysterectomy or supracervical

Vaginal adenosis

Therapy-induced metaplasia

Well-ordered atrophic cells

Goblet-like cells

Fallopian tube cells

Other, eg, endometriosis, fistula

Exclude: Well-differentiated AdCA

Metaplastic vaginal adenosis-like changes. These are common after radiation or chemotherapy, including Tamoxifen [Ganesan 1999, J Johnson 1999, Ramirez 2000, Tambouret 1998]. Radiation therapy may be the single most common explanation for finding benign appearing endocervical-like cells in the Pap test following hysterectomy for cancer.

The "glandular" cells actually are atrophic parabasal cells. These cells can have delicate (gland-like) cytoplasm and orderly cellular arrangements (mimicking a honeycomb pattern). Look for well-defined columnar cells, true honeycomb (with prominent cell borders), and intracytoplasmic mucin in genuine endocervical cells. Parabasal cells and metaplastic squamous cells can be indistinguishable.

The cells are goblet-like cells. These are relatively common in atrophy (~20% of cases). They occur as single, oval cells within parabasal "syncytia." They are mucin positive [Bewtra 1992, Koike 1990, 1993]. For purposes of determining specimen adequacy, these cells are not considered endocervical cells.

The glandular cells derive from the fallopian tube. The fallopian tube can granulate (prolapse) into the vaginal apex post-hysterectomy or it may be implanted deliberately during hysterectomy surgery to provide vaginal support [D Carmichael 1976, Hellen 1993, Silverberg 1974, Wolfendale 1980]. Some patients with fallopian tube prolapse have signs and symptoms of genital tract infection [Ponder 1997, Wolfendale 1980]. Occasional ciliated cells are possible clues to interpretation [Dudkiewicz 1968, 1970].

Other explanations: Endometriosis, mesonephric duct remnants/tumor, Bartholin glands/tumors, rectovaginal fistula are among other possible explanations for the presence of benign glandular cells in post-hysterectomy women [Angeles 1994, Dodson 1970, Ferrara 1997, Ganesan 1999, Ponder 1997, Sodhani 1999, Tambouret 1998, Welsh 2003].

Of course, it is important to rule out well-differentiated adenocarcinoma. Although well-differentiated tumor cells are not benign, they can be cytologically bland.

Ferning of the Cervical Mucus

As first noted by Papanicolaou in 1946, the cervical mucus tends to crystallize in an arborizing pattern, resembling ferns or palm leaves, near the time of ovulation [I5.39] [Papapanicolaou 1946]. This phenomenon correlates with spinnbarkeit, which refers to the ability of cervical mucus to form a thread. Ferning and spinnbarkeit peak at midcycle and are apparently associated with a peak in estrogen. Estrogen treatment can also induce ferning, while progestational agents inhibit it. The optimal time of sperm penetration is directly related to the degree of ferning [Zaneveld 1975]. Ferning is not observed in liquid-based cytology.

Curschmann Spirals

Although much more commonly present in sputum, Curschmann spirals are rarely detected in Pap tests (as well as in specimens from several other body sites [Canda 2001, Naylor 1990]

Curshmann Spirals

Rare finding

Identical to respiratory cytology

Intrinsic property of mucus

No special significance

[15.40a,b]. Their formation seems to be an intrinsic property of the mucus itself, rather than a foreign contaminant of the female genital tract, and is not related to cigarette smoking [Bornstein 1987, Demirezen 2003b, Novak 1984]. In the Pap test, Curshmann spirals have no special significance.

Fistulae

Rectovaginal Fistula

Rectovaginal fistula is associated with tall, columnar colorectal goblet cells, which may be reactive appearing [15.41a,b]. Colorectal cells normally form rosette-like glands and sheets of cells with crypt openings. Hyperkeratosis may occur as a reaction to chronic irritation. Caution: "Atypical" (reactive) intestinal cells forming rosettes in a dirty background could be mistaken for adenocarcinoma. Look for evidence of debris, bacteria (especially *Escherichia coli*), digested food, etc, (ie, caca) in the background [Angeles 1994, Ferrara 1997]. The differential of goblet-like cells includes: rectovaginal fistula, mucinous metaplasia in atrophy, vaginal adenosis, tubal metaplasia, intestinal variant of endocervical adenocarcinoma, adenoma malignum, and intestinal neovagina.

Vesicovaginal Fistula

Vesicovaginal fistula is associated with umbrella and other urothelial (transitional) cells [15.42a,b]. Degenerated cells containing cytoplasmic hyaline globules, common in voided urine specimens, may occur. Clinically, there may be a pale yellow watery discharge (ie, pee).

Neovagina

Grafts of colon, ileum, or skin can be used in constructing a vagina in females with congenital absence (agenesis) or therapeutic ablation of the organ, or in male-to-female transsexuals. The cytology depends upon the type of graft.

Following a skin graft operation, the cytology may resemble the normal vaginal squamous epithelium [Lellé 1990], with the maturation shifted to the right (toward superficial cells), but most patients exfoliate anucleate squames [Selvaggi 1995a, Takashina 1988a]. Neovaginal squamous epithelium can respond to hormones, and usually harbors lactobacilli, but infections, including human papillomavirus infection, can also occur [Belleannée 1998, Takashina 1988a]. In patients receiving intestinal grafts, intestinal-type (colonic or ileal) epithelium is seen in cytologic samples [15.43a,b]. Because "colitis," "ileitis," or neoplasia (squamous or glandular, depending on the type of graft) can occur in the neovagina, regular cytologic screening is recommended to detect these lesions in the graft [Lowe 2001, Munkarah 1994, Rotmensch 1983, Selvaggi 1995a, Steiner 2002, Toolenaar 1993, Wheelock 1986].

Spermatozoa

Spermatozoa, or sperm, are the male reproductive cells (gametes). They have oval heads, short necks, and long tails. The Dutch scientist, Anton van Leeuwenhoek and his student, Ham, first discovered spermatozoa, in 1677, using a simple (one lens) microscope.

Identification of sperm is important in cases of sexual assault [Allery 2001, M Costa 1991c]. In 1837, Rattier suggested that spermatozoa could be identified in seminal stain material and could be used in medicolegal investigations.

A century later, in 1939, Bayard published a paper on the use of the microscope to identify sperm in seminal stains. Further advances, including enzyme analysis, molecular, and cytogenetic techniques followed [Collins 2001, Roa 1995].

Spermatozoa begin to degenerate within hours after ejaculation [15.44a]. The first sign of degeneration is loss of the tail (flagellum), leaving only tiny sperm heads. Sperm heads are pear-shaped and show biphasic staining owing to the acrosomal cap. Sperm decrease in number over a period of a few days after intercourse, are found irregularly after the seventh day, and are rare after the tenth postcoital day, although exceptionally, they may remain for more than 3 weeks, and rarely as long as 2-3 months [Collins 2001]. Sperm can be detected within 3 days of coitus in only about 25% to 50% of cases [M Costa 1991c, B Randall 1987, Silverman 1978]. Intact sperm (with tails), or sperm heads only, may be present. Sperm heads could be mistaken for *Candida* spores (which have translucent cell walls) or isolated lobes of neutrophils (which are round and do not stain biphasically). The percentage of sperm with tails does not correlate significantly with time. Douching, pregnancy, oral contraceptives, coitus interruptus, condoms, and vasectomy reduce or eliminate sperm from the cytologic samples [Silverman 1978].

Seminal Vesicle Cells

Seminal vesicle cells derive from a male sexual partner. Particularly in elderly men, they can be large "ugly" cells, with big, hyperchromatic (polyploid) nuclei that can mimic high-grade malignancies, such as poorly-differentiated adenocarcinoma [15.44b]. Golden-brown lipochrome pigment in the cytoplasm may suggest metastatic melanoma. The cells are often degenerated or necrotic. The presence of cytoplasmic lipochrome pigment and sperm in the vicinity are the two best clues to a benign interpretation [Meisels 1976a]. Possible misinterpretation of these cells is one reason it is recommended women refrain from sexual intercourse the day before having a Pap test.

> **Seminal Vesicle Cells**
> Rare, partners = older men
> Columnar cells, "ugly" nuclei
>   vs Adenocarcinoma
> Clues: Golden brown pigment
>   Chromatin smudgy
>   Sperm in vicinity

Psammoma Bodies

Psammoma body is a term coined by Virchow, derived from the Greek, *psammos*, meaning sand, plus *-oma*, meaning tumor, hence "sand tumor." Psammoma bodies are microscopic, concentrically laminated, calcified structures, measuring about 10 µm-100 µm in diameter, and are often surrounded by cells [15.45]. Although classically associated with meningiomas and papillary carcinomas of thyroid and ovary, psammoma bodies occur in a wide variety of conditions from many different sites. They are also found rarely in Pap tests, estimated at roughly one in every 100,000 cases (range, 1 in 2,000 to 200,000 cases) [de Peralta –Venturino 2000, Kern 1991a, Nicklin 2001, Parkash 2002, Zreik 2001]. While raising the specter of malignancy, psammoma bodies in Pap tests are associ-

> **Psammoma Bodies**
> Rare finding
> Benign, eg, IUDs, BCPs, infection
>   Atypical cells may be present
> Malignant, eg, Papillary serous carcinoma
>   Cancer cells not always present
> Cause not found in many cases

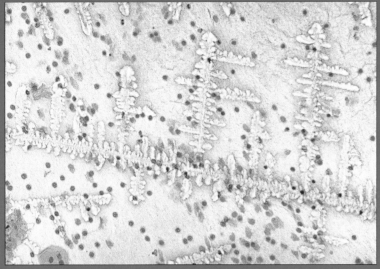

I5.39
Ferning, cervical mucus [C]

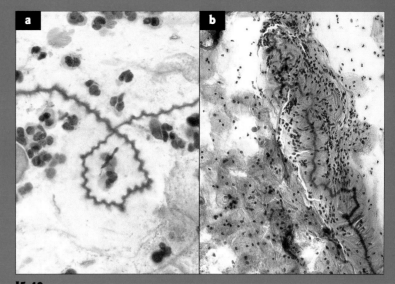

I5.40
a, Curschmann spiral [C]; **b**, Curschmann spiral [C]

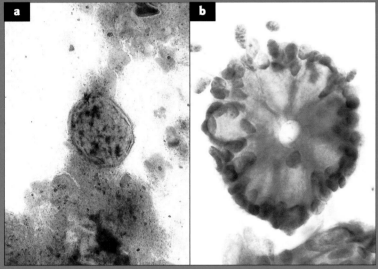

I5.41
a, Rectovaginal fistula, caca [C]; **b**, RV fistula, colorectal cells [C]

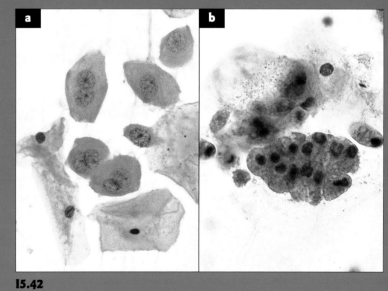

I5.42
a, Vesicovaginal fistula, urothelial cells [C]; **b**, V V fistula, hyaline globules [C]

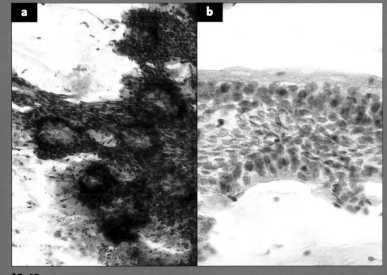

I5.43
a, Colonic neovagina [C]; **b**, Ileal neovagina [C]

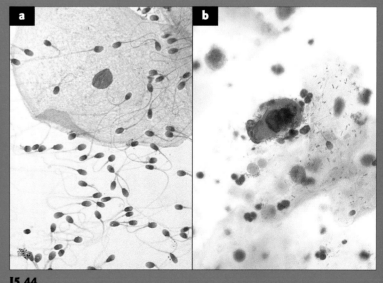

I5.44
a, Sperm [C]; **b**, Seminal vesicle cell [C]

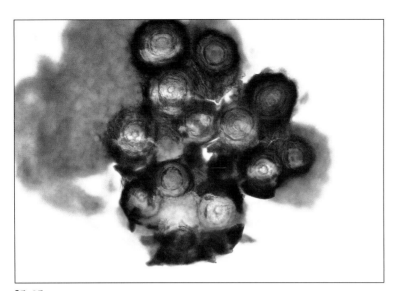

I5.45
Psammoma bodies [C]

ated with benign conditions in at least 50% of the cases [de Peralta–Venturino 2000, Kern 1991a, Nicklin 2001]. Malignancies associated with psammoma bodies occur over a wide age range (~20-85 years), but are relatively more common in post-menopausal women [Athavale 2002, Nicklin 2001, Zreik 2001].

Here are three key points regarding psammoma bodies in Pap tests. First, malignant cells are not always present in Pap tests of women ultimately found to have cancer [Nicklin 2001]. Second, atypical epithelial cells are commonly present in Pap tests of women who do not have cancer, which could result in false positive interpretations [Luzzatto 1981, Parkash 2002, Picoff 1970, Zreik 2001]. And third, in many women no cause is ever identified [Nicklin 2001].

The differential of psammoma bodies includes: "blue blobs" in atrophy, calcific debris, foreign material, inspissated mucus, and corpora amylacea [de Peralta–Venturino 2000, Martínez Girón 2004b]. Benign and malignant associations are outlined, below.

Benign Associations

Benign conditions associated with psammoma bodies include: use of deodorant powders [S Li 1999], benign fallopian tube [Grosen 1997], sexually transmitted disease [D Martin 1995], pregnancy [Zreik 2001], intrauterine contraceptive device [J Barter 1987, P Gupta 1982, Highman 1971], oral contraceptives [Valicenti 1977], benign ovarian cysts [Kern 1991, Luzzatto 1981], ovarian adenofibromas [Gould 1998, Kanbour 1980, Tutschka 1978], tubo-ovarian adhesions [Kern 1991], benign endometrium [Grosen 1997], tuberculous endometritis [DM Jenkins 1977], endometriosis [Zreik 2001], endosalpingiosis [de Peralta–Venturino 2000, Gould 1998, Hallman 1991, Seguin 2000], cervical polyp [Zreik 2001] and other benign gynecologic conditions [Kanbour 1980, S Li 1999, Luzzatto 1981, Picoff 1970].

Malignant Associations

Malignant conditions associated with psammoma bodies include: ovarian carcinoma (particularly serous carcinoma), ovarian borderline tumors [Ahsan 1998, P Benson 1973, Beyer–Boon 1974, Differding 1967, Fujimoto 1982, Kirkland 1979, DM Jenkins 1977, Qazi 1988, Qizilbash 1974b, Y Zhang 2003], fallopian tube carcinoma [Luzzatto 1996, Parkash 2002, Zreik 2001], endometrial malignancies (usually serous

morphology), including carcinosarcoma [An–Foraker 1985, Fugimoto 1982, Hidvegi 1982, Kuebler 1989, Parkash 2002, Spjut 1964, R Weaver 1967], cervical carcinoma (neuroendocrine [Russin 1987], papillary [Seltzer 1983]), primary peritoneal tumors [Shapiro 83], and metastases from nongynecologic cancers [Dance 1970, Fugimoto 1982, Kern 1991a].

Because psammoma bodies are such rare findings in Pap tests, management is not well established [Grosen 1997]. Pelvic ultrasonography, endometrial sampling, and possibly, laparoscopy may be considered to exclude the presence of a gynecologic malignancy [de Peralta–Venturino 2000, Nicklin 2001, Parkash 2002]. Women should also have regular follow-up examinations [Seguin 2000].

Ciliocytophthoria, Detached Ciliary Tufts

Ciliocytophthoria (*phthora*, Greek for destruction), in which the ciliary tufts detach from ciliated cells, was first noted in the female genital tract by Papanicolaou [Papanicolaou 1956] [I5.46]. Although undoubtedly a degenerative change, ciliocytophthoria has not been specifically associated with any disease in the female genital tract [Clocuh 1978, Hollander 1974b, 1979, Huisjes 1968, Kobold–Wolterbeck 1975]. However, these free little red "wigs" have been mistaken for protozoa, erroneously classified as *Polymastigina*, and unnecessarily treated with antibiotics! [Ashfaq–Drewett 1990, Cabanne 1975, Jabamoni 1977]. Easily overlooked and generally insignificant, the incidence is difficult to judge, but ciliocytophthoria is probably not extraordinarily rare if searched for diligently [Rilke 1976]. In the female genital tract, ciliocytophthoria is usually associated with cyclic physiologic shedding of fragments of ciliated epithelium. The source of the ciliated cells ranges from fallopian tube, normal ciliated endocervical cells, and tubal metaplasia. It is more common in premenopausal women [Rilke 1976]. Ovarian lesions can also exfoliate detached ciliary tufts detected in Pap tests [Kanbour 1980]. Ciliated cells or ciliocytophthoria can help distinguish benign reactive lesions from neoplasia.

Collagen Balls

Collagen balls, identical to those described in peritoneal washes, are very rare findings in Pap tests (0.006% of cases) [Sahoo 2004]. They are translucent blue-green, spheroid collagen bodies covered by a layer of flat to reactive mesothelium [I5.46a,b]. They probably arise from serosal surfaces in the pelvis or abdomen, and are transported via the fallopian tube into the uterine cavity, where they eventually find their way into Pap tests. Collagen balls could suggest malignancy, particularly adenocarcinoma. However, they are usually benign, although theoretically, they could also occur in mesothelioma [Sahoo 2004].

Other Artifacts

Plant cells [I5.48a] [Demirezen 1996], pollen [I5.48b] [Demirezen 2000a, Martinez–Girón 2004a], spores [I5.48c] [A–M Korhonen 2001], and algae [I5.48d] [Martínez –Girón 2001] as well as various fibers, eg, from tampons [van Hoeven 1996a], cardboard [I5.49a,b], various "dusts" [I5.49c], lubricants [I5.50a], spray fixation artifact [I5.50b], carpet beetle parts [I5.51a], glove powder (starch) [I5.51b], and even fluorescent dyes from foods and medications (the "glittering vagina") [M Hudson 1996], have been described as artifacts or contaminants of Pap tests. In some cases, these artifacts can mimic tumor cells. Most of these arrive as airborne contaminants. But, as my mentor used to say, *you never know what you might find in a Pap test!* [Ahmad 2002, Benjamin 1994, Jaluvka 1995, Meniru 1996, Puneet 2002].

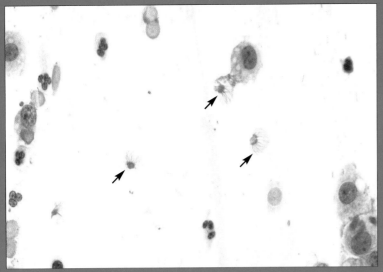

I5.46
Ciliocytophthoria (arrows) [C]

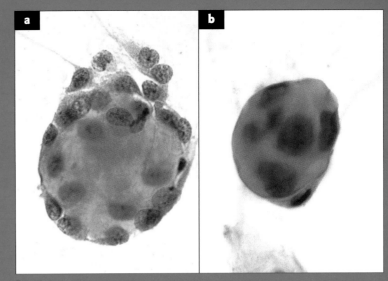

I5.47
a, Collagen ball [C]; **b**, Collagen ball [C]

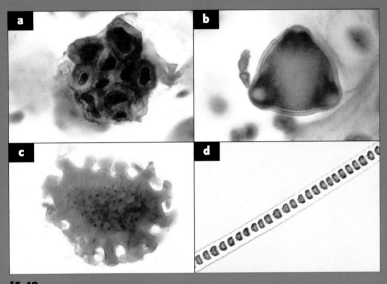

I5.48
a, Plant cells [C]; **b**, Pollen [C]; **c**, Sclereid [C]; **d**, Algae [C]

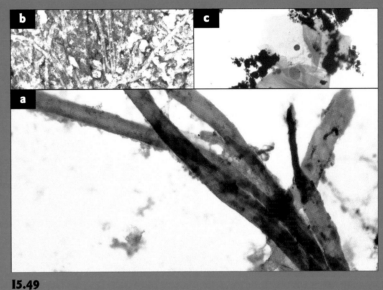

I5.49
a, Cardboard fibers [C]; **b**, Cardboard artifact [C]; **c**, Graphite pencil dust [C]

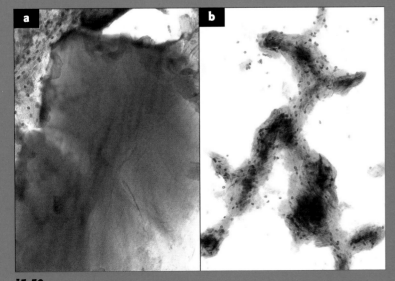

I5.50
a, Lubricant [C]; **b**, Spray fix artifact [C]

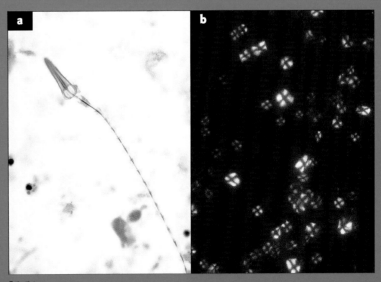

I5.51
a, Carpet beetle part [C]; **b**, Glove powder (starch), polarized [C]

VI. Clinical Considerations

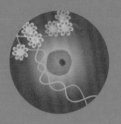

U nfortunately, the key question the clinician wants answered—which lesion will progress, and which will not—cannot be answered for an individual woman [Dupree 1998]. Although on average the behavior of dysplasia is predictable from the morphology, the grades of dysplasia/carcinoma in situ do not necessarily reflect the true biologic potential of a particular lesion [Koss 1978]. To put this problem into clinical perspective: at least 50,000,000 Pap tests are performed annually in the United States; at least 10-20 million women, possibly substantially more, are currently infected with HPV; at least 2.5 million women have squamous intraepithelial lesions; and a million or more women are treated for these lesions annually [Koutsky 1988, Kurman 1994, Morrow 1995, J Walsh 1998]. Yet, most women with SIL will never get cancer; in fact, most SILs disappear on their own, without therapy. Only a tiny fraction of those infected with HPV develop cervical cancer, and fewer still die of the disease (about 10,370 and 3,710 respectively, annually, in the US) [Jemal 2005]. Therefore, most women who are treated for SIL are overtreated, and the cost is currently measured in billions of dollars a year [Dupree 1998, Herbst 1990a,1992, H Jones 1995, Kurman 1994, Morrow 1995, Nobbenhuis 2001].

Any agent that can induce a high-grade lesion has the proven ability to induce cellular anaplasia. Because most cancers arise from the most advanced lesions, CIN 3 is a high- risk lesion. For women with CIN 3, it does not make any clinical difference *if* virus is present, let alone its *type:* the lesion must be destroyed [Crum 1989b]. On the other hand, millions of women are infected with HPV, but do not have lesions. Unfortunately, if there is no lesion to destroy, currently there is little that can be done therapeutically for the HPV-positive woman—even if she has an oncogenic virus. However, she is at high-risk and must be monitored closely.

Clinical Management

The management of precursor lesions has been modified by introduction of new terminology (ie, the Bethesda System), new outpatient therapeutic and screening procedures (such as loop electrosurgical excision procedure, viral testing, and cervicography [Autier 1999, S Costa 2000, Szarewski 1991]), and recognition of human papillomavirus as the cause of cervical neoplasia [Kurman 1994].

Dysplasia Management (4 D's)

Detect (cytology)
Delineate (colposcopy)
Diagnose (histology)
Destroy (LEEP, etc)

The prime objective of clinical management is to exclude the presence of invasive malignancy [Creasman 1981]. Once this has been accomplished, what remains is to determine the grade and distribution of an intraepithelial lesion (dysplasia) [ACOG 1993]. Under ideal conditions, there are four steps to clinical management of dysplasia, which can be summarized as the four D's: Detect, Delineate, Diagnose, and Destroy.

Detect

The first step is to detect the presence of a precursor lesion, in which the Pap test plays a key role. Of fundamental importance is procuring an adequate, representative sample of well-preserved cells. Cytology provides little or no information about the exact location or extent of the disease (although using "VCE" slides [denoting areas for vaginal, cervical, and endocervical samples], some guidance may be given [Wied 1959]).

Delineate

Once a significant lesion has been detected by cytology, the next step is to delineate the extent of the lesion by colposcopic examination of the cervix [JL Benedet 1992, DM Evans 1987, Singer 1984]. A "significant lesion" includes repeated cytologic findings of L SIL or ASC, or any finding of ASC-H, H SIL, atypical glandular cells, or cancer. Note that Pap tests repeated at the time of colposcopy have a high false-negative rate [Beeby 1993, Busseniers 1991, G Davis 1987, DE Jones 1987, Koss 1989a, Nyirjesy 1972, Panos 2001, Simsir 2001, Spitzer 1997, Wheelock 1989, Zardawi 2002]. Also note that colposcopy, like any other test, is subject to false results. The false-negative rate of colposcopy is probably *at least* 20% [Anonymous 2000, Belinson 2001,Cox 2003b, Hellberg 1994, Renshaw 2004a, Solomon 2001].

The colposcope is essentially a set of stereoscopic binoculars. Colposcopic diagnosis is based on evaluation of the surface contour, color (opacity), and outline of the lesion [R Reid 1980, 1984c, 1985]. In addition, stromal changes, often neglected in microscopy, are of primary importance in colposcopy [Stafl 1975]. In concert with abnormal epithelial changes, angiogenesis occurs in the stroma. The capillary network is normally flat, but with epithelial proliferation, it becomes tortuous, compressed, and extends close to the surface. The new blood vessels produce punctation (vessels grow vertically toward surface), mosaicism (vascular proliferation and interconnections), and abnormal vessels (neovascularization, associated with invasive cancer), which are important diagnostic features that can be seen with the colposcope. The vessels supply oxygen and nutrients for neoplastic growth. The stroma probably produces the basement membrane and definitely the vessels. White epithelium corresponds to surface keratosis and hypergranulosis (spiegelosis).

Diagnose

Diagnosis is based upon histologic evaluation of a colposcopically-directed biopsy, endocervical curettage, or conization biopsy. Using directed biopsies, samples of abnormal areas are obtained under direct visualization during colposcopy. Endocervical curettage is used to detect disease in the endocervical canal, but may inadvertently pick up a lesion on the ectocervix, near the external os, resulting in a false-positive curettage (ie, falsely indicating the endocervix is involved). Some clinicians consider a good cytologic sample of the endocervix using an endocervical brush the equivalent of endocervical curettage [Boardman 2003, Cox 1997b, Hoffman 1993, Klam 2000, Weitzman 1988]. Cone biopsy can be obtained surgically (cold knife cone) or by laser; more recently, loop electrocautery has become popular. The loop procedure (known as LEEP, for loop electrosurgical excision procedure, or LLETZ for large loop excision transformation zone) can be performed on an outpatient basis to destroy and diagnose cervical abnormalities detected by Pap test. With this procedure, the abnormal area is entirely excised (if possible) under colposcopic guidance, and the diagnosis is subsequently rendered on the removed tissue. The disadvantages include cautery artifact, which interferes with histologic interpretation. Also, there is a concern that this procedure will be overutilized because of its simplicity. Routine electroexcision of the transformation zone or of nonstaining areas with iodine (positive Schiller test) to evaluate an abnormal Pap test interpreted as low-grade squamous intraepithelial lesion or atypical squamous cells of undetermined significance is not recommended [Kurman 1994].

Destroy

The goal is outpatient treatment, avoiding hospitalization, if possible. If the entire lesion can be seen at colposcopy *and* there is no cytologic or colposcopic evidence of invasion *and* this is confirmed by tissue biopsy (ie, diagnosed), then the lesion can be destroyed on an outpatient basis by cryotherapy, laser ablation, or even by a thorough biopsy resection. Ablation without histologic confirmation of the cytologic interpretation is considered unacceptable [Kurman 1994], although using LEEP, the two processes (ablation, biopsy) can be combined into one procedure (see below).

Colposcopy has substantially reduced the need for conization biopsy [ACOG 1993]. However, if the colposcopy is inadequate, a cone biopsy or LEEP will likely be required [Richart 1981b]. The chance of missing an invasive cancer during colposcopy as well as the therapeutic failure rate is more closely related to the size of the lesion than its grade [Richart 1980a]. On the other hand, since many low-grade squamous intraepithelial lesions regress spontaneously, close follow-up, without cone biopsy, may be appropriate for those who are reliable to return for scheduled appointments [Kurman 1994].

Because it is not possible to predict which individual lesions will progress, many clinicians destroy any abnormality detected in an effort to prevent invasive cancer. However, many young women are diagnosed with transient, low-grade lesions, and therefore, some clinicians are now taking a more conservative approach to treatment. Women with high-grade lesions are usually treated with ablative therapy (cryotherapy or laser) or excisional therapy (LEEP or cone biopsy) [Cirisano 1999]. Other therapeutic approaches, including cytotoxic agents, such as 5-fluorouracil, trichloroacetic acid, and podophillin, are under investigation [Auborn 2000, Beutner 1997a].

Cryotherapy

Cryotherapy involves freezing the tissue below −22°C. The resulting ice formation dehydrates the cells, increasing their electrolyte concentrations, which releases lysosomal enzymes, killing the cells biochemically. The cervical epithelium sloughs, followed by a period of healing that usually lasts about 4-6 weeks. Failure and recurrence rates are low, and similar to cone biopsy.

Laser Ablation

Laser ablation, usually using a carbon dioxide laser, focuses a high-energy beam of infrared light on a small area. The energy is absorbed by intracellular water, causing it to boil and expand; this explodes the cells, literally vaporizing them [Ferenczy 1990]. This process causes less necrosis than cryotherapy, but the equipment is more expensive. Failure and recurrence are similar to cone biopsy or cryotherapy.

Loop Electrosurgery Excision Procedure

Loop electrosurgical excision procedure (LEEP) is currently popular, as mentioned above. A thin wire loop electrode cuts and coagulates the tissue.

This procedure is simultaneously diagnostic and therapeutic. Because it is performed under colposcopic guidance, it is up to the operator, not the pathologist, to determine the surgical margins and that the lesion was adequately excised.

Pap Test Basics

When it comes to Pap testing, even something as basic as whether or not to lubricate the vaginal speculum is controversial. The traditional teaching is that the speculum should be lubricated with warm water only [Koss 1989a, NCCLS 2001], because lubricants can interfere with both conventional Pap smears and liquid-based cytology [Zardawi 2002]. However, some studies have found that a small amount of water-soluble gel lubricant on the vaginal introitus and the outer inferior blade of speculum does not change the Pap test results and can make the procedure more comfortable [Amies 2002, Casselman 1997, Harer 2002, Tavernier 2003]. "Cleaning" the cervix (using a cotton swab) before taking the sample can reduce the number of specimens obscured by inflammation while increasing the number having endocervical cells [Kotaska 2002]; however, if overvigorous, this can remove abnormal cells possibly causing false negative-results [Rubio 1975b].

Endocervical cells (or metaplastic cells), indicative of sampling the transformation zone, are another area of controversy [Birdsong 2001]. Numerous studies have reported the importance of an endocervical, or transformation zone, component in the detection of cervical lesions [Alons–van Kordelaar 1988, Boon 1986, 1989a, Elias 1983, Frost 1969, Killough 1988, Mauney 1990, Mintzer 1999, H Mitchell 1992, NCI 1993a, b, Richart 1965b, J Robertson 1993, Vooijs 1985, 1986, Wied 1955c, CB Woodman 1989]. On the other hand, a few studies have failed to find a significant difference in detection rates for epithelial abnormalities between samples with and without endocervical cells [Baer 2002, Beilby 1982, Hislop 1994, Kivlahan 1986, Selvaggi 2002c, Szarewski 1990, 1993], and some have even demonstrated *more* abnormalities in samples *without* endocervical cells [Bos 2001, Siebers 2003, Vooijs 1985]. Also, longitudinal studies indicate little or no difference in rates of dysplasia or cancer in women with or without an endocervical component [Bos 2001, Kivlahan 1986, H Mitchell 1991, 2001, NCI 1993a, b, Vooijs 1985]. Moreover, the presence of endocervical cells may not be reported consistently [Klinkhamer 1989, H Mitchell 1994a]. The Bethesda System requires at least 10 endocervical or metaplastic cells, although some believe this number may be too small, particularly with regard to detecting endocervical glandular lesions [Frable 1999a, Mintzer 1999].

The presence of endocervical cells is related not only to method of collection, but also to the woman's age, day of the cycle, pregnancy, parity, method of contraception, and cervical disease, among other factors [Vooijs 1987a], including the performance of the person obtaining the sample [Celasun 2001]. The transformation zone recedes with age, making it more difficult to obtain endocervical cells in postmenopausal women [Gondos 1972, Mauney 1990]. Women who have had a previous Pap test with an inadequate endocervical component are more likely to have repeat samples with inadequate endocervical components [Sherman 1993]. At the

Factors Influencing Cellularity and Presence of Endocervical Cells

Anatomy
Skill of taking the sample
Sampling device
Slide preparation
Douching, lubricants, etc
Method of contraception
Age
Menstrual, pregnancy history
Cervical disease, eg, inflammation
Surgery, radiation, chemotherapy
Exogenous hormones (BCPs, HRT, etc)

other extreme, using the endocervical brush, it is possible to obtain Pap tests composed predominantly or exclusively of endocervical cells, without sufficient squamous cells; such specimens are unsatisfactory for evaluation. Note that the mere presence of endocervical or metaplastic cells does not guarantee adequate sampling of the transformation zone or that the Pap test is entirely satisfactory for evaluation. Furthermore, the presence of transformation zone cells in a "negative" Pap test does not completely exclude the possibility of an epithelial abnormality [F Gilbert 1974, Koss 1974]. On the other hand, abnormal cells can be present, even though endocervical cells are absent [Koss 1974]. Such specimens are not unsatisfactory, and the abnormality should be reported.

The sampling device significantly affects the composition of the sample [Boon 1989a, Kristensen 1989a, b]. Among the most commonly used devices today are the Ayre spatula (or a variation), endocervical brush, and the endocervical "broom" (Cervex Brush®). Endocervical aspiration is recommended, but seldom performed, to obtain good endocervical sampling. The use of a saline moistened cotton swab is not recommended due to low yield of endocervical cells. The nylon endocervical brush is much better, not only to increase the rate of recovery of endocervical cells [Boon 1986, Kawaguchi 1987, Kristensen 1989a, b, P Taylor 1987], but more to the point, to increase the rate of detection of dysplasia, especially the more advanced lesions that typically occur in the endocervical canal [Alons–van Kordelaar 1988]. The endocervical brush is more sensitive, although less specific, than endocervical curettage in evaluating the endocervical canal [Hoffman 1993, Weitzman 1988]. The brush should be used with another sampling device, usually an Ayre spatula, to obtain an ectocervical specimen.

The Ayre spatula used with an endocervical brush, or the endocervical broom used alone, are good sampling devices. The "broom" is easy to use and reduces technical artifacts, including air-drying [Cannon 1993, German 1994, Hutchinson 1991, Laverty 1989, Reissman 1988]. Although the brush or the broom add slightly to expense, the expense is more than offset by the increased yield of satisfactory specimens, thereby reducing the need for repeat examinations [Brink 1989, Harrison 1993]. New sampling devices continue to be developed [J du Plessis 2001, Kieswetter 2001, Longfield 1993, Monk 2002]. Note that the samples should be taken before application of acetic acid or Lugol solution (used for colposcopy) and before biopsy [Benda 1987, Cronjé 1997, Griffiths 1989, D Hammond 1980]. (See Technique, pg 199, for further discussion.)

Screening

Before the era of the Pap test, squamous cell carcinoma accounted for 95% of all cervical cancer [Hepler 1952]. So, in the past, "cervical cancer," for all practical purposes, meant squamous cancer. In many ways, squamous cell carcinoma of the cervix is an ideal disease to screen for. (Churchill to his editor, sarcastically, on ending a sentence with a preposition: "This is the sort of English up with which I will not put."). Squamous cell carcinoma was very common, and still is relatively common. It has a long preinvasive phase, so there is a long "window of opportunity" to detect disease. The lesions are usually visible, particularly using colposcopy. The site of occurrence is usually accessible to sampling. The precursor lesions are reasonably well-defined morphologically. And, finally, treating the precursor lesion will usually prevent the cancer. Note that many of these statements are *not* true of adenocarcinoma (not as common, unknown preinvasive phase, colposcopically invisible, not as accessible to sampling, less well-defined precursor lesions [the

very existence of glandular dysplasia is debated], and effect of therapy variable). Ideally, a screening test should have high sensitivity and reasonable specificity. It should be low cost, low risk, and readily acceptable.

While the value of Pap test screening is generally accepted [J Acs 1989, Brinton 1987a, Christopherson 1976, Herrero 1992, CJ Jones 1990, LaVecchia 1987], optimal screening practice is the subject of ongoing debate [S Feldman 2003, Foltz 1978, G Green 1978, Marx 1979, M Miller 2003, Sawaya 2000, 2001, Walton 1976, 1982]. Areas of concern include: the screening interval (most contentious), screening women who have had a hysterectomy, at what age should screening begin, and at what age, if any, can screening be stopped. There is a downside to screening. Screened women pay a price in overtreatment to minimize cervical cancer mortality [Bos 1997].

In the "well-duh" department, for a woman to get cervical cancer, she must have a cervix. Women who have had a hysterectomy are not "at risk" of cervical cancer and the risk of vaginal dysplasia/cancer after hysterectomy for benign disease is very low [J Miller 1987, H Mitchell 1990c, Pearce 1996, Piscitelli 1995, Sirovich 2004b]. (Carcinoma of the vagina accounts for only 0.3% of cancers in women [Sirovich 2004b].) Some women have had supracervical hysterectomies and may not be aware that they still should be screened for cervical cancer. Of course, women who have a history of malignancy require appropriate follow-up.

Most cancers, including cervical cancer, become more common with age. Although screening provides some measure of long-term (5, even 10 years) protection against cervical cancer [IARC 1986], frequent screening of women in their teens, 20s, and 30s does not confer much protection against cervical cancers that most commonly develop in the 50s or 60s [H Mitchell 1990c].

Central to the debate over screening interval is the level of protection offered by a Pap test (interval protection) [Sawaya 2000]. Traditionally, an annual Pap test has been the standard of practice. A single negative Pap test decreases the risk of cervical cancer by nearly 50% and nine lifetime screenings practically eliminates the risk of cervical cancer. The risk of developing invasive cervical cancer is approximately five to ten times higher in unscreened (risk range, 2.5% to 3.75%), compared with screened (risk range, 0.3% to 0.7%), populations [Cox 1998a, D Eddy 1990, Johannesson 1982, Shy 1989, C Walsh 1995]. On the other hand, even in the total absence of screening, a woman's risk of developing cervical cancer may be less than 5%; in other words, at least 95 out 100 women would never get cervical cancer, even if never screened [Cox 1998a, IARC 1986, A Miller 1995, H Mitchell 1990c].

Recently, increasing the interval to 2, or even 3, years has been recommended, largely based on cost-effectiveness studies. Such studies report that cancer screening programs add only about one month (32.4 days) to average life expectancy, compared with a gain of 46 days if cervical cancer were totally eliminated [van den Akker–van Marle 2002]. In an article published in a prestigious medical journal, it was estimated that the risk of cervical cancer changed from 2 cases per 100,000 women to "only" 5 per 100,000 women when the screening interval was increased from 1 to 3 years [Sawaya 2003]. Some organizations consider lengthening the screening interval to be associated with "small" and "reasonable" increased risk. There are several concerns about increasing the interval between screenings [Renshaw 2004a]. Most important, studies generally indicate that as the frequency of Pap screening decreases (from annual testing to less frequent testing), the incidence of cervical cancer increases [Austin 2003a,c, Colgan 2001a, Kinney 2001, McCrory 1999]. Moving from annual screening with conventional Pap smears to screening every three years could translate into an increased lifetime incidence of cervical cancer cases from 153,428 to 712,246, with increased mortality from 29,418 to 162,859 [Austin 2004]. Some people may not view this as "small" and "reasonable" increases! Just because less frequent screening is "cost-effective" does not mean that women, or the legal system, will accept it [Austin 2003c]. And here we come to the central issue of health care in America: what's best vs what's affordable. The gift of life is priceless...but who will pay the price? [Koss 1980].

The Pap test has a significant false-negative rate, as high as 50% [Fahey 1995, Franco 2000, Giard 2001, Hartman 2001, ML Hutchinson 1999, Martin-Hirsch 2002, McCrory 1999, Nanda 2000, Renshaw 2002b], including both sampling and interpretation errors, which are very variable among providers [D Eddy 1990, Koss 1989a, Richart 1981a]. Combining cytology and colposcopy, common in Europe, helps reduce the problem of false-negative results [Lozowski 1982]. Using "new technology" for cervical cancer screening, sensitivity can be improved. There are two points of view regarding the "new technology." Bean counters view the improved sensitivity as a means to increase the screening interval and save money. Patient advocates view the increased sensitivity as a way to decrease cervical cancer and save lives. Unfortunately, these views are diametrically opposed.

There are other arguments to maintain annual testing. Rapidly developing cancers probably exist, and could occur more commonly with an increased screening interval. Some women who actually have cervical lesions will be falsely reassured by "negative" Pap tests, and possibly lost to follow-up for a significant time. Also, the lengthened interval between screenings should be considered for low-risk women only. Because sexual histories are notoriously unreliable and difficult to obtain, it may be more cost-effective to simply take a Pap test. Furthermore, the annual Pap test serves as a reminder to many women to seek regular medical care, have medications reviewed, blood pressure checked, as well as have a physical examination, blood work, mammogram, colon cancer screening, etc [Twombly 2003]. And finally, with regard to increasing the time interval between Pap tests, there is a feeling among many that "if it ain't broke, don't fix it."

Low-risk women are virgins, women with total hysterectomies for benign disease, or women in a long-term monogamous relationship with a long history of negative Pap tests. Women considered to be *at risk* include those who are sexually active, began having intercourse after 20 years of age, and have had no more than two partners. *High-risk* women are defined as women who began having intercourse before 20 years of age or who have had more than two partners [Richart 1981a]. The number of recent (< 5 years) sexual partners is probably more important than the number of lifetime partners [R Burk 1996a,b, Fairley 1994, JP Figueroa 1995, Hildesheim 1993]. The number of sexual partners of the male is also an important risk factor [Brinton 1989b]. Since the "sexual revolution," there may be relatively few sexually active women who are not at risk or at high risk [Noller 1987]. Other important risk factors include history of abnormal Pap test, sexually transmitted diseases, immunosuppression including human immunodeficiency virus infection, and cigarette smoking.

The current Pap Test Screening recommendations, issued by the American Cancer Society, are summarized below [Saslow 2002].

ACS Pap Test Screening Recommendations

The American Cancer Society recommends that cervical cancer screening begin approximately three years after a woman begins having sexual (vaginal) intercourse, but no later than 21 years of age [T6.1]. Screening should be performed every year with conventional Pap smears or every two years using liquid-based cytology. Beginning at age 30, women who have had 3 consecutive normal tests may be screened every two to three years. However, health care providers may recommend more frequent testing if a woman has certain risk factors, such as HIV infection or a weak immune system. Beginning at age 70, women who have had three or more normal Pap tests and no abnormal Pap tests in the last 10 years may choose to stop cervical cancer screening. Screening after

T6.1 American Cancer Society Screening Recommendations

1. Begin screening 3 years after starting sexual intercourse, but no later than 21 years of age.
2. Screen every year with conventional Pap smear or every 2 years with liquid-based tests.
   After age 30, women with 3 normal tests in a row can be screened every 2-3 years.
3. Stop screening at age 70 with 3 or more normal Pap tests and no abnormal Pap tests in last 10 years.
4. Screening after total hysterectomy is not necessary, unless hysterectomy performed for cervical cancer or precancer.
5. More frequent screening in certain situations, eg, HIV infection or weak immune system, as determined by the health care provider and the woman.

total hysterectomy (with removal of the cervix) is not necessary unless the surgery was performed for treatment of cervical cancer or precancer. Women who have had a subtotal hysterectomy (leaving the cervix) should continue to be screened until at least age 70.

The American College of Obstetricians and Gynecologists (ACOG) has also issued recommendations that differ only slightly from the ACS recommendations [Anonymous 2003b]. For example, ACOG does not make a distinction between conventional Pap smears and liquid-based Pap tests, recommending annual screening with either until age 30 years. ACOG also does not set an upper age limit on screening, and leaves the choice to the clinician and the woman. Many clinicians may continue to recommend annual Pap tests. Even when annual examinations are recommended, up to 75% of women fail to return for a repeat in the second year [Wied 1981].

Sample Collection

General Instructions

The woman should not use vaginal medications, vaginal contraceptives, or douches for 48 hours before the test [T6.2]. Sexual intercourse should be avoided for 24 hours before the test (because cervicovaginal cells may be denuded by minor trauma, vaginal contraceptives or lubricants can interfere with interpretation, and seminal vesicle cells can be misleading). The sample should not be obtained during menstruation; days 15 to 25 are optimum. Pap tests should not be obtained until 6 to 8 weeks postpartum, if possible, to allow healing.

Technique

There are several acceptable methods of obtaining a Pap test. For conventional Pap tests, a combination of an Ayre spatula for ectocervical sampling plus a brush for endocervical sampling is recommended. Both samples can be placed on a single slide. Plastic spatulas are preferred over wooden spatulas, and cotton swabs are not recommend, because plant fibers trap cells. The broom samples both the ectocervix and endocervix simultaneously.

When using a spatula, the sample should be obtained by a *firm* scrape of the cervix, rotating it one full circle (360°). For conventional Pap smears, the spatula is used to spread, or literally smear, cells on the slide.

The endocervical brush is inserted into the cervical os, with some bristle still showing, and rotated between 90°-180°. Rotating the brush too much

T6.2 Procedure for Taking a Pap Test

Instructions for the woman:

No vaginal medications, contraceptive, or douches for 48 hours
No sexual intercourse for 24 hours
Optimum time, days 15-25; not during menstruation

Instructions for the clinician:

Use speculum lubricated with warm water
Cervix and adjacent vagina should be well-visualized
Sample ectocervix and endocervix separately (except with broom)
  Ectocervix: Rotate spatula with firm pressure over entire ectocervix (360°)
  Endocervix: Rotate brush 90° to 180°, no more
  [Broom: Rotate, clockwise, 3 to 5 full circles]
Prepare slides, fix immediately or place in LBC transport medium
Vaginal pool sample or cervical canal aspiration for detection of endometrial disease

T6.3: Recommended Follow-Up According to Specimen Adequacy

Unsatisfactory
• Repeat cytology in 2-4 months*

NILM with "quality indicators": No transformation zone component or partially obscured specimen
• For most women, repeat cytology in 12 months**
• For pregnant women, repeat postpartum

Consider 6 month repeat for:
• Previous squamous abnormality (≥ASC-US)
• Previous unexplained glandular abnormality
• Positive high-risk HPV test within 12 months
• Inability to visualize the cervix clearly or to sample the endocervical canal
• Immunosuppression
• Similar obscuring factor in consecutive screenings
• Inadequate frequency of previous screening

*additional evaluation may be indicated for some women
**assumes regular screening
Refs: Davey 2002, 2003b

can cause bleeding; inserting too deeply will obtain lower uterine segment/endometrial cells that can mimic H SIL or AIS, making interpretation difficult. Although originally not recommended for use during pregnancy, the endocervical brush has been found safe when properly used [Paraiso 1994]. The brush is not smeared or scrubbed on the slide; rather, the brush is gently rolled over an area about the size of a quarter (25¢ piece).

The broom is used by placing the longer central strips into the cervical os, with the lateral strips in contact with the ectocervix. It is then firmly rotated, *clockwise*, 3 to 5 full circles (1080° to 1800°). Clockwise rotation is important because the plastic strips are sharper on one side. Each side of the broom is then "painted" on the glass slide.

For conventional Pap smears, immediate fixation (< 10 seconds) is crucial to prevent air-drying artifacts. Commercial spray fixatives or immersion in 95% ethanol are recommended. For liquid-based Pap tests, recommendations vary with the manufacturer, but generally involve placing the cells in a transport medium instead of spreading the cells on a slide (see pg 214).

Pap Test Management Guidelines

Suggestions for follow up of women with inflammatory Pap test results are presented below. Recommendations from the American Society for Colposcopy and Cervical Pathology (ASCCP) for management of women with abnormal Pap test results are summarized (see pg 244ff) [Cox 2003a, Davey 2002, T Wright 2002a]. Consensus guidelines for management of women with cervical intraepithelial neoplasia have also been published [T Wright 2003a]. Consensus guidelines for following patients based on specimen adequacy are presented in tabular form [T6.3]. In making follow-up recommendations, lack of compliance is a serious issue that must be considered [Alanen 1998, Arora 2001, Bornstein 2004, Bucchi 2001, Quillet 1997, Suh–Burgmann 1998].

Inflammatory Change and Repair

Inflammatory change is a poor predictor of cervical infection, unless a specific pathogen is identified [Bertolino 1992, Kelly 1990, W Parsons 1993]. When the

lesion is apparently inflammatory, the woman can be treated appropriately for any specific infection and the Pap test repeated in a relatively short period of time ("treat and repeat"). If no specific infectious agent can be identified, sometimes a Betadine® douche or broad-spectrum antibiotics will be effective in clearing a nonspecific inflammatory process (not recommended for management of ASC-US). A rapidly repeated Pap test is not necessarily indicated in women with inflammatory changes (and rapidly repeated Pap test have high false-negatives rates). However, women with "only" inflammatory changes on Pap tests, particularly when the changes are persistent, are at increased risk (average, ~15% to 20%, range 3% to 50+%) of having squamous intraepithelial lesions [Busseniers 1991, Castle 2001, Cecchini 1990a, Creasman 1981, Cuzick 2001, Frisch 1990, Himmelstein 1989, Lawley 1990, Margolis 1999, McLachlan 1994, K Miller 1992, Neumoff 1987, Parashari 1995, Pearlstone 1992, Reiter 1986, Schwebke 1997, Seckin 1997, Sidawy 1993, Soofer 1997, Webb 2001b, J Wilson 1990]. Women with sexually transmitted diseases have a high risk of squamous intraepithelial lesions. Inflammatory change ("inflammatory atypia") can also mimic dysplasia.

To manage women with repair/regeneration, treat any identifiable infection/inflammation as specifically as possible, and repeat the Pap test within a short period of time. If cervical neoplasia cannot be excluded, refer the woman to colposcopy. Women who have a reparative process are at high risk of cervical neoplasia (squamous intraepithelial lesions) and should be monitored more closely.

Atypical Squamous Cells of Undetermined Significance (ASC-US)

There are three acceptable ways to manage a woman with a Pap test interpretation of ASC-US: 1. Repeat Pap test, 2. Colposcopy, or 3. Reflex HPV-DNA testing. Repeat Pap testing is widely used, but insensitive, and because it requires several return office or clinic visits, it is considered expensive (although, women should return for routine check-ups, regardless of their Pap test results). The disadvantage of immediate colposcopy is that it is relatively expensive, unpleasant, and anxiety provoking [Cox 1999]. Because HPV-DNA testing is highly sensitive and has a negative predictive value of >98% [*Cox 1995, 1999, 2000b, 2001, Crabtree 2002, Manos 1999, Schiffman 2003b*], reflex HPV testing on residual material from a liquid-based Pap test is currently the follow-up method preferred by the ASCCP. A concern, however, is that ASC-US rates, already high, could soar when using reflex HPV testing, since there will be medical, legal, and financial incentives to diagnose ASC-US with reflex HPV testing.

F6.1 DeMay Classification System

Happy Face: See you next time   Sad Face: Let's have a look

Atypical Squamous Cells, High-Grade Squamous Intraepithelial Lesion Cannot Be Excluded (ASC-H)

Because studies have shown that the subcategory of atypical squamous cells in which a high-grade squamous intraepithelial lesion cannot be excluded (ASC-H) has substantial predictive value for finding a high grade SIL on biopsy, averaging about 50% (range, 25% to 75%), the ASCCP recommends immediate colposcopy for women with an ASC-H interpretation. If any CIN is found, it is managed according to established protocol [*T Wright 2003a*]. If no lesion is identified, the ASCCP recommends reviewing all pertinent data (Pap test, colposcopic findings, and biopsies) to plan management. Because the prevalence of HPV diminishes with age, HPV testing could possibly be useful in women older than 35 years (though, currently, this is not an ASCCP recommendation).

Low-Grade Squamous Intraepithelial Lesion (L SIL)

Women with a Pap test interpretation of L SIL have at least a 15% to 20% chance of having H SIL (CIN 2,3) on biopsy. It had been hoped that HPV testing would be helpful in clinical management of women with L SIL interpretations, but it turned out that the large majority (>80%) of women with low-grade lesions have "high-risk" viral types. Therefore, HPV testing is not recommended for triage of women with L SIL.

Because of the risk of an underlying H SIL, the ASCCP recommends immediate colposcopy for women with a Pap test interpretation of L SIL. If no lesion is identified, endocervical sampling is recommended in non-pregnant women. Ordinarily, neither HPV testing nor repeat Pap testing is adequate for triage. However, in postmenopausal women, estrogen therapy *or* repeat Pap test at six months *or* HPV testing in one year are acceptable management alternatives. In teenagers, immediate colposcopy *or* repeat Pap test in six months *or* HPV testing in one year is acceptable.

High-Grade Squamous Intraepithelial Lesion (H SIL)

For women with a Pap test interpretation of H SIL, immediate colposcopy is recommended. For women with satisfactory colposcopy in whom CIN I or a less significant lesion is identified on biopsy, the ASCCP recommends reviewing all pertinent data to determine further management. Women with satisfactory colposcopy and a lesion worse than CIN I are managed according to established protocol [*T Wright 2003a*]. For women with unsatisfactory colposcopy, in whom no lesion is seen, all pertinent material is reviewed to determine further management. If any CIN is identified, it is managed according to protocol.

Atypical Glandular Cells (AGC)

Atypical glandular cells (AGC) is an irreproducible Pap test interpretation, but it nevertheless carries a significant risk of a significant underlying abnormality. HPV testing is not currently recommended by the ASCCP for triage of these women. For all categories of AGC, except atypical endometrial cells, the ASCCP recommends colposcopy plus endocervical sampling. For women older than 35 years or for those with abnormal bleeding at any age, endometrial sampling is also recommended. For women with a Pap test interpretation of atypical endometrial cells, endometrial sampling is recommended. Although HPV testing is not currently recommended by the ASCCP for triage of women with Atypical Glandular Cells, HPV negative women are highly unlikely to have cervical neoplasia (either glandular or squamous), although they could have endometrial carcinoma or some other lesion.

Summary of Management Guidelines

According to the Gary Larson Far Side School of Veterinary Medicine, the therapy for any malady of a horse, from a runny nose to a broken leg, is to shoot it. One could make an analogy to Pap test abnormalities: no matter what the abnormality, from ASC-US to ASC-H to AGC to L SIL to H SIL, immediate colposcopy is either acceptable or preferred management (the only exception being atypical endometrial cells, for which endometrial sampling is recommended—but then the Pap test is no good at screening for endometrial pathology anyway). So, based on this, the next iteration of Pap test terminology could be a happy face or a sad face. Women with "happy face" interpretations would return for their next regularly scheduled screening ("See you next time"); those with "sad face" interpretations could be considered for colposcopy ("Let's have a look") [F6.1, 6.2].

F6.2 Summary of Pap Test Terminology

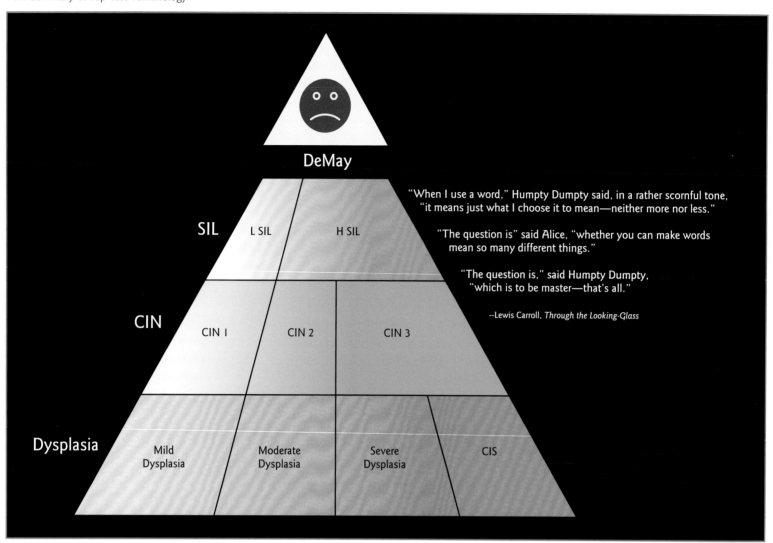

DeMay

"When I use a word," Humpty Dumpty said, in a rather scornful tone, "it means just what I choose it to mean—neither more nor less."

"The question is" said Alice, "whether you can make words mean so many different things."

"The question is," said Humpty Dumpty, "which is to be master—that's all."

--Lewis Carroll, *Through the Looking-Glass*

SIL | L SIL | H SIL

CIN | CIN 1 | CIN 2 | CIN 3

Dysplasia | Mild Dysplasia | Moderate Dysplasia | Severe Dysplasia | CIS

VII. Failure
of the Pap Test

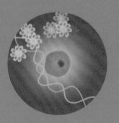

n the war on cancer, the Pap test has been our most effective weapon. No other test ever invented has been as successful as in eradicating cancer. Yet, in the past several years, the Pap test has gotten a lot of "bad press" [C Bedrossian 1994, Bogdanich 1987a, b, Koss 1989a, SE Wang 1994], including such sensational headlines as: "Homicide Charged in Lab Error on Pap Test" which appeared on the front page of newspapers nationwide in 1995. Because of its outstanding success in cancer prevention, expectations for the Pap test have been raised so high that any result short of perfection is likely to be considered malpractice and ominously, even criminal activity [Austin 1994b, 2003c, R Carr 1994, Koss 1978, 1993a, P Martin 1972, Robb 1993]. Unfortunately, despite its undeniable success,

---

The Pap Test

The Pap test is not perfect!!!

Can detect 50% to 90% precursor lesions

Fails to detect at least 10%–50%

Cannot detect all significant abnormalities

Problems:

·Sampling error: "no cells, no diagnosis"

·Diagnostic errors

Screening (failure to find)

Interpretation (failure to categorize)

---

the Pap test is not perfect.

The Pap test is a rather crude test with sensitivity as low as 50% [McCrory 1999]. Low sensitivity is obviously a bad thing for a screening test. But, specificity is also important. Because the overwhelming majority of women are normal, even small changes in specificity have profound effects on overall quality. To give an example, suppose 100,000 women, with a disease prevalence of 5000, are screened. A great improvement in sensitivity, from 50% to 85%, would mean that an additional 1750 cases of disease would be detected (true positives). But, a small loss of specificity, from 97% to 95%, would mean that an additional 1900 false positives would occur, more than offsetting the increase in true positives [Hartmann 2001].

What's more, Pap tests have never been proven effective in preventing adenocarcinomas, and yet, cervical adenocarcinomas are the basis of up to 80% of Pap test related lawsuits [Austin 2003a, b, Colgan 2001a, Cox 1998b, Renshaw 2004c, Richart 2000]. The failures of the Pap test were recognized from the very beginning of screening in the 1940s, investigated in the scientific literature since the 1970s, and trumpeted in lay press since the 1980s (Walt Bogdanich, front page Wall Street Journal, Pulitzer Prize; Diane Sawyer, Prime Time, etc etc etc). Every informed citizen, and certainly anyone providing health care for women, should know about the limitations of the Pap test by now. Missing, or misinterpreting, abnormal cells is *exactly* what is meant by these Pap test failures.

In theory, cervical carcinoma is preceded by a long prodrome of preinvasive disease that can be detected and treated, thereby preventing this cancer [Briggs 1979, Walton 1976, 1982]. In practice, although a remarkable reduction in cervical cancer has in fact occurred, cervical cancer has never been completely eradicated, in any population ever reported, no matter how thoroughly screened [Austin 2003a, c, J Carmichael 1984, M Costa 1991a, Devesa 1989, J Dunn 1981, Fidler 1968, Koss 1989a, 1993a, P Martin 1972, Rylander 1976, Walton 1982]. In the United States, despite half a century of screening, with at least 50 *million* Pap tests now performed annually [Austin 1993, Koss 1980, Davey 2000, Richart 1995, Stoler 2000c, 2003b, J Walsh 1998], 10,370 women are still expected to develop cervical cancer, and 3,710 die of it, in one year alone [Jemal 2005]. Moreover, cervical cancer remains a leading cause of cancer-related deaths in many countries [Parkin 1988, 1999a,b, Pisani 1999, 2002, Robles 1996]. Thus, in the real world, the goal of completely conquering cervical cancer is probably *impossible* to achieve through Pap test screening...and the question is: Why?

There is a chain of events that cannot be broken in order for the screening process to work in cancer prevention. First, the woman must come in to be screened. Then, the clinician must take an adequate, representative, well-preserved Pap test. Next, the cytologist must correctly identify any neoplastic lesion in the Pap test. Then, back to the clinician, who must act appropriately on the result. And finally, the woman must present herself either for therapy or her next regularly scheduled Pap test.

Although the Pap test can fail at many levels, ironically, the single most important error is failure to get women tested in the first place [P Martin 1972, A Miller 1995, H Mitchell 1993b, Slater 1994]. This can be because a woman—for whatever reason—fails to visit a health care provider or because the provider fails to obtain a Pap test. Unfortunately, other clinical errors, such as failure to follow up abnormal results, failure to perform a biopsy of suspicious lesions (the Pap test is not a substitute for biopsy), and failure to investigate suspicious symptoms (the Pap test is not a substitute for good clinical judgment), are also important factors in failure of prevention of cervical cancer morbidity and mortality. In addition, some cancers may progress so rapidly that they develop in the interval between screenings, precluding prevention by the Pap test.

---

2 Key Points in Management

1.*Biopsy any suspicious lesion*

2.*Investigate any suspicious symptoms*

Regardless of Pap test results!

Of course, problems in interpretation also occur (discussed in more detail below). However, many, if not most, problems relate to sampling errors, ie, few or no abnormal cells present on the glass slide, rather than errors of interpretation ("no cells, no diagnosis") [Dehner 1993, DiBonito 1993, Dodd 1993, Gay 1985, Husain 1974, M Joseph 1991, Joste 1995, Kristensen 1991, Lundberg 1989, Mobiüs 1993, Rohr 1990, Vooijs 1985]. Furthermore, the sensitivity of the Pap test has probably been grossly overestimated. Conventional Pap smears may have a sensitivity of as low as 50% in detection of H SIL [Fahey 1995, Franco 2000, Giard 2001, Hartman 2001, ML Hutchinson 1999, Martin-Hirsch 2002, McCrory 1999, Nanda 2000, Renshaw 2002b].

It must be clearly understood, by clinicians and the general public alike, that no cytology laboratory is completely free of error, the most important—for the present discussion—being false-negative results. False-negative results occur in every cytology laboratory, even the best [Austin 1994a, b, Beilby 1982, Bonfiglio 1993, Boon 1993, M Bosch 1992, J Carmichael 1984, Cecchini 1985, D Collins 1986, L Coppleson 1974, Davey 1993, JR Davis 1981, Davison 1994, Dehner 1993, Derman 1981, Fidler 1968, Gay 1985, Grosskopf 1978, Husain 1974, Janerich 1995, B Jones 1993, S Jordan 1981, Kierkegaard 1994, Klinkhamer 1988, Koss 1989a, b, 1993a, b, P Krieger 1994, Luthy 1978, H Mitchell 1988, Plott 1987, Richart 1964a, 1965b, Robb 1993, Sedlis 1974, Seybolt 1971, Shingleton 1975, Shulman 1974, Soost 1991, K Syrjänen 1992, Tabbara 1996, Tuncer 1967, van der Graaf 1987b, Wied 1981, Yobs 1985, Yule 1972]. Even when women are part of a study group, and the samples are taken with great care and thoroughness, and screened with exceptional attention, false-negative results still occur [Richart 1964a]. In meta-analysis of 28 published series, when reportedly "negative" Pap tests were reviewed following a "positive" interpretation, abnormal cells were in fact present in retrospect, in nearly half of cases [T7.1] [Allen 1994, Attwood 1985, Berkeley 1980, Berkowitz 1979, DiBonito 1993, Dodd 1993, Gay 1985, Hatem 1995, Husain 1974, Koss 1993a, Kristensen 1991, W Liu 1967a, LiVolsi 1984, Lundberg 1989, Macgregor 1993, P Martin 1972, H Mitchell 1990b, Morell 1982, Pairwuti 1991, M Paterson 1984, R Peters 1988, Richart 1964a, J Robertson 1993, 1994, Rylander 1976, 1977, Sherman 1992b, Slater 1994, Tuncer 1967, van der Graaf 1987a, b, Wain 1992, E Walker 1983]. What's more, the mistakes

Richard M DeMay

7

T7.1 False-Negative Results in the Pap Smear*

Study	Interval Preceding Positive Diagnosis	No. of Negative Smears Reviewed	No. (%) Reclassified as Abnormal
Tuncer 1967	Unknown	7	6 (85.7%)
P Martin 1972	Within 1 yr	13	10 (76.9%)
Hatem 1993	Averaged 9.3 mo	17	13 (76.5%)
Attwood 1985	Within 5 yr	28	20 (71.4%)
J Robertson 1993	Up to 12 yr	139	92 (66.2%)
Rylander 1977	4 to 5 yr	56	35 (62.5%)
Berkowitz 1979	Within 2 yr	13	8 (61.5%)
Pairwuti 1991	Unknown	70	43 (61.4%)
M Paterson 1984	Within 10 yr	58	34 (58.6%)
H Mitchell 1990b	Within 36 mo	136	75 (55.1%)
van der Graaf 1987b	3 yr	226	121 (53.5%)
Wain 1992	Within 2 yr	30	16 (53.3%)
Sherman 1992a	Median 93.5 mo	123	65 (52.8%)
LiVolsi 1984	Within 1 yr	10	5 (50.0%)
Kristensen 1991	Within 3 yr	96	39 (40.6%)
Gay 1985	Within 1 yr	63	24 (38.1%)
Husain 1974	3 mn	25	9 (36.0%)
Dodd 1993	Unknown	153	55 (35.9%)
DiBonito 1993	Unknown	59	21 (35.6%)
R Peters 1988	Within 3 yr	32	10 (31.3%)
E Walker 1983	Within 5 yr	11	3 (27.3%)
Schwartz 1988[†]	6 to 17 mo	22	5 (22.7%)
Slater 1994	1 to 8 yr	17	3 (17.6%)
Allen 1994	75% Within 2 yr	80	12 (15.0%)
Morell 1982	Within 3 yr	36	2 (5.6%)
W Liu 1967a	3.4 yr	16	0 (0.0%)
Richart 1964a	Unknown	9	0 (0.0%)
Total		1545	726 (47.0%)

- On average, nearly half of cases (47%) had abnormal cells on review.
- Many of the other cases were actually unsatisfactory or limited, rather than negative.
- A few cases may represent rapidly progressive cancers.

[†]Includes 10 cases from a previous report [Berkeley 1980].

often seem to be obvious errors on review in the "retrospectoscope" [M Bosch 1992, J Robertson 1993, 1994]. Many women with false-negative results only appear to have "negative" tests, when in reality the specimens were of limited quality (transformation zone not sampled, obscured by exudate, etc) or were entirely unsatisfactory for evaluation [Fetherston 1983, H Mitchell 1990b, Sherman 1992b]. Very low false-negative proportions may simply reflect poor sensitivity of rescreening [Naryshkin 2000].

Although the false-negative proportion (false-negatives compared with all positives, basically a quality assurance statistic [Lundberg 1989]) may seem alarmingly high, women can be reassured that the vast majority of *all* negative results (false-negatives compared with all tests, the discrepancy rate) are truly negative [G Anderson 1987, Austin 1994b, Lundberg 1989, Naryshkin 1996]. No one ever died of cervical dysplasia or carcinoma in situ. Even invasive carcinoma is rarely lethal when caught early (especially when microinvasive). Of clinical importance is that as many as 9 of 10 women with false-negative Pap test results have a history of abnormal Pap tests; therefore, the error is usually not

an isolated misleading event [Figge 1970, Hatem 1995, Hopkins 1991b, H Mitchell 1990b, M Paterson 1984, Sherman 1992b, Shulman 1974, Wain 1992]. In addition, most women have well-defined risk factors, and those with frank cancer are frequently symptomatic or have visible cervical lesions; yet too often, appropriate follow-up is not undertaken [Andersson–Ellström 2000, Fetherston 1983, Frable 1994, W Liu 1967a, P Martin 1972, Pretorius 1991, P Schwartz 1988, Tuncer 1967].

Clinically, many women have a lapse in screening [Sherman 1992b]. False-negative results may be more common in younger women [M Paterson 1984, Rylander 1977] and with more serious lesions [A Benoit 1984, Berkeley 1980, Berkowitz 1979, Richart 1965b, Rubio 1981b, Tuncer 1967, van der Graaf 1987b]. Unfortunately, Pap testing is simply less effective in preventing cancer in young women, exactly those who are most likely to sue [Gustafsson 1997, Macgregor 1994, Morrow 1995, Parkin 1985, Sasieni 1999, M Quinn 1999].

False-positive results also occur [MB Anderson 1997, P Levine 2003, McIntyre–Seltman 1995, Mount 2004]. They are of less medicolegal concern than false-negative results, because abnormal Pap test results should always be confirmed

205

histologically before major therapy (ablation, surgery, radiation, etc) is undertaken [Koss 1989a, 1993b, Kurman 1994, P Levine 2003, G–K Nguyen 1996]. In fact, cytology with a high false-positive rate lowers the risk of cancer [Ferenczy 1996b]. On the other hand, false-positive results can cause harm, which may take the form of increased evaluation, overtreatment, and psychologic distress [Hartmann 2001]. And because of the cost of investigating non-existent lesions, false-positive results may actually be *more* expensive than false-negatives, even factoring in the cost of litigation. Estimated costs per year of life saved by screening ranges from a few dollars in countries with no prior screening program to tens of thousands of dollars in the United States, where substantial resources are devoted to management of minor cytologic abnormalities [Crum 2002, Goldie 2001]. The cost of management of women with "atypical squamous cells" alone is estimated at several *billion* dollars a year in the United States [Titus 1996].

The false-positive rate for an interpretation of invasive carcinoma is conventionally thought to be on the order of 1% [D Eddy 1990, Yobs 1987]; however, it is probably substantially higher (although most will have H SILs) [Grubb 1967, Konikov 1969, P Levine 2003, Mount 2004, Uyar 2003]. The false positive rate for interpretations of SIL are also significant [Cox 1996]. False-positive interpretations can be divided into "true false-positives" and "false false-positives."

True false-positive results are usually due to interpretation errors. These include overinterpretation of benign changes due to inflammation, repair, degeneration, florid squamous metaplasia, radiation, etc [Davey 1993, Dodd 1993, Koss 1993b, Mount 2004, Sidawy 1992,1994]. Overinterpretations of H SIL and atypical repair are among the most common sources of false diagnoses of malignancy [Grubb 1967, Konikov 1969, P Levine 2003, Mount 2004].

False false-positives, ie, apparent false-positive results, can also occur. For example, a "false false-positive" could occur if the Pap test correctly identifies a lesion, but it regresses before colposcopic or biopsy confirmation [Crum 1998, D Eddy 1990, Husain 1974]. The spontaneous regression rate for dysplasia detected cytologically is as high as 60%-80% for low-grade SILs [Campion 1986, D Eddy 1990, C Fox 1967, Macgregor 1978a, Richart 1969b, J Robertson 1988]. False false-positive cytology results could also represent sampling error on the part of the biopsy; this is more likely if the biopsy is scant or the lesion is small or inaccessible [Frost 1969, Howell 2004a, Husain 1974, T Nichols 1968, Papanicolaou 1958, Sidawy 1994]. Squamous carcinoma precursor lesions of the cervix, especially when high-grade (CIN 3), can be easily dislodged, inadvertently, during sterile preparation of the biopsy site, dilatation and curettage preceding biopsy, or rough handling of the excised tissue [Frost 1969]. Rarely, even the minimal trauma of taking the Pap test itself can remove the dysplastic epithelium before biopsy [Berner 1980]. Small cervical lesions could be missed clinically, and overlooked, or occult vaginal or vulvar lesions could shed abnormal cells [Crum 1998]. Also, an apparent overinterpretation or "false-positive" of the Pap test may actually represent underinterpretation or misdiagnosis of the histology; this is probably not rare [Dodd 1993, Hellberg 1994, P Martin 1972, Seybolt 1971, Wadehra 2003]. Another important factor, which has not been well appreciated, is that colposcopy has a substantial false-negative rate, on the order of 20% to 40% for squamous lesions (glandular higher) [Anonymous 2000, Belinson 2001, Cox 2003b, Hellberg 1994, Renshaw 2004a, Solomon 2001]. Failure of colposcopy to identify the lesion to biopsy could make the Pap test interpretation seem to be a false-positive result, ie, a "false false-positive." (The Pap test can be right when the colposcopy is wrong, but clinicians tend to believe colposcopy results ["I did it myself!"] more than the Pap test results.) Of clinical importance is that many women with seemingly false-positive Pap tests will eventually have significant lesions on further follow-up [Dodd 1993].

Factors Related to Failure of Pap Test Screening

Reasons for failure of the Pap test in cervical cancer prevention are discussed in more detail below. In more than one way, the Pap test has been a victim of its own success. Mathematically, because the prevalence of cervical cancer has fallen so dramatically, the predictive value of the Pap test is correspondingly diminished, irrespective of the sensitivity and specificity of the test itself [Stelow 2004].

Factors related to failure of the Pap test in cervical cancer prevention can be divided into five groups: (1) patient, (2) clinician, (3) instrument and sample, (4) cytopreparation and interpretation, and (5) the lesion. These factors are, of course, interrelated.

Patient-Related Errors

The largest group of factors related to failure of Pap test screening are patient-related errors, including failure of women to get regular Pap tests or to seek any health care at all [J Carmichael 1984, Elkas 1998, Janerich 1995, Kinney 1998a, Koss 1989a, Macgregor 1993, P Martin 1972, Noller 1998, Rinas 1999, Sung 2000, Wied 1981, S Wilson 1992]. Up to 25% of American women 18 years of age and older, with an intact cervix, have not had a Pap test in the past 3 years, and as many as 10% have never had a Pap test [Hewitt 2002, Pretorius 1991, Sirovich 2004a, USHHS 1993]. These figures are even higher among poor, poorly educated, or older women [Brooks 1996, USHHS 1993]. Failure to get Pap tests has many explanations, ranging from inability to pay to distrust of doctors [P Martin 1972]. Some women are unaware of the importance of the Pap test and 1 in 25 has never even heard of it [NCHS 1987, USHHS 1993]. People frequently procrastinate, and put off having a Pap test, but in some cases, they simply refuse it, even when it is offered to them [P Martin 1972]. (Clinicians may also fail to offer the test—read on.)

In a study of 1000 cancer patients from the University of Chicago, of 500 women with squamous cell carcinoma of the cervix, 387 had not had a Pap test within the previous 10 years and an additional 63 had not had one in the previous 5 years (total = 450/500 cancer patients without a Pap test in at least 5 years). Of the remaining 50, 42 had "positive" Pap tests, but did not return for therapy. Therefore, more than 98% of cases (492 of 500) of invasive carcinoma could be considered patient-related errors. Of the remaining 8 patients, 3 had been treated for cervical intraepithelial neoplasia but developed invasive carcinoma later. In contrast, of another 500 women with squamous cell carcinoma detected by the Pap test, 453 were still alive at 10 years and only 3 had died of disease (the remaining 44 were lost to follow-up). Finally, of 1 million women, about one half did not return *at all* during the 27 years of the study. And only 3% had more than six Pap tests in the same period [Wied 1995].

In other studies, between 13% and 31% of women who develop cervical cancer had at least one negative Pap test within the preceding three years [Kristensen 1991, M Mitchell 1996]. Nearly 20% of women under 40 with cervical cancer had had a previous abnormal Pap test result, but were lost to follow-up [Anonymous 1989b, Cox 2001].

Other patient-related factors occur. For example, douching or coitus can mechanically remove the superficial cell layers that the Pap test samples, causing false-negative results due to sampling error [Rubio 1975b, 1981b, 1994]. Some women delay seeking medical attention even when they have symptoms that they know are suspicious, such as abnormal vaginal bleeding [P Martin 1972].

Clinical Errors

The next largest group of errors, unfortunately, comes from those who should "know better," the health care providers or clinicians [P Martin 1972, Rinas 1999]. Among the most common clinical errors are failure to take a Pap test at all [Koss 1989a, P Martin 1972, Mobiüs 1993, Slater 1994] or failure to take an adequate Pap test [Attwood 1985, Mobiüs 1993, Rubio 1981b]. Physician specialty, and to a lesser extent, gender also affect women's receipt of Pap tests (and other preventative services) [Cassard 1997].

Obtaining a Pap test is more complex than many people appreciate [Koss 1989a, Nasca 1991]. The sample must be obtained under direct visualization, with considerable pressure [Koss 1989a]. The speculum should not be lubricated excessively, if at all [Amies 2002]. Overzealous rubbing, swabbing, or "cleaning" the cervix before taking the sample can remove the abnormal cells, leading to false-negative results [Rubio 1975b]. Well-trained health care providers, not necessarily physicians, take better Pap tests; false-negative results are higher when students or untrained personnel obtain the sample [Brink 1989, Celasun 2001, Frost 1969, Husain 1974, Koss 1989a, Macgregor 1993, von Haam 1962, Wolfendale 1991]. Failure of the clinician to provide pertinent clinical data can severely compromise cytologic interpretation of the Pap test [Koss 1993a, Wain 1992].

Other common clinical errors include failure to follow-up abnormal Pap test results, failure to perform a biopsy of suspicious lesions, and failure to investigate suspicious clinical symptoms [J Carmichael 1984, Koss 1989a, P Martin 1972, Mobiüs 1993, E Walker 1983]. Unfortunately, some clinicians accept a "negative" report at face value, disregarding statements of specimen adequacy (quality indicators) [Attwood 1985]. Miscellaneous problems, such as clerical errors, also occur [Attwood 1985, P Martin 1972].

Instrument and Sample Errors

The instrument used to obtain the Pap test can also be a source of errors related to sampling [Rubio 1994]. The original Papanicolaou method of vaginal pool aspiration is much less efficient in obtaining cervical cells than the direct scrape method of Ayre [Ayre 1947, Richart 1965b, Wied 1955c]. However, vaginal pool samples are more useful in detecting cancer cells from the endometrium, fallopian tubes, and ovaries, cancers that become increasingly more common in women past 40 years of age [Husain 1974, Koss 1984, 1989a, Lundberg 1989]. An endocervical sample can be obtained by scrape, aspiration, brush, or broom. The endocervical brush may be more sensitive, though less specific, than formal endocervical curettage for diagnosis [Hoffman 1993, Weitzman 1988]. A combination of spatula and brush enhances sampling compared with either device used alone [Buntinx 1996].

The material from which the sampling device is made is important. Cotton swabs and wooden spatulas tend to trap cells so they unavailable for interpretation [L Katz 1979, Rubio 1977a]. Wooden spatulas collect between 600,000 and 1.2 million epithelial cells, but less than 20% are transferred to the glass slide when making a conventional Pap smear [Hutchinson 1994]. Furthermore, the transfer of cells to the slides is random and statistically prone to error because the abnormal cells are not homogeneously distributed in the sample [A Goodman 1996]. Endocervical samples taken by cotton swabs or with plastic spatulas obtain fewer atypical cells than do endocervical brushes [Rubio 1980a, b, c]. The shape of the sampling device is also important for obtaining an adequate sample, particularly of the endocervix.

The manner in which the conventional Pap smear is made is also important, including the smearing technique (zigzag, back and forth,

circular, etc) [Frost 1969, Rubio 1981c] and the pressure exerted while smearing [Rubio 1983]. In addition, once on the slide, the cells—"floaters"—may detach from the slide during processing (possibly causing a false-negative result) and can even reattach to another slide (possibly causing a false-positive result) [Rubio 1975a].

Sufficient numbers of well-preserved cells must be collected and the sample must be representative, including the transformation zone. A conventional Pap smear must be thinly spread and immediately and properly fixed [Frost 1969]. Hair spray is not an acceptable fixative; although some have high alcohol content, the composition can change without notice and the containers tend to disappear without explanation! [Holm 1988]. Thick specimens hamper or prevent microscopic examination, which may lead to false-negative results [Gay 1985, Rubio 1981b]. Air-drying due to delayed fixation causes cellular artifacts that can make it impossible to recognize atypical cells [Frost 1969, Gay 1985, Husain 1974, Koss 1974, Richart 1964a, Rubio 1981b]. As a cell air-dries, the air:water interface that passes through the cell exerts tremendous surface tension forces that denatures and disrupts proteins, forever altering the chromatin. This force has been calculated to be 320 tons/square inch (or 457 mg/μm^2) [G Gill 1998]. Liquid-based cytology avoids many of these sampling and preparation problems, eg, nonhomogeneous samples, air drying, etc [Hutchinson 1994]. However, other problems, such as clogging of filters, drop out of cells, and staining artifacts, can occur.

Cytopreparation and Interpretive Errors

Errors in Pap tests can arise in relation to cytopreparation, screening, or interpretation, as well as to general laboratory problems, such as mislabeling slides [Morell 1982, Rubio 1975a]. The Papanicolaou stain must be carefully monitored to prevent staining artifacts that can make interpretation difficult or impossible. Also, as previously mentioned, stains can become contaminated with "floaters," which can lead to false results [Husain 1974, Rubio 1975a]. Therefore, fresh preparation or frequent filtration of the stains is necessary [Koss 1989a, Rubio 1981b]. Pap tests should be stained separately from nongynecologic specimens [Lundberg 1989].

Screening a Pap test is like playing "Where's Waldo?" but more difficult. Waldo has consistent features and he's always around somewhere. Dysplasia varies from case to case and it's usually not present.

Pap Test Interpretive Problems:

Few abnormal cells (particularly <250)
Small abnormal cells (difficult to find)
Bland abnormal cells (difficult to interpret)
Hyperchromatic crowded groups (HCGs)
   (difficult: usually benign, can be malignant)
Certain tumor types
   Adenocarcinoma and adenosquamous CAs
   Minimal deviation tumors:
      Adenoma malignum; Verrucous CA
Also: lymphoma, sarcoma, other tumors
Obscuration: Excess exudate, blood;
   poorly preserved
Inadequate clinical information

Errors in cytologic interpretation are frequent even among experts, particularly when the quantity, preservation, or visualization of atypical cells is limited [Sherman 2001].

There are several points to be considered in assessing screening errors, ie, failure to detect abnormal cells that are present on the slide. Three of the most important sources of interpretive problems relate to the presence of *few* abnormal cells, *small* abnormal cells, and cytologically *bland*

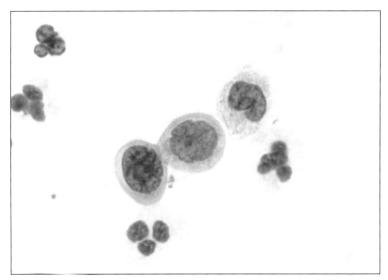

17.1
Few, small, bland cells (CIN 3) [C, oil]

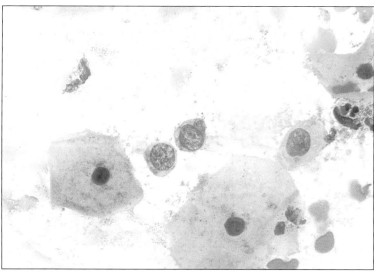

17.2
Few, small, bland cells (squamous cell carcinoma) [C]

abnormal cells [17.1, 17.2] [M Bosch 1992, Dressel 1992b, Fetherston 1983, Hatem 1995, Koss 1978, 1989a, 1993a, W Liu 1967a, Painwuti 1991, J Robertson 1993, Sherman 1992b, van der Graaf 1987a].

Conventional Pap smears typically have 50,000 to 300,000 normal epithelial cells, and liquid-based Pap tests have 50,000 to 75,000 cells. The number of abnormal cells is a *key* feature in reliability of the Pap test; this applies to both conventional Pap smears and liquid-based cytology [Renshaw 2004e]. When abnormal cells are sparse, they are more difficult to detect: it's like looking for a needle in a haystack. *The scientific evidence clearly shows that it is unreasonable to expect the Pap test to detect low numbers of abnormal cells in routine screening.* Although it is sometimes possible to detect even a single abnormal cell, especially in retrospective review, the presence of few abnormal cells (less than 50 to 250) has been well-documented as an important factor in false-negative results [R Baker 1999, M Bosch 1992, Hatem 1995, H Mitchell 1995b, 1998, O'Sullivan 1998b, Renshaw 2004c, Sherman 1992b]. The precise number of abnormal cells is of secondary importance. Slides containing thousands of abnormal cells can still be falsely interpreted as negative [R Baker 1999]. The ability to detect abnormal cells is influenced by many factors besides cellularity (see pg 207). Hyperchromatic crowded groups of cells pose unique interpretive difficulties not related to cellularity (see pg 182).

Paradoxically, low-grade lesions are often easier to detect than high-grade, serious lesions in the Pap test. Low-grade lesions tend to occur on the portio vaginalis, where they are readily sampled, and have the biggest, "ugliest" nuclei, which are found in the largest (most mature) cells. Therefore, these low-grade abnormal cells tend to be not only numerous, but also tend to stand out conspicuously in the Pap test ("outstanding...and they are mild"). Most of these low-grade lesions are clinically insignificant, and most of them will disappear on their own, even without treatment [M Brown 1985, Montz 1992, K Nasiell 1986, Patten 1978]. Respective review of "negative" Pap tests preceding invasive carcinoma rarely has only L SIL; more than 90% are re-interpreted as H SIL when abnormal cells are present [M Paterson 1984, Pinto 2000, Stanbridge 1992]. In other words, it is rare to be sued for missing L SIL.

On the other hand, high-grade dysplasias are significant precursor lesions that are more likely to progress to invasive cancer if left undetected. Unfortunately, high-grade dysplasias tend to be hidden in the endocervical canal, where they may be difficult to sample, and may be represented only by teeny-tiny

little cells with subtle cytologic abnormalities. Consequently, these small, bland—but serious—cells may be sparse and difficult to detect in the first place, and difficult to interpret once detected [M Bosch 1992, Hatem 1995, Montes 1999, J Robertson 1993, Sherman 1992b]. These small cells have high N/C ratios and minimal chromatin abnormalities, and may closely resemble ordinary immature squamous metaplasia, or even histiocytes [17.1] [M Bosch 1992, Dressel 1992b, Hatem 1995, O'Sullivan 2000, J Robertson 1993, Sherman 1992b]. A potential clue to the correct interpretation is that high-grade dysplastic cells usually have irregular nuclear membranes, resulting in characteristic "raisinoid" nuclei that look like shriveled up little raisins [17.1, 17.3]. (Interestingly, these cells that can look so bland in the microscope, can look far more ominous in photographs, especially when blown up to enormous proportions, which might lead a juror to think, "How could a qualified cytologist miss an abnormality that even I can see?" [O'Sullivan 2000].)

Another factor in misinterpretation is that high-grade lesions are usually accompanied by a low-grade component in the sample. The large and conspicuous, but low-grade cells may dominate and obscure a smaller, but more serious, high-grade component [Jarmulowicz 1989]. At least 15% to 20% (up to 40%) of cases suggestive of a low-grade lesion on Pap test will have a high-grade lesion on biopsy, and a few will have invasive cancer [Contreras–Melendez 1992, Crescini 1991, Duggan 1998a, Giles 1989, Greene 2001, S Hall 1994, Hanton 1966, J Hunt 1994, Jarmulowicz 1989, Kok 2000, Koss 1993b, Kremer 1955, Law 2001, K Lee 1997a, Lyall 1995, Maclean 1951, Montz 1992, Parazzini 1995, Pinto 2000, J Robertson 1988, Rohr 1990, Soutter 1986, K Syrjänen 1992, Tay 1987e, Tidbury 1992, E Walker 1986, Zuna 2002]. Some studies have found that up to 75% of biopsy-proven H SILs are preceded by negative, atypical, or low-grade SIL Pap test results [Howell 2004b, Kinney 1998b, Lonky 1999, Lyall 1995]. (A word of advice: when "on the fence" between L SIL and H SIL, diagnose aggressively, because these women have an increased risk of having H SIL on biopsy [Nasser 2003].) Conversely, up to 50% of Pap test interpretations of L SIL, and perhaps 15% of those of H SIL, will be not be confirmed on biopsy [Cioc 2002, Crum 1998, DiBonito 1993, B Jones 1996, Rasbridge 1995, Rohr 1990, Sidawy 1994]. These are not necessarily cytologic "overcalls." In most cases, the cytologic diagnosis is confirmed on review [Joste 1995]. Probably the most common source of discrepancy is sampling variation at the time of colposcopy [MB Anderson 1997, Cioc 2002, DiBonito 1993, B Jones 1996, Tritz 1995]. Re-evaluation of the histologic specimens, including reinterpretation of slides as well as reorientation and deeper sectioning

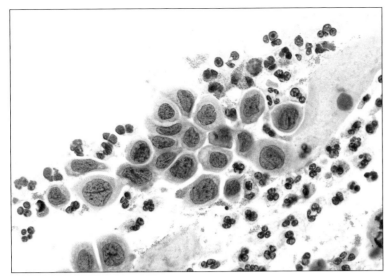

I7.3
Raisinoid nuclei, CIN 3 [C]

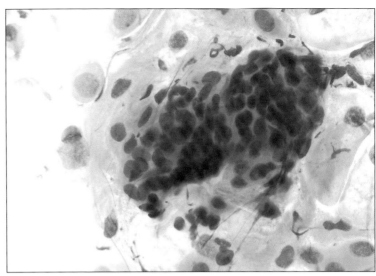

I7.4
HCG Atrophy [C]

of the blocks, will find many additional lesions [Bewtra 2003]. Also, many of these women harbor high risk HPVs [F Brown 1999, Joste 1995].

The results of histo-cyto-correlation in the *real world*, the actual outcomes of over 20,000 cases from nearly 350 laboratories, are shown in [T7.2] [B Jones 1996]. It is easy to see that the results are not perfect, with both overcalls and undercalls being common. Although biased in the sense that every woman was biopsied, the results clearly show that Negative or Reactive Pap test results do not guarantee absence of serious cervical disease, including invasive cancer!

HPV testing can help in two ways. Women who test positive for high-risk viral types are at risk, regardless of Pap test results: this is their safety net against false negative results. On the other hand, to help guard against false positive results, a possible guideline is that at least 15% to 50% of women with ASC-US, and 60% to 80% of those with L SIL, should test positive for HPV [Ferenczy 1995, Lörincz 1986, Sarode 2003, Sherman 1994, Stoler 2003a]. What the acceptable HPV positivity rate for women with negative Pap tests should be is unknown, but may be in the range of 10% to 40% [Stoler 2001b, 2003a].

As with precancerous lesions, fully malignant lesions can sometimes exfoliate cells with bland cytologic features, making recognition difficult or impossible [17.2] [Kok 2000, Koss 1989a, Seybolt 1971]. At the other end of the spectrum, accurately and reproducibly interpreting "atypical" findings is impossible [Koss 1993b, Robb 1994, Seybolt 1971]. Unfortunately, in some cases, "atypical cells" may be the only

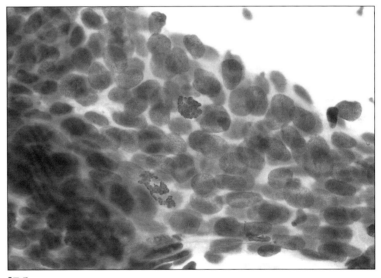

I7.5
HCG CIS, note mitoses [C]

identifiable cytologic abnormality during the early development of high-grade squamous intraepithelial lesions [Sherman 1992b].

Hyperchromatic crowded groups (HCGs), also known as tissue fragments or microbiopsies [Mravunac 1997, 1998, 2000], as has been emphasized throughout, can also present difficult problems in interpretation, and are well documented sources of false results [Boon 1991, Austin 2003b, DeMay 2000, M Harris 2000, Ramsanooj 2002, J Robertson 1993, Sherman 1992b, 1999, Stanbridge 1980]. Although hyperchromatic crowded groups are usually benign and include such entities as endometrial cells and severe atrophy [17.4], they can also represent a variety of serious lesions, eg, carcinoma in situ [17.5]. Look for disorderly arrangements of the cells (loss of nuclear polarity, chaotic architecture), coarse, dark chromatin, and mitotic figures—features that suggest carcinoma [Boon 1993, DeMay 2000]. Another helpful clue: squamous carcinoma in situ is usually accompanied by squamous

T7.2 Histo-Cyto Correlation in Real Life

Pap Test Result	Histologic Correlation (%)			
	Benign	L SIL	H SIL	Cancer
WNL/"Negative"	**65.7**	26.3	7.0	1.03
BCC/"Reactive"	**66.7**	24.3	8.4	0.61
L SIL/CIN 1	13.5	**67.0**	19.2	0.24
H SIL/CIN 2, 3	6.5	15.5	**75.9**	2.05
Cancer	4.2	3.2	16.7	**75.9**

Q-Probes Study: 22439 cases. 348 labs [B Jones 1996]

dysplasia. Other serious lesions, besides carcinoma in situ, that can present as hyperchromatic crowded groups include invasive squamous cell carcinoma and cervical adenocarcinoma, in situ and invasive [Boon 1991]. In glandular neoplasia, the hyperchromatic crowded groups, although generally similar to those of squamous carcinoma in situ, often have "feathery" edges, well-defined microacini, and elongated, oval nuclei with distinctively coarse, dark chromatin (see pg 182 for more discussion of HCGs) [DeMay 2000].

Other problems in Pap test interpretation include inflammatory changes, regeneration/repair, radiation effect, and atrophy [J Robertson 1993, Seybolt 1971]. Another error is rendering a negative interpretation on unsatisfactory material [Berkowitz 1979, Gay 1985, P Martin 1972, M Paterson 1984, P Schwartz 1988, Slater 1994, van der Graaf 1987b, Wain 1992]. This problem is specifically addressed in the Bethesda System by requiring a statement, in every case, regarding specimen adequacy. Inadequate clinical information can severely compromise cytologic interpretation [Koss 1993a, Wain 1992].

Probably the single most important source of diagnostic error is loss of concentration due to human fatigue, rather than inability to identify abnormal cells [Husain 1974, Koss 1993a, Pairwuti 1991, J Robertson 1993]. As mentioned before, screening is like searching for a needle in a haystack. It is an extremely tedious and mentally demanding chore [Husain 1974, Koss 1989a]. Compounding the tedium of screening is that most samples have no abnormal cells (most haystacks have no needles). Sustaining attention (maintaining vigilance) is difficult, particularly when the screener expects relatively few abnormalities to be present [Fowkes 1986]. Screeners need regular, short breaks, and it is best if they do not spend the entire day screening and can devote part of the day to other duties [Husain 1974]. Screening has also been compared to proofreading, with misspelled words being analogous to abnormal cells. Conventional Pap smears usually have on the order of 50,000 to 300,000 cells [Koss 1989a]. Imagine reading, say 50 books a day, each averaging approximately 100,000 words, looking for a few spelling errors in an occasional manuscript. Printed words, however, usually do not contain obscuring artifacts [Rinas 1999].

There is also a class of cells that have been designated "litigation cells" [Austin 1994b, Frable 1994]. (And now with the possibility of criminal charges in cases of misread Pap tests, these cells may well become known as "jail cells.") Litigation cells are important sources of false results, including both false-positive and false-negative readings [Frable 1994]. The clinical significance of these cells ranges from completely benign to frankly malignant. Here is a not quite tongue-in-cheek description of litigation cells. They can be found singly or in groups, including sheets or clusters. They are small, medium, or large cells, with low, intermediate, or high N/C ratios, smooth or irregular nuclear membranes, fine to coarse chromatin, which can range from pale to dark, and have inconspicuous to prominent nucleoli. The cytoplasm varies from squamoid to glandular or indeterminant, with smooth or irregular contours. The cells can be few or numerous, well preserved or degenerated, and obvious or obscured in the sample. Litigation cells can be mistaken for normal, reactive, or neoplastic conditions, including, but not limited to, metaplasia, parakeratosis, repair, human papillomavirus effect, dysplasia, endometrial cells, tubal metaplasia, and squamous or adenocarcinoma!

These are expensive cells [Frable 1994]. Found *prospectively*, litigation cells may lead to overcalling in order to prevent false-negative results and potential litigation, or even criminal prosecution. Such defensive medicine often results in unnecessary colposcopy, biopsy, conization, and even hysterectomy—all at enormous expense [Frable 1994, TJ Kline 1994]. These procedures cost billions of dollars annually [Herbst 1992, Kurman 1994]. Found *retrospectively*, in women with "bad outcomes," litigation cells can cost nearly a million dollars *each* in malpractice judgments [Frable 1994]. When Pap tests are reviewed for malpractice cases, experts cannot always agree on exactly which cells are abnormal, even though the same experts may testify that abnormal cells were present (they don't know which ones they are, but they're sure that they're there!) [Austin 1994b].

Ultimately, the idea that every cell in every Pap test can always be accurately identified is just plain wrong. The fact is that abnormal appearing cells can almost always be found in retrospective review of Pap tests [Hatem 1995], *even in women without cervical neoplasia* [W Sun 2002]. Because almost all Pap tests contain cells that mimic dysplasia or cancer, virtually any slide could be used by a plaintiff's expert witness to claim that a lesion was missed [W Sun 2002]! In fact, because the case is presented to a lay jury, any cell chosen *at random* could be said to be abnormal by an unscrupulous (or misinformed) expert. Fortunately, guidelines have been adopted for expert slide review in context of litigation [Fitzgibbons 2000].

Finally, to detemine that a cytologic interpretation is a false-negative result, it is usually compared against the "gold standard" of histologic diagnosis [Raab 1994]. But, histologic examination is itself well less than perfect [Clary 2003, DiBonito 1993, J Dunn 1981, Richart 1965b]. Few studies have challenged the histologic "gold standard" when evaluating apparant cytologic errors. Those that did, however, changed the histologic diagnosis in one-quarter to one-third of cases [Bewtra 2003, Dodd 1993]. In a histo-cyto correlation study, when a discrepancy occurred, the majority were attributable to histologic, rather than cytologic, misinterpretation [Clary 2002]. Moreover, there is a body of evidence that competent pathologists cannot agree with each other—or even with themselves from day to day—on the classification of the tissue biopsies, let alone the cytology [Cocker 1968, Confortini 1993, de Vet 1990, 1992, Duca 1988, Duggan 1999, Genest 1993, D Gupta 2001b, Hicklin 1984, Holmquist 1967b, Husain 1974, Ismail 1989, 1990, S Jones 1996, Klinkhamer 1988, 1989, Koss 1978, 1989a, Lambourne 1973, Llewellyn 2000, H Mitchell 1993b, O'Sullivan 1994, 1996, 1998a, Renshaw 2001a, A Robertson 1989b, Rohr 1990, Seybolt 1971, Siegler 1956, Willcox 1987, Woodhouse 1999, Yobs 1987, N Young 1994b]. Interobserver variation changes with the severity of the lesion. However, some studies find correlation is best for invasive cancer, intermediate for high-grade SIL, and poor for low-grade SIL, while other studies find the opposite, ie, better agreement for L SIL and less for H SIL and carcinomas [Renshaw 2003]. In the ALTS trial, a panel of experts reviewed 2237 cervical biopsies. Less than half (43%) of biopsies originally diagnosied as low-grade SIL were confirmed on review [Stoler 2001b]. The experts often downgraded L SIL to benign, reactive changes (but they did not have to worry about lawsuits for missed lesions). The dismal results for ASC-US and AGC correlations were previously discussed (see pgs 63 and 146).

How good a screener are you? There are four spelling errors in the preceding paragraph. Did you find all of them on the first reading? If you have to go back to look for them, armed with advanced knowledge, it is akin to the "special case" kind of rescreening that occurs with proficiency testing or legal case review. A test in the normal screening (reading) environment is completely different from a test in which one has been previously alerted. In the normal screening situation, abnormal cells (or spelling errors) are more commonly missed than in a known testing situation. This is why one should be skeptical of the value (or honesty) of rescreening Pap tests for proficiency testing (or malpractice litigation) [M Bosch 1992, TJ Kline 1994]. Moreover, when cases are reviewed under such conditions, although the false-negative cases may be "caught," the false-positive rates and screening times soar, which seriously compromises laboratory efficiency and cannot help but increase health care costs [M Bosch 1992].

Lesion-Related Errors

Certain problems in interpretation relate to the lesion itself, some of which have been discussed in the previous section. For various reasons, some lesions fail to exfoliate sufficient numbers of cells for detection [Felix 2003, Husain 1974, Koss 1989a, P Martin 1972, R Peters 1988, Richart 1964a]. "Nonshedding" lesions are extremely unlikely to be detected by the Pap test [Felix 2003]. Small or inaccessible lesions (eg, high in the endocervix) may be difficult to sample adequately [P Martin 1972, Morell 1982, Pinto 2002a, J Robertson 1993, Rylander 1977, Sherman 1992b]. False-negative cytology is more common with smaller lesions [Barton 1989b, Giles 1988, Jarmulowicz 1989]. Interestingly, the shape of the cell [Rubio 1981c] and the quality of the cervical mucus also affect the sampling [Rubio 1983]. Unfortunately, Pap tests are more often inadequate in women with advanced epithelial abnormalities [A Benoit 1984, Berkeley 1980, Berkowitz 1979, Richart 1965b, Rubio 1981b, Tuncer 1967, van der Graaf 1987b]. Necrosis, inflammation, or bleeding may obscure, alter, or dilute the abnormal cells, making interpretation difficult [Gay 1985, Husain 1974, Koss 1989a, Pairwuti 1991, J Robertson 1993, Rubio 1977b, Seybolt 1971, van der Graaf 1987a]. Hence, another paradox: the Pap test is less efficient in detecting invasive carcinoma than of finding preinvasive disease, with false-negative results occurring in up to 75% of cases of squamous cell carcinoma (average, ~50%) [A Benoit 1984, Gay 1985, Gondos 1972, Husain 1974, Jafari 1978, SJ Johnson 2001, Konikov 1969, Koss 1989b, 1993a, Pairwuti 1991, Richart 1964a, Rubio 1981b, van der Graaf 1987a, b]. Certain types of tumors are more difficult to identify in the Pap test, particularly adenocarcinoma and adenosquamous carcinoma, but also lymphoma and sarcoma, leading to increased false-negative rates for these tumors [A Benoit 1984, M Bosch 1992, J Carmichael 1984, Gay 1985, Jafari 1978, Kristensen 1991, W Liu 1967a, P Martin 1972, H Mitchell 1988, 1993a, Nieminen 1995, Rylander 1977, P Schwartz 1988, Wain 1992]. Some tumors (eg, verrucous carcinoma, adenoma malignum) are composed of normal, or nearly normal-appearing cells, making cytologic recognition difficult or impossible.

Pap tests repeated within a short time (up to several weeks) have a particularly high false-negative rate, up to 80⁺%, even when carefully obtained at the time of colposcopy [Beeby 1993, Busseniers 1991, G Davis 1987, DE Jones 1987, Koss 1989a, Nyirjesy 1972, Panos 2001, Simsir 2001, Spitzer 1997, Wheelock 1989, Zardawi 2002]. Apparently it takes some time for the lesion to regenerate sufficient cells to be detected in the cytologic sample. A "negative" following a "positive" interpretation can mislead the clinician into thinking the lesion has regressed or the previous positive report was wrong. It is also possible that some tumors progress so rapidly that they develop in between Pap test screenings (see rapidly progressing tumors, pg 75).

Standard of Practice

Most societies accept failure as an unfortunate, but inevitable, result of the imperfect nature of any test. Not the United States. Here medicolegal pressure to "name and blame" for any unfortunate result, plus a genuine desire by all to eliminate every preventable death, has led to the intense (read, costly) investigation of even the most minimally atypical (read, essentially normal) Pap test [Cox 1996]. Historically, there was a desire to avoid overdiagnosis that kept the number of abnormal test results within reason. This has been superseded by the fear of being held responsible for missing any abnormality [Scheiden 2003]. In the past, cytologists were reluctant to make a diagnosis unless they had *all* the criteria; now they feel pressured to make an interpretation if they have *any* of the criteria. There has been a fundamental change from diagnosing what you think it *is*, to what you're afraid it *could be*. The financial, physical, and psychological costs of this change from diagnostic conservatism to liberalism are enormous.

A zero screening error rate for Pap test interpretation is an impossible standard of practice. It is both unreasonable and unachievable [Austin 1994b, M Bosch 1992, R Carr 1994, Koss 1989a, Robb 1993, 1994, Valente 1994a]. Unfortunately, however, acceptable practice standards have not been well defined in cytology [Dehner 1993]. It is probably impossible to define an acceptable screening error rate. Blinded review of slides involved in litigation has been promoted as a reasonable method of determining if the standard of care has been met (see Chapter 10) [Frable 2004, Renshaw 2004f]. This is, of course, retrospective. Even if a standard could be defined, it would not be meant to condone sloppy work or incompetence, but rather to acknowledge the reality of significant errors by competent, conscientious cytologists [R Carr 1994]. Cytology practice guidelines, which provide an encapsulation of expert opinion, have been adopted by the American Society of Cytopathology [Anonymous 2001].

Probably owing to its remarkable success in cancer prevention, the sensitivity of the Pap smear has been highly overestimated in the past. It has now been documented that the sensitivity of the conventional Pap test in detecting high-grade lesions is as low as 50% [Fahey 1995, Franco 2000, Giard 2001, Hartman 2001, ML Hutchinson 1999, Martin-Hirsch 2002, McCrory 1999, Nanda 2000, Renshaw 2002b]. Even with the advent of LBC, there may still be an irreducible 20% false-negative rate in actual practice [Nanda 2000]. Anyone who suggests that the Pap test performs perfectly or that errors are tantamount to negligence is being unscientific, at best, or just plain lying. And because everyone makes mistakes, errors must be judged not as individual cases, but in the context of overall laboratory performance. Laboratories that are in substantial compliance with pertinent rules and regulations, eg, CLIA '88, and pass inspections (eg, CAP), are *ipso facto* practicing high quality cytopathology, by definition meeting "standard of care" expectations.

Although it is a common assumption that screening errors are usually the result of professional incompetence, poor supervision, inadequate continuing education, or excessive number of cases, this is not the case in most accredited laboratories. *Most errors occur because screeners are human and humans make mistakes.* This simple, obvious fact cannot be remedied by rules and regulations, proficiency testing, or malpractice litigation. Any system that relies upon perfect human performance, all of the time, is doomed to failure, at least some of the time, even if the penalty for error is severe.

The ability of the Pap test to prevent cervical cancer is inversely related to its cost [Austin 1994b, Helfand 1992]. Quality assurance measures and application of "new technology" [Boon 1993, Koss 1994, Ouwerkerk-Noordam 1994], take time and cost money [Austin 1991, Davila 1994, Koss 1993a]. For example, it has been estimated that complying with a *single* CLIA regulation can cost as much as 40 *million* dollars annually [Allen 1995]. Therefore, the unintended consequence of efforts by the "cytobureaucracy" to reduce the false-negative rate could actually be to *increase* the number of invasive cancers by reducing access to this life-saving test for the very women (low-income, high-risk) who are most likely to benefit from it [Austin 1994a]. More women, by far, develop cervical cancer owing to failure to get regular Pap tests than to errors in cytologic interpretation [Attwood 1985, J Carmichael 1984, E Clarke 1979, Janerich 1995, P Martin 1972, Mobius 1993, Morell 1982, Nasca 1991, Noller 1998, M Paterson 1984, Rinas 1999, MA Quinn 1989, Tuncer 1967, E Walker 1983, S Wilson 1992]. It may well be that keeping the price of the Pap test low, encouraging more frequent Pap tests, casting the screening net wider to encompass as many women at risk as possible, and/or public education regarding the importance of the Pap test are more cost-effective than some of the other quality assurance measures [Bachner 1991, JL Benedet 1992, Helfand 1992, Holland 1993, Sherlaw-Johnson 1994, MA Quinn 1989]. The value of regulatory proficiency testing, in particular, has been questioned [Austin 1994a, Bachner 1991, M Bosch 1992, CL Collins 1994]. In fact, some evidence suggests that such regulations cause more harm than good [Austin 1991, 1994a]. Because regulatory policies directly affect health care, perhaps they should be subjected to the same standards required of medical tests and pharmaceuticals, such as proof of efficacy, safety, etc [Helfand 1992].

The Pap test is a screening test, not a diagnostic test [Robb 1993]. Although the Pap test is a critical component in cancer detection, it is not the only important component [Koss 1989a]. Clinicians must guard against a false sense of security generated by negative Pap test results [D Ashley 1966a, Berkowitz 1979, Koss 1989a, P Martin 1972, P Schwartz 1988, Sherman 1992b]. A "negative" report does not guarantee the absence of significant cervical disease [Hadjimichael 1989, P Martin 1972, P Schwartz 1988]. The Pap test is not a replacement for careful clinical evaluation [Berkowitz 1979]. The clinician must decide whether to follow or treat the woman according to the clinical findings and level of risk for disease [Robb 1993]. A biopsy must be taken of suspicious visible lesions, and clinical symptoms cannot be ignored, even if the Pap test is completely normal. The Pap test is not a good a screening test for glandular cancers of the female genital tract, which are increasingly common despite widespread screening [Andersson 2003, Austin 2003b,c, A Benoit 1984, Bergström 1999, Bjersing 1991, Boddington 1976, Boon 1987, Brinton 1987b, J Burk 1974, Canavan 2000, Christopherson 1979, Colgan 2001a, Crum 2002, Erzen 2002, Etherington 2001, Franco 2003, Fry 1969, Fu 1987, Hayes 1997, Herbert 2001, Herrero 1992, Janerich 1995, Jaworski 1990, Keyhani-Rofagha 1995, H-S Kim 1991, Kinney 2003, Krane 2002, K Lee 1997b, 1998, 1999, 2002, S Liu 2001, Makino 1995, A Miller 1995, H Mitchell 1988, 1990c, 1993a, 1995a, Mody 1999, Moriarty 2003a, G-K Nguyen 1993, Nieminen 1995, Ollayos 1997, Parkin 1985, R Peters 1986a, Renshaw 2004c, Ruba 2004, Sasieni 2001, Schoolland 2002a,b, H Smith 2000, Stockton 1997, Vizcaino 1998, SS Wang 2004, Zappa 2004, T Zheng 1996].

In summary, the Pap test has been remarkably effective in reducing cervical cancer mortality. In fact, it bears repeating, no other test has been so successful in eradicating cancer. But this must be tempered by realizing that the Pap test is far from perfect. It is simply impossible to avoid all false-negative reporting [M Bosch 1992]. It is thought that at least 10% of cervical cancers are just not preventable [P Martin 1972]. Therefore, unfortunately, some women will develop cervical cancer in spite of appropriate screening [Kurman 1994, P Martin 1972]. But most women who develop cervical cancer have not been adequately screened, rather than cytologically misinterpreted [Attwood 1985, J Carmichael 1984, E Clarke 1979, Janerich 1995, P Martin 1972, Mobius 1993, Morell 1982, Nasca 1991, MA Quinn 1989, Tuncer 1967, E Walker 1983, S Wilson 1992].

There are some important steps that can be taken to help prevent a tragic outcome [Koss 1989a]. First and foremost, women should get regular Pap tests, even if they have a long history of "normals" [R Peters 1988, Sandmire 1976, Sherman 1992b]. Women should also be informed of the fallibility of the Pap test and the availability of more sensitive screening tests, such as HPV-DNA testing [M Bosch 1992]. Women should have at least three consecutive, satisfactory, negative Pap tests before being reassured. Close surveillance of high-risk women, including those with multiple infections and heavy inflammation, is important [Pairwuti 1991, Sherman 1992b]. All abnormal Pap test results should be followed-up, even if the abnormality is "only" atypical squamous cells of undetermined significance [J Carmichael 1984, Sherman 1992b]. And, of great importance, suspicious lesions should be biopsied and suspicious symptoms investigated, even when the Pap test is negative [Berkeley 1980, Koss 1989a].

A parting thought: misread Pap tests do not cause cancer—think about it.

VIII. Liquid-Based Cytology, Death of the Pap Smear, and Primary Prevention

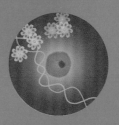

Liquid-Based Pap Tests

Liquid-based, or thin-layer, technology has revolutionized the Pap test and now accounts for as much as 80% of all collection methods [Noller 2003]. This technology was developed to overcome some of the problems with conventional Pap smears, namely, trapping of cells by collection devices, poor fixation, cell distribution, obscuring elements, and technical variability of smear quality [Bur 1995]. Transferring the cells from the collection device into the liquid medium addresses the first two problems. The cells are fixed immediately and nearly all of them are released into the medium. Problems with physical cell distortion and air-drying are minimized. The specimen is mechanically mixed, providing a uniform distribution of abnormal cells; therefore, the sample is theoretically more representative than a conventional Pap smear.

There are two basic slide preparation systems currently in use, although other systems are being developed. One uses a filter (such as ThinPrep®) and the other that uses gravity sedimentation (such as SurePath®). Both systems concentrate epithelial cells and dilute extraneous elements. Both systems provide between 50,000 and 75,000 cells for analysis (compared with 50,000 to 300,000 or more cells in conventional Pap smears). The viewing field is limited to a small circle (ranging from 13mm for SurePath® to 20mm for ThinPrep®). Because cells are present on less than half the slide area, CLIA had originally allowed LBC cases to be counted as one-half slide; however, the 2003 modification now counts LBC slides as whole slides [Voytek 2003]. In fact, LBC slides require meticulous screening because abnormal cells can be sparse and widely dispersed.

The sample is placed in a preservative solution, rather than smeared on a glass slide. Consequently, nearly the entire specimen is collected in the liquid, compared with about 20% transferred to a glass slide [Hutchinson 1999]. The liquid-based technique improves slide quality by reducing obscuring blood (>99%) and inflammatory exudate (95%) [Franco 2001]. Ancillary testing and automated screening can also be performed [Akpolat 2004, D Cohn 2001, Stoler 2000, Yoshida 2004].

In the ThinPrep® filter system, the specimen is collected either with a combination of plastic spatula and endocervical brush, or with the broom, and rinsed in a vial of methanol-based solution (PreservCyt®). In the laboratory, the vial containing the specimen is placed in the ThinPrep® Processor along with a plastic cylinder with an attached polycarbonate filtration membrane. The processor automatically immerses the filter in the vial and rotates the cell sample (either by spinning the filter [T2000] or the vial [T3000]). This creates gentle shear forces that can disaggregate loose cell clusters (true clusters remain intact) and disperse mucus, blood, and debris, homogenizing the cell sample in the process. Then, using a vacuum, the specimen is drawn through the TransCyt® Filter. Epithelial cells and organisms attach to the filter, but much of the obscuring debris, mucus, blood, and inflammation pass through and are removed. When a pressure sensor determines that the filter is sufficiently "full," the suction is automatically discontinued, and a "touch prep" of the filter, facilitated by a slight puff of air, is made on a specially manufactured slide, producing a 20 mm disc of thinly layered cells. The slide is immediately and automatically fixed with 95% ethanol and is ready for staining. The advantages include elimination of air-drying artifact and excessively thick specimens [Bishop 2000, Hutchinson 1994].

In the SurePath® system, the specimen is collected using a broom, the head of which can be detached and left in the collection vial, which contains an ethanol-based solution. In the laboratory, the sampled is vortexed and strained to break up mucus and large cell clusters. The sample is then layered onto a liquid density gradient, vortexed, and then centrifuged. The gradient concentrates epithelial cells preferentially over debris, blood, and inflammation. An aliquot of the filtrate is then placed in a chamber and allowed to sediment by gravity onto a coated slide forming a 13 mm disc of cells [Bishop 2000].

Cytology of Liquid-Based Cytology

The cytology of liquid-based Pap tests is more or less the same as conventional Pap smears, but there are some important differences. In conventional Pap smears, the cells are non-randomly distributed, there are thick and thin areas, and air-drying and smearing artifacts are common. In liquid–based cytology (LBC), the cells are randomly, evenly, and thinly distributed, and concentrated in a limited area of the slide; drying and smearing artifacts are minimized. However, LBC has its own set of artifacts [Kurtycz 2000]. For example, in ThinPrep®, the cells at the periphery of the circle are frequently distorted (crushed) which can make them look abnormal. Other artifacts are discussed below.

Basic cytomorphology, including architectural arrangements and individual cellular features, as well as microbiological agents, are generally similar in conventional Pap smears and LBC [T8.1]. In LBC, squamous cells still look like squamous cells [I8.1], glandular cells look like glandular cells [I8.2], and inflammatory cells look like inflammatory cells [I8.3b]. Intermediate cell nuclei remain key references in evaluating nuclear size and chromatin quality. The morphology of squamous intraepithelial lesions is more or less similar to that of conventional Pap smears, but—unfortunately—interpretive difficulties increase with grade of the lesion. Low-grade squamous intraepithelial lesions, and particularly koilocytes, are usually fairly easy to identify in liquid-based cytology. However, the interpretation of high-grade squamous intraepithelial lesions can be more difficult in liquid-based Pap tests than in conventional Pap smears. Glandular lesions also present certain difficulties, discussed below. The ability to perform HPV-DNA testing may help compensate for the interpretive difficulties in liquid-based cytology. In addition, other special studies, ranging from infectious disease testing to immunocytochemistry to detect oncoprotein expression or for tumor classification, can be performed on the residual material [Yoshida 2004].

T8.1 LBC and CPS: Similar with Differences

Conventional Pap Smear	Liquid-Based Cytology
Cells nonrandomly distributed	Cells randomly distributed
Thick and thin areas	Even, thin distribution
Spread over slide	Concentrated small area
Drying, smearing artifacts	Other artifacts, eg, crushed border

In liquid-based cytology (LBC), the cells are suspended in the fixative solution instead of being "smeared" on a slide and in some proprietary systems, the initial fixative is different (eg, ThinPrep® uses methanol instead of ethanol) and its concentration is lower. This leads to some important cytologic changes. First, because all cells tend to round up in fluids, cells and their nuclei tend to be smaller and more uniform in LBC than in conventional Pap smears. Second, nuclear staining is frequently less intense, so that dysplastic nuclei may be less hyperchromatic, and in some cases, hypochromatic. Therefore, two key interpretive clues to dysplasia—big and dark nuclei—may be less apparent, or even absent, in LBC (although, of course, these are useful when present). Third, in contrast with conventional Pap smears, small or indistinct nucleoli are commonly seen in dysplasia/carcinoma in situ in LBC, which could be mistaken for reactive changes [18.3a]. (Even neutrophils can have nucleoli in LBC! [18.3b]) Fourth, because specimens are mechanically agitated during preparation, loosely aggregated cells tend to disaggregate; single cells are more prominent; and the cells are randomly dispersed on the slide in LBC. This eliminates the "smear pattern" that can be helpful in interpretation of conventional Pap tests. For example, dysplastic cells do not line up in strings in LBC, as they frequently do in conventional Pap smears. Cell dispersion also makes cell-to-cell comparisons difficult. Fifth, true tissue fragments (eg, hyperchromatic crowded groups) remain intact, but may appear more three-dimensional. Evaluation of cells at the edges of these groups, often the best clue to their nature, is more difficult in LBC. Finally, because the liquid-based specimen represents a sample of a sample (ie, a subsample), not only are there fewer total cells to examine, but naturally, there are also fewer *abnormal* cells. Because abnormal cells can be sparse, even a single atypical cell can be highly significant. On the other hand, the background is "cleaned up" in LBC, so it is theoretically easier to find a few abnormal cells, because they are not obscured by inflammation or thick areas. Although blood, mucus, inflammation, and diathesis are still present in LBC, they may have a different appearance. For example, fresh blood is lyzed in LBC, leaving pale ghosts; old blood does not completely lyze and stains variably red. Tumor diathesis, inflammation, and atrophy can give a "ratty" (dirty, tattered) background, often "clinging" to cells. Mucus, lubricant, etc, can also clog filters, such as used in the ThinPrep® system, limiting the adequacy of the sample. (Specimen adequacy is covered under the Bethesda System, see pg 236.)

Atrophy in LBC is generally similar to atrophy in conventional Pap smears [18.4, 8.5, 8.6, 8.7]. Atrophy may show a granular background of degenerative cellular debris (which tends to clump and may cling to cells), an inflammatory response is common ("atrophy with inflammation"), and sometimes bleeding occurs. Three-dimensional clusters of basal/parabasal cells ("hyperchromatic crowded groups"), slight irregularities of nuclear contour, and naked nuclei occurring in atrophy could mimic a neoplastic process. Absence of marked nuclear membrane irregularities, abnormal chromatin patterns, and mitotic figures favor a benign interpretation. Glycogenated cells, which can be seen in atrophy (androgenic atrophy) or pregnancy (navicular cells), could mimic koilocytes; however, the nuclei are not abnormal ("dysplastic") and the vacuoles are not as sharply defined, but contain glycogen, which stains golden yellow [18.8].

LBC vs Conventional Pap Smears

  More alike than different

  Changes include:

  1. Cells round up in fluid

  2. Nuclear staining may be less intense

  3. Nucleoli more conspicuous

  4. Disaggregation (due to agitation)

    More single cells

    No "smear pattern"

  5. Groups more difficult to evaluate

  6. Subsample ⇒ fewer abnormal cells

    but easier to see in clean background

Squamous metaplasia exfoliates loose sheets of cells in cobble-stone arrangements or single cells [18.9, 8.10]. . The cells appear smaller and rounder than conventional Pap smears, but still have dense, homogeneous cytoplasm. Hyperkeratosis is characterized by anucleate squames; parakeratosis by miniature squamous cells that tend to stain more eosinophilic than orangeophilic in LBC [18.11]. As usual, these keratotic reactions can be associated with significant underlying lesions. Intermediate cell predominance, with numerous bare nuclei, and lactobacilli (often overlying cells or trapped in mucus [18.12]) characterize cytolysis.

Organisms are usually apparent in LBC, and some cases, such as *Candida*, stand out [18.13]. The spearing, or "shish kebab," effect of *Candida* is particularly prominent in LBC. However, mucus strands in LBC can mimic *Candida* pseudohyphae (look for budding, like strings of sausages; mucus strands are nonbudding and have variable diameters) [11.94a,b]. Trichomonads occur singly, in groups, or attached to squamous cells, but appear smaller than in conventional Pap smears [18.14]. Although the *Trichomonas* nucleus must still be identified, red granules may be more difficult to appreciate, but flagella can sometimes be seen in LBC. *Herpes* changes are similar in both conventional and liquid-based specimens, consisting of multinucleation, molding, margination of chromatin with ground glass effect, and presence of intranuclear inclusions (which tend to stand out in LBC) [18.15]. Other organisms, too, have similar morphologic features in LBC. *Actinomyces* forms dense clusters of filamentous bacteria [18.16]. "Shift in vaginal flora" can look like a granular blue background of small coccobacilli, although this tends to diminish in LBC. However, clue cells (squamous cells coated with coccobacilli) may still be apparent [18.17], and lactobacilli and inflammation are absent by definition. Follicular cervicitis may present as small, three-dimensional clusters of lymphoid cells; these aggregates can mimic endometrial cells, for example (look for tingible body macrophages) [18.18].

Reactive cellular changes are characterized by slight nuclear enlargement (usually <2 times an intermediate cell nucleus), smooth nuclear membranes, fine chromatin, nucleoli, and frequently, degenerated or vacuolated cytoplasm in both conventional Pap smears and LBC [18.19]. Inflammatory perinuclear halos are to be distinguished from koilocytotic halos [18.20]. Repair/regeneration also has the usual features, including cohesive, sheets of orderly cells (like a "school of fish"), with smooth nuclear membranes, fine chromatin, prominent nucleoli, and occasional mitoses often accompanied by inflammation and organisms [8.22, 8.23]. However, the sheets may be more rounded up or folded, with greater depth of focus, and streaming may be less apparent in LBC [18.24]. Radiation change (macrocytes, multinucleation, vacuolization, polychromasia, etc) in LBC is similar to conventional Pap smears [18.25]. Pregnancy changes, such as decidual cells [18.26] and Arias-Stella reaction, can also be seen in LBC, and are similar to conventional Pap smears.

Background inflammatory material may be evenly distributed in LBC, but has a tendency to clump or to cling to epithelial cells [18.21]. Sometimes, an inflammatory background has a "ratty" appearance comprising dirty, tattered looking material mixed with poorly preserved epithelial cells. In "atrophy with inflammation" the background inflammation and granular debris forms small clumps often "clinging" to parabasal cells [18.6]. (See squamous cell carcinoma, below, for further discussion.)

Dysplasia, in conventional Pap smears, is recognized using an intermediate cell nucleus as a reference: "if it's big and it's dark, it's dysplasia," and this still hold true in LBC. Unfortunately, however, in LBC, nuclear hyperchromasia can be minimal and the nuclei tend to be smaller and more uniform, particularly in high-grade lesions. Hyperchromasia related to degeneration is reduced or eliminated in LBC, although hyperchromasia related to polyploidy or aneuploidy is maintained. In consequence, however, other interpretive criteria, especially nuclear membrane irregularities, assume increased importance, particularly for high-grade lesions.

Low-grade SILs are practically identical, morphologically, in LBC and conventional Pap smears [18.27, 8.28, 8.29]. In fact, L SIL in general, and koilocytes in particular, tend to stand out like **STOP** signs in LBC [18.30, 8.31]. LBC enhances nuclear irregularities and chromatin pattern, and highlights the cytoplasmic cavity of koilocytes. L SIL is characterized by mature intermediate to superficial cells, with nuclear enlargement (>3 times the area of a normal intermediate cell nucleus), irregular nuclear membranes, and chromatin abnormalities, including hyperchromasia (which ranges from minimal to marked compared with an intermediate cell nucleus). As in conventional Pap tests showing L SIL, macrocytes, abnormal keratinization, including parakeratosis, binucleation or multinucleation, pyknotic nuclei, etc, can also be seen in LBC. Small or indistinct nucleoli are more commonly seen in dysplasia in LBC than in conventional Pap smears.

High-grade SILs are generally similar in appearance to those in conventional Pap smears, but can sometimes be very subtle in LBC [18.32-8.37]. H SIL is generally characterized by parabasal-sized cells, with high N/C ratios, irregular nuclear membranes, and chromatin abnormalities. Sheets and clusters ("hyperchromatic crowded groups") may be present, but streaks of cells are absent in LBC. Single abnormal cells are more common in LBC because the specimen is mechanically agitated during processing. As in conventional Pap smears, some cases of H SIL are characterized by marked cellular pleomorphism and keratinization. Although marked hyperchromasia can occur, it is frequently diminished and sometimes absent in LBC. H SIL cells with small, pale nuclei can easily be overlooked or misinterpreted. Other nuclear abnormalities, which can be very subtle in some cases, become critically important in evaluating dysplasia in LBC. Look carefully for small cells with high N/C ratios, increased depth of focus, irregular nuclear membranes, and subtle chromatin abnormalities (speckled chromatin) in H SIL. A key interpretive clue to H SIL in LBC is the presence highly irregular nuclear membranes (like little "brains in bottles"). Note that binucleation can mimic irregular membranes at low power (examine carefully at high power). The presence of nucleoli can also be misleading. As in conventional Pap smears, the N/C ratio is a measure of cell maturity and degree of dysplasia (ie, higher N/C ratio, more advanced dysplasia). Abnormal cells, singly or in small groups, often sit exposed in a small clear space, but strings of cells are absent. The differential of H SIL includes atrophy, benign immature metaplasia, atypical metaplasia, histiocytes, and small glandular cells, and it can be quite difficult to distinguish among these possibilities in some cases.

Carcinoma in situ exfoliates three-dimensional syncytial-like aggregates of abnormal cells showing chaotic architecture or loss of nuclear polarity (ie, hyperchromatic crowded groups) [18.38, 8.39]. Irregular nuclear membranes, chromatin abnormalities, mitotic figures, and an accompanying squamous dysplasia are typical findings. Naked abnormal nuclei are common in carcinoma in situ. In some cases, nuclear membranes are unexpectedly smooth. The differential is wide, ranging from benign endometrial cells to adenocarcinoma (see hyperchromatic crowded groups, pg 182).

Squamous cell carcinoma (SCC), still the most common cervical cancer, shows similar features in both LBC and conventional Pap smears

[18.40-8.47]. The cells have malignant appearing nuclei (enlarged, variably hyperchromatic, irregular nuclear membranes, abnormal chromatin structure, prominent nucleoli) and squamoid (dense) cytoplasm. Although LBC tends to clear the background, a tumor diathesis can still be appreciated in the majority (50% to 80%) of cases of invasive carcinoma (described below). However, the diathesis can plug filters, making tumor cells sparse or absent.

Non-keratinizing SCC, the most common form, is characterized by relatively uniform, medium to large squamous cells, present singly, in small sheets, or syncytial-like aggregates [18.40, 8.41, 8.42]. The nuclei typically have irregular membranes, coarse, irregular chromatin, prominent or irregular nucleoli, and moderately elevated N/C ratios. The cytoplasm is dense and cyanophilic. A tumor diathesis is usually present. Degenerative cytoplasmic vacuolization can occur, mimicking secretory vacuolization of glandular cells. Furthermore, rounding up of clusters of cells (often with prominent nucleoli) in LBC may suggest adenocarcinoma. However, no true glandular features, such as rosettes, feathering, columnar cells with elongated nuclei and nucleo-cytoplasmic polarity, or mucin production occurs in pure SCC. Flatter sheets of cells with distinct cell borders suggest squamous differentiation. Look for dyskeratotic cells to suggest squamous origin of poorly-differentiated tumors. Repair is another classic differential of non-keratinizing SCC in both conventional Pap smears and LBC. Orderliness, cohesion, and fine chromatin are key features favoring repair in either specimen type.

Keratinizing SCC is characterized by marked pleomorphism, including bizarre cells (spindle, tadpole, etc), and marked keratinization, including dense orangeophilia, and pearls [18.43, 8.44, 8.45]. Cytoplasmic blebs of keratin are common in LBC, and usually not seen in conventional Pap smears of SCC [18.45]. Single abnormal cells are prominent. Keratinization as well as pleomorphism stands out in LBC. Nuclear hyperchromasia, including ink dot nuclei, as well as nuclear ghosts, can still be appreciated in LBC. Tumor diathesis is less common than in non-keratinizing SCC.

Individual squamous cancer cells have dense cytoplasm with well-defined cell borders, and can mimic squamous metaplasia or dysplasia. Atrophy can shed hyperchromatic crowded groups and can have a granular tumor diathesis-like background, mimicking malignancy. Critical high power evaluation of the nuclei is the key to correct interpretation.

Small cell squamous carcinoma is characterized by relatively uniform, small cells with very high N/C ratios and scant cytoplasm [18.46]. Syncytial-like aggregates and naked nuclei are common. The nuclei have relatively smooth membranes, and coarse, dark chromatin; the small nucleoli may be more easily appreciated in LBC. The differential includes endometrial cells, carcinoma in situ, and small cell neuroendocrine carcinoma.

A tumor diathesis is an important feature of invasive squamous cell carcinoma that is present in the majority of cases [18.47]. In LBC, the diathesis has a "ratty" appearance, composed of blood, fibrin, protein, necrosis, and cell debris. It tends to clump, have a fibrillar or frayed appearance, and may cling to tumor cells ("clinging diathesis"). Fresh blood is lysed (to red blood cell stroma, or "ghosts") in LBC, although old blood does not lyse completely. The differential of a ratty background includes: infection, cytolysis, and atrophy with inflammation.

Atypical squamous cells (ASC), as defined by the Bethesda System, are similar in conventional Pap smears and LBC. Criteria used for recognition of ASC are similar in either specimen type. Briefly, ASC-undetermined significance is characterized by mature intermediate or superficial cells with minimal nuclear enlargement (2-3 times normal intermediate nucleus) [18.48,

8.49]. Changes suggestive, but not diagnostic of koilocytes, can also be interpreted as ASC-US [18.50]. ASC-cannot exclude H SIL is characterized by by immature metaplastic cells with minimal nuclear enlargement [18.51]. Both forms of ASC have minimal chromatin abnormalities and nuclear membrane irregularities. On the one hand, ASC rates may diminish since air-drying and smear artifacts that make cells difficult to interpret are eliminated in LBC, but on the other hand, ASC rates may increase because cells may be better preserved and nuclear detail may be overinterpreted.

Endocervical cells can occur in small and large groups, honeycomb sheets, palisades, or as isolated columnar cells [18.52-8.55]. Groups of endocervical cells tend to "round up" or fold in LBC, forming three-dimensional, tight clusters, which can be confused with endometrial cells or other, more ominous, hyperchromatic crowded groups, such as carcinoma in situ. The nuclei can look more "reactive" in LBC, compared with conventional Pap smears. Endocervical cells have larger nuclei and more abundant cytoplasm than endometrial cells. Look for honeycombing and palisading at the edge of endocervical clusters; this helps distinguish endocervical clusters from both endometrial cells and neoplastic HCGs. Single endocervical cells, which are more common in LBC, can be difficult to identify, particularly when trapped in mucus or in clumps of leukocytes. Endocervical cells from high in the endocervix can have dense cytoplasm, mimicking squamous metaplasia. At least 10 endocervical (or metaplastic) cells must be present as one measure of specimen adequacy.

Endometrial cells usually exfoliate as tight, three-dimensional aggregates of small glandular cells with or without central cores of stroma [18.56, 8.57]. Nuclei have crisp, distinct chromatin, prominent chromocenters, and micronucleoli, and may stain pale. Endometrial nuclei are normally about the same size as intermediate cell nuclei. However, in LBC, endometrial nuclei are slightly larger and more variable in size and shape, the chromatin details are accentuated, and nucleoli may be visible, which could lead to unnecessary interpretations of atypical endometrial cells in LBC. The cytoplasm is often more distinctly vacuolated in LBC. Also, apoptosis (single cell necrosis) may be more obvious. The background looks cleaner, especially in menstrual samples, compared with conventional Pap smears. Other endometrial cell features, such as double contour cell balls and small crowded groups, are similar in LBC, although the aggregates tend to focus above the plane of the squamous cells, particularly in gradient-based methods such as SurePath®.

Superficial stromal cells are indistinguishable from histiocytes ("sticky histiocytes"); they tend to have bean-shaped nuclei and foamy, vacuolated cytoplasm [18.58]. It can be difficult to distinguish dense, three-dimensional clusters of endometrial stromal histiocytes from endometrial glandular cells in LBC; bean-shaped nuclei and more abundant, finely vacuolated cytoplasm suggest stromal histiocytes. Deep endometrial stromal cells have elongated to spindle-shaped nuclei, longitudinal nuclear grooves, fine, even chromatin, occasional chromocenters, and scant cytoplasm. The Bethesda System recommends reporting normal-appearing, spontaneously exfoliated, endometrial cells in women 40 years of age or older. Directly sampled endometrium need not be mentioned in the report. Of course, abnormal appearing endometrial cells should always be reported, regardless of the woman's age or menstrual status.

Atypical glandular cells refers to endocervical or endometrial cells showing cytologic abnormalities, such as nuclear crowding, enlargement, hyperchromasia, chromocenters, or nucleoli, beyond normal/reactive but insufficient to be certain of adenocarcinoma. In LBC, there is an unfortunate

tendency of the morphology of benign and malignant glandular cells to overlap. Benign glandular cells appear more "reactive" in LBC, with seemingly larger nuclei, more open chromatin, and more prominent nucleoli. On the other hand, malignant nuclear features, particularly hyperchromasia, may be diminished in adenocarcinomas, which can make malignant cells look benign/reactive. This convergence of cytologic features can lead to false-negative or positive results, or to interpretations of atypical glandular cells. On the other hand, better preservation of cells can lead to a decrease in AGC rates, with a corresponding increase in the proportion of abnormalities confirmed by biopsy.

Atypical endocervical cells are characterized by somewhat disorderly sheets or crowded groups of glandular cells, with abundant cytoplasm, low-to-moderate N/C ratios, round to oval nuclei, with smooth to slightly irregular nuclear membranes, granular chromatin, and single or multiple, small to prominent nucleoli. Not all need be present. Three-dimensional crowding, rosette formation, and mitoses are three key features [18.59]. Remember, normal endocervical cells commonly have nucleoli in LBC.

Atypical endometrial cells are characterized by three-dimensional loose or tight aggregates of small glandular cells, with high N/C ratios, enlarged, round to oval nuclei, with smooth to irregular membranes, coarse chromatin, variable nucleoli, and more abundant, distinctly vacuolated cytoplasm. Not all of these findings need to be present for an interpretation of atypical endometrial cells. Nuclear enlargement and prominent nucleoli are two key features [18.60].

The differential of atypical glandular cells includes endocervical repair (cohesive sheets of orderly cells, round nuclei, fine chromatin, low N/C ratios), tubal metaplasia (which can closely mimic adenocarcinoma in situ in some cases; look for cilia) [18.61], lower uterine segment and directly sampled endometrium [18.62] (look for tissue fragments, tightly packed, but well-ordered, small uniform glandular cells, with high N/C ratios, regular round nuclei, bland chromatin, and possibly nucleoli, as well as associated endometrial stroma [biphasic pattern]), IUD changes (single or clustered glandular cells, mimicking CIN 3 [18.63] and adenocarcinoma, respectively), and of course, adenocarcinoma (endometrial, endocervical, in situ and invasive). Squamous lesions, particularly carcinoma in situ, can mimic atypical glandular cells (look for flatter sheets, rounder nuclei [vs elongated], more and denser cytoplasm, and accompanying dysplastic squamous cells, as well as absence of true glandular structures such as well-formed rosettes).

Endocervical adenocarcinoma in situ typically exfoliates numerous, variably-sized, disorderly hyperchromatic crowded groups of abnormal glandular cells that may be apparent at low scanning power [18.64-8.67]. At high power, architectural abnormalities, such as marked crowding, stratification, and rosette formation, and nuclear abnormalities, such as high N/C ratios, nuclear elongation, membrane irregularities, and mitotic figures can be appreciated in LBC, findings similar to conventional Pap smears. However, in LBC, feathering may be less conspicuous, the chromatin pattern is more variable (ie, the distinctive coarse dark chromatin may be lacking), and nucleoli are more common, ranging from inconspicuous to prominent. The cytoplasm is finely vacuolated with indistinct cell borders in both types of specimens, although remnants of the honeycomb pattern are sometimes seen in LBC. The differential includes endocervical repair (loose for orderly sheets with rounded nuclei and fine chromatin); tubal metaplasia (look for cilia); lower uterine segment (look for closely packed, but uniform, orderly cells and endometrial stroma); and invasive adenocarcinoma (look for more nuclear abnormalities, including more nuclear membrane irregularities, more abnormal chromatin, and more prominent nucleoli, as well as more single cells and a tumor diathesis).

Endocervical adenocarcinoma, in LBC, ranges from well-differentiated adenocarcinoma, which closely resembles in situ adenocarcinoma (see above), to poorly-differentiated tumors, characterized by rounder nuclei, more open chromatin, more prominent nucleoli, and somewhat more abundant cytoplasm [I8.68-8.70]. The cells show typical malignant criteria, which may include nuclear enlargement, hyperchromasia, irregular nuclear membranes, abnormal irregular chromatin, and prominent or irregular nucleoli. The cytoplasm is finely vacuolated and N/C ratios are elevated. Although sheet-like groups are typical in conventional Pap smears, in LBC, endocervical adenocarcinoma tends to exfoliate aggregates that are more three dimensional, making it more difficult to distinguish from endometrial adenocarcinoma. Single abnormal cells are present in both conventional Pap smears and LBC. A tumor diathesis points to an invasive process. However, because the background is cleared of obscuring inflammation and blood, identification of a tumor diathesis can be more difficult in LBC. The diathesis tends to be less pronounced and to clump in an otherwise clean background. It appears similar to the diathesis present in invasive squamous carcinoma, and in some cases, it is closely associated with cells ("clinging diathesis"). The differential is similar to that described under endocervical adenocarcinoma in situ.

Endometrial adenocarcinoma, the most common invasive gynecologic malignancy, occurs in two clinical settings as previously described (see pg 119) [I8.71-8.73]. Briefly, type I carcinomas, associated with endometrial hyperplasia and estrogen stimulation, usually occur perimenopausally, are well-differentiated, and have a favorable prognosis. These tumors may shed few (or no) cells. The cells are cytologically bland and typically found in a background of high squamous maturation ("estrogen effect"). Type II carcinomas occur spontaneously in older, postmenopausal women, are poorly-differentiated, and have a worse prognosis. These tumors tend to shed more cells, which are more cytologically atypical, in an atrophic background. Nuclear abnormalities, such enlargement, membrane irregularities, chromatin abnormalities, and nucleoli, increase with the grade of the tumor. Neutrophil engulfment is typical of endometrial carcinoma, but is not specific. The watery diathesis characteristic of endometrial adenocarcinoma is less apparent, but may be present as finely granular or clumped debris in the background or associated with tumor cells. The differential includes endocervical adenocarcinoma and squamous carcinoma in situ or poorly-differentiated squamous cell carcinoma. LBC may help increase detection of endometrial carcinomas by reducing obscuring background blood and inflammation.

As in conventional Pap smears, a wide variety of rare tumors, ranging from primary sarcomas to metastatic malignancies, can sometimes be detected in LBC [I8.74-8.78]. The morphology of these lesions in LBC is generally similar to that seen in conventional Pap smears, with the usual caveats, such as rounding up of cells, previously discussed. Sarcomas look like sarcomas; metastases look like floaters; unusual morphology suggests extrauterine primary tumor. History, as always, is paramount in interpretation.

Performance of Liquid-Based Cytology

The conventional wisdom holds that the majority of false-negative results are due to sampling errors. The benefits of the liquid-based technology include not only providing a "prettier," easier to screen sample, with fewer, though better preserved cells, but more importantly, a sample that is more representative than a conventional Pap smear. There is evidence that LBC can increase the sensitivity and specificity of interpretations of squamous lesions [J Baker 2002, Belinson 2001, SJ Bernstein 2001, Colgan 2003, Fremont-Smith 2004, Hartmann 2001, Klinkhamer 2003, McCrory 1999, Pan 2003, Sass 2004]. In biopsy-controlled studies, ThinPrep®, for example, increased detection of SIL up to 80% compared with conventional Pap smears [Díaz-Rosario 1999, Papillo 1998, Renshaw 2002b]. In a large study, ThinPrep® was associated with significantly lower error rates than conventional Pap smears [Renshaw 2004c]. Although the absolute number of ASCUS cases also tends to increase, the ASCUS/SIL rate may remain unchanged or even diminish [Cheung 2003, Davey 2004, Quddus 2004]. There is inconclusive evidence that LBC can increase the sensitivity and specificity of glandular interpretations [Ashfaq 1999, Bai 2000, Eltabbakh 2000b, Guidos 2000, Hecht 2002, Schorge 2002, N Wang 2002]. When used in conjunction with thin-layer slides, computer-assisted screening holds tremendous promise for the future. And one of the biggest benefits of liquid-based technology is the ability to perform, from a single sample, multiple tests, including not only a Pap test, but also testing for infectious agents, including HPV, *Chlamydia, Herpes*, and gonorrhea. DNA ploidy and molecular testing, including oncogene expression, can be analyzed on the residual specimen [Altiok 2003, Bollmann 2003, W Lin 2000, Wang-Johanning 2002, E Weaver 2000]. It is also possible to prepare cell blocks from the residual material in the vials, creating a "histologic" sample on which any number of special procedures can then be performed [Freitas 2001, Kabbani 2002, Keyhani-Rofagha 2002, K Richard 1999, Rowe 2001].

HPV testing has become an important part of screening for cervical cancer and its precursor lesions. Primary screening with an HPV test, with reflex Pap testing, reversing the current screening test order, is a possible consideration for the future [Cuzick 2000, 2001, Herrington 2001, Hillemanns 1999, Kulasingam 2002, Mandelblatt 2002, Schiffman 2000b]. In fact, the combination of HPV and Pap testing could lead to the demise of the false-negative cervical cancer-screening test.

The Demise of the False-Negative Cervical Cancer Screen

We'll have fun, fun, fun
'til the lawyers take the Pap test away...

Who would have thought in the 1940s, certainly not Papanicolaou, that today we would be spending *billions* of dollars annually for cervical cancer screening, more than half of that spent on minor atypia alone? Who would have thought that we would be diagnosing cervical abnormalities in up to 10,000 women per 100,000 annually, when the incidence of cervical cancer never exceeded 50 women per 100,000? And, who would have thought that multimillion dollar malpractice judgments would become common, and account for 40% of pathology malpractice claims? Or that homicide would be charged for a misread Pap test?

Because of its remarkable success, the public now expects that the Pap test can and should prevent all cervical cancer. The obvious corollary is that since cervical cancer is completely preventable (in the public imagination), then every single case is someone's fault. Who would have thought that the public's unrealistic expectations might now be achievable?

The "Holy Grail" in cervical cancer screening is a cervical cancer-screening test with 100% sensitivity (and reasonable specificity) This seemingly impossible dream has now been substantially realized [Renshaw 2002a]. We now know the cause of cervical cancer, human papillomavirus [Crum 2000]. Highly sensitive tests to detect HPV have been available for several years, ie, HPV-DNA tests (eg, Hybrid Capture, PCR) [Qureshi 2003]. When combined with liquid-based Pap testing, the double "HPV-Pap test" has an ability to detect clinically significant cervical lesions with sensitivity for H SIL between 90% and 100% in published studies [Austin 2003b, Belinson 2001, Clavel 1999, 2001, Ferenczy 1996a, K-J Lee 2004, Pan 2003].

Holy Grail

100% sensitive screening test

HPV-Pap Test comes close

A "double negative" test

1. HPV-DNA test

2. Liquid-based Pap test

Practically guarantees absence

of HPV-related cervical disease

Risk of CxCA for several years is very low

The sensitivity of the HPV-Pap test for H SIL was studied in 1997 women who had both HPV-DNA testing and a proprietary liquid-based Pap test (ThinPrep®) [Belinson 2001]. The unique feature of this study was that *every single woman* was biopsied (cervical biopsies, endocervical sampling), including those with a negative HPV tests and negative Pap tests. The sensitivity and specificities from this study are shown in [T8.2].

T8.2 HPV-Pap Test in Detection of H SIL

	Sensitivity	Specificity
HPV Test	95%	85%
TP* (ASCUS threshold)	94%	78%
TP (H SIL threshold)	77%	98%
Colposcopy	81%	77%
TP + HPV achieved 100% sensitivity!		

*TP=ThinPrep® [Belinson 2001]

The key finding was that the combination of a liquid-based Pap test (ThinPrep® in this study) and HPV-DNA test achieved 100% sensitivity (!) in the detection of H SIL, confirmed by biopsy. Another interesting finding was that colposcopy, often considered a gold standard test, had a sensitivity of only 81%. According to the US Food and Drug Administration, women who have a normal Pap test and no HPV infection are at very low risk (1 in 500) for developing cervical cancer; those who have an abnormal Pap test and a positive high-risk HPV test are at higher risk (1 in 15) of developing cervical cancer if not treated.

Yet, some have been reluctant to embrace this double test [Herbst 2001]. The clinical concern is how to manage women who have a positive HPV-DNA test, but negative Pap test, which is a relatively common occurrence [A Miller 2001]. (Women with positive Pap tests can be managed according to established protocols [Cox 2000a, T Wright 2003a].) Some clinicians view this combination (positive HPV test, negative Pap test) as false positive test results, since these women apparently have no lesions and few will develop cancer [Cain 2000]. But, others

What About Positive HPV Test

...With Negative Pap Test?

False Positive?

Most will not develop CxCA

True Positive?

Identifies high-risk women

Up to 100x increased risk CIN 3

contend that these are not false positives results. These women are infected with a DNA tumor virus that causes nearly all cervical cancers [T Wright 2002b, 2003b]. HPV positive, Pap test negative women are at increased risk of subsequently developing SILs [Castle 2002b, Clavel 2000a, Coker 2001, Liaw 1999, Moscicki 1998, 2001, Rozendaal 1996, Schiffman 1995a, Sherman 2003, Tachezy 2003, Zielinski 2001]. (One study found a 100 *times* increased risk of CIN 3 [Rozendaal 1996].) HPV-positive, cytology-negative women should be carefully followed [Castle 2002b, Sherman 2003]. However, cytologically negative women who clear their HPV infections are at very low risk of cervical neoplasia. Therefore, conservative management is probably indicated. HPV positivity also warns of possible false-negative Pap test interpretations [Moscicki 1991, A Schneider 1988b, Wagner 1985, Zielinski 2001].

Conventional Pap smears are approximately 50% to 70% sensitive to detection of H SIL; sensitivity increases to as high as 95% using liquid-based Pap tests [Austin 2003a, Fahey 1995, McCrory 1999, Renshaw 2002a]. Meta-analysis supports the contention that thin layer technology is superior to the conventional Pap smear for detecting cytologic abnormalities [Austin 1998, S Bernstein 2001, Nanda 2000, Sulik 2001]. Large series report increased detection of H SIL by liquid-based technology [Díaz-Rosario 1999, Hutchinson 1999, Limaye 2003]. Finally, two biopsy-controlled studies also report that liquid-based preparations are superior to conventional Pap smears [Belinson 1999, Hutchinson 1999].

From the "no test is perfect" file, the detection of HPV-DNA is better using a direct cervical scrape than vaginal lavage or vaginal pool aspirate. Using direct cervical scrapes, HPV testing can detect >90% of CIN 3 [Cuzick 1999, Schiffman 2000b, Solomon 2001]. Detection is enhanced when there is a good sample of the T zone. Detection rate (sensitivity) diminishes with age, perhaps because the T zone recedes and is more difficult to sample adequately [Sherman 2003]. The phase of the menstrual cycle can affect detection of HPV [A Schneider 1992a]. Note also that not every HPV type is tested for in these routine tests.

The implication is that nearly perfect (~95%) sensitivity in the detection of clinically significant HPV-related cervical disease, including SIL and cancer, can *theoretically* be approached using the combination of HPV-DNA testing and liquid-based Pap testing [Belinson 2001, Hutchinson 1999, Schiffman 2000b, Solomon 2001]. Women who score a "double negative" on their HPV-Pap test can almost be guaranteed of the absence of any current, clinically significant HPV-related cervical disease [Lörincz 2003, Sherman 2003, Stoler 2001a]. One "double negative" HPV-Pap test gives a better assurance against the risk of CIN 3 than *three* negative conventional Pap smears [Lörincz 2003]. And, what's more, the risk of developing cervical cancer in the next several years (5, possibly 10) is very low (~1/1000) [Sherman 2003], *but not zero* [Muñoz 2003]. No woman can be truly informed about her cervical cancer screening options without her provider telling her about this double test [Austin 2003a]. The FDA has approved the use of HPV-DNA testing as an adjunct to the Pap test for women over age 30 [Goldie 2004]. Interim guidelines for use of HPV-DNA testing have been published [T Wright 2004]. It is possible that the HPV-DNA test will eventually supplant the Pap test for primary cervical cancer screening.

Other new methods, in addition to HPV testing, are being investigated. Location guided screening holds promise for the future of cytologic screening [A Chang 2002, Wilbur 2002]. In addition, various biomarkers, including p16^{INK4a} (cyclic kinase inhibitor), PCNA (proliferating cell nuclear antigen), Ki-67 (nuclear antigen), MCM proteins (members of the pre-replication complex, replicated once per cell cycle), telomerase (necessary for cell immortalization), microsatellite alterations (loss of heterozygosity is seen on several chromosomes), are under investigation to improve cervical cancer screening [Baldwin 2003].

Since HPV testing is now being incorporated into cervical cancer screening, it is important that women be informed about HPV. Unfortunately, the news media does not always fulfill these educational needs, and indeed, the coverage is often incomplete, and sometimes misleading [Anhang 2004]. Here are 5 take home points about HPV for women. I. HPV infection is a sexually transmitted disease. 2. HPV infection is extremely common, in fact, the most common sexually transmitted disease. 3. The vast majority of HPV infected women, even those with so-called "high risk" viral types, will never get cervical cancer (although follow-up is important). 4. Most HPV infections resolve spontaneously. 5. The Pap test is used to detect HPV-related cancers and precursor lesions [Monk 2004].

Primary Prevention of Cervical Cancer

Primary prevention is considered the optimal approach to cancer prevention when the causative agent(s) is known and can be controlled or eliminated [Braun 1999, Fernández – Esquer 2000]. The cause of virtually every case of cervical cancer is known: it is a virus, human papillomavirus. It follows that this disease can be prevented by controlling HPV infection [CS Morrison 1997]. The single greatest predictor of HPV infection is the lifetime number of sexual partners. Thus, avoiding high-risk sexual behaviors, delaying onset of intercourse, and practicing long-term monogamy, could largely prevent cervical cancer [Anonymous 1996]. Yet many young, sexually active women have never heard of HPV and few know the risk factors for acquiring this potentially deadly infection, even though most report sexual behaviors that place them at risk [Anonymous 1997, D Dell 2000, Mays 2000, Ramirez 1997, J Reid 2001, Vail–Smith 1992, Yacobi 1999].

Primary Prevention of Cervical CA

Controlling HPV infection can prevent cancer

Risk factors:

- *Age of first*
- *Number of sexual partners*
- *Method of contraception*
- *Cigarette smoking*

Life style profoundly affects risk

Education can save lives!

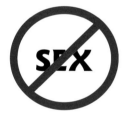

Life style factors profoundly influence the risk of developing cervical cancer [Brinton 1992, Morrow 1995]. Key lifestyle risk factors for cervical cancer that are important in primary prevention include: age at first intercourse, number of sexual partners, method of contraception, and cigarette smoking [Averette 1993, Barber 1981, Braun 1999, Davtyan 2000, Devesa 1989]. It is important to educate women about these risk factors [Ferrera 2000, Furniss 2000, Shepherd 2000a,b]. The target population is primarily adolescents and young adults who are most susceptible to potential carcinogens. It is important to reach socially and economically disadvantaged women. Educational efforts directed at delaying the initiation of intercourse, reducing the number of sexual partners, teaching "safer sex" negotiation skills, and increasing the use of condoms could be effective in reducing the risk of cervical cancer [Jastreboff 2002, CS Morrison 1997, Rock 2000, Shepherd 2000a,b, Suris 1999]. Dietary adjustment, chemoprevention, and vaccines are also potentially important preventative measures [Tewari 2002].

The risk of cervical cancer is probably more closely related to sexual practices than to differences in Pap test screening [de Vet 1994, Kjær 1989, H–q Li 2000a]. Education about the risks of smoking, early and indiscriminate sexual behavior, and the advantages of barrier contraceptives can save lives [Crowther 1995]. The prevention of cervical cancer may become a fortuitous side benefit of "safer sex" campaigns aimed at preventing AIDS and other sexually transmitted diseases [Pontén 1995].

In summary, the risk of HPV infection and, consequently, cervical cancer, can be substantially reduced or even totally eliminated by lifestyle choices. HPV negative women have no practical risk of developing cervical cancer. Women cannot make informed lifestyle decisions without knowing the facts [Braun 1999]. Should these facts be "trade secrets" [Littell 2000]?

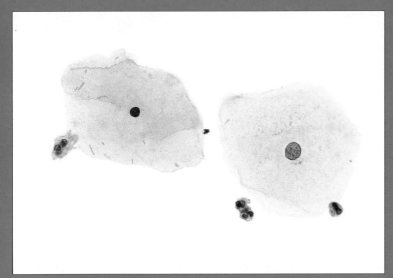

18.1 Squamous cells still look like squamous cells in LBC. The intermediate cell nucleus remains a key reference for nuclear size and chromatin quality

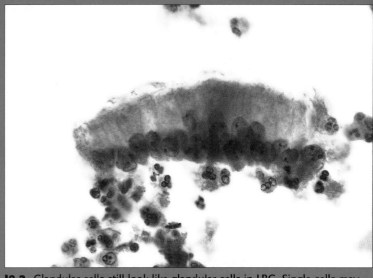

18.2 Glandular cells still look like glandular cells in LBC. Single cells may be more prominent because the specimen is agitated during processing

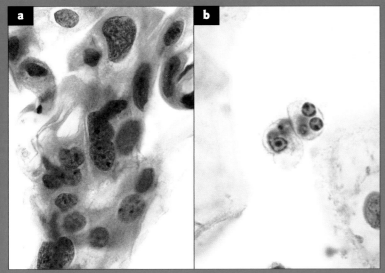

18.3 a, Cells tend to look more "reactive" in LBC (L SIL with nucleoli) ; **b**, even neutrophils can have nucleoli in LBC! (oil)

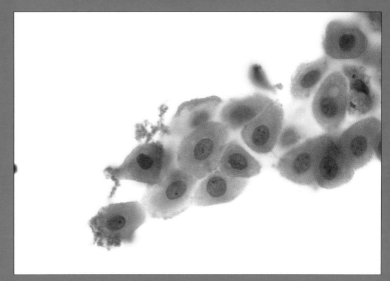

18.4 Atrophy: parabasal cell predominant maturation index

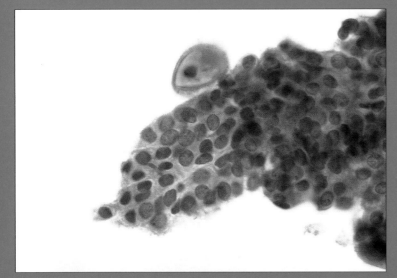

18.5 Atrophy: syncytial-like sheets, 3D clusters of hyperchromatic basal/parabasal cells, slightly irregular nuclear contours could mimic a neoplastic process

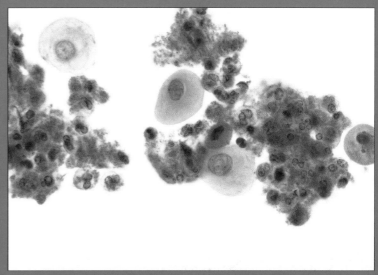

18.6 Atrophy with inflammation has a granular background of leukocytes and cell debris (pseudodiathesis), which tends to clump and cling to cells

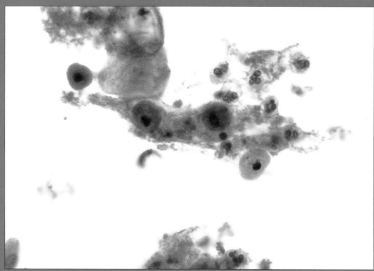

18.7 Atrophy, pseudokeratinization and pseudodiathesis

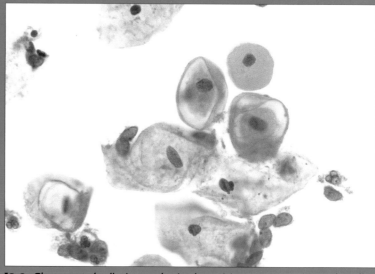

18.8 Glycogenated cells, in atrophy (androgenic) or pregnancy (navicular cells), can mimic koilocytes, but have normal nuclei and yellow cytoplasmic glycogen

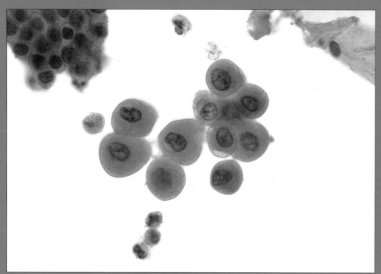

18.9 Squamous metaplasia: rounded parabasal-sized cells with dense cytoplasm in cobblestone arrangements or single cells

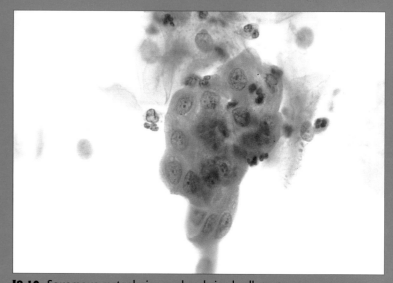

18.10 Squamous metaplasia: parabasal-sized cells may appear more "reactive" in LBC, possibly leading to unnecessary "atypical" interpretations

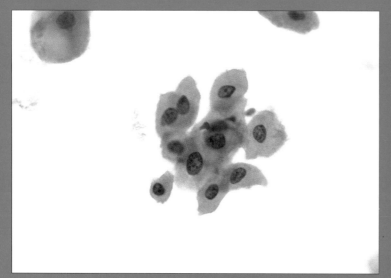

18.11 Parakeratosis: akin to miniature superficial cells (and hyperkeratosis ~ anucleate superficial cells). Surface keratotic reactions can mask significant underlying lesions, in this case, squamous cell carcinoma

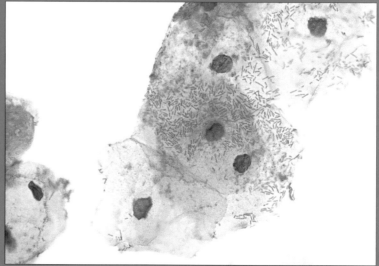

18.12 Intermediate cells with characteristic lactobacilli (often overlying cells or trapped in mucus). Other organisms also maintain their characteristic morphology in LBC

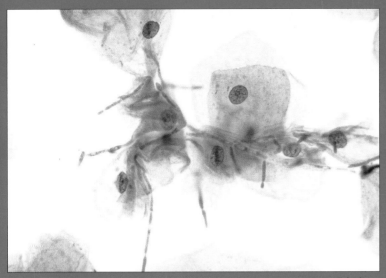

18.13 Some organisms, eg, *Candida*, stand out in LBC. Note prominent "shish kebab" effect. Mucus strands can mimic *Candida* (look for budding, like sausages)

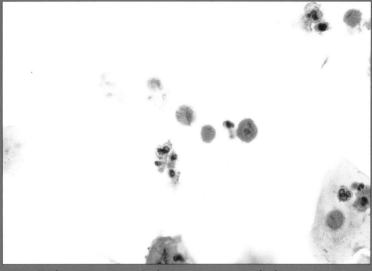

18.14 *Trichomonas* occurs singly, in groups, or attached to squamous cells, but appears smaller in LBC. The nucleus must be identified, red granules can be subtle, but flagella can sometimes be seen in LBC

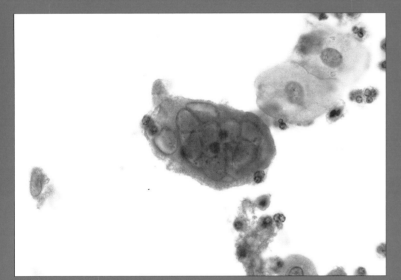

18.15 *Herpes* changes are similar in LBC, consisting of the 3 Ms: multinucleation, molding, margination of chromatin, with ground glass effect. Intranuclear inclusions tend to stand out in LBC

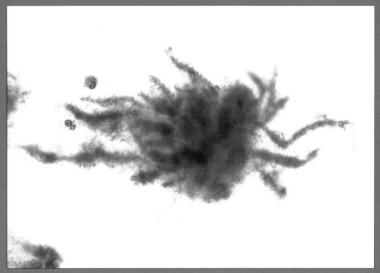

18.16 *Actinomyces* forms dense clusters of filamentous bacteria with colonies of nonfilamentous bacteria; often associated with IUDs

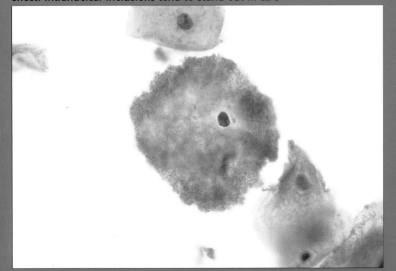

18.17 "Shift in vaginal flora": granular blue coccobacillary background diminishes, but clue cells (squamous with velvety coats) may be seen; lactobacilli and inflammation are absent by definition

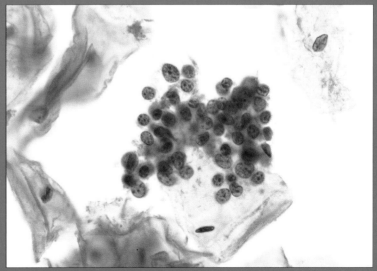

18.18 Follicular cervicitis presents as small, three-dimensional clusters of lymphoid cells that can mimic endometrial cells or other HCGs (look for tingible body macrophages)

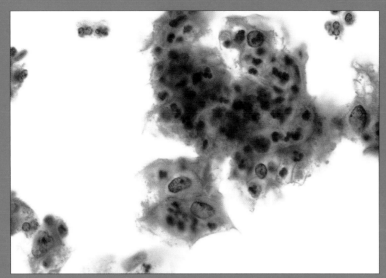

18.19 Inflammatory change: Characterized by slight nuclear enlargement (usually <2×), smooth membranes, fine chromatin, nucleoli, degenerated or vacuolated cytoplasm, and inflammation

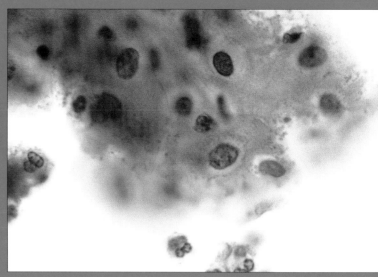

18.20 Inflammatory change with perinuclear halos can mimic koilocytotic halos

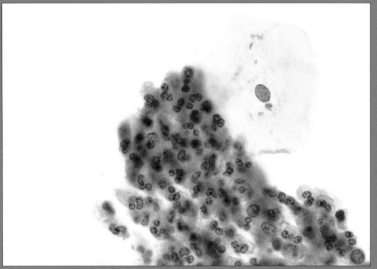

18.21 Inflammatory exudate has a tendency to clump or to cling to epithelial cells

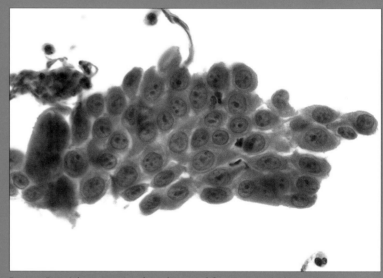

18.22 Repair/regeneration has the usual features, including cohesive sheets of orderly cells

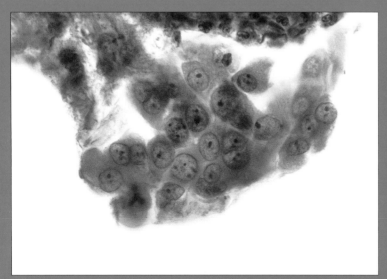

18.23 Repair/regeneration has smooth nuclear membranes, fine chromatin, and prominent nucleoli; normal mitotic figure may occur

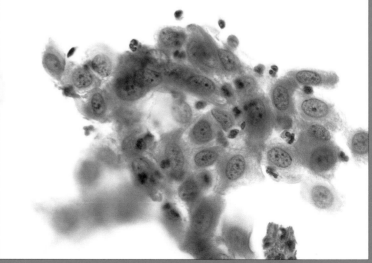

18.24 Repair/regeneration: The sheets may be more rounded up or folded, with greater depth of focus, and streaming may be less apparent in LBC

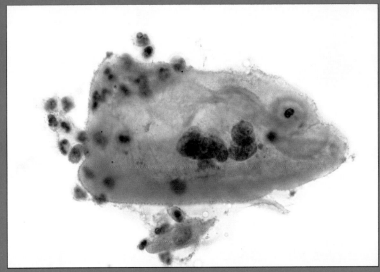

18.25 Radiation change: Macrocytes, multinucleation, vacuolization, polychromasia, etc; chemotherapy can produce similar changes

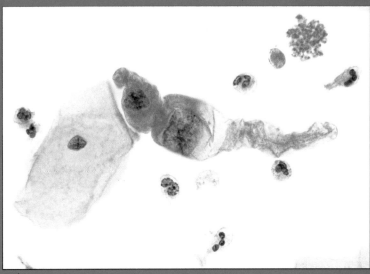

18.26 Pregnancy changes, such as decidual cells (illustrated) and Arias-Stella reaction, can also be seen in LBC

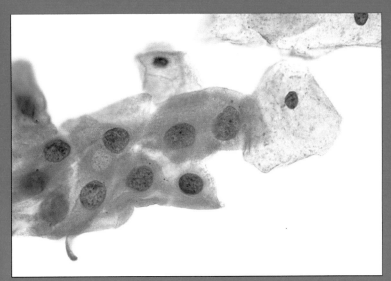

18.27 Mild dysplasia (L SIL): "If it's big and it's dark, it's dysplasia" still holds true in LBC

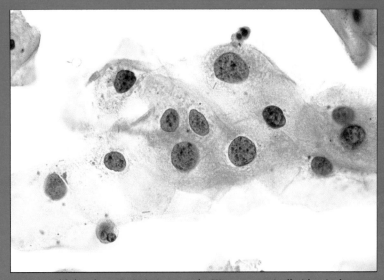

18.28 Mild dysplasia (L SIL): Low-grade SILs are practically identical, morphologically, in LBC and conventional Pap smears. Mature cells, big nuclei (>3×), hyperchromasia, mild increase N/C ratio

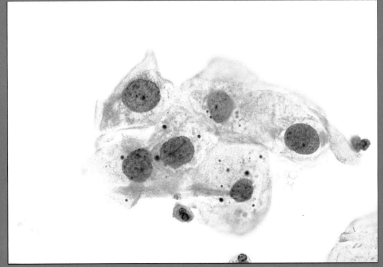

18.29 Mild dysplasia (L SIL): Small or indistinct nucleoli are more commonly seen in dysplasia in LBC

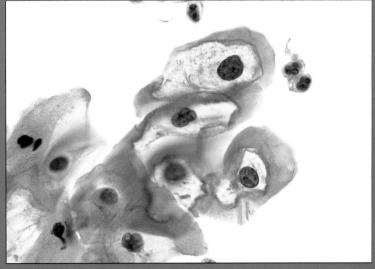

18.30 Koilocytes (L SIL): L SIL in general, and koilocytes in particular, tend to stand out like **STOP** signs in LBC

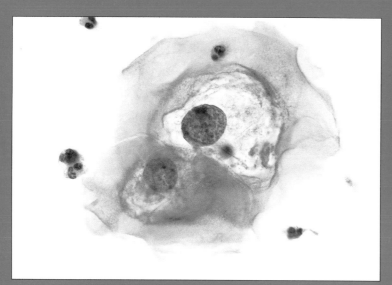

18.31 Koilocytes (L SIL): LBC enhances nuclear detail and highlights the cytoplasmic cavity of koilocytes

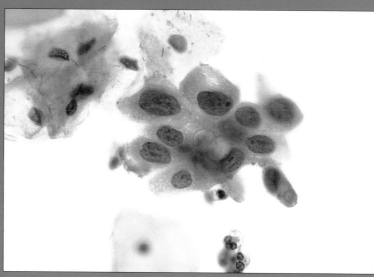

18.32 Moderate dysplasia (H SIL): Generally similar in appearance to conventional Pap smears

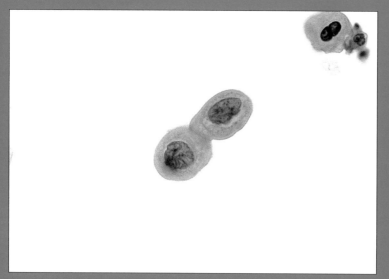

18.33 Moderate dysplasia (H SIL): Parabasal-sized cells, with moderately high N/C ratios, nuclear enlargement, irregular nuclear membranes, and hyperchromasia

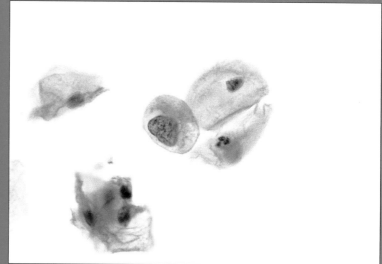

18.34 Moderate dysplasia (H SIL): Nuclear enlargement and hyperchromasia may be less apparent in LBC; other features, eg. irregular nuclear membranes (like little "brains") assume increased importance in interpretation

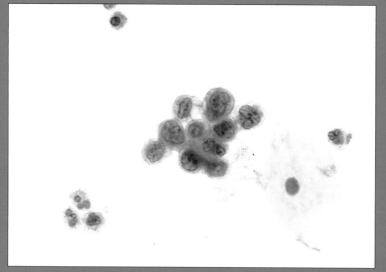

18.35 Severe dysplasia (H SIL): Small cells, high N/C ratios, and irregular nuclear membranes

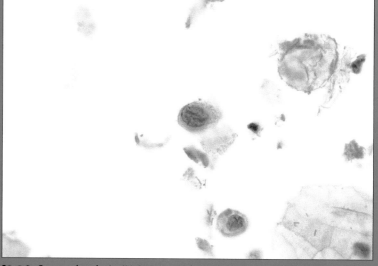

18.36 Severe dysplasia (H SIL): Irregular, "raisinoid" nuclei and high N/C ratios are characteristic

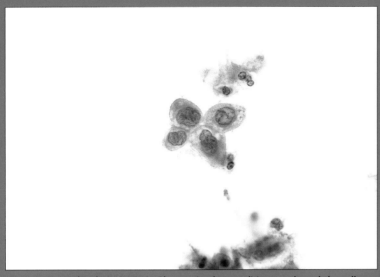

18.37 Severe dysplasia (H SIL): Chromatin abnormalities may be subtle; cells can mimic histiocytes or squamous metaplasia. Note irregular nuclear membranes

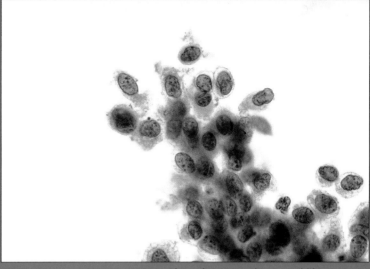

18.38 Carcinoma in situ (H SIL): Three-dimensional syncytial-like aggregates of abnormal cells showing chaotic architecture or loss of nuclear polarity (ie, hyperchromatic crowded groups)

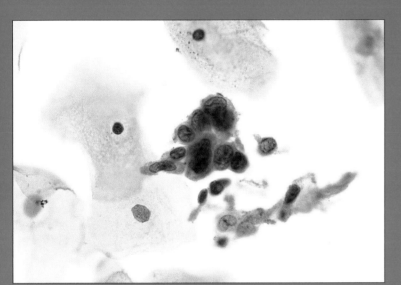

18.39 Carcinoma in situ (H SIL): HCGs can mimic benign entities; irregular nuclear membranes, chromatin abnormalities, mitotic figures, and squamous dysplasia are possible clues

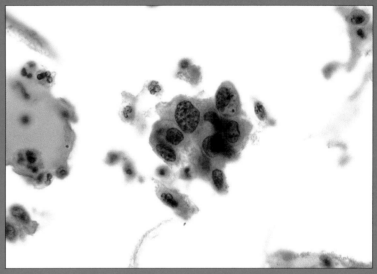

18.40 Nonkeratinizing squamous carcinoma: Still looks like cancer in LBC; note malignant appearing nuclei and dense, squamoid cytoplasm

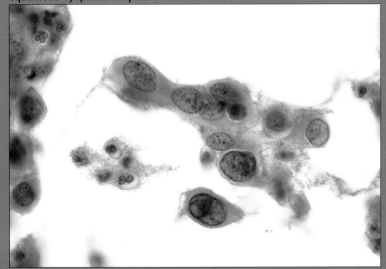

18.41 Nonkeratinizing squamous carcinoma: Relatively uniform, medium to large malignant squamous cells, present singly, in small sheets, or syncytial-like aggregates

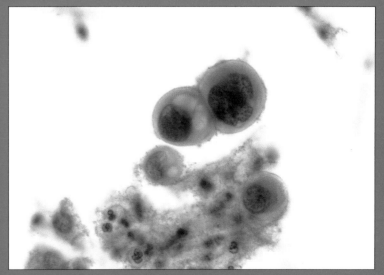

18.42 Nonkeratinizing squamous carcinoma: Tumor diathesis tends to clump and cling to cells

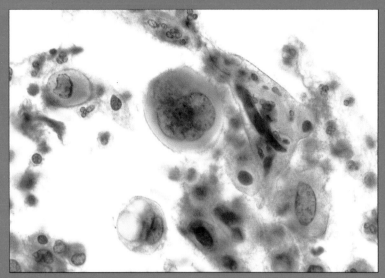

18.43 Keratinizing squamous carcinoma: Marked pleomorphism, orangeophilia (some cells). Note diathesis clinging to cells

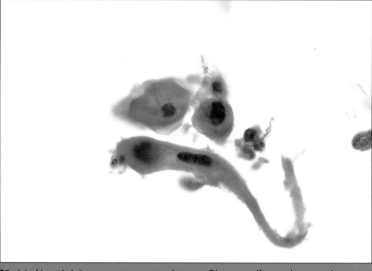

18.44 Keratinizing squamous carcinoma: Bizarre cells, such as snakes, tadpoles

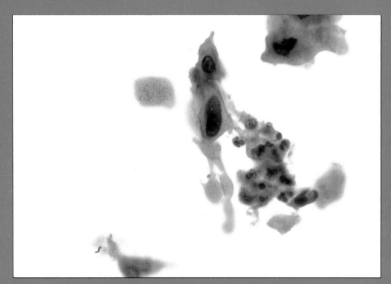

18.45 Keratinizing squamous carcinoma: Heavy cytoplasmic keratinization with cytoplasm keratin blebs

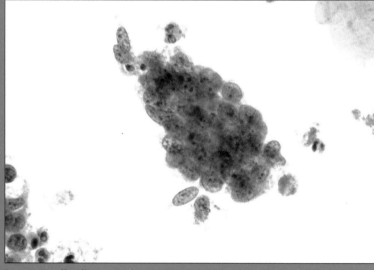

18.46 Small cell squamous carcinoma: Relatively uniform, small cells, with very high N/C ratios, coarse chromatin, small nucleoli, and scant cytoplasm. Differential includes other HCGs

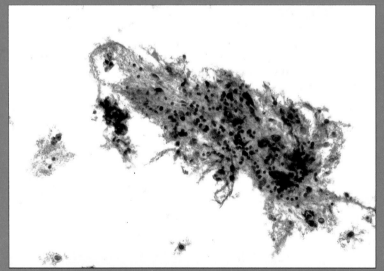

18.47 Tumor diathesis: Has a "ratty" appearance, composed of blood, fibrin, protein, necrosis, and cell debris. It tends to clump, have a fibrillar or frayed appearance, and may cling to tumor cells ("clinging diathesis")

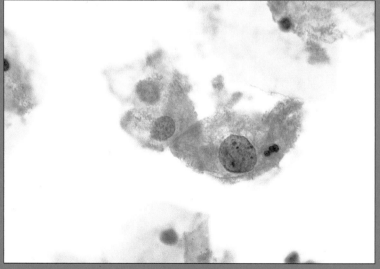

18.48 ASC-US: Mature intermediate or superficial cells with minimal nuclear enlargement (2-3×)

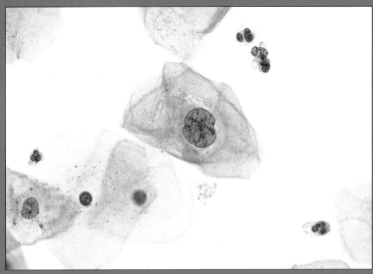

18.49 ASC-US: "US" means undetermined significance; this woman was HPV negative, despite the cytologic atypia

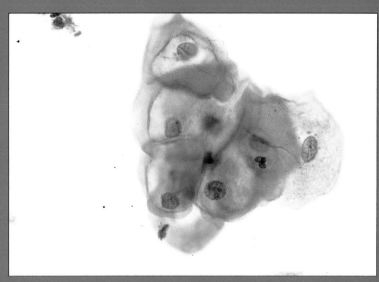

18.50 ASC-US: Changes suggestive, but not diagnostic of koilocytes, can also be interpreted as ASC-US

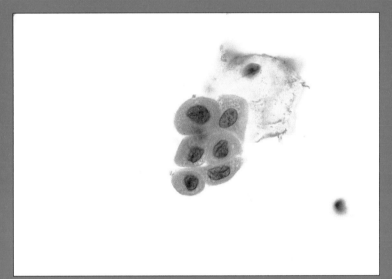

18.51 ASC-cannot exclude H SIL (ASC-H): Immature metaplastic cells with minimal nuclear enlargement and minimal nuclear atypia. Differential is benign metaplasia vs H SIL; this woman was HPV negative

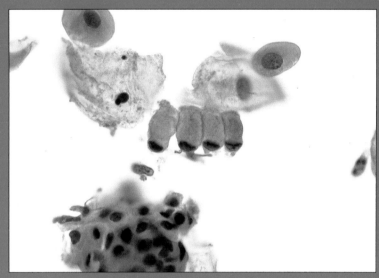

18.52 Endocervical cells: Nuclear cytoplasmic polarity, palisade

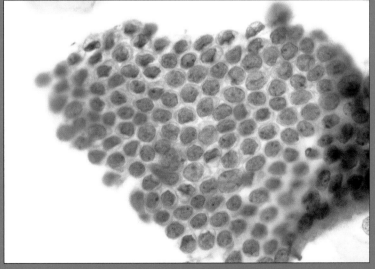

18.53 Endocervical cells: Honeycomb; endocervical cells are one measure of specimen adequacy

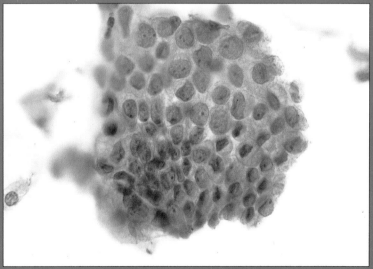

18.54 Endocervical cells: Endocervical cells may appear more "reactive" in LBC

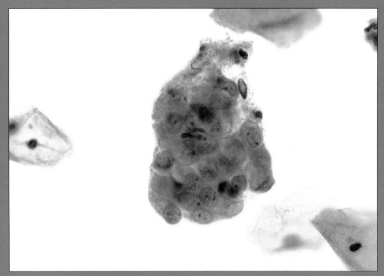

18.55 Endocervical cells: Endocervical cells and groups may "round up" in LBC making them more difficult to distinguish from endometrial cells

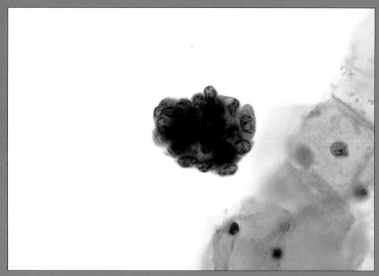

18.56 Endometrial cells: Tight, three-dimensional aggregates of small glandular cells; chromatin detail may be accentuated in LBC

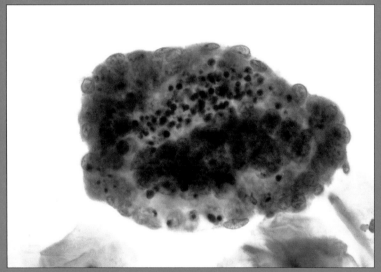

18.57 Endometrial cells: Double contour cell ball with central stroma; note apoptosis which is normal for endometrial cells, but abnormal for endocervical cells

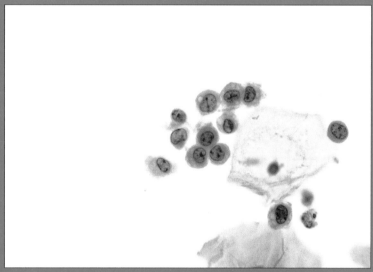

18.58 Stromal histiocytes: Indistinguishable from ordinary histiocytes, but tend to aggregate ("sticky histiocytes"); typically have bean-shaped nuclei and foamy cytoplasm

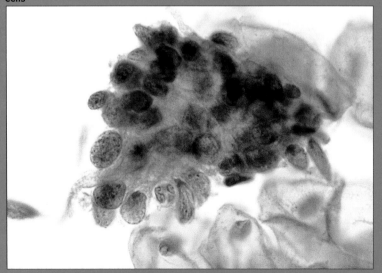

18.59 Atypical endocervical cells: Crowding, rosettes, and mitosis/apoptosis are key features

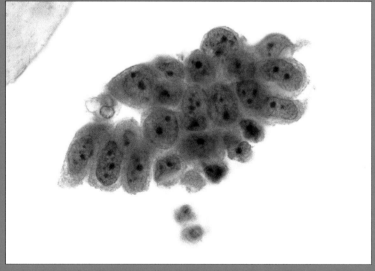

18.60 Atypical endometrial cells: Nuclear enlargement and prominent nucleoli are two key features

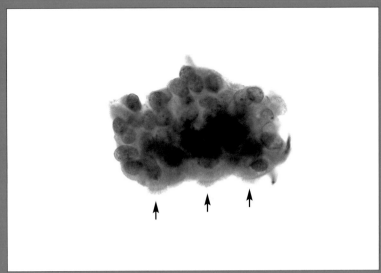

18.61 Tubal metaplasia: Hyperchromatic crowded group (HCG); note cilia (arrows)

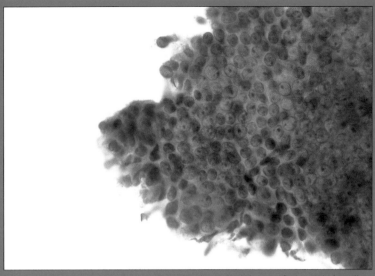

18.62 Lower uterine segment: HCG; closely packed, but uniform, orderly cells; associated endometrial stroma (biphasic pattern), when present, provides clue

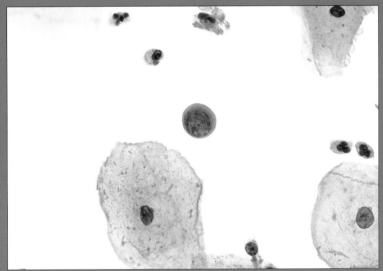

18.63 IUD effect: Single "IUD cells" can mimic CIN 3. No aggregates; no associated low-grade dysplasia

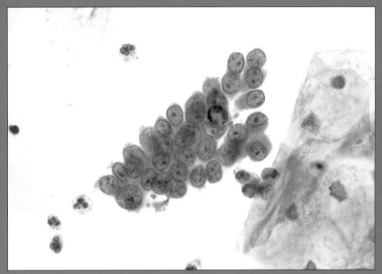

18.64 Adenocarcinoma in situ: Typically exfoliates numerous, variably-sized, disorderly hyperchromatic crowded groups of abnormal glandular cells

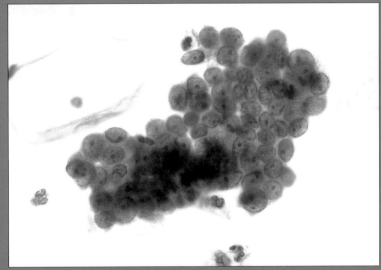

18.65 Adenocarcinoma in situ: Architectural abnormalities, eg, marked crowding, and nuclear abnormalities are similar in LBC, although nucleoli tend to be more conspicuous

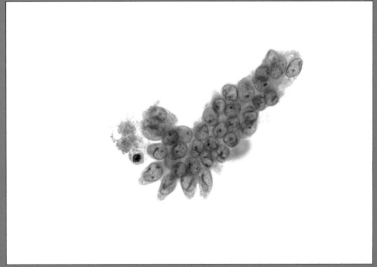

18.66 Adenocarcinoma in situ: Feathering and nuclear elongation may be less apparent, but nuclear membrane irregularities are more apparent, in LBC

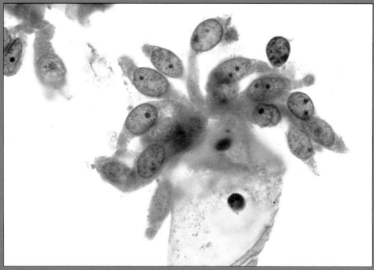

18.67 Adenocarcinoma in situ: The chromatin pattern is more variable (ie, the distinctive coarse dark chromatin may be lacking), and nucleoli are more common in LBC

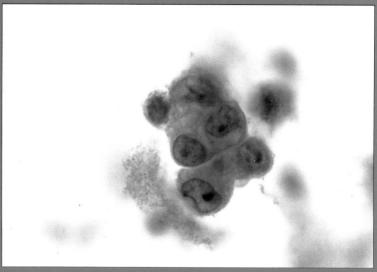

18.68 Endocervical adenocarcinoma: Typical malignant criteria, eg, nuclear enlargement, hyperchromasia, irregular membranes, abnormal chromatin, and prominent nucleoli

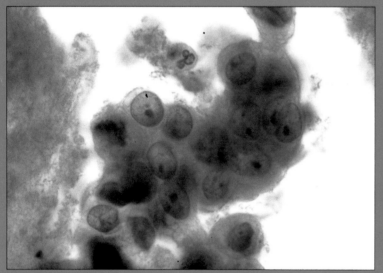

18.69 Endocervical adenocarcinoma: Three dimensional aggregates are more difficult to distinguish from endometrial carcinoma in LBC; note tumor diathesis

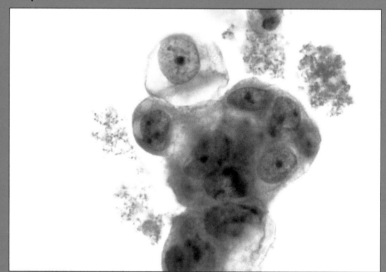

18.70 Endocervical adenocarcinoma: High grade tumor with large nuclei, prominent nucleoli, and vacuolated cytoplasm

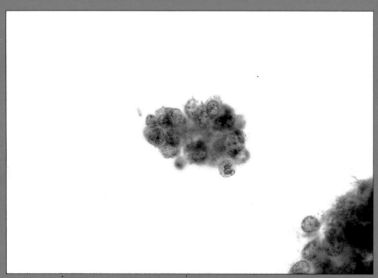

18.71 Endometrial carcinoma: Well differentiated, cytologically bland, can mimic benign endometrial cells; associated with clinical risk factors

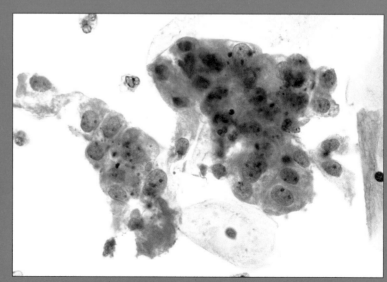

18.72 Endometrial carcinoma: Poorly differentiated with more obvious nuclear abnormalities; not all high grade endometrial cancers occur in background of atrophy

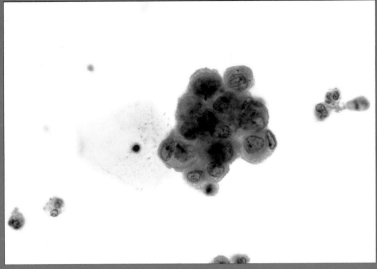

I8.73 Endometrial carcinoma: Watery diathesis less apparent, but clean background may help detect tumor cells

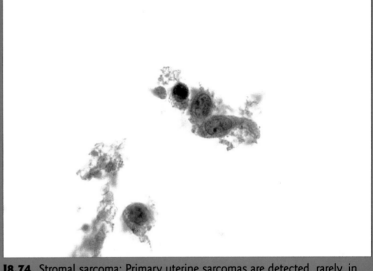

I8.74 Stromal sarcoma: Primary uterine sarcomas are detected, rarely, in Pap tests; the morphology is similar in LBC

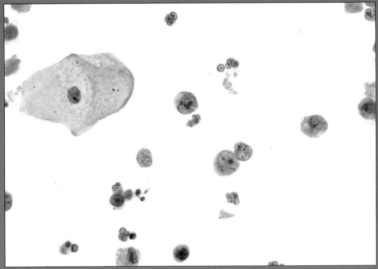

I8.75 Lymphoma: Single atypical lymphoid cells. Differential includes follicular cervicitis, which is far more common. Clinical history and presence of mass aid interpretation

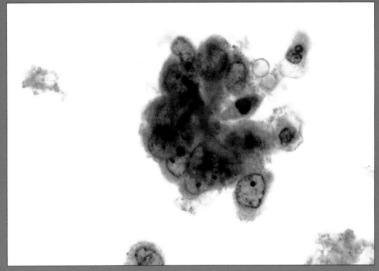

I8.76 Colon carcinoma: Direct extension with necrotic background. Differential includes primary uterine adenocarcinoma; clinical history paramount in interpretation

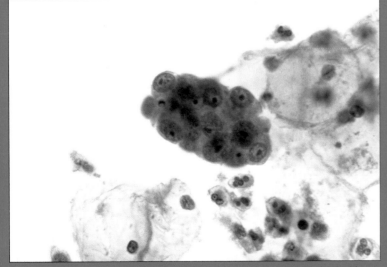

I8.77 Metastatic carcinoma: Classically, metastatic carcinoma looks like a "floater" in a clean background (papillary serous ovarian carcinoma)

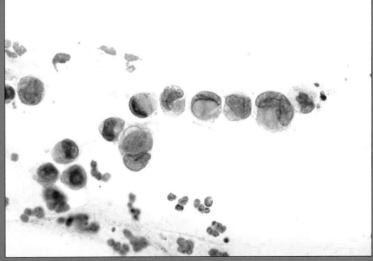

I8.78 Metastatic carcinoma: Unusual patterns, such as signet ring cells, suggest extrauterine primary, but can occur in primary tumors

IX. An Overview
of the Bethesda System

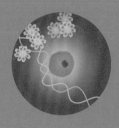

National Cancer Institute workshop developed the Bethesda System for reporting cervical/vaginal cytology in 1988, with revisions in 1991, and again in 2001 **[T9.1]** [Berek 2003, NCI 1989a, b, c, 1992, 1993a, b, Solomon 2002]. The Bethesda System, or TBS, was the work of a large committee (with representatives from many different groups interested in cervical cancer) reaching a consensus opinion. In an interesting innovation, worldwide participation in discussions before the TBS 2001 meeting was made possible via the Internet. Since its introduction, TBS has received widespread, but not universal support [Herbst 1990a, Kühler-Obbarius 1994a, Schenck 1998, K Syrjänen 1992, 1994], and is used by over 90% of American cytology laboratories [Davey 1992b].

The goal of TBS is to provide a uniform system of cytopathology reporting [MR Henry 2003, Koss 1990]. Effective communication between the pathologist and the clinician is essential for patient care, and the basis for this is a report that clearly conveys the significant cytologic findings. The irreproducible Papanicolaou system was discarded, as were loosely defined terms such as "atypia." Communication is a two-way street, however, and the health care provider is expected to provide relevant clinical information to the cytologist. TBS addresses several key points, including a standardized system of nomenclature; a clear statement of specimen adequacy; a general categorization for triage; and educational notes and suggestions for further evaluation if clinically indicated.

The new millennium was taken as an opportunity to re-evaluate TBS in light of new Pap test technologies and recent research as well as to remove ambiguous terminology. In TBS 2001, cervical cytology is recognized as a screening test, not a diagnostic test. Accordingly, the words "interpretation" or "report" replace the term "diagnosis." The woman's final *diagnosis* integrates cytology results with clinical findings and other laboratory or radiologic studies *by the clinician* [Noller 2002]. Although the squamous intraepithelial lesion terminology is gaining acceptance among histopathologists, no specific recommendations for its use in histology were made in TBS 2001. TBS 2001 replaced some terms from older versions of TBS, eg, Negative for Intraepithelial Lesion or Malignancy (NILM) replaced Within Normal Limits (WNL) and Benign Cellular Changes (BCC), added some new terms, eg, "atypical squamous cells cannot exclude high-grade squamous intraepithelial lesion," and eliminated others, eg, "favor reactive" associated with "atypical" [N Young 2002]. There were minor changes to the list of organisms. No separate document for anal/rectal cytology was produced.

An official list of non-neoplastic findings was added to the NILM category. These include: Reactive changes associated with inflammation, radiation, or intrauterine contraceptive device (IUD); Glandular cells status post-hysterectomy; and Atrophy. The list is optional and not all-inclusive, but can be helpful in explaining findings. Reporting atrophy, for example, might help explain why an endocervical component is not apparent or to document an interpretation of hyperchromatic crowded groups as clusters of benign basal/parabasal cells [N Young 2002].

The basic categories in the TBS 2001 report include: Specimen type (new); Specimen Adequacy; General Category (Optional); Ancillary Testing and Automated Review (both new); Interpretation/Result; and Educational Notes and Suggestions. Specimen Adequacy includes Satisfactory, with or without quality indicators, and Unsatisfactory. The General Category includes: Negative for Intraepithelial Lesion or Malignancy; Epithelial Cell Abnormalities; and Other. The Interpretation/Result includes Negative for Intraepithelial Lesion or Malignancy (organisms and other non-neoplastic findings [optional]); Other (eg, endometrial cells in women age 40 or older); Epithelial Cell Abnormalities; and Other Malignant Neoplasms. Epithelial Cell Abnormalities includes Squamous Cell Abnormalties (Atypical Squamous Cells, Squamous Intraepithelial Lesions; and Squamous Cell Carcinoma) and Glandular Cell Abnormalities (Atypical Glandular Cells and Adenocarcinoma). Finally, an optional section for Educational Notes and Suggestions is provided. These are discussed in more detail below.

Specimen Type

Because there is now more than one way to process Pap tests, a new category, Specimen Type, was introduced in TBS 2001. In this section the type of specimen, ie, conventional Pap smear, liquid-based cytology, or other, is specified.

Specimen Adequacy

One of the most important contributions of TBS is the requirement of a statement, in every case, regarding the adequacy of the specimen for evaluation. In the previous versions of TBS, there were three categories, Satisfactory for evaluation, Unsatisfactory for evaluation, and an intermediate category (for specimens that were not entirely satisfactory for evaluation). In 1988, the intermediate category was termed "less than optimal," but clinicians did not like their specimens being so labeled; therefore, in 1991, this category was changed to "satisfactory, but limited by [specify]" (commonly abbreviated, "SBLB"). Clinicians did not like their specimens being labeled "limited," either. It was also felt that the "SBLB" term was confusing, led to many unnecessary repeat tests, and criteria were difficult to apply reproducibly [G Gill 2000, MR Henry 2003, Renshaw 1999, Valente 1991]. So, in TBS 2001, the intermediate adequacy category was officially dropped, leaving only two specimen adequacy categories (Satisfactory and Unsatisfactory), but "quality indicators" could be added to Satisfactory specimens in TBS 2001. So, now there are Satisfactory, Unsatisfactory, and Satisfactory with quality indicators. The "quality indicators" are remarkably similar to what used to render a specimen "less than optimal" or "limited." And, "quality indicators" still indicate the same thing as the older terms, ie, that an interpretation may be given; however, the result may be compromised for the reason(s) stated. In other words, what so-called quality indicators indicate is not quality, but rather lack of it. With apologies to Jeremy Bentham, the idea that clinicians should not be clearly informed about the adequacy of the specimen is nonsense; the idea that women don't deserve to know that their cancer-screening test may have been compromised is nonsense on stilts.

The goal of reporting specimen adequacy is to obtain better samples by providing feedback to the clinician regarding the quality of the specimen [M Nielsen 1993]. The statement of adequacy may be the single most important feature of TBS for quality improvement. There is generally good reproducibility of the Bethesda criteria for adequacy, particularly in designating a specimen "satisfactory" [Spires 1995]. Most laboratories now report specimen adequacy [Davey 1992b]. The American Society for Colposcopy and Cervical Pathology (ASCCP) has published patient management guidelines relating to specimen adequacy and quality indicators (see table, pg 242) [Davey 2002, 2003b]. Longitudinal studies indicate that women with unsatisfactory specimens are more likely to be "high risk," and significantly more

T 9.1 The Bethesda System 2001

Specimen Type
Indicate conventional Pap smear vs liquid-based preparation vs other

Specimen Adequacy
- Satisfactory for evaluation *(describe presence or absence of endocervical/transformation zone component and any other quality indicators, eg, partially obscuring blood, inflammation, etc)*
- Unsatisfactory for evaluation ... *(specify reason)*
  - Specimen rejected/not processed *(specify reason)*
  - Specimen processed and examined, but unsatisfactory for evaluation of epithelial abnormality because of *(specify reason)*

General Categorization *(optional)*
- Negative for Intraepithelial Lesion or Malignancy
- Other: See Interpretation/Result
  (eg, endometrial cells in a woman ≥ 40 years of age)
- Epithelial Cell Abnormality: See Interpretation/Result
  (specify 'squamous' or 'glandular' as appropriate)

Interpretation/Result
Negative for Intraepithelial Lesion or Malignancy
(when there is no cellular evidence of neoplasia, state this in the General Categorization above and/or in the Interpretation/Result section of the report—whether or not there are organisms or other non-neoplastic findings)

Organisms
- *Trichomonas vaginalis*
- Fungal organisms morphologically consistent with *Candida* spp
- Shift in flora suggestive of bacterial vaginosis
- Bacteria morphologically consistent with *Actinomyces* spp.
- Cellular changes consistent with Herpes simplex virus

Other Non-Neoplastic Findings *(Optional to report; list not inclusive)*
- Reactive cellular changes associated with
- inflammation (includes typical repair)
- radiation
- intrauterine contraceptive device (IUD)
- Glandular cells status posthysterectomy
- Atrophy

Other
- Endometrial cells *(in a woman ≥ 40 years of age)*

(Specify if 'negative for squamous intraepithelial lesion')

Epithelial Cell Abnormalities
Squamous Cell
- Atypical squamous cells
- of undetermined significance (ASC-US)
- cannot exclude H SIL (ASC-H)
- Low-grade squamous intraepithelial lesion (L SIL)
  (encompassing: HPV/mild dysplasia/CIN 1)
- High-grade squamous intraepithelial lesion (H SIL)
  (encompassing: moderate and severe dysplasia, CIS; CIN 2 and CIN 3)
  with features suspicious for invasion *(if invasion is suspected)*
- Squamous cell carcinoma

Glandular Cell
- Atypical
- endocervical cells (NOS *or specify in comments*)
- endometrial cells (NOS *or specify in comments*)
- glandular cells (NOS *or specify in comments*)
- Atypical
- endocervical cells, favor neoplastic
- glandular cells, favor neoplastic
- Cervical adenocarcinoma in situ
- Adenocarcinoma
- endocervical
- endometrial
- extrauterine
- not otherwise specified (NOS)

Other Malignant Neoplasms *(specify)*

Ancillary Testing
Provide a brief description of the test methods and report the result so that it is easily understood by the clinician.

Automated Review
If case examined by automated device, specify device and result.

Educational Notes and Suggestions *(optional)*
Suggestions should be concise and consistent with clinical follow-up guidelines published by professional organizations (references to relevant publications may be included).

likely to have abnormalities on follow-up than women with satisfactory index specimens [Davey 2003b, Ransdell 1997].

There are four important elements in evaluation of specimen adequacy: (1) patient and specimen identification, and (2) pertinent clinical information, and (3) technical interpretability (eg, adequate fixation without air drying), and (4) cellular composition and sampling of the endocervical/transformation zone (eg, presence of squamous and endocervical cells in the Pap test) [NCI 1993a, b].

All four individual elements must each be satisfactory for a specimen to be entirely satisfactory. Reports from satisfactory specimens should describe the presence or absence of endocervical/transformation zone component and note any other quality indicators, eg, partially obscuring blood, inflammation, etc. The clinician *must* provide appropriate clinical history (including age, pregnancy and menstrual history, use of oral contraceptives or other hormones or drugs, use of intrauterine contraceptive device, previous abnormal cytology or histology, history of neoplasia, therapy, cigarette smoking, and any other pertinent information, including high-risk sexual behavior). Specimens received without pertinent clinical information may be considered "Satisfactory with quality indicators." In cases with "quality indicators" it is the responsibility of the clinician to correlate the findings from the individual woman to determine whether the Pap test should be repeated immediately or at the next regular examination.

A specimen may be considered entirely unsatisfactory for evaluation if (1) there is lack of proper identification or no requisition form or (2) the slide is technically unacceptable (eg, irreparably broken, inadequate preservation) or (3) there is scant cellularity or (4) more than 75% of the cells are obscured (excess blood, exudate, etc). In prior TBS iterations, "limited" or "SBLB" slides included those in which 50% to 75% of the epithelial cells are obscured, lack of endocervical cells/T zone, etc.

Any one of these is sufficient to render a specimen unsatisfactory for evaluation. The most common reasons for unsatisfactory specimens are scant cellularity followed by obscuration of the cells. Unsatisfactory specimens that cannot be accessioned by the laboratory, eg, unlabelled or badly damaged slides, are distinguished from specimens that have been processed by the laboratory and determined to be "unsatisfactory" after microscopic review [Solomon 2002].

An unsatisfactory specimen is unreliable for interpretation. However, unsatisfactory specimens are more likely among high-risk women; significantly more women have SIL or cancer on follow-up compared to those with satisfactory specimens [Davey 2000, Ransdell 1997]. Therefore, it is important to carefully scrutinize apparently unsatisfactory slides for abnormal cells before dismissing the case as unsatisfactory for evaluation. A corollary is that *if abnormal cells are present, the specimen is not unsatisfactory* [NCI 1993a, b]. Furthermore, even though unreliable for cervical cancer prevention, unsatisfactory specimens may provide other useful information, such as presence of organisms, endometrial cells in women ≥ 40 years of age, etc. Finally, the report should indicate why the specimen was unsatisfactory (cells obscured by excess blood, exudate, etc or simply low cellularity).

Cellular composition, which in the Pap test encompasses endocervical and squamous cells, is influenced by many factors. The sample must include an adequate number of cells that are representative of the anatomic site.

Adequate Squamous Cellularity

In TBS 1991, adequate squamous cellularity was defined as: well-preserved and well-visualized squamous cells should cover more than 10% of the slide surface [NCI 1993a, b, Renshaw 1999, Valente 1991]. However, in TBS 2001, new numeric criteria were proposed and the number depends on specimen type.

Conventional Pap tests usually have on the order of 50,000 to 300,000 epithelial cells [Koss 1989a]. Liquid-based Pap tests average about 50,000 to 75,000 cells. In TBS 2001, conventional Pap smears should have a minimum of 8,000 to 12,000 well-preserved, well-visualized squamous cells to be considered satisfactory. For liquid-based cytology, there should be a minimum of 5,000 such (good-looking) cells based on preliminary scientific evidence [Geyer 2000, Solomon 2002, Studeman 2003]. Note that there is a numerical *range* for conventional Pap smears, but a *single number* for liquid-based Pap tests. Note also that there is no longer any requirement regarding how much of the slide is covered with cells. Pap tests with fewer than the recommended number of cells are considered "unsatisfactory" for evaluation (unless an abnormality is identified). A slight increase in "unsatisfactory" cases was expected using these new criteria, from the old figure of slightly less than 1% to a new figure of slightly more than 2%, although much higher unsatisfactory rates have been reported using the TBS 2001 [Fidda 2004]. Also note that adequate cellularity alone does not guarantee the overall adequacy of the specimen [Bishop 2002].

When assessing specimen cellularity, there are two points to be emphasized [MR Henry 2003]. First, adequate squamous cellularity is usually obvious; in only a small minority of cases will it be necessary to estimate cellularity. Second, *do not try to count all the cells on the slide!* Instead, compare the slide with "reference images" of known cellularity or, for liquid-based cytology, a few fields of cells can be counted, and then extrapolated using a chart. Squamous metaplastic cells, but not endocervical cells, are included in the evaluation of squamous cellularity. Cellularity can be difficult to estimate owing to such factors as cell clustering, atrophy, cytolysis, or obscuration. Only well-visualized cells are included in estimating cellularity. Interobserver agreement in assessing squamous adequacy on conventional smears is only fair, but is improved using TBS 2001 adequacy criteria along with reference images [Haroon 2002, Sheffield 2003]. In LBC, the specimen is within a standard-sized circle and the cells are evenly distributed (in theory). Thus, cellularity can be estimated by counting cells in a few fields using this formula, which accounts for the ocular field number, the objective magnification, and the diameter of the cellular preparation.

Formula

Number of cells required per field = 5000 cells/[(area of circle)/(area of ocular)]

The number of cells per field in a minimum of 10 fields should be counted along a diameter of the circle (that includes the center). The average number of cells per field is then calculated. Holes or empty areas must be accounted for in the estimations. [T9.2] shows the average number of cells per field needed at various magnifications and ocular areas (field number, FN) to achieve a minimum of 5000 total cells on the slide. (The magnification and field number are usually engraved on the lens casing.) SurePath®'s circle is 13mm; ThinPrep®'s circle is 20mm. For example, for ThinPrep®, using a 10X objective and an ocular with a field number of 20, there must be an average of 50 cells per field (or 500 cells in ten fields), to achieve a minimum of 5000 cells on the slide.

In practice, cells can be difficult to count owing to clustering, atrophy, cytolysis, etc. In some cases, a technical problem can be identified and reprocessing the specimen may yield adequate cellularity. A little-known factoid, however, is that (as of this writing) the FDA only approves the "first off" liquid-based specimen for analysis (see package insert for up-to-date information). The report should state the reason for unsatisfactory specimens, eg, excess blood, mucus, exudate, etc vs simple low squamous cellularity.

T9.2 Average number cells per field for adequate squamous cellularity in LBC for minimum 5000 cells

Preparation diameter (mm)	Area mm²	FN20 ocular/10× objective		FN20 ocular/40× objective		FN22 ocular/10× objective		FN22 ocular/40× objective	
		# fields	# cells/field	# fields	#cells/field	#fields	# cells/field	#fields	# cells/field
13mm (SurePath®)	132.7	42.3	118.3	676	7.4	34.9	143.2	559	9.0
20mm (ThinPrep®)	314.2	100	50.0	1600	3.1	82.6	60.5	1322	3.8

Notes:
Microscopic field diameter (in mm) = Ocular field number/Objective magnification
Field radius = field diameter ÷ 2
Area of microscopic field = (πr²) = π × (field radius)²
Ocular magnification does not affect calculation

Adequate Endocervical/Transformation Zone Component

The transformation zone is theoretically the key site to sample, since this is where most precursor lesions and cervical cancers arise. However, the practical importance of an endocervical cell/transformation zone (EC/TZ) component is controversial [Birdsong 2001, MR Henry 2003]. Briefly (see pg 197 for more discussion), several studies support the importance of sampling the transformation zone, reporting that squamous abnormalities (SILs) are more likely to be detected in slides containing endocervical cells [Elias 1983, Kristensen 1991, Martin–Hirsch 1999, Mintzer 1999, Vooijs 1985]. However, retrospective cohort studies have indicated that women whose samples lack endocervical cells are *not* more likely to have squamous lesions on follow-up than those whose samples do have endocervical cells [Bos 2001, Kivlahan 1986, H Mitchell 1991, 2001]. Also, retrospective case-control studies failed to find an association between false-negative results and lack of endocervical cells [H Mitchell 1995b, O'Sullivan 1998a]. Nevertheless, even though the data are conflicting, the consensus was that an EC/TZ component is an important measure of adequate sampling and that its absence should be reported with any other comments on quality indicators [MR Henry 2003]. Furthermore, it is quite possible that an EC/TZ component is important in detecting *glandular* neoplasia, which is increasing in incidence.

In TBS 2001 the presence or absence of an endocervical/transformation zone component is described. The numeric criterion for a transformation zone component is unchanged. There should be at least 10 well-preserved endocervical cells or squamous metaplastic cells. However, clusters of cells are no longer required [Solomon 2002]. Also, specimens need not have an adequate EC/TZ component to be classified as "satisfactory" for evaluation. However, the presence or absence of an EC/TZ component should be clearly stated in the report; those without an adequate EC/TZ sample are reported as "satisfactory," but with quality indicators.

The Bethesda System accepts both actual endocervical cells and squamous metaplastic cells as being indicative of a transformation zone component. Endocervical mucus is insufficient evidence of an endocervical sample. The definition applies to both premenopausal and postmenopausal women with a cervix. However, parabasal cells in atrophy, as can be seen in menopause, postpartum, or progestational therapy, can closely resemble metaplastic or endocervical cells. Therefore, the absence of an identifiable EC/TZ zone component in the setting of atrophy does not affect the specimen adequacy [NCI 1993a, b]. If the specimen shows a high-grade lesion or cancer, it is not necessary to comment on the presence or absence of a transformation zone component.

Technical Interpretability

Technical interpretability can usually be determined by a quick scan at low power. Limiting factors can be divided into three groups: cellularity, distortion (eg, air-drying, spray fixative artifact, extensive cytolysis), and obscuration

(eg, excess exudate, foreign material). The Pap test itself must be adequately prepared. This means an abundance of representative cells must be forcefully scraped (not gently swabbed) during collection. Conventional Pap smears are thinly smeared on a properly labeled slide (or slides), and immediately fixed (<10 seconds), either by immersion in 95% ethanol or with commercial spray fixative. Liquid-based Pap tests are prepared according to the manufacturer's directions. For proper evaluation, there should not be an excess of blood or exudate diluting or obscuring the cells.

The presence of air-drying, excess blood or exudate, thick smears, marked degeneration, poor stain, extraneous material, or other artifacts should be visually assessed. For a satisfactory specimen, at least 75% of the epithelial cells should be well preserved and well visualized. If more than 75% of the epithelial cells are obscured or distorted, the specimen is "unsatisfactory," unless abnormal cells are present. A specimen is considered "partially obscured" when 50% to 75% of the epithelial cells cannot be properly visualized [Solomon 2002]. This is reported as "satisfactory with quality indicators." Slides that are apparently unsatisfactory should be carefully scrutinized for abnormal cells, because, eg, a few indubitable cancer cells may be found in blood or inflammation [M Costa 1991b]. Pap tests in which abnormal cells can be identified should not be designated "unsatisfactory."

A specimen reported as "unsatisfactory" should be repeated. However, those with quality indicators do not necessarily require an immediately repeated examination (see pg 200). Individual factors, such as location of the transformation zone, age, pregnancy, and previous therapy, may limit the clinician's ability to obtain an endocervical sample. *Ultimately, the clinician must determine what is "adequate sampling" for an individual woman, based on integrating information from the clinical history, visual inspection of the cervix, and the cytopathology report* [NCI 1993a, b].

General Categorization

TBS 2001 provides for a "general categorization" of the specimen. The general categorization is optional, but may be included to aid clinicians or their staff in triaging reports as well as in compiling statistics. The general categories are: (1) Negative for Intraepithelial Lesion or Malignancy (2) Epithelial Cell Abnormality, and (3) Other. The previous categories, "within normal limits" and "benign cellular changes" have been combined into a single new category, "negative for intraepithelial lesion or malignancy," (NILM). Although "NILM" can be used as an interpretation without further explanation, the general categorization is *not* to be used as a substitute for a descriptive interpretation/result. If there is more than one finding, the general category is based on the most clinically significant result [Solomon 2002].

Negative for Intraepithelial Lesion or Malignancy

Negative for Intraepithelial Lesion or Malignancy (NILM) is used as the general category for Pap tests that lack cytologic evidence of a squamous intraepithelial lesion or malignancy. It combines the former general categories, "within normal limits" and "benign cellular changes." Many conditions formerly classified as "benign cellular changes," including infection and reactive changes (including typical repair, atrophy with inflammation, radiation, IUD changes, other nonspecific causes), are now included in the NILM category. Important note: although the category of reactive changes has been deleted from the TBS 2001, federal rules and regulations (CLIA) and the College of American Pathologists (CAP) still require pathologist review of Pap tests with reactive changes. Reactive changes (and other non-neoplastic findings) can be described in the interpretation/results section. Additional information can also be provided in the interpretation/result portion of the report (see below).

Epithelial Cell Abnormality

Epithelial Cell Abnormality is for potentially premalignant or malignant lesions (including "suspicious," "dysplastic," or "positive" cases). Epithelial Cell Abnormality includes abnormalities of both squamous and glandular cells, which should be specified as appropriate. More information should be provided under Interpretation/Result.

Other (Under General Category)

The "Other" category was added to the general categorization for cases in which there are no abnormalities of the cells themselves, but the findings may indicate some increased risk of neoplasia, eg, benign-appearing "endometrial cells in a woman ≥40 years of age" [Solomon 2002]. Additional information can be provided under Interpretation/Result. ("Other" is also a major heading for Interpretation Result other than NILM, Epithelial Cell Abnormalities, and Other Malignant Neoplasms (see pg 241).

Automated Review

When using an automated slide review system, the instrumentation used and the result should be specified in the report (reporting raw data is not recommended). No individual's name should be included on the report *if no manual review was performed* because this could be misconstrued as identifying a person who examined the slide. However, the name of the medical director may be required as part of laboratory identification according to local custom or regulatory requirement. As with any automated laboratory equipment, the results should be reviewed and verified by qualified laboratory personnel, and records maintained per regulatory requirements [MR Henry 2003].

Ancillary Testing

TBS 2001 does not recommend any particular additional testing [MR Henry 2003]. However, TBS recognizes that ancillary tests are increasingly used to complement cervical cytology and makes recommendations for reporting the results. A brief description of the ancillary test methods should be provided and the result should be reported so that it is easily understood by the clinician [Raab 2003]. Ideally, the cytology and ancillary testing result are reported concurrently; this is *integrated reporting*. If this is not possible, then the separate cytology and ancillary testing results can be *cross-referenced*. Probabilistic and interpretive styles are two methods for integrated reporting of cytology and ancillary testing results. In the probabilistic method, the cytology result is reported with the molecular test result, along with a summary risk statement. For example: the Pap test result may be ASC-US; oncogenic HPV-DNA not detected. A probabilistic report could note "these findings suggest a 1% to 2% risk of underlying H SIL." In the interpretive method, the cytology and molecular test results are considered together in arriving at a summary result. For the same example (ASC-US; HPV negative), an interpretive report could note "The cytologic interpretation is ASC-US. Oncogenic HPV-DNA is not detected. In combination, these findings favor a reactive process." Laboratories are encouraged to review cytology cases in conjunction with the HPV results as a quality improvement tool; however, be cautious changing the cytology interpretation based on HPV results [Davey 2003a].

Interpretation/Result

In TBS 2001, the word "diagnosis" was replaced by "interpretation" or "result" to emphasize that the Pap test is a screening test, not a diagnostic test. The woman's *diagnosis* is based upon integration of Pap test results, clinical findings, laboratory tests, etc, and is made by the clinician.

TBS 2001 includes four categories under Interpretation/Result. These are: Negative for Intraepithelial Lesion or Malignancy; Other; Epithelial Cell Abnormality; and Other Malignant Neoplasm. The terminology of "squamous intraepithelial lesion," divided into low-grade and high-grade categories (encompassing dysplasia/carcinoma in situ or cervical intraepithelial neoplasia, as previously discussed), was introduced in 1988 and remains unchanged in TBS 2001. However, the categories of atypical squamous cells and atypical glandular cells were modified somewhat (see pg 241). For most other diagnoses, the Bethesda System incorporates previously existing terminology.

Negative for Intraepithelial Lesion or Malignancy

Specimens for which no neoplastic abnormality is identified are reported as "negative for intraepithelial lesion or malignancy." There are two subcategories in NILM: Organisms and Other Non-Neoplastic Findings.

Organisms

In TBS 2001, the term "organisms" replaces "infection" because the mere presence of organisms does not necessarily indicate clinical infection. The list of organisms is unchanged from TBS 1991, except that "predominance of coccobacilli consistent with shift in vaginal flora" was replaced by "shift in vaginal flora suggestive of bacterial vaginosis" in TBS 2001. Although identification of organisms is not the primary mission of the Pap test, providing such information can be clinically helpful [N Young 2002].

Other Non-Neoplastic Findings

The reporting of "other non-neoplastic findings" under the NILM category is optional [Solomon 2002]. Included in this optional subcategory are reactive cellular changes and atrophy. Reactive cellular changes encompasses such entities as inflammation (including typical repair), radiation effect, and IUD effect. Another phrase, added in TBS 2001, is "benign glandular cells status post hysterectomy." Studies have reported that these women rarely develop neoplastic lesions, regardless of history of prior malignancy [Ponder 1997, Ramirez 2000, Tambouret 1998]. The origin of these glandular cells can be perplexing, but possibilities include vaginal adenosis, glandular metaplasia associated with prior radiation or chemotherapy, prolapse of fallopian tube, endometriosis, and fistula (see pg 188). These cases usually do not warrant an interpretation of Atypical Glandular Cells.

The clinical significance of inflammatory (reactive/reparative) changes is controversial in regard to its predictive value for either a gynecologic infection or an epithelial abnormality. Although several studies have reported a correlation between sexually transmitted diseases and the presence of inflammatory changes on Pap test [Eckert 1995, S Edwards 1998, Kelly 1990, Mali 1993, Singh 1995, 1999, J Wilson 1990], others do not [Bertolino 1992, Dimian 1992, W Parsons 1993] probably because many factors besides infection can cause inflammation. On the other hand, numerous studies report an increased risk of SIL in women with inflammatory Pap tests [Busseniers 1991, Castle 2001, Cecchini 1990a, Creasman 1981, Cuzick 2001, Frisch 1990, Himmelstein 1989, Lawley 1990, Margolis 1999, McLachlan 1994, K Miller 1992, Noumoff 1987, Parashari 1995, Pearlstone 1992, Reiter 1986, Schwebke 1997, Seckin 1997, Sidawy 1993, Soofer 1997, Webb 2001b, J Wilson 1990]. Reactive/reparative changes are common in estrogen deficiency, IUD, coitus, or tampon use, following surgery, radiation therapy, and the list goes on.

Because the significance of "benign cellular changes" was unclear, its predictive value unknown, and the term itself ambiguous, it was dropped from TBS 2001. Note again, however, that CLIA regulations still require pathologist review of cases thought to be "reactive cellular changes" even though this category is no longer recognized in the Bethesda System.

Other

In previous versions of TBS, the finding of endometrial cells was reported only in postmenopausal women and was considered a glandular abnormality. In TBS 2001, however, the presence of benign appearing endometrial cells is reported in *all* women 40 years of age or older, *regardless* of menstrual status, hormone therapy, etc. Age was selected as the best determining factor, because other clinical data and risk factors are often unclear or unknown to the clinician or the pathologist [MR Henry 2003]. Although usually a benign finding, there is a risk of an underlying endometrial abnormality. However, it is recognized that cervical cytology is an inaccurate test for endometrial pathology, and so this finding was placed in the "Other" category, neither epithelial cell abnormality nor negative for intraepithelial lesion (NILM). It is up to the clinician to determine whether shedding endometrial cells is abnormal, or not, for the individual woman and to determine follow-up of the result. Of course, the presence of *abnormal*-appearing endometrial cells should be reported as a glandular abnormality.

The terminology provided for the above finding is: "Endometrial cells in a women ≥40 years of age" [Solomon 2002]. This can be applied regardless of menstrual or menopausal status or exogenous hormonal therapy. There are two points worth noting. First, the wording, "endometrial cells," does not differentiate between endometrial glandular and stromal cells, because it can be difficult to distinguish these cell types in practice. However, it is primarily abnormally shed endometrial glandular cells that increase the risk of endometrial pathology. Second, this interpretive category is exclusively for spontaneously shed endometrial cells, not directly sampled lower uterine segment or endometrium. A comment regarding the "Other" category is optional. For example: "Endometrial cells after age 40, particularly out-of-phase or after menopause, may be associated with benign endometrium, hormonal alterations, and less commonly, endometrial abnormalities. Suggest clinical correlation." When using this category, it still should be specified if the specimen is "negative for squamous intraepithelial lesion."

A crystal ball may be needed to determine, *a priori,* that the endometrial cells are benign, since it is well known that endometrial cancer can shed cytologically benign-*appearing* endometrial cells. Because neoplastic lesions can exfoliate as hyperchromatic crowded groups mimicking endometrial cells, some laboratories *always* report endometrial cells, regardless of age or menstrual status. While this is not required by TBS, neither is it prohibited. Clinicians rarely question this simple statement ("endometrial cells present") on the report.

Epithelial Cell Abnormalities

Epithelial cell abnormalities are divided into three groups—squamous, glandular, and other. These can then be further subdivided.

Squamous Cell Abnormalities

Squamous cell abnormalities include: atypical squamous cells; squamous intraepithelial lesions (low-grade and high-grade); and squamous cell carcinoma. Low-grade squamous intraepithelial lesion (L SIL) includes both mild dysplasia (CIN 1) and cellular changes associated with human papillomavirus (HPV). High-grade squamous intraepithelial lesion (H SIL) includes moderate dysplasia (CIN 2), well as severe dysplasia and carcinoma in situ (which together constitute CIN 3).

Atypical Squamous Cells

In the Bethesda System, the use of word "atypia" is discouraged unless specifically defined. In the past, the word "atypia" was used to describe everything from completely benign to frankly malignant cells. Moreover, "atypia," according to the dictionary, also means "abnormal" and therefore, medicolegally, could be construed as *requiring* significant medical intervention. Changes that are purely reactive in nature should not be classified as "atypical." For example, use of the terms "radiation atypia" or "inflammatory atypia" is discouraged; they should be replaced with radiation effect or inflammatory change, or the like.

In TBS 1991, atypical squamous cells were reported as "atypical squamous cells of undetermined significance" or "ASCUS" as it became widely known. The term, ASCUS, was defined as "cellular abnormalities that are more marked than those attributable to reactive changes, but that quantitatively or qualitatively fell short of a definitive diagnosis of 'squamous intraepithelial lesion.'" In TBS 1991, ASCUS could be further subclassified as "favor reactive" or "favor SIL." In practice, ASCUS was usually used unqualified. ASCUS became far and away the most common cytologic interpretation on Pap tests, at least 2 to 3 *times* the number of SILs detected.

In TBS 2001, the "favor reactive" and "favor SIL" subcategories were dropped. In fact, there was discussion about dropping ASCUS altogether. Some felt that ASCUS was too subjective, irreproducible, and over-utilized; that it had become a wastebasket diagnosis; and furthermore, created anxiety for women and management problems for clinicians, not to mention the cost to the health care system. However, this equivocal category was maintained because: experience with eliminating ASCUS was limited to only a few cytology laboratories; there might be an increase in reporting of L SIL with a decrease in reporting of H SIL; there is a 10% to 20% risk an underlying H SIL, and 1 in 1000 risk of cancer in cases interpreted as ASCUS [Solomon 2001, 2002]. Furthermore, there is a limit to the ability to make a definitive microscopic interpretation [MR Henry 2003]. Finally, eliminating this category was judged imprudent owing to the high expectations for very sensitive cytological screening in the United States [MR Henry 2003, Solomon 2002].

In TBS 2001 the basic category was changed to Atypical Squamous Cells (ASC), but two subcategories are defined: ASC-undetermined significance (ASC-US) and ASC-cannot exclude high-grade squamous intraepithelial lesion (ASC-H). For cellular alterations that are less than diagnostic of a squamous intraepithelial lesion, but thought to be noninflammatory in nature (eg, squamous atypia or minimal dysplasia, see pg 59), the terminology of "atypical squamous cells-undetermined significance" (ASC-US) can be used (note that hyphen). This terminology can also be used for other squamous cell changes that are less than diagnostic or of uncertain nature, in each case qualifying as best as possible the nature of the change, to aid the clinician in proper management. An interpretation of ASC-US carries a significant risk of an underlying H SIL. Because the number of ASC cases is so high, it is the most common interpretation preceding a biopsy diagnosis of H SIL.

The new category, ASC-H, reflects a mixture of true H SIL and its mimics [Solomon 2002]. Like ASC-US, this designation is also irreproducible among cytologists, but studies suggest that ASC-H has a predictive value for CIN 2 or CIN 3 that is intermediate between ASC-US and H SIL [Solomon 2002]. Roughly 50% of women (range 25% to 75%) with ASC-H on Pap test have H SIL on biopsy (compared with about 10%-20% for ASC-US).

Hyperkeratosis and parakeratosis are not included in the category of ASC, although atypical parakeratosis or dyskeratocytes may be categorized as ASC or squamous intraepithelial lesion, depending on the degree of nuclear abnormality [NCI 1993a,b]. A diagnosis of ASC is expected for about 5% of women in most populations. However, in high-risk populations, with a high prevalence of squamous intraepithelial lesions, there will be a correspondingly higher prevalence of ASC (generally about 2 to 3 times the rate of squamous intraepithelial lesions) [Kurman 1994].

Squamous Intraepithelial Lesions

In 1988, the Bethesda System introduced a two-tiered terminology for precursor lesions, low-grade and high-grade squamous intraepithelial lesions. This has remained unchanged in TBS 2001. This dichotomous division of SIL reflects the current belief that L SIL is usually a transient HPV infection, while H SIL is more often associated with persistence or progression of the lesion [Einstein 2001, Ho 1998a, T Park 1996, T Wright 1994b, zur Hausen 2000]. The ALTS trial data indicate that distinguishing L SIL from H SIL is fairly well reproducible, that distinguishing CIN 2 from CIN 3 is not very reproducible, and that distinguishing HPV cytopathic effect ("koilocytosis") from CIN 1 is not reproducible [Solomon 2002]. Nevertheless, the three-tiered system (CIN 1, 2, 3)

may be helpful in managing some women; in correlating cytology and histology findings; and is preferred in many countries outside the United States. Perhaps underappreciated, however, is that the CIN or dysplasia/carcinoma in situ terminology can be used in addition to, *or instead of,* the SIL terminology in TBS [Solomon 2002]. Still, most American cytology laboratories use the SIL terminology, with or without further description.

One new addition to the SIL category is "High-grade squamous intraepithelial lesion with features suspicious for invasion." This interpretation, or one similar to it, has been in wide use for many years, but did not have a specific entry in TBS lexicon.

Squamous Cell Carcinoma

For the purposes of the Bethesda System, squamous cell carcinoma can be used without further qualification. However, at the discretion of the cytologist, this category can be further specified, eg, nonkeratinizing, keratinizing, or small cell squamous carcinoma.

Glandular Cell Abnormalities

Glandular cell abnormalities also encompass a spectrum of lesions, ranging from atypical glandular cells to invasive adenocarcinoma. In cases of adenocarcinoma, an attempt can be made to classify by site. Although the Bethesda System now reports, "benign appearing endometrial cells in women 40 or older," regardless of menstrual status or hormonal therapy, this is no longer considered a glandular cell abnormality. This category has also been controversial, and may change, since many women in their 40s have not entered menopause, and cyclic endometrial shedding would be normal for them. However, the presence of spontaneously exfoliated endometrial cells *out-of-cycle* may be significant, particularly after 40 years of age, though this is not the current usage in TBS 2001. Of course, *atypical* endometrial cells are always abnormal, regardless of age or menstrual status, and are reported as a glandular cell abnormality.

In TBS 1991, atypical glandular cells of undetermined significance (AGUS) could be subdivided into AGUS, Endocervical Origin; AGUS, Endometrial Origin, or AGUS, not otherwise specified. Except for AGUS, endometrial origin, the other two AGUS categories could be further subdivided into "favor reactive" or "favor neoplastic." Endocervical adenocarcinoma in situ (AIS) would have been placed into the "AGUS, endocervical origin, favor neoplastic" group.

In TBS 2001, the terminology of atypical glandular cells of uncertain significance (AGUS) was deleted, to avoid confusion with ASC-US. TBS 2001 now uses the term "atypical glandular cells" (AGC). ("AGUS" had a nice ring to it when spoken [ay-gus]; try to say "AGC" and it sounds like a cat coughing up a fur ball.) Glandular abnormalities can be subdivided into "atypical endocervical cells," "atypical endometrial cells," or simply, "atypical glandular cells." Atypical endocervical cells or atypical glandular cells can be used either without further specification or with the term, "favor neoplastic." However, the qualifier, "favor reactive," was dropped because it could lead to a false sense of security in women who actually have underlying high-grade squamous or glandular lesions [R Cheng 1999, Chhieng 2003, MR Henry 2003, K Lee 1995]. "Atypical endometrial cells" is not further divided. An effort should be made to distinguish atypical endocervical cells from atypical endometrial cells, because the clinical follow-up is different, but this is not always possible. TBS 2001 also allows the term "atypical epithelial cells" when it cannot be determined whether the atypical cells are glandular or squamous in origin [Solomon 2002].

TBS 2001 now includes the term, "cervical adenocarcinoma in situ" because studies have indicated favorable positive predictive value and reproducibility for this interpretation [Betsill 1986, Biscotti 1997, K Lee 1991]. The category, "atypical endocervical cells, favor neoplastic" remains in TBS 2001, and is perhaps a more realistic interpretation than a cytologic designation of *in situ* adenocarcinoma (AIS). Cytology cannot exclude invasion since the morphologic features of AIS and well-differentiated invasive adenocarcinoma are similar. Because endocervical glandular dysplasia is controversial, no separate category was included for this interpretation [Farnsworth 1989, MR Henry 2003].

The finding of AGC is important because the percentage of cases associated with underlying high-grade lesions is generally higher than for ASC-US. High-grade squamous or glandular lesions are found in ~10% to 40% of cases on follow-up (see pg 145). Unfortunately, the AGC interpretation is poorly reproducible and potentially includes "atypical" glandular cells from diverse entities, such as polyps, IUDs, endometriosis, cone biopsy artifact, tubal metaplasia, reactive changes, microglandular hyperplasia, pregnancy changes, SIL involving glands, glandular dysplasia and adenocarcinoma in situ, endometrial hyperplasia, and various cancers that do not look fully malignant. AGC is not a rare interpretation, and although there is a high rate of underlying abnormalities, it performs poorly in specifically identifying adenocarcinoma. Most of the significant lesions identified are squamous, not glandular. Furthermore, invasive cervical adenocarcinoma sometimes have *less* marked cytologic abnormalities than glandular precursor lesions owing to smaller size, endocervical origin, deep location of the lesion, and unpredictable shedding of cells. It is worthwhile noting again that, to date, the Pap test has not reduced the incidence of adenocarcinoma.

Other Malignant Neoplasms

Other malignant neoplasms have a separate category in recognition of the fact that not all lesions are epithelial in origin. If possible, indicate the specific type of tumor.

Educational Notes, Suggestions

An optional section for recommendations, comments, and educational notes is provided in TBS 2001. These are the responsibility of the pathologist and should be directed to the health care provider who requested the test. Communicating results directly to the woman should be avoided, unless specifically requested by the provider. Suggestions should be concise and consistent with follow-up guidelines published by professional organizations. References to relevant publications may be included.

Suggestions or recommendations are generally provided only as a guide to further *diagnostic*, as opposed to *therapeutic*, management of the woman, and generally include a phrase such as "if clinically indicated". Notes can also be used to clarify ambiguous findings, improve specimen quality, etc [MR Henry 2003]. In addition, notes can be used to educate the provider about the limited accuracy of the Pap test and the availability of more sensitive tests, such as HPV-DNA tests.

Be aware that making specific recommendations may essentially force clinicians to do procedures that are not actually indicated or go to great lengths to document why they were not performed, due to the possible medicolegal consequences of not following recommendations. However, many health care providers, particularly nongynecologists, appreciate having specific recommendations for further evaluation. Furthermore, including suggestions for further evaluation increases the likelihood that appropriate follow-up actually occurs [Austin 2000, B Jones 2000]. Management guidelines for women with abnormal cytology results, based on TBS 2001, have been developed at a consensus conference sponsored by the American Society for Colposcopy and Cervical Pathology (see pg 244) [T Wright 2002a].

An educational note for a negative cervical cytology report has suggested by a task force of the Papanicolaou Society of Cytopathology [Anonymous 2003a].

Cervical cytology is a screening test with limited sensitivity [Fahey 1995, Franco 2000, Giard 2001, Hartman 2001, ML Hutchinson 1999, Martin–Hirsch 2002, McCrory 1999, Nanda 2000, Renshaw 2002b]. Regular screening is critical for cancer prevention [Janerich 1995]. Pap tests are primarily effective for the detection/prevention of squamous cell carcinoma, not adenocarcinoma or other cancers [H Smith 2000, H Mitchell 1995a].

Report Format

TBS does not prescribe a specific report format or the order in which information is presented. However, it is recommended that the "Interpretation/Results" field be highlighted for easy identification. The most clinically significant findings should be listed first if several findings are included in the report. Acronyms, eg, ASC-H, should not be used as stand-alone interpretations.

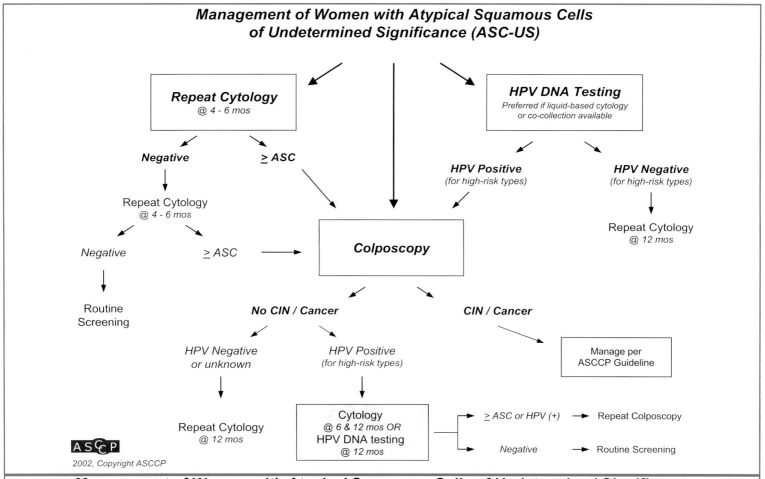

Management of Women with Atypical Squamous Cells of Undetermined Significance (ASC-US)

Repeat Cytology
@ 4 - 6 mos

HPV DNA Testing
Preferred if liquid-based cytology or co-collection available

Negative   *≥ ASC*

HPV Positive
(for high-risk types)

HPV Negative
(for high-risk types)

Repeat Cytology
@ 4 - 6 mos

Repeat Cytology
@ 12 mos

Negative   ≥ ASC   **Colposcopy**

Routine Screening

No CIN / Cancer   *CIN / Cancer*

HPV Negative or unknown   *HPV Positive (for high-risk types)*

Manage per ASCCP Guideline

Repeat Cytology
@ 12 mos

Cytology
@ 6 & 12 mos OR
HPV DNA testing
@ 12 mos

≥ ASC or HPV (+) → Repeat Colposcopy

Negative → Routine Screening

ASCCP
2002, Copyright ASCCP

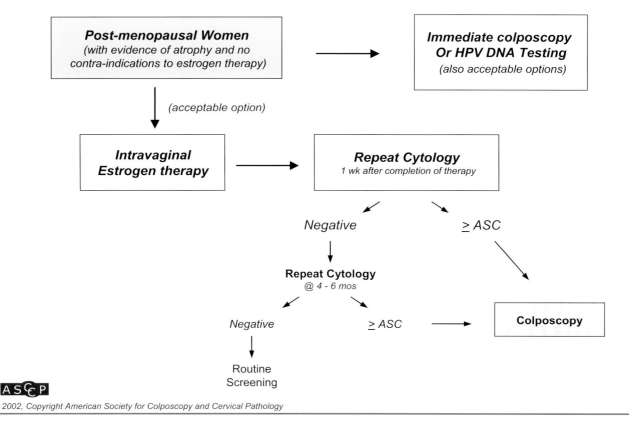

Management of Women with Atypical Squamous Cells of Undetermined Significance (ASC-US) In Special Circumstances

Post-menopausal Women
(with evidence of atrophy and no contra-indications to estrogen therapy)

**Immediate colposcopy
Or HPV DNA Testing**
(also acceptable options)

(acceptable option)

**Intravaginal
Estrogen therapy**

Repeat Cytology
1 wk after completion of therapy

Negative   *≥ ASC*

Repeat Cytology
@ 4 - 6 mos

Negative   *≥ ASC* → **Colposcopy**

Routine Screening

ASCCP
2002, Copyright American Society for Colposcopy and Cervical Pathology

Management of Women with Atypical Squamous Cells: Cannot Exclude High-grade SIL (ASC - H)

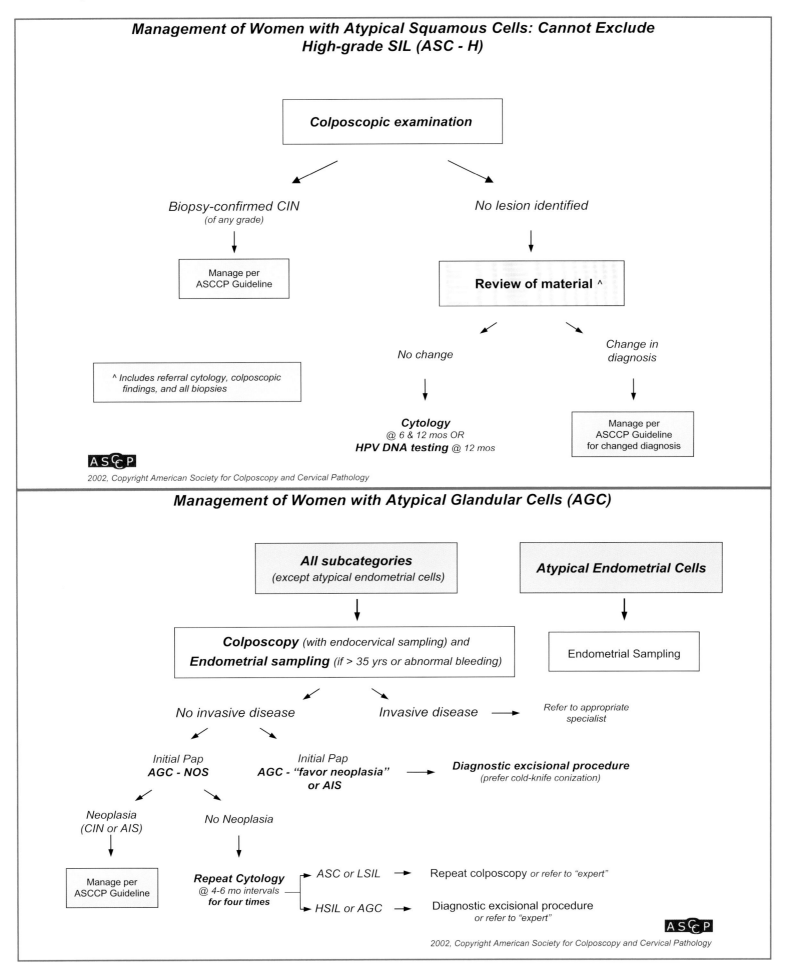

Colposcopic examination

Biopsy-confirmed CIN
(of any grade)

No lesion identified

Manage per
ASCCP Guideline

Review of material ^

^ *Includes referral cytology, colposcopic findings, and all biopsies*

No change

Change in diagnosis

Cytology
@ 6 & 12 mos OR
HPV DNA testing @ 12 mos

Manage per
ASCCP Guideline
for changed diagnosis

Management of Women with Atypical Glandular Cells (AGC)

All subcategories
(except atypical endometrial cells)

Atypical Endometrial Cells

Colposcopy *(with endocervical sampling)* and
Endometrial sampling *(if > 35 yrs or abnormal bleeding)*

Endometrial Sampling

No invasive disease

Invasive disease → Refer to appropriate specialist

Initial Pap
AGC - NOS

Initial Pap
**AGC - "favor neoplasia"
or AIS** → **Diagnostic excisional procedure**
(prefer cold-knife conization)

Neoplasia
(CIN or AIS)

No Neoplasia

Manage per
ASCCP Guideline

Repeat Cytology
@ 4-6 mo intervals
for four times

→ ASC or LSIL → Repeat colposcopy *or refer to "expert"*

→ HSIL or AGC → Diagnostic excisional procedure
or refer to "expert"

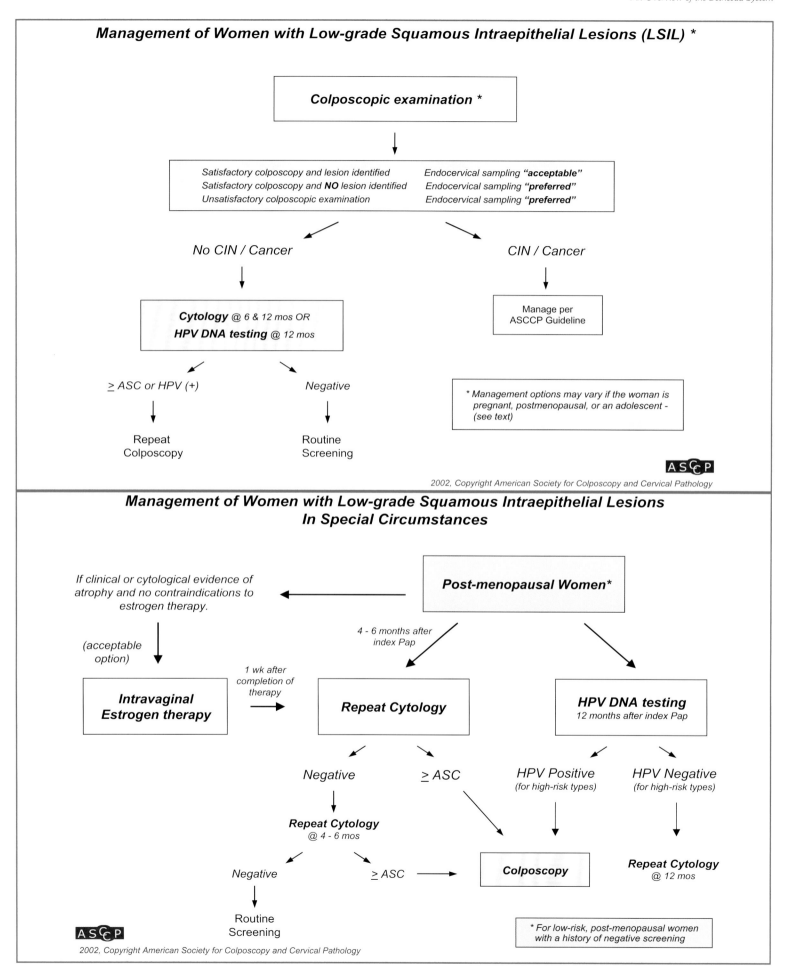

Management of Women with Low-grade Squamous Intraepithelial Lesions (LSIL) *

Colposcopic examination *

Satisfactory colposcopy and lesion identified	*Endocervical sampling "acceptable"*
Satisfactory colposcopy and NO lesion identified	*Endocervical sampling "preferred"*
Unsatisfactory colposcopic examination	*Endocervical sampling "preferred"*

No CIN / Cancer

CIN / Cancer

Cytology *@ 6 & 12 mos OR*
HPV DNA testing *@ 12 mos*

Manage per
ASCCP Guideline

≥ ASC or HPV (+)

Negative

Repeat
Colposcopy

Routine
Screening

* Management options may vary if the woman is pregnant, postmenopausal, or an adolescent - (see text)

A S C C P

2002, Copyright American Society for Colposcopy and Cervical Pathology

Management of Women with Low-grade Squamous Intraepithelial Lesions In Special Circumstances

If clinical or cytological evidence of atrophy and no contraindications to estrogen therapy.

Post-menopausal Women*

(acceptable option)

4 - 6 months after index Pap

Intravaginal Estrogen therapy

1 wk after completion of therapy

Repeat Cytology

HPV DNA testing
12 months after index Pap

Negative

≥ ASC

HPV Positive (for high-risk types)

HPV Negative (for high-risk types)

Repeat Cytology
@ 4 - 6 mos

Negative

≥ ASC

Colposcopy

Repeat Cytology
@ 12 mos

Routine
Screening

A S C C P

* For low-risk, post-menopausal women with a history of negative screening

2002, Copyright American Society for Colposcopy and Cervical Pathology

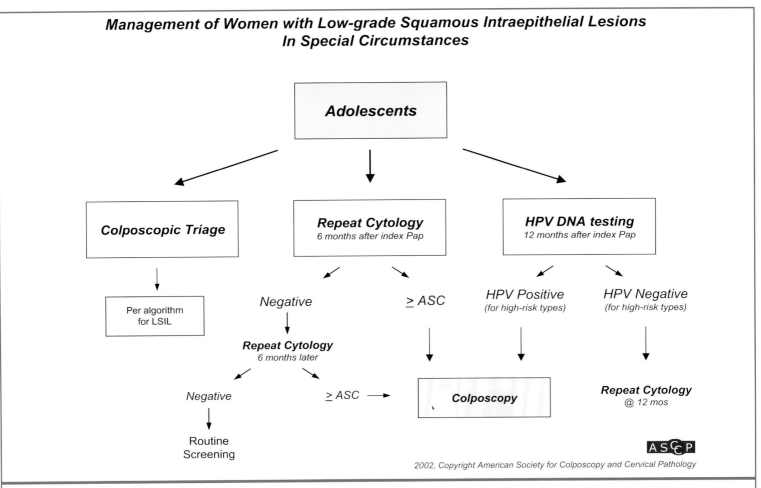

Management of Women with Low-grade Squamous Intraepithelial Lesions In Special Circumstances

Adolescents

- **Colposcopic Triage**
  - Per algorithm for LSIL

- **Repeat Cytology**
  6 months after index Pap
  - *Negative*
    - **Repeat Cytology** *6 months later*
      - *Negative*
        - Routine Screening
      - *≥ ASC* → **Colposcopy**
  - *≥ ASC* → **Colposcopy**

- **HPV DNA testing**
  12 months after index Pap
  - *HPV Positive* *(for high-risk types)* → **Colposcopy**
  - *HPV Negative* *(for high-risk types)* → **Repeat Cytology** *@ 12 mos*

A S C C P

2002, Copyright American Society for Colposcopy and Cervical Pathology

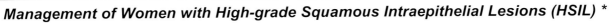

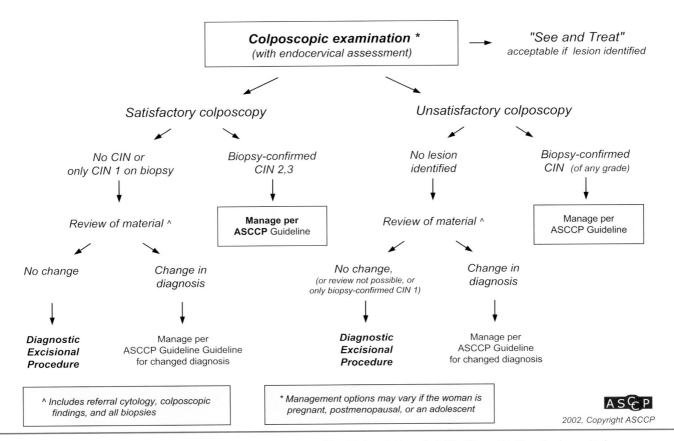

Management of Women with High-grade Squamous Intraepithelial Lesions (HSIL) *

Colposcopic examination * *(with endocervical assessment)* → *"See and Treat"* *acceptable if lesion identified*

Satisfactory colposcopy
- *No CIN or only CIN 1 on biopsy*
  - *Review of material ^*
    - *No change* → ***Diagnostic Excisional Procedure***
    - *Change in diagnosis* → Manage per ASCCP Guideline Guideline for changed diagnosis
- *Biopsy-confirmed CIN 2,3*
  - **Manage per ASCCP** Guideline

Unsatisfactory colposcopy
- *No lesion identified*
  - *Review of material ^*
    - *No change,* *(or review not possible, or only biopsy-confirmed CIN 1)* → ***Diagnostic Excisional Procedure***
    - *Change in diagnosis* → Manage per ASCCP Guideline for changed diagnosis
- *Biopsy-confirmed CIN* *(of any grade)*
  - Manage per ASCCP Guideline

^ Includes referral cytology, colposcopic findings, and all biopsies

* Management options may vary if the woman is pregnant, postmenopausal, or an adolescent

A S C C P

2002, Copyright ASCCP

X. Lessons from Litigation

by R Marshall Austin, MD, PhD and E Blair Holladay, PhD

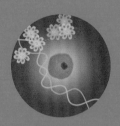

here are many difficult challenges in comparing Papanicolaou (Pap) test screening accuracy among laboratories and assessing adherence to "the standard of practice." Despite the remarkable effectiveness of the Pap test in reducing cervical carcinoma by >70%, public expectations of 100% effectiveness have never been achieved [Devesa 1989, Koss 1989a]. Consequently, there is a gap between the capability of the Pap test to prevent cancer and the expectations of the public. The unrealistically high expectations of the public are reflected in the legal system.

A trial lawyer's newsletter opined that a claim for medical malpractice against some health care provider almost certainly exists in any case in which a woman develops cervical carcinoma and undergoes a hysterectomy or dies, unless the woman utterly failed to obtain even periodic Pap tests [Perey 1997]. The expectation expressed here is that the Pap test is essentially a cervical cancer insurance policy that will pay a substantial monetary award to any woman who ever had a Pap test and develops cervical cancer. Unfortunately, expert witnesses have compounded the problem by giving testimony based on biased review of Pap test slides studied with knowledge of patient outcome [Holladay 2003]. Lay juries must ultimately assess adherence to "the standard of practice," based on such testimony. Yet, the scientific evidence clearly indicates that the Pap test has significant limits for effectiveness.

With these issues in mind, this chapter will focus on insights from Pap test litigation in the hope of further reducing the risk of similar problems occurring in the future. The emphasis will be on clinically significant lesions repeatedly seen in Pap litigation case material, most often in forms that are difficult to detect or interpret, eg, non-classic manifestations of high-grade lesions (H SIL & AIS) and cancer (especially, adenocarcinoma). In addition, an unbiased adjudication system of "blinded" review of slides will be presented as a more appropriate method than biased retrospective review as an objective basis for any assertion that an original Pap test interpretation was "below the standard of practice." Thus far, roughly 150 litigated cases have passed through this system of analysis.

How to Minimize the Laboratory's Risk for Failing to Identify Cancer

Litigation cases alleging interpretive or screening errors involving L SIL are rare to nonexistent. Also rare are cases with cytologic evidence of widespread classic H SIL.

1. L SIL: "The Dog That Didn't Bark"

Missed L SIL cases have been strikingly absent in retrospective reviews of litigated Pap slides [I10.1]. This is consistent with our current understanding that L SIL is generally non-progressive or slowly progressive. Moreover, "state of Texas" sized cells of CIN 1 or HPV effect are usually readily detected. Although detection of L SIL is still important as approximately 20% of women with L SIL reported on Pap tests actually harbor H SIL when biopsied. Still, L SIL is rarely associated with cervical cancer within the 5-year period of federally mandated Pap slide retention. As in a mystery novel where something that did not happen may be the most significant clue ("the dog that didn't bark"), absence of missed L SIL cases in litigation reflects the dominant clinical significance of failure to detect cases of high-grade intraepithelial lesions (H SIL, AIS) and invasive cancer.

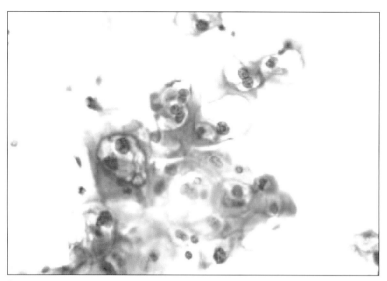

I10.1
L SIL: CIN1, HPV effect [C]

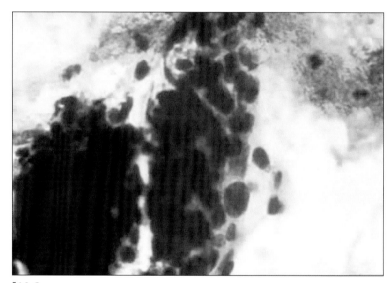

I10.2
Hyperchromatic crowded group [C]

2. Overlooked or Difficult to Interpret Manifestations of High-Grade Intraepithelial Lesions, Especially Carcinoma In Situ and Adenocarcinoma In Situ

Difficult-to-interpret variations of H SIL (particularly, carcinoma in situ) and adenocarcinoma in situ (AIS) are the most commonly missed abnormalities detected in retrospective slide reviews of litigated cases. Many cases present as **hyperchromatic crowded groups** (HCGs) of cells that can be very difficult to interpret ([I10.2], see also pg 182). Careful high-power review of such overlapping cell groups is often essential to detect occasional abnormal nuclei and to distinguish these clusters from menstrual endometrial shedding. In some cases, it may be difficult or impossible even to determine whether HCGs represent squamous or glandular lesions, only that a high-grade lesion is in the differential. AIS, for example, often lacks classic features of "feathering" or rosette formation [I10.3]. In cases for which a definitive interpretation cannot be made, cytologic reporting may be of "atypical squamous cells, cannot exclude a high-grade lesion" (ASC-H); "atypical immature

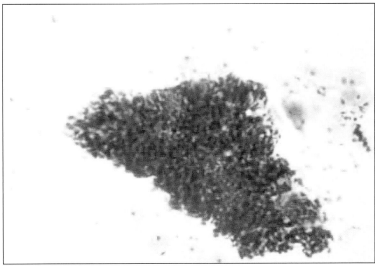

I10.3
HCG: Adenocacinoma in situ [C]

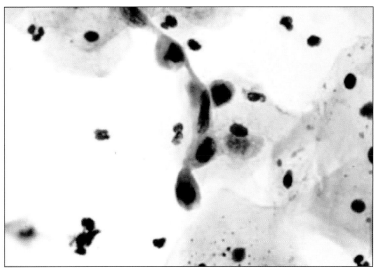

I10.5
Nondiagnostic findings [C]

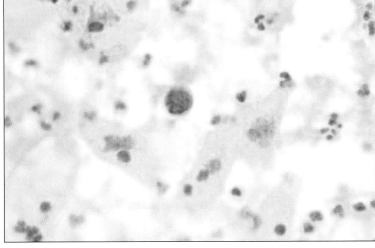

I10.4
Rare small, bland cell [C]

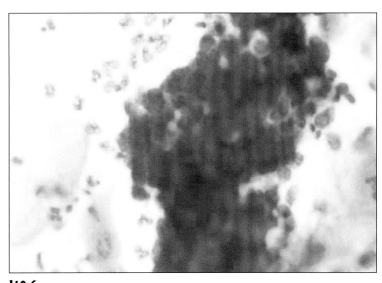

I10.6
HCG: Endometrial cells vs small cell carcinoma [C]

transformation zone cells, cannot rule out a high-grade intraepithelial lesion"; or "atypical squamous cells, cannot exclude a high-grade glandular intraepithelial lesion." Any such report should be formulated to encourage or suggest an appropriately aggressive diagnostic evaluation (colposcopy, cervical biopsy, endocervical sampling, and (for glandular abnormalities in women over 35) endometrial sampling [see pg 244ff]).

Also common among litigated Pap cases are slides with only a few H SIL cells [I10.4]. This field shows only around a dozen H SIL cells overlooked on a conventional Pap smear of a middle-aged woman 4 years before she presented with cervical cancer. These cells may be small and bland and easily overlooked in routine screening. Conventional pap smears with fewer than 50 H SIL cells have been estimated to be 25 times more likely to be read as false negatives than H SIL smears with over 50 cells. Hypocellular H SIL cases are also more likely to be overlooked than more cellular H SIL cases on manually screened liquid-based cytology preparations. Also common on Pap litigation reviews are nondiagnostic manifestations of H SIL (ASC-H) [I10.5].

This field shows an isolated group of atypical immature metaplastic squamous cells probably reflecting a nondiagnostic manifestation of H SIL in a "negative" conventional Pap smear obtained a year before another Pap smear reported as H SIL (CIS) and a follow-up cervical biopsy revealing microinvasive squamous carcinoma.

3. Difficult to Interpret or Overlooked Manifestations of Carcinoma

Other frequently encountered patterns of misinterpreted or overlooked abnormality in litigated Pap tests are those that, when viewed retrospectively, may be realized to have been manifestations of invasive cancer. Several examples are illustrated. The first example is of hyperchromatic crowded cell groups thought to represent endometrial cells in a woman later documented to have a rare small cell neuroendocrine carcinoma [I10.6]. Only careful, time-consuming, high-power, up-and-down focusing on such crowded groups may

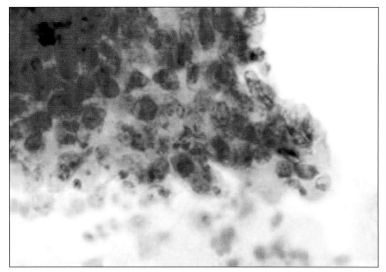

110.7
Atypical repair vs invasive cancer [C]

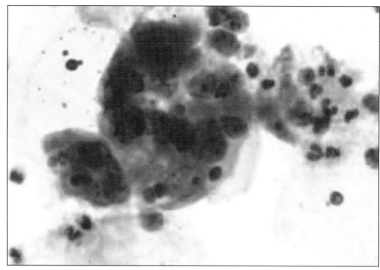

110.9
Atypical repair vs invasive cancer [L]

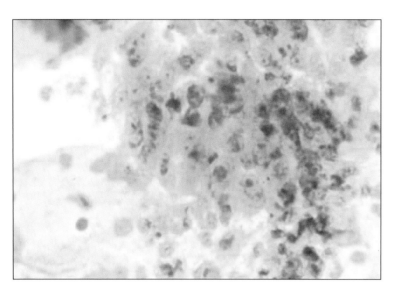

110.8
Atypical repair vs invasive cancer [C]

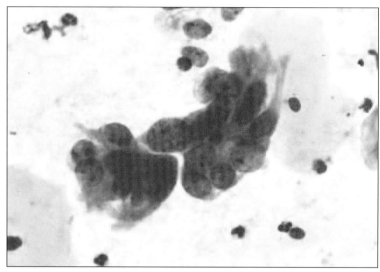

110.10
Atypical repair vs invasive cancer [L]

detect suspicious nuclear features. Invasive cancer cases misinterpreted as atypical repair in conventional Pap smears [110.7,10.8], or liquid-based cytology [110.9] are a well-recognized subgroup in litigated cervical cancer cases. Because of the well-documented difficulty in distinguishing all cases of atypical repair from cancer, our practice has been to recommend colposcopic and cervical biopsy evaluations on Pap test reports of "atypical repair." Such cases are reported as ASC-H along with the admonition that "neoplasia must be considered in the differential. Recommend colposcopically directed diagnostic tissue studies." Conventional Pap smears misinterpreted on successive occasions at atypical repair in [110.7,10.8] preceded clinical diagnosis of advanced and ultimately fatal cervical squamous carcinoma. Liquid-based cytology shows a rare cell group interpreted as atypical repair in a young woman who several years later presented with clinically diagnosed cervical squamous carcinoma [110.9]. In our opinion extreme caution and strong follow-up recommendations in such cases can minimize the likelihood of a tragic outcome [110.10] .

4. Endocervical Lesions

Nowhere is the gap between what is expected and what is achievable wider than in the interpretation of endocervical glandular neoplasia. Although cervical adenocarcinoma still represents a minority (25%-33%) of cervical cancers [Janerich 1995, HO Smith 2000], endocervical glandular lesions represent up to 80% of litigated Pap test cases [Cox 1998b]. Yet, the Pap test has never been proven effective in lowering the incidence or mortality of adenocarcinoma [Bergstrom 1999, Brinton 1987b, H Mitchell 1995a]. Liquid-based Pap tests [Bai 2000] and HPV testing [Hildesheim 1999, Ronnett 1999] may offer hope for the future.

Questions to Bear in Mind When Analyzing Equivocal Cells
• Could this be a difficult-to-recognize form of H SIL or AIS?
• Could this be a difficult-to-recognize form of invasive cancer?

This is the proper "mind set" when evaluating Pap tests, because these are the clinically significant lesions that when missed, or misinterpreted, may well cause harm.

Reporting and Risk Management

The Bethesda System (2001) is recommended for reporting Pap tests. Particular attention is suggested for those lesions that are more likely to progress to cancer, or those for which the sensitivity of cytology could be improved, either through DNA testing or appropriate follow-up management recommendations. Reporting the level of risk associated with the laboratory's final interpretation is an excellent way to communicate to the clinician the most appropriate follow-up for the Pap test result. Making follow-up management recommendations is not only helpful, but also makes it more likely that appropriate follow-up will actually occur [B Jones 2000].

Recommendations are particularly important with endocervical glandular lesions (AGC, adenocarcinoma in situ, adenocarcinoma) due to the often more rapid progression of these lesions and their frequently equivocal cytomorphology. Unfortunately, clinicians have often underestimated the importance of AGC and offered follow up similar to that for ASC-US. Current management recommendations suggest that all atypical glandular interpretations should be followed up with colposcopy, endocervical sampling,, and endometrial sampling in women over 35 (see pg 244ff) [T Wright 2002a].

An educational note may be included on the report. This statement may reference the sensitivity of the Pap test, communicate the limitations of negative Pap test reports, stress that the test is a screening procedure rather than diagnostic test, and focus on follow up recommendations for abnormal results, reflecting consensus guidelines. Some may want to add a statement such as "100% sensitivity in the detection of clinically significant lesions can be approached by adding HPV-DNA testing (FDA approved from residual ThinPrep® vial fluid up to 3 weeks after collection) as a co-test to the ThinPrep® Pap test [Belinson 2001]." Although there should be no expectation that such statements "disclaim" or reduce the laboratory's legal risk, they can help to remind and educate the clinician as to realistic expectations from the Pap test and provide information on the availability of advanced testing options.

Any tool that facilitates better communication is not only helpful to the clinician, but also to the woman. Always put the woman first, and that in turn will reduce the risk for the laboratory and the clinician. Communication is a two-way street, however. Clinicians also need to provide relevant clinical information to assist optimal Pap test interpretation. In our laboratory, whenever clinical findings of suspicious signs or symptoms such as post-coital bleeding or any lesion are noted by the clinician, an additional comment is made. "The Pap test is a screening test, not a diagnostic test. Suspicious signs or symptoms may warrant follow-up diagnostic studies regardless of Pap test findings."

Theories of Standard of Practice

Pap Test Adjudication

- Zero error standard = public
- Biased expert standard = problem of biased retrospective review by experts with financial incentives
- Multiple slide blinded rescreening standard [F10.1,10.2]

Multiple Slide Blinded Rescreening (Overview)

- Simulates prospective screening

F10.1 Biased Expert Standard

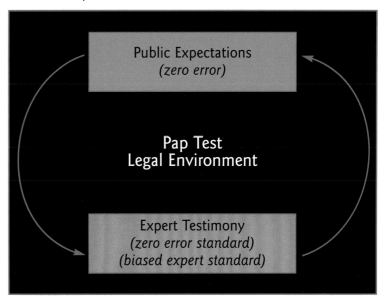

F10.2 Blinded Screening Standard

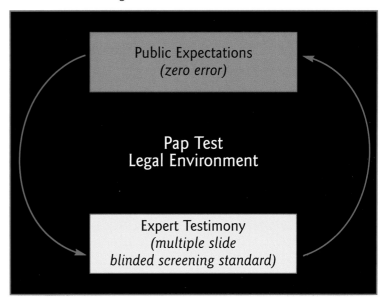

F10.3 Blinded Rescreening Overview

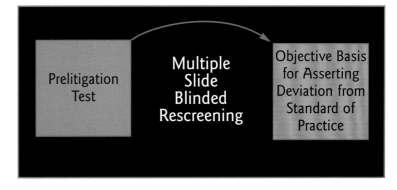

- 50-60 slides are read in one 8-hour period
- 10 cytotechnologists are used
- Standard: slides are evaluated "regularly and reliably" by reasonably prudent practitioners as "significantly abnormal" [F10.3]

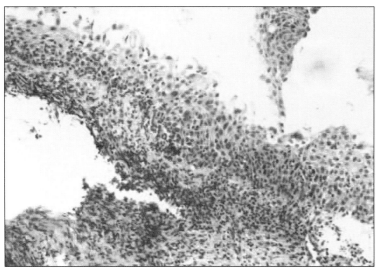

I10.11
Case I [C]

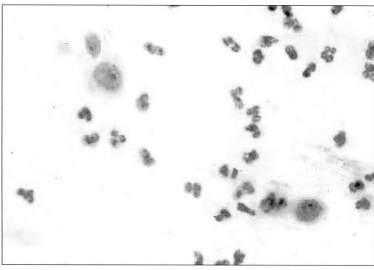

I10.13
Expert: "ASC-US-border on mild dysplasia"

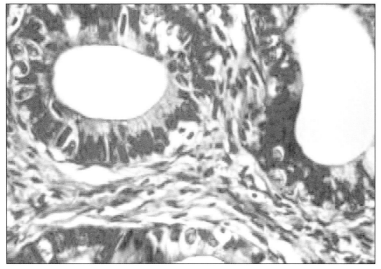

I10.12
Case I [C]

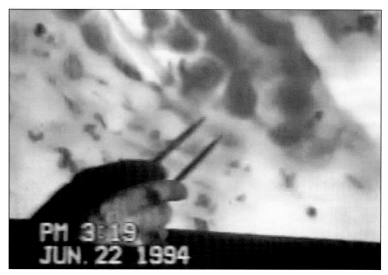

I10.14
Expert: "Atypical, significance unknown"

Adjudication of Litigated Cases

Case One [I10.11-12]

Original laboratory diagnosis: Benign, no significant abnormalities seen.

- Expert Diagnosis I: ASC-US, border on mild dysplasia, failure to correctly diagnose, below the standard of care [I10.13].

- Expert Diagnosis II: ASC-US, immature squamous cells, favor reactive, failure to detect cellular changes, below the standard of care.

- Expert Diagnosis III: Atypical, significance unknown, failure to correctly diagnose, below the standard of care [I10.14].

Multiple Slide Blinded Rescreening (MSBR)

Philosophy

Multiple slide blinded rescreening (MSBR) is a method that provides an unbiased and objective assessment of how a specific Pap slide(s) would be interpreted in an actual screening environment. Whereas retrospective analysis of litigation slides by experts is prone to the effects of outcome and context bias, MSBR is an objective, unbiased and impartial method that is fair to both the patient and the health care provider. To date, it is the only unbiased basis for asserting that the specific reading of a slide was "below the standard of practice." MSBR indicates what could reasonably be expected of a well-trained competent and prudent practitioner under similar circumstances. Blinded rescreening results indicate below standard performance when the slides in question are regularly read as significantly more abnormal than the original interpretation. MSBR has been endorsed by key national organizations associated with cytopathology (ASC, ASCP, CAP, and ASCT) and by the overwhelming majority of state and local pathology and cytology societies [R Austin 1997, Frable 1998].

Goal of MSBR

The environment for the blinded review should be similar to that at the time the case in question was initially screened. Adjudication must be provided by peers who routinely perform the function of "screening" or "interpretation". If a mistake was allegedly made by a cytotechnologist, the blinded review panel should consist solely of cytotechnologists, ie, practitioners who routinely perform this job function. Similarly, should the alleged mistake be made by a pathologist, the peer review should be performed by pathologists in a blinded setting.

In our experience, the majority of allegations are based on cytotechnologist "error" resulting in false-negative interpretations [T10.1].

T10.1 Types of Allegations Against Cytotechnologists

Allegations against cytotechnologists include:

Abnormality not detected
Abnormality detected, but not forwarded to pathologist
Failure to forward reactive cases to pathologist

Allegations based on pathologist "error" usually involve:

Abnormality significantly undergraded or downgraded to benign
  resulting in lack of appropriate patient management

Methodology

I. Preliminary Preparation
  a. Copy of the original test requisition that was received from the referring clinician
  b. 59 additional slides
    1) reproduce a typical daily workload
    2) necessary to match slide/coverslip specifics
    3) varying slide types (square vs round edges)
    4) varying coverslips (glass, tape)

II. Slide Selection
The goal is to prevent the valuator from "clueing in" and performing enhanced or focused reviewing of any particular slide. One should make an attempt to recreate the laboratory's abnormal rate by randomly inserting known abnormal slides (validation slides). This can be achieved by using a "typical" percentage which would be expected by the cytotechnologist reviewers in their respective laboratories, eg, by randomly inserting between one and four abnormals. This creates a mixture of both normal and abnormal gynecologic cases. In addition, using the validation slides helps to document the CT's performance and document the competence of the reviewers. Validation slides serve as an internal quality control for the blinded study. In any instance where reviewers miss any of the validation slides, their results are not included, and additional CTs must be used in the study. The assumption here is that if the CTs successfully identify the seeded abnormal slides, they would be expected to locate any abnormal cells that might have been on the seeded litigation slides as well.

III. Preparing the Slides for Evaluation
a. Remove Dots
  1) A photocopy (or computer scan) of the litigation slide(s) should be made in the event that there are identifying marks (dots, circles, etc.) on the glass. This documents the original location of dots and notes other attributes peculiar to the slide(s) in question.
  2) Slide Labels: A removable label should be placed on top of the slide label and a second "fixed" label should be placed on the removable label. This prevents the evaluator from seeing the original laboratory label and allows for successful removal of label after study is completed.

IV. Study Methodologies
a. **Methodology I** (slide insertion into laboratory workload and reviewed by 10 cytotechnologists)
  1) Expedited review
  2) More administrative effort
  This method does not work well for litigation slides with air bubbles under the coverslip. Should the slide in question have air bubble(s) under the coverslip (or the coverslip is different from that which the laboratory uses), it may become necessary for the cytopreparatory staff person to prevent any of the cytotechnologists from re-coverslipping the litigation slide (may be considered altering physical evidence) or use Methodology II
b. **Methodology II** (slide insertion into simulated workload and reviewed by 10 cytotechnologists)
  1) Time consuming
  2) Less administrative effort
  3) Must perform consistent QC studies to avoid suspicion. Slides are reviewed as part of other Quality Control work performed in the laboratory by the external personnel.
    a) Limitation: cytotechnologists may be reviewing the slide(s) in somewhat of a "suspicious" fashion with a more "focused" effort. However, the cytotechnologists are prevented from having the opportunity to perform an "enhanced" review because they are evaluating 60 slides in one 8-hour sitting. Moreover, because abnormals and negatives are mixed into the workload, no "alarm" is set off when they identify an abnormality.

V. Diagnostic Forms
CT diagnostic forms are coded such that all identifiers (name, initials, CT#) are not on the diagnostic forms. This protects cytotechnologist anonymity and maintains the "blinded" nature of the study. If the cytotechnologists do not know they are reviewing litigation slides, they cannot be subpoenaed by the opposing council. If they could be subpoenaed, one would have to tell them they are reviewing litigation slides—and few would want to review the slides under such circumstances. Withholding their identity both maintains the blinded nature of the study and allows for future reviews to be conducted.

VI. Statistical Significance
  a. Cumulative Binomial Distribution Function:
    1) Out of ten trials, with each trial having 5% probability of being "positive," the likelihood of $N \leq x$ number of positive events. In this case a "positive" event is defined as an alleged "abnormal slide" being interpreted as normal [T10.2].

T10.2 Cumulative Binomial Distribution Function

X	P(X ≤ x)
0.00	0.5987
1.00	0.9139
2.00	0.988t
3.00	0.9990
4.00	0.9999
5.00	1.0000
6.00	1.0000
7.00	1.0000
8.00	1.0000
9.00	1.0000
10.00	1.0000

2) If an allegedly "abnormal slide" is given to 10 people and 2 or more call it negative, that is a statistically significantly higher proportion than would be expected with an "irreducible" false-negative rate of 5%. Such findings would not support the contention that any reasonable prudent practitioner would have interpreted the slide as abnormal. However, to

show a significant difference from a smaller acceptable false-negative rate, for example, 0.01% (essentially a zero-error rate), the slide would have to be reviewed by approximately 369,000 cytotechnologists.

b. Using Statistical Analysis to Define Appropriate Thresholds [*Renshaw 2004f*]
   1) May need to increase the number of reviews to 15-20, depending upon the ease of interpretation (EOI)
      EOI = 80% for cases that are almost always identified,
      EOI = 40% for cases that are routinely missed
   2) If case was missed twice no further review is required

VII. The Report

An interpretation of ASC-US is by definition an uncertain assessment (ASC-H favor high-grade squamous intraepithelial lesion is a possible exception due to the ASCCP guidelines for following these patients). Interpretations of ASC-US are not emphasized: ASC-US cases are not included in most proficiency testing formats. Guidelines for review of litigation slides emphasize the poor interobserver reproducibility of ASC-US. Below is an example of both a positive [F10.4] and a negative [F10.5] review.

F10.4 Positive Review

Dear Mr. Attorney (1):

The following information serves as the report for the "Multiple Slide Blinded Rescreening Study" for cytology case **P04-12345**. The study was conducted in a manner described in the study protocol previously submitted. Additional information related to this process may be requested if necessary.

Please find the enclosure that represents the diagnostic findings for the blinded review study. The following information represents a summary of these results:

P04-12345

7 Diagnoses
Negative for Squamous Intraepithelial Lesion

2 Diagnoses
Atypical Squamous Cells of Undetermined Significance (ASC-US)

1 Diagnosis
Atypical Glandular Cells of Undetermined Significance (AGUS)

The diagnosis of ASC-US or AGUS would have been sent to a pathologist for review. However, the term ASC-US or AGUS indicates "Undetermined Significance"; therefore, at the time the cytotechnologist located the alleged cells, the individual was unsure as to the degree of their abnormality. The diagnoses of ASC-US or AGUS **may or may not be representative of a definitive significant abnormality**. This philosophy has also been adopted by all of the national cytopathology organizations. Find attached to this report a copy of the *Guidelines for Review of GYN Cytology Samples in the Context of Litigation or Potential Litigation* (note item #2). Because of the poor reproducibility of this diagnosis and the interobserver variability amongst practitioners, any diagnosis of ASC-US or AGUS is not reproducible, and **failure of a cytotechnologist to render this diagnosis is not considered to be below the standard of care**.

Multiple Slide Blinded Rescreening (MSBR) is the only method that provides an unbiased and objective assessment of how a specific Pap slide(s) would be interpreted in a simulated, typical screening environment. Whereas retrospective analysis of litigation slides is prone to the effects of outcome and context bias, MSBR is an objective, unbiased and impartial method that is fair to both the patient and the health care provider. It remains as the only unbiased basis for asserting that the specific reading of a slide (or slides) is "below the standard of practice." It indicates what could reasonably be expected of a well-trained competent and prudent practitioner under similar circumstances. Blinded rescreening results indicate below standard performance only when a slide (or slides) in question is interpreted *regularly and reliably as clinically significantly more abnormal than the original interpretation*.

Multiple Slide Blinded Rescreening has been endorsed by all of the national cytopathology-associated organizations (American Society of Cytopathology, American Society for Clinical Pathology, College of American Pathologists, and American Society for Cytotechnology) and by the overwhelming majority of state and local pathology and cytology societies.

As for case P04-12345, seven of the ten reviewers rendered a diagnosis of Negative for Squamous Intraepithelial Lesion or Unsatisfactory for Evaluation. Two additional reviewers diagnosed the case as ASC-US (for which the patient does not generally receive clinical intervention, ie, colposcopy and biopsy, to determine cervical disease based solely on the Pap interpretation. Please note: HPV testing was not offered at the time this case was originally reviewed). Therefore, the blinded review for this slide was read **regularly and reliably** as negative or clinically significantly the same as negative nine of ten times. The study reveals this slide is **not clinically significantly different** from an original diagnosis of negative. Therefore, the original diagnosis by your client for this slide was **within the standard of care**. This review was statistically validated using the cumulative binomial distribution factor ($p < 0.05$) and the EOI factor.

F10.5 Negative Review

Dear Ms. Attorney (2):

The following information serves as the report for the "Multiple Slide Blinded Rescreening Study" for cytology case **P04-67890**. The study was conducted in a manner described in the study protocol previously submitted. Additional information related to this process may be requested if necessary.

Please find the enclosure that represents the diagnostic findings for the blinded review study. The following information represents a summary of these results:

P04-67890

2 Diagnoses
Atypical Glandular Cells of Undetermined Significance (AGUS)

3 Diagnoses
High-Grade Squamous Intraepithelial Lesion (H SIL)

2 Diagnoses
Adenocarcinoma In Situ (AIS)

3 Diagnoses
Adenocarcinoma (Endocervical Type)

Multiple Slide Blinded Rescreening (MSBR) is the only method that provides an unbiased and objective assessment of how a specific Pap slide(s) would be interpreted in a simulated, typical screening environment.

Whereas retrospective analysis of litigation slides is prone to the effects of outcome and context bias, MSBR is an objective, unbiased and impartial method that is fair to both the patient and the health care provider. It remains as the only unbiased basis for asserting that the specific reading of a slide (or slides) is "below the standard of practice." It indicates what could reasonably be expected of a well-trained competent and prudent practitioner under similar circumstances. Blinded rescreening results indicate below standard performance only when a slide (or slides) in question is interpreted *regularly and reliably as clinically significantly more abnormal than the original interpretation.*

Multiple Slide Blinded Rescreening has been endorsed by all of the national cytopathology-associated organizations (American Society of Cytopathology, American Society for Clinical Pathology, College of American Pathologists, and American Society for Cytotechnology) and by the overwhelming majority of state and local pathology and cytology societies.

As for case P04-67890, eight of the ten reviewers rendered a diagnosis of H SIL, AIS or cancer. Therefore, the blinded review for this slide was read **regularly and reliably** as a significant abnormality. The study reveals this slide is **clinically significantly different** from an original diagnosis of negative. Therefore, the original diagnosis by your client for this slide was **below the standard of care**. This review was statistically validated using the cumulative binomial distribution factor ($p < 0.05$) and the EOI factor.

Multiple Slide Blinded Rescreening (MSBR)

- So called "flag waving" or "egregious" errors alleged by experts are generally not confirmed by blinded review
- The "missed" cells consist of a few scattered cells seen singly or in rare groups [I10.15a]
- The "missed" cells are often immature metaplastic cells [I10.15b]
- Obscuring blood or exudate is a common finding [I10.15b]
- The "missed" cells are often cells which possess marginal histiocytic features [I10.15c]
- The chromatin of the "questionable" cells is often pale, washed out
- The "missed" cells are often air-dried clumps of overlapping cells (HCG's) [I10.15d]
- Most (75%) of the time, the slide(s) are not interpreted consistently as abnormal
- Represent slides that would be "thrown out" under proficiency testing or self-assessment testing due to poor performance

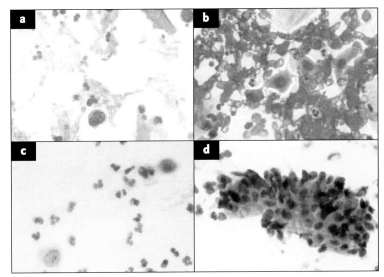

I10.15
a, Few scattered cells [C]; **b**, Immature metaplastic cells [C]; **c**, Histiocyte-like cells [C] **d**, Air-dried HCGs [C]

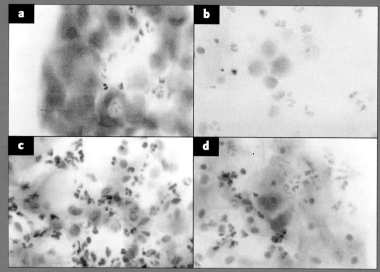

Case 40
- Requested by defense attorney
- Blinded review finding
  8 WNL
  2 ASC-US
- Supported defendant

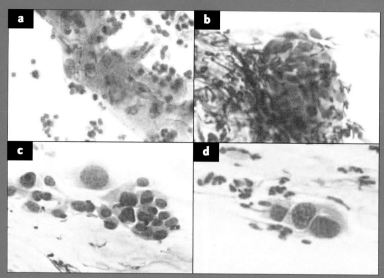

Case 42
- Requested by defense attorney
- Blinded review finding
  I L SIL
  7 H SIL
  2 Carcinoma
- Supported plaintiff

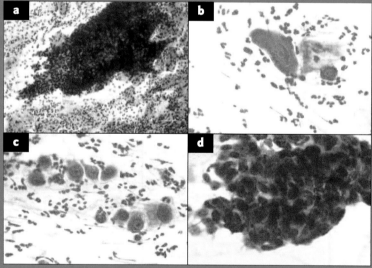

Case 58
- Requested by plaintiff attorney
- Blinded review finding
  7 H SIL
  3 Carcinoma
- Supported plaintiff

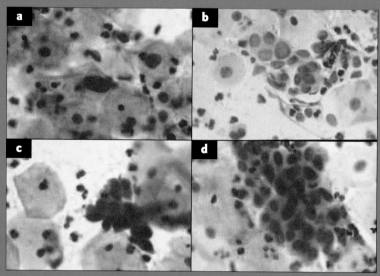

Case 69
- Requested by defense attorney
- Blinded review finding
  5 WNL
  3 BCC with reactive endocervical cells
  2 ASC-US
- Supported defendant

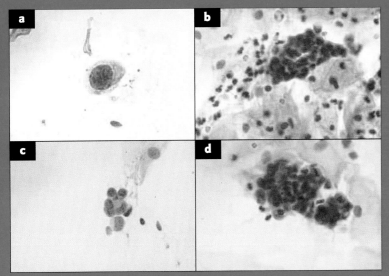

Case 70
- Requested by defense attorney
- Blinded review finding
  10 WNL
- Supported defendant

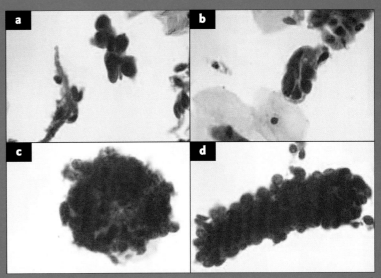

Case 73: TP Case
- Requested by defense attorney
- Blinded review finding
  2 WNL
  3 ASC-US; R/O H SIL
  2 L SIL
  3 H SIL
- Supported plaintiff

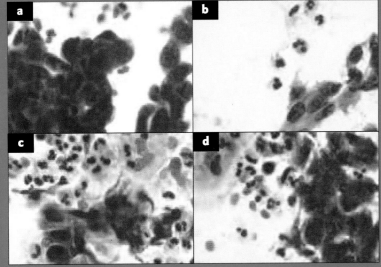

Case 76
- Requested by defense attorney
- Blinded review finding
  2 H SIL
  5 AGUS/AIS
- Supported plaintiff

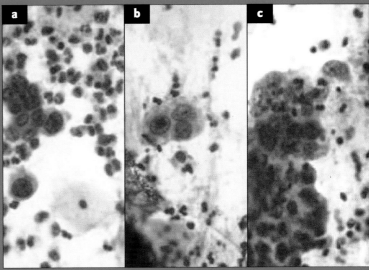

Case 83
- Requested by plaintiff attorney
- Blinded review finding
  I BCC
  I ASC-US
  2 AGUS
  4 H SIL
  I Squamous cell carcinoma
  I Adenocarcinoma
- Supported plaintiff

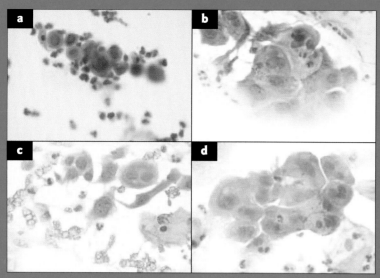

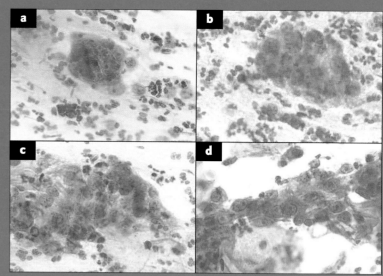

Case 84
- Requested by defense attorney
- Blinded review finding
  5 WNL
  3 BCC/Repair
  3 ASC-US
- Supported defendant

Case 100
- Requested by plaintiff attorney
- Blinded review finding
  5 WNL
  5 AGUS
- Equivocal

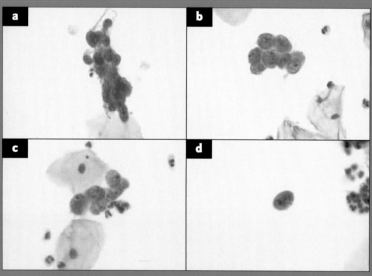

Case 104: TP Case
- Requested by plaintiff attorney
- Blinded review finding
  7 H SIL
  3 Squamous cell carcinoma
- Supported plaintiff

References

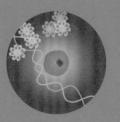

A

Abadi MA, Barakat RE, Saigo PE: Effects of Tamoxifen on Cervicovaginal Smears from Patients With Breast Cancer. *Acta Cytol* 44: 141-146, 2000.

Abati A, Jaffurs W, Wilder AM: Squamous Atypia in the Atrophic Cervical Vaginal Smear: A New Look at an Old Problem. *Cancer (Cancer Cytopathol)* 85: 218-225, 1998.

Abdul-Karim FW, Fu YS, Regan JW, et al: Morphometric Study of Intraepithelial Neoplasia of the Uterine Cervix. *Obstet Gynecol* 60: 210-214, 1982.

Abdulla M, Hombal S, Kanbour A, et al: Characterizing "Blue Blobs": Immunohistochemical Staining and Ultrastructural Study. *Acta Cytol* 44: 547-550, 2000.

Abeler VM, Holm R, Nesland JM, et al: Small Cell Carcinoma of the Cervix: A Clinicopathologic Study of 26 Patients. *Cancer* 73: 672-677, 1994.

Abell MR, Gosling JRG: Gland Cell Carcinoma (Adenocarcinoma) of the Uterine Cervix. *Am J Obstet Gynecol* 83: 729-755, 1962.

Abell MR, Ramirez JA: Sarcomas and Carcinosarcomas of the Uterine Cervix. *Cancer* 31: 1176-1192, 1973.

Abitbol MM, Davenport JH: The Irradiated Vagina. *Obstet Gynecol* 44: 249-256, 1974.

Abramovich CM, Wasman JK, Siekkinen P, et al: Histopathologic Correlation of Atypical Parakeratosis Diagnosed on Cervicovaginal Cytology. *Acta Cytol* 47: 405-409, 2003.

Abrams HL, Spiro R, Goldstein N: Metastases in Carcinoma: Analysis of 1000 Autopsied Cases. *Cancer* 3: 74-85, 1950.

Abu-Jawdeh GM, Trawinski G, Wang HH: Histocytological Study of Squamous Atypia on Pap Smears. *Mod Pathol* 7: 920-924, 1994.

Ackerman LV: Verrucous Carcinoma of the Oral Cavity. *Surgery* 23: 670-678, 1948.

Acladious NN, Sutton C, Mandal D, et al: Persistant Human Papillomavirus Infection and Smoking Increase Risk of Failure of Treatment of Cervical Intraepithelial Neoplasia (CIN). *Int J Cancer* 98: 435-439, 2002.

[ACOG] American College of Obstetricians and Gynecologists: Cervical Cytology: Evaluation and Management of Abnormalities. *ACOG Technical Bulletin* No. 183: 1-8, August, 1993. (*Int J Gynecol Obstet* 43: 212-219, 1993).

Acs G, Gupta PK, Baloch ZW: Glandular and Squamous Atypia and Intraepithelial Lesions in Atrophic Cervicovaginal Smears: One Institution's Experience. *Acta Cytol* 44: 611-617, 2000.

Acs J, Hildesheim A, Reeves WC, et al: Regional Distribution of Human Papillomavirus DNA and Other Risk Factors for Invasive Cervical Cancer in Panama. *Cancer Res* 49: 5725-5729, 1989.

Adachi A, Fleming I, Burk RD, et al: Women With Human Immunodeficiency Virus Infection and Abnormal Papanicolaou Smears: A Prospective Study of Colposcopy and Clinical Outcome. *Obstet Gynecol* 81: 372-377, 1993.

Adam E, Kaufman RH, Berkova Z, et al: Is Human Papillomavirus Testing an Effective Triage Method for Detection of High-Grade (Grade 2 or 3) Cervical Intraepithelial Neoplasia? *Am J Obstet Gynecol* 178: 1235-1244, 1998.

Adam E, Berkova Z, Daxnerova Z, et al: Papillomavirus Detection: Demographic and Behavioral Characteristics Influencing the Identification of Cervical Disease. *Am J Obstet Gynecol* 182: 257-264, 2000.

Adami H-O, Pontén J, Sparén P, et al: Survival Trend After Invasive Cervical Cancer Diagnosis in Sweden Before and After Cytologic Screening. 1960-1984. *Cancer* 73: 140-147, 1994.

Adami H-O, Trichopoulos D: Cervical Cancer and the Elusive Male Factor (Editorial). *N Engl J Med* 346: 1160-1161, 2002.

Adcock LL, Julian TM, Okagaki T, et al: Carcinoma of the Uterine Cervix FIGO Stage I-B. *Gynecol Oncol* 14: 199-208, 1982.

Addiss DG, Vaughn ML, Golubjatnikov R, et al: *Chlamydia trachomatis* Infection in Women Attending Urban Midwestern Family Planning and Community Health Clinics: Risk Factors, Selective Screening, and Evaluation of Non-Culture Techniques. *Sex Transm Dis* 17: 138-146, 1990.

Adeniran A, Dimashkieh H, Nikiforov Y: Schistosomiasis of the Cervix. *Arch Pathol Lab Med* 127: 1637-1638, 2003.

Affandi MZ, Doctor V, Jhaveri K: The Endocervical Smear as a Simple and Quick Method for the Determination of Ovulation. *Acta Cytol* 29: 638-641, 1985.

Affandi MZ, Dun T, Mantuano V, et al: Epidemiology of Cervical Carcinoma in Brunei Darussalam: Analysis of Data on 27,208 Women Screened With Cytologic Examinations. *Acta Cytol* 37: 175-180, 1993.

Agarwal S, Sharma S: Localization of Carcinoembryonic Antigen in Uterine Cervical Neoplasia. *Ind J Med Res* 92: 452-455, 1990.

Agarwal SS, Sehgal A, Sardana S, et al: Role of Male Behavior in Cervical Carcinogenesis Among Women With One Lifetime Sexual Partner. *Cancer* 72: 1666-1669, 1993.

Agoff SN, Lamps LW, Philip AT, et al: Thyroid Transcription Factor-1 Is Expressed in Extrapulmonary Small Cell Carcinomas But Not in Other Extrapulmonary Neuroendocrine Tumors. *Mod Pathol* 13: 238-242, 2000.

Ahdoot D, Van Nostrand KM, Nguyen NJ, et al: The Effect of Route of Delivery on Regression of Abnormal Cervical Cytologic Findings in the Postpartum Period. *Am J Obstet Gynecol* 178: 1116-1120, 1998.

Ahmad M: Intravaginal Vibrator of Long Duration. *Eur J Emerg Med* 9: 61-62, 2002.

Ahrné S, Nobaek S, Jeppsson B, et al: The Normal *Lactobacillus* Flora of Healthy Human Rectal and Oral Mucosa. *J Appl Microbiol* 85: 88-94, 1998.

Ahsan S, Manyonda I, Spencer T, et al: Psammoma Bodies in a Cervical Smear in Association With Borderline Ovarian Epithelial Malignancy. *J Pakistan Med Assn* 48: 52-53, 1998.

Aitken-Swan J, Baird D: Cancer of the Uterine Cervix in Aberdeenshire: Aetiological Aspects. *Br J Cancer* 20: 642-659, 1966.

Ajit D, Dighe S, Gujral S: Cytologic Features of Villoglandular Adenocarcinoma of the Cervix (Letter). *Acta Cytol* 48: 288-289, 2004.

Akin M-R, Nguyen G-K: Cytologic Manifestations of Advanced Endometrial Adenocarcinomas in Cervical-Vaginal Smears (Letter). *Diagn Cytopathol* 20: 108-110, 1999.

Akkad AA, Habiba MA, Ismail N, et al: Abnormal Uterine Bleeding on Hormone Replacement: The Importance of Intrauterine Structural Abnormalities. *Obstet Gynecol* 86: 330-334, 1995.

Akpolat I, Smith DA, Ramzy I, et al: The utility of p16^{INK4a} and Ki-67 Staining on Cell Blocks Prepared from Residual Thin-Layer Cervicovaginal Material. *Cancer (Cancer Cytopathol)* 102: 142-149, 2004.

Alanen KW, Elit LM, Molinaro PA, et al: Assessment of Cytologic Follow-Up as the Recommended Management for Patients With Atypical Squamous Cells of Undetermined Significance or Low-Grade Squamous Intraepithelial Lesions. *Cancer (Cancer Cytopathol)* 84: 5-10, 1998.

Alani RM, Münger K: Human Papillomaviruses and Associated Malignancies. *J Clin Oncol* 16: 330-337, 1998.

Albert A: Estimated Cervical Cancer Disease State and Incidence and Transition Rates. *J Natl Cancer Inst* 67: 571-576, 1981.

Albores-Saavedra J, Larraza O, Poucell S, et al: Carcinoid of the Uterine Cervix, Additional Observations on a New Tumor Entity. *Cancer* 38: 2328-2342, 1976.

Albores-Saavedra J, Rodríguez-Martínez HA, Larraza-Hernández O: Carcinoid Tumors of the Cervix. *Pathol Annu* 14(Pt 2): 273-291, 1979.

Albores-Saavedra J, Gersell D, Gilks CB, et al: Terminology of Endocrine Tumors of the Uterine Cervix: Results of a Workshop Sponsored by the College of American Pathologists and the National Cancer Institute. *Arch Pathol Lab Med* 121: 34-39, 1997.

Albukerk J: False-Positive Cytology in Ectopic Pregnancy (Letter). *N Engl J Med* 291: 1142, 1974.

Albukerk JN, Gnecco CA: Atypical Cytology in Tubal Pregnancy. *J Reprod Med* 19: 273-276, 1977.

Alexander LL, ed: *Sexually Transmitted Diseases in America: How Many Cases and at What Cost?* American Social Health Association for the Kaiser Family Foundation, Research Triangle Park, NC, 1-27, 1998.

Alexander NJ, Andersen DJ: Immunology of Semen. *Fertility Sterility* 47: 192-205, 1987.

Alfsen GC, Thoresen SO, Kristensen GB, et al: Histopathologic Subtyping of Cervical Adenocarcinoma Reveals Increasing Incidence Rates of Endometrioid Tumors in all Age Groups. A Population Based Study With Review of All Nonsquamous Cervical Carcinomas in Norway from 1966 to 1970, 1976 to 1980, and 1986 to 1990. *Cancer* 89: 1291-1299, 2000.

Allen KA, Zaleski S, Cohen MB: Review of Negative Papanicolaou Tests: Is the Retrospective 5-Year Review Necessary? *Am J Clin Pathol* 101: 19-21, 1994.

Allen KA, Zaleski S, Cohen MB: Laboratory Use of the Diagnosis "Reactive/Reparative" in Gynecologic Smears: Impact of CLIA '88. *Mod Pathol* 8: 266-269, 1995.

Allerding TJ, Jordan SW, Boardman RE: Association of Human Papillomavirus and Chlamydia Infections With Incidence Cervical Neoplasia. *Acta Cytol* 29: 653-660, 1985.

Allery J-P, Telmon N, Mieusset R, et al: Cytological Detection of Spermatozoa: Comparison of Three Staining Methods. *J Forensic Sci* 46: 349-351, 2001.

Alli PM, Ali SZ: Atypical Squamous Cells of Undetermined Significance—Rule Out High-Grade Squamous Intraepithelial Lesion: Cytopathologic Characteristics and Clinical Correlates. *Diagn Cytopathol* 28: 308-312, 2003.

Alloub MI, Barr BBB, McLaren KM, et al: Human Papillomavirus Infection and Cervical Intraepithelial Neoplasia in Women With Renal Allografts. *Br Med J* 298: 153-156, 1989.

Almoujahed MO, Briski LE, Prysak M, et al: Uterine Granulomas: Clinical and Pathologic Features. *Am J Clin Pathol* 117: 771-775, 2002.

Al-Nafussi A, Rahilly M: The Prevalence of Tubo-Endometrial Metaplasia and Adenomatoid Proliferation. *Histopathology* 22: 177-179, 1993.

Al-Nafussi A, Rebello G, Al-Yusif R, et al: The Borderline Cervical Smear: Colposcopic and Biopsy Outcome. *J Clin Pathol* 53: 439-444, 2000.

Alonio LV, Picconi MA, Dalbert D, et al: Ha-*ras* Oncogene Mutation Associated to Progression of Papillomavirus Induced Lesions of Uterine Cervix. *J Clin Virol* 27: 263-269, 2003.

Alons-van Kordelaar JJM, Boon ME: Diagnostic Accuracy of Squamous Cervical Lesions Studied in Spatula-Cytobrush Smears. *Acta Cytol* 32: 801-804, 1988.

Al-Talib RK, Sworn MJ, Ramsay AD, et al: Primary Cervical Lymphoma: The Role of Cervical Cytology. *Cytopathology* 7: 173-177, 1996.

Altekruse SF, Lacey JV, Brinton LA, et al: Comparison of Human Papillomavirus Genotypes, Sexual, and Reproductive Risk Factors of Cervical Adenocarcinoma and Squamous Cell Carcinoma: Northeastern United States. *Am J Obstet Gynecol* 188: 657-663, 2003.

Altiok S: Molecular Markers in Cervical Cytology. *Clin Lab Med* 23: 709-728, 2003.

Alva J, Lauchlan SC: The Histogenesis of Mixed Cervical Carcinomas: The Concept of Endocervical Columnar-Cell Dysplasia. *Am J Clin Pathol* 64: 20-25, 1975.

Alvarez-Santin C, Sica A, Rodriquez MC, et al: Microglandular Hyperplasia of the Uterine Cervix: Cytologic Diagnosis in Cervical Smears. *Acta Cytol* 43: 110-113, 1999.

Ambros RA, Kurman RJ: Current Concepts in the Relationship of Human Papillomavirus Infection to the Pathogenesis and Classification of Precancerous Squamous Lesions of the Uterine Cervix. *Semin Diagn Pathol* 7: 158-172, 1990.

Ambros RA, Park J-S, Shah KV, et al: Evaluation of Histologic, Morphometric, and Immunochemical Criteria in the Differential Diagnosis of Small Cell Carcinomas of the Cervix With Particular Reference to Human Papillomavirus Type 16 and 18. *Mod Pathol* 4: 586-593, 1991.

Amies A-M, Miller L, Lee S-J, et al: The Effect of Vaginal Speculum Lubrication on the Rate of Unsatisfactory Cervical Cytology Diagnosis. *Obstet Gynecol* 100: 889-892, 2002.

Amsel R, Totten PA, Spiegel CA, et al: Nonspecific Vaginitis: Diagnostic Criteria and Microbial and Epidemiologic Associations. *Am J Med* 74: 14-22, 1983.

Anciaux D, Lawrence WD, Gregoire L: Glandular Lesions of the Uterine Cervix: Prognostic Implications of Human Papillomavirus Status. *Int J Gynecol Pathol* 16: 103-110, 1997.

Andersch B, Forssman L, Lincoln K, et al: Treatment of Bacterial Vaginosis With an Acid Cream: A Comparison Between the Effect of Lactate-Gel and Metronidazole. *Gynecol Obstet Invest* 21: 19-25, 1986.

Andersen ES, Arffmann E: Adenocarcinoma In Situ of the Uterine Cervix: A Clinico-Pathologic Study of 36 Cases. *Gynecol Oncol* 35: 1-7, 1989.

Andersen ES, Nielsen K, Pedersen B: The Reliability of Preconization Diagnostic Evaluation in Patients With Cervical Intraepithelial Neoplasia and Microinvasive Carcinoma. *Gynecol Oncol* 59: 143-147, 1995.

Andersen W, Frierson H, Barber S, et al: Sensitivity and Specificity of Endocervical Curettage and the Endocervical Brush for the Evaluation of the Endocervical Canal. *Am J Obstet Gynecol* 159: 702-707, 1988.

Anderson DG, Eaton CJ, Galinkin LJ, et al: The Cytologic Diagnosis of Endometrial Adenocarcinoma. *Am J Obstet Gynecol* 125: 376-383, 1976.

Anderson GH, Matisic JP, Thomas BA: Confirmation of Genital Herpes Simplex Viral Infection by an Immunoperoxidase Technique. *Acta Cytol* 29: 695-700, 1985.

Anderson GH, Flynn KJ, Hickey LA, et al: A Comprehensive Internal Quality Control System for a Large Cytology Laboratory. *Acta Cytol* 31: 895-899, 1987.

Anderson GH, Boyes DA, Benedet JL, et al: Organisation and Results of the Cytology Screening Programme in British Columbia, 1955-1985. *Br Med J* 296: 975-978, 1988.

Anderson GH, Benedet JL, Le Riche JC, et al: Invasive Cancer of the Cervix in British Columbia: A Review of the Demography and Screening Histories of 437 Cases Seen from 1985-1988. *Obstet Gynecol* 80: 1-4, 1992.

Anderson MB, Jones BA: False Positive Cervicovaginal Cytology: A Follow-Up Study. *Acta Cytol* 41: 1697-1700, 1997.

Anderson MC: The Pathology of Cervical Cancer. *Clin Obstet Gynaecol* 12: 87-119, 1985.

Anderson MC, Brown CL, Buckley CH, et al: Current Views on Cervical Intraepithelial Neoplasia. *J Clin Pathol* 44: 969-978, 1991.

Anderson MC: Glandular Lesions of the Cervix: Diagnostic and Therapeutic Dilemmas. *Baillieres Clin Obstet Gynaecol* 9: 105-109, 1995.

Anderson SM: Human Papillomavirus and Cervical Cancer. *Advance Lab*, June, 90-94, 2001.

Andersson S, Larson B, Hjerpe A: Adenocarcinoma of the Uterine Cervix: The Presence of Human Papillomavirus and the Method of Detection. *Acta Obstet Gynecol Scand* 82: 960-965, 2003.

Andersson-Ellström A, Hagmar BM, Johansson B, et al: Human Papillomavirus Deoxyribonucleic Acid in Cervix Only Detected in Girls After Coitus. *Int J STD AIDS* 7: 333-336, 1996.

Andersson-Ellström A, Seidal T, Grannas M, et al: The Pap-Smear History of Women With Invasive Cervical Squamous Carcinoma: A Case-Control Study from Sweden. *Acta Obstet Gynecol Scand* 79: 221-226, 2000.

Andrews S, Hernandez E, Miyazawa K: Paired Papanicolaou Smears in the Evaluation of Atypical Squamous Cells. *Obstet Gynecol* 73: 747-750, 1989a.

Andrews S, Miyazawa K: The Significance of a Negative Papanicolaou Smear With Hyperkeratosis or Parakeratosis. *Obstet Gynecol* 73: 751-753, 1989b.

Andrews SJ, Hernandez E, Woods J, et al: Burkitt's-Like Lymphoma Presenting as a Gynecologic Tumor. *Gynecologic Oncol* 30: 131-136, 1988.

Anello C, Lao C: U.S. Trends in Mortality from Carcinoma of Cervix (Letter). *Lancet* (i): 1038, 1979.

An-Foraker SH, Kawada CY: Cytodiagnosis of Endometrial Malignant Mixed Mesodermal Tumor. *Acta Cytol* 29: 137-141, 1985.

Angel C, DuBeshter B, Lin JY. Clinical Presentation and Management of Stage I Cervical Adenocarcinoma: A 25 Year Experience. *Gynecol Oncol* 44: 71-78, 1992.

Angeles MA, Saigo PE: Cytologic Findings in Rectovaginal Fistulae. *Acta Cytol* 38: 373-376, 1994.

Angrish K, Verma K: Cytologic Detection of Tuberculosis of the Uterine Cervix. *Acta Cytol* 25: 160-162, 1981.

Anhang R, Stryker JE, Wright TC Jr, et al: News Media Coverage of Human Papillomavirus. *Cancer* 100: 308-314, 2004.

Anonymous: New Pap Tests Suggested for Air Force Dependents. *U.S. Medicine*, 14, 16-17, August 1, 1978.

Anonymous: Update on Toxic Shock Syndrome. *FDA Drug Bull* 10: 17-19, 1980.

Anonymous: Human Papillomaviruses and Cervical Cancer: A Fresh Look at the Evidence. *Lancet* (i): 725-726, 1987.

Anonymous: Human Papillomaviruses and the Polymerase Chain Reaction. *Lancet* (i): 1051-1052, 1989a.

Anonymous: Leads from the MMWR. Chronic Disease Reports: Mortality Trends—United States, 1979-1986. *JAMA* 5: 2495, 1989b.

Anonymous: 1993 Revised Classification System for HIV Infection and Expanded Surveillance Case Definition for AIDS Among Adolescents and Adults. *JAMA* 10: 729-730, 1993a.

Anonymous: Invasive Squamous-Cell Cervical Carcinoma and Combined Oral Contraceptives: Results from a Multinational Study. WHO Collaborative Study of Neoplasia and Steroid Contraceptives. *Int J Cancer* 55: 228-236, 1993b.

Anonymous: Risk of Cervical Dysplasia in Users of Oral Contraceptives, Intrauterine Devices or Depot-Medroxyprogesterone Acetate: The New Zealand Contraception and Health Study Group. *Contraception* 50: 431-441, 1994a.

Anonymous: History of Long-Term Use of Depot-Medroxyprogesterone Acetate in Patients With Cervical Dysplasia; Case Control Analysis Nested in a Cohort Study: The New Zealand Contraception and Health Study Group. *Contraception* 50: 443-449, 1994b.

Anonymous: Cervical Cancer: Behavioral Changes Could Save Most Women. *Oncology* 10: 862, 1996.

Anonymous: Summary of the NIH Consensus Development Conference on Cervical Cancer. *Oncology* 11: 672, 674, 1997.

Anonymous: Human Papillomavirus Testing for Triage of Women With Cytologic Evidence of Low-Grade Squamous Intraepithelial Lesions: Baseline Data from a Randomized Trial. *J Natl Cancer Inst* 92: 397-402, 2000.

Anonymous: Cervical Cytology Practice Guidelines: American Society of Cytopathology. *Acta Cytol* 45: 201-226, 2001.

Anonymous: Trends in Sexual Risk Behaviors Among High School Students—United States, 1991-2001. *MMWR* 51: 856-859, 2002.

Anonymous: Papanicolaou Society of Cytopathology Guidelines for Educational Notes, Disclaimers, and Similar Comments on Reports of Cervical Cytology Specimens. *Diagn Cytopathol* 28: 282-285, 2003a.

Anonymous: Cervical Cytology Screening: Clinical Management Guidelines for Obstetrician-Gynecologists (reprint of ACOG Practice Bulletin, No. 45, 2003). *Obstet Gynecol* 102: 417-427, 2003b.

Anonymous: Cervical Cancer Screening: Testing Can Start Later and Occur Less Often Under New ACOG Recommendations. ACOG News Release, August 11, 2003. [http://www.acog.com/from_home/publications/press_releases/nr07-31-1.cfm?=03]

Anton RC, Ramzy I, Schwartz MR, et al: Should the Cytologic Diagnosis of "Atypical Squamous Cells of Undetermined Significance" Be Qualified? *Cancer (Cancer Cytopathol)* 93: 93-99, 2001.

Antonio MAD, Hawes SE, Hillier SL: The Identification of Vaginal *Lactobacillus* Species and the Demographic and Microbiologic Characteristics of Women Colonized by These Species. *J Infect Dis* 180: 1950-1956, 1999.

Antonioli DA, Burke L: Vaginal Adenosis: Analysis of 325 Biopsy specimens from 100 Patients. *Am J Clin Pathol* 64: 625-638, 1975.

Antonioli DA, Rosen S, Burke L, et al: Glandular Dysplasia in Diethylstilbestrol-Associated Vaginal Adenosis: A Case Report and Review of the Literature. *Am J Clin Pathol* 71: 715-721, 1979.

Anttila T, Saikku P, Koskela P, et al: Serotypes of *Chlamydia trachomatis* and Risk for Development of Cervical Squamous Cell Carcinoma. *JAMA* 285: 47-51, 2001.

Apple RJ, Erlich HA, Klitz W, et al: HLA DR-DQ Associations With Cervical Carcinoma Show Papillomavirus-Type Specificity. *Nature (Genetics)* 6: 157-162, 1994.

Apple RJ, Becker TM, Wheeler CM, et al: Comparison of Human Leukocyte Antigen DR-DQ Disease Associations Found With Cervical Dysplasia and Invasive Cervical Carcinoma. *J Natl Cancer Inst* 87: 427-436, 1995.

Arbeit JM, Howley PM, Hanahan D: Chronic Estrogen-Induced Cervical and Vaginal Squamous Carcinogenesis in Human Papillomavirus Type 16 Transgenic Mice. *Proc Natl Acad Sci (USA)* 93: 2930-2935, 1996.

Archer DF, Pickar JH, Bottiglioni F: Bleeding Patterns in Postmenopausal Women Taking Continuous Combined or Sequential Regimens of Conjugated Estrogens With Medroxyprogesterone Acetate: Menopause Study Group. *Obstet Gynecol* 83: 686-692, 1994.

Archer DF, Pickar JH: Hormone Replacement Therapy: Effect of Progestin Dose and Time Since Menopause on Endometrial Bleeding. *Obstet Gynecol* 96: 899-905, 2000.

Arends MJ, Donaldson YK, Duvall E, et al: Human Papillomavirus Type 18 Associates With More Advanced Cervical Neoplasia Than Human Papillomavirus Type 16. *Hum Pathol* 24: 432-437, 1993.

Arends MJ, Buckley CH, Wells M: Aetiology, Pathogenesis, and Pathology of Cervical Neoplasia. *J Clin Pathol* 51: 96-103, 1998.

Arias-Stella J: Atypical Endometrial Changes Associated With the Presence of Chorionic Tissue. *Arch Pathol* 58: 112-128, 1954.

Armstrong B, Holman D: Increasing Mortality from Cancer of the Cervix in Young Australian Women. *Med J Aust* 1: 460-462, 1981.

Armstrong BK: The Falling, Rising Incidence of Invasive Cancer of the Cervix. *Med J Aust* 1: 147-148, 1983.

Arora CD, Schmidt DS, Rader AE, et al: Adolescents With ASCUS: Are They a High Risk Group? *Clin Pediatr (Phila)* 40: 133-138, 2001.

Aroutcheva A, Gariti D, Simon M, et al: Defense Factors of Vaginal Lactobacilli. *Am J Obstet Gynecol* 185: 375-379, 2001.

Arrighi AA: Cytology of Endometrial Hyperplasia (Symposium on Endometrial Cytology. C: Endometrial Cytology in Endocrinology). *Acta Cytol* 2: 613, 1958.

Arroyo G, Elgueta R: Squamous Cell Carcinoma Associated With Amoebic Cervicitis: Report of a Case. *Acta Cytol* 33: 301-304, 1989a.

Arroyo G, Linnemann C, Wesseler T: Role of the Papanicolaou Smear in Diagnosis of Chlamydial Infections. *Sex Transm Dis* 16: 11-14, 1989b.

Arroyo G, Quinn JA Jr: Association of Amoebae and Actinomyces in an Intrauterine Contraceptive Device User. *Acta Cytol* 33: 298-300, 1989c.

Arsenault GM, Kalman CF, Sorensen KW, et al: The Papanicolaou Smear as a Technique for Gonorrhea Detection: A Feasibility Study. *J Am Vener Dis Assoc* 2: 35-38, 1976.

Ashfaq R, Gibbons D, Vela C, et al: ThinPrep Pap Test: Accuracy for Glandular Disease. *Acta Cytol* 43: 81-85, 1999.

Ashfaq R, Sharma S, Dulley T, et al: Clinical Relevance of Benign Endometrial Cells in Postmenopausal Women. *Diagn Cytopathol* 25: 235-238, 2001.

Ashfaq-Drewett R, Allen C, Harrison, RL: Detached Ciliary Tufts: Comparison With Intestinal Protozoa and a Review of the Literature. *Am J Clin Pathol* 93: 541-545, 1990.

Ashley DJB: The Biological Status of Carcinoma In-Situ of the Uterine Cervix. *J Obstet Gynaecol Br Commonw* 73: 372-381, 1966a.

Ashley DJB: Evidence for the Existence of Two Forms of Cervical Carcinoma. *J Obstet Gynaecol Br Commonw* 73: 382-389, 1966b.

Ashley RL: Laboratory Techniques in the Diagnosis of Herpes Simplex Infection. *Genitourin Med* 69: 174-183, 1993.

Ashworth CT, Luibel FJ, Sanders E: Epithelium of Normal Cervix Uteri Studied With Electon Microscopy and Histochemistry. *Am J Obstet Gynecol* 79: 1149-1160, 1960.

Athanassiadou PP, Kyrkou KA, Antoniades LG, et al: Cytological Evaluation of the Effect of Tamoxifen in Premenopausal and Post-Menopausal Women With Primary Breast Cancer by Analysis of the Karyopyknotic Indices of Vaginal Smears. *Cytopathology* 3: 203-208, 1992.

Athavale RD, Chia KV: Psammoma Bodies on Postmenopausal Cervical Smear—A Rare Sinister Finding. *J Obstet Gynaecol* 22: 328-329, 2002.

Attwood ME, Woodman CBJ, Luesley D, et al: Previous Cytology in Patients With Invasive Carcinoma of the Cervix. *Acta Cytol* 29: 108-110, 1985.

Auborn KJ, Woodworth C, DiPaolo JA, et al: The Interaction Between HPV Infection and Estrogen Metabolism in Cervical Carcinogenesis. *Int J Cancer* 49: 867-869, 1991.

Auborn KJ, Carter TH: Treatment of Human Papillomavirus Gynecologic Infections. *Clin Lab Med* 20: 407-422, 2000.

Auger M, Charbonneau M, Arseneau J: Atypical Squamous Cells of Undetermined Significance: A Cytohistologic Study of 52 Cases. *Acta Cytol* 41: 1671-1675, 1997.

August N: Cervicography for Evaluating the "Atypical" Papanicolaou Smear. *J Reprod Med* 36: 89-94, 1991.

Aurelian L: Persistence and Expression of the Herpes Simplex Virus Type 2 Genome in Cervical Tumor Cells. *Cancer Res* 34: 1126-1135, 1974.

Austin RM: Why CLIA '88 Will Increase Cervical Cancer Deaths. *CAP Today* 5: 15-18, 1991.

Austin RM: The Future of Cytology: Prospects for the Nonprofit Hospital Cytology Laboratory. *Diagn Cytopathol* 9: 130-132, 1993.

Austin RM: Can Regulatory Proficiency Testing by the Cytobureaucracy Decrease Both False Negatives and Cervical Cancer Deaths? *Diagn Cytopathol* 11: 109-112, 1994a.

Austin RM: In Search of a "Reasonable Person Standard" for Gynecologic Cytologists. *Diagn Cytopathol* 11: 216-218, 1994b.

Austin RM, Ramzy I: Increased Detection of Epithelial Cell Abnormalities by Liquid-Based Gynecologic Cytology Preparations: A Review of Accumulated Data. *Acta Cytol* 42: 178-184, 1998.

Austin RM: Follow-Up of Abnormal Gynecologic Cytology: A College of American Pathologists Q-Probes Study of 16312 Cases from 306 Laboratories. *Arch Pathol Lab Med* 124: 1113-1114, 2000.

Austin RM: The Detection of Precancerous Cervical lesions Can Be Significantly Increased: Who Cares and Who Should Know? (Editorial) *Arch Pathol Lab Med* 127: 143-145, 2003a.

Austin RM: Human Papillomavirus Reporting: Minimizing Patient and Laboratory Risk. *Arch Pathol Lab Med* 127: 973-977, 2003b.

Austin RM: Public Expectations, Achievable Cervical Screening Sensitivity, and the Standard of Practice (Editorial). *Cancer (Cancer Cytopathol)* 99: 1-3, 2003c.

Austin RM: New Cervical Cancer Screening Guidelines: The Other Side of Group Health Care "Rights." *Diagn Cytopathol* 30: 208-210, 2004.

Autier P, Coibion M, Huet F, et al: Transformation Zone Location and Intraepithelial Neoplasia of the Cervix Uteri. *Br J Cancer* 74: 488-490, 1996.

Autier P, Coibion M, De Sutter P, et al: Cytology Alone Versus Cytology and Cervicography for Cervical Cancer Screening: A Randomized Study. *Obstet Gynecol* 93: 353-358, 1999.

Averette HE, Weinstein GD, Frost P: Autoradiographic Analysis of Cell Proliferation Kinetics in Human Genital Tissues: I. Normal Cervix and Vagina. *Am J Obstet Gynecol* 108: 8-17, 1970.

Averette HE, Steren A, Nguyen HN: Screening in Gynecologic Cancers. *Cancer* 72: 1043-1049, 1993.

Avonts D, Sercu M, Heyerick P, et al: Incidence of Uncomplicated Genital Infections in Women Using Oral Contraception or an Intrauterine Device: A Prospective Study. *Sex Transm Dis* 17: 23-29, 1990.

Avram E, Yakovlevitz M, Schachter A: Cytologic Detection of *Enterobius vermicularis* and *Strongyloides stercoralis* in Routine Cervicovaginal Smears and Urocytograms. *Acta Cytol* 28: 468-470, 1984.

Axiotis CA, Merino MJ, Duray PH: Langerhans Cell Histocytosis of the Female Genital Tract. *Cancer* 67: 1650-1660, 1991.

Ayer B, Pacey F, Greenberg M: The Cytologic Diagnosis of Adenocarcinoma In Situ of the Cervix Uteri and Related Lesions: I. Adenocarcinoma In Situ. *Acta Cytol* 31: 397-411, 1987.

Ayer B, Pacey F, Greenberg M: The Cytologic Diagnosis of Adenocarcinoma In Situ of the Cervix Uteri and Related Lesions: II. Microinvasive Carcinoma. *Acta Cytol* 32: 318-324, 1988.

Ayer B, Pacey FN, Greenberg ML: The Cytological Features of Invasive Adenocarcinoma of the Cervix Uteri. *Cytopathology* 2: 181-191, 1991.

Ayre JE: A Simple Office Test for Uterine Cancer Diagnosis. *CMAJ* 51:17-22, 1944.

Ayre JE: Vaginal and Cervical Cytology in Uterine Cancer Diagnosis. *Am J Obstet Gynecol* 51: 743-750, 1946.

Ayre JE: Selective Cytology Smear for Diagnosis of Cancer. *Am J Obstet Gynecol* 53: 609-617, 1947.

Ayre JE: Cervical Cytology in the Diagnosis of Early Cancer. *JAMA* 136: 513-517, 1948.

Ayre JE: The Vaginal Smear. "Precancer" Cell Studies Using A Modified Technique. *Am J Obstet Gynecol* 58: 1205-1219, 1949.

Ayre JE, Berger J, Graham RM, et al: Opinion Poll on Gynecological Terminology. *Acta Cytol* 2: 112-114, 1958.

Ayre JE: Role of the Halo Cell in Cervical Cancerigenesis: A Virus Manifestation in Premalignancy? *Obstet Gynecol* 15: 481-491, 1960.

Azocar J, Acosta H, Hernandez R, et al: Prevalence of Cervical Dysplasia and HPV Infection According to Sexual Behavior. *Int J Cancer* 45: 622-625, 1990.

Azodi M, Chambers SK, Rutherford TJ, et al: Adenocarcinoma In Situ of the Cervix: Management and Outcome. *Gynecol Oncol* 73: 348-353, 1999.

Azzopardi JG, Hou LT: Intestinal Metaplasia With Argentaffin Cells in Cervical Adenocarcinoma. *J Pathol Bacteriol* 90: 686-690, 1965.

B

Baay MFD, Smits E, Wiebren AA, et al: Can Cervical Cancer Screening Be Stopped at 50? The Prevalence of HPV in Elderly Women. *Int J Cancer* 108: 258-261, 2004.

Babès A: Diagnostic du Cancer du Col Utérin par les Frottis. *La Presse Medicale* 36: 451-454, 1928.

Babès A: Sur le Cancer Superficiel du Col Utérin. *Gynecologie et Obstetrique* 23: 417-433, 1931.

Babkowski RC, Rutkowski MA, Wilbur DC, et al: The Effects of Endocervical Canal Topography, Tubal Metaplasia, and High Canal Sampling on the Cytologic Presentation of Nonneoplastic Endocervical Cells. *Am J Clin Pathol* 105: 403-410, 1996.

Bachner P: Can Cytology Proficiency Testing Programs Discriminate Between Competent and Incompetent Practitioners? *Qual Rev Bull (QRB)* 17: 150-151, 1991.

Baekelandt M, Nesbakken AJ, Kristensen GB, et al: Carcinoma of the Fallopian Tube: Clinicopathologic Study of 151 Patients Treated at the Norwegian Radium Hospital. *Cancer* 89: 2076-2084, 2000.

Baer A, Kiviat NB, Kulasingam S, et al: Liquid-Based Papanicolaou Smears Without a Transformation Zone Component: Should Clinicians Worry? *Obstet Gynecol* 99: 1053-1059, 2002.

Baggish MS, Woodruff JD: Adenoid-Basal Carcinoma of the Cervix. *Obstet Gynecol* 28: 213-218, 1966.

Bahamondes L, Trevisan M, Andrade L, et al: The Effect Upon the Human Vaginal Histology of the Long-Term Use of the Injectable Contraceptive Depo-Provera®. *Contraceptive* 62: 23-27, 2000.

Bai H, Sung CJ, Steinhoff MM: ThinPrep Pap Test Promotes Detection of Glandular Lesions of the Endocervix. *Diagn Cytopathol* 23: 19-22, 2000.

Bain RW, Crocker DW: Rapid Onset of Cervical Cancer in an Upper Socioeconomic Group. *Am J Obstet Gynecol* 146: 366-371, 1983.

Baird PJ, Russell P, Laverty CR: Clear Cell Adenocarcinoma of the Uterine Cervix: A Histological and Histochemical Study. *Pathology* 9: 257-262, 1977.

Bajardi F, Gompel CM, Tsanov K, et al: European Comment on Statement of Caution in Reference to Human Papillomavirus Infection. *Acta Cytol* 30: 445-446, 1986.

Baker JJ: Conventional and Liquid-Based Cervicovaginal Cytology: A Comparison Study With Clinical and Histologic Follow-Up. *Diagn Cytopathol* 27: 185-188, 2002.

Baker RW, O'Sullivan JP, Hanley J, et al: The Characteristics of False Negative Cervical Smears—Implications for the UK Cervical Cancer Screening Programme. *J Clin Pathol* 52: 358-362, 1999.

Baldwin P, Laskey R, Coleman N: Translational Approaches to Improving Cervical Screening. *Nature Rev (Cancer)* 3: 1-10, 2003.

Balega J, Michael H, Hurteau J, et al: The Risk of Nodal Metastasis in Early Adenocarcinoma of the Uterine Cervix. *Int J Gynecol Cancer* 14: 104-109, 2004.

Ballo MS, Silverberg SG, Sidawy MK: Cytologic Features of Well-Differentiated Villoglandular Adenocarcinoma of the Cervix. *Acta Cytol* 40: 536-540, 1996.

Bamford PN, Beilby JOW, Steele SJ, et al: The Natural History of Cervical Intraepithelial Neoplasia as Determined by Cytology and Colposcopic Biopsy. *Acta Cytol* 27: 482-484. 1983.

Band V, Zajchowski D, Kulesa V, et al: Human Papilloma Virus DNAs Immortalize Normal Human Mammary Epithelial Cells and Reduce Their Growth Factor Requirements. *Proc Natl Acad Sci (USA)* 87: 463-467, 1990.

Baquet C, Ringen K: Health Policy: Gaps in Access, Deliver, and Utilization of the Pap Smear in the United States. *Milbank Q* 65: 322-347, 1987.

Barber HRK: Uterine Cancer (Prevention). *Cancer* 47: 1126-1132, 1981.

Barbone F, Austin H, Louv WC, et al: A Follow-Up Study of Methods of Contraception, Sexual Activity, and Rates of Trichomoniasis, Candidiasis, and Bacterial Vaginosis. *Am J Obstet Gynecol* 163: 510-514, 1990.

Bardales RH, Valente PT, Stanley MW: Cytology of Suture Granulomas in Post-Hysterectomy Vaginal Smears. *Diagn Cytopathol* 13: 336-338, 1995.

Barnes W, Delgado G, Kurman RJ, et al: Possible Prognostic Significance of Human Papillomavirus Type in Cervical Cancer. *Gynecol Oncol* 29: 267-273, 1988.

Barnes W, Woodworth C, Waggoner S, et al: Rapid Dysplastic Transformation of Human Genital Cells by Human Papillomavirus Type 18. *Gynecol Oncol* 38: 343-346, 1990.

Barr ML, Bertram EG: A Morphological Distinction Between Neurones of the Male and Female, and the Behaviour of the Nucleolar Satellite During Accelerated Nucleoprotein Synthesis. *Nature* 163: 676-677, 1949.

Barrasso R, De Brux J, Croissant O, et al: High Prevalence of Papillomavirus-Associated Penile Intraepithelial Neoplasia in Sexual Partners of Women With Cervical Intraepithelial Neoplasia. *N Engl J Med* 317: 916-923, 1987.

Barrett RJ II, Davos I, Leuchter RS, et al: Neuroendocrine Features in Poorly Differentiated and Undifferentiated Carcinomas of the Cervix. *Cancer* 60: 2325-2330, 1987.

Barrett TJ, Silbar JD: Genital Warts—A Venereal Disease. *JAMA* 154: 333-334, 1954.

Barron BA, Richart RM: A Statistical Model of the Natural History of Cervical Carcinoma Based on a Prospective Study of 557 Cases. *J Natl Cancer Inst* 41: 1343-1353, 1968.

Barron BA, Richart RM: An Epidemiologic Study of Cervical Neoplastic Disease: Based on a Self-Selected Sample of 7,000 Women in Barbados, West Indies. *Cancer* 27: 978-986, 1971.

Barron BA, Cahill MC, Richart RM: A Statistical Model of the Natural History of Cervical Neoplastic Disease: The Duration of Carcinoma In Situ. *Gynecol Oncol* 6: 196-205, 1978.

Barter JF, Orr JW, Holloway RW, et al: Psammoma Bodies in a Cervicovaginal Smear Associated With an Intrauterine Device. *J Reprod Med* 32: 147-148, 1987.

Barter JF: The Life and Contributions of Doctor George Nicholas Papanicolaou. *Surg Gynecol Obstet* 174: 530-532, 1992.

Barter RA, Waters ED: Cyto- and Histo-Morphology of Cervical Adenocarcinoma In Situ. *Pathology* 2: 33-40, 1970.

Bartlett JG, Onderdonk AB, Drude E, et al: Quantitative Bacteriology of the Vaginal Flora. *J Infect Dis* 136: 271-277, 1977.

Bartlett JG, Moon NE, Goldstein PR, et al: Cervical and Vaginal Bacterial Flora: Ecologic Niches in the Female Lower Genital Tract. *Am J Obstet Gynecol* 130: 658-661, 1978.

Bartlett JG, Polk BF: Bacterial Flora of the Vagina: Quantitative Study. *Rev Infect Dis* 6(Suppl 1): S67-S72, 1984.

Barton SE, Jenkins D, Cuzick J, et al: Effect of Cigarette Smoking on Cervical Epithelial Immunity: A Mechanism for Neoplastic Change? *Lancet* (ii): 652-654, 1988.

Barton SE, Hollingsworth A, Maddox PH, et al: Possible Cofactors in the Etiology of Cervical Intraepithelial Neoplasia: An Immunopathologic Study. *J Reprod Med* 34: 613-616, 1989a.

Barton SE, Jenkins D, Hollingsworth A, et al: An Explanation for the Problem of False Negative Cervical Smears. *Br J Obstet Gynaecol* 96: 482-485, 1989b.

Barua R, Matthews CD: Verrucous Carcinoma of the Uterine Cervix: A Case Report. *Acta Cytol* 27: 540-542, 1983.

Barwick KW, LiVolsi VA: Malignant Mixed Müllerian Tumors of the Uterus. A Clinicopathologic Assessment of 34 Cases. *Am J Surg Pathol* 3: 125-135, 1979.

Baschinsky D, Keyhani-Rofagha S, Hameed A: Exfoliative Cytology of Atypical Polypoid Adenomyoma: A Case Report. *Acta Cytol* 43: 637-640, 1999.

Bateman H, Yazici Y, Leff L, et al: Increased Cervical Dysplasia in Intravenous Cyclophosphamide-Treated Patients with SLE: A Preliminary Study. *Lupus* 9: 542-544, 2000.

Batrinos M, Eustratiades M: The Diagnostic Significance of Parabasal Cells: I. Correlation With the Clinical Diagnosis in 209 Patients. *Acta Cytol* 19: 97-99, 1975a.

Batrinos M, Eustratiades M: The Diagnostic Significance of Parabasal Cells: II. Rate of Their Disappearance and Reappearance Under Estrogen Administration and Withdrawal. *Acta Cytol* 19: 100-102, 1975b.

Bauer G: Lactobacilli-Mediated Control of Vaginal Cancer Through Specific Reactive Oxygen Species Interaction. *Med Hypotheses* 57: 252-257, 2001.

Bauer HM, Ting Y, Greer CE, et al: Genital Human Papillomavirus Infection in Female University Students as Determined by PCR-Based Method. *JAMA* 265: 472-477, 1991.

Bauer HM, Hildesheim A, Schiffman MH, et al: Determinants of Genital Human Papillomavirus Infection in Low-Risk Women in Portland, Oregon. *Sex Transm Dis* 20: 274-278, 1993.

Beaudenon S, Kremsdorf D, Croissant O, et al: A Novel Type of Human Papillomavirus Associated With Genital Neoplasias. *Nature* 321: 246-249, 1986.

Bechtold E, Reicher NB: The Relationship of Trichomonas Infestations to False Diagnoses of Squamous Carcinoma of the Cervix. *Cancer* 5: 442-457, 1952.

Becker E Jr, Edelweiss MI, Nonnenmacher B, et al: Prevalence and Epidemiologic Correlates of Atypical Squamous Cells of Undetermined Significance in Women at Low Risk for Cervical Cancer. *Diagn Cytopathol* 24: 276-282, 2001.

Becker SN: Keratin Bodies and Pseudokeratin Bodies Endometrial Adenocanthroma Versus "Ligneous" Vaginitis. *Acta Cytol* 20: 486-488, 1976.

Becker SN, Wong JY: Detection of Endometrial Stromal Sarcoma in Cervicovaginal Smears: Reports of Three Cases. *Acta Cytol* 25: 272-276, 1981.

Becker TM, Wheeler CM, McGough NS, et al: Contraceptive and Reproductive Risks for Cervical Dysplasia in Southwestern Hispanic and Non-Hispanic White Women. *Int J Epidemiol* 23: 913-922, 1994a.

Becker TM, Wheeler CM, McGough NS, et al: Sexually Transmitted Diseases and Other Risk Factors for Cervical Dysplasia Among Southwestern Hispanic and Non-Hispanic White Women. *JAMA* 271: 1181-1188, 1994b.

Bedrossian CWM, Gupta PK: Cytology in the Headlines. *Diagn Cytopathol* 11: 1-3, 1994.

Bedrossian UK, Fairfax MR, Ayers M: Pap Smear Follow-Up of Possible Role of Mucopurulent Exudate as a Prognosticator of a Negative Pregnancy Outcome. *Diagn Cytopathol* 21: 4-6, 1999.

Beeby AR, Wadehra V, Keating PJ, et al: A Retrospective Analysis of 94 Patients With CIN and False Negative Cervical Smears Taken at Colposcopy. *Cytopathology* 4: 331-337, 1993.

Beilby JOW, Bourne R, Guillebaud J, et al: Paired Cervical Smears: A Method of Reducing the False-Negative Rate in Population Screening. *Obstet Gynecol* 60: 46-48, 1982.

Belinson J, Qiao YL, Pretorius R, et al: Shanxi Province Cervical Cancer Screening Study: A Cross-Sectional Comparative Trial of Multiple Techniques to Detect Cervical Neoplasia. *Gynecol Oncol* 83: 439-444, 2001; erratum appears in *Gynecol Oncol* 84: 355, fig. 1, 2002.

Belleannée G, Brun JL, Trouette H, et al: Cytologic Findings in a Neovagina Created With Vecchietti's Technique for Treating Vaginal Aplasia. *Acta Cytol* 42: 945-948, 1998.

Bellina JH, Seto YJ: Pathological and Physical Investigations in CO_2 Laser—Tissue Interactions With Specific Emphasis on Cervical Intraepithelial Neoplasm. *Lasers Surg Med* 1: 47-69, 1980.

Benard VB, Lee NC, Piper M, et al: Race-Specific Results of Papanicolaou Testing and the Rate of Cervical Neoplasia in the National Breast and Cervical Cancer Early Detection Program, 1991-1998 (United States). *Cancer Causes Control* 12: 61-68, 2001.

Ben-Baruch G, Rothenberg D, Modan M, et al: Abnormal Cervical Cytologic, Colposcopic and Histologic Findings in Exposed DES Young Israeli Jewish Women. *Clin Exp Obstet Gynaecol* 18: 71-74, 1991.

Benda JA, Platz CE, Buchsbaum H, et al: Mucin Production in Defining Mixed Carcinoma of the Uterine Cervix: A Clinicopathologic Study. *Int J Gynecol Pathol* 4: 314-327, 1985.

Benda JA, Lamoreaux J, Johnson SR: Artifact Associated With the Use of Strong Iodine Solution (Lugol's) in Cone Biopsies. *Am J Surg Pathol* 11: 367-374, 1987.

Benda JA: Pathology of Cervical Carcinoma and Its Prognostic Implications. *Semin Oncol* 21: 3-11, 1994.

Bender S: Carcinoma In-Situ of Cervix in Sisters. *Br Med J* 1:502, 1976.

Benedet JH, Bender H, Jones H III, et al: FIGO Staging Classifications and Clinical Practice Guidelines in the Management of Gynecologic Cancers. *Int J Gynecol Obstet* 70: 209-262, 2000.

Benedet JL, Anderson GH: Cervical Intraepithelial Neoplasia in British Columbia: A Comprehensive Program for Detection, Diagnosis and Treatment. *Gynecol Oncol* 12(2 Pt 2): S280-S291, 1981.

Benedet JL, Selke PA, Nickerson KG: Colposcopic Evaluation of Abnormal Papanicolaou Smears in Pregnancy. *Am J Obstet Gynecol* 157: 932-937, 1987.

Benedet JL, Anderson GH, Matisic JP: A Comprehensive Program for Cervical Cancer Detection and Management. *Am J Obstet Gynecol* 166: 1254-1259, 1992.

Benjamin F, Guillaume AJ, Chao LP, et al: Vaginal Smuggling of Illicit Drug: A Case Requiring Obstetric Forceps for Removal of the Drug Container. *Am J Obstet Gynecol* 171: 1385-1387, 1994.

Benoit AG, Krepart GV, Lotocki RJ: Results of Prior Cytologic Screening in Patients With a Diagnosis of Stage I Carcinoma of the Cervix. *Am J Obstet Gynecol* 148: 690-694, 1984.

Benoit JL, Kini SR: "Arias-Stella Reaction"-Like Changes in Endocervical Glandular Epithelium in Cervical Smears During Pregnancy and Postpartum States—A Potential Diagnostic Pitfall. *Diagn Cytopathol* 14: 349-355, 1996.

Benoit MF, Hannigan EV, Smith RP, et al: Primary Gastrointestinal Cancers Presenting as Gynecologic Malignancies. *Gynecol Oncol* 95: 388-392, 2004.

Benson PA: Psammoma Bodies Found in Cervico-Vaginal Smears: Case Report. *Acta Cytol* 17: 64-66, 1973.

Benson PA: Cytologic Diagnosis in Primary Carcinoma of Fallopian Tube: Case Report and Review. *Acta Cytol* 18: 429-434, 1974.

Benson WL, Norris HJ: A Critical Review of the Frequency of Lymph Node Metastasis and Death from Microinvasive Carcinoma of the Cervix. *Obstet Gynecol* 49: 632-638, 1977.

Beral V: Cancer of the Cervix: A Sexually Transmitted Infection? *Lancet* (i): 1037-1040, 1974.

Beral V, Booth M: Predictions of Cervical Cancer Incidence and Mortality in England and Wales (Letter). *Lancet* (i): 495, 1986.

Beral V, Hannaford P, Kay C: Oral Contraceptive Use and Malignancies of the Genital Tract: Results from the Royal College of General Practitioners' Oral Contraception Study. *Lancet* (ii): 1331-1335, 1988.

Bercovici B, Diamant Y, Polishuk WZ: A Simplified Evaluation of Vaginal Cytology in Third Trimester Pregnancy Complications. *Acta Cytol* 17: 67-72, 1973.

Berek JS, Hacker NF, Fu Y-S, et al: Adenocarcinoma of the Uterine Cervix: Histologic Variables Associated With Lymph Node Metastasis and Survival. *Obstet Gynecol* 65: 46-52, 1985.

Berek JS: Simplification of the New Bethesda 2001 Classification System. *Am J Obstet Gynecol* 188: S2-S5, 2003.

Berg JW, Durfee GR: The Cytological Presentation of Endometrial Carcinoma. *Cancer* 11: 158-172, 1958.

Bergeron C, Ferenczy A, Shah KV, et al: Multicentric Human Papillomavirus Infections of the Female Genital Tract: Correlations of Viral Types With Abnormal Mitotic Figures, Colposcopic Presentation and Location. *Obstet Gynecol* 69: 736-742, 1987.

Bergeron C, Ferenczy A, Richart R: Underwear: Contamination by Human Papillomavirus. *Am J Obstet Gynecol* 162: 25-29, 1990.

Bergeron C, Barrasso R, Beaudenon S, et al: Human Papillomaviruses Associated With Cervical Intraepithelial Neoplasia: Great Diversity and Distinct Distribution in Low- and High-Grade Lesions. *Am J Surg Pathol* 16: 641-649, 1992.

Bergström R, Sparén P, Adami H-O: Trends in Cancer of the Cervix Uteri in Sweden Following Cytological Screening. *Br J Cancer* 81: 159-166, 1999.

Berkeley AS, LiVolsi VA, Schwartz PE: Advanced Squamous Cell Carcinoma of the Cervix With Recent Normal Papanicolaou Tests. *Lancet* (ii): 375-376, 1980.

Berkow SG: A Visit With Dr. George N. Papanicolaou. *Obstet Gynecol* 16: 243-252, 1960.

Berkowitz RS, Ehrmann RL, Lavizzo-Mourey R, et al: Invasive Cervical Carcinoma in Young Women. *Gynecol Oncol* 8: 311-316, 1979.

Bernal JN, Martinez MA, Dabancens A: Evaluation of Proposed Cytomorphologic Criteria for the Diagnosis of *Chlamydia trachomatis* in Papanicolaou Smears. *Acta Cytol* 33: 309-313, 1989.

Bernard HU: Coevolution of Papillomaviruses With Human Populations. *Trends Microbiol* 2: 140-143, 1994.

Berner A, Hoeg K, Oppedal BR: Smear Biopsies. A Cause of Negative Follow-up Biopsies in Patients With Premalignant Conditions of the Uterine Cervix. *Diagn Gynecol Obstet* 2: 99-102, 1980.

Bernstein A, Harris B: The Relationship of Dietary and Serum Vitamin A to the Occurrence of Cervical Intraepithelial Neoplasia in Sexually Active Women. *Am J Obstet Gynecol* 148: 309-312, 1984.

Bernstein SG, Voet RL, Guzick DS, et al: Prevalence of Papillomavirus Infection in Colposcopically Directed Cervical Biopsy Specimens in 1972 and 1982. *Am J Obstet Gynecol* 151: 577-581, 1985.

Bernstein SJ, Sanchez-Ramos L, Ndubisi B: Liquid-Based Cervical Cytologic Smear Study and Conventional Papanicolaou Smears: A Meta-Analysis of Prospective Studies Comparing Cytologic Diagnosis and Sample Adequacy. *Am J Obstet Gynecol* 185: 308-317, 2001.

Berry A: A Cytopathological and Histopathological Study of Bilharziasis of the Female Genital Tract. *J Pathol Bacteriol* 91: 325-338, 1966.

Berry A: Multispecies Schistosomal Infections of the Female Genital Tract Detected in Cytology Smears. *Acta Cytol* 20: 361-365, 1976.

Berry AV, Livni NM, Epstein N: Some Observations on Cell Morphology in the Cytodiagnosis of Endometrial Carcinoma. *Acta Cytol* 13: 530-533, 1969.

Bertini-Oliveira AM, Keppler MM, Luisi A, et al: Comparative Evaluation of Abnormal Cytology, Colposcopy and Histopathology in Preclinical Cervical Malignancy During Pregnancy. *Acta Cytol* 26: 636-644, 1982.

Bertolino JG, Rangel JE, Blake RL Jr, et al: Inflammation on the Cervical Papanicolaou Smear: The Predictive Value for Infection in Asymptomatic Women. *Family Medicine* 24: 447-452, 1992.

Bertolissi A, Cartei D, Turrin D, et al: Behaviour of Vaginal Epithelial Maturation and Sex Hormone Binding Globulin in Post-Menopausal Breast Cancer Patients During the First Year of Tamoxifin Therapy. *Cytopathology* 9: 263-270, 1998.

Bertrand M, Lickrish GM, Colgan TJ: The Anatomic Distribution of Cervical Adenocarcinoma In Situ: Implications for Treatment. *Am J Obstet Gynecol* 157: 21-25, 1987.

Besharov DJ, Gardiner KN: Trends in Teen Sexual Behavior. *Child Youth Serv Rev* 12: 341-367, 1997.

Besserer G: Was leistet die Zytodiagnostik bei der Erkennung des primären Tubenkarzinoms? [What Is the Value of Cytodiagnosis in Detection of Primary Carcinoma of the Fallopian Tube?] *Geburtsh u. Frauenk* 13: 660-671, 1953.

Betsill WL Jr, Clark AH: Early Endocervical Glandular Neoplasia. I. Histomorphology and Cytomorphology. *Acta Cytol* 30: 115-126, 1986.

Beutner KR: Therapeutic Approaches to Genital Warts. *Am J Med* 102(5A): 28-37, 1997a.

Beutner KR, Tyring S: Human Papillomavirus and Human Disease. *Am J Med* 102(5A): 9-15, 1997b.

Bevan IS, Blomfield PI, Johnson MA, et al: Oncogenic Viruses and Cervical Cancer. *Lancet* (i): 907-908, 1989.

Bewtra C: Columnar Cells in Posthysterectomy Vaginal Smears. *Diagn Cytopathol* 8: 342-345, 1992.

Bewtra C, Pathan M, Hashish H: Abnormal Pap Smears With Negative Follow-Up Biopsies: Improving Cytohistologic Correlations. *Diagn Cytopathol* 29: 200-202, 2003.

Beyer-Boon ME: Psammoma Bodies in Cervicovaginal Smears: An Indicator of the Presence of Ovarian Carcinoma. *Acta Cytol* 18: 41-44, 1974.

Beyer-Boon ME, Verdonk GW: The Identification of Atypical Reserve Cells in Smears of Patients With Premalignant and Malignant Changes in the Squamous and Glandular Epithelium of the Uterine Cervix. *Acta Cytol* 22: 305-311, 1978.

Bhagavan BS, Weinberg T: Cytopathologic Diagnosis of Metastatic Cancer by Cervical and Vaginal Smears With Report of a Case. *Acta Cytol* 13: 377-381, 1969.

Bhagavan BS, Gupta PK: Genital Actinomycosis and Intrauterine Contraceptive Devices: Cytopathologic Diagnosis and Clinical Significance. *Hum Pathol* 9: 567-578, 1978.

Bhagavan BS, Ruffier J, Shinn B: Pseudoactinomycotic Radiate Granules in the Lower Female Genital Tract: Relationship to the Splendore-Hoeppli Phenomenon. *Hum Pathol* 13: 898-904, 1982.

Bhambhani S: Egg of *Ascaris lumbricoides* in Cerviovaginal Smear (Letter). *Acta Cytol* 28: 92, 1984.

Bhambhani S, Milner A, Pant J, et al: Ova of *Taenia* and *Enterobius vermicularis* in Cervicovaginal Smears (Letter). *Acta Cytol* 29: 913-914, 1985.

Bhambhani S, Kashyap V: Amoebiasis: Diagnosis by Aspiration and Exfoliative Cytology. *Cytopathology* 12: 329-333, 2001.

Bibbo M, Bartels PH, Bahr GF, et al: Data Bank for Endometrial Cells: Operation of the TICAS File Project. *Acta Cytol* 14: 574-582, 1970.

Bibbo M, Keebler CM, Wied GL: Prevalence and Incidence Rates of Cervical Atypia: A Computerized File Analysis on 148,735 Patients. *J Reprod Med* 6: 184-188, 1971a.

Bibbo M, Keebler CM, Wied GL: The Cytologic Diagnosis of Tissue Repair in the Female Genital Tract. *Acta Cytol* 15: 133-137, 1971b.

Bibbo M, Harris MJ: Leptothrix. *Acta Cytol* 16: 2-4, 1972.

Bibbo M, Rice AM, Wied GL, et al: Comparative Specificity and Sensitivity of Routine Cytologic Examination and the Gravlee Jet Wash Technic for Diagnosis of Endometrial Changes. *Obstet Gynecol* 43: 253-256, 1974.

Bibbo M, Ali I, Al-Naqeeb M, et al: Cytologic Findings in Female and Male Offspring of DES Treated Mothers. *Acta Cytol* 19: 568-572, 1975.

Bibbo M: What You Should Know About Papanicolaou Smears. *Diagn Cytopathol* 5: 104-107, 1989a.

Bibbo M, Dytch HE, Alenghat E, et al: DNA Ploidy Profiles as Prognostic Indicators in CIN Lesions. *Am J Clin Pathol* 92: 261-265, 1989b.

Bibbo M, Klump WJ, DeCecco J, et al: Procedure for Immunocytochemical Detection of p16^{INK4a} Antigen in Thin-Layer, Liquid-Based Specimens. *Acta Cytol* 46: 25-29, 2002.

Bibbo M, DeCecco J, Kovatich AJ: p16^{INK4a}: an Adjunct Test in Liquid-Based Cytology. *Analy Quant Cytol Histol* 25 9-11, 2003.

Bibel DJ, Aly R, Lahti L, et al: Microbial Adherence to Vulvar Epithelial Cells. *J Med Microbiol* 23: 75-82, 1987.

Binder MA, Cates GW, Emson HE, et al: The Changing Concepts of Condyloma: A Retrospective Study of Colposcopically Directed Cervical Biopsies. *Am J Obstet Gynecol* 151: 213-219, 1985.

Birdsong GG: Pap Smear Adequacy: Is Our Understanding Satisfactory...Or Limited? *Diagn Cytopathol* 24: 79-81, 2000.

Bing Z, Levine L, Lucci JA, et al: Primary Small Cell Neuroendocrine Carcinoma of the Vagina: A Clinicopathologic Study. *Arch Pathol Lab Med* 128: 857-862, 2004.

Birch PK: Hormonal Cytology of Pregnancy. *Clin Obstet Gynecol* 4: 1062-1074, 1961.

Biscotti CV, Gero MA, Toddy SM, et al: Endocervical Adenocarcinoma In Situ: An Analysis of Cellular Features. *Diagn Cytopathol* 17: 326-332, 1997.

Biscotti CV, Hart WR: Apoptotic Bodies: A Consistent Morphologic Feature of Endocervical Adenocarcinoma In Situ. *Am J Surg Pathol* 22: 434-439, 1998.

Bishop JW, Marshall CJ, Bemtz JS: New Technologies in Gynecologic Cytology. *J Reprod Med* 45: 701-719, 2000.

Bishop JW: Cellularity of Liquid-Based, Thin-Layer Cervical Cytology Slides. *Acta Cytol* 46: 633-636, 2002.

Biswas LN, Manna B, Maiti PK, et al: Sexual Risk Factors for Cervical Cancer Among Rural Indian Women: A Case-Control Study. *Int J Epidemiol* 26: 491-495, 1997.

Bitterman P, Chun B, Kurman RJ: The Significance of Epithelial Differentiation in Mixed Mesodermal Tumors of the Uterus. A Clinicopathologic and Immunohistochemical Study. *Am J Surg Pathol* 14: 317-328, 1990.

Bjersing L, Rogo K, Evander M, et al: HPV 18 and Cervical Adenocarcinomas. *Anticancer Res* 11: 123-127, 1991.

Blackett AD, Conyers MG, Sharp F: The Incidence of HPV and EBV DNA in Normal, Koilocytic, and Dysplastic Cervical Tissue (Abstract). *Br J Obstet Gynecol* 101: 814, 1994.

Blackledge D, Russell R: "HPV Effect" in the Female Lower Genital Tract: A Community Study. *J Reprod Med* 43: 929-932, 1998.

Blandamura S, Boccato P, Spadaro M, et al: Endometrial Hyperplasia With Berrylike Squamous Metaplasia and Pilomatrixomalike Shadow Cells: Report of an Intriguing Cytohistologic Case. *Acta Cytol* 46: 887-892, 2002.

Block GB, Patterson B, Subar A: Fruit, Vegetables, and Cancer Prevention: A Review of the Epidemiologic Evidence. *Nutr Cancer* 18: 1-29, 1992.

Blohmer J-U, Schmalisch G, Klette I, et al: Increased Incidence of Cervical Intraepithelial Neoplasia in Young Women in the Mitte District, Berlin, Germany. *Acta Cytol* 43: 195-200, 1999.

Blumenfeld W, Holly EA, Mansur DL, et al: Histiocytes and the Detection of Endometrial Adenocarcinoma. *Acta Cytol* 29: 317-322, 1985.

Boardman LA, Adams AE, Peipert JF: Clinical Predictors of Cervical Intraepithelial Neoplasia 2 or Greater in Women With Mildly Abnormal Pap Smears. *J Reprod Med* 47: 891-896, 2002.

Boardman LA, Meinz H, Steinhoff MM et al: A Randomized Trial of the Sleeved Cytobrush and the Endocervical Curette. *Obstet Gynecol* 101: 426-430, 2003.

Boccardo F, Bruzzi P, Rubagotti A, et al: Estrogen-Like Action of Tamoxifen on Vaginal Epithelium in Breast Cancer Patients. *Oncology* 38: 281-285, 1981.

Böcking A, Hilgarth M, Auffermann W, et al: DNA-Cytometric Diagnosis of Prospective Malignancy in Borderline Lesions of the Uterine Cervix. *Acta Cytol* 30: 608-615, 1986.

Boddington MM, Spriggs AI, Cowdell RH: Adenocarcinoma of the Uterine Cervix: Cytological Evidence of a Long Preclinical Evolution. *Br J Obstet Gynecol* 83: 900-903, 1976.

Bogdanich W: The Pap Test Misses Much Cervical Cancer Through Lab's Errors. *The Wall Street Journal* 88: 1, 20, November 2, 1987a.

Bogdanich W: Physician's Carelessness With Pap Tests Is Cited in Procedure's High Failure Rate. *The Wall Street Journal* 88: 17, December 29, 1987b.

Bokhman JV: Two Pathogenetic Types of Endometrial Carcinoma. *Gynecol Oncol* 15: 10-17, 1983.

Bokhman JV, Urmancheyeva AF: Cervix Uteri Cancer and Pregnancy. *Eur J Gynaecol Oncol* 10: 406-411, 1989.

Bokun R, Perkovic M, Milasinovic D, et al: Cytology and Histopathology of Metastatic Malignant Melanoma Involving a Polyp on the Uterine Cervix: A Case Report. *Acta Cytol* 29: 612-615, 1985.

Bolla M, Berland E, Salvat J, et al: Fast Growing Cervical Carcinomas: A Retrospective Analysis of 20 IB-IIB FIGO. *Eur J Obstet Gynecol Reprod Biol* 90: 81-85, 2000.

Bollen LJ, Tjong-A-Hung SP, van der Velden J, et al: Human Papillomavirus DNA After Treatment of Cervical Dysplasia: Low Prevalence in Normal Cytologic Smears. *Cancer* 77: 2538-2543, 1996.

Bollen LJ, Tjong-A-Hung SP, van der Velden J, et al: Prediction of Recurrent and Residual Cervical Dysplasia by Human Papillomavirus Detection Among Patients With Abnormal Cytology. *Gynecol Oncol* 72: 199-201, 1999.

Bollmann R, Bollmann M, Henso D, et al: DNA Cytometry Confirms the Utility of the Bethesda System for the Classification of Papanicolaou Smears. *Cancer (Cancer Cytopathol)* 93: 222-228, 2001.

Bollmann R, Méhes G, Torka R, et al: Human Papillomavirus Typing and DNA Ploidy Determination of Squamous Intraepithelial Lesions in Liquid-Based Cytologic Samples. *Cancer (Cancer Cytopathol)* 99: 57-62, 2003a.

Bollmann R, Méhes G, Torka R, et al: Determination of Features Indicating Progression in Atypical Squamous Cells With Undetermined Significance. *Cancer (Cancer Cytopathol)* 99: 113-117, 2003b.

Bonacho I, Pita S, Gómez-Besteiro MI: The Importance of the Removal of the Intrauterine Device in Genital Colonization by *Actinomyces*. *Gynecol Obstet Invest* 52: 119-123, 2001.

Bonfiglio TA, Patten SF Jr, Woodworth FE: Fibroxanthosarcoma of the Uterine Cervix: Cytopathologic and Histopathologic Manifestations. *Acta Cytol* 20: 501-504, 1976.

Bonfiglio TA: Diagnostic Cytology of the Uterine Cervix: A Major Contribution and Classic Reference in Gynecologic Cytopathology. *Cancer (Cancer Cytopathol)* 81: 324-327, 1997.

Bonfiglio TA: Atypical Squamous Cells of Undetermined Significance: A Continuing Controversy (Editorial). *Cancer (Cancer Cytopathol)* 96: 125-127, 2002.

Bonfiglio TR, cited by Voelker R: Cytology Proficiency Testing Has Stumped the Experts. *JAMA* 270: 2779-2780, 1993.

Bonte J, Decoster JM, Ide P: Vaginal Cytological Evaluation as a Practical Link Between Hormone Blood Levels and Tumor Hormone Dependency in Exclusive Medroxyprogesterone Treatment of Recurrent or Metastatic Endometrial Adenocarcinoma. *Acta Cytol* 21: 218-224, 1977.

Boon ME, Baak JPA, Kurver PJH, et al: Adenocarcinoma In Situ of the Cervix: An Underdiagnosed Lesion. *Cancer* 48: 768-773, 1981a.

Boon ME, Kirk RS, Rietveld-Scheffers PEM: The Morphogenesis of Adenocarcinoma of the Cervix— A Complex Pathological Entity. *Histopathology* 5: 565-577, 1981b.

Boon ME, Kirk RS, De Graff GJC: Psammoma Bodies and Some Opportunistic Infections Detected in Cervical Smears of Women Fitted With an IUD. *Adv Contracep Deliv Syst* 2: 231-236, 1981c.

Boon ME, Hogewoning CJ, Tjiam KH, et al: Cervical Cytology and *Chlamydia trachomatis* Infection. *Arch Gynecol* 233: 131-140, 1983.

Boon ME, Alons-van Kordelaar JJM, Rietveld-Scheffers PEM: Consequences of the Introduction of Combined Spatula and Cytobrush Sampling for Cervical Cytology: Improvements in Smear Quality and Detection Rates. *Acta Cytol* 30: 264-270, 1986.

Boon ME, deGraaff Guilloud JC, Kob LP, et al: Efficacy of Screening for Cervical Squamous and Adenocarcinoma: The Dutch Experience. *Cancer* 59: 862-866, 1987.

Boon ME, Schneider A, Hogewoning CJA, et al: Penile Studies and Heterosexual Partners: Peniscopy, Cytology, Histology, and Immunocytochemistry. *Cancer* 61: 1652-1659, 1988.

Boon ME, deGraaff Guilloud JC, Rietveld WJ: Analysis of Five Sampling Methods for the Preparation of Cervical Smears. *Acta Cytol* 33: 843-848, 1989a.

Boon ME, Susanti I, Tasche MJA, et al: Human Papillomavirus (HPV)-Associated Male and Female Genital Carcinomas in a Hindu Population. *Cancer* 64: 559-565, 1989b.

Boon ME, Zeppa P, Ouwerkerk-Noordam E, et al: Exploiting the "Toothpick Effect" of the Cytobrush by Plastic Embedding of Cervical Samples. *Acta Cytol* 35: 57-63, 1991.

Boon ME, Kok LP: Neural Network Processing Can Provide Means to Catch Errors That Slip Through Human Screening of Pap Smears. *Diagn Cytopathol* 9: 411-416, 1993.

Boon ME, van Dunne FM, Vardaxis NJ: Recognition of Atypical Reserve Cell Hyperplasia in Cervical Smears and Its Diagnostic Significance. *Mod Pathol* 8: 786-794, 1995.

Boon ME, Suurmeijer AJH: *The Pap Smear*. 3rd ed. Harwood Academic Publishers, The Netherlands, 1996.

Boon ME, Ouwerkerk-Noordam E, van Leeuwen AW, et al: How to Improve Cytologic Screening for Endocervical Adenocarcinoma? *Eur J Gynaecol Oncol* 23: 481-485, 2002.

Boon ME, Ouwerkerk-Noordam E, van Leeuwen AWMF: Clinical and Diagnostic Significance of Blood in Cervical Smears. *Diagn Cytopathol* 28: 181-185, 2003.

Boon ME, Vinkestein A, van Binsbergen-Ingelse A, et al: Significance of MiB-1 Staining in Smears With Atypical Glandular Cells. *Diagn Cytopathol* 31: 77-82, 2004.

Boone CW, Kelloff GJ, Steele VE: Natural History of Intraepithelial Neoplasia in Humans With Implications for Cancer Chemoprevention Strategy. *Cancer Res* 52: 1651-1659, 1992.

Boquet-Jiménez E, San Cristóbal AA: Cytologic and Microbiologic Aspects of Vaginal Torulopsis. *Acta Cytol* 22: 331-334, 1978.

Boram LH, Eklandson RA, Hajdu SI: Mesodermal Mixed Tumor of the Uterus: A Cytologic, Histologic, and Electron Microscopic Correlation. *Cancer* 30: 1295-1306, 1972.

Boras VF, Duggan MA: Cervical Dyskeratotic Cells as Predictors of Condylomatous Changes on Biopsy. *Acta Cytol* 33: 223-227, 1989.

Borg AJ, Medley G, Garland SM: Polymerase Chain Reaction: A Sensitive Indicator of the Prevalence of Human Papillomavirus DNA in a Population With Sexually Transmitted Disease. *Acta Cytol* 39: 654-658, 1995.

Boring C, Silverberg SG: Annual Cancer Statistics. *CA: Cancer J Clin* Volumes 20-44, years 1970-1994.

Boris S, Barbés C: Role Played by Lactobacilli in Controlling the Population of Vaginal Pathogens. *Microbes Infection* 2: 543-546, 2000.

Bornstein J, Stinson-Carter T, Kaufman RH: Curschmann's Spiral in an Endocervical Brushing. *Acta Cytol* 31: 530-531, 1987.

Bornstein J, Rahat MA, Abramovici H: Etiology of Cervical Cancer: Current Concepts. *Obstet Gynecol* 50: 146-154, 1995.

Bornstein J, Bahat-Steremsus J: Predictive Factors for Noncompliance With Follow-Up Among Women Treated for Cervical Intraepithelial Neoplasia. *Gynecol Obstet Invest* 58: 202-206, 2004.

Boronow RC: Death of the Papanicolaou Smear? A Tale of Three Reasons. *Am J Obstet Gynecol* 179: 391-396, 1998.

Borst M, Butterworth CE, Baker V, et al: Human Papillomavirus Screening for Women With Atypical Papanicolaou Smears. *J Reprod Med* 36: 95-99, 1991.

Bos AB, van Ballegooijen M, van Oortmarssen GJ, et al: Non-Progression of Cervical Intraepithelial Neoplasia Estimated from Population-Screening Data. *Br J Cancer* 75: 124-130, 1997.

Bos AB, van Ballegooijen M, Elske van den Akker-van Marle M, et al: Endocervical Status Is Not Predictive of the Incidence of Cervical Cancer in the Years After Negative Smears. *Am J Clin Pathol* 115: 851-855, 2001.

Bosch FX, Muñoz N, de Sanjosé S, et al: Risk Factors for Cervical Cancer in Columbia and Spain. *Int J Cancer* 52: 750-758, 1992.

Bosch FX, Manos MM, Muñoz N, et al: Prevalence of Human Papillomavirus in Cervical Cancer: A Worldwide Perspective. International Biological Study on Cervical Cancer (IBSCC) Study Group. *J Natl Cancer Inst* 87: 796-802, 1995.

Bosch FX, Castellsagué X, Muñoz N, et al: Male Sexual Behavior and Human Papillomavirus DNA: Key Risk Factors for Cervical Cancer in Spain. *J Natl Cancer Inst* 88: 1060-1067, 1996.

Bosch FX, Lorincz A, Muñoz N, et al: The Causal Relation Between Human Papillomavirus and Cervical Cancer. *J Clin Pathol* 55: 244-265, 2002a.

Bosch FX, de Sanjosé S: Human Papillomavirus in Cervical Cancer. *Curr Oncol Reports* 4: 175-183, 2002b.

Bosch MMC, Rietveld-Scheffers PEM, Boon ME: Characteristics of False-Negative Smears Tested in the Normal Screening Situation. *Acta Cytol* 36: 711-716, 1992.

Boschann H-W: Cytometry on Normal and Abnormal Endometrial Cells (Symposium on Endometrial Cytology. A: Endometrial Cancer Cytology). *Acta Cytol* 2: 520-522. 1958.

Bose S, Kannan V, Kline TS: Abnormal Endocervical Cells: Really Abnormal? Really? *Am J Clin Pathol* 101: 708-713, 1994.

Boshart M, Gissmann L, Ikenberg H, et al: A New Type of Papillomavirus DNA, Its Presence in Genital Cancer Biopsies and in Cell Lines Derived from Genital Cancer. *EMBO J* 3: 1151-1157, 1984.

Boskey ER, Cone RA, Whaley KH, et al: Origins of Vaginal Acidity: High D/L Lactate Ratio Is Consistent With Bacteria Being the Primary Source. *Hum Reprod* 16: 1809-1813, 2001.

Bottles K: Pap Smear Classification: A Tricky Business. *Cytopathology Annual* (1991): 81-87, 1991.

Bottles K, Reiter RC, Steiner AL, et al: Problems Encountered With the Bethesda System: The University of Iowa Experience. *Obstet Gynecol* 78: 410-414, 1991.

Bourgain C, Amy J-J, Wallon J, et al: A Tale of Medical Shopping or the Hazards of Repetitious Cytological Screening of the Cervix (Case Report). *Gynecol Obstet Invest* 59: 41-42, 2005.

Bourne RG, Grove WD: Invasive Carcinoma of the Cervix in Queensland: Change in Incidence and Mortality, 1959-1980. *Med J Aust* 1: 156-158, 1983.

Bousfield L, Pacey F, Young Q, et al: Expanded Cytologic Criteria for the Diagnosis of Adenocarcinoma In Situ of the Cervix and Related Lesions. *Acta Cytol* 24: 283-296, 1980.

Boutselis JG, Thompson JN: Clinical Aspects of Primary Carcinoma of the Fallopian Tube. *Am J Obstet Gynecol* 111: 98-101, 1971.

Boutselis JG: Intraepithelial Carcinoma of the Cervix Associated With Pregnancy. *Obstet Gynecol* 40: 657-666, 1972.

Bowen JT: Precancerous Dermatoses: A Study of Two Cases of Chronic Atypical Epithelial Proliferation. *J Cutaneous Dis* 30: 241-255, 1912.

Boyce JG, Lu T, Nelson JH Jr, et al: Oral Contraceptives and Cervical Carcinoma. *Am J Obstet Gynecol* 128: 761-766, 1977.

Boyd JT, Doll R: A Study of the Aetiology of Carcinoma of the Cervix Uteri. *Br J Cancer* 18: 419-434, 1964.

Boyes DA, Fidler KH, Lock DR: Significance of In Situ Carcinoma of the Uterine Cervix. *Br Med J* 1: 203-205, 1962.

Boyle DCM, Smith JR: Infection and Cervical Intraepithelial Neoplasia. *Int J Gynecol Cancer* 9: 177-186, 1999.

Brainard JA, Hart WR: Adenoid Basal Epitheliomas of the Uterine Cervix: A Reevaluation of Distinctive Cervical Basaloid Lesions Currently Classified as Adenoid Basal Carcinoma and Adenoid Basal Hyperplasia. *Am J Surg Pathol* 22: 965-975, 1998.

Branca M, Migliore G, Giuliani M, et al: Using the Number of Koilocytes to Predict HIV Serostatus in Women With HPV-Associated SIL. *Acta Cytol* 44: 1000-1004, 2000.

Brand E, Berek JS, Hacker NF: Controversies in the Management of Cervical Adenocarcinoma. *Obstet Gynecol* 71: 261-269, 1988.

Braun V, Gavey N: Exploring the Possibility of Sexual-Behavioural Primary Prevention Interventions for Cervical Cancer. *Aust NZ J Public Health* 22: 353-359, 1998.

Braun V, Gavey N: 'With the Best of Reasons': Cervical Cancer Prevention Policy and the Suppression of Sexual Risk Factor Information. *Soc Sci Med* 48: 1463-1474, 1999.

Breathnach CS: Biographical Sketches No. 29—Papanicolaou. *Irish Med J* 76: 220, 1983.

Brenner RW, Gehring SW II: Pelvic Actinomycosis in the Presence of an Endocervical Contraceptive Device: Report of a Case. *Obstet Gynecol* 29: 71-73, 1967.

Brescia RJ, Jenson AB, Lancaster WD, et al: Progress in Pathology: The Role of Human Papillomaviruses in the Pathogenesis and Histologic Classification of Precancerous Lesions of the Cervix. *Hum Pathol* 17: 552-559, 1986.

Brewer JI, Guderian AM: Diagnosis of Uterine-Tube Carcinoma by Vaginal Cytology. *Obstet Gynecol* 8: 664-672, 1956.

Briggs RM: Dysplasia and Early Neoplasia of the Uterine Cervix: A Review. *Obstet Gynecol Surv* 34: 70-99, 1979.

Brink A, DuToit JP, Deale CJC: In Search of More Representative Cervical Cytology: A Preliminary Prospective Study. *S Afr Med J* 76: 55-57, 1989.

Brinton LA, Huggins GR, Lehman HF, et al: Long-Term Use of Oral Contraceptives and Risk of Invasive Cervical Cancer. *Int J Cancer* 38: 339-344, 1986a.

Brinton LA, Schairer C, Haenszel W, et al: Cigarette Smoking and Invasive Cervical Cancer. *JAMA* 255: 3265-3269, 1986b.

Brinton LA, Fraumeni JF Jr: Epidemiology of Uterine Cervical Cancer. *J Chronic Dis* 39: 1051-1065, 1986c.

Brinton LA, Hamman RF, Huggins GR, et al: Sexual and Reproductive Risk Factors for Invasive Squamous Cell Cervical Cancer. *J Natl Cancer Inst* 79: 23-30, 1987a.

Brinton LA, Tashima KT, Lehman HF, et al: Epidemiology of Cervical Cancer by Cell Type. *Cancer Res* 47: 1706-1711, 1987b.

Brinton LA, Reeves WC, Brenes MM, et al: Parity as a Risk Factor for Cervical Cancer. *Am J Epidemiol* 130: 486-496, 1989a.

Brinton LA, Reeves WC, Brenes MM, et al: The Male Factor in the Etiology of Cervical Cancer Among Sexually Monogamous Women. *Int J Cancer* 44: 199-203, 1989b.

Brinton LA: Oral Contraceptive and Cervical Neoplasia. *Contraception* 43: 581-595, 1991.

Brinton LA: Epidemiology of Cervical Cancer—Overview. In: Bosch, FX, Shah KV, Meheus A, eds. *The Epidemiology of Cervical Cancer and Human Papillomavirus.* Vol. 3. International Agency for Research on Cancer, Lyon, 3-23, 1992.

Brinton LA, Herrero R, Reeves WC, et al: Risk Factors for Cervical Cancer by Histology. *Gynecol Oncol* 51: 301-306, 1993.

Briselli MF: Trying to Drain the "ASCUS" Swamp (Letter). *Diagn Cytopathol* 13: 278-279, 1995.

Brisson J, Morin c, Fortier M, et al: Risk Factor for Cervical Intraepithelial Neoplasia: Differences between Low- and High- Grade Lesions. *Am J Epidemiol* 140: 700-710, 1994.

Britsch CJ, Azar HA: Estrogen Effect in Exfoliated Vaginal Cells Following Treatment With Digitalis: A Case Report With Experimental Observations in Mice. *Am J Obstet Gynecol* 85: 989-993, 1963.

Brock KE, MacLennan R, Brinton LA, et al: Smoking and Infectious Agents and Risk of In Situ Cervical Cancer in Sydney, Australia. *Cancer Res* 49: 4925-4928, 1989.

Broders AC: Carcinoma In Situ Contrasted With Benign Penetrating Epithelium. *JAMA* 99: 1670-1674, 1932.

Brogi E, Tambouret R, Bell DA: Classification of Benign Endometrial Glandular Cells in Cervical Smears from Postmenopausal Women. *Cancer (Cancer Cytopathol)* 96: 60-66, 2002.

Brooks SE: Cervical Cancer Screening and the Older Woman. *Cancer Practice* 4: 125-129. 1996.

Broso PR, Buffetti G: George Nicholas Papanicolaou. *Minerva Ginecologica* 45: 511-516, 1993.

Brotzman GL, Julian TM: The Minimally Abnormal Papanicolaou Smear. *Am Family Physician* 53: 1154-1162, 1996.

Brown FM, Faquin WC, Sun D, et al: LSIL Biopsies After HSIL Smears: Correlation With High-Risk HPV and Greater Risk of HSIL on Follow-Up. *Am J Clin Pathol* 112: 765-768, 1999.

Brown J: Nutrition During and After Cancer Treatment: A Guide for Informed Choices by Cancer Survivors. *CA: Cancer J Clin* 51: 153-187, 2001.

Brown LJR, Wells M: Cervical Glandular Atypia Associated With Squamous Intraepithelial Neoplasia: A Premalignant Lesion? *J Clin Pathol* 39: 22-28, 1986.

Brown LJR, Griffin NR, Wells M: Cytoplasmic Reactivity With the Monoclonal Antibody HMFG1 as a Marker of Cervical Glandular Atypia. *J Pathol* 151: 203-208, 1987.

Brown MS, Phillips GL Jr: Management of the Mildly Abnormal Pap Smear: A Conservative Approach. *Gynecol Oncol* 22: 149-153, 1985.

Brown ST, Nalley JF, Kraus SJ: Molluscum Contagiosum. *Sex Transm Dis* 8: 227-234, 1981.

Bruner KS, Davey DD: ASC-US and HPV Testing in Women Aged 40 Years and Over. *Diagn Cytopathol* 31: 358-361, 2004.

Brunham RC, Paavonen J, Stevens CE, et al: Mucopurulent Cervicitis—The Ignored Counterpart in Women of Urethritis in Men. *N Engl J Med* 311: 1-6, 1984.

Bucchi L, Zani J, Pierri C, et al: Cervical Screening Behavior of Women With Atypical Squamous Cells of Underminded Significance (ASCUS). *Diagn Cytopathol* 24: 21-27, 2001.

Buckley CH, Butler EB, Fox H: Cervical Intraepithelial Neoplasia. *J Clin Pathol* 35: 1-13, 1982.

Buckley CH, Beards CS, Fox H: Pathological Prognostic Indicators in Cervical Cancer With Particular Reference to Patients Under the Age of 40 Years. *Br J Obstet Gynaecol* 95: 47-56, 1988.

Buckley CH, Fox H: Carcinoma of the Cervix. In: Anthony PP, Woolf N, eds. *Recent Advances in Histopathology.* Vol 14. Churchill Livingstone, Edinburgh, 63-78, 1989.

Buckley CH, Herbert A, Johnson J, et al: Borderline Nuclear Changes in Cervical Smears: Guidelines on Their Recognition and Management. *J Clin Pathol* 47: 481-492, 1994.

Buckley JD, Harris RW, Doll R: Case-Control Study of the Husbands of Women With Dysplasia or Carcinoma of the Cervix Uteri. *Lancet* (ii): 1010-1015, 1981.

Buckovsky A, Zidovsky J: Cytologic Phenomena Accompaning Uterine Cervix Electrocoagulation. *Acta Cytol* 29: 353-362, 1985.

Bulten J, de Wilde PCM, Boonstra H, et al: Proliferation in "Atypical" Atrophic Pap Smears. *Gynecol Oncol* 79: 225-229, 2000a.

Bulten J, de Wilde PC, Schijf C, et al: Decreased Expression of Ki-67 in Atrophic Cervical Epithelium of Post-Menopausal Women. *J Pathol* 190: 545-553, 2000b.

Buntinx F, Brouwers M: Relation Between Sampling Device and Detection of Abnormality in Cervical Smears: A Meta-Analysis of Randomised and Quasi-Randomised Studies. *Br Med J* 313: 1285-1290, 1996.

Bur M, Knowles K, Pekow P, et al: Comparison of ThinPrep Preparations With Conventional Cervicovaginal Smears: Practical Considerations. *Acta Cytol* 39: 631-642, 1995.

Burger MP, Hollema H, Gouw AS: Cigarette Smoking and Human Papillomavirus in Patients With Reported Cervical Cytological Abnormality. *Br Med J* 306: 749-752, 1993.

Burger MP, Hollema H, Pieters WJ, et al: Epidemiological Evidence of Cervical Intraepithelial Neoplasia Without the Presence of Human Papillomavirus. *Br J Cancer* 73: 831-836, 1996.

Burger RA, Monk BJ, Kurosaki T, et al: Human Papillomavirus Type 18: Association With Poor Prognosis in Early Stage Cervical Cancer. *J Natl Cancer Inst* 88: 1361-1368, 1996.

Burghardt E: Latest Aspects of Precancerous Lesions in Squamous and Columnar Epithelium of the Cervix. *Int J Gynecol Obstet* 8: 573-580, 1970.

Burghardt E: *Early Histological Diagnosis of Cervical Cancer.* Saunders, Philadelphia, pp. 319-362, 1973.

Burghardt E: Premalignant Conditions of the Cervix. *Clin Obstet Gynaecol* 3: 257-294, 1976.

Burghardt E, Östör AG: Site and Origin of Squamous Cervical Cancer: A Histomorphologic Study. *Obstet Gynecol* 62: 117-127, 1983.

Burghardt E, Girardi F, Lahousen M, et al: Microinvasive Carcinoma of the Uterine Cervix (International Federation of Gynecology and Obstetrics IA). *Cancer* 67: 1037-1045, 1991.

Burja IT, Thompson SK, Sawyer WL Jr, et al: Atypical Glandular Cells of Undetermined Significance on Cervical Smears: A Study With Cytohistologic Correlation. *Acta Cytol* 43: 351-356, 1999.

Burja IT, Shurbaji MS: Clinical Impact of Identifying *Trichomonas vaginalis* on Cervicovaginal (Papanicolaou) Smears. *Diagn Cytopathol* 24: 195-199, 2001.

Burk JR, Lehman HF, Wolf FS: Inadequacy of Papanicolaou Smears in the Detection of Endometrial Cancer. *N Engl J Med* 291: 191-192, 1974.

Burk RD, Kadish AS, Calderin S: Human Papillomavirus Infection of the Cervix Detected by Cervicovaginal Lavage and Molecular Hybridization: Correlation With Biopsy Results and Papanicolaou Smear. *Am J Obstet Gynecol* 154: 982-989, 1986.

Burk RD, Ho GY, Beardsley L, et al: Sexual Behavior and Partner Characteristics Are the Predominant Risk Factors for Genital Human Papillomavirus Infection in Young Women. *J Infect Dis* 174: 679-689, 1996a.

Burk RD, Kelly P, Feldman J, et al: Declining Prevalence of Cervicovaginal Human Papillomavirus Infection With Age Is Independent of Other Risk Factors. *Sex Transm Dis* 23: 333-341, 1996b.

Burk RD: Pernicious Papillomavirus Infection (Editorial). *N Engl J Med* 341: 1687-1688, 1999.

Burkett BJ, Peterson CM, Birch LM, et al: The Relationship Between Contraceptives, Sexual Practices, and Cervical Human Papillomavirus Infection Among a College Population. *J Clin Epidemiol* 45: 1295-1302, 1992.

Burks RT, Schwartz AM, Wheeler JE, et al: Late Recurrence of Clear-Cell Adenocarcinoma of the Cervix: Case Report. *Obstet Gynecol* 76: 525-527, 1990.

Burkman R, Schlesselman S, McCaffrey L, et al: The Relationship of Genital Tract Actinomycetes and the Development of Pelvic Inflammatory Disease. *Am J Obstet Gynecol* 143: 585-589, 1982.

Burnett AF: Atypical Glandular Cells of Undetermined Significance Pap Smears: Appropriate Evaluation and Management. *Curr Opin Obstet Gynecol* 12: 33-37, 2000.

Burns DA: 'Warts and All'— the History and Folklore of Warts: A Review. *J R Soc Med* 85: 37-40, 1992.

Burrows DA, Howell LP, Hinrichs S, et al: Cytomorphologic Features in the Diagnosis of Human Papillomavirus Infection of the Uterine Cervix. *Acta Cytol* 34: 737-738, 1990.

Burton J, Cadieux PA, Reid G: Improved Understanding of the Bacterial Vaginal Microbiota of Women Before and After Probiotic Instillation. *Appl Environ Microbiol* 69: 97-101, 2003.

Burton JL, Wells M: The Effect of Phytoestrogens on the Female Genital Tract. *J Clin Pathol* 55: 401-407, 2002.

Buscema J, Woodruff JD: Significance of Neoplastic Atypicalities in Endocervical Epithelium. *Gynecol Oncol* 17: 356-362, 1984.

Buschmann C, Hergenrader M, Porter D: Keratin bodies—A Clue in the Cytological Detection of Endometrial Adenoacanthoma: Report of Two Cases. *Acta Cytol* 18: 297-299, 1974.

Busnach G, Civati G, Brando B, et al: Viral and Neoplastic Changes of the Lower Genital Tract in Women With Renal Allografts. *Transplant Proc* 25: 1389-1390, 1993.

Busseniers AE, Sidawy MK: Inflammatory Atypia on Cervical Smears: A Diagnostic Dilemma for the Gynecologist. *J Reprod Med* 36: 85-88, 1991.

Butler EB, Taylor DS: The Postnatal Smear. *Acta Cytol* 17: 237-240, 1973.

Buttenberg D, Stoll P: Cyto- and Histomorphology of Carcinoma of the Gartnerian Duct. *Acta Cytol* 4: 344-346, 1960.

Butterworth CE Jr, Hatch KD, Gore H, et al: Improvement in Cervical Dysplasia Associated With Folic Acid Therapy in Users of Oral Contraceptives. *Am J Clin Nutr* 35: 73-82, 1982.

Butterworth CE Jr: Effect of Folate on Cervical Cancer: Synergism Among Risk Factors. *Ann NY Acad Sci* 669: 293-299, 1992a.

Butterworth CE Jr, Hatch KD, Macaluso M, et al: Folate Deficiency and Cervical Dysplasia. *JAMA* 267: 528-533, 1992b.

Butterworth CE Jr, Hatch KD, Soong S-J, et al: Oral Folic Acid Supplementation for Cervical Dysplasia: A Clinical Intervention Trial. *Am J Obstet Gynecol* 166: 803-809, 1992c.

Byrne MA, Turner MJ, Griffiths M: Evidence That Patients Presenting With Dyskaryotic Cervical Smears Should Be Screened for Genital-Tract Infections Other Than Human Papillomavirus Infection. *Eur J Obstet Gynecol Reprod Biol* 41: 129-133, 1991.

C

Cabanne F, Michiels R, Mottot C, et al: Ciliated Bodies in Gynecologic Cytopathology: Parasite or Cellular Debris? *Acta Cytol* 19: 407-410, 1975.

Cahill LA, Stastny JF, Frable WJ: Primary Lymphoma of the Endometrium: A Report of Two Cases Diagnosed on Cervicovaginal Smears. *Acta Cytol* 41: 533-538, 1997.

Cahill LA, Brainard JA, Frable WJ: Life Without ASCUS. The Cytotechnologist's and Cytopatholgist's Perspective (Abstract). *Acta Cytol* 44: 853-854, 2000.

Cain JM, Howett MK: Preventing Cervical Cancer. *Science* 288: 1753-1755, 2000.

Calore EE, Cavaliere MJ, Calore NMP: Squamous Intraepithelial Lesions in Cervical Smears of Human Immunodeficiency Virus-Seropositive Adolescents. *Diagn Cytopathol* 18: 91-92, 1998.

Calore EE, Pereira SMM, Cavaliere MJ: Progression of Cervical Lesions in HIV-Seropositive Women: A Cytological Study. *Diagn Cytopathol* 24: 117-119, 2001.

Campbell WC: A Historic Photomicrograph of a Parasite (*Trichomonas vaginalis*). *Trends Parasitol* 17: 499-500, 2001.

Campion MJ, Singer A, Clarkson PK, et al: Increased Risk of Cervical Neoplasia in Consorts of Men With Penile Condylomata Acuminata. *Lancet* (i): 943-946, 1985.

Campion MJ, Cuzick J, McCance DJ: Progressive Potential of Mild Cervical Atypia: Prospective Cytological, Colposcopic, and Virological Study. *Lancet* (ii): 237-240, 1986.

Campion MJ, McCance DJ, Mitchell HS, et al: Subclinical Penile Human Papillomavirus Infection and Dysplasia in Consorts of Women With Cervical Neoplasia. *Genitourin Med* 64: 90-99, 1988.

Campo MS: HPV and Cancer: The Story Unfolds. *Trends in Microbiol* 6: 424-426, 1998.

Campos R de C J: Persistent Tumor Cells in the Vaginal Smears and Prognosis of Cancer of the Radiated Cervix. *Acta Cytol* 14: 519-522, 1970.

Canavan TP, Doshi NR: Cervical Cancer. *Am Fam Physician* 61: 1369-1376, 2000.

Canda T, Ozkal S, Ozer E: Curschmann's Spirals in Cyst Fluid Associated With a Teratoma of the Ovary: A Case Report. *Acta Cytol* 45: 441-444, 2001.

Cangiarella JF, Chhieng DC: Atypical Glandular Cells—An Update. *Diagn Cytopathol* 29: 271-279, 2003.

Cannistra SA, Niloff JM: Cancer of the Uterine Cervix. *N Engl J Med* 334: 1030-1038, 1996.

Cannon JM, Blythe JG: Comparison of the Cytobrush Plus Plastic Spatula With the Cervex Brush for Obtaining Endocervical Cells. *Obstet Gynecol* 82: 569-572, 1993.

Caorsi J, Figueroa CD: Langerhans' Cell Density in the Normal Exocervical Epithelium and in the Cervical Intraepithelial Neoplasia. *Br J Obstet Gynaecol* 93: 993-998, 1986.

Capaldo G, LeGolvan DP, Dramczyk JE: Hematoidin Crystals in Cervicovaginal Smears: Review of 27 Cases Seen in One Year. *Acta Cytol* 27: 237-240, 1983.

Capasso LL: Antiquity of Cancer. *Int J Cancer* 113: 2-13, 2005.

Cardillo M, Hagan R, Abadi J, et al: CD4 T-Cell Count, Viral Load, and Squamous Intraepithelial Lesions in Women Infected With the Human Immunodeficiency Virus. *Cancer (Cancer Cytopathol)* 93: 111-114, 2001.

Cardillo MR, Forte F: The Diagnostic Value of Citology [sic] in a Case of Lymphoma of the Uterine Cervix. *Eur J Gynaecol Oncol* 8: 597-602, 1987.

Cariani DJ, Guderian AM: Gestational Atypia in Endocervical Polyps—The Arias-Stella Reaction. *Am J Obstet Gynecol* 95: 589-590, 1966.

Carmichael DE: *The Pap Smear: Life of George N. Papanicolaou.* Charles C Thomas, Publisher, Springfield, Illinois, 1973.

Carmichael DE: Prolapse of the Fallopian Tube into the Vaginal Vault. *Am J Obstet Gynecol* 15: 266-267, 1976.

Carmichael E: Dr. Papanicolaou and the Pap Smear. *Alab J Med Sci* 21: 101-104, 1984.

Carmichael JA, Jeffrey JF, Steele HD, et al: The Cytologic History of 245 Patients Developing Invasive Cervical Carcinoma. *Am J Obstet Gynecol* 148: 685-690, 1984.

Carmichael JA, Clarke DH, Moher D, et al: Cervical Carcinoma in Women Aged 34 and Younger. *Am J Obstet Gynecol* 154: 264-269, 1986.

Carmichael R, Jeaffreson BL: Basal Cells in the Epithelium of the Human Cervical Canal. *J Pathol Bacteriol* 49: 63-69, 1939.

Carmichael R, Jeaffreson BL: Squamous Metaplasia of the Columnar Epithelium in the Human Cervix. *J Pathol* 52: 173-186, 1941.

Carozzi FM, Cariaggi MP, Bonardi L, et al: Clinical Impact (Cost-Effectiveness) of Qualifying Atypical Squamous Cells of Undetermined Significance (ASCUS) in Cases Favoring a Reactive or Dysplastic Process. *Diagn Cytopathol* 29: 4-7, 2003.

Carr J, Gyorfi T: Human Papillomavirus: Epidemiology, Transmission, and Pathogenesis. *Clin Lab Med* 20: 235-255, 2000.

Carr RF: Response to Editorial on the Pap Smear as a Cancer Screening Test (Letter). *Diagn Cytopathol* 10: 95, 1994.

Carson HJ: Unpublished observations. 1990.

Carson HJ, DeMay RM: The Mode Ages of Women With Cervical Dysplasia. *Obstet Gynecol* 82: 430-434, 1993.

Carter JJ, Koutsky LA, Wipf GC, et al: The Natural History of Human Papillomavirus Type 16 Capsid Antibodies Among a Cohort of University Women. *J Infect Dis* 174: 927-936, 1996.

Casas-Cordero M, Morin C, Roy M, et al: Origin of the Koilocyte in Condylomata of the Human Cervix: Ultrastructural Study. *Acta Cytol* 25: 383-392, 1981.

Case TC: Primary Adenocarcinoma of the Fallopian Tube. *NY State J Med* 51:1429-1432, 1951.

Casey MB, Caudill JL, Salomão DR: Cervicovaginal (Papanicolaou) Smear Findings in Patients With Malignant Mixed Müllerian Tumors. *Diagn Cytopathol* 28: 245-249, 2003.

Casper GR, Östör AG, Quinn MA: A Clinicopathologic Study of Glandular Dysplasia of the Cervix. *Gynecol Oncol* 64: 166-170, 1997.

Casper MJ, Clarke AE: Making the Pap Smear into the 'Right Tool' for the Job: Cervical Cancer Screening in the USA, Circa 1940-95. *Soc Studies Sci* 28: 255-290, 1998.

Cassano PA, Saigo PE, Hajdu SI: Comparison of Cytohormonal Status of Postmenopausal Women With Cancer to Age-Matched Controls. *Acta Cytol* 30: 93-98, 1986.

Cassard SD, Weisman CS, Plichta SB, et al: Physician Gender and Women's Preventive Services. *J Women's Health* 6: 199-207, 1997.

Casselman CW, Crutcher RA, Jadusingh IH: Use of Water-Soluble Gel in Obtaining the Cervical Cytologic Smear (Letter). *Acta Cytol* 41: 1861-1862, 1997.

Castellsagué X, Bosch FX, Muñoz N, et al: Male Circumcision, Penile Human Papillomavirus Infection, and Cervical Cancer in Female Partners. *N Engl J Med* 346: 1105-1112, 2002.

Castle PE, Hillier SL, Rabe LK, et al: An Association of Cervical Inflammation With High-Grade Cervical Neoplasia in Women Infected With Oncogenic Human Papillomavirus (HPV). *Cancer Epidemiol Biomarkers Prev* 10: 1021-1027, 2001.

Castle PE, Wacholder S, Lorincz A, et al: A Prospective Study of High-Grade Cervical Neoplasia Risk Among Human Papillomavirus-Infected Women. *J Natl Cancer Inst* 94: 1406-1414, 2002a.

Castle PE, Wacholder S, Sherman ME, et al: Absolute Risk of a Subsequent Abnormal Pap Among Oncogenic Human Papillomavirus DNA-Positive, Cytologically Negative Women. *Cancer* 95: 2145-2151, 2002b.

Cauci S, Guaschino S, Driussi S, et al: Correlation of Local Interleukin-8 With Immunoglobulin A Against *Gardnerella vaginalis* Hemolysin and With Prolidase and Sialidase Levels in Women With Bacterial Vaginosis. *J Infect Dis* 185: 1614-1620, 2002.

Caudill JL, Humphrey SK, Goellner JR: Cervicovaginal Cytology and the Diagnosis of *Chlamydia trachomatis*: A Comparison With Immunofluorescent Results. *Diagn Cytopathol* 11: 20-22, 1994.

[CDC] Centers for Disease Control and Prevention: *Condyloma acuminatum*—United States, 1966-1981. *MMWR* 32: 306-308, 1983.

[CDC] Centers for Disease Control and Prevention: Black-White Differences in Cervical Cancer Mortality—United States, 1980-1987. *MMWR* 39: 245-248, 1990.

[CDC] Centers for Disease Control and Prevention: Premarital Sexual Experience Among Adolescent Women—United States, 1970-1988. *MMWR* 39: 929-932, 1991.

[CDC] Centers for Disease Control and Prevention: 1993 Revised Classification System for HIV Infection and Expanded Surveillance Case Definition for AIDS Among Adolescents and Adults. *JAMA* 269: 729-730, 1993.

[CDC] Centers for Disease Control and Prevention: Results from the National Breast and Cervical Cancer Early Detection Program, October 31, 1991-September 30, 1993. *MMWR* 43: 530-534, 1994.

[CDC] Centers for Disease Control and Prevention: Trends in Self-Reported Use of Mammograms (1989-1997)—and Papanicolaou Tests (1991-1997)—Behavioral Risk Factor Surveillance System. *MMWR (CDC Surveillance Summaries)* 48: 1-22, 1999.

Cecchini S: Cervical Intraepithelial Neoplasia in Younger Women. *Lancet* (ii): 926-927, 1982.

Cecchini S, Palli D, Casini A: Cervical Intraepithelial Neoplasia III: An Estimate of Screening Error Rates and Optimal Screening Interval. *Acta Cytol* 29: 329-333, 1985.

Cecchini S, Confortini M, Bonardi L, et al: "Nonclassic" Cytologic Signs of Cervical Condyloma: A Case-Control Study. *Acta Cytol* 34: 781-784, 1990a.

Cecchini S, Iossa A, Ciatto S: Routine Colposcopic Survey of Patients With Squamous Atypia: A Method for Identifying Cases With False-Negative Smears. *Acta Cytol* 34: 778-780, 1990b.

Cecchini S, Iossa A, Ciatto S, et al: Colposcopic Survey of Papanicolaou Test-Negative Cases With Hyperkeratosis or Parakeratosis. *Obstet Gynecol* 76: 857-859, 1990c.

Ceelen GH, Sakurai M: Vaginal Cytology in Leukemia. *Acta Cytol* 6: 370-372, 1962.

Ceelen GH: Persistent Radiation Changes in Vaginal Smears and Their Meaning for the Prognosis of Squamous Cell Carcinoma of the Cervix. *Acta Cytol* 10: 350-352, 1966.

Celasun B: Presence of Endocervical Cells and Number of Slides in Cervicovaginal Smears: Differences in Performance Between Gynecologists. *Acta Cytol* 45: 730-734, 2001.

Cenci M, Mancini R, Nofroni I, et al: Endocervical Atypical Glandular Cells of Undetermined Significance. I. Morphometric and Cytologic Characterization of Cases That "Cannot Rule Out Adenocarcinoma In Situ". *Acta Cytol* 44: 319-325, 2000a.

Cenci M, Mancini R, Nofroni I, et al: Endocervical Atypical Glandular Cells of Undetermined Significance: II. Morphometric and Cytologic Analysis of Nuclear Features Useful in Characterizing Differently Correlated Subgroups. *Acta Cytol* 44: 327-331, 2000b.

Cerilli J, Hattan D: Immunosuppression and Oncogenesis. *Am J Clin Pathol* 62: 218-223, 1974.

Cerqueira EMM, Santoro CL, Donozo NF, et al: Genetic Damage in Exfoliated Cells of the Uterine Cervix: Association and Interaction Between Cigarette Smoking and Progression to Malignant Transformation? *Acta Cytol* 42: 639-649, 1998.

Ces-Blanco JA: Sarcoma of the Vagina: An Unusual Cytologic Diagnosis. *Acta Cytol* 21: 547-549, 1977.

Cevenini R, Costa R, Rumpianesi F, et al: Cytological and Histopathological Abnormalities of the Cervix in Genital *Chlamydia trachomatis* Infections. *Br J Vener Dis* 57: 334-337, 1981.

Chacho MS, Mattie ME, Schwartz PE: Cytohistologic Correlation Rates Between Conventional Papanicolaou Smears and ThinPrep Cervical Cytology: A Comparison. *Cancer (Cancer Cytopathol)* 99: 135-140, 2003.

Chagpar A, Kanthan SC: Vaginal Metastasis of Colon Cancer. *Am Surg* 67: 171-172, 2001.

Chakrabarti S, Guijon FB, Paraskevas M: Brush vs Spatula for Cervical Smears. Histologic Correlation With Concurrent Biopsies. *Acta Cytol* 38: 315-318, 1994.

Chan E, Thakur A, Farid L, et al: Pemphigus Vulgaris of the Cervix and Upper Vaginal Vault: A Cause of Atypical Papanicolaou Smears. *Arch Dermatol* 134: 1485-1486, 1998.

Chan EL, Brandt K, Stoneham H, et al: Comparison of the Effectiveness of Polymerase Chain Reaction and Enzyme Immunoassay in Detecting *Chlamydia trachomatis* in Different Female Genitourinary Specimens. *Arch Pathol Lab Med* 124: 840-843, 2000.

Chan JKC, Tsui WMS, Tung SY, et al: Endocrine Cell Hyperplasia of the Uterine Cervix: A Precursor of Neuoendocrine Carcinoma of the Cervix? *Am J Clin Pathol* 92: 825-830, 1989.

Chan WK, Klock G, Bernard H-U: Progesterone and Glucocorticoid Response Elements Occur in the Long Control Regions of Several Human Papillomaviruses Involved in Anogenital Neoplasia. *J Virol* 63: 3261-3269, 1989.

Chandra K, Annousamy R: An Unusual Finding in the Vaginal Smear (Letter). *Acta Cytol* 19: 403, 1975.

Chandra M: Cervical Smear With Intracellular Organisms from a Case of Granuloma Venereum (Donovanosis). *Acta Cytol* 35: 143-145, 1991.

Chang A, Sandweiss L, Bose S: Cytologically Benign Endometrial Cells in the Papanicolaou Smears of Postmenopausal Women. *Gynecol Oncol* 80: 37-43, 2001.

Chang AR: Health Screening: An Analysis of Abnormal Cervical Smears at Dunedin Hospital 1963-82. *N Z Med J* 98: 104-107, 1985.

Chang AR: Carcinoma In Situ of the Cervix and Its Malignant Potential: A Lesson from New Zealand. *Cytopathology* 1: 321-328, 1990.

Chang AR, Lin WF, Chang A, et al: Can Technology Expedite the Cervical Cancer Screening Process? A Hong Kong Experience Using the AutoPap Primary Screening System With Location-Guided Screening Capability. *Am J Clin Pathol* 117: 437-443, 2002.

Chang F: Role of Papillomaviruses. *J Clin Pathol* 43: 269-276, 1990.

Chang JH, Rutkowski MA, Phillips MA, et al: The Potential Biological and Clinical Signifiance of Reactive/Reparative Cellular Changes in Cervical Smears (Abstract). *Acta Cytol* 40: 1038, 1996.

Chang RJ, Judd HL: The Ovary After Menopause. *Clin Obstet Gynecol* 24: 181-191, 1981.

Chang SH, Maddox WA: Adenocarcinoma Arising Within Cervical Endometriosis and Invading the Adjacent Vagina. *Am J Obstet Gynecol* 110: 1015-1017, 1971.

Chang WC, Matisic JP, Zhou C, et al: Cytologic Features of Villoglandular Adenocarcinoma of the Uterine Cervix: Comparison With Typical Endocervical Adenocarcinoma With a Villoglandular Component and Papillary Serous Carcinoma. *Cancer (Cancer Cytopathol)* 87: 5-11, 1999.

Chang YC, Craig JM: Vaginal-Smear Assessment of Estrogen Activity in Endometrial Carcinoma. *Obstet Gynecol* 21: 170-174, 1963.

Chaouki N, Bosch FX, Muñoz N, et al: The Viral Origin of Cervical Cancer in Rabat, Morocco. *Int J Cancer* 75: 546-554, 1998.

Chapman GW Jr, Abreo F, Thompson HE: Carcinoma of the Cervix in Young Females (35 Years, and Younger). *Gynecol Oncol* 31: 430-434, 1988.

Chattopadhyay I, Cruckshank DJ, Packer M: Non Diethylstilbesterol Induced Vaginal Adenosis—A Case Series and Review of Literature. *Eur J Gynaecol Oncol* 22: 260-262, 2001.

Chatwani A, Amin-Hanjani S: Incidence of Actinomycosis Associated With Intrauterine Devices. *J Reprod Med* 39: 585-587, 1994.

Chavez LR, Hubbell FA, McMullin JM, et al: Structure and Meaning in Models of Breast and Cervical Cancer Risk Factors: A Comparison of Perceptions Among Latinas, Anglo Women, and Physicians. *Med Anthropol Q* 9: 40-74, 1995.

Chen KTK, Hendricks EJ: Malakoplakia of the Female Genital Tract. *Obstet Gynecol* 65 (Suppl 3): 84S-87S, 1985.

Chen YC, Chen JH, Richard K, et al: Lung Adenocarinoma and Human Papillomavirus Infection. *Cancer* 101: 1428-1436, 2004.

Cheng RF, Hernandez E, Anderson LL, et al: Clinical Significance of a Cytologic Diagnosis of Atypical Glandular Cells of Undetermined Significance. *J Reprod Med* 44: 922-928, 1999.

Cheng W-F, Chen C-A, Lee C-N, et al: Vascular Endothelial Growth Factor in Cervical Carcinoma. *Obstet Gynecol* 93: 761-765, 1999.

Chenoy R, Billingham L, Irani S, et al: The Effect of Directed Biopsy on the Atypical Cervical Transformation Zone: Assessed by Digital Imaging Colposcopy. *Br J Obstet Gynecol* 103: 457-462, 1996.

Cherkis RC, Patten SF Jr, Dickinson JC, et al: Significance of Atypical Endometrial Cells Detected by Cervical Cytology. *Obstet Gynecol* 69: 786-789, 1987.

Cherkis RC, Patten SF Jr, Andrews TJ, et al: Significance of Normal Endometrial Cells Detected by Cervical Cytology. *Obstet Gynecol* 71: 242-244, 1988.

Cheuk W, Kwan MY, Suster S, et al: Immunostaining for Thyroid Transcription Factor 1 and Cytokeratin 20 Aids the Distinction of Small Cell Carcinoma from Merkel Cell Carcinoma, but not Pulmonary from Extrapulmonary Small Cell Carcinomas. *Arch Pathol Lab Med* 125: 228-231, 2001.

Cheung AN, Szeto EF, Leung BS, et al: Liquid-Based Cytology and Conventional Cervical Smears. *Cancer* 99: 331-335, 2003.

Chhieng DC, Elgert PA, Cangiarella JF, et al: Clinical Significance of Atypical Glandular Cells of Undetermined Significance: A Follow-Up Study from an Academic Medical Center. *Acta Cytol* 44: 557-566, 2000a.

Chhieng DC, Elgert PA, Cangiarella JF, et al: Cytology of Polypoid Adenomyomas: A Report of Two Cases. *Diagn Cytopathol* 22: 176-180, 2000b.

Chhieng DC, Elgert P, Cohen J-M, et al: Clinical Significance of Atypical Glandular Cells of Undetermined Significance in Postmenopausal Women. *Cancer (Cancer Cytopathol)* 93: 1-7, 2001a.

Chhieng DC, Elgert P, Cohen J-M, et al: Clinical Implications of Atypical Glandular Cells of Undetermined Significance, Favor Endometrial Origin. *Cancer (Cancer Cytopathol)* 93: 351-356, 2001b.

Chhieng DC, Elgert P, Cangiarella JF, et al: Variation in the Incidence of AGUS Between Different Patient Populations. *Acta Cytol* 45: 287-293, 2001c.

Chhieng DC, Elgert P, Cangiarella JF, et al: Significance of AGUS Pap Smears in Pregnant and Postpartum Women. *Acta Cytol* 45: 294-299, 2001d.

Chhieng DC, Talley LI, Roberson J, et al: Interobserver Variability: Comparison Between Liquid-Based and Conventional Preparations in Gynecologic Cytology. *Cancer (Cancer Cytopathol)* 96: 67-73, 2002.

Chhieng DC, Cangiarella JF: Atypical Glandular Cells. *Clin Lab Med* 23: 633-657, 2003.

Chhieng DC, Gallaspy S, Yang H, et al: Women With Atypical Glandular Cells: A Long-Term Follow-Up Study in a High-Risk Population. *Am J Clin Pathol* 122: 575-579, 2004.

Chichareon S, Herrero R, Muñoz N, et al: Risk Factors for Cervical Cancer in Thailand: A Case-Control Study. *J Natl Cancer Inst* 90: 50-57, 1998.

Chilvers C, Mand D, Pike MC: Cervical Adenocarcinoma and Oral Contraceptives. *Br Med J (Clin Res Edit)* 295: 1446-1447, 1987.

Chin AB, Bristow RE, Korst LM, et al: The Significance of Atypical Glandular Cells on Routine Cervical Cytologic Testing in a Community-Based Population. *Am J Obstet Gynecol* 182: 1278-1282, 2000.

Chin KM, Sidhu JS, Janssen RS, et al: Invasive Cervical Cancer in Human Immunodeficiency Virus-Infected and Uninfected Hospital Patients. *Obstet Gynecol* 92: 83-87, 1998.

Cho NH, Joo HJ, Ahn HJ, et al: Detection of Human Papillomavirus in Warty Carcinoma of the Uterine Cervix: Comparison of Immunohistochemistry, In Situ Hybridization and In Situ Polymerase Chain Reaction Methods. *Pathol Res Pract* 194: 713-720, 1998.

Chong S-M, Wee A, Yeoh S-C, et al: Retroperitoneal Endodermal Sinus Tumor. Report of a Case With an Abnormal Cervicovaginal Smear. *Acta Cytol* 38: 562-567, 1994.

Choo YC, Mak KC, Hsu C, et al: Postmenopausal Uterine Bleeding of Nonorganic Cause. *Obstet Gynecol* 66: 225-228, 1985.

Chorlton I, Karnei RF Jr, King FM, et al: Primary Malignant Reticuloendothelial Disease Involving the Vagina, Cervix, and Corpus Uteri. *Obstet Gynecol* 44: 735-748, 1974.

Chowdhury TR, Chowdhury JR: Significance of the Occurrence and Distribution of Glycogen in Cervical Cells Exfoliated Under Different Physiologic and Pathologic Conditions. *Acta Cytol* 25: 557-565, 1981.

Chretien MF, Levouvier B, Denis A, et al: Cytomorphometric Analysis of Vaginal Cells During Normal Cycle, Under Oral Contraceptive Therapy or In-Vitro Fertilization Stimulation Protocol. *Hum Reprod* 13: 2767-2771, 1998.

Christ ML, Haja J: Cytologic Changes Associated With Vaginal Pessary Use: With Special Reference to the Presence of *Actinomyces*. *Acta Cytol* 22: 146-149, 1978.

Christie AJ, Krieger HA: Indolent Necrotizing Granulomas of the Uterine Cervix, Possibly Related to Chlamydial Infection. *Am J Obstet Gynecol* 136: 958-960, 1980.

Christopherson WM, Parker JE: Microinvasive Carcinoma of the Uterine Cervix. *Cancer* 17: 1123-1131, 1964.

Christopherson WM, Mendez WM, Ahuja EM, et al: Cervix Cancer Control in Louisville, Kentucky. *Cancer* 26: 29-38, 1970a.

Christopherson WM, Parker JE, Mendez WM, et al: Cervix Cancer Death Rates and Mass Cytologic Screening. *Cancer* 26: 808-811, 1970b.

Christopherson WM, Mendez WM, Parker JE, et al: Carcinoma of the Endometrium: A Study of Changing Rates Over a 15-Year Period. *Cancer* 27: 1005-1008, 1971.

Christopherson WM, Lundin FE, Mendez WM, et al: Cervical Cancer Control: A Study of Morbidity and Mortality Trends Over A Twenty-One-Year Period. *Cancer* 38: 1357-1366, 1976.

Christopherson WM: Dysplasia, Carcinoma In Situ, and Microinvasive Carcinoma of the Uterine Cervix. *Hum Pathol* 8: 489-501, 1977a.

Christopherson WM, Scott MA: Trends in Mortality from Uterine Cancer in Relation to Mass Screening. *Acta Cytol* 21: 5-9, 1977b.

Christopherson WM, Nealon N, Gray LA: Noninvasive Precursor Lesions of Adenocarcinoma and Mixed Adenosquamous Carcinoma of the Cervix Uteri. *Cancer* 44: 975 983, 1979.

Chu J, White E: Decreasing Incidence of Invasive Cervical Cancer in Young Women. *Am J Obstet Gynecol* 157: 1105-1107, 1987.

Chu TY, Shen CY, Chiou YS, et al: HPV-Associated Cervical Cancers Show Frequent Allelic Loss at 3p14 But No Apparent Aberration of FHIT mRNA. *Int J Cancer* 75: 199-204, 1998.

Chua KL, Hjerpe A: Persistence of Human Papillomavirus (HPV) Infections Preceding Cervical Carcinoma. *Cancer* 77: 121-127, 1996.

Chumas JC, Nelson B, Mann WJ, et al: Microglandular Hyperplasia of the Uterine Cervix. *Obstet Gynecol* 66: 406-409, 1985.

Chung HR, Riccio JA Jr, Gerstung RA, et al: Discovery Rate of Dysplasia and Carcinoma of the Uterine Cervix in an Urban Medical Center Serving Patients at High Risk. *Int J Gynaecol Obstet* 20: 449-454, 1982.

Chung J-H, Koh J-S, Lee-SS, et al: Glassy Cell Carcinoma of the Uterine Cervix: Cytologic Features and Expression of Estrogen and Progesterone Receptors. *Acta Cytol* 44: 551-556, 2000.

Cibley LJ, Cibley LJ: Cytolytic Vaginosis. *Am J Obstet Gynecol* 165: 1245-1249, 1991.

Ciesla MC, Guidos BJ, Selvaggi SM: Cytomorphology of Small-Cell (Neuroendocrine) Carcinoma on ThinPrep® Cytology as Compared to Conventional Smears. *Diagn Cytopathol* 24: 46-52, 2001.

Cina SJ, Richardson MS, Austin RM, et al: Immunohistochemical Staining for Ki-67 Antigen, Carcinoembryonic Antigen, and p53 in the Differential Diagnosis of Glandular Lesions of the Cervix. *Mod Pathol* 10: 176-180, 1997.

Cioc AM, Julius CJ, Proca DM: Cervical Biopsy/Cytology Correlation Data Can Be Collected Prospectively and Shared Clinically. *Diagn Cytopathol* 26: 49-52, 2002.

Cirisano FD: Management of Pre-Invasive Disease of the Cervix. *Semin Surg Oncol* 16: 222-227, 1999.

Ciuffo G: Innesto Positivo Con Filtrato di Verruca Volgare. *Giorn Ital Mal Venereol* 48: 12, 1907.

Claas EC, Melchers WJ, Niesters HG, et al: Infections of the Cervix Uteri With Human Papillomavirus and *Chlamydia trachomatis*. *J Med Virol* 37: 54-57, 1992.

Claas HC, Melchers WJ, de Bruijn IH, et al: Detection of *Chlamydia trachomatis* in Clinical Specimens by the Polymerase Chain Reaction. *Eur J Clin Microbiol Infect Dis* 9: 864-868, 1990.

Clark AH, Betsill WL Jr: Early Endocervical Glandular Neoplasia. II. Morphometric Analysis of the Cells. *Acta Cytol* 30: 127-134, 1986a.

Clark AH, Betsill WL Jr: A Morphometric Study of Primary Adenocarcinoma of the Vagina. *Acta Cytol* 30: 323-333, 1986b.

Clark MA, Rakowski W, Ehrich B: Breast and Cervical Cancer Screening: Associations With Personal, Spouse's, and Combined Smoking Status. *Cancer Epidemiol Biomarkers Prev* 9: 513-516, 2000.

Clark RB, Schneider V, Gentile FG, et al: Cervical Chlamydial Infections: Diagnostic Accuracy of the Papanicolaou Smear. *South Med J* 78: 1301-1303, 1985.

Clark SB, Dawson AE: Invasive Squamous-Cell Carcinoma in ThinPrep Specimens: Diagnostic Clues in the Cellular Pattern. *Diagn Cytopathol* 26: 1-4, 2002.

Clarke AE, Casper MJ: From Simple Technology to Complex Arena: Classification of Pap Smears, 1917-90. *Med Anthropol Quart* 10: 601-623, 1996.

Clarke B, Chetty R: Postmodern Cancer: The Role of Human Immunodeficiency Virus in Uterine Cervical Cancer. *J Clin Pathol Mol Pathol* 55: 19-24, 2002.

Clarke EA, Anderson TW: Does Screening by "Pap" Smears Help Prevent Cervical Cancer? A Case-Control Study. *Lancet* (ii): 1-4, 1979.

Clarke EA, Morgan RW, Newman AM: Smoking as a Risk Factor in Cancer of the Cervix: Additional Evidence from a Case-Control Study. *Am J Epidemiol* 115: 59-66, 1982.

Clarke EA, Hatcher J, McKeown-Eyssen GE, et al: Cervical Dysplasia: Association With Sexual Behavior, Smoking and Oral Contraceptive Use? *Am J Obstet Gynecol* 151: 612-616, 1985.

Clarke MC, DeMay RM, Spiegel GW: Pseudoparakeratosis in Uterine Endocervical Pap Smears (Abstract). *Mod Pathol* 6: 28A, 1993.

Clary KM, Silverman JF, Liu Y, et al: Cytohistologic Discrepancies: A Means to Improve Pathology Practice and Patient Outcomes. *Am J Clin Pathol* 117: 567-573, 2002.

273

Clavel C, Masure M, Putaud I, et al: Hybrid Capture II, A New Sensitive Test for Human Papillomavirus Detection: Comparison With Hybrid Capture I and PCR Results in Cervical Lesions. *J Clin Pathol* 51: 737-740, 1998.

Clavel C, Masure M, Bory, et al: Hybrid Capture II-Based Human Papillomavirus Detection, a Sensitive Test to Detect in Routine High-Grade Cervical Lesions: A Preliminary Study on 1518 Women. *Br J Cancer* 80: 1306-1311, 1999.

Clavel C, Masure M, Levert M, et al: Human Papillomavirus Detection by the Hybrid Capture II Assay: A Reliable Test to Select Women With Normal Cervical Smears at Risk for Developing Cervical Lesions. *Diagn Mol Pathol* 9: 145-150, 2000a.

Clavel C, Nawrocki B, Bosseaux B, et al: Detection of Human Papillomavirus DNA in Bronchopulmonary Carcinomas by Hybrid Capture II: A Study of 185 Tumors. *Cancer* 88: 1347-1352, 2000b.

Clavel C, Masure M, Bory J-P, et al: Human Papillomavirus Testing in Primary Screening for the Detection of High-Grade Cervical Lesions: A Study of 7932 Women. *Br J Cancer* 88: 1616-1623, 2001.

Cleaves MA: Radium, Its Physics, Physiological Action and Therapeutic Effects. American Electro-Therapeutic Association, September 1903, cited In: Cleaves MA Light Energy: Its Physics, Physiological Action and Therapeutic Applications. Rebman Co., New York, 718, 744, 1904.

Clement PB, Young RH, Keh P, et al: Malignant Mesonephric Neoplasms of the Uterine Cervix: A Report of Eight Cases, Including Four With a Malignant Spindle Cell Component. *Am J Surg Pathol* 19: 1158-1171, 1995.

Clement PB, Zubovits JT, Young RH, et al: Malignant Müllerian Mixed Tumors of the Uterine Cervix: A Report of Nine Cases of a Neoplasm With Morphology Often Different from Its Counterpart in the Corpus. *Int J Gynecol Pathol* 17: 211-222, 1998.

Clocuh YP: Ciliocytophrhorie im Zervikalabstrich. [Cilicytophthoria in the Cervical Smear.] *Geburtshilfe Frauenheilkd* 38: 229-230, 1978.

Coach S, Cason Z, Benghuzzi H: An Evaluation of Infectious Diseases in Cervicovaginal Smears from Patients With Atypical Cells of Undetermined Significance. *Biomed Sci Instrum* 37: 167-172, 2001.

Cocchi V, Carretti D, Franti S, et al: Intralaboratory Quality Assurance in Cervical/Vaginal Cytology: Evaluation of Intercytologist Diagnostic Reproducibility. *Diagn Cytopathol* 16: 87-92, 1997.

Cocker J, Fox H, Langley FA: Consistency in the Histological Diagnosis of Epithelial Abnormalities of the Uterine Cervix. *J Clin Pathol* 21: 67-70, 1968.

Cohen C: Three Cases of Amoebiasis of the Cervix Uteri. *J Obstet Gynaecol Br Commonw* 80: 476-479, 1973.

Cohen C, Shulman G, Budgeon LR: Endocervical and Endometrial Adenocarcinoma: An Immunoperoxidase and Histochemical Study. *Am J Surg Pathol* 6: 151-157, 1982.

Cohen CR, Duerr A, Pruithithada N, et al: Bacterial Vaginosis and HIV Seroprevalence Among Female Commerical Sex Workers in Chiang Mai, Thailand. *AIDS* 9: 1093-1097, 1995.

Cohen L: Influence of pH on Vaginal Discharges. *Br J Vener Dis* 45: 241-247, 1969.

Cohen ML, Ducatman BS, Stock RJ: Differential Staining Techniques in Amniotic Fluid Cytology of Neural Tube Defects: A Prospective Study of 129 Pregnancies. *Diagn Cytopathol* 3: 271-277, 1987.

Cohn DE, Herzog TJ: New Innovations in Cervical Cancer Screening. *Clin Obstet Gynecol* 44: 538-549, 2001.

Cohn, JA, Gagnon S, Spence MR: The Role of Human Papillomavirus Deoxyribonucleic Acid Assay and Repeated Cervical Cytologic Examination in the Detection of Cervical Intraepithelial Neoplasia Among Human Immunodeficiency Virus-Infected Women. *Am J Obstet Gynecol* 184: 322-330, 2001.

Coker AL, Rosenberg AJ, McCann MF, et al: Active and Passive Cigarette Smoke and Cervical Intraepithelial Neoplasia. *Cancer Epidemiol Biomarkers Prev* 1: 349-356, 1992.

Coker AL, Gerasimova T, King MR, et al: High-Risk HPVs and Risk of Cervical Neoplasia: A Nested Case-Control Study. *Exp Mol Pathol* 70: 90-95, 2001.

Coleman DV: A Case of Tuberculosis of the Cervix. *Acta Cytol* 13: 104-107, 1969.

Coleman DV, Russell WJ, Hodgson J, et al: Human Papovavirus in Papanicolaou Smears of Urinary Sediment Detected by Transmission Electron Microscopy. *J Clin Pathol* 30: 1015-1020, 1977.

Coleman DV: Cytological Diagnosis of Virus-Infected Cells in Papanicolaou Smears and Its Application in Clinical Practice. *J Clin Pathol* 32: 1075-1089, 1979.

Coleman DV: Cytological Diagnosis of Virus-Infected Cells in Cervical Smears. *Diagn Gynecol Obstet* 4: 363-373, 1982.

Colgan TJ, Lickrish GM: The Topography and Invasive Potential of Cervical Adenocarcinoma In Situ, With and Without Associated Squamous Dysplasia. *Gynecol Oncol* 36: 246-249, 1990.

Colgan TJ, Austin RMA, Davey DD: The Annual Papanicolaou Test: Women's Safety and Public Policy. *Cancer (Cancer Cytopathol)* 93: 81-85, 2001a.

Colgan TJ, Woodhouse SL, Styer PE, et al: Reparative Changes and the False-Positive/False-Negative Papanicolaou Test: A Study from the College of American Pathologists Interlaboratory Comparison Program in Cervicovaginal Cytology. *Arch Pathol Lab Med* 125: 134-140, 2001b.

Colgan TJ, Clarke A, Hakh N, et al: Screening for Cervical Disease in Mature Women: Strategies for Improvement. *Cancer (Cancer Cytopathol)* 96: 195-203, 2002.

Colgan TJ: Programmatic Assessments of the Clinical Effectiveness of Gynecologic Liquid-Based Cytology: The Ayes Have It. *Cancer (Cancer Cytopathol)* 99: 259-262, 2003.

Colino GD, Rua deCorrao IJ, Martinez EA: Unusual Mycotic Findings in Cytodiagnosis. *Acta Cytol* 20: 288-289, 1976.

Collinet P, Prolongeau JF, Vaneecloo S: Villoglandular Papillary Adenocarcinoma of the Uterine Cervix. *Eur J Obstet Gynecol Reprod Biol* 86: 101-103, 1999.

Collins C, Dhurandhan N: Cervical Biopsy Findings in Women With Benign Cellular Atypia on a Routine Pap Smear (Abstract). *Am J Clin Pathol* 97: 442, 1992.

Collins CL: The Challenge of Cytology Proficiency Testing. *Laboratory Medicine* 25: 219-220, 1994.

Collins DN, Patacsil DP: Proficiency Testing in Cytology in New York: Analysis of a 14-Year State Program. *Acta Cytol* 30: 633-642, 1986.

Collins KA, Bennett AT: Persistence of Spermatozoa and Prostatic Acid Phosphatase in Specimens from Deceased Individuals During Varied Postmortem Intervals. *Am J Forensic Med Pathol* 22: 228-232, 2001.

Collins LC, Wang HH, Abu-Jawdeh GM: Qualifiers of Atypical Squamous Cells of Undetermined Significance Help in Patient Management. *Mod Pathol* 9: 677-681, 1996.

Coman DR: Decreased Mutual Adhesiveness, a Property of Cells from Squamous Cell Carcinomas. *Cancer Res* 4: 625-629, 1944.

Condel JL, Mahood LK, Grzybicki DM, et al: Papanicolaou Tests Diagnosed as Atypical by a Cytotechnologist and Downgraded to Benign by a Pathologist: A Measure of Laboratory Quality. *Am J Clin Pathol* 117: 534-540, 2002.

Confortini M, Biggeri A, Cariaggi MP, et al: Intralaboratory Reproducibility in Cervical Cytology: Results of the Application of a 100-Slide Set. *Acta Cytol* 37: 49-54, 1993.

Confortini M, Carozzi F, Dalla Palma P, et al: Interlaboratory Reproducibility of Atypical Squamous Cells of Undetermined Significance Report: A National Survey. *Cytopathology* 14: 263-268, 2003.

Conner MG, Richter H, Moran CA, et al: Small Cell Carcinoma of the Cervix: A Clinicopathologic and Immunohistochemical Study of 23 Cases. *Ann Diagn Pathol* 6: 345-348, 2002.

Connor JP, Ferrer K, Kane JP, et al: Evaluation of Langerhans' Cells in the Cervical Epithelium of Women With Cervical Intraepithelial Neoplasia. *Gynecol Oncol* 75: 130-135, 1999.

Connor JP, Elam G, Goldberg JM: Empiric Vaginal Metronidazole in the Management of the ASCUS Papanicolaou Smear: A Randomized Controlled Trial. *Obstet Gynecol* 99: 183-187, 2002.

Contreras-Melendez L, Herbert A, Millward-Sadler GH, et al: Assessment of the Accuracy of Cytology in Women Referred for Colposcopy and Biopsy: The Results of a 1 Year Audit. *Cytopathology* 3: 267-274, 1992.

Cook GA, Draper GJ: Trends in Cervical Cancer and Carcinoma In Situ in Great Britain. *Br J Cancer* 50: 367-375, 1984.

Cooper K, Herrington CS, Lo ES, et al: Integration of Human Papillomavirus Types 16 and 18 in Cervical Adenocarcinoma. *J Clin Pathol* 45: 382-384, 1992.

Cooper K, McGee J: Human Papillomavirus, Integration and Cervical Carcinogenesis: A Clinicopathological Perspective. *Mol Pathol* 50: 1-3, 1997.

Cooper P, Russell G, Wilson B: Adenocarcinoma of the Endocervix—A Histochemical Study. *Histopathology* 11: 1321-1330, 1987.

Coppleson LW, Brown B: Estimation of the Screening Error Rate from the Observed Detection Rates in Repeated Cervical Cytology. *Am J Obstet Gynecol* 119: 953-958, 1974.

Coppleson M, Reid B: The Etiology of Squamous Carcinoma of the Cervix (Editorial). *Obstet Gynecol* 32: 432-436, 1968.

Coppleson M: The Origin and Nature of Premalignant Lesions of the Cervix Uteri. *Int J Gynecol Obstet* 8: 539-550, 1970.

Corey L: The Diagnosis and Treatment of Genital Herpes. *JAMA* 248: 1041-1049, 1982.

Corey L, Adams HG, Brown ZA, et al: Genital Herpes Simplex Virus Infections: Clinical Manifestations, Course, and Complications. *Ann Intern Med* 98: 958-972, 1983a.

Corey L, Holmes KK: Genital Herpes Simplex Virus Infections: Current Concepts in Diagnosis, Therapy, and Prevention. *Ann Intern Med* 98: 973-983, 1983b.

Correa P: Vitamins and Cancer Prevention. *Cancer Epidemiol Biomarkers Prev* 1: 241-243, 1992.

Coscia-Porrazzi LO, Maiello FM, de Falco ML: The Cytology of the Normal Cyclic Endometrium. *Diagn Cytopathol* 2: 198-203, 1986.

Costa MJ, Grimes C, Tackett E: Cervicovaginal Cytology in an Indigent Population: Comparison of Results for 1964, 1981 and 1989. *Acta Cytol* 35: 51-56, 1991a.

Costa MJ, Kenny MB, Naib ZM: Cervicovaginal Cytology in Uterine Adenocarcinoma and Adenosquamous Carcinoma: Comparison of Cytologic and Histologic Findings. *Acta Cytol* 35: 127-134, 1991b.

Costa MJ, Tadros T, Tackett E, et al: Vaginocervical Cytology in Victims of Sexual Assault. *Diagn Cytopathol* 7: 337-340, 1991c.

Costa MJ, Tidd C, Willis D: Cervicovaginal Cytology in Carcinosarcoma (Malignant Mixed Müllerian [Mesodermal] Tumor) of the Uterus. *Diagn Cytopathol* 8: 33-40, 1992.

Costa S, Sideri M, Syrjanen K, et al: Combined Pap Smear, Cervicography and HPV DNA Testing in the Detection of Cervical Intraepithelial Neoplasia and Cancer. *Acta Cytol* 44: 310-318, 2000.

Costello TJ, Wang HH, Schnitt SJ, et al: Paget's Disease With Extensive Involvement of the Female Genital Tract Initially Detected by Cervical Cytosmear. *Arch Pathol Lab Med* 112: 941-944, 1988.

Coursaget P, Muñoz N: Vaccination Against Infectious Agents Associated With Human Cancer. *Cancer Surveys: Infections and Human Cancer* 1999: 335-381, 1999.

Cove H: The Arias-Stella Reaction Occurring in the Endocervix in Pregnancy: Recognition and Comparison With an Adenocarcinoma of the Endocervix. *Am J Surg Pathol* 3: 567-568, 1979.

Covell JL, Frierson HF: Intraepithelial Neoplasia Mimicking Microinvasive Squamous-Cell Carcinoma in Endocervical Brushings. *Diagn Cytopathol* 8: 18-22, 1992.

Cox JT, Lorincz AT, Schiffman MH, et al: Gynecology: Human Papillomavirus Testing by Hybrid Capture Appears to Be Useful in Triaging Women With a Cytologic Diagnosis of Atypical Squamous Cells of Undetermined Significance. *Am J Obstet Gynecol* 172: 946-954, 1995.

Cox JT: Clinical Role of HPV Testing. *Obstet Gynecol Clin North Am* 23: 811-815, 1996.

Cox JT: ASCCP Practice Guidelines: Management of Glandular Abnormalities in the Cervical Smear. *J Low Genital Tract Dis* 1: 41-45, 1997a.

Cox JT: ASCCP Practice Guidelines: Endocervical Curettage. *J Low Genital Tract Dis* 1: 251-256, 1997b.

Cox JT: HPV Testing: Is It Useful in Triage of Minor Pap Abnormalities? *J Family Pract* 46: 121-124, 1998a.

Cox JT: AGUS Pap Smears: A Follow-Up Strategy. *OBG Management* 7: 74-81, 85-87, 1998b.

Cox JT: Evaluating the Role of HPV Testing for Women With Equivocal Papanicolaou Test Findings. *JAMA* 281: 1645-1647, 1999.

Cox JT, Massad LS, Lonky N, et al: ASCCP Practice Guidelines Management Guidelines for the Follow-Up of Cytology Read as Low-Grade Squamous Intraepithelial Lesion. *J Low Genital Tract Dis* 2: 83-92, 2000a.

Cox JT, Wilkinson EJ, Lonky N, et al: ASCCP Practice Guidelines Management Guidelines for the Follow-Up of Atypical Squamous Cells of Undetermined Significance (ASCUS). *J Low Genital Tract Dis* 4: 99-105, 2000b.

Cox JT: Management of Atypical Squamous Cells of Undetermined Significance and Low-Grade Squamous Intraepithelial Lesion by Human Papillomavirus Testing. *Best Prac Res Clin Obstet Gynaecol* 15: 715-741, 2001.

Cox JT: Role of Human Papillomavirus Testing in the American Society for Colposcopy and Cervical Pathology Guidelines for the Management of Abnormal Cervical Cytology and Cervical Cancer Precursors. *Arch Pathol Lab Med* 127: 950-958, 2003a.

Cox JT, Schiffman M, Solomon D, et al: Prospective Follow-Up Suggests Similar Risk of Subsequent Cervical Intraepithelial Neoplasia Grade 2 or 3 Among Women With Cervical Intraepithelial Neoplasia Grade 1 or Negative Colposcopy and Directed Biopsy. *Am J Obstet Gynecol* 188: 1406-1412, 2003b.

Crabtree D, Unkraut A, Cozens D, et al: Role for HPV Testing in ASCUS: A Cytologic-Histologic Correlation. *Diagn Cytopathol* 27: 382-386, 2002.

Cramer DW: The Role of Cervical Cytology in the Declining Morbidity and Mortality of Cervical Cancer. *Cancer* 34: 2018-2027, 1974a.

Cramer DW, Cutler SJ: Incidence and Histopathology of Malignancies of the Female Genital Organs in the United States. *Am J Obstet Gynecol* 118: 443-460, 1974b.

Cramer HM, Skinner-Wannemuehler SE, Brown DR, et al: Cytomorphologic Correlates of Human Papillomavirus Infection in the "Normal" Cervicovaginal Smear. *Acta Cytol* 41: 261-268, 1997.

Creasman WT, Rutledge F: Carcinoma In Situ of the Cervix: An Analysis of 861 Patients. *Obstet Gynecol* 39: 373-380, 1972.

Creasman WT, Weed JC Jr: Screening Techniques in Endometrial Cancer. *Cancer* 38: 436-440, 1976.

Creasman WT, Clarke-Pearson DL, Ashe C, et al: The Abnormal Pap Smear—What to Do Next? *Cancer* 48: 515-522, 1981.

Creasman WT, Fetter BF, Clarke-Pearson DL, et al: Management of Stage IA Carcinoma of the Cervix. *Am J Obstet Gynecol* 153: 164-172, 1985.

Creasman WT, Zaino RJ, Major FJ, et al: Early Invasive Carcinoma of the Cervix (3 to 5 mm Invasion): Risk Factors and Prognosis—A Gynecologic Oncology Group Study. *Am J Obstet Gynecol* 178: 62-65, 1998.

Creasman WT: Cancer and Pregnancy. *Ann NY Acad Sci* 943: 281-286, 2001.

Crescini C, Pezzica E, Artuso A, et al: Esito colposcopico-istologico in 97 pazienti con displasia lieve al pap-test. [Colposcopy and Biopsy in 97 Patients With Pap-Test Mild Dysplasia. Eng. Abstr.] *Minerva Ginecologica* 43:509-512, 1991.

Crissman JD, Makuch R, Budhraja M: Histopathologic Grading of Squamous Cell Carcinoma of the Uterine Cervix: An Evaluation of 70 Stage Ib Patients. *Cancer* 55: 1590-1596, 1985.

Critchlow CW, Wolner-Hanssen P, Eschenbach DA, et al: Determinants of Cervical Ectopia and of Cervicitis: Age, Oral Contraception, Specific Cervical Infection, Smoking, and Douching. *Am J Obstet Gynecol* 173: 534-543, 1995.

Cronjé HS, Divall P, Bam RH, et al: Effects of Dilute Acetic Acid on the Cervical Smear. *Acta Cytol* 41: 1091-1094, 1997.

Crook T, Tidy JA, Vousden KH: Degradation of p53 Can Be Targeted by HPV E6 Sequences Distinct from Those Required for p53 Binding and Trans-Activation. *Cell* 67: 547-556, 1991a.

Crook T, Wrede D, Vousden KH: p53 Point Mutation in HPV Negative Human Cervical Carcinoma Cell Lines. *Oncogene* 6: 873-875, 1991b.

Crook T, Wrede D, Tidy JA, et al: Clonal p53 Mutation in Primary Cervical Cancer: Association With Human-Papillomavirus-Negative Tumours. *Lancet* 339: 1070-1073, 1992.

Crowther ME, Lowe DG, Shepherd JH: Verrucous Carcinoma of the Female Genital Tract: A Review. *Obstet Gynecol Surv* 43: 263-280, 1988.

Crowther ME: Is the Nature of Cervical Carcinoma Changing in Young Women? *Obstet Gynecol Surv* 50: 71-82. 1995.

Crum CP, Egawa K, Barron B, et al: Human Papilloma Virus Infection (Condyloma) of the Cervix and Cervical Intraepithelial Neoplasia: A Histopathologic and Statistical Analysis. *Gynecol Oncol* 15: 88-94, 1983a.

Crum CP, Egawa K, Fu Y-S, et al: Atypical Immature Metaplasia (AIM): A Subset of Human Papilloma Virus Infection of the Cervix. *Cancer* 51: 2214-2219, 1983b.

Crum CP, Levine RU: Human Papillomavirus Infection and Cervical Neoplasia: New Perspectives. *Int J Gynecol Pathol* 3: 376-388, 1984a.

Crum CP, Ikenberg H, Richart RM, et al: Human Papillomavirus Type 16 and Early Cervical Neoplasia. *N Engl J Med* 310: 880-883, 1984b.

Crum CP, Mitao M, Winkler B, et al: Localizing Chlamydial Infection in Cervical Biopsies With the Immunoperoxidase Technique. *Int J Gynecol Pathol* 3: 191-197, 1984c.

Crum CP, Mitao M, Levin RU, et al: Cervical Papillomaviruses Segregate Within Morphologically Distinct Precancerous Lesions. *J Virol* 54: 675-681, 1985.

Crum CP, Fu Y-S, Kurman RJ, et al: Practical Approach to Cervical Human Papillomavirus-Related Intraepithelial Lesions. *Int J Gynecol Pathol* 8: 388-399, 1989a.

Crum CP: Identifying High-Risk Precursors of Cervical Cancer: How and Why. *Am J Clin Pathol* 92: 379-382, 1989b.

Crum CP, McLachlin CM: Cervical Intraepithelial Neoplasia. *J Cell Biochem* Supplement 23: 71-79, 1995.

Crum CP: Detecting Every Genital Papilloma Virus Infection. What Does It Mean? (Commentary). *Am J Pathol* 153: 1667-1671, 1998.

Crum CP, Genest DR, Krane J, et al: Subclassifying Atypical Squamous Cells in Thin-Prep Cervical Cytology Correlates With Detection of High-Risk Human Papillomavirus DNA. *Am J Clin Pathol* 112: 384-390, 1999.

Crum CP: Contemporary Theories of Cervical Carcinogenesis: The Virus, the Host, and the Stem Cell. *Mod Pathol* 13: 243-251, 2000.

Crum CP: The Beginning of the End for Cervical Cancer? (Editorial). *N Engl J Med* 347: 1703-1705, 2002.

Crum CP: Symposium Part I: Should the Bethesda System Terminology Be Used in Diagnostic Surgical Pathology?: Point. *Int J Gynecol Pathol* 22: 5-12, 2003.

Cubilla AL, Meijer CJLM, Young RH: Morphological Features of Epithelial Abnormalities and Precancerous Lesions of the Penis. *Scand J Urol Nephrol* 34(Suppl 205): 215-219, 2000.

Cui S, Lespinasse P, Cracchiolo B, et al: Large Cell Neuroendocrine Carcinoma of the Cervix Associated With Adenocarcinoma In Situ: Evidence of a Common Origin (Letter). *Int J Gynecol Pathol* 20: 311-312, 2001.

Cullen AP, Reid R, Campion M, et al: Analysis of the Physical State of Different Human Papillomavirus DNAs in Intraepithelial and Invasive Cervical Neoplasm. *J Virol* 65: 606-612, 1991.

Cullimore JE, Luesley DM, Rollason TP, et al: A Case of Glandular Intraepithelial Neoplasia Involving the Cervix and Vagina. *Gynecol Oncol* 34: 249-252, 1989a.

Cullimore JE, Rollason TP, Marshall T: Nucleolar Organiser Regions in Adenocarcinoma In Situ of the Endocervix. *J Clin Pathol* 42: 1276-1280, 1989b.

Cullimore JE, Leusley DM, Rollason TP, et al: A Prospective Study of Conization of the Cervix in the Management of Cervical Intraepithelial Glandular Neoplasia (CIGN)—A Preliminary Report. *Br J Obstet Gynaecol* 99: 314-318, 1992.

Cunnane MF, Rothblat IP: Atypical Squamous Cells in Women Over 50: Histologic Correlations (Abstract). *Acta Cytol* 37: 784, 1993.

Currie MM, Casm Z, Balign M, et al: The Significance of Atypical Glandular Cells on Papanicolaou Smears: An Eight-Year Follow-Up Study (Abstract). *Acta Cytol* 38: 810, 1994.

Curtin JP, Saigo P, Slucher B, et al: Soft-Tissue Sarcoma of the Vagina and Vulva: A Clinicopathologic Study. *Obstet Gynecol* 86: 269-272, 1995.

Cuschieri KS, Cubie HA, Whitley MW, et al: Multiple High Risk HPV Infections Are Common in Cervical neoplasia and Young Women in a Cervical Screening Population. *J Clin Pathol* 57: 68-72, 2004.

Cuzick J, De Stavola BL, Russell MJ, et al: Vitamin A, Vitamin E and the Risk of Cervical Intraepithelial Neoplasia. *Br J Cancer* 62: 651-652, 1990.

Cuzick J, Terry G, Ho L, et al: Type-Specific Human Papillomavirus DNA in Abnormal Smears as a Predictor of High-Grade Cervical Intraepithelial Neoplasia. *Br J Cancer* 69: 167-171, 1994.

Cuzick J, Sasieni P, Singer A: Risk Factors for Invasive Cervix Cancer in Young Women. *Eur J Cancer* 32A: 836-841, 1996.

Cuzick J: Screening for Cancer: Future Potential. *Eur J Cancer* 35: 685-692, 1999.

Cuzick J: Human Papillomavirus Testing for Primary Cervical Cancer Screening. *JAMA* 283: 108-109, 2000.

Cuzick J: Time to Consider HPV Testing in Cervical Screening. *Ann Oncol* 12: 1511-1514, 2001.

D

Dabbs DJ, Geisinger KR, Norris H: Intermediate Filaments in Endometrial and Endocervical Carcinomas: The Diagnostic Utility of Vimentin Patterns. *Am J Surg Pathol* 10: 568-576, 1986.

Dabbs DJ, Sturtz K, Zaino RJ: The Immunohistochemical Discrimination of Endometrioid Adenocarcinomas. *Hum Pathol* 27: 172-177, 1996.

Daling JR, Sherman KJ, Weiss NS: Risk Factors for *Condyloma acuminatum* in Women. *Sex Transm Dis* 13: 16-18, 1986.

Daling JR, Sherman KJ, Hislop TG, et al: Cigarette Smoking and the Risk of Anogenital Cancer. *Am J Epidemiol* 135: 180-189, 1992.

Dallenbach-Hellweg G: On the Origin and Histological Structure of Adenocarcinoma of the Endocervix in Women Under 50 Years of Age. *Pathol Res Pract* 179: 38-50, 1984.

Daly SF, Doyle M, English J, et al: Can the Number of Cigarettes Smoked Predict High-Grade Cervical Intraepithelial Neoplasia Among Women With Mildly Abnormal Pap Smears? *Am J Obstet Gynecol* 179: 399-402, 1998.

Dance EF, Fullmer CD: Extrauterine Carcinoma Cells Observed in Cervico-Vaginal Smears. *Acta Cytol* 14: 187-191, 1970.

Daneshbod Y, Monabati A, Bedayat GR: *Strongyloides stercoaralis* as a Contaminant in a Cervicovaginal Smear (Letter). *Acta Cytol* 48: 768-769, 2004.

Danos M, Holmquist ND: Cytologic Evaluation of Decidual Cells: A Report of Two Cases With False Abnormal Cytology. *Acta Cytol* 11: 325-330, 1967.

Danos ML: Post Partum Cytology: Observations Over a Four Year Period. *Acta Cytol* 12: 309-312, 1968.

Darne JF, Polacarz SV, Sheridan E, et al: Nucleolar Organiser Regions in Adenocarcinoma In Situ and Invasive Adenocarcinoma of the Cervix. *J Clin Pathol* 43: 657-660, 1990.

Daroca PJ, Dhurandhar HN: Basaloid Carcinoma of Uterine Cervix. *Am J Surg Pathol* 4: 235-239, 1980.

Daron F, Wright TC Jr, Litaker MS, et al: Comparison of Two Tests for Detecting Carcinogenic HPV in Women With Papanicolaou Smear Reports of ASCUS and LSIL. *J Fam Pract* 46: 136-141, 1998.

Das DK, Pathan SK, Hira PR, et al: Pelvic Abscess from *Enterobius vermicularis*: Report of a Case with Cytologic Detection of Eggs and Worms. *Acta Cytol* 45: 425-429, 2002.

Das Gupta T, D'Urso J: Melanoma of Female Genitalia. *Surg Gynecol Obstet* 119: 1074-1078, 1964.

Davey DD, Gallion H, Jennings CD: DNA Cytometry in Postirradiation Cervical-Vaginal Smears. *Hum Pathol* 23: 1027-1031, 1992a.

Davey DD, Nielsen ML, Rosenstock W, et al: Terminology and Specimen Adequacy in Cervicovaginal Cytology. The College of American Pathologists Interlaboratory Comparison Program Experience. *Arch Pathol Lab Med* 116: 903-907, 1992b.

Davey DD, Nielsen ML, Frable WJ, et al: Improving Accuracy in Gynecologic Cytology: Results of the College of American Pathologists Interlaboratory Comparison Program in Cervicovaginal Cytology. *Arch Pathol Lab Med* 117: 1193-1198, 1993.

Davey DD, Naryshkin S, Nielsen ML, et al: Atypical Squamous Cells of Undetermined Significance: Interlaboratory Comparison and Quality Assurance Monitors. *Diagn Cytopathol* 11: 390-396, 1994.

Davey DD, Nielsen ML, Naryshkin S, et al: Atypical Squamous Cells of Undetermined Significance: Current Laboratory Practices of Participants in the College of American Pathologists Interlaboratory Comparison Program in Cervicovaginal Cytology. *Arch Pathol Lab Med* 120: 440-444, 1996.

Davey DD, Zaleski S, Sattich M, et al: Prognostic Significance of DNA Cytometry of Postirradiation Cervicovaginal Smears. *Cancer (Cancer Cytopathol)* 84: 11-16, 1998.

Davey DD, Woodhouse S, Styer P, et al: Atypical Epithelial Cells and Specimen Adequacy: Current Laboratory Practices of Participants in the College of American Pathologists Interlaboratory Comparison Program in Cervicovaginal Cytology. *Arch Pathol Lab Med* 124: 203-211, 2000.

Davey DD, Austin RM, Birdsong G, et al: ASCCP Patient Management Guidelines: Pap Test Specimen Adequacy and Quality Indicators. *Am J Clin Pathol* 118: 714-718, 2002.

Davey DD: Reflex Human Papillomavirus Testing: Leave the Cytology Interpretation Alone (Editorial). *Cancer (Cancer Cytopathol)* 99: 187-190, 2003a.

Davey DD: Cervical Cytology Classification and the Bethesda System. *Cancer J* 9: 327-334, 2003b.

Davey DD, Neal MH, Wilbur DC, et al: Bethesda 2001 Implementation and Reporting Rates: 2003 Practices of Participants in the College of American Pathologists Interlaboratory Comparison Program in Cervicovaginal Cytology. *Arch Pathol Lab Med* 128: 1224-1229, 2004.

David ALM, Taylor GM, Gokhale D, et al: HLA-DQB1*03 and Cervical Intraepithelial Neoplasia Type III (Letter). *Lancet* 340: 52, 1992.

Davies SW, Kelly RM: Intraepithelial Carcinoma of the Cervix Uteri in Women Aged Under 35 Years. *Br Med J* 4: 525-526, 1971.

Davila RM: Cervicovaginal Smear, True or False? *Am J Clin Pathol* 102: 1-2, 1994.

Davis GL, Hernandez E, Davis JL, et al: Atypical Squamous Cells in Papanicolaou Smears. *Obstet Gynecol* 69: 43-46, 1987.

Davis JD, Connor EE, Clark P, et al: Correlation Between Cervical Cytologic Results and Gram Stain as Diagnostic Tests for Bacterial Vaginosis. *Am J Obstet Gynecol* 177: 532-535, 1997.

Davis JR, Moon LB: Increased Incidence of Adenocarcinoma of Uterine Cervix. *Obstet Gynecol* 45: 79-83, 1975.

Davis JR, Hindman WM, Paplanus SH, et al: Value of Duplicate Smears in Cervical Cytology. *Acta Cytol* 25: 533-538, 1981.

Davis JR, Aristizabal S, Way DL, et al: DNA Ploidy, Grade, and Stage in Prognosis of Uterine Cervical Cancer. *Gynecol Oncol* 32: 4-7, 1989.

Davison JM, Marty JJ: Detecting Premalignant Cervical Lesions. Contributions of Screening Colposcopy to Cytology. *J Reprod Med* 39: 388-392, 1994.

Davtyan C: Contraception for Adolescent. *West J Med* 172: 166-171, 2000.

Daw E: Extragenital Adenocarcinoma Metastatic to the Cervix Uteri. *Am J Obstet Gynecol* 114: 1104-1105, 1972.

Dawagne MP, Silverberg SG: Foam Cells in Endometrial Carcinoma—A Clinicopathologic Study. *Gynecol Oncol* 13: 67-75, 1982.

Dayton V, Henry M, Stanley MW, et al: Adenoid Cystic Carcinoma of the Uterine Cervix: Cytologic Features. *Acta Cytol* 34: 125-128, 1990.

de Alvarez RR, Figge DC: Diagnosis of Ovarian Carcinoma by Vaginal Cytology. *Obstet Gynecol* 8: 655-663, 1956.

de Boer, A-L, de Bope F, Van der Merwe JV: Cytologic Identification of Donovan Bodies in *Granuloma inquinale*. *Acta Cytol* 28: 126-128, 1984.

de Borges R: Findings of Microfilarial Larval Stages in Gynecologic Smears. *Acta Cytol* 15: 476-478, 1971.

de Borges RJ, Carmona O, Machado H, et al: Chlamydial Infection in Papanicolaou-Stained Cervical Smears. *Acta Cytol* 28: 471-476, 1984.

de Borges RJ, Garcia-Tamayo J, Zaitzman M: Cytologic and Ultrastructural Findings of a Peculiar Alteration in Cervical Cells from Patients With Human Papillomavirus Infections. *Acta Cytol* 33: 314-318, 1989.

de Brux J, Froment- Dupré J: Cytology of Endometrial Hyperplasia (Symposium on Endometrial Cytology. C: Endometrial cytology in Endocrinology). *Acta Cytol* 2: 613-617, 1958.

de Brux J, Froment- Dupré J: Exfoliative Cytology of Reserve Cell Hyperplasia, Basal Cell Hyperplasia and Dysplasia. *Acta Cytol* 5: 142-149, 1961.

Deden C: Cancer I Tuba Uterina: Diagnostigeret ad Cytologisk Vej. [Cytodiagnosis of Carcinoma of the Fallopian Tube.] *Ugesk Laeger* 117: 790-791, 1955.

Degefu S, O'Quinn AG, Lacey CG, et al: Verrucous Carcinoma of the Cervix: A Report of Two Cases and Literature Review. *Gynecol Oncol* 25: 37-47, 1986.

De Girolami E: Perinuclear Halo Versus Koilocytotic Atypia. *Obstet Gynecol* 29: 479-487, 1967.

Dehner LP: Cervicovaginal Cytology, False-Negative Results, and Standards of Practice. *Am J Clin Pathol* 99: 45-47, 1993.

de Jesus M, Tang W, Sadjadi M, et al: Carcinoma of the Cervix With Extensive Endometrial and Myometrial Involvement. *Gynecol Oncol* 36: 263-270, 1990.

Dekel A, van Iddekinge B, Leiman G: Invasive Squamous Carcinoma of the Cervix in a 15-Year-Old Girl: A Case Report and Review of the Literature. *S Afr Med J* 61: 628-629, 1982.

Delaflor-Weiss E, Zauber NP, Kintiroglou M, et al: Acute Myelogenous Leukemia Relapsing as Granulocytic Sarcoma of the Cervix: A Case Report. *Acta Cytol* 43: 1124-1130, 1999.

de la Monte SM, Gupta PK, White CL 3rd: Systemic *Actinomyces* Infection: A Potential Complication of Intrauterine Contraceptive Devices. *JAMA* 248: 1876-1877, 1982.

Delgado G, Smith JP, Luis D, et al: Reticulum-Cell Sarcoma of the Cervix. *Am J Obstet Gynecol* 125: 691-694, 1976.

Delgado-Rodriguez M, Sillero-Arenas M, Martin-Moreno JM, et al: Oral Contraceptives and Cancer of the Cervix Uteri: A Meta-Analysis. *Acta Obstet Gynecol Scand* 71: 368-376, 1992.

Deligdisch L, Escay-Martinez, Cohen CJ: Endocervical Carcinoma: A Study of 23 Patients With Clinical-Pathological Correlation. *Gynecol Oncol* 18: 326-333, 1984.

Dell DL, Chen H, Ahmad F, et al: Knowledge About Human Papillomavirus Among Adolescents. *Obstet Gynecol* 96: 653-656, 2000.

Dell G, Gaston K: Contributions in the Domain of Cancer Research: Review. Human Papillomaviruses and Their Role in Cervical Cancer. *Cell Mol Life Sci (CMLS)* 58: 1923-1942, 2001.

DeLuca L, Maestri N, Bonanni F: Maintenance of Epithelial Cell Differentiation: The Mode of Action of Vitamin A. *Cancer* 30: 1326-1331, 1972.

DeMay RM: Should We Abandon Pap Smear Testing? *Am J Clin Pathol (Pathology Patterns Reviews)* 114: S48-S51, 2000.

Demian SDE, Bushkin FL, Echevarria RA: Perineural Invasion and Anaplastic Transformation of Verrucous Carcinoma. *Cancer* 32: 395-401, 1973.

DeMille PA, Bourquin P, Sun C-CJ: Cytologic Diagnosis of *Schistosoma haematobium* in Routine Cervicovaginal Smear from an Infertile Woman (Letter). *Diagn Cytopathol* 13: 181-182, 1995.

Demirezen S, Bozcuk S, Özcan M: Unusual Plant Cell Contamination in a Vaginal Smear (Letter). *Acta Cytol* 40: 841-842, 1996.

Demirezen S: Pinus Pollen in a Vaginal Smear (Letter). *Acta Cytol* 44: 481-482, 2000a.

Demirezen S, Safi Z, Beksac S: The Interaction of *Trichomonas vaginalis* With Epithelial Cells, Polymorphonuclear Leucocytes and Erythrocytes on Vaginal Smears: Light Microscopic Observation. *Cytopathology* 11: 326-332, 2000b.

Demirezen S: Phagocytosis of Erythrocytes by *Trichomonas vaginalis:* Examination of a Cervicovaginal Smear (Letter). *Diagn Cytopathol* 24: 425, 2001.

Demirezen S: Cytolytic Vaginosis: Examination of 2947 Vaginal Smears. *Cent Eur J Public Health* 11: 23-24, 2003a.

Demirezen S: Curschmann's Spiral in an 8-Year-Old Patient's Gynecologic Smear (Images in Cytopathology). *Diagn Cytopathol* 28: 212. 2003b.

Demirezen S: Review of Cytologic Criteria of Bacterial Vaginosis: Examination of 2,841 Papanicolaou-Stained Vaginal Smears. *Diagn Cytopathol* 29: 156-159, 2003c.

Demirkiran F, Arvas M, Erkun E, et al: The Prognostic Significance of Cervico-Vaginal Cytology in Endometrial Cancer. *Eur J Gynaecol Oncol* 16: 403-409, 1995.

DeMoraes-Ruehsen M, McNeill RE, Gupta PK, et al: Amebae Resembling *Entamoeba gingivalis* in the Genital Tracts of IUD Users. *Acta Cytol* 24: 413-420, 1980.

Denehy TR, Gregori CA, Breen JL: Endocervical Curettage, Cone Margins, and Residual Adenocarcinoma In Situ of the Cervix. *Obstet Gynecol* 90: 1-6, 1997.

de Peralta-Venturino M, Purslow MJ, Kini SR: Endometrial Cells of the "Lower Uterine Segment" (LUS) in Cervical Smears Obtained by Endocervical Brushings: A Source of Potential Diagnostic Pitfall. *Diagn Cytopathol* 12: 263-268; discussion 268-271, 1995.

de Peralta-Venturino M: Clinical Significance of Psammoma Bodies (PS) in Cervicovaginal Smears (CVS): A 5-Year Experience (Abstract). *Laboratory Investigation* 80: 43A, 2000.

DePetrillo AD, Townsend DE, Morrow CP, et al: Colposcopic Evaluation of the Abnormal Papanicolaou Test in Pregnancy. *Am J Obstet Gynecol* 121: 441-445, 1975.

Derman H, Koss LG, Hyman MP, et al: Cervical Cytopathology I: Peers Compare Performance. *Pathologist* 35: 317-325, 1981.

de Roda Husman A-M, Walboomers JMM, Meijer CJLM, et al: Analysis of Cytomorphologically Abnormal Cervical Scrapes for the Presence of 27 Mucosotropic Human Papillomavirus Genotypes, Using Polymerase Chain Reaction. *Int J Cancer* 56: 802-806, 1994.

de Sanjosé S, Muñoz N, Bosch FX, et al: Sexually Transmitted Agents and Cervical Neoplasia in Colombia and Spain. *Int J Cancer* 56: 358-363, 1994.

Deshpande AH, Munshi MM: Primary Malignant Melanoma of the Uterine Cervix: Report of a Case Diagnosed by Cervical Scrape Cytology and Review of the Literature. *Diagn Cytopathol* 25: 108-111, 2001.

De Torres EF, Benitez-Bribiesca L: Cytologic Detection of Vaginal Parasitosis. *Acta Cytol* 17: 252-257, 1973.

Devesa SS, Silverman DT, Young JL Jr, et al: Cancer Incidence and Mortality Trends Among Whites in the United States, 1947-1984. *J Natl Cancer Inst* 79: 701-770, 1987.

Devesa SS. Young JL Jr, Brinton LA, et al: Recent Trends in Cervix Uteri Cancer. *Cancer* 64: 2184-2190, 1989.

de Vet HC, Knipschild PG, Schouten HJ, et al: Interobserver Variation in Histopathological Grading of Cervical Dysplasia. *J Clin Epidemiol* 43: 1395-1398, 1990.

de Vet HC, Knipschild PG, Schouten HJ, et al: Sources of Interobserver Variation in Histopathological Grading of Cervical Dysplasia. *J Clin Epidemiol* 45: 785-790, 1992.

de Vet HC, Knipschild PG, Sturmans F: The Role of Sexual Factors in the Aetiology of Cervical Dysplasia. *Int J Epidemiol* 22: 798-803, 1993.

de Vet HC, Sturmans F: Risk Factors for Cervical Dysplasia: Implications for Prevention. *Public Health* 108: 241-249, 1994.

de Villiers E-M, Schneider A, Miklaw H, et al: Human Papillomavirus Infections in Women With and Without Abnormal Cervical Cytology. *Lancet* (ii): 703-706, 1987.

de Villiers E-M, Wagner D, Schneider A, et al: Human Papillomavirus DNA in Women Without and With Cytological Abnormalities: Results of a 5-Year Follow-up Study. *Gynecol Oncol* 44: 33-39, 1992.

de Villiers E-M: Taxonomic Classification of Papillomaviruses. *Papillomavirus Report* 12: 57-63, 2001.

Dhar JP, Kmak D, Bhan R, et al: Abnormal Cervicovaginal Cytology in Women With Lupus: A Retrospective Cohort Study. *Gynecol Oncol* 82: 4-6, 2001.

Dhimes P, Alberti N, De Agustin P, et al: Primary Malignant Lymphoma of the Uterine Cervix: Report of a Case With Cytologic and Immunohistochemical Diagnosis. *Cytopathology* 7: 204-210, 1996.

Diamandopoulos GT: Cancer: An Historial Perspective. *Anticancer Res* 16: 1595-1602, 1996.

Díaz-Rosario LA, Kabawat SE: Performance of a Fluid-Based, Thin-Layer Papanicolaou Smear Method in the Clinical Setting of an Independent Laboratory and an Outpatient Screening Population in New England. *Arch Pathol Lab Med* 123: 817-821, 1999.

DiBonito L, Falconieri G, Tomasic G, et al: Cervical Cytopathology: An Evaluation of Its Accuracy Based on Cytohistologic Comparison. *Cancer* 72: 3002-3006, 1993.

Dickersin GR, Welch WR, Erlandson R, et al: Ultrastructure of 16 Cases of Clear Cell Adenocarcinoma of the Vagina and Cervix in Young Women. *Cancer* 45: 1615-1624, 1980.

Dieckmann WJ, Davis ME, Rynkiewicz LM, et al: Does the Administration of Diethylstilbestrol During Pregnancy Have Therapeutic Value? *Am J Obstet Gynecol* 181: 1572-1573, 1999.

Differding JT: Psammoma Bodies in a Vaginal Smear. *Acta Cytol* 11: 199-201, 1967.

Di Luca D, Rotola A, Pilotti S, et al: Simultaneous Presence of Herpes Simplex and Human Papilloma Virus Sequences in Human Genital Tumors. *Int J Cancer* 40: 763-768, 1987.

Di Luca D, Costa S, Monini P, et al: Search for Human Papillomavirus, Herpes Simplex Virus and c-myc Oncogene in Human Genital Tumors. *Int J Cancer* 43: 570-577, 1989.

Dimian C, Nayagam M, Bradbeer C: The Association Between Sexually Transmitted Diseases and Inflammatory Cervical Cytology. *Genitourin Med* 68: 305-306, 1992.

DiTomasso JP, Ramzy I, Mody DR: Glandular Lesions of the Cervix. Validity of Cytologic Criteria Used to Differentiate Reactive Changes, Glandular Intraepithelial Lesions and Adenocarcinoma. *Acta Cytol* 40: 1127-1135, 1996; erratum appears in *Acta Cytol* 41: 619-620, 1997.

Dodd LG, Sneige N, Villarreal Y, et al: Quality-Assurance Study of Simultaneously Sampled, Non-Correlating Cervical Cytology and Biopsies. *Diagn Cytopathol* 9: 138-144, 1993.

Döderlein A: III. Die Scheidensekretuntersuchungen. *Zentralbl Gynäcologie* 18: 10-14, 1894.

Dodson MG, O'Leary JA, Averette HE: Primary Carcinoma of Bartholin's Gland. *Obstet Gynecol* 35: 578-584, 1970.

Doherty MG, Payne D, Tyring SK, et al: Chronic Plasma Cell Cervicitis Simulating a Cervical Malignancy: A Case Report. *Obstet Gynecol* 82: 646-650, 1993.

Doll R: Cancers Weakly Related to Smoking. *Br Med Bull* 52: 35-49, 1996.

Donders GG, van Straeten D, Hooft P, et al: Detection of Candida Cell Forms in Pap Smears During Pregnancy *Eur J Obstet Gynecol Reprod Biol* 43: 13-18, 1992.

Donders GGG: Microscopy of the Bacterial Flora on Fresh Vaginal Smears. *Infect Dis Obstet Gynecol* 7:126-127; erratum appears in *Infect Dis Obstet Gynecol* 7: 177-179, 1999.

Donders GGG, Vereecken A, Bosmans E, et al: Definition of a Type of Abnormal Vaginal Flora that Is Distinct from Bacterial Vaginosis: Aerobic Vaginitis. *Br J Obstet Gynecol* 109: 34-43, 2002.

Doornewaard H, Sie-Go DMD, Woudt JMC, et al: De betekenis van endometriumcellen in de cervixuitstrijk (Dutch). [The Significance of Endometrial Cells in the Cervical Smear.] *Ned Tijdschr v. Geneeskunde* 137: 868-872, 1993.

Dorman SA, Danos LM, Wilson DJ, et al: Detection of Chlamydial Cervicitis by Papanicolaou Stained Smears and Culture. *Am J Clin Pathol* 79: 421-425, 1983.

Doss BJ, DeMay RM, Larson RA et al: Chemotherapy Induced Epithelial Atypia in the Female Lower Genital Tract (Abstract). *Mod Pathol* 8: 89A. 1995.

Douglass LE: A Further Comment on the Contributions of Aurel Babès to Cytology and Pathology. *Acta Cytol* 11: 217-224, 1967.

Douglass LE: Odorico Viana and His Contribution to Diagnostic Cytology. *Acta Cytol* 14: 544-549, 1970.

Drake M: Nomenclature of Precancerous Lesions of the Uterine Cervix: A Position Paper. *Acta Cytol* 28: 527-534, 1984.

Draper GJ, Cook GA: Changing Patterns of Cervical Cancer Rates. *Br Med J* 287: 510-512, 1983.

Dressel DM, Dressel IJ, Wilbur DC: Stromal Histiocytes in Routine Papanicolaou Smears: Histopathologic and Clinical Significance (Abstract). *Acta Cytol* 36: 629, 1992a.

Dressel DM, Wilber DC: Atypical Immature Squamous Metaplastic Cells in Cervical Smears: Association With High-Grade Squamous Intraepithelial Lesions and Carcinoma of the Cervix (Abstract). *Acta Cytol* 36: 630, 1992b.

Drijkoningen M, Meertens B, Lauweryns J: High-Grade Squamous Intraepithelial Lesion (CIN 3) With Extension into the Endocervical Clefts: Difficulty of Cytologic Differentiation from Adenocarcinoma In Situ. *Acta Cytol* 40: 889-894, 1996.

DuBeshter B, Warshal DP, Angel C, et al: Endometrial Carcinoma: The Relevance of Cervical · Cytology. *Obstet Gynecol* 77: 458-462, 1991.

DuBeshter B: Endometrial Cancer: Predictive Value of Cervical Cytology (Editorial). *Gynecol Oncol* 72: 271-272, 1999.

DuBeshter B, Deuel C, Gillis S, et al: Endometrical Cancer: The Potential Role of Cervical Cytology in Current Surgical Staging. *Obstet Gynecol* 101: 445-450, 2003.

Duca P, Braga M, Chiappa L, et al: Intralaboratory Reproducibility of Interpretation of Pap Smears: Results of an Experiment. *Tumori* 74: 737-744, 1988.

Ducan ME, Tibaux G, Pelzer A, et al: First Coitis Before Menarche and Risk of Sexually Transmitted Disease. *Lancet* 335: 338-340, 1990.

Ducatman BS, Wang HH, Jonasson JG, et al: Tubal Metaplasia: A Cytologic Study With Comparison to Other Neoplastic and Non-Neoplastic Conditions of the Endocervix. *Diagn Cytopathol* 9: 98-105, 1993.

Dudding N: Pale Dsykaryosis in Cervical Smears (Letter). *Cytopathology* 7: 221-222, 1996a.

Dudding N, Sutton J, Lane S: Koilocytosis; an Indication for Conservative Management. *Cytopathology* 7: 32-37, 1996b.

Dudkiewicz J: Cytomorphology of Epithelial Cells of Fallopian Tubes Obtained by Aspiration from Operative Specimens. *Am J Obstet Gynecol* 102: 82-90, 1968.

Dudkiewicz J: Quantitative and Qualitative Changes of Epithelial Cells of Fallopian Tubes in Women According to the Phase of Menstrual Cycle: A Cytologic Study. *Acta Cytol* 14: 531-537, 1970.

Duensing S, Duensing A, Crum CP, et al: Human Papillomavirus Type 16 E7 Oncoprotein–Induced Abnormal Centrosome Synthesis Is an Early Event in the Evolving Malignant Phenotype. *Cancer Res* 61: 2356-2360, 2001.

Duerr A, Kieke B, Warren D, et al: Human Papillomavirus-Associated Cervical Cytologic Abnormalities Among Women With or at Risk of Infection With Human Immunodeficiency Virus. *Am J Obstet Gynecol* 184: 584-590, 2001.

Duffy BJ: Papanicolaou Testing: Are We Screening the Wrong Women? (Massachusetts Department of Health) (Letter). *New Engl J Med* 294: 223, 1976.

Duggan MA, Benoit JL, McGregor SE, et al: The Human Papillomavirus Status of 114 Endocervical Adenocarcinoma Cases by Dot Blot Hybridization. *Hum Pathol* 24: 121-125, 1993.

Duggan MA, Benoit JL, McGregor SE, et al: Adenocarcinoma In Situ of the Endocervix-Human Papillomavirus Determination by Dot Blot Hybridization and Polymerase Chain Reaction Amplification. *Int J Gynecol Pathol* 13: 143-149, 1994.

Duggan MA, McGregor SE, Benoit JL, et al: The Human Papillomavirus Status of Invasive Cervical Adenocarcinoma: A Clinicopathological and Outcome Analysis. *Hum Pathol* 26: 319-325, 1995.

Duggan MA, McGregor SE, Stuart GCE, et al: Predictors of Co-Incidental CIN II/III Amongst a Cohort of Women With CIN I Detected by a Screening Pap Test. *Eur J Gynaecol Oncol* 19: 209-214, 1998a.

Duggan MA, McGregor SE, Stuart GCE, et al: The Natural History of CIN I Lesions. *Eur J Gynaecol Oncol* 19: 338-344, 1998b.

Duggan MA, Brasher PMA: Accuracy of Pap Tests Reported as CIN I. *Diagn Cytopathol* 21: 129-136, 1999.

Duggan MA: Cytologic and Histologic Diagnosis and Significance of Controversial Squamous Lesions of the Uterine Cervix. *Mod Pathol* 13: 252-260, 2000.

Duggan-Keen MF, Brown MD, Stacey SN, et al: Papillomavirus Vaccines. *Frontiers Biosci* 3: d1192-d1208, 1998.

Duguid HL, Parratt D, Traynor RT: Actinomyces-Like Organisms in Cervical Smears from Women Using Intrauterine Contraceptive Devices. *Br Med J* 281: 534-537, 1980.

Dunn AEG, Ogilvie MM: Intranuclear Virus Particles in Human Genital Wart Tissue: Observations on the Ultrastructure of the Epidermal Layer. *J Ultrastruct Res* 22: 282-295, 1968.

Dunn JE Jr, Martin PL: Morphogenesis of Cervical Cancer. Findings from San Diego County Cytology Registry. *Cancer* 20: 1899-1906, 1967.

Dunn JE Jr, Schweitzer V: The Relationship of Cervical Cytology to the Incidence of Invasive Cervical Cancer and Mortality in Alameda County, California, 1960 to 1974. *Am J Obstet Gynecol* 139: 868-876, 1981.

Dunn TB: Cancer of the Uterine Cervix in Mice Fed a Liquid Diet Containing an Antifertility Drug. *J Natl Cancer Inst* 43: 671-692, 1969.

Du Plessis EM, Dicks LM: Evaluation of Random Amplified Polymorphic DNA (RAPD)-PCR as a Method to Differentiate *Lactobacillus acidophilus, Lactobacillus crispatus, Lactobacillus amylovorus, Lactobacillus gallinarium, Lactobacillus gasseri,* and *Lactobacillus johnsonnii. Curr Microbiol* 31: 114-118, 1995.

du Plessis JM, Schaetzing AE, Wrantz PA: Aylesbury and Cervitula Spatulas: A Comparative Study to Assess the Adequacy of Cervical Smears. *Acta Cytol* 45: 675-678, 2001.

Dupree WB, Suprun HZ, Beckwith DG, et al: The Promise and Risk of a New Technology: The Lehigh Valley Hospital's Experience With Liquid-Based Cervical Cytology. *Cancer (Cancer Cytopathol)* 84: 202-207, 1998; erratum with editorial counterpoint by RM Austin appearing under Beckwith DG, Shane JJ, Dupree WB, *Cancer (Cytopathol)* 84: 317-318, 1998.

Dürst M, Gissmann L, Ikenberg H, et al: A Papillomavirus DNA from a Cervical Carcinoma and Its Prevalence in Cancer Biopsy Samples from Different Geographic Regions. *Proc Natl Acad Sci (USA)* 80: 3812-3815, 1983.

Dürst M, Kleinheinz A, Hotz M, et al: The Physical State of Human Papillomavirus Type 16 DNA in Benign and Malignant Genital Tumours. *J Gen Virol* 66: 1515-1522, 1985.

Dürst M, Croce CM, Gissmann L, et al: Papillomavirus Sequences Integrate Near Cellular Oncogenes in Some Cervical Carcinomas. *Proc Natl Acad Sci (USA)* 84: 1070-1074, 1987a.

Dürst M, Dzarlieva-Petrusevska RT, Boukamp P, et al: Molecular and Cytogenetic Analysis of Immortalized Primary Keratinocytes Obtained after Transfection With Human Papillomavirus Type 16 DNA. *Oncogene* 1: 251-256, 1987b.

Duska LR, Flynn CF, Chen A, et al: Clinical Evaluation of Atypical Glandular Cells of Undetermined Significance on Cervical Cytology. *Obstet Gynecol* 91: 278-282, 1998.

Dvorak KA, Finnemore M, Maksem JA: Histology Correlation With Atypical Squamous Cells of Undetermined Significance (ASCUS) and Low-Grade Squamous Intraepithelial Lesion (LSIL) Cytology Diagnoses: An Argument to Ensure ASCUS Follow-Up That Is as Aggressive as That for LSIL. *Diagn Cytopathol* 21: 292-295, 1999.

Dvoretsky PM, Bonfiglio TA, Patten SF Jr, at al: Pemphigus Vulgaris and Microinvasive Squamous-Cell Carcinoma of the Uterine Cervix. *Acta Cytol* 29: 403-410, 1985.

Dybdahl H, Hastrup J, Baandrup U: The Clinical Significance of *Actinomyces* Colonization as Seen in Cervical Smears. *Acta Cytol* 35: 142-143, 1991.

Dyer ML, Young TL, Kattine AA, et al: Blastomycosis in a Papanicolaou Smear: Report of a Case With Possible Venereal Transmission. *Acta Cytol* 27: 285-287, 1983.

Dyson N, Howley PM, Münger K, et al: The Human Papilloma Virus-16 E7 Oncoprotein Is Able to Bind to the Retinoblastoma Gene Product. *Science* 243: 934-937, 1989.

E

Ebrahim S, Daponte A, Smith TH, et al: Primary Mucinous Adenocarcinoma of the Vagina. *Gynecol Oncol* 80: 89-92, 2001.

Eckert LO, Koutsky LA, Kiviat NB, et al: The Inflammatory Papanicolaou Smear: What Does It Mean? *Obstet Gynecol* 86: 360-366, 1995.

Economos K, Veridiano NP, Delke I, et al: Abnormal Cervical Cytology in Pregnancy: A 17-Year Experience. *Obstet Gynecol* 81: 915-918, 1993.

Economos K, Perez-Veridiano N, Mann M, et al: Abnormal Cervical Cytology in Adolescents: A 15-Year Experience. *J Reprod Med* 39: 973-976, 1994.

Eddy DM: Screening for Cervical Cancer. *Ann Intern Med* 113: 214-226, 1990.

Eddy GL, Spiegel GW, Creasman WT: Adverse Effect of Electrosurgical Loop Excision on Assignment of FIGO Stage in Cervical Cancer: Report of Two Cases. *Gynecol Oncol* 55: 313-317, 1994.

Eddy GL, Strumpf KB, Wojtowycz MA, et al: Biopsy Findings in Five Hundred Thirty-One Patients With Atypical Glandular Cells of Uncertain Significance as Defined by the Bethesda System. *Am J Obstet Gynecol* 177: 1188-1195, 1997a.

Eddy GL, Ural SH, Strumpf KB, et al: Incidence of Atypical Glandular Cells of Uncertain Significance in Cervical Cytology Following Introduction of the Bethesda System. *Gynecol Oncol* 67: 51-55, 1997b.

Eddy GL, Wojtowycz MA, Piraino PS, et al: Papanicolaou Smears by the Bethesda System in Endometrial Malignancy: Utility and Prognostic Importance. *Obstet Gynecol* 90: 999-1003, 1997c.

Edebiri AA: Cervical Intraepithelial Neoplasia: The Role of Age at First Coitus in Its Etiology. *J Reprod Med* 35: 256-259, 1990.

Edelman M, Fox A, Alderman EM, et al: Cervical Papanicolaou Smear Abnormalities in Inner City Bronx Adolescents. Prevalence, Progression, and Immune Modifiers. *Cancer (Cancer Cytopathol)* 87: 184-189, 1999.

Edelman M, Fox A, Alderman E, et al: Cervical Papanicolaou Smear Abnormalities and *Chlamydia trachomatis* in Sexually Active Adolescent Females. *J Pediatr Adolesc Gynecol* 13: 65-69, 2000.

Edwards SK, Sonnex C: Influence of Genital Infection on Cervical Cytology. *Sex Transm Inf* 74: 271-273, 1998.

Eells TP, Alpern HD, Grzywacz C, et al: The Effect of Tamoxifen on Cervical Squamous Maturation in Papanicolaou Stained Cervical Smears of Post-Menopausal Women. *Cytopathology* 1: 263-268, 1990.

Efstratiades M, Tamvakopoulou E, Papatheodorou B, et al: Postmenopausal Vaginal Cytohormonal Pattern in 597 Healthy Women and 301 Patients With Genital Cancer. *Acta Cytol* 26: 126-130, 1982.

Egan AJ, Russel P: Transitional (Urothelial) Cell Metaplasia of the Uterine Cervix: Morphological Assessment of 31 Cases. *Int J Gynecol Pathol* 16: 89-98, 1997.

Egan ME, Lipsky MS: Diagnosis of Vaginitis. *Am Fam Physician* 62: 1095-1104, 2000.

Ehrmann RL, Younge PA, Lerch VL: The Exfoliative Cytology and Histogenesis of an Early Primary Malignant Melanoma of the Vagina. *Acta Cytol* 6: 245-254, 1962.

Ehrmann RL: Atypical Endometrial Cells and Stromal Breakdown: Two Case Reports. *Acta Cytol* 19: 463-469, 1975.

Ehrmann RL, Dwyer IM, Yavner D, et al: An Immunoperoxidase Study of Laminin and Type IV Collagen Distribution in Carcinoma of the Cervix and Vulva. *Obstet Gynecol* 72: 257-262, 1988.

Ehrmann RL: Benign to Malignant Progression in Cervical Squamous Epithelium. *Comprehensive Therapy* 22: 67-75, 1996.

Eichhorn JH, Young RH: Neuroendocrine Tumors of the Genital Tract. *Am J Clin Pathol (Pathology Patterns Reviews)* 115: S94-S112, 2001.

Einstein MH, Burk RD: Persistent Human Papillomavirus Infection: Definitions and Clinical Implications. *Papillomavirus Report* 12: 119-123, 2001.

Eisenstein R, Battifora H: Lymph Follicles in Cervical Smears. *Acta Cytol* 9: 344-346, 1965.

Ejersbo D, Jensen HA, Holund B: Efficacy of Ki-67 Antigen Staining in Papanicolaou (Pap) Smears in Post-Menopausal Women With Atypia—An Audit. *Cytopathology* 10: 369-374, 1999.

Elfgren K, Kalantari M, Moberger B, et al: a Population-Based Five-Year Follow-up Study of Cervical Human Papillomavirus Infection. *Am J Obstet Gynecol* 183: 561-567, 2000.

El Hamidi A, Kocjan G, Du M-Q: Clonality Analysis of Archival Cervical Smears: Correlation of Monoclonality With Grade and Clinical Behavior of Cervical Intraepithelial Neoplasia. *Acta Cytol* 47: 117-123, 2003.

Elias A, Linthorst G, Bekker B, et al: The Significance of Endocervical Cells in the Diagnosis of Cervical Epithelial Changes. *Acta Cytol* 27: 225-229, 1983.

Elkas J, Farias-Eisner R: Cancer of the Uterine Cervix. *Curr Opin Obstet Gynecol* 10: 47-50, 1998.

Ellerbrock TV, Chiasson MA, Bush TJ, et al: Incidence of Cervical Squamous Intraepithelial Lesions in HIV-Infected Women. *JAMA* 283: 1031-1037, 2000.

Elliott PM, Tattersall MHN, Coppleson M, et al: Changing Character of Cervical Cancer in Young Women. *Br Med J* 298: 288-290, 1989.

Elnashar AM, Aboelea A, Tantawy TA: Cytologic, Coloscopic, and Virologic Detection of Cervical Herpes Simplex Virus. *Int J Gynecol Obstet* 81: 69-70, 2003.

el Tabbakh G, Hamza MA: Carcinoma of the Uterine Cervix and Schistosomiasis. *Int J Gynaecol Obstet* 29: 263-268, 1989.

Eltabbakh GH, Lipman JN, Mount ST, et al: Significance of Atypical Squamous Cells of Undetermined Significance on ThinPrep Papanicolaou Smears. *Gynecol Oncol* 79: 44-49, 2000a.

Eltabbakh GH, Lipman JN, Mount SL, et al: Significance of Atypical Glandular Cells of Undetermined Significance on ThinPrep Papanicolaou Smears. *Gynecol Oncol* 78: 245-250, 2000b.

Eluf-Neto J, Booth M, Muñoz N, et al: Human Papillomavirus and Invasive Cervical Cancer in Brazil. *Br J Cancer* 69: 114-119, 1994.

Emerson RE, Puzanov A, Brunnemer C, et al: Long-Term Follow-Up of Women With Atypical Squamous Cells of Undetermined Significance (ASCUS). *Diagn Cytopathol* 27: 153-157, 2002.

Engineer AD, Misra JS, Tandon P: Long-Term Cytologic Studies of Copper-IUD Users. *Acta Cytol* 25: 550-556, 1981.

Enhörning G, Huldt L, Melén B: Ability of Cervical Mucus to Act as a Barrier Against Bacteria. *Am J Obstet Gynecol* 108: 532-537, 1970.

Epstein NA: The Significance of Cellular Atypia in the Diagnosis of Malignancy in Ulcers of the Female Genital Tract. *Acta Cytol* 16: 483-489, 1972.

Epstein NA: Cytologic Presentation of Transitional Cell Carcinoma Metastatic to Uterus. *Acta Cytol* 20: 283-285, 1976.

Eren F, Savci D, Erbarut Í, et al: Benign Glandular Cells in Posthysterectomy Vaginal Smears: The Incidence Is Higher Than Expected. *Cytopathology* 15: 195-199, 2004.

Erzen M, Mozina A, Bertole J, et al: Factors Predicting Disease Outcome in Early Stage Adenocarcinoma of the Uterine Cervix. *Eur J Obstet Gynecol Reprod Biol* 101: 185-191, 2002.

Eschenbach DA, Hillier S, Critchlow C, et al: Diagnosis of Clinical Manifestations of Bacterial Vaginosis. *Am J Obstet Gynecol* 158: 819-828, 1988.

Eschenbach DA, Davick PR, Williams BL, et al: Prevalence of Hydrogen Peroxide-Producing *Lactobacillus* Species in Normal Women and Women With Bacterial Vaginosis. *J Clin Microbiol* 27: 251-256, 1989.

Eschenbach DA: History and Review of Bacterial Vaginosis. *Am J Obstet Gynecol* 169: 441-445, 1993.

Eschenbach DA, Patton DL, Hooton TM, et al: Influence of Normal Menstrual Cycle on Vaginal Tissue, Discharge, and Microflora. *Clin Infect Dis* 30: 901-907, 2000.

Eschenbach DA, Patton DL, Hooton TM, et al: Effects of Vaginal Intercourse With and Without a Condom on Vaginal Flora and Vaginal Epithelium. *J Infect Dis* 183: 913-918, 2001.

Eskenazi B, Warner ML: Epidemiology of Endometriosis. *Obstet Gynecol Clin North Am* 24: 235-258, 1997.

Etherington IJ, Ellis JR, Luesley DM, et al: Histologic and Immunologic Associations of an HPV16 Variant in LoSIL Smears. *Gynecol Oncol* 72: 56-59, 1999.

Etherington IJ, Luesley DM: Adenocarcinoma In situ of the Cervix—Controversies in Diagnosis and Treatment. *J Low Genital Tract Dis* 5: 94-98, 2001.

Ettler HC, Joseph MG, Downing PA, et al: Atypical Squamous Cells of Undetermined Significance: A Cytohistological Study in a Colposcopy Clinic. *Diagn Cytopathol* 21: 211-216, 1999.

Evander M, Frazer IH, Payne E, et al: Identification of the Alpha 6 Integrin as a Candidate Receptor for Papillomaviruses. *J Virol* 71: 2449-2456, 1997.

Evans AS, Monaghan JM: Spontaneous Resolution of Cervical Warty Atypia: The Relevance of Clinical and Nuclear DNA Features: A Prospective Study. *Br J Obstet Gynaecol* 92: 165-169, 1985.

Evans AS, Mueller NE: Viruses and Cancer: Causal Associations. *Ann Epidemiol* 1: 71-92, 1990.

Evans CS, Klein HZ, Goldman R, et al: Necrobiotic Granulomas of the Uterine Cervix: A Probable Postoperative Reaction. *Am J Surg Pathol* 8: 841-844, 1984.

Evans DM, Hudson EA, Brown CL, et al: Terminology in Gynaecological Cytopathology: Report of the Working Party of The British Society for Clinical Cytology. *J Clin Pathol* 39: 933-944, 1986.

Evans DM, Hudson EA, Brown CL, et al: Management of Women With Abnormal Cervical Smears: Supplement to Terminology in Gynaecological Cytopathology. *J Clin Pathol* 40: 530-531, 1987.

Evans DT: *Actinomyces israelii* in the Female Genital Tract: A Review. *Genitourin Med* 69: 54-59, 1993.

Evans S, Dowling K: The Changing Prevalence of Cervical Human Papilloma Virus Infection. *Aust N Z J Obstet Gynaecol* 30: 375-377, 1990.

Ezra D, Baithun SI, Dodd SM, et al: Ethnic Factors in the Pathology of the Uterine Cervix Cervical Screening: A Population at Variance With National Targets. *Cytopathology* 11: 480-487, 2000.

F

Fahey MT, Irwig L, Macaskill P: Meta-Analysis of Pap Test Accuracy. *Am J Epidemiol* 141: 680-689, 1995.

Fairley CK, Chen S, Tabrizi SN, et al: The Absence of Genital Human Papillomavirus DNA in Virginal Women. *Int J STD AIDS* 3: 414-417, 1992.

Fairley CK, Chen S, Ugoni A, et al: Human Papillomavirus Infection and Its Relationship to Recent and Distant Sexual Partners. *Obstet Gynecol* 84: 755-759, 1994.

Falcón-Escobedo R, Mora-Tiscareno A, Puebilitz-Peredo S: Malakoplakia of the Uterine Cervix: Histologic, Cytologic and Ultrastructural Study of a Case. *Acta Cytol* 30: 281-284, 1986.

Falls RK: Spontaneous Resolution Rate of Grade 1 Cervical Intraepithelial Neoplasia in a Private Practice Population. *Am J Obstet Gynecol* 181: 278-282, 1999.

Faquin WC, Brown FM, Krane JF, et al: Extensively Keratinized Squamous Intraepithelial Lesions of the Cervix Are Difficult to Grade. *Am J Clin Pathol* 115: 80-84, 2001.

Farnsworth A, Laverty C, Stoler MH: Human Papillomavirus Messenger RNA Expression in Adenocarcinoma In Situ of the Uterine Cervix. *Int J Gynecol Pathol* 8: 321-330, 1989.

Fasal E, Simmons ME, Kampert JB: Factors Associated With High- and Low-Risk of Cervical Neoplasia. *J Natl Cancer Inst* 66: 631-636, 1981.

Fechner RE, Bossart MI, Spjut HJ: Ultrastructure of Endometrial Stromal Foam Cells. *Am J Clin Pathol* 72: 628-633, 1979.

Feeley KM, Wells M: Hormone Replacement Therapy and the Endometrium. *J Clin Pathol* 54: 435-440, 2001.

Fehr PE, Prem KA: Malignancy of the Uterine Corpus Following Irradiation Therapy for Squamous Cell Carcinoma of the Cervix. *Am J Obstet Gynecol* 119: 685-692, 1974.

Feichter G, Curschellas E, Gobat S, et al: Malignant Melanoma of the Uterine Cervix: Case Report Including Cytology, Histology and Immunocytochemistry. *Cytopathology* 6: 196-200, 1995.

Feingold AR, Vermund SH, Burk RD, et al: Cervical Cytologic Abnormalities and Papillomavirus in Women Infected With Human Immunodeficiency Virus. *J Acquir Immune Defic Syndr* 3: 896-903, 1990.

Feingold ML, Koss LG: Effects of Long-Term Administration of Busulfan: Report of a Patient With Generalized Nuclear Abnormalities, Carcinoma of Vulva, and Pulmonary Fibrosis. *Arch Intern Med* 124: 66-71, 1969.

Feldman D, Feldman SH, Covell JL, et al: Retrospective Study of *Chlamydia trachomatis* Using the Polymerase Chain Reaction on Archival Papanicolaou-Stained Cytologic Smears. *Acta Cytol* 45: 985-989, 2001.

Feldman MJ, Linzey EM, Srebnik E, et al: Abnormal Cervical Cytology in the Teenager: A Continuing Problem. *Am J Obstet Gynecol* 126: 418-421, 1976.

Feldman S, Cook EF, Harlow BL, et al: Predicting Endometrial Cancer Among Older Women Who Present With Abnormal Vaginal Bleeding. *Gynecol Oncol* 56: 376-381, 1995.

Feldman S: How Often Should We Screen for Cervical Cancer? (Perspective) *N Engl J Med* 349: 1495-1496, 2003.

Feldmeier H, Helling-Giese G, Poggensee G: Unreliability of PAP Smears to Diagnose Female Genital Schistosomiasis. *Tropical Medicine* 6: 31-33, 2001.

Felix JC: The Science Behind the Effectiveness of In Vivo Screening. *Am J Obstet Gynecol* 188(Suppl 3): S8-S12, 2003.

Felman YM, Nikitas JA: Trichomoniasis, Candidiasis, and *Corynebacterium vaginale* vaginitis. *NY State J Med* 79: 1563-1566, 1979.

Fels E: Endometriose der Portico. *Zentralbl Gynäkol* 52: 285-288, 1928.

Fennell RH Jr: Carcinoma In Situ of the Cervix With Early Invasive Changes. *Cancer* 8: 302-309, 1955.

Fenoglio CM: Viruses in the Pathogenesis of Cervical Neoplasia: An Update. *Hum Pathol* 13: 785-787, 1982.

Fentanes deTorres E, Mora A: Verrucous Carcinoma of the Cervix Uteri: Report of a Case. *Acta Cytol* 25: 307-309, 1981.

Fenton J, Chevret S, Asselain B, et al: Le cancer invasive du col utérin de la femme jeune: étude rétrospective de 236 cas. [Invasive Cancer of the Uterine Cervix in Young Women: Retrospective Study of 236 Cases.] *Bull Cancer* 77: 109-116, 1990.

Ferenczy A, Richart RM, Okagaki T: Endometrial Involvement by Cervical Carcinoma In Situ. *Am J Obstet Gynecol* 110: 590-592, 1971.

Ferenczy A, Braun L, Shah KV: Human Papillomavirus (HPV) in Condylomatous Lesions of Cervix: A Comparative Ultrastructural and Immunohistochemical Study. *Am J Surg Pathol* 5: 661-670, 1981.

Ferenczy A, Kohn I, Shore M: Evaluating Male Partners of Condyloma Patients. *Contemp OB-Gyn* 6: 183-190; 193-196, 1983.

Ferenczy A, Gelfand MM: Outpatient Endometrial Sampling With Endocyte: Comparative Study of Its Effectiveness With Endometrial Biopsy. *Obstet Gynecol* 63: 295-302, 1984.

Ferenczy A, Mitao M, Nagai N, et al: Latent Papillomavirus and Recurring Genital Warts. *N Engl J Med* 313: 784-788, 1985.

Ferenczy A, Bergeron C, Richart R: Human Papillomavirus DNA in Fomites on Objects for the Management of Patients With Genital Human Papillomavirus Infections. *Obstet Gynecol* 74: 950-954, 1989.

Ferenczy A, Bergeron C, Richart R: Human Papillomavirus DNA in CO_2 Laser-Generated Plume of Smoke and Its Consequences to the Surgeon. *Obstet Gynecol* 75: 114-118, 1990.

Ferenczy A: Viral Testing for Genital Human Papillomavirus Infections: Recent Progress and Clinical Potentials. *Int J Gynecol Cancer* 5: 321-328, 1995.

Ferenczy A, Franco E, Arseneau J, et al: Diagnostic Performance of Hybrid Capture Human Papillomavirus Deoxyribonucleic Acid Assay Combined With Liquid-Based Cytologic Study. *Am J Obstet Gynecol* 175: 651-656, 1996a.

Ferenczy A, Jenson AB: Tissue Effects and Host Response: The Key to the Rational Triage of Cervical Neoplasia. *Obstet Gynecol Clin North Am* 23: 759-782, 1996b.

Ferenczy A, Gelfand MM, Franco E, et al: Human Papillomavirus Infection in Postmenopausal Women With and Without Hormone Therapy. *Obstet Gynecol* 90: 7-11, 1997.

Ferguson AW, Svoboda-Newman SM, Frank TS: Analysis of Human Papillomavirus Infection and Molecular Alterations in Adenocarcinoma of the Cervix. *Mod Pathol* 11: 11-8, 1998.

Ferguson JH: Positive Cancer Smears in Teenage Girls. *JAMA* 178: 365-368, 1961.

Fernández-Esquer ME, Ross MW, Torres I: The Importance of Psychosocial Factors in the Prevention of HPV Infection and Cervical Cancer. *Int J STD AIDS* 11: 701-713, 2000.

Ferrante JM, Mayhew DY, Goldberg S, et al: Empiric Treatment of Minimally Abnormal Papanicolaou Smears With 0.75% Metronidazole Vaginal Gel. *J Am Board Fam Pract* 15: 347-354, 2002; erratum appears in *J Am Board Fam Pract* 15: 456, 2002.

Ferrara G, Goglia P: Recognition of Rectal Glandular Cells in Vaginal Smears (Letter). *Acta Cytol* 41: 1860-1861, 1997.

Ferrara G, Cannone M, Guadagnino A, et al: Nested Polymerase Chain Reaction on Vaginal Smears of Tuberculous Cervicitis: A Case Report. *Acta Cytol* 43: 308-312, 1999.

Ferrazzi E, Cartei G, Mattarazzo R, et al: Oestrogen-Like Effect of Tamoxifen on Vaginal Epithelium. *Br Med J* 1: 1351-1352, 1977.

Ferreira do Amaral C: Cytology of Endometrial Hyperplasia (Symposium on Endometrial Cytology. C: Endometrial Cytology in Endocrinology). *Acta Cytol* 2: 617, 1958.

Ferrera A, Velema JP, Figueroa M, et al: Co-Factors Related to the Causal Relationship Between Human Papillomavirus and Invasive Cervical Cancer in Honduras. *Int J Epidemiol* 29: 817-825, 2000.

Ferris DG, Krumholz BA, Jester DM et al: Atypical Glandular Cells of Undetermined Significance and Adenocarcinoma In Situ: Summoning Colposcopic Expertise? *J Fam Pract* 43: 181-187, 1996.

Ferris DG, Wright TC Jr, Litaker MS, et al: Triage of Women With ASCUS and LSIL on Pap Smear Reports: Management by Repeat Pap Smear, HPV DNA Testing, or Colposcopy. *J Fam Pract* 46: 125-134, 1998.

Ferry JA, Scully RE: "Adenoid Cystic" Carcinoma and Adenoid Basal Carcinoma of the Uterine Cervix: A Study of 28 Cases. *Am J Surg Pathol* 12: 134-144, 1988.

Ferry JA, Scully RE: Mesonephric Remnants, Hyperplasia, and Neoplasia in the Uterine Cervix: A Study of 49 Cases. *Am J Surg Pathol* 14: 1100-1111, 1990a.

Ferry JA, Young RH: Malignant Lymphoma, Pseudolymphoma, and Hematopoietic Disorders of the Female Genital Tract. *Pathol Annu* 26(Pt 1): 227-263, 1990b.

Fetherston WC: False-Negative Cytology in Invasive Cancer of the Cervix. *Clin Obstet Gynecol* 26: 929-937, 1983.

Fetissof F, Serres G, Arbeille B, et al: Argyrophilic Cells and Ectocervical Epithelium. *Int J Gynecol Pathol* 10: 177-190, 1991.

Fidda N, Miron J, Rodgers WH, et al: Impact of the New Bethesda System 2001 on Specimen Adequacy of Conventional Cervicovaginal Smears. *Diagn Cytopathol* 30: 235-239, 2004.

Fidler HK, Lock DR, Vancouver BC: Carcinoma of the Fallopian Tube Detected by Cervical Smear. *Am J Obstet Gynecol* 67: 1103-1111, 1954.

Fidler HK, Boyes DA: Patterns of Early Invasion from Intraepithelial Carcinoma of the Cervix. *Cancer* 12: 673-680, 1959.

Fidler HK, Boyes DA, Worth AJ: Cervical Cancer Detection in British Columbia: A Progress Report. *J Obstet Gynaecol Br Commonw* 75: 392-404, 1968.

Fife KH, Coplan PM, Jansen KU, et al: Poor Sensitivity of Polymerase Chain Reaction Assays of Genital Skin Swabs and Urine to Detect HPV 6 and 11 DNA in Men. *Sex Transm Dis* 30: 246-248, 2003.

Figge DC, Bennington JL, Schweid AI: Cervical Cancer After Initial Negative and Atypical Vaginal Cytology. *Am J Obstet Gynecol* 108: 422-428, 1970.

FIGO Cancer Committee [International Federation of Gynecology and Obstetrics]: Staging Announcement. *Gynecol Oncol* 25: 383-385, 1986.

Figueroa JM, Huffaker AK, Diehl EJ: Malignant Plasma Cells in Cervical Smear. *Acta Cytol* 22: 43-45, 1978.

Figueroa JP, Ward E, Luthi TE et al: Prevalence of Human Papillomavirus Among STD Clinic Attenders in Jamaica: Association of Younger Age and Increased Sexual Activity. *Sex Transm Dis* 22: 114-118, 1995.

Filho AL, Maeda MYS, Oyafuso MS, et al: Cytomorphologic Evidence of Human Papillomavirus Infection in Smears from the Irradiated Uterine Cervix. *Acta Cytol* 41: 1079-1084, 1997.

Finan RR, Irani-Hakime N, Tamim H, et al: Molecular Diagnosis of Human Papillomavirus: Comparison Between Cervical and Vaginal Sampling. *Infect Dis Obstet Gynecol* 9: 119-122, 2001.

Fink DJ: Change in American Cancer Society Checkup Guidelines for Detection of Cervical Cancer. *CA: Cancer J Clin* 38: 127-128, 1988.

Fink MJ, Fruchter RG, Maiman M, et al: The Adequacy of Cytology and Colposcopy in Diagnosing Cervical Neoplasia in HIV-Seropositive Women. *Gynecol Oncol* 55: 133-137, 1994.

Fiorella RM, Cheng J, Kragel PJ: Papanicolaou Smears in Pregnancy. Positivity of Exfoliated Cells for Human Chorionic Gonadotropin and Human Placental Lactogen. *Acta Cytol* 37: 451-456, 1993a.

Fiorella RM, Beckwith LG, Miller LK, et al: Metastatic Signet Ring Carcinoma of the Breast as a Source of Positive Cervicovaginal Cytology: A Case Report. *Acta Cytol* 37: 948-952, 1993b.

Fiorella RM, Casafrancisco D, Yokota S, et al: Artifactual Endocervical Atypia Induced by Endocervical Brush Collection. *Diagn Cytopathol* 11: 79-84, 1994.

Fiorino AS: Intrauterine Contraceptive Device—Associated Actinomycotic Abscess and *Actinomyces* Detection on Cervical Smear. *Obstet Gynecol* 87: 142-149, 1996.

Fischer EG, Bocklage TJ, Rabinowitz I, et al: Primary Plasmacytoma Arising in an Endocervical Polyp With Detection of Neoplastic Cells on Papanicolaou Test: A Case Report and Review of the Literature. *Arch Pathol Lab Med* 127: e28-e31, 2003.

Fish EN, Tobin SM, Cooter NBE, et al: Update on the Relation of Herpesvirus Hominis Type II to Carcinoma of the Cervix. *Obstet Gynecol* 59: 220-224, 1982.

Fitzgibbons PL, Austin RM: Expert Review of Histologic Slides and Papanicolaou Tests in the Context of Litigation or Potential Litigation. *Arch Pathol Lab Med* 124: 1717-1719, 2000.

Fleming H, Mein P: Primary Melanoma of the Cervix. A Case Report. *Acta Cytol* 38: 65-69, 1994.

Fletcher S: Histopathology of Papilloma Virus Infection of the Cervix Uteri: The History, Taxonomy, Nomenclature and Reporting of Koilocytic Dysplasias. *J Clin Pathol* 36: 616-624, 1983.

Fleury FJ: Diagnosis of *Trichomonas vaginalis* Infection. *JAMA* 242: 2556-2557, 1979.

Fluhmann CF: The Nature and Development of the So-Called Glands of the Cervix Uteri. *Am J Obstet Gynecol* 74: 753-768, 1957.

Fluhmann CF: The Squamocolumnar Transitional Zone of the Cervix Uteri. *Obstet Gynecol* 14: 133-148, 1959.

Flynn K, Rimm DL: Diagnosis of "ASCUS" in Women Over Age 50 Is Less Likely to Be Associated with Dysplasia. *Diagn Cytopathol* 24: 132-136, 2001.

Folkman J: Tumor Angiogenesis: Therapeutic Implications. *N Engl J Med* 285: 1182-1186, 1971.

Foltz AM, Kelsey JL: The Annual Pap Test: A Dubious Policy Success. *Milbank Memorial Fund Quarterly—Health and Society* 56: 426-462, 1978.

Foote FW, Li K: Smear Diagnosis of In Situ Carcinoma of the Cervix. *Am J Obstet Gynecol* 56: 335-339, 1948a.

Foote FW, Stewart FW: The Anatomical Distribution of Intraepithelial Epidermoid Carcinomas of the Cervix. *Cancer* 1: 431-440, 1948b.

Footer W: Kaiser Permanente Medicine 50 years Ago: The Gynecological Cancer Detection Clinic. *Permanente Foundation Med Bull* 2: 165-174, 1944.

Fornander T, Rutqvist LE, Cedermark B, et al: Adjuvant Tamoxifen in Early Breast Cancer: Occurrence of New Primary Cancers. *Lancet* (i): 117-120, 1989.

Fornari ML: Cellular Changes in the Glandular Epithelium of Patients Using IUCD—A Source of Cytologic Error. *Acta Cytol* 18: 341-343, 1974.

Forster GE, Cookey I, Mandray PE, et al: Investigation into the Value of Papanicolaou Stained Cervical Smears for the Diagnosis of Chlamydial Cervical Infection. *J Clin Pathol* 38: 399-402, 1985.

Forsum U, Jakobsson T, Larsson PG, et al: An International Study of the Interobserver Variation Between Interpretations of Vaginal Smear Criteria of Bacterial Vaginosis. *APMIS* 110: 811-818, 2002.

Fouts AC, Kraus SJ: *Trichomonas vaginalis*: Reevaluation of Its Clinical Presentation and Laboratory Diagnosis. *J Infect Dis* 141: 137-143, 1980.

Fowkes FGR: Diagnostic Vigilance. *Lancet* (i): 493-494, 1986.

Fowler WC Jr, Walton LA, Edelman DA: Cervical Intraepithelial Neoplasia During Pregnancy. *South Med J* 73: 1180-1185, 1980.

Fowler WC Jr, Schmidt G, Edelman DA, et al: Risks of Cervical Intraepithelial Neoplasia Among DES-Exposed Women. *Obstet Gynecol* 58: 720-724, 1981.

Fox CH: Biologic Behavior of Dysplasia and Carcinoma In Situ. *Am J Obstet Gynecol* 99: 960-974, 1967.

Fox CH: Time Necessary for Conversion of Normal to Dysplastic Cervical Epithelium. *Obstet Gynecol* 31: 749-754, 1968.

Fox CH: Adenxal Malignancy Detected by Cervical Cytology. *Am J Obstet Gynecol* 132: 148-150, 1978.

Fox H, Kazzaz B, Langley FA: Argyrophil and Argentaffin Cells in the Female Genital Tract and in Ovarian Mucinous Cysts. *J Pathol Bacteriol* 88: 479-488, 1964.

Fox H, More JRS: Primary Malignant Lymphoma of the Uterus. *J Clin Pathol* 18: 723-728, 1965.

Fox H, Wells M, Harris M, et al: Enteric Tumours of the Lower Female Genital Tract: A Report of Three Cases. *Histopathology* 12: 167-176, 1988.

Frable WJ, Smith JH, Perkins J, et al: Vaginal Cuff Cytology: Some Difficult Diagnostic Problems. *Acta Cytol* 17: 135-140, 1973.

Frable WJ: Litigation Cells: Definition and Observations on a Cell Type in Cervical Vaginal Smears Not Addressed by the Bethesda System. *Diagn Cytopathol* 11: 213-215, 1994.

Frable WJ: Integration of Surgical and Cytopathology: A Historial Perspective. *Diagn Cytopathol* 13: 375-378, 1995.

Frable WJ: Reflections on Adequacy in Cervical/Vaginal Cytology (Editorial). *Cancer (Cancer Cytopathol)* 87: 103-104, 1999a.

Frable WJ: ASCUS! ASCUS! Down the Rabbit Hole (Editorial). *Cancer (Cancer Cytopathol)* 87: 319-321, 1999b.

Frable WJ: Blinded Review of Papanicolaou Smears (Editorial). *Cancer (Cancer Cytopathol)* 102: 133-135, 2004.

Fraenkel L, Papanicolaou GN: Growth, Desquamation and Involution of the Vaginal Epithelium of Fetuses and Children With a Consideration of the Related Hormonal Factors. *Am J Anat* 62: 427-441, 1938.

Franchi R, Signaroldi A, Croce P, et al: Gastric Carcinoma Detected by Cervical Cytology. *Anti-Cancer Drugs* 11: 645-648, 2000.

Franco EL, Rohan TE, Villa LL: Epidemiologic Evidence and Human Papillomavirus Infection as a Necessary Cause of Cervical Cancer. *J Natl Cancer Inst* 91: 506-511, 1999.

Franco EL: Statistical Issues in Human Papillomavirus Testing and Screening. *Clin Lab Med* 20: 345-367, 2000.

Franco EL, Duarte-Franco E, Ferenczy A: Cervical Cancer: Epidemiology, Prevention and the Role of Human Papillomavirus Infection. *CMAJ* 164: 1017-1025, 2001.

Franco EL, Schlecht NE, Saslow D: The Epidemiology of Cervical Cancer. *Cancer J* 9: 348-359, 2003.

Frank TS, Bhat N, Noumoff JS, et al: Residual Trophoblastic Tissue as a Source of Highly Atypical Cells in the Postpartum Cervicovaginal Smear. *Acta Cytol* 35: 105-108, 1991.

Frankel A: Primary Carcinoma of the Fallopian Tube. *Am J Obstet Gynecol* 72: 131-142, 1956.

Frankel K: Formal Proposal to Combine the Papanicolaou Numerical System With Bethesda Terminology for Reporting Cervical/Vaginal Cytologic Diagnoses. *Diagn Cytopathol* 10: 395-396, 1994.

Franklin RD, Kutteh WH: Characterization of Immunoglobulins and Cytokines in Human Cervical Mucus: Influence of Exogenous and Endogenous Hormones. *J Reprod Immunol* 42: 93-106, 1999.

Franquemont DW, Ward BE, Andersen WA, et al: Prediction of 'High-Risk' Cervical Papillomavirus Infection by Biopsy Morphology. *Am J Clin Pathol* 92: 577-582, 1989.

Fraser RC, Cudmore DC, Melanson J, et al: The Metabolism and Production Rates of Estradiol-17ß in Premenopausal Women With Cervical Carcinoma. *Am J Obstet Gynecol* 98: 509-515, 1967.

Frauchiger WL, De Frias DVS, Cajulis RS, et al: The Immediate Postconization Endocervical Smear: Evaluation of Its Utility in the Detection of Residual Dysplasia. *Acta Cytol* 42: 1139-1143, 1998.

Frech HC: Adenocarcinoma of the Ovary Diagnosed by Vaginal Smears. *Am J Obstet Gynecol* 57: 802-804, 1949.

Free K, Roberts S, Bourne R, et al: Cancer of the Cervix: Old and Young, Now and Then. *Gynecol Oncol* 43: 129-136, 1991.

Freeman C, Berg JW, Cutler SJ: Occurrence and Prognosis of Extranodal Lymphomas. *Cancer* 29: 252-260, 1972.

Freitas C, Milanezi F, Dias AJ, et al: Use of Cell Block Preparation for Morphological, Immunocytochemstry, and Ploidy Analysis in ThinPrep® Monolayer Preparations (Letter). *Diagn Cytopathol* 25: 415-416, 2001.

Fremont-Smith M, Graham RM, Meigs JV: Vaginal Smears as an Aid in the Diagnosis of Early Carcinoma of the Cervix. *N Engl J Med* 237: 302-304, 1947.

Fremont-Smith M, Marino J, Griffin B, et al: Comparison of the SurePath™Liquid-Based Papanicolaou Smear With the Conventional Papanicolaou Smear in a Multsite Direct-to-Vial Study. *Cancer (Cancer Cytopathol)* 102: 269-279, 2004.

French PW, Coppleson M, Reid BL: Effects of Sperm Protamine on Human Cervical Epithelial Cells and BHK 21 Cells In Vitro. *J R Soc Med* 80: 434-437, 1987.

Freund KM, Buttlar CA, Giampalo C, et al: The Use of Cervical Cytology to Identify Women at Risk for Chlamydial Infection. *Am J Prev Med* 8: 292-297, 1992.

Frick HC II, Munnell EW, Richart RM, et al: Carcinoma of the Endometrium. *Am J Obstet Gynecol* 115: 663-676, 1973.

Friedell GH, McKay DG: Adenocarcinoma In Situ of the Endocervix. *Cancer* 6: 887-897, 1953.

Friedell GH, Parsons L: Late Manifestation of Cancer of the Cervix After Irradiation Therapy: Report of Two Cases. *Obstet Gynecol* 17: 582-586, 1961.

Friedman D, Haim S, Paldi E: Refractory Involvement of Cervix Uteri in a Case of Pemphigus Vulgaris. *Am J Obstet Gynecol* 110: 1023-1024, 1971.

Friedman HD, Adelson MD, Elder RC, et al: Granulocytic Sarcoma of the Uterine Cervix: Literature Review of Granulocytic Sarcoma of the Female Genital Tract. *Gynecol Oncol* 46: 128-137, 1992.

Friedrich M, Mink D, Villena-Heinsen C, et al: The Influence of Tamoxifin on the Maturation Index of Vaginal Epithelium. *Clin Exp Obstet Gynecol* 25: 121-124, 1998.

Frierson HF Jr, Covell JL, Anderson WA: Radiation Changes in Endocervical Cells in Brush Specimens. *Diagn Cytopathol* 6: 243-247, 1990.

Frisch LE: Inflammatory Atypia: An Apparent Link With Subsequent Cervical Intraepithelial Neoplasia Explained by Cytologic Underreading. *Acta Cytol* 31: 869-872, 1987a.

Frisch LE: Inflammatory Atypia and the False-Negative Smear in Cervical Intraepithelial Neoplasia. *Acta Cytol* 31: 873-877, 1987b.

Frisch LE, Parmar H, Buckley LD, et al: Colposcopy of Patients With Cytologic Inflammatory Epithelial Changes. *Acta Cytol* 34: 133-135, 1990.

Frost JK: *Trichomonas vaginalis* and Cervical Epithelial Changes. *Ann NY Acad Sci* 97: 792-799, 1962.

Frost JK: Diagnostic Accuracy of "Cervical Smears." *Obstet Gynecol Surv* 24: 893-908, 1969.

Fruchter RG, Maiman M, Sillman FH, et al: Characteristics of Cervical Intraepithelial Neoplasia in Women Infected With the Human Immunodeficiency Virus. *Am J Obstet Gynecol* 17: 531-537, 1994.

282

Fry R, Linder AM: The Value of Exfoliative Cytology During Pregnancy. *S Afr Med J* 43: 1231-1232, 1969.

Fu YS, Reagan JW, Richart RM: Definition of Precursors. *Gynecol Oncol* 12(2 Pt2): S220-S231, 1981.

Fu YS, Reagan JW, Hsiu JG, et al: Adenocarcinoma and Mixed Carcinoma of the Uterine Cervix. I. A Clinicopathologic Study. *Cancer* 49: 2560-2570, 1982.

Fu YS, Braun L, Shah KV, et al: Histologic, Nuclear DNA, and Human Papillomavirus Studies of Cervical Condylomas. *Cancer* 52: 1705-1711, 1983.

Fu YS, Berek JS, Hilborne LH: Diagnostic Problems of In Situ and Invasive Adenocarcinoma of the Uterine Cervix. *Appl Pathol* 5: 47-56, 1987.

Fu YS, Huang I, Beaudenon S, et al: Correlative Study of Human Papillomavirus DNA, Histopathology, and Morphometry in Cervical Condyloma and Intraepithelial Neoplasia. *Int J Gynecol Pathol* 7: 297-307, 1988.

Fu YS, Cheng L, Huang I, et al: DNA Ploidy Analysis of Cervical Condyloma and Intraepithelial Neoplasia in Specimens Obtained by Punch Biopsy. *Anal Quant Cytol Histol* 11: 197-195, 1989.

Fuchs PG, Girardi F, Pfister H: Human Papillomavirus DNA in Normal, Metaplastic, Preneoplastic and Neoplastic Epithelia of the Cervix Uteri. *Int J Cancer* 41: 41-45, 1988.

Fugimoto I, Masubuchi S, Miwa H, et al: Psammoma Bodies Found in Cervicovaginal and/or Endometrial Smears. *Acta Cytol* 26: 317-322, 1982.

Fujii S, Konishi I, Ferenczy A, et al: Small Cell Undifferentiated Carcinoma of the Uterine Cervix: Histology, Ultrastructure, and Immunohistochemistry of Two Cases. *Ultrastruct Pathol* 10: 337-346, 1986.

Fujimoto I, Masubuchi S, Miwa H, et al: Psammoma Bodies Found in Cervicovaginal and/or Endometrial Smears. *Acta Cytol* 26: 317-322, 1982.

Fujiwara H, Mitchell MF, Arseneau J, et al: Clear Cell Adenosquamous Carcinoma of the Cervix: An Aggressive Tumor Associated With Human Papillomavirus-18. *Cancer* 76: 1591-1600, 1995.

Fukazawa I, Iwasaki H, Endo N, et al: A Case Report of Adenoma Malignum of the Uterine Cervix (Abstract). *Acta Cytol* 36: 780, 1992.

Fukuda K, Hachisuga T, Nakamura S, et al: Local Immune Response in Persistent Cervical Dysplasia. *Obstet Gynecol* 82: 941-945, 1993.

Fukuda K, Mori M, Uchiyama M, et al: Preoperative Cervical Cytology in Endometrial Carcinoma and Its Clinicopathologic Relevance. *Gynecol Oncol* 72: 273-277, 1999.

Fukushima M, Shimano S, Yamakawa Y, et al: The Detection of Human Papillomavirus (HPV) in a Case of Minimal Deviation Adenocarcinoma of the Uterine Cervix (Adenoma Malignum) Using In Situ Hybridization. *Jpn J Clin Oncol* 20: 407-412, 1990.

Funk JO, Waga S, Harry JB, et al: Inhibition of CDK Activity and PCNA-Dependent DNA Replication by p21 Is Blocked by Interaction With the HPV-16 E7 Oncoprotein. *Genes Dev* 11: 2090-2100, 1997.

Furgyik S, Grubb R, Kullander S, et al: Familial Occurrence of Cervical Cancer, Stages 0-IV. *Acta Obstet Gynecol Scand* 65: 223-227, 1986.

Furniss K: Tomatoes, Pap Smears, and Tea? Adopting Behaviors that May Prevent Reproductive Cancers and Improve Health. *J Obstet Gynecol Neonatal Nurs* 29: 641-652, 2000.

G

Gad C: The Management and Natural History of Severe Dysplasia and Carcinoma In Situ of the Uterine Cervix. *Br J Obstet Gynecol* 83: 554-559, 1976.

Gagnon F: Contribution to the Study of the Etiology and Prevention of Cancer of the Cervix of the Uterus. *Am J Obstet Gynecol* 60: 516-522, 1950.

Galera-Davidson H, Fernandez A, Navarro J, et al: Mucinous Metaplasia to Neoplastic Lesions in Endometrial Samples With Cytohistoloic Correlation. *Diagn Cytopathol* 5: 150-153, 1989.

Gallagher B, Wang Z, Schymura MJ et al: Cancer Incidence in New York State Acquired Immunodeficiency Syndrome Patients. *Am J Epidiol* 154: 544-556, 2001.

Galloway DA, McDougall JK: The Oncogenic Potential of Herpes Simplex Viruses: Evidence for a 'Hit-and-Run' Mechanism. *Nature* 302: 21-24, 1983.

Galloway DA: Is Vaccination Against Human Papillomavirus a Possibility? *Lancet* 351: 22-24, 1998.

Gallup DG, Abell MR: Invasive Adenocarcinoma of the Uterine Cervix. *Obstet Gynecol* 49: 596-603, 1977.

Ganesan R, Ferryman SR, Waddell CA: Vaginal Adenosis in a Patient on Tamoxifen Therapy: A Case Report. *Cytopathology* 10: 127-130; discussion, 131, 1999.

Garcia-Valdecasas R, Rodriguez-Rico L, Linares J, et al: Malignant Melanoma of the Vagina: A Case Diagnosed Cytologically. *Acta Cytol* 18: 535-537, 1974.

Gardner H, Dukes CD: *Haemophilus vaginalis* Vaginitis: A Newly Defined Specific Infection Classified "Nonspecific" Vaginitis. *Am J Obstet Gynecol* 69: 962-976, 1955.

Gardner HL: Cervical and Vaginal Endometriosis. *Clin Obstet Gynecol* 9: 358-372, 1966.

Gardner JW, Lyon JL: Cancer of the Cervix: A Sexually Transmitted Infection? *Lancet* (ii): 470-471, 1974.

Gardner JW, Schuman KL, Slattery ML, et al: Is Vaginal Douching Related to Cervical Carcinoma? *Am J Epidemiol* 133: 368-375, 1991.

Gardner JW, Sandorn JS, Slattery ML: Behavioral Factors Explaining the Low Risk for Cervical Carcinoma in Utah Mormon Women. *Epidemiology* 6: 187-189, 1995.

Gardner WA Jr, Culberson DE, Bennett BD: *Trichomonas vaginalis* in the Prostate Gland. *Arch Pathol Lab Med* 110: 430-432, 1986.

Garland SM: Human Papillomavirus Update With a Particular Focus on Cervical Disease. *Pathology* 34: 213-224, 2002.

Garret R: Extrauterine Tumor Cells in Vaginal and Cervical Smears. *Obstet Gynecol* 14: 21-27, 1959.

Garud MA, Saraiya U, Paraskar M, et al: Vaginal Parasitosis. *Acta Cytol* 24: 34-35, 1980.

Gatscha RM, Abadi M, Babore S, et al: Smears Diagnosed as ASCUS: Interobserver Variation and Follow-Up. *Diagn Cytopathol* 25: 138-140, 2001.

Gay JD, Donaldson LD, Goellner JR: False-Negative Results in Cervical Cytologic Studies. *Acta Cytol* 29: 1043-1046, 1985.

Geerling S, Nettum JA, Lindner LE, et al: Sensitivity and Specificity of the Papanicolaou-Stained Cervical Smear in the Diagnosis of *Chlamydia trachomatis* Infection. *Acta Cytol* 29: 671-675, 1985.

Geier CS, Wilson M, Creasman W: Clinical Evaluation of Atypical Glandular Cells of Undetermined Significance. *Am J Obstet Gynecol* 184: 64-69, 2001.

Geirsson G, Woodworth FE, Patten SF Jr, et al: Epithelial Repair and Regeneration in the Uterine Cervix I: An Analysis of the Cells. *Acta Cytol* 21: 371-378, 1977.

Geisinger KR, Teot LA, Richter JE: A Comparative Cytopathologic and Histologic Study of Atypia, Dysplasia, and Adenocarcinoma in Barrett's Esophagus. *Cancer* 69: 8-16, 1992.

Genadry R, Olson J, Parmley T, et al: The Morphology of the Earliest Invasive Cell in Low Genital Tract Epidermoid Neoplasia. *Obstet Gynecol* 51: 718-722, 1978.

Genest DR, Stein L, Cibas E, et al: A Binary (Bethesda) System for Classifying Cervical Cancer Precursors: Criteria, Reproducibility, and Viral Correlates. *Hum Pathol* 24: 730-736, 1993.

Genest DR, Dean B, Lee KR, et al: Qualifying the Cytologic Diagnosis of "Atypical Squamous Cells of Undetermined Significance" Affects the Predictive Value of a Squamous Intraepithelial Lesion on Subsequent Biopsy. *Arch Pathol Lab Med* 122: 338-341, 1998.

Geng L, Connolly DC, Isacson C, et al: Atypical Immature Metaplasia (AIM) of the Cervix: Is It Related to High-Grade Squamous Intraepithelial Lesion (HSIL)? *Hum Pathol* 30: 345-351, 1999.

Genvert GI, Drusin LM, Seybolt JF, et al: Evaluation of the Papanicolaou-Stained Cytological Smear as a Screening Technique for Asymptomatic Gonorrhoea. *Br J Vener Dis* 56: 400-403, 1980.

German M, Heaton R, Erickson D, et al: A Comparison of the Three Most Common Papanicolaou Smear Collection Techniques. *Obstet Gynecol* 84: 168-173, 1994.

Gero MA, Toddy SM, Biscotti CV, et al: Endocervical Adenocarcinoma In Situ: An Analysis of Cytologic Features (Abstract). *Am J Clin Pathol* 105: 500-501, 1996.

Gersell DJ, Mazoujian G, Mutch DG, et al: Small-Cell Undifferentiated Carcinoma of the Cervix: A Clinicopathologic, Ultrastructural, and Immunocytochemical Study of 15 Cases. *Am J Surg Pathol* 12: 684-698, 1988.

Ghazizadeh S, Lessan-Pezeshki M, Einollahi B, et al: Uterine Cervical Intraepithelial Neoplasia in Renal Transplantation (Brief Report). *Transplant Proc* 33: 2817, 2001.

Ghirardini C, Boselli F, Messi P, et al: *Chlamydia trachomatis* Infections in Asymptomatic Women: Results of a Study Employing Different Staining Techniques. *Acta Cytol* 33: 115-119, 1989.

Ghirardini C, Ghinosi P, Raisi O, et al: Detection of *Chlamydia trachomatis* in Papanicolaou-Stained Cervical Smears: Control Study by In Situ Hybridization. *Diagn Cytopathol* 7: 211-214, 1991.

Ghorab Z, Mahmood S, Schinella R: Endocervical Reactive Atypia: A Histologic-Cytologic Study. *Diagn Cytopathol* 22: 342-346, 2000.

Ghoussoub RAD, Rimm DL: Degree of Dysplasia Following Diagnosis of Atypical Squamous Cells of Undetermined Significance Is Influenced by Patient History and Type of Follow-Up. *Diagn Cytopathol* 17: 14-19, 1997.

Giacomini G, Simi U: CIN or Not CIN. *Acta Cytol* 27: 543-545, 1983.

Giacomini G, Reali D, Vita D, et al: The Diagnostic Cytology of Nonspecific Vaginitis. *Diagn Cytopathol* 3: 198-205, 1987.

Giacomini G, Paavonen J, Rilke F: Microbiologic Classification of Cervicovaginal Flora in Papanicolaou Smears (Letter). *Acta Cytol* 33: 276-278, 1989.

Giacomini G, Simi U: Nomenclature for the Cytodiagnosis of Cervical Intraepithelial Lesions. *Acta Cytol* 35: 657-658, 1991.

Giacomini G, Schnadig VJ: The Cervical Papanicolaou Smear: Bacterial Infection and the Bethesda System. *Acta Cytol* 36: 109-110, 1992.

Giacomini G, Calcinai A, Moretti D, et al: Accuracy of Cervical/Vaginal Cytology in the Diagnosis of Bacterial Vaginosis. *Sex Transm Dis* 25: 24-27, 1998.

Giacomini G: Permanent Diagnosis of Bacterial Vaginosis: Gram Stain or Papanicolaou Stain? (Letter) *Diagn Cytopathol* 23: 292-293, 2000.

Giannoudis A, Herrington CS: Differential Expression of p53 and p21 in Low-Grade Cervical Squamous Intraepithelial Lesions Infected With Low, Intermediate, and High Risk Human Papillomaviruses. *Cancer* 89: 1300-1207, 2000.

Giannoudis A, Herrington CS: Human Papillomavirus Variants and Squamous Neoplasia of the Cervix. *J Pathol* 193: 295-302, 2001.

Giard RWM: False-Negative Rate of Cervical Cytology: Sense and Sensitivity (Editorial). *Diagn Cytopathol* 25: 275-277, 2001.

Gideon K, Zaharopoulos P: Cytomegalovirus Endocervicitis Diagnosed by Cervical Smear. *Diagn Cytopathol* 7: 625-627, 1991.

Gilbert FE, Hicklin MD, Inhorn SL, et al: Standards of Adequacy of Cytologic Examination of the Female Genital Tract. *Am J Clin Pathol* 61: 285-286, 1974.

Gilbert LK, Alexander L, Grosshans JF, et al: Answering Frequently Asked Questions About HPV. *Sex Transm Dis* 30: 193-194, 2003.

Giles JA, Hudson E, Crow J, et al: Colposcopic Assessment of the Accuracy of Cervical Cytology Screening. *Br Med J* 296: 1099-1102, 1988.

Giles JA, Deery A, Crow J, et al: The Accuracy of Repeat Cytology in Women With Mildly Dyskaryotic Smears. *Br J Obstet Gynaecol* 96: 1067-1070, 1989.

Gilks CB, Young RH, Aguirre P, et al: Adenoma Malignum (Minimal Deviation Adenocarcinoma) of the Uterine Cervix: A Clinicopathological and Immunohistochemical Analysis of 26 Cases. *Am J Surg Pathol* 13: 717-729, 1989.

Gilks CB, Clement PB: Papillary Serous Adenocarcinoma of the Uterine Cervix: A Report of Three Cases. *Mod Pathol* 5: 426-431, 1992.

Gilks CB, Young RH, Gersell DJ, et al: Large Cell Neuroendocrine [Corrected] Carcinoma of the Uterine Cervix: A Clinicopathologic Study of 12 Cases. *Am J Surg Pathol* 21: 905-914, 1997; erratum appears in *Am J Surg Pathol* 21:1260, 1977.

Gill BL, Simpson JF, Somlo G, et al: Effects of Tamoxifen on the Cytology of the Uterine Cervix in Breast Cancer Patients. *Diagn Cytopathol* 19: 417-422, 1998.

Gill GW: Air-Dried/Rehydrated CV Smears Are Different (Letter). *Diagn Cytopathol* 18: 381-382, 1998.

Gill GW: Pap Smear Cellular Adequacy: What does 10% Coverage Look Like?—What Does It Mean? (Abstract) *Acta Cytol* 44:873, 2000.

Gillison ML, Koch WM, Capone RB, et al: Evidence for a Causal Association Between Human Papillomavirus and a Subset of Head and Neck Cancers. *J Natl Cancer Inst* 92: 709-720, 2000.

Gillison ML, Shah KV: Human Papillomavirus-Associated Head and Neck Squamous Cell Carcinoma: Mounting Evidence for an Etiologic Role for Human Papillomavirus in a Subset of Head and Neck Cancers. *Curr Opin Oncol* 13: 183-188, 2001.

Giorgi A, Torriani S, DeHaglio F, et al: Identification of Vaginal Lactobacilli from Asymptomatic Women. *Microbiologica* 10: 377-384, 1987.

Gissmann L, zur Hausen H: Partial Characterization of Viral DNA from Human Genital Warts (Condylomata Acuminata). *Int J Cancer* 25: 605-609, 1980.

Gissmann L, De Villiers E-M, zur Hausen H: Analysis of Human Genital Warts (Condylomata Acuminata) and other Genital Tumors for Human Papillomavirus Type 6 DNA. *Int J Cancer* 29: 143-146, 1982.

Gissmann L, Wolnik L, Ikenberg H, et al: Human Papillomavirus Types 6 and 11 DNA Sequences in Genital and Laryngeal Papillomas and in Some Cervical Cancers. *Proc Natl Acad Sci (USA)* 80: 560-563, 1983.

Gitsch G, Kainz C, Reinthaller A, et al: Cervical Neoplasia and Human Papillomavirus Infection in Prostitutes. *Genitourin Med* 67: 478-480, 1991.

Giudice LC, Tazuke SI, Swiersz L: Status of Current Research on Endometriosis. *J Reprod Med* 43(Suppl 3): 252-262, 1998.

Giuliano AR, Gapstur S: Can Cervical Dysplasia and Cancer Be Prevented With Nutrients? *Nutr Rev* 56: 9-16, 1998.

Giuliano AR: The Role of Nutrients in the Prevention of Cervical Dysplasia and Cancer. *Nutrition* 16: 570-572, 2000.

Giuliano AR, Harris R, Sedjo RL, et al: Incidence, Prevalence, and Clearance of Type-Specific Human Papillomavirus Infections: The Young Women's Health Study. *J Infect Dis* 186: 462-469, 2002.

Giuliano AR, Siegel EM, Roe DJ, et al: Dietary Intake and Risk of Persistent Human Papillomavirus (HPV) Infection: The Ludwig-McGill HPV Natural History Study. *J Infect Dis* 188: 1508-1516, 2003.

Giuntoli R, Yeh IT, Bhuett N, et al: Conservative Management of Cervical Intraepithelial Neoplasia During Pregnancy. *Gynecol Oncol* 42: 68-73, 1991.

Gius D, Laimins LA: Activation of Human Papillomavirus Type 18 Gene Expression by Herpes Simplex Virus Type 1 Viral Transactivators and a Phorbol Ester. *J Virol* 63: 555-563, 1989.

Gladwell P, Duncan P, Barham K, et al: Amnioscopy of Late Pregnancy With Fetal Membrane and Decidual Cytology. *Acta Cytol* 18: 333-337, 1974.

Gloor E, Ruzicka J: Morphology of Adenocarcinoma In Situ of the Uterine Cervix: A Study of 14 Cases. *Cancer* 49: 294-302, 1982.

Gloor E, Hurlimann J: Cervical Intraepithelial Glandular Neoplasia (Adenocarcinoma In Situ and Glandular Dysplasia). A Correlative Study of 23 Cases With Histologic Grading, Histochemical Analysis of Mucins, and Immunohistochemical Determination of the Affinity for Four Lectins. *Cancer* 58: 1272-1280, 1986.

Gloss B, Bernard HU, Seedorf K, et al: The Upstream Regulatory Region of the Human Papilloma Virus-16 Contains an E2 Protein-Independent Enhancer Which Is Specific for Cervical Carcinoma Cells and Regulated by Glucocorticoid Hormones. *EMBO J* 6: 3735-3743, 1987.

Glücksmann A, Cherry CP: Incidence, Histology, and Response to Radiation of Mixed Carcinomas (Adenocathomas) of the Uterine Cervix. *Cancer* 9: 971-979, 1956.

Goff BA, Atanasoff P, Brown E, et al: Endocervical Glandular Atypia in Papanicolaou Smears. *Obstet Gynecol* 79: 101-104, 1992.

Goff BA, Muntz HG, Bell DA, et al: Human Papillomavirus Typing in Patients With Papanicolaou Smears Showing Squamous Atypia. *Gynecol Oncol* 48: 384-388, 1993.

Goellner JR: Carcinoma of the Cervix: Clinicopathologic Correlation of 196 Cases. *Am J Clin Pathol* 66: 775-785, 1976.

Goldie SJ, Kuhn L, Denny K, et al: Policy Analysis of Cervical Cancer Screening Strategies in Low-Resource Settings: Clinical Benefits and Cost-Effectiveness. *JAMA* 283: 3107-3115, 2001.

Goldie SJ, Kim JJ, Wright TC: Cost-Effectiveness of Human Papillomavirus DNA Testing for Cervical Cancer Screening in Women Aged 30 years or More. *Obstet Gynecol* 103: 619-631, 2004.

Goldman RL, Friedman NB: Blue Nevus of the Uterine Cervix. *Cancer* 20: 210-214, 1967.

Goldstein NS, Ahmad E, Hussain M, et al: Endocervical Glandular Atypia: Does a Preneoplastic Lesion of Adenocarcinoma In Situ Exist? *Am J Clin Pathol* 110: 200-209, 1998a.

Goldstein NS, Mani A: The Status and Distance of Cone Biopsy Margins as a Predictor of Excision Adequacy for Endocervical Adenocarcinoma In Situ. *Am J Clin Pathol* 109: 727-732, 1998b.

Gomez-Fernández CR, Ganjei-Azar P, Capote-Dishaw J, et al: Reporting Normal Endometrial Cells in Pap Smears: An Outcome Appraisal. *Gynecol Oncol* 74: 381-384, 1999.

Gomez-Fernández CR, Ganjei-Azar P, Behshid K, et al: Normal Endometrial Cells in Papanicolaou Smears: Prevalence in Women With and Without Endometrial Disease. *Obstet Gynecol* 96: 874-878, 2000.

Gomousa-Michael M, Deligeorgi-Politi H, Condi-Paphiti A, et al: Human Papillomavirus Identification and Typing of Both Sexual Partners. *Acta Cytol* 41: 244-250, 1997.

Gompel C, Spetchinsky A: Dépistage Systématique du Cancer Utérin par la Cytologie Exfoliative: Bilan de 8 Années d'activité du Laboratoire de Cytologie de l'Institut Jules Bordet. [Systematic Screening for Uterine Cancer by Exfoliative Cytology: An Account of 8 Years Activity in the Cytology Laboratory of the Jules Bordet Institute.] *Rev Franç Gynec Obstet* 69: 473-478, 1974.

Gompel C, Horanyl Z, Simone ML: Ultrastructure of Clear Cell Carcinoma of the Vagina and the Cervix: Report of a Case With Unusual Ultrastructural Findings. *Acta Cytol* 20: 262-265, 1976.

Gondos B, Smith LR, Townsend DE: Cytologic Changes in Cervical Epithelium Following Cryosurgery. *Acta Cytol* 14: 386-389, 1970.

Gondos B, Marshall D, Ostergard DR: Endocervical Cells in Cervical Smears. *Am J Obstet Gynecol* 114: 833-834, 1972.

Gondos B, King EB: Significance of Endometrial Cells in Cervicovaginal Smears. *Ann Clin Lab Sci* 7: 486-490, 1977.

Gonzalez D, Hernandez E, Anderson L, et al: Clinical Significance of a Cervical Cytologic Diagnosis of Atypical Squamous Cells of Undetermined Significance: Favoring a Reactive Process or Low-Grade Squamous Intraepithelial Lesion. *J Reprod Med* 41: 719-723, 1996.

González-Merlo J, Ausín J, Lejárcegui JA, et al: Regeneration of the Ectocervical Epithelium after Its Destruction by Electrocauterization. *Acta Cytol* 17: 366-371, 1973.

González-Oliver A, Echeverria OM, Hernández-Pando R: Ultrastructural Study of the Nuclei of Normal, Dysplastic, and Carcinomatous Epithelial Cells of the Human Cervix Uteri. *Ultrastruct Pathol* 21: 379-392, 1997.

Goodman A, Hutchinson ML: Cell Surplus on Sampling Devices After Routine Cervical Cytologic Smears: A Study of Residual Cell Populations. *J Reprod Med* 41: 239-241, 1996.

Goodman A, Wilbur DC: Case 32-2003: A 37-Year-Old Woman With Atypical Squamous Cells on a Papanicolaou Smear. *N Engl J Med* 349: 1555-1564, 2003.

Goodman HM, Buttlar CA, Niloff JM, et al: Adenocarcinoma of the Uterine Cervix: Prognostic Factors and Patterns of Recurrence. *Gynecol Oncol* 33: 241-247, 1989.

Goodman MT, McDuffie K, Hernandez B, et al: Association of Methylenetetrahydrofolate Reductase Polymorphims C677T and Dietary Folate With the Risk of Cervical Dysplasia. *Cancer Epidemiol Biomarkers Prev* 10: 1275-1280, 2001.

Goodman ZD, Gupta PK, Frost JK, et al: Cytodiagnosis of Viral Infections in Body Cavity Fluids. *Acta Cytol* 23: 204-208, 1979.

Gorbach SL, Menda KG, Thadepalli H, et al: Anaerobic Microflora of the Cervix in Healthy Women. *Am J Obstet Gynecol* 15: 1053-1055, 1973.

Gorham H, Yoshida K, Sugino T, et al: Telomerase Activity in Human Gynaecological Malignancies. *J Clin Pathol* 50: 501-504, 1997.

Gornall RJ, Singh N, Noble W, et al: Glandular Abnormalities on Cervical Smear: A Study to Compare the Accuracy of Cytological Diagnosis With Underlying Pathology. *Eur J Gynaecol Oncol* 21: 49-52, 2000.

Gostout BS, Poland GA, Calhoun ES, et al: TAP1, TAP2, and HLA-DR2 Alleles are Predictors of Cervical Cancer Risk. *Gynecol Oncol* 88: 326-332, 2003.

Gould DA, Butler-Manuel SA, Carter PG, et al: Psammoma Bodies on Routine Cervical Smear. *J Roy Soc Med* 91: 383-385, 1998.

Grace A, O'Connell NO, Byrne P, et al: Malignant Lymphoma of the Cervix: An Unusual Presentation and a Rare Disease. *Eur J Gynaecol Oncol* 20: 26-28, 1999.

Grafton WD, Kamm RC, Cowley LH: Cytologic Characteristics of Adenoid Cystic Carcinoma of the Uterine Cervix. *Acta Cytol* 20: 164-166, 1976.

Graham RM: The Effect of Radiation on Vaginal Cells in Cervical Carcinoma: I. Description of Cellular Changes. *Surg Gynecol Obstet* 84: 153-165, 1947a.

Graham RM: The Effect of Radiation on Vaginal Cells in Cervical Carcinoma. II. The Prognostic Significance. *Surg Gynecol Obstet* 84: 166-173, 1947b.

Graham RM, Graham JB: Cytological Prognosis in Cancer of the Uterine Cervix Treated Radiologically. *Cancer* 8: 59-70, 1955.

Graham RM, Nuovo VM, Rauy A, et al: Cytology of Uterine Sarcoma and Chorionepithelioma. *Acta Cytol* 2: 555-562; discussion 563-565, 1958a.

Graham RM, Papanicolaou GN, Pundel JP: Definition of Spindle-Shaped Squamoid Cells. *Acta Cytol* 2: 208-216, 1958b.

Graham RM: Cytomorphology of Carcinoma In Situ. *Acta Cytol* 5: 425-426, 1961.

Graham RM, van Niekerk WA: Vaginal Cytology in Cancer of the Ovary. *Acta Cytol* 6: 496-499, 1962.

Graham RM: Accuracy of Cytologic Diagnosis in the Treated Cancer Patient. *Acta Cytol* 8: 3-10, 1964.

Graham S, Priore R, Graham M, et al: Genital Cancer in Wives of Penile Cancer Patients. *Cancer* 44: 1870-1874, 1979a.

Graham S, Schotz W: Epidemiology of Cancer of the Cervix in Buffalo, New York. *J Natl Cancer Inst* 63: 23-27, 1979b.

Graham S, Rawls W, Swanson M, et al: Sex Partners and Herpes Simplex Virus Type 2 in the Epidemiology of Cancer of the Cervix. *Am J Epidemiol* 115: 729-735, 1982.

Gram IT, Austin H, Stalsberg H: Cigarette Smoking and the Incidence of Cervical Intraepithelial Neoplasia, Grade III, and Cancer of the Cervix Uteri. *Am J Epidemiol* 135: 341-346, 1992a.

Gram IT, Macaluso M, Churchill J, et al: *Trichomonas vaginalis* (TV) and Human Papillomavirus (HPV) Infection and the Incidence of Cervical Intraepithelial Neoplasia (CIN) Grade III. *Cancer Causes Control* 3: 231-236, 1992b.

Gram IT, Macaluso M, Stalsberg H: Oral Contraceptive Use and the Incidence of Cervical Intraepithelial Neoplasia. *Am J Obstet Gynecol* 167: 40-44, 1992c.

Granter SR, Lee KR: Cytologic Finding in Minimal Deviation Adenocarcinoma (Adenoma Malignum) of the Cervix: A Report of Seven Cases. *Am J Clin Pathol* 105: 327-333, 1996.

Graves WP: The Detection of the Clinically Latent Cancer of the Cervix: With a Report on Schiller's Lugol Test. *Surg Gynecol Obstet* 56: 317-322, 1933.

Gray, HJ, Garcia R, Tamimi HK, et al: Glassy Cell Carcinoma of the Cervix Revisited. *Gynecol Oncol* 85: 274-277, 2002.

Gray J-A, Nguyen G-K: Cytologic Detection of Endometrial Pathology by Pap Smears (Letter). *Diagn Cytopathol* 20: 181-182, 1999.

Gray J-A, Nguyen G-K: Can Glassy Cell Carcinoma of the Cervix Be Diagnosed by Pap Smear? *Acta Cytol* 46: 1168-1170, 2002.

Grayson W, Taylor L, Cooper K: Detection of Integrated High Risk Human Papillomavirus in Adenoid Cystic Carcinoma of the Uterine Cervix. *J Clin Pathol* 49: 805-809, 1996.

Grayson W, Taylor LF, Cooper K: Adenoid Cystic and Adenoid Basal Carcinoma of the Uterine Cervix: Comparative Morphologic, Mucin, and Immunohistochemical Profile of Two Rare Neoplasms of Putative 'Reserve Cell' Origin. *Am J Surg Pathol* 23: 448-458, 1999.

Greeley C, Schroeder S, Silverberg SG: Microglandular Hyperplasia of the Cervix: A True "Pill" Lesion? *Int J Gynecol Pathol* 14: 50-54, 1995.

Green GH, Donovan JW: The Natural History of Cervical Carcinoma In Situ. *J Obstet Gynaecol Br Commonw* 77: 1-9, 1970.

Green GH: Cervical Cancer and Cytology Screening in New Zealand. *Br J Obstet Gynaecol* 85: 881-886, 1978.

Green GH: Rising Cervical Cancer Mortality in Young New Zealand Women. *NZ Med J* 89: 89-91, 1979.

Green TH Jr, Scully RE: Tumors of the Fallopian Tube. *Clin Obstet Gynecol* 5: 886-906, 1962.

Greenberg ER, Vessey M, McPherson K, et al: Cigarette Smoking and Cancer of the Uterine Cervix. *Br J Cancer* 51: 139-141, 1985.

Greenberg MD, Reid R, Schiffman M, et al: A Prospective Study of Biopsy-Confirmed Cervical Intraepithelial Neoplasia Grade I: Colposcopic, Cytological, and Virological Risk Factors for Progression. *J Low Genital Tract Dis* 3: 104-110, 1999.

Greene A, Heatley MK: The Appropriateness of Examining the Entire Cervix Histologically in Hysterectomy Specimens from Women With a Previous History of Cervical Intraepithelial Neoplasia or Dyskaryosis. *J Clin Pathol* 54: 155-157, 2001.

Greene JF, Kuehl TJ, Allen SR: The Papanicolaou Smear: Inadequate Screening Test for Bacterial Vaginosis During Pregnancy. *Am J Obstet Gynecol* 182: 1048-1049, 2000.

Greer BE, Figge DC, Tamimi HK, et al: Stage IB Adenocarcinoma of the Cervix Treated by Radical Hysterectomy and Pelvic Lymph Node Dissection. *Am J Obstet Gynecol* 160: 1509-1514, 1989.

Grenko RT, Abendroth CS, Frauenhoffer ES, et al: Variance in the Interpretation of Cervical Biopsy Specimens Obtained for Atypical Squamous Cells of Undetermined Significance. *Am J Clin Pathol* 114: 735-740, 2000.

Griffin NR, Wells M, Fox H: Modulation of the Antigenicity of Amylase in Cervical Glandular Atypia, Adenocarcinoma In Situ and Invasive Adenocarcinoma. *Histopathology* 15: 267-279, 1989.

Griffin NR, Bevan IS, Lewis FA, et al: Demonstration of Multiple HPV Types in Normal Cervix and in Cervical Squamous Cell Carcinoma Using the Polymerase Chain Reaction on Paraffin Wax Embedded Material. *J Clin Pathol* 43: 52-56, 1990.

Griffin NR, Wells M: Characterisation of Complex Carbohydrates in Cervical Glandular Intraepithelial Neoplasia and Invasive Adenocarcinoma. *Int J Gynecol Pathol* 13: 319-329, 1994.

Griffiths M, Turner MJ, Partington CK, et al: Should Smears in a Colposcopy Clinic Be Taken After the Application of Acetic Acid? *Acta Cytol* 33: 324-326, 1989.

Griffiths M: "Nuns, Virgins, and Spinsters." Rigoni-Stern and Cervical Cancer Revisited. *Br J Obstet Gynaecol* 98: 797-802, 1991.

Groben P, Reddick R, Askin F: The Pathologic Spectrum of Small Cell Carcinoma of the Cervix. *Int J Gynecol Pathol* 4: 42-57. 1985.

Gronroos M, Tyrkko J, Siiteri PK, et al: Cytolysis and Karyopyknosis in Postmenopausal Vaginal Smears as Markers of Endometrial Cancer, Diabetes and Obesity: Studies Based on a Ten-Year Follow-up. *Acta Cytol* 30: 628-632, 1986.

Grosen E: How Do You Evaluate an Atypical Glandular Cell Papanicolaou Smear With Psammoma Bodies Present? *J Low Genital Tract Dis* 1: 276-281, 1997.

Gross G, Pfister H: Role of Human Papillomavirus in Penile Cancer, Penile Intraepithelial Squamous Cell Neoplasias and in Genital Warts. *Med Microbiol Immunol* 193: 35-44, 2004.

Grosskopf SK: Cytopathology: Past, Present, and Future. *J Am Med Womens Assoc* 33: 415-418, 1978.

Grubb C, Janota I: Squamous Differentiation in Carcinoma In Situ of the Cervix Uteri: A Cyto-Histological Correlation of Malignant Intraepithelial Lesions With Invasive Carcinoma. *J Clin Pathol* 20: 7-14, 1967.

Grunbaum JA, Kann L, Kinchen SA, et al: Youth Risk Behavior Surveillance—United States, 2001. *J Sch Health* 72: 313-328, 2002.

Gu M, Jacobsen J, Erroll M, et al: Pap Smears of Patients on Tamoxifen (Letter). *Diagn Cytopathol* 16: 96-97, 1997.

Gu M, Shi W, Barakat RR, et al: Pap Smears in Women With Endometrial Carcinoma. *Acta Cytol* 45: 555-560, 2001.

Guarino M, Giordano F, Pallotti F, et al: Malignant Mixed Müllerian Tumor of the Uterus: Features Favoring Its Origin from a Common Cell Clone and an Epithelial-To-Mesenchymal Transformation Mechanism of Histogenesis. *Tumori* 84: 391-397, 1998.

Guerrini L, Sama D, Visani M, et al: Is It Possible to Define a Better ASCUS Class in Cervicovaginal Screening? A Review of 187 Cases. *Acta Cytol* 45: 532-536, 2001.

Guidos BJ, Selvaggi SM: Detection of Endometrial Adenocarcinoma With the ThinPrep® Pap Test™. *Diagn Cytopathol* 23: 260-265, 2000.

Guijon FB, Paraskevas M, Rand F, et al: Vaginal Microbial Flora as a Cofactor in the Pathogenesis of Uterine Cervical Intraepithelial Neoplasia. *Int J Gynaecol Obstet* 37: 185-191, 1992.

Gunn SA, Gould TC: Reliability of Negative Gynecologic Cytologic Findings (Letter). *JAMA* 223: 326, 1973.

Gupta D, Balsara G: Extrauterine Malignancies: Role of Pap Smears in Diagnosis and Management. *Acta Cytol* 43: 806-813, 1999.

Gupta D, Kannan V, Komaromy-Hiller G, et al: ASCUS, Mature Metaplastic Type: Cytologic Diagnosis and Follow-Up. *Acta Cytol* 45: 192-196, 2001a.

Gupta D, Komaromy-Hillar G, Raab, et al: Interobserver and Intraobserver Variability in the Cytologic Diagnosis of Normal and Abnormal Metaplastic Squamous Cells in Pap Smears. *Acta Cytol* 45: 697-703, 2001b.

Gupta K, Hillier SL, Hooton TM, et al: Effects of Contraceptive Method on the Vaginal Microbial Flora: A Prospective Evaluation. *J Infect Dis* 181: 595-601, 2000.

Gupta PK, Pinn VM, Taft PD: Cervical Dysplasia Associated With Azathiprine (Imuran) Therapy. *Acta Cytol* 13: 373-376, 1969.

Gupta PK, Hollander DH, Frost JK: *Actinomyces* in Cervico-Vaginal Smears: An Association With IUD Usage. *Acta Cytol* 20: 295-297, 1976.

Gupta PK, Burroughs F, Luff RD, et al: Epithelial Atypias Associated With Intrauterine Contraceptive Devices (IUD). *Acta Cytol* 22: 286-291, 1978.

Gupta PK, Lee EF, Erozan YS, et al: Cytologic Investigations in Chlamydia Infection. *Acta Cytol* 23: 315-320, 1979.

Gupta PK: Intrauterine Contraceptive Devices: Vaginal Cytology, Pathologic Changes and Clinical Implications. *Acta Cytol* 26: 571-613, 1982.

Gupta PK, Shurbaji MS, Mintor LJ, et al: Cytopathologic Detection of *Chlamydia trachomatis* in Vaginopancervical (Fast) Smears. *Diagn Cytopathol* 4: 224-229, 1988.

Gupta RK, Naran S, Lallu S, et al: Diagnosis of *Entamoeba histolytica* in a Routine Cervical Smear (Images in Cytology). *Diagn Cytopathol* 29: 13, 2003.

Gupta S, Gupta YN, Sanyal B: Radiation Changes in Vaginal and Cervical Cytology in Carcinoma of the Cervix Uteri. *J Surg Oncol* 19: 71-73, 1982.

Gupta S, Mukherjee K, Gupta YN, et al: Sequential Radiation Changes in Cytology of Vaginal Smears in Carcinoma of Cervix Uteri During Radiotherapy. *Int J Gynaecol Obstet* 25: 303-308, 1987.

Gupta S, Sodhani P: Nuclear Grooves in Intermediate Cells in Cervical Smears. *Cytopathology* 11: 91-95, 2000.

Gupta S, Sodhani P, Jain S: Macroconidia of *Fusarium* Species: An Unusual Finding in Cervical Smears. *Acta Cytol* 47: 41-44, 2003a.

Gupta S, Sodhani P, Jain S: Primary Malignant Melanoma of Uterine Cervix: A Rare Entity Diagnosed on Fine Needle Aspiration Cytology: Report of a Case. *Cytopathology* 14: 153-156, 2003b.

Gupta S, Sodhani P, Jain S: Acantholytic Cells Exfoliated from Pemphigus Vulgaris of the Uterine Cervix: A Case Report. *Acta Cytol* 47: 795-798, 2003c.

Gureli N, Denham SW, Root SW: Cytologic Dysplasia Related to Busulfan (Myleran) Therapy. *Obstet Gynecol* 21: 466-470. 1963.

Gusberg SB: The Rise and Fall of Endometrial Cancer (Editorial). *Gynecol Oncol* 35: 124, 1989a.

Gusberg SB: Precursors of Corpus Carcinoma: Estrogens and Adenomatous Hyperplasia. 1947. *CA: Cancer J Clin* 39: 179-192, 1989b.

Gusserow ALS: Ueber Sarcome des Uterus. *Arch Gynäkol* 1: 240-251, 1870.

Gustafsson L, Sparen P, Gustafsson M, et al: Low Efficiency of Cytologic Screening for Cancer In Situ of the Cervix in Older Women. *Int J Cancer* 63: 804-809, 1995.

Gustafsson L, Pontén J, Zack M, et al: International Incidence Rates of Invasive Cervical Cancer After Introduction of Cytological Screening. *Cancer Causes Control* 8: 755-763, 1997.

Gutmann EJ: Syphilitic Cervicitis Simulating Stage II Cervical Cancer: Report of Two Cases With Cytologic Findings. *Am J Clin Pathol* 104: 643-647, 1995.

Gwinn ML, Lee NC, Rubin GL: Trends in the Incidence of Endometrial and Ovarian Cancers. *MMWR* 35 (CDC Surveillance Summaries): 23SS-27SS, 1986.

H

Haas JF: Pregnancy in Association With a Newly Diagnosed Cancer: A Population-Based Epidemiologic Assessment. *Int J Cancer* 34: 229-235, 1984.

Hachisuga T, Fukuda K, Kawarabayashi T: Local Immune Response in Squamous Cell Carcinoma of the Uterine Cervix. *Gynecol Obstet Invest* 52: 3-8, 2001.

Hadjimichael O, Janerich D, Lowell DM, et al: Histologic and Clinical Characteristics Associated With Rapidly Progressive Invasive Cervical Cancer: A Preliminary Report from the Yale Cancer Control Research Unit. *Yale J Biol Med* 62: 345-350, 1989.

Hafez ES: Structural and Ultrastructural Parameters of the Uterine Cervix. *Obstet Gynecol Surv* 37: 507-516, 1982.

Hafiz MA, Kragel PJ, Toker C: Carcinoma of the Uterine Cervix Resembling Lymphoepithelioma. *Obstet Gynecol* 66: 829-831, 1985.

Hajdu SI, Koss Lg: Cytologic Diagnosis of Metastatic Myosarcomas. *Acta Cytol* 13: 545-551, 1969.

Hajdu SI, Savino A: Cytologic Diagnosis of Malignant Melanoma. *Acta Cytol* 17: 320-327, 1974.

Hajdu SI: The Discovery of *Trichomonas vaginalis* (Historical sketch). *Acta Cytol* 42: 1075, 1998.

Hajdu SI: Greco-Roman Thought About Cancer. *Cancer* 100: 2048-2050, 2004a.

Hajdu SI: Medieval Pathfinders in Surgical Oncology. *Cancer* 101: 879-882, 2004b.

Hakama M, Louhivuori K: A Screening programme for Cervical Cancer that Worked. *Cancer Surv* 7: 403-416, 1988.

Halbert CL, Demers GW, Galloway DA: The E7 Gene of Human Papillomavirus Type 16 Is Sufficient for Immortalization of Human Epithelial Cells. *J Virol* 65: 473-478, 1991.

Halford JA: Cytological Features of Chronic Follicular Cervicitis in Liquid-Based Specimens: A Potential Diagnostic Pitfall. *Cytopathology* 13: 364-370, 2002.

Hall DJ, Schneider V, Goplerud DR: Primary Malignant Melanoma of the Uterine Cervix. *Obstet Gynecol* 56: 525-529, 1980.

Hall EJ: Radiation Biology. *Cancer* 55: 2051-2057, 1985.

Hall JE, Walton L: Dysplasia of the Cervix: A Prospective Study of 206 Cases. *Am J Obstet Gynecol* 100: 662-671, 1968.

Hall S, Wu TC, Soudi N, et al: Low-Grade Squamous Intraepithelial Lesions: Cytologic Predictors of Biopsy Confirmation. *Diagn Cytopathol* 10: 3-9, 1994.

Hall TE, Stapleton JJ, McCance JM: The Isolated Finding of Histiocytes in Papanicolaou Smears from Postmenopausal Women. *J Reprod Med* 27: 647-650, 1982.

Hall WS, Goto-Mandeville R, Shih HA, et al: Molecular Analysis of Episomal Human Papillomavirus Type 16 DNA in a Cervical Carcinoma Cell Line. *Virus Res* 51: 183-195, 1997.

Hallman KB, Nahhas WA, Connelly PJ: Endosalpingiosis as a Source of Psammoma Bodies in a Papanicolaou Smear: Report of a Case. *J Reprod Med* 36: 675-678, 1991.

Halpert R, Fruchter RG, Sedlis A, et al: Human Papillomavirus and Lower Genital Neoplasia in Renal Transplant Patients. *Obstet Gynecol* 68: 251-258, 1986.

Halpin TF, Hunter RE, Cohen MB: Lymphoepithelioma of the Uterine Cervix. *Gynecol Oncol* 34: 101-105, 1989.

Hamazaki K, Fujita H, Arata T, et al: [Medullary Carcinoma With Lymphoid Infiltration of the Uterine Cervix—A Pathological Picture of a Case of Cervix Cancer With a Favorable Prognosis.] (Japanese Journal Article) *Jpn J Cancer Clin (Gan No Rinsho)* 14: 787-792, 1968.

Hamilton SR, Smith RR: The Relationship Between Columnar Epithelial Dysplasia and Invasive Adenocarcinoma Arising in Barrett's Esophagus. *Am J Clin Pathol* 87: 303-312, 1987.

Hammerschlag MR, Alpert S, Onderdonk AB: Anaerobic Microflora of the Vagina in Children. *Am J Obstet Gynecol* 131: 853-856, 1978.

Hammond DO, Seckinger D, Keefe C: Effects of Dilute Acetic Acid on Cancer Cytology. I. Effects on Normal Tissue. *J Reprod Med* 25: 97-100, 1980.

Hammond EC, Burns EL, Seidman H, et al: Detection of Uterine Cancer. High and Low Risk Groups. *Cancer* 22: 1096-1107, 1968.

Hammoud MM, Haefner HK, Michael CW, et al: Atypical Glandular Cells of Undetermined Significance: Histologic Findings and Proposed Management. *J Reprod Med* 47: 266-270, 2002.

Hanau CA, Begley N, Bibbo M: Cervical Endometriosis: A Potential Pitfall in the Evaluation of Glandular Cells in Cervical Smears. *Diagn Cytopathol* 16: 274-280, 1997.

Handsfield HH: Clinical Presentation and Natural Course of Anogenital Warts. *Am J Med* 102(5A): 16-20, 1997.

Hannigan EV: Cervical Cancer in Pregnancy. *Clin Obstet Gynecol* 33: 837-845, 1990.

Hanselaar AG, Vooijs GP, Oud PS, et al: DNA Ploidy Patterns in Cervical Intraepithelial Neoplasia Grade III, With and Without Synchronous Invasive Squamous Cell Carcinoma: Measurements in Nuclei Isolated from Paraffin-Embedded Tissue. *Cancer* 62: 2537-2545, 1988.

Hanselaar AG, Van Leusen ND, De Wilde PC, et al: Clear Cell Adenocarcinoma of the Vagina and Cervix: A Report of the Central Netherlands Registry With Emphasis on Early Detection and Prognosis. *Cancer* 67: 1971-1978, 1991.

Hanselaar AGJM, Boss EA, Massuger LFAG, et al: Cytologic Examination to Detect Clear Cell Adenocarcinoma of the Vagina or Cervix. *Gynecol Oncol* 75: 338-344, 1999.

Hanselaar AGJM, Böcking A, Gundlach H, et al: Summary Statement on Quantitative Cytochemistry (DNA and Molecular Biology): Task Force 8. *Acta Cytol* 45: 499-501, 2001.

Hanton EM, Malkasian GD Jr, Dahlin D, et al: Primary Carcinoma of the Fallopian Tube. *Am J Obstet Gynecol* 94: 832-839, 1966.

Hare AA, Duncan AR, Sharp AJ: Cytology Suggestive of Glandular Neoplasia: Outcomes and Suggested Management. *Cytopathology* 14: 12-18, 2003.

Hare MJ, Toone E, Taylor-Robinson D, et al: Follicular Cervicitis—Colposcopic Appearances and Association With *Chlamydia trachomatis*. *Br J Obstet Gynaecol* 88: 174-180, 1981.

Hare MJ, Taylor-Robinson D, Cooper P: Evidence for an Association Between *Chlamydia trachomatis* and Cervical Intraepithelial Neoplasia. *Br J Obstet Gynaecol* 89: 489-492, 1982.

Harer WB Jr, el-Dawakhly Z: Peseshet—The First Female Physician? *Obstet Gynecol* 74:960-961, 1989.

Harer WB, Valenzuela G Jr, Lebo D: Lubrication of the Vaginal Introitus and Speculum Does Not Affect Papanicolaou Smears. *Obstet Gynecol* 100: 887-888, 2002.

Harington JS: Epidemiology and Aetiology of Cancer of the Uterine Cervix Including the Detection of Carcinogenic N-Nitrosamines in the Human Vaginal Vault. *S Afr Med J* 49: 443-445, 1975.

Harlan LC, Bernstein AB, Kessler LG: Cervical Cancer Screening: Who Is Not Screened and Why? *Am J Public Health* 81: 885-891, 1991.

Harmsel BT, Smedts F, Kuijpers J, et al: Relationship Between Human Papillomavirus Type 16 in the Cervix and Intraepithelial Neoplasia. *Obstet Gynecol* 93: 46-50, 1999.

Harnden P, Kennedy W, Andrew AC, et al: Immunophenotype of Transitional Metaplasia of the Uterine Cervix. *Int J Gynecol Pathol* 18: 125-129, 1999.

Haroon S, Samayoa L, Witzke D, et al: Reproducibility of Cervicovaginal ThinPrep Cellularity Assessment. *Diagn Cytopathol* 26: 19-21, 2002.

Harper DM, Hildesheim A, Cobb JL, et al: Collection Devices for Human Papillomavirus. *J Fam Pract* 48: 531-535, 1999.

Harper JM, Levine AJ, Rosenthal DL, et al: Erythrocyte Folate Levels, Oral Contraceptive Use and Abnormal Cervical Cytology. *Acta Cytol* 38: 324-330, 1994.

Harris M: Spindle Cell Squamous Carcinoma: Ultrastructural Observations. *Histopathology* 6: 197-210, 1982.

Harris MV, Cason Z, Benghuzzi H, et al: Cytomorphological Assessment of Benign and Malignant Dense Hyperchromatic Groups in Cervicovaginal Smears. *Biomed Sci Instrum* 36: 349-354, 2000.

Harris NL, Scully RE: Malignant Lymphoma and Granulocytic Sarcoma of the Uterus and Vagina. *Cancer* 53: 2530-2545, 1984.

Harris RW, Scott WA: Vasectomy and Cancer of the Cervix (Letter). *N Engl J Med* 301: 1064-1065, 1979.

Harris RW, Brinton LA, Codell RH, et al: Characteristics of Women With Dysplasia or Carcinoma In Situ of the Cervix Uteri. *Br J Cancer* 42: 359-369, 1980.

Harrison DD, Hernandez E, Dunton CJ: Endocervical Brush Versus Cotton Swab for Obtaining Cervical Smears at a Clinic: A Cost Comparison. *J Reprod Med* 38: 285-288, 1993.

Hart WR, Townsend DE, Aldrich JO, et al: Histopathologic Spectrum of Vaginal Adenosis and Related Changes in Stilbestrol-Exposed Females. *Cancer* 37: 763-775, 1976a.

Hart WR, Zaharov I, Kaplan BJ, et al: Cytological Findings in Stilbestrol-Exposed Females With Emphasis on Detection of Vaginal Adenosis. *Acta Cytol* 20: 7-14, 1976b.

Hart WR: Symposium II: Special Types of Adenocarcinoma of the Uterine Cervix. *Int J Gynecol Pathol* 21: 327-346, 2002.

Hartmann KE, Nanda K, Hall S, et al: Technologic Advances for Evaluation of Cervical Cytology: Is Newer Better? *Obstet Gynecol Surv* 56: 765-774, 2001.

Harty DW, Oakey HJ, Patrikakis M, et al: Pathogenic Potential of Lactobacilli. *Int J Food Microbiol* 24: 179-189, 1994.

Hasegawa T, Tsutsui F, Kurihara S: Cytomorphologic Study on the Atypical Cells Following Cryosurgery for Treatment of Chronic Cervicitis. *Acta Cytol* 19: 533-537, 1975.

Hashi A, Yasumizu T, Yoda I, et al: A Case of Small Cell Carcinoma of the Uterine Cervix Presenting Cushing's Syndrome. *Gynecol Oncol* 61: 427-431, 1996.

Hasumi K, Sugano H, Sakamoto G, et al: Circumscribed Carcinoma of the Uterine Cervix, With Marked Lymphocytic Infiltration. *Cancer* 39: 2503-2507, 1977.

Hasumi K, Ehrmann RL: Clear Cell Carcinoma of the Uterine Endocervix With an In Situ Component. *Cancer* 42: 2435-2438, 1978.

Haswani P, Arseneau J, Ferenczy A: Primary Signet Ring Cell Carcinoma of the Uterine Cervix: A Clinicopathologic Study of Two Cases With Review of the Literature. *Int J Gynecol Cancer* 8: 374-379, 1998.

Hata S, Mikami Y, Manabe T: Diagnostic Significance of Endocervical Glandular Cells With "Golden-Yellow" Mucin on Pap Smear. *Diagn Cytopathol* 27: 80-84, 2002.

Hatch EE, Herbst AL, Hoover RN, et al: Incidence of Squamous Neoplasia of the Cervix and Vagina in DES-Exposed Daughters (Abstract). *Ann Epidemiol* 10: 467, 2000.

Hatch EE, Herbst AL, Hoover RN, et al: Incidence of Squamous Neoplasia of the Cervix and Vagina in Women Exposed Prenatally to Diethylstilbestrol (United States). *Cancer Causes Control* 12: 837-845, 2001.

Hatem F, Wilbur DC: High-Grade Sqamous Cervical Lesions Following Negative Papanicolaou Smears: False-Negative Cervical Cytology or Rapid Progression. *Diagn Cytopathol* 12:135-141, 1995.

Hausdorfer GS, Chandrasoma P, Pettross BR, et al: Cytologic Diagnosis of Mesonephric Adenocarcinoma of the Urinary Bladder. *Acta Cytol* 29: 823-826, 1985.

Hauser G: Zur Histogenese des Krebses. *Virchows Archiv (Path Anat)* 138: 482-499, 1894.

Hawes SE, Hillier SL, Benedetti J, et al: Hydrogen Peroxide-Producing Lactobacilli and Acquisition of Vaginal Infections. *J Infect Dis* 174: 1058-1063, 1996.

Hayes MMM, Matisic JP, Chen C-H: Cytological Aspects of Uterine Cervical Adenocarcinoma, Adenosquamous Carcinoma and Combined Adenocarcinoma-Squamous Carcinoma: Appraisal of Diagnostic Criteria for In Situ Versus Invasive Lesions. *Cytopathology* 8: 397-408, 1997.

Heard I, Tassie J-M, Schmitz V, et al: Increased Risk of Cervical Disease Among Human Immunodeficiency Virus-Infected Women With Severe Immunosuppression and High Human Papillomavirus Load. *Obstet Gynecol* 96: 403-409, 2000.

Heaton RB Jr, Harris TF, Larson DM, et al: Glandular Cells Derived from Direct Sampling of the Lower Uterine Segment in Patients Status Post-Cervical Cone Biopsy: A Diagnostic Dilemma. *Am J Clin Pathol* 106: 511-516, 1996.

Heber KR: The Effect of Progestogens on Vaginal Cytology. *Acta Cytol* 19: 103-109, 1975.

Hecht JL, Sheets EE, Lee KR: Atypical Glandular Cells of Undetermined Significance in Conventional Cervical/Vaginal Smears and Thin-Layer Preparations: A Follow-Up Comparison Study. *Cancer (Cancer Cytopathol)* 96: 1-4, 2002.

Heck DV, Yee CL, Howley PM, et al: Efficiency of Binding the Retinoblastoma Protein Correlates With the Transforming Capacity of the E7 Oncoproteins of the Human Papillomaviruses. *Proc Natl Acad Sci (USA)* 89: 4442-4446, 1992.

Heimann A, Scanlon R, Gentile J, et al: Measles Cervicitis. Report of a Case With Cytologic and Molecular Biologic Analysis. *Acta Cytol* 36: 727-730, 1992.

Hein K, Schreiber K, Cohen MI, et al: Cervical Cytology: The Need for Routine Screening in the Sexually Active Adolescent. *J Pediatr* 91: 123-126, 1977.

Heinzl S, Szalmay G, Jochum L, et al: Observations on the Development of Dysplasia. *Acta Cytol* 26: 453-456, 1982.

Helfand M, O'Connor GY, Zimmer-Gembec M, et al: Effect of Clinical Laboratory Improvement Amendments of 1988 (CLIA '88) on the Incidence of Invasive Cervical Cancer. *Med Care* 30: 1067-1082, 1992.

Hellberg D, Valentin J, Nilsson S: Smoking as Risk Factor in Cervical Neoplasia (Letter). *Lancet* (ii): 1497, 1983.

Hellberg D, Axelsson O, Gad A, et al: Conservative Management of the Abnormal Smear During Pregnancy: A Long-Term Follow-Up. *Acta Obstet Gynaecol Scand* 66: 195-199, 1987.

Hellberg D, Nilsson S, Haley NJ, et al: Smoking and Cervical Intraepithelial Neoplasia: Nicotine and Cotinine in Serum and Cervical Mucus in Smokers and Nonsmokers. *Am J Obstet Gynecol* 158: 910-913, 1988.

Hellberg D, Nilsson S, Valentin J: Positive Cervical Smear With Subsequent Normal Colposcopy and Histology—Frequency of CIN in a Long-Term Follow-Up. *Gynecol Oncol* 53: 148-151, 1994.

Hellberg D, Nilsson S, Mårdh, P-A: Bacterial Vaginosis and Smoking. *Int J STD AIDS* 11: 603-606, 2000.

Hellberg D, Nilsson S, Mårdh, P-A: The Diagnosis of Bacterial Vaginosis and Vaginal Flora Changes. *Arch Gynecol Obstet* 265: 11-15, 2001.

Hellen EA, Coghill SB, Clark JV: Prolapsed Fallopian Tube After Abdominal Hysterectomy: A Report of the Cytological Findings. *Cytopathology* 4: 181-185, 1993.

Heller C, Hoyt V: Squamous Cell Changes Associated With the Presence of *Candida sp*. In Cervical-Vaginal Papanicolaou Smears. *Acta Cytol* 15: 379-384, 1971.

Heller CJ: Neisseria Gonorrhoeae in Papanicolaou Smears. *Acta Cytol* 18: 338-340, 1974.

Helmerhorst TJM, Meijer CJLM: Cervical Cancer Should Be Considered as a Rare Complication of Oncogenic HPV Infection Rather than a STD. *Int J Gyecol Cancer* 12: 235-236, 2002.

Henderson SR: Pelvic Actinomycosis Associated With an Intrauterine Device. *Obstet Gynecol* 41: 726-732, 1973.

Hendricks DT, Taylor R, Reed M, et al: FHIT Gene Expression in Human Ovarian, Endometrial, and Cervical Cancer Cell Lines. *Cancer Res* 57: 2112-2115, 1997.

Hendrickson M, Ross J, Eifel P, et al: Uterine Papillary Serous Carcinoma: A Highly Malignant Form of Endometrial Adenocarcinoma. *Am J Surg Pathol* 6: 93-108, 1982.

Hendsch SA, Glover SD, Otis CN: Atypical Glandular Cells of Undetermined Significance from Extramammary Paget's of the Bladder. *Obstet Gynecol* 99: 912-914, 2002.

Henriksen E: Precancerous and Carcinoid Lesions of the Cervix Uteri: With Comments on the Schiller Test. *Surg Gynecol Obstet* 60: 635-644, 1935.

Henry MJ, Stanley MW, Cruikshank S, et al: Association of Human Immunodeficiency Virus-Induced Immunosuppression With Human Papillomavirus Infection and Cervical Intrapithelial Neoplasia. *Am J Obstet Gynecol* 160: 352-353, 1989.

Henry MR, Jensen KL deM, Skoglund CD, et al: *Chlamydia trachomatis* in Routine Cervical Smears: A Microscopic and Ultrastructural Analysis. *Acta Cytol* 37: 343-352, 1993.

Henry MR: The Bethesda System 2001: An Update of New Terminology for Gynecologic Cytology. *Clin Lab Med* 23: 585-603, 2003.

Henry-Stanley MJ, Stanley MW, Burton LG, et al: Cytologic Diagnosis of Cytomegalovirus in Cervical Smears. *Diagn Cytopathol* 9: 364-365, 1993a.

Henry-Stanley MJ, Simpson M, Stanley MW: Cervical Cytology Findings in Women Infected With the Human Immunodeficiency Virus. *Diagn Cytopathol* 9: 508-509, 1993b.

Hepler TK, Dockerty MB, Randall LM: Primary Adenocarcinoma of the Cervix. *Am J Obstet Gynecol* 63: 800-808, 1952.

Herbert A, Smith JAE: Cervical Intraepithelial Neoplasia Grade III (CIN III) and Invasive Cervical Carcinoma: The Yawning Gap Revisited and the Treatment of Risk. *Cytopathology* 10: 161-170, 1999.

Herbert A: Cervical Screening in England and Wales: Its Effect Has Been Underestimated. *Cytopathology* 11: 471-479, 2000.

Herbert A, Singh N, Smith JAE: Adenocarcinoma of the Uterine Cervix Compared With Squamous Cell Carcinoma: A 12-Year Study in Southampton and South-West Hampshire. *Cytopathology* 12: 26-36, 2001.

Herbst AL, Green TH Jr, Ulfelder H: Primary Carcinoma of the Vagina: An Analysis of 68 Cases. *Am J Obstet Gynecol* 106: 210-218, 1970a.

Herbst AL, Scully RE: Adenocarcinoma of the Vagina in Adolescence: A Report of 7 Cases Including 6 Clear-Cell Carcinomas (So-Called Mesonephromas). *Cancer* 25: 745-757, 1970b.

Herbst AL, Ulfelder H, Poskanzer DC: Adenocarcinoma of the Vagina: Association of Maternal Stilbestrol Therapy With Tumor Appearance in Young Women. *N Engl J Med* 284: 878-881, 1971.

Herbst AL, Kurman RJ, Scully RE: Vaginal and Cervical Abnormalities After Exposure to Stilbestrol *in utero*. *Obstet Gynecol* 40: 287-298, 1972.

Herbst AL, Robboy SJ, Scully RE, et al: Clear-Cell Adenocarcinoma of the Vagina and Cervix in Girls: Analysis of 170 Registry Cases. *Am J Obstet Gynecol* 119: 713-724, 1974.

Herbst AL, Scully RE, Robboy SJ: The Significance of Adenosis and Clear-Cell Adenocarcinoma of the Genital Tract in Young Females. *J Reprod Med* 15: 5-11, 1975.

Herbst AL, Cole P, Norusis MJ, et al: Epidemiologic Aspects and Factors Related to Survival in 384 Registry Cases of Clear Cell Adenocarcinoma of the Vagina and Cervix. *Am J Obstet Gynecol* 135: 876-886, 1979a.

Herbst AL, Noruses MJ, Rosenow PJ, et al: An Analysis of 346 Cases of Clear Cell Adenocarcinoma of the Vagina and Cervix With Emphasis on Recurrence and Survival. *Gynecol Oncol* 7: 111-122, 1979b.

Herbst AL: The Bethesda System for Cervical/Vaginal Cytologic Diagnoses: A Note of Caution. *Obstet Gynecol* 76: 449-450, 1990a.

Herbst AL, Anderson D: Clear Cell Adenocarcinoma of the Vagina and Cervix Secondary to Intrauterine Exposure to Diethylstilbestrol. *Sem Surg Oncol* 6: 343-346, 1990b.

Herbst AL: The Bethesda System for Cervical/Vaginal Cytologic Diagnoses. *Clin Obstet Gynecol* 35: 22-27, 1992.

Herbst AL, Pickett KE, Follen M, et al: The Management of ASCUS Cervical Cytologic Abnormalities and HPV Testing: A Cautionary Note. *Obstet Gynecol* 98: 849-851, 2001.

Hering B, Horn L-C, Nenning H, et al: Predictive Value of DNA Cytometry in CIN 1 and 2: Image Analysis of 193 Cases. *Anal Quant Cytol Histol* 22: 333-337, 2000.

Hermonat PL, Daniel RW, Shah KV: The Spermicide Nonoxynol-9 does Not Inactivate Papillomavirus. *Sex Transm Dis* 19: 203-205, 1992.

Hermonat PL, Han L, Wendel PJ, et al: Human Papillomavirus Is More Prevalent in First Trimester Spontaneously Aborted Products of Conception Compared to Elective Specimens. *Virus Genes* 14: 13-17, 1997.

Hernandez-Avila M, Lazcano-Ponce EC, Berumen-Campos J, et al: Human Papilloma Virus 16-18 Infection and Cervical Cancer in Mexico: A Case-Control Study. *Arch Med Res* 28: 265-271, 1997.

Herrero R, Brinton LA, Reeves WC, et al: Invasive Cervical Cancer and Smoking in Latin America. *J Natl Cancer Inst* 81: 205-211, 1989.

Herrero R, Brinton LA, Reeves WC, et al: Sexual Behavior, Venereal Diseases, Hygiene Practices, and Invasive Cervical Cancer in a High-Risk Population. *Cancer* 65: 380-386, 1990.

Herrero R, Brinton LA, Reeves WC, et al: Screening for Cervical Cancer in Latin America: A Case-Control Study. *Int J Epidemiol* 21: 1050-1056, 1992.

Herrero R, Muñoz N: Human Papillomavirus and Cancer. *Cancer Surv* 33: 75-98, 1999.

Herrero R, Hildesheim A, Bratti C, et al: Population-Based Study of Human Papillomavirus Infection and Cervical Neoplasia in Rural Costa Rica. *J Natl Cancer Inst* 92: 464-474, 2000.

Herrero R, Castellsagué X, Pawlita M, et al: Human Papillomavirus and Oral Cancer: The International Agency for Research on Cancer Multicenter Study. *J Natl Cancer Inst* 95: 1772-1783, 2003.

Herrington CS: Human Papillomaviruses (HPV) in Gynaecological Cytology: From Molecular Biology to Clinical Testing. *Cytopathology* 6: 176-189, 1995a.

Herrington CS: Human Papillomaviruses and Cervical Neoplasia. II. Interaction of HPV and Other Factors. *J Clin Pathol* 48: 1-6, 1995b.

Herrington CS: Do HPV-Negative Cervical Carcinomas Exist?—Revisited (Editorial). *J Pathol* 189: 1-3, 1999.

Herrington CS: Does HPV Testing Have a Role in Primary Cervical Screening? (Invited Editorial). *Cytopathology* 12: 71-74, 2001.

Herzberg AJ, Silverman JF: Detection of *Trichomonas vaginalis* in Endocervical and Ectocervical Smears. *Diagn Cytopathol* 14: 273-276, 1996.

Heselmeyer K, Schrock E, du Manoir S, et al: Gain of Chromosome 3q Defines the Transition from Severe Dysplasia to Invasive Carcinoma of the Uterine Cervix. *Proc Natl Acad Sci (USA)* 93: 479-484, 1996.

Hess RA, Bunick D, Bahr J: Oestrogen, Its Receptors and Function in the Male Reproductive Tract—A Review. *Mol Cell Endocrinol* 178: 29-38, 2001.

Hewitt M, Devesa S, Breen N: Papanicolaou Test Use Among Reproductive-Age Women at High Risk for Cervical Cancer: Analyses of the 1995 National Survey of Family Growth. *Am J Public Health* 92: 666-669, 2002.

Hicklin MD, Watts JC, Plott AE, et al: Retrospective Evaluation of Gynecologic Cytodiagnosis. I. Reproducibility Using an Experimental Diagnostic Scale. *Acta Cytol* 28: 58-71, 1984.

Hidvegi DF, DeMay RM, Sorensen K: Uterine Müllerian Adenosarcoma With Psammoma Bodies: Cytologic, Histologic and Ultrastructural Studies of a Case. *Acta Cytol* 26: 323-326, 1982.

Higgins GD, Davy M, Roder D, et al: Increased Age and Mortality Associated With Cervical Carcinomas Negative for Human Papillomavirus RNA. *Lancet* 338: 910-913, 1991.

Higgins GD, Phillips GE, Smith LA, et al: High Prevalence of Human Papillomavirus Transcripts in All Grades of Cervical Intraepithelial Glandular Neoplasia. *Cancer* 70: 136-146, 1992.

Highman WJ: Calcified Bodies and the Intrauterine Device. *Acta Cytol* 15: 473-475, 1971.

Hilders CG, Houbiers JG, Krul EJ, et al: The Expression of Histocompatibility-Related Leukocyte Antigens in the Pathway to Cervical Carcinoma. *Am J Clin Pathol* 101: 5-12, 1994.

Hildesheim A, Brinton LA, Mallin K, et al: Barrier and Spermicidal Contraceptive Methods and Risk of Invasive Cervical Cancer. *Epidemiology* 1: 266-272, 1990a.

Hildesheim A, Reeves WC, Brinton LA, et al: Association of Oral Contraceptive Use and Human Papillomaviruses in Invasive Cervical Cancers. *Int J Cancer* 45: 860-864, 1990b.

Hildesheim A, Mann V, Brinton LA, et al: Herpes Simplex Virus Type 2: Possible Interaction With Human Papillomavirus Types 16/18 in the Development of Invasive Cervical Cancer. *Int J Cancer* 49: 335-340, 1991.

Hildesheim A, Gravitt P, Schiffman MH, et al: Determinants of Genital Human Papillomavirus Infection in Low-Income Women in Washington. DC. *Sex Transm Dis* 20: 279-285, 1993.

Hildesheim A, Schiffman MH, Gravitt PE, et al: Persistence of Type-Specific Human Papillomavirus Infection Among Cytologically Normal Women. *J Infect Dis* 169: 235-240, 1994.

Hildesheim A, Schiffman M, Scott DR, et al: Human Leukocyte Antigen Class I/II Alleles and Development of Human Papillomavirus-Related Cervical Neoplasia: Results from a Case-Control Study Conducted in the United States. *Cancer Epidemiol Biomarkers Prev* 7: 1035-1041, 1998.

Hildesheim A, Hadjimichael O, Schwartz PE, et al: Risk Factors for Rapid-Onset Cervical Cancer. *Am J Obstet Gynecol* 180: 571-577, 1999.

Hildesheim A, Schiffman M, Bromley C, et al: Human Papillomavirus Type 16 Variants and Risk of Cervical Cancer. *J Natl Cancer Inst* 93: 315-318, 2001.

Hill GB: *Eubacterium nodatum* Mimics Actinomyces in Intrauterine Device-Associated Infections and Other Settings Within the Female Genital Tract. *Obstet Gynecol* 79: 534-538, 1992.

Hill GB: The Microbiology of Bacterial Vaginosis. *Am J Obstet Gynecol* 169: 450-454, 1993.

Hillemanns P, Kimmig R, Hüttemann U, et al: Screening for Cervical Neoplasia by Self-Assessment for Human Papillomavirus DNA (Letter). *Lancet* 354: 1970.

Hillier SL: Diagnostic Microbiology of Bacterial Vaginosis. *Am J Obstet Gynecol* 169: 455-459, 1993a.

Hillier SL, Krohn MA, Rabe LK, et al: The Normal Vaginal Flora, H_2O_2–Producing Lactobacilli, and Bacterial Vaginosis in Pregnant Women. *Clin Infect Dis* 16(Suppl 4): S273-S281, 1993b.

Hillier SL, Nugent RP, Eschenbach DA, et al: Association Between Bacterial Vaginosis and Preterm Delivery of a Low-Birth-Weight Infant: The Vaginal Infections and Prematurity Study Group. *N Engl J Med* 333: 1737-1742, 1995.

Hillier SL: The Vaginal Microbial Ecosystem and Resistance to HIV. *AIDS Res Hum Retroviruses* 14(Suppl 1): S17-S21, 1998.

Hills E, Laverty CR: Electron Microscopic Detection of Papilloma Virus Particles in Selected Koilocytotic Cells in a Routine Cervical Smear. *Acta Cytol* 23: 53-56, 1979.

Hilrich NM, Hipke MM: Endometrial and Cytologic Atypism in the Postabortal State. *Obstet Gynecol* 6: 452-454, 1955.

Himmelstein LR: Evaluation of Inflammatory Atypia: A Literature Review. *J Reprod Med* 34: 634-637, 1989.

Hines JF, Ghim S-j, Schlegel R, et al: Prospects for a Vaccine Against Human Papillomavirus. *Obstet Gynecol* 86: 860-866, 1995.

Hines JF, Ghim S-j, Jenson AB: Prospects for Human Papillomavirus Vaccine Development: Emerging HPV Vaccines. *Curr Opin Obstet Gynecol* 10: 15-19, 1998.

Hinsey JC: George Nicholas Papanicolaou, M.D., Ph.D., D.Sc.: May 13, 1883-February 19, 1962. *Acta Cytol* 6: 483-486, 1962.

Hirahatake K, Hareyama H, Kure R, et al: Cytologic and Hormonal Findings in a Carcinoid Tumor of the Uterine Cervix. *Acta Cytol* 34: 119-124, 1990.

Hirai Y, Chen J-T, Hamada T, et al: Clinical and Cytologic Aspects of Primary Fallopian Tube Carcinoma: A Report of Ten Cases. *Acta Cytol* 31: 834-840, 1987.

Hirai Y, Takeshima N, Haga A, et al: A Clinicopathologic Study of Adenoma Malignum of the Uterine Cervix. *Gynecol Oncol* 70: 219-223, 1998.

Hirokawa M, Shimizu M, Nakamura E, et al: Basement Membrane Material and Tigroid Background in a Fine Needle Aspirate of Clear Cell Adenocarcinoma of the Cervix: A Case Report. *Acta Cytol* 44: 251-254, 2000.

Hirschowitz L, Raffle AE, Mackenzie EFD, et al: Long Term Follow Up of Women With Borderline Cervical Smear Test Results: Effects of Age and Viral Infections on Progression to High-Grade Dyskaryosis. *Br Med J* 304: 1209-1212, 1992.

Hirschowitz L, Eckford D, Phillpotts B, et al: Cytological Changes Associated With Tubo-Endometrioid Metaplasia of the Uterine Cervix. *Cytopathology* 5: 1-8, 1994.

Hislop TG, Band PR, Deschamps M, et al: Cervical Cancer Screening in Canadian Native Women: Adequacy of the Papanicolaou Smear. *Acta Cytol* 38: 29-32, 1994.

Hitchcock A, Johnson J, McDowell K, et al: A Retrospective Study into the Occurrence of Cervical Glandular Atypia in Cone Biopsy Specimens 1977-1978 With Clinical Follow-Up. *Int J Gynecol Cancer* 3: 164-168, 1993.

Ho GY, Burk RD, Fleming I, et al: Risk of Genital Human Papillomavirus Infection in Women With Human Immunodeficiency Virus-Induced Immunosuppression. *Int J Cancer* 56:788-792, 1994.

Ho GY, Burk RD, Klein S, et al: Persistent Genital Human Papillomavirus Infection as a Risk Factor for Persistent Cervical Dysplasia. *J Natl Cancer Inst* 87: 1365-1371, 1995.

Ho GY, Bierman R, Beardsley L, et al: Natural History of Cervicovaginal Papillomavirus Infection in Young Women. *N Engl J Med* 338: 423-428, 1998a.

Ho GY, Kadish AS, Burk RD, et al: HPV 16 and Cigarette Smoking as Risk Factors for High-Grade Cervical Intra-Epithelial Neoplasia. *Int J Cancer* 78: 281-285, 1998b.

Hocking GR, Hayman JA, Östör AG: Adenocarcinoma In Situ of the Uterine Cervix Progressing to Invasive Adenocarcinoma. *Aust N Z J Obstet Gynaecol* 36: 218-220, 1996.

Hoda RS, Madory H, Jones JB, et al: Metastatic Merkel Cell Carcinoma Diagnosed on a Pap Smear (Letter, Case Report). *Acta Cytol* 48: 586-588, 2004.

Hoerl HD, Schink J, Hartenbach E, et al: Exfoliative Cytology of Primary Poorly Differentiated (Small-Cell) Neuroendocrine Carcinoma of the Uterine Cervix in ThinPrep® Material: A Case Report. *Diagn Cytopathol* 23: 14-18, 2000.

Hoerl HD, Roth-Cline MD, Shalkham JE, et al: Rare Atypical Squamous Cells of Undetermined Significance (ASCUS): A Clinically Significant Diagnosis? *Diagn Cytopathol* 27: 5-9, 2002.

Hoffman MS, Sterghos S Jr, Gordy LW, et al: Evaluation of the Cervical Canal With the Endocervical Brush. *Obstet Gynecol* 82: 573-577, 1993.

Holcomb K, Maiman M, Dimaio T, et al: Rapid Progression to Invasive Cervix Cancer in a Woman Infected With the Human Immunodeficiency Virus. *Obstet Gynecol* 91: 848-850, 1998.

Holland BK, Foster JD, Louria DB: Cervical Cancer and Health Care Resources in Newark, New Jersey, 1970 to 1988. *Am J Public Health* 83: 45-48, 1993.

Hollander DH, Gupta PK: Hematoidin Cockleburrs in Cervico-Vaginal Smears. *Acta Cytol* 18: 268-269, 1974a.

Hollander DH, Gupta PK: Detached Ciliary Tufts in Cervico-Vaginal Smears. *Acta Cytol* 18: 367-369, 1974b.

Hollander DH, Gupta PK: DCT, CCP and Pseudoprotozoa (Letter). *Acta Cytol* 23: 258-259, 1979.

Hollander DH: Curschmann's Spirals in Cervicovaginal Smears (Letter), *Acta Cytol* 28: 518, 1984.

Holloway RW, Farrell MP, Castellano C, et al: Identification of Human Papillomavirus Type 16 in Primary and Recurrent Cervical Cancer Following Radiation Therapy. *Gynecol Oncol* 41: 123-128, 1991.

Holly EA, Petrakis NL, Friend NF, et al: Mutagenic Mucus in the Cervix of Smokers. *J Natl Cancer Inst* 76: 983-986, 1986.

Holly EA: Cervical Intraepithelial Neoplasia, Cervical Cancer, and HPV. *Ann Rev Public Health* 17: 69-84, 1996.

Holm K, Grinsted P, Poulsen EF, et al: Can Hairspray Be Used as a Smear Fixative? A Comparison Between Two Types of Coating Fixatives. *Acta Cytol* 32: 422-424, 1988.

Holmes EJ, Lyle WH: How Early in Pregnancy Does the Arias-Stella Reaction Occur? *Arch Pathol Lab Med* 95: 302-303, 1973.

Holmquist ND: The Exfoliative Cytology of Mixed Mesodermal Tumors of the Uterus. *Acta Cytol* 6: 373-375, 1962.

Holmquist ND, Danos M: The Cytology of Early Abortion. *Acta Cytol* 11: 262-266, 1967a.

Holmquist ND, McMahan CA, Williams OD: Variability in Classification of Carcinoma In Situ of the Uterine Cervix. *Arch Pathol* 84: 334-345, 1967b.

Holmquist ND, Bellina JH, Danos ML: Vaginal and Cervical Cytologic Changes Following Laser Treatment. *Acta Cytol* 20: 290-294, 1976.

Holmquist ND, Torres J: Malignant Melanoma of the Cervix: A Report of a Case. *Acta Cytol* 32: 252-256, 1988.

Holmquist ND: Revisiting the Effect of the Pap Test on Cervical Cancer. *Am J Public Health* 90: 620-623, 2000.

Holowaty P, Miller AB, Rohan T, et al: Natural History of Dysplasia of the Uterine Cervix. *J Natl Cancer Inst* 91: 252-258, 1999.

Hong IS, Marshalleck J, Williams RH, et al: Comparative Analysis of a Liquid-Based Pap Test and Concurrent HPV DNA Assay of Residual Samples: A Study of 608 Cases. *Acta Cytol* 46: 828-834, 2002.

Hong SR, Park JS, Kim HS: Atypical Glandular Cells of Undetermined Significance in Cervical Smears After Conization: Cytologic Features Differentiating Them from Adenocarcinoma In Situ. *Acta Cytol* 45: 163-168, 2001.

Hopfel-Kreiner I, Mikuz G: Accidental Cytological Findings in Routine Vaginal Smear in Primary Carcinoma of the Fallopian Tube. *Pathol Res Pract* 163: 163-167, 1978.

Hopkins MP, Roberts JA, Schmidt RW: Cervical Adenocarcinoma In Situ. *Obstet Gynecol* 71: 842-844, 1988.

Hopkins MP, Morley GW: A Comparison of Adenocarcinoma and Squamous Cell Carcinoma of the Cervix. *Obstet Gynecol* 77: 912-917, 1991a.

Hopkins MP, Morley GW: Stage IB Squamous Cell Cancer of the Cervix: Clinicopathologic Features Related to Survival. *Am J Obstet Gynecol* 164: 1520-1529, 1991b.

Hopman EH, Rozendaal L, Voorhorst FJ, et al: High Risk Human Papillomavirus in Women With Normal Cervical Cytology Prior to the Development of Abnormal Cytology and Colposcopy. *Br J Obstet Gynaecol* 107: 600-604, 2000.

Hori S, Itoh H, Tsutsumi Y, et al: Immunoelectron Microscopic Detection of Chlamydial Antigens in Papanicolaou-Stained Routine Vaginal Smears (Letter). *Acta Cytol* 39: 835-837, 1995.

Horowitz BJ, Mårdh P-A, Nagy E, et al: Vaginal Lactobacillosis. *Am J Obstet Gynecol* 170: 857-861, 1994.

Horowitz IR, Jacobson LP, Zucker PK, et al: Epidemiology of Adenocarcinoma of the Cervix. *Gynecol Oncol* 31: 25-41, 1988.

Hoskins PJ, Wong F, Swenerton KD, et al: Small Cell Carcinoma of the Cervix Treated With Concurrent Radiotherapy, Cisplatin, and Etoposide. *Gynecol Oncol* 56: 218-225, 1995.

Houghton SJ, Shafi MI, Rollason TP, et al: Is Loop Excision Adequate Primary Management of Adenocarcinoma In situ of the Cervix? *Br J Obstet Gynecol* 104: 325-329, 1997.

Houissa-Vuong S, Catanzano-Laroudie M, Baviera E, et al: Primary Squamous Cell Carcinoma of the Endometrium: Case History, Pathologic Findings, and Discussion. *Diagn Cytopathol* 27: 291-293, 2002.

Howard L Jr, Erickson CC, Stoddard LD: Study of Incidence and Histogenesis of Endocervical Metaplasia and Intraepithelial Carcinoma: Observations of 400 Uteri Removed for Noncervical Disease. *Cancer* 4: 1210-1223, 1951.

Howard M, Sellors J, Lytwyn A: Cervical Intraepithelial Neoplasia in Women Presenting With External Genital Warts. *CMAJ* 166: 598-599, 2002.

Howdon WM, Howdon A, Frost JK, et al: Cyto- and Histopathologic Correlation in Mixed Mesenchymal Tumors of the Uterus. *Am J Obstet Gynecol* 89: 670-679, 1964.

Howell LP, Davis RL: Follow-Up of Papanicolaou Smears Diagnosed as Atypical Squamous Cells of Undetermined Significance. *Diagn Cytopathol* 14: 20-24, 1996.

Howell LP, Tabnak F, Tudury AJ, et al: Role of Pap Test Terminology and Age in the Detection of Carcinoma Invasive and Carinoma In Situ in Medically Underserved California Women. *Diagn Cytopathol* 30: 227-234, 2004a.

Howell LP, Zhou H, Wu W, et al: Significance of Subclassifying High-Grade Squamous Intraepithelial Lesions into Moderate Dysplasia/CIN II Versus Severe Dysplasia/CIN III/CIS in the Bethesda System Terminology. *Diagn Cytopathol* 30: 362-366, 2004b.

Hsiu J-G, Stawicki ME: The Cytologic Findings in Two Cases of Stromal Sarcoma of the Uterus. *Acta Cytol* 23: 487-489, 1979.

Hu CY, Taymor ML, Hertig AT: Primary Carcinoma of the Fallopian Tube. *Am J Obstet Gynecol* 59: 58-67, 1950.

Huang JC, Naylor B: Cytomegalovirus Infection of the Cervix Detected by Cytology and Histology: A Report of Five Cases. *Cytopathology* 4: 237-241, 1993.

Huang L-W, Chao S-L, Hwang J-L: Human Papillomavirus-31-Related Types Predict Better Survival in Cervical Carcinoma. *Cancer* 100: 327-334, 2004.

Hubbard RA: Human Papillomavirus Testing Methods. *Arch Pathol Lab Med* 127: 940-945, 2003.

Hudock J, Hanau CA, Hawthorne C, et al: Predictors of Human Papilloma Virus in Patients With Keratinization. *Diagn Cytopathol* 12: 28-31, 1995.

Hudson AP: What Is the Evidence for a Relationship Between *Chlamydia pneumoniae* and Late-Onset Alzheimer's Disease. *Laboratory Medicine* 32: 680-685, 2001.

Hudson MMT, Windle H, Kinghorn GR: The Glittering Vagina—A Seasonal Phenomenon? (Letter) *Genitourin Med* 72: 227, 1996.

Huettner PC, Gerhard DS, Li L, et al: Loss of Heterozygosity in Clinical State IB Cervical Carcinoma: Relationship With Clinical and Histopathologic Features. *Hum Pathol* 29: 364-370, 1998.

Hughes JH, Cohen MB: Is the Cytologic Diagnosis of Esophageal Glandular Dysplasia Feasible? *Diagn Cytopathol* 18: 312-316, 1998.

Huijssoon A, ter Harmsel B: Papillary Adenocarcinoma of the Ovary Presenting in a PAP-Smear. *Acta Obstet Gynecol Scand* 80: 659-660, 2001.

Huisjes HJ: Cast-Off Endometrial Cilia in Vaginal Smears (Letter). *Obstet Gynecol* 32: 587, 1968.

Hulka BS: Cytologic and Histologic Outcome Following an Atypical Cancer Smear. *Am J Obstet Gynecol* 101: 190-199, 1968.

Hunt JL, Baloch Z, Judkins A, et al: Unique Cytomegalovirus Intracytoplasmic Inclusions in Ectocervical Cells on a Cervical/Endocervical Smear. *Diagn Cytopathol* 18: 110-112, 1998.

Hunt JM, Irwig LM, Towler BP: The Management of Women With Initial Minor Pap Smear Abnormalities. *Med J Aust* 160: 558-563, 1994.

Hurlimann J, Gloor E: Adenocarcinoma In Situ and Invasive Adenocarcinoma of the Uterine Cervix: An Immunohistologic Study With Antibodies Specific for Several Epithelial Markers. *Cancer* 54: 103-109, 1984.

Hurt WG, Silverberg SG, Frable WJ, et al: Adenocarcinoma of the Cervix: Histopathologic and Clinical Features. *Am J Obstet Gynecol* 129: 304-315, 1977.

Husain OAN, Butler EB, Evans DMD, et al: Quality Control in Cervical Cytology. *J Clin Pathol* 27: 935-944, 1974.

Hutchinson M, Fertitta L, Goldbaum B, et al: Cervex-Brush and Cytobrush: Comparison of Their Ability to Sample Abnormal Cells for Cervical Smears. *J Reprod Med* 36: 581-586, 1991.

Hutchinson ML, Isenstein LM, Goddman A, et al: Homogeneous Sampling Accounts for the Increased Diagnostic Accuracy Using the ThinPrep Processor. *Am J Clin Pathol* 101: 215-219, 1994.

Hutchinson ML, Zahniser DJ, Sherman ME, et al: Utility of Liquid-Based Cytology for Cervical Carcinoma Screening: Results of a Population-Based Study Conducted in a Region of Costa Rica With a High Incidence of Cervical Carcinoma. *Cancer (Cancer Cytopathol)* 87: 48-55, 1999.

Hutter RVP: Arthur I Holleb, M.D. (Tribute) *Cancer* 88: 2653-2654, 2000.

Hutti MH, Hoffman C: Cytolytic Vaginosis: An Overlooked Cause of Cyclic Vaginal Itching and Burning. *J Am Acad Nurse Pract* 12: 55-57, 2000.

I

[IAC] Interntional Academy of Cytology: Opinion Poll on Cytological Definitions. *Acta Cytol* 2: 26-62, 1958a.

[IAC] Interntional Academy of Cytology: Opinion Poll on Cytological Terminology. *Acta Cytol* 2: 63-139, 1958b.

[IARC] Working Group on the Evaluation of Cervical Cancer Screening Programs. "Screening for Squamous Cervical Cancer: Duration of Low Risk After Negative Results of Cervical Cytology and Its Implication for Screening Policies." *Br Med J* 293: 659-664, 1986.

[IARC] International Agency for Research on Cancer, Working Group: Evaluation of Carcinogenic Risks to Humans: Human Papillomaviruses. *IARC Monograph* 64: 381-409. World Health Organization, Lyon, 1995.

[IARC] International Agency for Research on Cancer, Working Group: Evaluation of Carcinogenic Risks to Humans: Some Pharmaceutical Drugs. *IARC Monograph* 66: 35-445. World Health Organization, Lyon, 1996.

Iezzoni JC, Gaffey MJ, Weiss LM: The Role of Epstein-Barr Virus in Lymphoepithelioma-Like Carcinomas. *Am J Clin Pathol* 103: 308-315, 1995.

Ikenberg H, Spitz C, Schmitt B, et al: Human Papillomavirus DNA in Locally Recurrent Cervical Cancer. *Gynecol Oncol* 52: 332-336, 1994.

Im DD, Duska LR, Rosenshein NB: Adequacy of Conization Margins in Adenocarcinoma In Situ of the Cervix as a Predictor of Residual Disease. *Gynecol Oncol* 59: 179-182, 1995.

Imai H, Kitamura H, Nananura T, et al: Müllerian Carcinofibroma of the Uterus: A Case Report. *Acta Cytol* 43: 667-674, 1999.

Inaba N, Fukazawa I, Iwasaki H, et al: Cervical Verrucous Carcinoma: A Case Report (Abstract). *Acta Cytol* 36: 790, 1992.

Inman GJ, Cook ID, Lau RK: Human Papillomaviruses, Tumour Suppressor Genes and Cervical Cancer. *Int J STD AIDS* 4: 128-134, 1993.

Inserra P, Abrahamsen M, Papenfuss M, et al: Ethnic Variation of the p53 Codon 72 Polymorphism, HPV Persistence, and Cervical Cancer Risk. *Int J STD AIDS* 14: 800-804, 2003.

Ioffe OB, Brooks SE, Bueno de Rezende R, et al: Artifact in Cervical LLETZ Specimens: Correlation With Follow-Up. *Int J Gynecol Pathol* 18: 115-121, 1999.

Ioffe OB, Sagae S, Moritani S, et al: Symposium Part 3: Should Pathologists Diagnose Endocervical Preneoplastic Lesions "Less Than" Adenocarcinoma In Situ?: Point. *Int J Gynecol Oncol* 22: 18-21, 2003.

Ionescu DN, Mohan D, Carter G, et al: Epidermoid Metaplasia of the Cervix (Case Report). *Arch Pathol Lab Med* 128: 1052-1053, 2004.

Irwin KL, Rosero-Bixby L, Oberle MW, et al: Oral Contraceptives and Cervical Cancer Risk in Costa Rica. *JAMA* 259: 59-64, 1988.

Isaacs JH: Verrucous Carcinoma of the Female Genital Tract. *Gynecol Oncol* 4: 259-269, 1976.

Isbell NP, Jewett JF, Allan MS, et al: A Correlation Between Vaginal Smear and Tissue Diagnosis in 1045 Operated Gynecologic Cases. *Am J Obstet Gynecol* 54: 576-583, 1947.

Ishi K, Suzuki F, Saito A, et al: Cytodiagnosis of Vaginal Endodermal Sinus Tumor: A Case Report. *Acta Cytol* 42: 399-402, 1998a.

Ishi K, Suzuki F, Saito A, et al: Cytodiagnosis of Placental Site Trophoblastic Tumor: Report of Two Cases. *Acta Cytol* 42: 745-750, 1998b.

Ishibashi-Ueda H, Imakita M, Yutani C, et al: Small Cell Carcinoma of the Uterine Cervix With Syndrome of Inappropriate Antidiuretic Hormone Secretion. *Mod Pathol* 9: 397-400, 1996.

Ishii K, Hosaka N, Toki T, et al: A New View of the So-Called Adenoma Malignum of the Uterine Cervix. *Virchows Archiv (Path Anat)* 432: 315-322, 1998.

Ishii K, Katsuyama T, Ota H, et al: Cytologic and Cytochemical Features of Adenoma Malignum of the Uterine Cervix. *Cancer (Cancer Cytopathol)* 87: 245-253, 1999.

Ishii Y, Fujii M: Criteria for Differential Diagnosis of Complex Hyperplasia or Beyond in Endometrial Cytology. *Acta Cytol* 41: 1095-1102, 1997.

Ismail SM, Colclough AB, Dinnen JS, et al: Observer Variation in Histopathological Diagnosis and Grading of Cervical Intraepithelial Neoplasia. *Br Med J* 298: 707-710, 1989.

Ismail SM, Colclough AB, Dinnen JS, et al: Reporting Cervical Intra-Epithelial Neoplasia (CIN): Intra- and Interpathologist Variation and Factors Associated With Disagreement. *Histopathology* 16: 371-376, 1990.

Ismail SM: Cone Biopsy Causes Cervical Endometriosis and Tubo-Endometrioid Metaplasia. *Histopathology* 18: 107-114, 1991.

Israel SL, Crisp WE, Adrian DC: Preoperative Diagnosis of Primary Carcinoma of the Fallopian Tube. *Am J Obstet Gynecol* 68: 1589-1593, 1954.

Issa PY, Salem PA, Brihi E, et al: Eosinophilic Granuloma With Involvement of the Female Genitalia. *Am J Obstet Gynecol* 137: 608-612, 1980.

Ito E, Kudo R: Scanning Electron Microcopy of Normal Cells, Dyskaryotic Cells and Malignant Cells Exfoliated from the Uterine Cervix. *Acta Cytol* 26: 457-465, 1982.

Ito E, Saito T, Suzuhi T, et al: Cytology of Vaginal and Uterine Sarcomas. *Acta Cytol* 48: 601-607, 2004.

Iwasaka T, Yokoyama M, Hayashi Y, et al: Combined Herpes Simplex Virus Type 2 and Human Papillomavirus Type 16 or 18 Deoxyribonucleic Acid Leads to Oncogenic Transformation. *Am J Obstet Gynecol* 159: 1251-1255, 1988.

Iwasawa A, Nieminen P, Lehtinen M, et al: Human Papillomavirus DNA in Uterine Cervix Squamous Cell Carcinoma and Adenocarcinoma Detected by Polymerase Chain Reaction. *Cancer* 77: 2275-2279, 1996.

Izumi S, Hasegawa T, Tsutsui F, et al: Carcinosarcoma of the Uterus: Cytologic and Ultrastructural Features. *Acta Cytol* 29: 602-606, 1985.

J

Jabamoni R, Dodson MG, Blecka LJ, et al: Unusual Protozoal Infestation of the Cervical Mucus. *Obstet Gynecol* 50: 224-227, 1977.

Jackson S, Harwood C, Thomas M, et al: Role of BAK in UV-Induced Apoptosis in Skin Cancer and Abrogation by HPV E6 Proteins. *Genes Dev* 14: 3065-3073, 2000.

Jackson SR, Hollingworth TA, Anderson MC, et al: Glandular Lesions of the Cervix—Cytological and Histological Correlation. *Cytopathology* 7: 10-16, 1996.

Jacobs MV, Snijders PJ, van den Brule AJ, et al: A General Primer GP5+/GP6(+)-Mediated PCR-Enzyme Immunoassay Method for Rapid Detection of 14 High-Risk and 6 Low-Risk Human Papillomavirus Genotypes in Cervical Scrapings. *J Clin Microbiol* 35: 791-795, 1997.

Jacobs MV, Walboomers JMM, Snijders PJF, et al: Distribution of 37 Mucosotropic HPV Types in Women With Cytologically Normal Cervical Smears: The Age-Related Patterns for High-Risk and Low-Risk Types. *Int J Cancer* 87: 221-227, 2000.

Jacobson DL, Peralta L, Graham NM, et al: Histologic Development of Cervical Ectopy: Relationship to Reproductive Hormones. *Sex Transm Dis* 27: 252-258, 2000a.

Jacobson DL, Womack SD, Peralta L, et al: Concordance of Human Papillomavirus in the Cervix and Urine Among Inner City Adolescents. *Pediatr Infect Dis J* 19: 722-728, 2000b.

Jafari K: False-Positive Pap Smear in Uterine Malignancy. *Gynecol Oncol* 6: 76-82, 1978.

Jakobsen A, Kristensen PB, Poulsen HK: Flow Cytometric Classification of Biopsy Specimens from Cervical Intraepithelial Neoplasia. *Cytometry* 4: 166-169, 1983.

Jaluvka V, Novak A: Vaginal Foreign Bodies in Women in Postmenopause and in Senium. *Eur J Obstet Gynecol Reprod Biol* 61: 167-169, 1995.

Janerich DT, Hadjimichael O, Schwartz P, et al: The Screening Histories of Women With Invasive Cancer, Connecticut. *Am J Public Health* 85: 791-794, 1995.

Janicek MF, Averette HE: Cervical Cancer: Prevention, Diagnosis and Therapeutics. *CA: Cancer J Clin* 51: 92-114, 2001.

Japaze H, Van Dinh T, Woodruff JD: Verrucous Carcinoma of the Vulva: Study of 24 Cases. *Obstet Gynecol* 60: 462-466, 1982.

Jarmulowicz MR, Jenkins D, Bartons SE, et al: Cytological Status and Lesion Size: A Further Dimension in Cervical Intraepithelial Neoplasia. *Br J Obstet Gynaecol* 96: 1061-1066, 1989.

Jarvis D: Isolation and Identification of Actinomycetes from Women Using Intrauterine Contraceptive Devices. *J Infect* 10: 121-125, 1985.

Jastreboff AM, Cymet T: Role of the Human Papilloma Virus in the Development of Cervical Intraepithelial Neoplasia and Malignancy. *Postgrad Med J* 78: 225-228, 2002.

Jaworski RC, Pacey NF, Greenberg ML, et al: The Histologic Diagnosis of Adenocarcinoma In Situ and Related Lesions of the Cervix Uteri: Adenocarcinoma In Situ. *Cancer* 61: 1171-1181, 1988.

Jaworski RC: Endocervical Glandular Dysplasia, Adenocarcinoma In Situ and Early (Microinvasive) Adenocarcinoma of the Uterine Cervix. *Semin Diagn Pathol* 7: 190-204, 1990.

Jay N, Moscicki A-B: Human Papillomavirus Infections in Women With HIV Disease: Prevalence, Risk, and Management. *AIDS Reader* 10: 659-668, 2000.

Jayant K: Additive Effect of Two Risk Factors in the Aetiology of Cancer of the Cervix Uteri. *Br J Cancer* 56: 685-686, 1987.

Jemal A, Murray T, Wood E, et al: Cancer Statistics, 2005. *CA: Cancer J Clin* 55: 10-30, 2005.

Jenkins D, Tay SK, McCance DJ, et al: Histological and Immunocytochemical Study of Cervical Intraepithelial Neoplasia (CIN) With Associated HPV 6 and HPV 16 Infections. *J Clin Pathol* 39: 1177-1180, 1986.

Jenkins DM, Goulden R, Psammoma Bodies in Cervical Cytology Smears. *Acta Cytol* 21: 112-113, 1977.

Jeppsson S, Johansson ED, Ljungberg O, et al: Endometrial Histology and Circulating Levels of Medroxyprogesterone Acetate (MPAS), Estradiol, FSH and LH in Women With MPA Induced Amenorrhoea Compared With Women With Secondary Amenorrhoea. *Acta Obstet Gynecol Scand* 56: 43-48, 1977.

Jha PK, Beral V, Peto J, et al: Antibodies to Human Papillomavirus and to Other Genital Infectious Agents and Invasive Cervical Cancer Risk. *Lancet* 341: 1116-1118, 1993.

Jiji V: Blue Nevus of the Endocervix: Review of the Literature. *Arch Pathol Lab Med* 92: 203-205, 1971.

Jiménez-Ayala M, Martínez-Cabruja R, Casado MLE: Serous Surface Papillary Carcinoma of the Ovary Metastatic to a Cervical Polyp: A Case Report. *Acta Cytol* 40: 765-769, 1996.

Jin XW, Xu H: Cervical Cancer Screening from Pap Smear to Human Papillomavirus DNA Testing. *Comp Ther* 27: 202-208, 2001.

Jobo T, Arai T, Sato R, et al: Clinicopathologic Relevance of Asymptomatic Endometrial Carcinoma. *Acta Cytol* 47: 611-615, 2003.

Johannesson G, Geirsson G, Day N, et al: Screening for Cancer of the Uterine Cervix in Iceland 1965-1978. *Acta Obstet Gynecol Scand* 61: 199-203, 1982.

Johnson CE, Soule EH: Malignant Lymphoma as a Gynecologic Problem: Report of Five Cases Including One Primary Lymphosarcoma of the Cervix Uteri. *Obstet Gynecol* 9: 149-157, 1957.

Johnson J: Commentary on the Presence of Glandular Cells in Vault Smears. *Cytopathology* 10: 131, 1999.

Johnson JC, Burnett AF, Willet GD, et al: High Frequency of Latent and Clinical Human Papillomavirus Cervical Infections in Immunocompromised Human Immunodeficiency Virus-Infected Women. *Obstet Gynecol* 79: 321-327, 1992.

Johnson JE, Rahemtulla A: Endocervical Glandular Neoplasia and Its Mimics in ThinPrep Pap Tests: A Descriptive Study. *Acta Cytol* 43: 369-375, 1999.

Johnson LD, Easterday CL, Gore H, et al: The Histogenesis of Carcinoma In Situ of the Uterine Cervix: A Preliminary Report of the Origin of Carcinoma In Situ in Subcylindrical Cells of Anaplasia. *Cancer* 17: 213-229, 1964.

Johnson LD, Nickerson RJ, Easterday CL, et al: Epidemiologic Evidence for the Spectrum of Change from Dysplasia Through Carcinoma In Situ to Invasive Cancer. *Cancer* 22: 901-914, 1968.

Johnson LD: The Histopathological Approach to Early Cervical Neoplasia. *Obstet Gynecol Surv* 24: 735-767, 1969.

Johnson MA, Blomfield PI, Bevan IS, et al: Analysis of Human Papillomavirus Type 16 E6-E7 Transcription in Cervical Carcinomas and Normal Cervical Epithelium Using the Polymerase Chain Reaction. *J Gen Virol* 71: 1473-1479, 1990.

Johnson S: The Multifaceted and Widespread Pathology of Magnesium Deficiency. *Med Hypotheses* 56: 163-170, 2001.

Johnson SJ, Wadehra V: How Predictive Is a Cervical Smear Suggesting Invasive Squamous Cell Carcinoma? *Cytopathology* 12: 144-150, 2001.

Johnson TL, Joseph CLM, Caison-Sorey TJ, et al: Prevalence of HPV 16 and 18 DNA Sequences in CIN III Lesions of Adults and Adolescents. *Diagn Cytopathol* 10: 276-283, 1994.

Johnson TL, Kini SR: Endometrial Metaplasia as a Source of Atypical Glandular Cells in Cervicovaginal Smears. *Diagn Cytopathol* 14: 25-31, 1996.

Johnston C: Mild Cytological Atypia in Women With HIV Infection (Comment). *Lancet* 358: 837-838, 1996.

Johnston C: Quantitative Tests for Human Papillomavirus. (Commentary) *Lancet* 355: 2179-2180, 2000.

Johnston M, Benrubi GI, Nuss RC, et al: Age and Cervical Dysplasia. *South Med J* 81: 1458-1459, 1988.

Johnston WW, Goldston WR, Montgomery MS: Clinicopathologic Studies in Feminizing Tumors of the Ovary: III. The Role of Genital Cytology. *Acta Cytol* 15: 334-338, 1971.

Johnston WW, Myers B, Creasman WT, et al: Cytopathology and the Management of Early Invasive Cancer of the Uterine Cervix. *Obstet Gynecol* 60: 350-353, 1982.

Jonasson JG, Wang HH, Antonioli DA, et al: Tubal Metaplasia of the Uterine Cervix: A Prevalence Study in Patients With Gynecologic Pathology Findings. *Int J Gynecol Pathol* 11: 89-95, 1992.

Jones BA, Heard NV: Pap Smear Rescreening Data Analysis and Critique. *College of American Pathologists Q-Probe Study* 3: 1-16, 1993.

Jones BA, Novis DA: Cervical Biopsy—Cytology Correlation: A College of American Pathologists Q-Probes Study of 22439 Correlations in 348 Laboratories. *Arch Pathol Lab Med* 120: 523-531, 1996.

Jones BA: Follow-Up of Abnormal Gynecologic Cytology: A College of American Pathologists Q-Probes Study of 16,132 Cases from 306 Laboratories. *Arch Pathol Lab Med* 124: 665-671, 2000.

Jones CA, Neustaedter T, Mackenzie LL: The Value of Vaginal Smears in the Diagnosis of Early Malignancy. *Am J Obstet Gynecol* 49: 159-168, 1945.

Jones CJ, Brinton LA, Hamman RF, et al: Risk Factors for In Situ Cervical Cancer: Results from a Case-Control Study. *Cancer Res* 50: 3657-3662, 1990.

Jones DED, Creasman WT, Dombroski RA, et al: Evaluation of the Atypical Pap Smear. *Am J Obstet Gynecol* 157: 544-549, 1987.

Jones DL, Alani RM, Münger K: The Human Papillomavirus E7 Oncoprotein Can Uncouple Cellular Differentiation and Proliferation in Human Keratinocytes by Abrogating p21[CIP1]-Mediated Inhibtion of cdk2. *Genes Dev* 11: 2101-2111, 1997.

Jones DM, Davson J: *Mycoplasma hominis* in Ayre's Smears. *Nature* (i): 828-829, 1967.

Jones EG, MacDonald I, Breslow L: A Study of Epidemiologic Factors in Carcinoma of the Uterine Cervix. *Am J Obstet Gynecol* 76: 1-10, 1958.

Jones HW III, Droegemueller W, Makowski EL: A Primary Melanocarcinoma of the Cervix. *Am J Obstet Gynecol* 111: 959-963, 1971.

Jones HW III: Impact of the Bethesda System. *Cancer* 76: 1914-1918, 1995.

Jones HW III: Clinical Treatment of Women With Atypical Squamous Cells of Undetermined Significance or Atypical Glandular Cells of Undetermined Significance Cervical Cytology. *Clin Obstet Gynecol* 43: 381-393, 2000.

Jones MA, Andrews J, Tarraza HM: Mesonephric Remnant Hyperplasia of the Cervix: A Clinicopathologic Analysis of 14 Cases. *Gynecol Oncol* 49: 41-47, 1993.

Jones MA, Young RH: Endocervical Type A (Noncystic) Tunnel Clusters With Cytologic Atypia: A Report of 14 Cases. *Am J Surg Pathol* 20: 1312-1318, 1996.

Jones MA, Young RH: Atypical Oxyphilic Metaplasia of the Endocervical Epithelium: A Report of Six Cases. *Int J Gynecol Pathol* 16: 99-102, 1997.

Jones MA: Transitional Cell Metaplasia and Neoplasia in the Female Genital Tract: An Update. *Adv Anat Pathol* 5: 106-113, 1998.

Jones MC, Buschmann BO, Dowling EA, et al: The Prevalence of Actinomycetes-Like Organisms Found in Cervicovaginal Smears of 300 IUD Wearers. *Acta Cytol* 23: 282-286, 1979.

Jones MH, Jenkins D, Cuzick J, et al: Mild Cervical Dyskaryosis: Safety of Cytological Surveillance. *Lancet* 339: 1440-1443, 1992.

Jones MW, Silverberg SG: Cervical Adenocarcinoma in Young Women: Possible Relationship to Microglandular Hyperplasia and Use of Oral Contraceptives. *Obstet Gynecol* 73: 984-989, 1989.

Jones MW, Silverberg SG, Kurman RJ: Well-Differentiated Villoglandular Adenocarcinoma of the Uterine Cervix: A Clinicopathologic Study of 24 Cases. *Int J Gynecol Pathol* 12: 1-7, 1993.

Jones MW, Kounelis S, Papadaki H, et al: The Origin and Molecular Characterization of Adenoid Basal Carcinoma of the Uterine Cervix. *Int J Gynecol Pathol* 16: 301-306, 1997.

Jones MW, Kounelis S, Papadaki H, et al: Well-Differentiated Villoglandular Adenocarcinoma of the Uterine Cervix: Oncogene/Tumor Suppressor Gene Alterations and Human Papillomavirus Genotyping. *Int J Gynecol Pathol* 19: 110-117, 2000.

Jones OV: Primary Carcinoma of the Uterine Tube. *Obstet Gynecol* 26: 122-129, 1965.

Jones S, Thomas GD, Williamson P: Observer Variation in the Assessment of Adequacy and Neoplasia in Cervical Cytology. *Acta Cytol* 40: 226-234, 1996.

Jones WB, Saigo PE: The "Atypical" Papanicolaou Smear. *CA: Cancer J Clin* 36: 237-242, 1986.

Jones WB, Shingleton HM, Russell A, et al: Cervical Carcinoma and Pregnancy. A National Patterns of Care Study of the American College of Surgeons. *Cancer* 77: 1479-1488, 1996.

Jordan MJ, Bader GM, Day E: A Rational Approach to the Management of Atypical Lesions of the Cervix. *Am J Obstet Gynecol* 72: 725-739, 1956.

Jordan MJ, Bader GM, Day E: Carcinoma In Situ of the Cervix and Related Lesions. An 11 Year Prospective Study. *Am J Obstet Gynecol* 89: 160-182, 1964.

Jordan SW, Smith NL, Dike LS: The Significance of Cervical Cytologic Dysplasia (Abstract). *Acta Cytol* 24: 65, 1980.

Jordan SW, Smith NL, Dike LS: The Significance of Cervical Cytologic Dysplasia. *Acta Cytol* 25: 237-244, 1981.

Josefsson AM, Magnusson PK, Ytalo N, et al: Viral Load of Human Papilloma Virus 16 as a Determinant for Development of Cervical Carcinoma In Situ: A Nested Case-Control Study. *Lancet* 355: 2189-2193, 2000.

Joseph MG, Cragg F, Wright VC, et al: Cyto-Histological Correlates in a Colposcopic Clinic: A 1-Year Prospective Study. *Diagn Cytopathol* 7: 477-481, 1991.

Joseph RE, Enghardt MH, Doering DL, et al: Small Cell Neuroendocrine Carcinoma of the Vagina. *Cancer* 70: 784-789, 1992.

Josey WE, Nahmias AJ, Naib ZM: Viruses and Cancer of the Lower Genital Tract. *Cancer* 38: 526-533, 1976.

Joste NE, Crum CP, Cibas ES: Cytologic/Histologic Correlation for Quality Control in Cervicovaginal Cytology. *Am J Clin Pathol* 103: 32-34, 1995.

Jovanovic AS, McLachlin CM, Shen L, et al: Postmenopausal Squamous Atypia: A Spectrum Including "Pseudo-Koilocytosis". *Mod Pathol* 8: 408-412, 1995.

Junor EJ, Symonds RP, Watson ER, et al: Survival of Younger Cervical Carcinoma Patients Treated by Radical Radiotherapy in the West of Scotland 1964-1984. *Br J Obstet Gynaecol* 96: 522-528, 1989.

Juskevicius R, Zou KH, Cibas ES: An Analysis of Factors That Influence the ASCUS/SIL Ratio of Pathologists. *Am J Clin Pathol* 116: 331-335, 2001.

K

Kabbani W, Raisanen J, Thomas S, et al: Cell Block Findings from Residual PreservCyt Samples in Unsatisfactory ThinPrep Paps: No Additional Benefit. *Diagn Cytopathol* 27: 238-243, 2002.

Kadish AS, Burk RD, Kress Y, et al: Human Papillomaviruses of Different Types in Precancerous Lesions of the Uterine Cervix: Histologic, Immunocytochemical and Ultrastructural Studies. *Hum Pathol* 17: 384-392, 1986.

Kadish AS, Hagan RJ, Ritter DB, et al: Biologic Characteristics of Specific Human Papillomavirus Types Predicted from Morphology of Squamous Lesions. *Hum Pathol* 23: 1262-1269, 1992.

Kadish AS: Biology of Anogenital Neoplasia. *Cancer Treat Res* 104: 267-286, 2001.

Kahn JA, Emans SJ: Pap Smears in Adolescents: To Screen or Not to Screen? *Pediatrics* 103: 673-674, 1999.

Kahn JA: An Update on Human Papillomavirus Infection and Papanicolaou Smears in Adolescents. *Curr Opin Pediatrics* 13: 303-309, 2001.

Kaku T, Enjoji M: Extremely Well-Differentiated Adenocarcinoma ("Adenoma Malignum") of the Cervix. *Int J Gynecol Pathol* 2: 28-41, 1983.

Kaku T, Kamura T, Sakai K: Early Adenocarcinoma of the Uterine Cervix. *Gynecol Oncol* 65: 281-285, 1997.

Kalantari M, Karlsen F, Johansson B, et al: Human Papillomavirus Findings in Relation to Cervical Intraepithelial Neoplasia Grade: A Study on 476 Stockholm Women, Using PCR for Detection and Typing of HPV. *Hum Pathol* 28: 899-904, 1997.

Kalayoglu MV, Libby P, Byrne GI: *Chlamydia pneumoniae* as an Emerging Risk Factor in Cardiovascular Disease. *JAMA* 288: 2724-2731, 2002.

Kalo-Klein A, Witkin SS: *Candida albicans*: Cellular Immune System Interactions During Different Stages of Menstrual Cycle. *Am J Obstet Gynecol* 161: 1132-1136, 1989.

Kaminetzky HA: Methylocholanthrene-Induced Cervical Dysplasia and the Sex Steroids. *Obstet Gynecol* 27: 489-498, 1966.

Kaminski PF, Maier RC: Clear Cell Adenocarcinoma of the Cervix Unrelated to Diethylstilbestrol Exposure. *Obstet Gynecol* 62: 720-727, 1983.

Kaminski PF, Norris HJ: Coexistence of Ovarian Neoplasms and Endocervical Adenocarcinoma. *Obstet Gynecol* 64: 553-556, 1984

Kaminski PF, Sorosky JI, Wheelock JB, et al: The Significance of Atypical Cervical Cytology in an Older Population. *Obstet Gynecol* 73: 13-15, 1989a.

Kaminski PF, Stevens CW Jr, Wheelock JB: Squamous Atypia on Cytology: The Influence of Age. *J Reprod Med* 34: 617-620, 1989b.

Kaminski PF, Lyon DS, Soroky JI, et al: Significance of Atypical Cervical Cytology in Pregnancy. *Am J Perinatol* 9: 340-343, 1992.

Kamiya M, Uei Y, Higo Y, et al: Immunocytochemical Diagnosis of Small Cell Undifferentiated Carcinoma of the Cervix. *Acta Cytol* 37: 131-134, 1993.

Kanai M, Shiozawa T, Xin L, et al: Immunohistochemical Detecton of Sex Steroid Receptors, Cyclins, and Cyclin-Dependent Kinases in the Normal and Neoplastic Squamous Epithelia of the Uterine Cervix. *Cancer* 82: 1709-1719, 1998.

Kanbour A, Stock RJ: Squamous Cell Carcinoma In Situ of the Endometrium and Fallopian Tube as Superficial Extension of Invasive Cervical Carcinoma. *Cancer* 42: 570-580, 1978.

Kanbour A, Doshi N: Psammoma Bodies and Detached Ciliary Tufts in a Cervicovaginal Smear Associated With Benign Ovarian Cystadenofibroma. *Acta Cytol* 24: 549-552, 1980.

Kaneko C, Shamoto M, Kobayashi TK: Nuclear Grooves in Vaginal Cells (Letter). *Acta Cytol* 42: 823-824, 1998.

Kapila K, Verma K: Intracellular Bacilli in Vaginal Smears in a Case of Malakoplakia of the Uterine Cervix (Letter). *Acta Cytol* 33: 410-411, 1989.

Kaplan AL, Kaufman RH: Diagnosis and Management of Dysplasia and Carcinoma In Situ of the Cervix in Pregnancy. *Clin Obstet Gynecol* 10: 871-878, 1967.

Kaplan B, Orvieto R, Hirsch M, et al: The Impact of Intrauterine Contraceptive Devices on Cytological Findings from Routine Pap Smear Testing. *Eur J Contracept Reprod Health Care* 3: 75-77, 1998.

Kaplan KJ, Dainty LA, Dolinsky B, et al: Prognosis and Recurrence Risk for Patients With Cervical Squamous Intraepithelial Lesions Diagnosed During Pregnancy. *Cancer (Cancer Cytopathol)* 102: 228-232, 2004.

Kaptain S, Bloom LI, Weir MM: Hormonal Effects of Depo-Provera in Cervical Smears: A Comparison With Triphasil and Postmenopausal Effects. *Cancer (Cancer Cytopathol)* 96: 74-82, 2002.

Karamanidis D, Tamiolakis D, Koutsougeras G, et al: Cigarette Smoking and the Degree of Maturation of the Vaginal Squamous Epithelium in Postmenopausal Women. *Clin Exp Obstet Gynecol* 28: 274-276, 2001.

Kardinal CG, Yarbro JW: A Conceptual History of Cancer. *Seminars Oncology* 6: 396-408, 1979.

Karim BO, Burroughs FH, Rosenthal DL, et al: Endometrial-Type Cells in Cervico-Vaginal Smears: Clinical Significance and Cytopathologic Correlates. *Diagn Cytopathol* 26: 123-127, 2002.

Karlsson R, Jonsoon M, Edlund K, et al: Lifetime Number of Partners as the Only Independent Risk Factor for Human Papillomavirus Infection: A Population-Based Study. *Sex Transm Dis* 22: 119-127, 1995.

Karpas CM, Bridge MF: Endometrial Adenocarcinoma With Psammomatous Bodies. *Am J Obstet Gynecol* 87: 935-341, 1963.

Kase H, Kodama S, Tanaka K: Observations of High Iron Diamine-Alcian Blue Stain in Uterine Cervical Glandular Lesions. *Gynecol Obstet Invest* 48: 56-60, 1999.

Kashima HK, Shah F, Lyles A, et al: A Comparison of Risk Factors in Juvenile-Onset and Adult-Onset Recurrent Respiratory Papillomatosis. *Laryngoscope* 102: 9-13, 1992.

Kashimura M, Kashimura Y, Matsuyama T, et al: Adenocarcinoma of the Uterine Cervix Metastatic from Primary Stomach Cancer: Cytologic Findings in Six Cases. *Acta Cytol* 27: 54-58, 1983.

Kashimura M, Tsukamoto N, Matsukuma K, et al: Verrucous Carcinoma of the Uterine Cervix: Report of a Case With follow-Up of 6 1/2 Years. *Gynecol Oncol* 19: 204-215, 1984.

Kashimura M, Baba S, Nakamura S, et al: Short-Term Estrogen Test for Cytodiagnosis in Postmenopausal Women. *Diagn Cytopathol* 3: 181-184, 1987.

Kashimura M, Baba S, Shinohara M, et al: Cytologic Findings in Endometrial Hyperplasia. *Acta Cytol* 32: 335-340, 1988.

Kashimura M, Shinohara M, Oikawa K, et al: An Adenocarcinoma In Situ of the Uterine Cervix that Developed into Invasive Adenocarcinoma after 5 Years. *Gynecol Oncol* 36: 128-133, 1990.

Kashimura M, Matsuura Y, Shinohara M, et al: Comparative Study of Cytology and Punch Biopsy in Cervical Intraepithelial Neoplasia During Pregnancy: A Preliminary Report. *Acta Cytol* 35: 100-104, 1991.

Kasnic G Jr, Sayeed A, Azar HA: Nuclear and Cytoplasmic Inclusions in Disseminated Human Cytomegalovirus Infection. *Ultrastruct Pathol* 3: 229-235, 1982.

Kaspar HG, Dinh TV, Doherty MG, et al: Clinical Implications of Tumor Volume Measurement in Stage I Adenocarcinoma of the Cervix. *Obstet Gynecol* 81: 296-300, 1993.

Kataja V, Syrjänen K, Mäntyjärvi R, et al: Prospective Follow-up of Cervical HPV Infections: Life-Table Analysis of Histopathological, Cytological and Colposcopic Data. *Eur J Epidemiol* 5: 1-7, 1989.

Kataja V, Syrjänen S, Mäntyjärvi R, et al: Prognostic Factors in Cervical Human Papillomavirus Infections. *Sex Transm Dis* 19: 154-160, 1992.

Katayama I, Hajian G, Evjy JT: Cytologic Diagnosis of Reticulum Cell Sarcoma of the Uterine Cervix. *Acta Cytol* 17: 498-501, 1973.

Katz L, Hinberg I, Weber F: False-Negative Smears in Gynaecological Cytology (Letter). *Lancet* (i): 562, 1979.

Katz RL, Veanattukalathil S, Weiss KM: Human Papillomavirus Infection and Neoplasia of the Cervix and Anogenital Region in Women With Hodgkin's Disease. *Acta Cytol* 31: 845-854, 1987.

Kaufman R, Koss LG, Kurman RJ, et al: Statement of Caution in the Interpretation of Papillomavirus-Associated Lesions of the Epithelium of the Uterine Cervix. *Acta Cytol* 27: 107-108, 1983a.

Kaufman R, Koss LG, Kurman RJ, et al: Statement of Caution in the Interpretation of Papillomavirus-Associated Lesions of the Epithelium of Uterine Cervix (Editorial). *Am J Obstet Gynecol* 146: 125, 1983b.

Kaufman RH, Topek NH, Wall JA: Late Irradiation Changes in Vaginal Cytology. *Am J Obstet Gynecol* 81: 859-866, 1961.

Kaufman RH, Watts JM, Gardner HL: Pemphigus Vulgaris Genital Involvement: Report of Two Cases. *Obstet Gynecol* 33: 264-266, 1969.

Kaufman RH, Burmeister RE, Spjut HJ: Cervical Cytology in the Teen-Age Patient. *Am J Obstet Gynecol* 108: 515-519, 1970.

Kaufman RH: Atypical Squamous Cells of Undetermined Significance and Low-Grade Squamous Intraepithelial Lesion: Diagnostic Criteria and Management. *Am J Obstet Gynecol* 175: 1120-1128, 1996.

Kaufman RH, Adam E, Vonka V: Human Papillomavirus Infection and Cervical Carcinoma. *Clin Obstet Gynecol* 43: 363-380, 2000.

Kaufman RH, Adam E: Findings in Female Offspring of Women Exposed *in utero* to Diethylstilbestrol. *Obstet Gynecol* 99: 197-200, 2002.

Kaur AC, Paksoy N, Kara M: Charcot-Leyden Crystals in Cervical Smear (Letter). *Diagn Cytopathol* 21: 433-434, 1999.

Kawaguchi K, Nogi M, Ohya M, et al: The Value of the Cytobrush for Obtaining Cells from the Uterine Cervix. *Diagn Cytopathol* 3: 262-267, 1987.

Kawai K, Yaginuma H, Tsuruoka M, et al: Telomerase Activity and Human Papillomavirus (HPV) Infection in Human Uterine Cervical Cancers and Cervical Smears. *Eur J Cancer* 34: 2082-2086, 1998.

Kay S, Frable WJ, Hume DM: Cervical Dysplasia and Cancer Developing in Women on Immunosuppression Therapy for Renal Homotransplantation. *Cancer* 26: 1048-1052, 1970.

Keane FEA, Ison CA, Taylor-Robinson D: A Longitudinal Study of the Vaginal Flora Over a Menstrual Cycle. *Int J STD AIDS* 8: 489-494, 1997.

Kearns PR, Gray JE: Mycotic Vulvovaginitis: Incidence and Persistence of Specific Yeast Species During Infection. *Obstet Gynecol* 22: 621-625, 1963.

Keating JT, Cviko A, Riethdorf S, et al: Ki-67, Cyclin E, and p16^{INK4a} Are Complimentary Surrogate Biomarkers for Human Papilloma Virus-Related Cervical Neoplasia. *Am J Surg Pathol* 25: 884-891, 2001a.

Keating JT, Ince T, Crum CP: Surrogate Biomarkers of HPV Infection in Cervical Neoplasia Screening and Diagnosis. *Adv Anat Pathol* 8: 83-92, 2001b.

Keating JT, Wang HH: Significance of a Diagnosis of Atypical Squamous Cells of Undetermined Significance for Papanicolaou Smears in Perimenopausal and Postmenopausal Women. *Cancer (Cancer Cytopathol)* 93: 100-105, 2001c.

Kedzia W, Gozdzika-Jozefiak A, Kwasniewska A, et al: Relationship Between HPV Infection of the Cervix and Blood Serum Levels of Steroid Hormones Among Pre- and Postmenopausal Women. *Eur J Gynaecol Oncol* 21: 177-179, 2000.

Keebler C, Wied GL: The Estrogen Test: An Aid in Differential Cytodiagnosis. *Acta Cytol* 18: 482-493, 1974.

Keebler C, Chatwani A, Schwartz R: Actinomycosis Infection Associated With Intrauterine Contraceptive Devices. *Am J Obstet Gynecol* 145: 596-599, 1983.

Keighley E: Carcinoma of the Cervix Among Prostitutes in a Women's Prison. *Br J Vener Dis* 44: 254-255, 1968.

Kelly BA, Black AS: The Inflammatory Cervical Smear: A Study in General Practice. *Br J Gen Pract* 40: 238-240, 1990.

Kemna ME, Neri RC, Ali R, et al: *Cokeromyces recurvatus*, a Mucoraceous Zygomycete Rarely Isolated in Clinical Laboratories. *J Clin Microbiol* 32: 843-845, 1994.

Kennedy AW, Salmieri SS, Wirth SL, et al: Results of Clinical Evaluation of Atypical Glandular Cells of Undetermined Significane (AGCUS) Detected on Cervical Cytology Screening. *Gynecol Oncol* 63: 14-18, 1996.

Kenny MB, Under ER, Chenggis ML, et al: In Situ Hybridization for Human Papillomavirus DNA in Uterine Adenosquamous Carcinoma With Glassy Cell Features ("Glassy Cell Carcinoma"). *Am J Clin Pathol* 98: 180-187, 1992.

Kenter GG, Schoonderwald EM, Koelma IA, et al: The Cytological Screening History of 469 Patients With Squamous Cell Carcinoma of the Cervix Uteri; Does Interval Carcinoma Exist? *Acta Obstet Gynecol Scand* 75: 400-403, 1996.

Kern SB: Prevalence of Psammoma Bodies in Papanicolaou-Stained Cervicovaginal Smears. *Acta Cytol* 35: 81-88, 1991a.

Kern SB: Significance of Anucleated Squames in Papanicolaou-Stained Cervicovaginal Smears. *Acta Cytol* 35: 89-93, 1991b.

Kernodle JR, Cuyler WK, Thomas WL: The Diagnosis of Genital Malignancy by Vaginal Smears. *Am J Obstet Gynecol* 56: 1083-1089, 1948.

Kerpsack JT, Finan MA, Kline RC: Correlation Between Endometrial Cells on Papanicolaou Smear and Endometrial Carcinoma. *Southern Med J* 91: 749-752, 1998.

Kersemaekers AM, Hermans J, Fleuren GJ, et al: Loss of Heterozygosity for Defined Regions on Chromosomes 3, 11 and 17 in Carcinomas of the Uterine Cervix. *Br J Cancer* 77:192-200, 1998.

Kessler II: Perspectives on the Epidemiology of Cervical Cancer With Special Reference to the Herpesvirus Hypothesis. *Cancer Res* 34: 1091-1110, 1974a.

Kessler II, Kulcar Z, Zimolo A, et al: Cervical Cancer in Yugoslavia. II. Epidemiologic Factors of Possible Etiologic Significance. *J Natl Cancer Inst* 53: 51-60, 1974b.

Kessler II: Human Cervical Cancer as a Venereal Disease. *Cancer Res* 36: 783-791, 1976.

Kessler II: Venereal Factors in Human Cervical Cancer: Evidence from Marital Clusters. *Cancer* 39: 1912-1919, 1977.

Kessler II: Etiological Concepts in Cervical Carcinogenesis. *Gynecol Oncol* 12(2 Pt 2): S7-S24, 1981.

Kessler II: Etiological Concepts in Cervical Carcinogenesis. *Appl Pathol* 5: 57-75, 1987.

Keyhani-Rofagha S, Brewer J, Prokorym P: Comparative Cytologic Findings of In Situ and Invasive Adenocarcinoma of the Uterine Cervix. *Diagn Cytopathol* 12: 120-125, 1995.

Keyhani-Rofagha S, Vesey-Shecket M: Diagnostic Value, Feasibility, and Validity of Preparing Cell Blocks from Fluid-Based Gynecologic Cytology Specimens. *Cancer* 96: 204-209, 2002.

Khanna M, Brooks SE, Chen TT, et al: Human Papillomavirus Absence Predicts Normal Cervical Histopathologic Findings With Abnormal Papanicolaou Smears: A Study of a University-Based Inner City Population. *J Human Virol* 4: 283-287, 2001.

Khunamornpong S, Siraunkgul S, Suprasert P: Well-Differentiated Villoglandular Adenocarcinoma of the Uterine Cervix: Cytomorphologic Observation of Five Cases. *Diagn Cytopathol* 26: 10-14, 2002.

Kierkegaard O, Byrjalsen C, Frandsen KH, et al: Diagnostic Accuracy of Cytology and Colposcopy in Cervical Squamous Intraepithelial Lesions. *Acta Obstet Gynecol Scand* 73: 648-651, 1994.

Kieswetter C, Hernandez E, Anderson L, et al: Evaluation of a Cervical Cytology Device (Cell-Sweep) Based on Comparison to Colposcopic Findings. *J Natl Med Assoc* 93: 436-439, 2001.

Kiguchi K, Bibbo M, Hasegawa T, et al: Dysplasia During Pregnancy: A Cytologic Follow-Up Study. *J Reprod Med* 26: 66-72, 1981.

Killackey MA, Hakes TB, Pierce VK: Endometrial Adenocarcinoma in Breast Cancer Patients Receiving Antiestrogens. *Cancer Treat Rep* 69: 237-238, 1985.

Killough BV, Clark AH, Garvin J: Correlation Between Cytodiagnosis and the Presence of Endocervical or Squamous Metaplastic Cells in Gynecologic Smears (Abstract). *Acta Cytol* 32: 758, 1988.

Kim H-S, Underwood D: Adenocarcinoma in the Cervicovaginal Papanicolaou Smear: Analysis of a 12 Year Experience. *Diagn Cytopathol* 7: 119-124, 1991.

Kim JJ, Wright TC, Goldie SJ: Cost-Effectiveness of Alternative Triage Strategies for Atypical Squamous Cells of Undetermined Significance. *JAMA* 287: 2382-2390, 2002.

Kim TJ, Kim HS, Park CT, et al: Clinical Evaluation of Follow-Up Methods and Results of Atypical Glandular Cells of Undetermined Significance (AGUS) Detected on Cervicovaginal Pap Smears. *Gynecol Oncol* 73: 292-298, 1999.

Kim Y, Ha HJ, Kim JS, et al: Significance of Cytologic Smears in the Diagnosis of Small Cell Carcinoma of the Uterine Cervix. *Acta Cytol* 46: 637-644, 2002.

Kimura J, Okamoto H, Yamamoto H, et al: Cytologic Features of Atypical Polypoid Adenomyoma of the Endometrium: A Case Report. *Acta Cytol* 47: 287-292, 2003.

King JAC, Elkhalifa MY, Michael C: Malignant Lymphoma Identified on a Cervical Cytologic Smear, With Immunophenotypic Analysis (Letter). *Acta Cytol* 41: 1228-1230, 1997.

Kinlen LJ, Spriggs AI: Women With Positive Cervical Smears but Without Surgical Intervention: A Follow-Up Study. *Lancet* (ii): 463-465, 1978.

Kinney W, Sung HY, Kearney KA, et al: Missed Opportunities for Cervical Cancer Screening of HMO Members Developing Invasive Cervical Cancer (ICC). *Gynecol Oncol* 71: 428-430, 1998a.

Kinney W, Manos MM, Hurley LB, et al: Where's the High-Grade Cervical Neoplasia? The Importance of Minimally Abnormal Papanicolaou Diagnoses. *Obstet Gynecol* 91: 973-976, 1998b.

Kinney W, Miller M, Sung H-Y, et al: Risk of Invasive Squamous Carcinoma of the Cervix Associated With Screening Intervals of 1, 2, and 3 Years: A Case-Control Study (Abstract). *Obstet Gynecol* 97(Suppl 4): 3S, 2001.

Kinney W, Sawaya GF, Sung H-Y, et al: Stage at Diagnosis and Mortality in Patients With Adenocarcinoma and Adenosquamous Carcinoma of the Uterine Cervix Diagnosed as a Consequence of Cytologic Screening. *Acta Cytol* 47: 167-171, 2003.

Kirkland N, Hardy N: Psammoma Bodies Found in Cervicovaginal Smears: A Case Report. *Acta Cytol* 23: 131-133, 1979.

Kirkup W, Singer A: Colposcopy in the Management of the Pregnant Patient With Abnormal Cervical Cytology. *Br J Obstet Gynaecol* 87: 322-325, 1980.

Kitay DZ, Wentz WB: Cervical Cytology in Folic Acid Deficiency of Pregnancy. *Am J Obstet Gynecol* 104: 931-938, 1969.

Kittrich M: Zytodiagnostik des Fruchtwasserablfusses mit Hilfe von Niblau. *Geburshilfe Frauenheilkd* 23: 156-163, 1963.

Kiviat NB, Paavonen JA, Brockway J, et al: Cytologic Manifestations of Cervical and Vaginal Infections. I. Epithelial and Inflammatory Cellular Changes. *JAMA* 253: 989-996, 1985a.

Kiviat NB, Peterson M, Kinney-Thomas E, et al: Cytologic Manifestations of Cervical and Vaginal Infections. II. Confirmation of *Chlamydia trachomatius* Infection by Direct Immunofluorescence Using Monoclonal Antibodies. *JAMA* 253: 997-1000, 1985b.

Kiviat NB: Natural History of Cervical Neoplasia: Overview and Update. *Am J Obstet Gynecol* 175: 1099-1104, 1996.

Kiviat NB, Koutsky LA, Paavonen JA, et al: Prevalence of Genital Papillomavirus Infection Among Women Attending a College Student Health Clinic or a Sexually Transmitted Disease Clinic. *J Infect Dis* 159: 293-302, 1989.

Kiviat NB, Critchlow CW, Kurman RJ: Reassessment of the Morphological Continuum of Cervical Intraepithelial Lesions: Does It Reflect Different Stages in the Progression to Cervical Carcinoma? In: Muñoz N, Bosch FX, Shah KV, et al, eds. *The Epidemiology of Cervical Cancer and Human Papillomavirus.* Vol 3. International Agency for Research on Cancer, Lyon, 59-66, 1992a.

Kiviat NB, Koutsky LA, Critchlow MS: Prevalence and Cytologic Manifestations of Human Papillomavirus (HPV) Types 6, 11, 16, 18, 31, 33, 35, 42, 43, 44, 45, 51, 52, and 56 Among 500 Consecutive Women. *Int J Gynecol Pathol* 11: 197-203, 1992b.

Kivlahan C, Ingram E: Papanicolaou Smears Without Endocervical Cells: Are They Inadequate? *Acta Cytol* 30: 258-260, 1986.

Kiyono T, Foster SA, Koop JK: Both Rb/p16^{INK4a} Inactivation and Telomerase Activity Are Required to Immortalize Human Epithelial Cells (Letter). *Nature* 396: 84-88, 1998.

Kjær SK, de Villiers E-M, Haugaard BJ, et al: Human Papillomavirus, Herpes Simplex Virus and Cervical Cancer Incidence in Greenland and Denmark. A Population-Based Cross-Sectional Study. *Int J Cancer* 41: 518-524, 1988.

Kjær SK, Teisen C, Haugaard BJ, et al: Risk Factors for Cervical Cancer in Greenland and Denmark: A Population-Based Cross-Sectional Study. *Int J Cancer* 44: 40-47, 1989.

Kjær SK, Engholm G, Teisen C, et al: Risk Factors for Cervical Human Papillomavirus and Herpes Simplex Virus Infections in Greenland and Denmark: A Population-Based Study. *Am J Epidemiol* 131: 669-682, 1990.

Kjær SK, de Villiers EM, Dahl C, et al: Case-Control Study of Risk Factors for Cervical Neoplasia in Denmark. I: Role of the "Male Factor" in Women With One Lifetime Sexual Partner. *Int J Cancer* 48: 39-44, 1991.

Kjær SK Dahl C, Engholm G, et al: Case-Control Study of Risk Factors for Cervical Neoplasia in Denmark. II. Role of Sexual Activity, Reproductive Factors, and Venereal Infections. *Cancer Causes Control* 3: 339-348, 1992.

Kjær SK, Brinton LA: Adenocarcinomas of the Uterine Cervix: The Epidemiology of an Increasing Problem. *Epidemiol Rev* 15: 486-498, 1993a.

Kjær SK, Engholm G, Dahl C, et al: Case-Control Study of Risk Factors for Cervical Squamous Cell Neoplasia in Denmark. III. Role of Oral Contraceptive Use. *Cancer Causes Control* 4: 513-519, 1993b.

Kjær SK, Engholm G, Dahl C, et al: Case-Control Study of Risk Factors for Cervical Squamous Cell Neoplasia in Denmark. IV: Role of Smoking Habits. *Eur J Cancer Prev* 5: 359-365, 1996a.

Kjær SK, van den Brule AJC, Bock JE, et al: Human Papillomavirus—The Most Significant Risk Determinant of Cervical Intraepithelial Neoplasia. *Int J Cancer* 65: 601-606, 1996b.

Kjær SK, van den Brule AJC, Bock JE, et al: Determinants for Genital Human Papillomavirus (HPV) Infection in 1000 Randomly Chosen Young Danish Women With Normal Pap Smear: Are There Different Risk Profiles for Oncogenic and Nononcogenic HPV Types? *Cancer Epidemiol Biomarkers Prev* 6: 799-805, 1997.

Kjær SK: Risk Factors for Cervical Neoplasia in Denmark. *APMIS* 60(Suppl 80): 1-41, 1998.

Kjær SK, Chackerian B, van den Brule AJ, et al: High-Risk Human Papillomavirus Is Sexually Transmitted: Evidence from a Follow-up Study of Virgins Starting Sexual Activity (Intercourse). *Cancer Epidemiol Biomarkers Prev* 10: 101-106, 2001.

Kjellberg L, Wang Z, Wiklund F, et al: Sexual Behaviour and Papillomavirus Exposure in Cervical Intraepithelial Neoplasia: A Population-Based Case-Control Study. *J Gen Virology* 80: 391-398, 1999.

Kjellberg L, Hallmans G, Ahren AM, et al: Smoking, Diet, Pregnancy and Oral Contraceptive Use as Risk Factors for Cervical Intra-Epithelial Neoplasia in Relation to Human Papillomavirus Infection. *Br J Cancer* 82: 1332-1338, 2000.

Klaes R, Ridder R, Schaefer U, et al: No Evidence of p53 Allel-Specific Predisposition in Human Papillomavirus-Associated Cervical Cancer. *J Mol Med* 77: 299-302, 1999.

Klaes R, Friedrich T, Spitkovsky D, et al: Overexpression of p16^{INK4a} as a Specific Marker for Dyplastic and Neoplastic Epithelial Cells of the Cervix Uteri. *Int J Cancer* 92: 276-284, 2001.

Klam S, Arseneau J, Mansour N, et al: Comparison of Endocervical Curettage and Endocervical Brushing. *Obstet Gynecol* 96: 90-94, 2000.

Klaus H: Quantitative Criteria of Folate Deficiency in Cervico-Vaginal Cytograms, With Report of a New Parameter. *Acta Cytol* 15: 50-53, 1971.

Klebanoff SJ, Hillier SL, Eschenbach DA, et al: Control of the Microbial Flora of the Vagina by H_2O_2-Generating Lactobacilli. *J Infect Dis* 164: 94-100, 1991.

Klimov E, Vinokourova S, Moisjak E, et al: Human Papilloma Viruses and Cervical Tumours: Mapping of Integration Sites and Analysis of Adjacent Cellular Sequences. *BMC Cancer* 2: 24, 2002. [http://www.biomedcentral.com/1471-2407/2/24]

Kline MJ, Davey DD: Atypical Squamous Cells of Undetermined Significance Qualified: A Follow-Up Study. *Diagn Cytopathol* 14: 380-384, 1996.

Kline TJ: Cytopathology: Negligence and a Lawyer's Opinion (Editorial). *Diagn Cytopathol* 11: 219, 1994.

Kline TS, Holland M, Wemple D: Atypical Cytology With Contraceptive Hormone Medication. *Am J Clin Pathol* 53: 215-222, 1970.

Kline TS: The Papanicolaou Smear: A Brief Historical Perspective and Where We Are Today. *Arch Pathol Lab Med* 121: 205-209, 1997.

Kling TG, Buchsbaum HJ: Cervical Carcinoma in Women Under Twenty-One Years of Age. *Obstet Gynecol* 42: 205-207, 1973.

Klingelhutz AJ, Foster SA, McDougall JK: Telomerase Activation by the E6 Gene Product of Human Papillomavirus Type 16. *Nature* 380: 79-82, 1996.

Klinkhamer PJJM, Vooijs GP, de Haan AFJ: Intraobserver and Interobserver Variability in the Diagnosis of Epithelial Abnormalities in Cervical Smears. *Acta Cytol* 32: 794-800, 1988.

Klinkhamer PJJM, Vooijs GP, de Haan AFJ: Intraobserver and Interobserver Variability in the Quality Assessment of Cervical Smears. *Acta Cytol* 33: 215-218, 1989.

Klinkhamer PJJM, Meerding WJ, Rosier PFWM, et al: Liquid-Based Cervical Cytology: A Review of the Literature With Methods of Evidence-Based Medicine. *Cancer (Cancer Cytopathol)* 99: 263-271, 2003.

Knapp VJ: How Old Is Endometriosis? Late 17th- and 18th-Century European Descriptions of the Disease. *Fertility Sterility* 72: 10-14, 1999.

Knight R van D: Superficial Noninvasive Intraepithelial Tumors of the Cervix. *Am J Obstet Gynecol* 46: 333-349, 1943.

Knudsen UB, Uldbjerg N, Rechberger T, et al: Eosinophils in Human Cervical Ripening. *Eur J Obstet Gynecol Reprod Biol* 72: 165-168, 1997.

Kobayashi TK, Yuasa M, Fujimoto T, et al: Cytologic Findings in Postpartum and Postabortal Smears. *Acta Cytol* 24: 328-334, 1980.

Kobayashi TK, Fujimoto T, Okamoto H, et al: Cytologic Evaluation of Atypical Cells in Cervicovaginal Smears from Women With Tubal Pregnancies. *Acta Cytol* 27: 28-32, 1983a.

Kobayashi TK, Fujimoto T, Okamoto H, et al: Association of Mast Cells With Vaginal Trichomoniasis in Endocervical Smears. *Acta Cytol* 27: 133-137, 1983b.

Kobayashi TK, Ueda M, Araki H, et al: Immunocytochemical Demonstration of Chlamydia Infection in the Urogenital Tracts. *Diagn Cytopathol* 3: 303-306, 1987.

Kobayashi TK, Okamoto H: Arias-Stella Changes in Cervicovaginal Specimens (Letter). *Cytopathology* 8: 289-290, 1997.

Kobayashi TK, Okamoto H: Cytopathology of Pregnancy-Induced Cell Patterns in Cervicovaginal Smears. *Am J Clin Pathol (Pathology Patterns Reviews)* 114: S6-S20, 2000.

Kobayashi TK, Ueda M, Nishino T, et al: Cellular Changes Following Uterine Artery Embolization for the Treatment of Adenomyosis (Letter). *Cytopathology* 12: 270-272, 2001.

Kobayashi TK, Ueda M, Nishino T, et al: Cytology of High-Grade Squamous Intraepithelial Lesion in Japanese-Brazilian Women With HIV Infection With Polymerase Chain Reaction-Assisted Human Papilloma Virus Detection. *Diagn Cytopathol* 26: 268-271, 2002.

Kobayashi-Kawata T, Harami K: Tuberculous Cervicitis. *Acta Cytol* 22: 193-194, 1978.

Kobelin MH, Kobelin CG, Burke L, et al: Incidence and Predictors of Cervical Dysplasia in Patients With Minimally Abnormal Papanicolaou Smears. *Obstet Gynecol* 92: 356-359, 1998.

Kobold-Wolterbeck AC, Beyer-Boon ME: Ciliocytophthoria in Cervical Cytology (Letter). *Acta Cytol* 19: 89-91, 1975.

Koch CA, Azumi N, Furlong MA, et al: Carcinoid Syndrome Caused by an Atypical Carcinoid of the Uterine Cervix. *J Clin Endocrinol Metab* 84: 4209-4213, 1999.

Kohan S, Beckman EM, Bigelow B, et al: The Role of Colposcopy in the Management of Cervical Intraepithelial Neoplasia During Pregnancy and Postpartum. *J Reprod Med* 25: 279-284, 1980.

Kohan S, Noumoff J, Beckman EM, et al: Colposcopic Screening of Women With Atypical Papanicolaou Smears. *J Reprod Med* 30: 383-387, 1985.

Koike N, Higuchi T, Sakai Y: Goblet-Like Cells in Atrophic Vaginal Smears and Their Histologic Correlation: Possible Confusion With Endocervical Cells. *Acta Cytol* 34: 785-788, 1990.

Koike N, Kobayashi TK: Appearance of Goblet Cells in Atrophic Vaginal Smears. *Diagn Cytopathol* 9: 475-476, 1993.

Koike N, Kasamatsu T: Efficacy of the Cytobrush Method in Aged Patients. *Diagn Cytopathol* 10: 311-314, 1994.

Koizumi JH: Nipplelike Protrusions in Endocervical and Other Cells: Further Observations. *Acta Cytol* 40: 519-528, 1996.

Kok MR, Boon ME, Schreiner-Kok PG, et al: Cytological Recognition of Invasive Squamous Cancer of the Uterine Cervix: Comparison of Conventional Light-Microscopical Screening and Neural Network-Based Screening. *Hum Pathol* 31: 23-28, 2000.

Kokawa K, Shikone T, Otani T, et al: Apoptosis and the Expression of Bax and Bcl-2 in Squamous Cell Carcinoma and Adenocarcinoma of the Uterine Cervix. *Cancer* 85: 1799-1809, 1999.

Kokelj F, Baraggino E, Stinco G, et al: Study of the Partners of Women With Human Papillovirus Infection. *Int J Dermatol* 32: 661-663, 1993.

Kolstad P: Follow-up Study of 232 Patients With Stage Ia1 and 411 Patients With Stage Ia2 Squamous Cell Carcinoma of the Cervix (Microinvasive Carcinoma). *Gynecol Oncol* 33: 265-272, 1989.

Komaki R, Cox JD, Hansen PM, et al: Malignant Lymphoma of the Uterine Cervix. *Cancer* 54: 1699-1704, 1984.

Konikov NF, Kempson RL, Piskie V: Cytohistologic Correlation in Dysplasia, Carcinoma In Situ, and Invasive Carcinoma of the Uterine Cervix. *Am J Clin Pathol* 51: 463-469, 1969.

Konishi I, FujiiS, Nanbu Y, et al: Mucin Leakage Into the Cervical Stroma May Increase Lymph Node Metastasis in Mucin-Producing Cervical Adenocarcinomas. *Cancer* 65: 229-237, 1990.

Konishi I, Fujii S, Nonogaki H, et al: Immunohistochemical Analysis of Estrogen Receptors, Progesterone Receptors, Ki-67 Antigen, and Human Papillomavirus DNA in Normal and Neoplastic Epithelium of the Uterine Cervix. *Cancer* 68: 1340-1350, 1991.

Koonings PP, Price JH: Evaluation of Atypical Glandular Cells of Undetermined Significance: Is Age Important? *Am J Obstet Gynecol* 184: 1457-1461, 2001.

Koprowska I: Early Use of the Vaginal Smear for Cervical Cancer Detection (Letter). *Acta Cytol* 25: 202, 1981.

Koprowska I: Concurrent Discoveries of the Value of Vaginal Smears for Diagnosis of Uterine Cancer. *Diagn Cytopathol* 1: 245-248, 1985.

Korhonen A-M, Issakainen J, Ekfors T, et al: Summer Spores of Birch Rust Fungus in Papanicolaou Smears from Healthy Mass Screening Participants. *Acta Cytol* 45: 679-682, 2001.

Korhonen MO: Adenocarcinoma of the Uterine Cervix: An Evaluation of the Available Diagnostic Methods. *Acta Pathol Microbiol Scand* Suppl 264: 1-59, 1978.

Korhonen MO: Epidemiological Differences Between Adenocarcinoma and Squamous Cell Carcinoma of the Uterine Cervix. *Gynecol Oncol* 10: 312-317, 1980.

Korn AP, Autry M, DeRemer PA, et al: Sensitivity of the Papanicolaou Smear in Human Immunodeficiency Virus-Infected Women. *Obstet Gynecol* 83: 401-404, 1994.

Korn AP, Judson PL, Zaloudek CJ: Importance of Atypical Glandular Cells of Uncertain Significance in Cervical Cytologic Smears. *J Reprod Med* 43: 774-778, 1998.

Korn AP: Gynecologic Care of Women Infected With HIV. *Clin Obstet Gynecol* 44: 226-242, 2001.

Koss LG, Durfee GR: Unusual Patterns of Squamous Epithelium of the Uterine Cervix: Cytologic and Pathologic Study of Koilocytotic Atypia. *Ann NY Acad Sci* 63: 1245-1261, 1956.

Koss LG, Wolknska WH: *Trichomonas vaginalis* Cervicitis and Its Relationship to Cervical Cancer: A Histocytological Study. *Cancer* 12: 1171-1193, 1959.

Koss LG, Melamed MR, Daniel WW: In Situ Epidermoid Carcinoma of the Cervix and Vagina Following Radiotherapy for Cervical Cancer. *Cancer* 14: 353-360, 1961.

Koss LG, Durfee GR: Cytologic Diagnosis of Endometrial Carcinoma: Result of Ten Years of Experience. *Acta Cytol* 6: 519-531, 1962.

Koss LG, Stewart FW, Foote FW, et al: Some Histological Aspects of Behavior of Epidermoid Carcinoma In Situ and Related Lesions of the Uterine Cervix: A Long-Term Prospective Study. *Cancer* 16: 1160-1211, 1963.

Koss LG, Melamed MR, Mayer K: The Effect of Busulfan on Human Epithelia. *Am J Clin Pathol* 44: 385-397, 1965.

Koss LG, Hicklin MD: Standards of Adequacy of Cytologic Examination of the Female Genital Tract: Conclusions of Study Group on Cytology. *Obstet Gynecol* 43: 792-793, 1974.

Koss LG: A Quarter of a Century of Cytology. *Acta Cytol* 21: 639-642, 1977.

Koss LG: Dysplasia: A Real Concept or a Misnomer? *Obstet Gynecol* 57: 374-379, 1978.

Koss LG: The Attack on the Annual 'Pap Smear' (Editorial). *Acta Cytol* 24: 181-183, 1980.

Koss LG, Schreiber K, Oberlander SG, et al: Screening of Asymptomatic Women for Endometrial Cancer. *Obstet Gynecol* 57: 681-691, 1981.

Koss LG, Schreiber K, Oberlander SG, et al: Detection of Endometrial Carcinoma and Hyperplasia in Asymptomatic Women. *Obstet Gynecol* 64: 1-11, 1984.

Koss LG: Current Concepts of Intraepithelial Neoplasia in the Uterine Cervix (CIN). *Appl Pathol* 5: 7-18, 1987a.

Koss LG: Cytologic and Histologic Manifestations of Human Papillomavirus Infection of the Female Genital Tract and Their Clinical Significance. *Cancer* 60: 1942-1950, 1987b.

Koss LG: The Papanicolaou Test for Cervical Cancer Detection: A Triumph and a Tragedy. *JAMA* 261: 737-743, 1989a.

Koss LG: Cytology. Accuracy of Diagnosis. *Cancer* 64 (Suppl 1): 249-252; discussion 253-257, 1989b.

Koss LG: The New Bethesda System for Reporting Results of Smears of the Uterine Cervix. *J Natl Cancer Inst* 82: 988-991, 1990.

Koss LG: Cervical (Pap) Smear: New Directions. *Cancer* 71: 1406-1412, 1993a.

Koss LG: Diagnostic Accuracy in Cervicovaginal Cytology. *Arch Pathol Lab Med* 117: 1240-1242, 1993b.

Koss LG, Lin E, Schreiber K, et al: Evaluation of the PAPNET™ Cytologic Screening System for Quality Control of Cervical Smears. *Am J Clin Pathol* 101: 220-229, 1994.

Koss LG: Traditional [sic] Cell Metaplasia of the Cervix: A Misnomer (Letter). *Am J Surg Pathol* 22: 774-776, 1998a.

Koss LG: Transitional Cell Metaplasia (Letter). *Adv Anat Pathol* 5: 202-203, 1998b.

Koss LG: Correspondence re: Sherman ME, Tabbara SO, Scott DR, Kurman RJ, Glass AG, Manos MM, et al "ASCUS, Rule Out HSIL": Cytologic Features, Histologic Correlates, and Human Papillomavirus Detection (Letter). *Mod Pathol* 12: 335-342, 1999.

Koss LG: Correspondence re: Sherman ME, Tabbara SO, Scott DR, Kurman RJ, Glass AG, Mano MM, et al: "ASCUS, Rule Out HSIL": Cytologic Features, Histologic Correlates, and Human Papillomavirus Detection. [*Mod Pathol* 12: 335-342, 1999]. *Mod Pathol* 13: 208-209, 2000a.

Koss LG: Evolution in Cervical Pathology and Cytology: A Historical Perspective. *Eur J Gynaecol Oncol* 21: 550-554, 2000b.

Koss LG: George Papanicolaou (1883-1962) (Letter). *Cytopathology* 11: 355-356, 2000c.

Koss LG: Correspondence re Tasca L, Östör AG, Babes' V: History of Gynecologic Pathology. XII, Aurel Babes'. *Int J Gynecol Pathol* 22: 101-102, 2002.

Kotaska AJ, Matisic JP: Cervical Cleaning Improves Pap Smear Quality. *CMAJ* 169: 666-669, 2003.

Kottmeier HL: Evolution et Traitment des Epitheliomas. *Rev Fr Gynecol Obstet* 56: 821-826, 1961.

Koutsky L, Galloway DA, Holmes KK: Epidemiology of Genital Human Papillomavirus Infection. *Epidemiol Rev* 10: 122-163, 1988.

Koutsky L, Holmes KK, Critchlow CW, et al: A Cohort Study of the Risk of Cervical Intraepithelial Neoplasia Grade 2 or 3 in Relation to Papillomavirus Infection. *N Engl J Med* 327: 1272-1278, 1992a.

Koutsky L, Stevens CE, Holmes KK, et al: Underdiagnosis of Genital Herpes by Current Clinical and Viral-Isolation Procedures. *N Engl J Med* 326: 1533-1539, 1992b.

Koutsky L: Epidemiology of Genital Human Papillomavirus Infection. *Am J Med* 102 (5A): 3-8, 1997.

Koutsky L, Ault KA, Wheeler CM, et al: A Controlled Trial of a Human Papillomavirus Type 16 Vaccine. *N Engl J Med* 347: 1645-1651, 2002.

Kovi J, Tillman L, Lee SM: Malignant Transformation of *Condyloma acuminatum*. A Light Microscopic and Ultrastructural Study. *Am J Clin Pathol* 61: 702-710, 1974.

Krain LS, Rosenthal L, Newcomer VD: Pemphigus Vulgaris Involving the Cervix Associated With Endometrial Carcinoma of the Uterus: A Case Report With Immunofluorescent Findings. *Int J Dermatol* 12: 220-228, 1973.

Krane JF, Granter SR, Trask CE, et al: Papanicolaou Smear Sensitivity for the Detection of Adenocarcinoma of the Cervix: A Study of 49 Cases. *Cancer (Cancer Cytopathol)* 93: 8-15, 2001.

Krane JF, Lee KR, Sun D, et al: Atypical Glandular Cells of Undetermined Significance: Outcome Predictions Based on Human Papillomavirus Testing. *Am J Clin Pathol* 121: 87-92, 2004.

Krantz KE, Atkinson JP: Pediatric and Adolescent Gynecology. Part I. Fundamental Considerations: Gross Anatomy. *Ann NY Acad Sci* : 551-575, 1967.

Kraus FT, Perezmesa C: Verrucous Carcinoma: Clinical and Pathologic Study of 105 Cases Involving Oral Cavity, Larynx and Genitalia. *Cancer* 19: 26-38, 1966.

Kraus H, Schuhmann R, Ganal M, et al: Cyologic Findings in Vaginal Smears from Patients Under Treatment With Cyclophosphamide. *Acta Cytol* 21: 726-730, 1977.

Kraus H, Schuhmann R: Cytologic Presentation of Recurrent Carcinoma of the Uterine Cervix and Corpus After Radiotherapy. *Acta Cytol* 23: 114-118, 1979.

Krcmar M, Suchánková A, Kanka J, et al: Prospective Study on the Relationship Between Cervical Neoplasia and Herpes Simplex Type 2 Virus. III. Presence of Herpes Simplex Type 2 Antibody in Sera of Subjects Who Developed Cervical Neoplasia Later in the Study. *Int J Cancer* 38: 161-165, 1986.

Krebs H-B, Schneider V, Hurt WG, et al: Genital Condylomas in Immunosuppressed Women: A Therapeutic Challenge. *South Med J* 79: 183-187, 1986.

Krebs H-B, Helmkamp BF: Does the Treatment of Genital Condylomata in Men Decrease the Treatment Failure Rate of Cervical Dysplasia in the Female Sexual Partner? *Obstet Gynecol* 76: 660-663, 1990.

Krebs H-B, Helmkamp BF: Treatment Failure of Genital Condylomata Acuminata in Women: Role of the Male Sexual Partner. *Am J Obstet Gynecol* 165: 337-340, 1991.

Kreider JW, Howett MK, Stoler MH, et al: Susceptibility of Various Human Tissues to Transformation In Vivo With Human Papillomavirus Type 11. *Int J Cancer* 39: 459-465, 1987.

Kremer H, Ulm R: Zur Problemtik des primären Tubencrcinomas. *Archiv Gynäk* 185: 609-623, 1955.

Krieger JN: Urologic Aspects of Trichomoniasis. *Invest Urol* 18: 411-417, 1981.

Krieger JN: Diagnosis of Trichomoniasis: Comparison of Conventional Wet-Mount Examination With Cytologic Studies, Cultures, and Monoclonal Antibody Staining of Direct Specimens. *JAMA* 259: 1223-1227, 1988.

Krieger P, Naryshkin S: Random Rescreening of Cytologic Smears: A Practical and Effective Component of Quality Assurance in Both Large and Small Cytology Laboratories (Editorial). *Acta Cytol* 38: 291-298, 1994.

Krishnamoorthy A, De Sai M, Simanowitz M: Primary Malignant Melanoma of the Cervix: Case Report. *Br J Obstet Gynaecol* 93: 84-86, 1986.

Kristensen GB, Jensen LK, Ejersbo D, et al: The Efficiency of the Cytobrush and Cotton Swab in Obtaining Endocervical Cells in Smears Taken After Conization of the Cervix. *Arch Gynecol Obstet* 246: 207-210, 1989a.

Kristensen GB, Holund B, Grinsted P: Efficacy of the Cytobrush Versus the Cotton Swab in the Collection of Endocervical Cells. *Acta Cytol* 33: 849-851, 1989b.

Kristensen GB, Skyggebjerg K-D, Holund B, et al: Analysis of Cervical Smears Obtained Within Three Years of the Diagnosis of Invasive Cervical Cancer. *Acta Cytol* 35: 47-50, 1991.

Krivak TC, Retherford B, Voskuil S, et al: Recurrent Invasive Adenocarcinoma After Hysterectomy for Cervical Adenocarcinoma In Situ. *Gynecol Oncol* 77: 334-335, 2000.

Krivak TC, McBroom JW, Sundborg M, et al: Large Cell Neuroendocrine Cervical Carcinoma: A Report of Two Cases and Review of the Literature. *Gynecol Oncol* 82: 187-191, 2001.

Krüger-Kjær S, van den Brule AJC, Svare EI, et al: Different Risk Factor Patterns for High-Grade and Low-Grade Intraepithelial Lesions on the Cervix Among HPV-Positive and HPV-Negative Young Women. *Int J Cancer* 76: 613-619, 1998.

Krul EJ, Schipper RE, Schreuder GM, et al: HLA and Susceptibility to Cervical Neoplasia. *Hum Immunol* 60: 337-342, 1999.

Krumerman MS, Chung A: Solitary Reticulum Cell Sarcoma of the Uterine Cervix With Initial Cytodiagnosis. *Acta Cytol* 22: 46-50, 1978.

Krumins I, Young Q, Pacey F, et al: The Cytologic Diagnosis of Adenocarcinoma In Situ of the Cervix Uteri. *Acta Cytol* 21: 320-329, 1977.

Kuberski T: *Trichomonas vaginalis* Associated With Nongonococcal Urethritis and Prostatitis. *Sex Transm Dis* 7: 135-136, 1980.

Kudo R, Sagae S, Hayakawa O, et al: The Cytological Features and DNA Content of Cervical Adenocarcinoma. *Diagn Cytopathol* 3: 191-197, 1987.

Kudo R, Sagae S, Hayakawa O, et al: Morphology of Adenocarcinoma In Situ and Microinvasive Adenocarcinoma of the Uterine Cervix: A Cytologic and Ultrastructural Study. *Acta Cytol* 35: 109-116, 1991.

Kudo R: Cervical Adenocarcinoma. *Curr Topics Pathol* 85: 81-111, 1992.

Kuebler DL, Nikrui N, Bell DA: Cytologic Features of Endometrial Papillary Serous Carcinoma. *Acta Cytol* 33: 120-126, 1989.

Kühler-Obbarius C, Milde-Langosch K, Löning T, et al: Polymerase Chain Reaction-Assisted Evaluation of Low and High-Grade Squamous Intraepithelial Lesion Cytology and Reappraisal of the Bethesda System. *Acta Cytol* 38: 681-686, 1994a.

Kühler-Obbarius C, Milde-Langosch K, Helling-Giese G, et al: Polymerase Chain Reaction-Assisted Papillomavirus Detection in Cervicovaginal Smears: Stratification by Clinical Risk and Cytology Reports. *Virchows Archiv (Path Anat)* 425: 157-163, 1994b.

Kuhn L, Sun X-W, Wright TC: Human Immunodeficiency Virus Infection and Female Lower Genital Tract Malignancy. *Curr Opin Obstet Gynecol* 11: 35-39, 1999.

Kulasingam SL, Hughes JP, Kiviat NB, et al: Evaluation of Human Papillomavirus Testing in Primary Screening for Cervical Abnormalities: Comparson of Sensitivity, Specificity, and Frequency of Referral. *JAMA* 288: 1749-1757, 2002.

Kumar NB, Hart WR: Metastases to the Uterine Corpus from Extragenital Cancer: A Clinicopathologic Study of 63 Cases. *Cancer* 50: 2163-2169, 1982.

Kumar PV, Bedayat GR, Mousavi A, et al: *Vorticella* in Pap Smears as a Contaminant (Letter). *Acta Cytol* 45: 655-656, 2001.

Kumar V, Abbas AK, Fausto N, eds: *Robbins and Cotran Pathologic Basis of Disease*, 7th ed, Elsevier Saunders, Philadelphia, PA, 2005.

Kuo CC, Wang SP, Grayston JT, et al: TRIC Type K, a New Immunologic Type of *Chlamydia trachomatis*. *J Immunol* 113: 591-596, 1974.

Kurian K, Al-Nafussi A: Relation of Cervical Glandular Intraepithelial Neoplasia to Microinvasive and Invasive Adenocarcinoma of the Uterine Cervix: A Study of 121 Cases. *J Clin Pathol* 52: 112-117, 1999.

Kurita T, Cunha GR: Roles of p63 in Differentiation of Müllerian Duct Epithelial Cells. *Ann NY Acad Sci* 948: 9-12, 2001.

Kurman RJ, Scully RE: The Incidence and Histogenesis of Vaginal Adenosis. An Autopsy Study. *Hum Pathol* 5: 265-276, 1974.

Kurman RJ, Shah KH, Lancaster WD, et al: Immunoperoxidase Localization of Papillomavirus Antigens in Cervical Dysplasia and Vulvar Condylomas. *Am J Obstet Gynecol* 140: 931-935, 1981.

Kurman RJ, Jenson AB, Lancaster WD: Papillomavirus Infection of the Cervix. II: Relationship to Intraepithelial Neoplasia Based on the Presence of Specific Viral Structural Proteins. *Am J Surg Pathol* 7: 39-52, 1983.

Kurman RJ, Kaminski PF, Norris HJ: The Behavior of Endometrial Hyperplasia: A Long-Term Study of "Untreated Hyperplasia" in 170 Patients. *Cancer* 56: 403-412, 1985.

Kurman RJ, Schiffman MH, Lancaster WD, et al: Analysis of Individual Human Papillomavirus Types in Cervical Neoplasia: A Possible Role for Type 18 in Rapid Progression. *Am J Obstet Gynecol* 159: 293-296, 1988.

Kurman RJ, Malkasian GD, Sedlis A, et al: Clinical Commentary: From Papanicolaou to Bethesda: The Rationale for a New Cervical Cytologic Classification. *Obstet Gynecol* 77: 779-782, 1991.

Kurman RJ, Norris HJ, Wilkinson EJ: *Tumors of the Cervix, Vagina, and Vulva.* (Atlas of Tumor Pathology, 3rd Ser. Fasc 4), Armed Forces Institute of Pathology, Washington DC, 1-255, 1992.

Kurman RJ, Henson DE, Herbst AL, et al: Interim Guidelines for Management of Abnormal Cervical Cytology. *JAMA* 271: 1866-1869, 1994.

Kurtycz D, Nuñez M, Arts T, et al: Use of Fluorescent In Situ Hybridization to Detect Aneupoloidy in Cervical Dysplasia. *Diagn Cytopathol* 15: 46-51, 1996.

Kurtycz DF, Hoerl HD: Thin-Layer Technology: Tempered Enthusiasm. *Diagn Cytopathol* 23: 1-5, 2000.

Kusuyama Y, Yoshida M, Imai H, et al: Secretory Carcinoma of the Endometrium. *Acta Cytol* 33: 127-130, 1989.

Kutteh WH, Hatch KD: Case Report: Primary Vaginal Tuberculosis After Vaginal Carcinoma. *Gynecol Oncol* 44: 113-115, 1992.

Kyle RA, Shampo MA: [Philatelic Vignette] *JAMA* 238: 1636, 1977.

Kyo S, Inoe M, Koyama M, et al: Detection of High-Risk Human Papillomavirus in the Cervix and Semen of Sex Partners. *J Infect Dis* 170: 682-685, 1994.

Kyriakos M, Kempson RL, Perez CA: Carcinoma of the Cervix in Young Women. I. Invasive Carcinoma. *Obstet Gynecol* 38: 930-944, 1971.

L

Läärä E, Day NE, Hakama M: Trends in Mortality from Cervical Cancer in the Nordic Countries: Association With Organised Screening Programmes. *Lancet* (i): 1247-1249, 1987.

Lacey JV Jr, Brinton LA, Abbas FM, et al: Oral Contraceptives as Risk Factors for Cervical Adenocarcinomas and Squamous Cell Carcinomas. *Cancer Epidemiol Biomarkers Prev* 8: 1079-1085, 1999.

Lacey JV Jr, Brinton LA, Barnes WA, et al: Use of Hormone Replacement Therapy and Adenocarcinomas and Squamous Cell Carcinomas of the Uterine Cervix. *Gynecol Oncol* 77: 149-154, 2000.

Lacey JV Jr, Swanson CA, Brinton LA, et al: Obesity as a Potential Risk Factor for Adenocarcinomas and Squamous Cell Carcinomas of the Uterine Cervix. *Cancer* 98: 814-821, 2003.

Lachman MF, Cavallo-Calvanese C: Qualification of Atypical Squamous Cells of Undetermined Significance in an Independent Laboratory: Is It Useful or Significant? *Am J Obstet Gynecol* 179: 421-429, 1998.

Lambourne A, Lederer H: Effects of Observer Variation in Population Screening for Cervical Carcinoma. *J Clin Pathol* 26: 564-569, 1973.

Lambropoulos AF, Agorastos T, Foka ZJ, et al: Methylenetetrahydrofolate Reductase Polymorphism C677T Is Not Associated to the Risk of Cervical Dysplasia. *Cancer Letters* 191: 187-191, 2003.

Lammens L, Fenton D: Abnormal Glandular Smear: First Evidence of Ovarian Malignancy (Case Report). *J Obstet Gynaecol* 22: 702, 2002.

Lancaster WD, Castellano C, Santos C, et al: Human Papillomavirus Deoxyribonucleic Acid in Cervical Carcinoma from Primary and Metastatic Sites. *Am J Obstet Gynecol* 154: 115-119, 1986.

Lane DP: Cancer: p53, Guardian of the Genome. *Nature* 358: 15-16, 1992.

Lane V, Lawler J: Pap Smear Brochures, Misogyny and Language: A Discourse Analysis and Feminist Critique. *Nurs Inquiry* 4: 262-267, 1997.

Lang G, Dallenbach-Hellweg G: The Histogenetic Origin of Cervical Mesonephric Hyperplasia and Mesonephric Adenocarcinoma of the Uterine Cervix Studied With Immunohistochemical Methods. *Int J Gynecol Pathol* 9: 145-157, 1990.

Langlois NEI, Miller ID, Mann EMF: Adenoid Basal Carcinoma of the Cervix: An Unusual Cytological Appearance. *Cytopathology* 6: 104-109, 1995.

LaPolla JP, O'Neill C, Wetrich D: Colposcopic Management of Abnormal Cervical Cytology in Pregnancy. *J Reprod Med* 33: 301-306, 1988.

Lara-Torre E, Pinkerton JS: Accuracy of Detection of *Trichomonas vaginalis* Organisms on a Liquid-Based Papanicolaou Smear. *Am J Obstet Gynecol* 188: 354-356, 2003.

Larsen B, Galask RP: Vaginal Microbial Flora: Practical and Theoretic Relevance. *Obstet Gynecol* 55(Suppl 5): S100-113S, 1980.

Larsen B, Galask RP: Vaginal Microbal Flora: Composition and Influences of Host Physiology. *Ann Intern Med* 96: 926-930, 1982a.

Larsen B, Goplerud CP, Petzold CR, et al: Effect of Estrogen Treatment on the Genital Tract Flora of Postmenopausal Women. *Obstet Gynecol* 60: 20-24, 1982b.

Larson AA, Kern S, Curtiss S, et al: High Resolution Analysis of Chromosome 3p Alterations in Cervical Carcinoma. *Cancer Res* 57: 4082-4090, 1997a.

Larson AA, Liao S-Y, Stanbridge EJ, et al: Genetic Alterations Accumulate During Cervical Tumorigenesis and Indicate a Common Origin for Multifocal Lesions. *Cancer Res* 57: 4171-4176, 1997b.

Larson DM, Johnson KK, Reyes CN, et al: Prognostic Significance of Malignant Cervical Cytology in Patients With Endometrial Cancer. *Obstet Gynecol* 84: 399-403, 1994.

Larson NS: Invasive Cervical Cancer Rising in Young White Females. *J Natl Cancer Inst* 86: 6-7, 1994.

Larsson E, Schooley JL: Positive Vaginal Cytology in Primary Carcinoma of the Fallopian Tubes. *Am J Obstet Gynecol* 72: 1364-1366, 1956.

Larsson G, Alm P, Gullberg B, et al: Prognostic Factors in Early Invasive Carcinoma of the Uterine Cervix: A Clinical, Histopathologic, and Statistical Analysis of 343 Cases. *Am J Obstet Gynecol* 146: 145-153, 1983.

Laskey PW, Meigs JW, Flannery JT: Uterine Cervical Carcinoma in Connecticut, 1935-1973: Evidence for Two Classes of Invasive Disease. *J Natl Cancer Inst* 57: 1037-1043, 1979.

Lassise DL, Savitz DA, Hamman RF, et al: Invasive Cervical Cancer and Intrauterine Device Use. *Int J Epidemiol* 20: 865-870, 1991.

Lauchlan SC, Penner DW: Simultaneous Adenocarcinoma In Situ and Epidermoid Carcinoma In Situ: Report of Two Cases. *Cancer* 20: 2250-2254, 1967.

Lauer E, Helming C, Kandler O: Heterogeneity of the Species *Lactobacillus acidophilus* (Moro) Hansen and Mocquot as Revealed by Biochemical Characteristics and DNA-DNA Hybridization. *Zentbl Bakt Microbiol Hyg* Abt I Orig C1: 150-168, 1980.

LaVecchia C, Franceschi S, DeCarli A, et al: Invasive Cervical Cancer in Young Women. *Br J Obstet Gynaecol* 91: 1149-1155, 1984a.

LaVecchia C, Franceschi S, DeCarli A, et al: Dietary Vitamin A and the Risk of Invasive Cervical Cancer. *Int J Cancer* 34: 319-322, 1984b.

LaVecchia C, Franceschi S, DeCarli A, et al: Cigarette Smoking and the Risk of Cervical Neoplasia. *Am J Epidemiol* 123: 22-29, 1986a.

LaVecchia C, Franceschi S, DeCarli A, et al: Sexual Factors, Venereal Diseases, and the Risk of Intraepithelial and Invasive Cervical Neoplasia. *Cancer* 58: 935-941, 1986b.

LaVecchia C, Decali A, Fasoli M, et al: Oral Contraceptives and Cancers of the Breast and of the Female Genital Tract: Interim Results from a Case-Control Study. *Br J Cancer* 54: 311-317, 1986c.

LaVecchia C, DeCarli A, Gallus G: Epidemiological Data on Cervical Carcinoma Relevant to Cytopathology. *Appl Pathol* 5: 25-32, 1987.

LaVecchia C, Altieri A, Franceschi S, et al: Oral Contraceptives and Cancer: An Update. *Drug Safety* 24: 741-754, 2001.

Laverty CR, Russell P, Black J: Adenovirus Infection of the Cervix. *Acta Cytol* 21: 114-117, 1977.

Laverty CR, Russell P, Hills E, et al: The Significance of Noncondylomatous Wart Virus Infection of the Cervical Transformation Zone: A Review With Discussion of Two Illustrative Cases. *Acta Cytol* 22: 195-201, 1978.

Laverty CR, Farnsworth A, Thurloe JK, et al: The Reliability of a Cytological Prediction of Cervical Adenocarcinoma In Situ. *Aust NZ J Obstet Gynaecol* 28: 307-312, 1988.

Laverty CR, Farnsworth A, Thurloe JK, et al: The Importance of the Cell Sample in Cervical Cytology: A Controlled Trial of a New Sampling Device. *Med J Aust* 150: 432-436, 1989.

Law KS, Chang TC, Hsueh S, et al: High Prevalence of High-Grade Squamous Intraepithelial Lesions and Microinvasive Carcinoma in Women With a Cytologic Diagnosis of Low-Grade Squamous Intraepithelial Lesions. *J Reprod Med* 46: 61-64, 2001.

Lawing LF, Hedges SR, Schwebke JR: Detection of Trichomonosis in Vaginal and Urine Specimens from Women by Culture and PCR. *J Clin Microbiol* 38: 3585-3588, 2000.

Lawley TB, Lee RB, Kapela R: The Significance of Moderate and Severe Inflammation on Class I Papanicolaou Smear. *Obstet Gynecol* 76: 997-999, 1990.

Lawrence WD: Advances in the Pathology of the Uterine Cervix. Current Concepts in Cervical Pathology. *Hum Pathol* 22: 792-806, 1991.

Lawson HW, Lee NC, Thames SF, et al: Cervical Cancer Screening Among Low-Income Women: Results of a National Screening Program, 1991-1995. *Obstet Gynecol* 92: 745-752, 1998.

Lazo PA: The Molecular Genetics of Cervical Carcinoma. *Br J Cancer* 80: 2008-2018, 1999.

Learmonth GM, Murray MM: Helminths and Protozoa as an Incidental Finding in Cytology Specimens. *Cytopathology* 1: 163-170, 1990.

Leary J, Jaworski R, Houghton R: In-Situ Hybridization Using Biotinylated DNA Probes to Human Papillomavirus in Adenocarcinoma-In-Situ and Endocervical Glandular Dysplasia of the Uterine Cervix. *Pathology* 23: 85-89, 1991.

Lederer H, Lambourne A: The Results of Screening by Cervical Cytology and of Histological Examination of Gynaecological Operation Specimens. *J Obstet Gynaecol Br Commonw* 80: 67-71, 1973.

Lee K-J, Lee J-K, Saw H-S: Can Human Papillomavirus DNA Testing Substitute for Cytology in the Detection of High-Grade Cervical Lesions? *Arch Pathol Lab Med* 128: 298-302, 2004.

Lee KR, Ayer B: False-Positive Diagnosis of Adenocarcinoma In Situ of the Cervix. *Acta Cytol* 32: 276-277, 1988.

Lee KR, Trainer TD: Adenocarcinoma of the Uterine Cervix of Small Intestinal Type Containing Numerous Paneth Cells. *Arch Pathol Lab Med* 114: 731-733, 1990.

Lee KR, Manna EA, Jones MA: Comparative Cytologic Features of Adenocarcinoma In Situ of the Uterine Cervix. *Acta Cytol* 35: 117-126, 1991.

Lee KR: Atypical Glandular Cells in Cervical Smears from Women Who Have Undergone Cone Biopsy: A Potential Diagnostic Pitfall. *Acta Cytol* 37: 705-709, 1993a.

Lee KR, Howard P, Heintz NH, Collins CC: Low Prevalence of Human Papillomavirus Types 16 and 18 in Cervical Adenocarcinoma In Situ, Invasive Adenocarcinoma, and Glandular Dysplasia by Polymerase Chain Reaction. *Mod Pathol* 6: 433-437, 1993b.

Lee KR, Manna EA, St. John T: Atypical Endocervical Glandular Cells: Accuracy of Cytologic Diagnosis. *Diagn Cytopathol* 13: 202-208, 1995.

Lee KR, Minter LJ, Crum, CP: Koilocytotic Atypia in Papanicolaou Smears: Reproducibility and Biopsy Correlations. *Cancer* 81: 10-15, 1997a.

Lee KR, Minter LJ, Granter SR: Papanicolaou Smear Sensitivity for Adenocarcinoma In Situ of the Cervix: A Study of 34 Cases. *Am J Clin Pathol* 107: 30-35, 1997b.

Lee KR, Genest DR, Minter LJ, et al: Adenocarcinoma In Situ in Cervical Smears With a Small Cell (Endometrioid) Pattern: Distinction from Cells Directly Sampled from the Upper Endocervical Canal or Lower Segment of the Endometrium. *Am J Clin Pathol* 109: 738-742, 1998.

Lee, KR: Adenocarcinoma In Situ With a Small Cell (Endometrioid) Pattern in Cervical Smears. *Cancer (Cancer Cytopathol)* 87: 254-258, 1999.

Lee KR, Flynn CE: Early Invasive Adenocarcinoma of the Cervix: A Histopathologic Analysis of 40 Cases With Observations Concerning Histogenesis. *Cancer* 89: 1048-1055, 2000a.

Lee KR, Sun D, Crum CP: Endocervical Intraepithelial Glandular Atypia (Dysplasia): A Histopathologic, Human Papillomavirus, and MIB-1 Analysis of 25 Cases. *Hum Pathol* 31: 656-664, 2000b.

Lee KR, Darragh TM, Joste NE, et al: Atypical Glandular Cells of Undetermined Significance (AGUS): Interobserver Reproducibility in Cervical Smears and Corresponding Thin-Layer Preparations. *Am J Clin Pathol* 117: 96-102, 2002.

Lee KR: Symposium Part 4: Should Pathologists Diagnose Endocervical Preneoplastic "Less Than" Adenocarcinoma In Situ?: Counterpoint. *Int J Gynecol Pathol* 22: 22-24, 2003.

Lee SJ, Rollason TP: Argyrophilic Cells in Cervical Intraepithelial Glandular Neoplasia. *Int J Gynecol Pathol* 13: 131-132, 1994.

Lee WY: Exfoliative Cytology of Large Cell Neuroendocrine Carcinoma of the Uterine Cervix. *Acta Cytol* 46: 1176-1179, 2002.

Lee Y-C, Holcomb K, Buhl A, et al: Rapid Progression of Primary Vaginal Squamous Cell Carcinoma in a Young HIV-Infected Woman. *Gynecol Oncol* 78: 380-382, 2000.

Leeson SC, Inglis TCM, Salman WD: A Study to Determine the Underlying Reason for Abnormal Glandular Cytology and the Formulation of a Management Protocol. *Cytopathology* 8: 20-26, 1997.

Lehmann F: Zur Frage der diagnostischen Verwertbarkeit des Scheidenabstriches, ein Beitrag zum Mikrobismus der Scheide. *Zentrabl f. Gyn* 45:647-656, 1921.

Lehmann M, Groh A, Rödel J, et al: Detection of *Chlamydia trachomatis* DNA in Cervical Samples With Regard to Infection by Human Papillomavirus. *J Infect* 38: 12-17, 1999.

Lehn H, Krieg P, Sauer G: Papillomavirus Genomes in Human Cervical Tumors: Analysis of Their Transcriptional Activity. *Proc Natl Acad Sci (USA)* 82: 5540-5544, 1985.

Lehn H, Villa LL, Marziona F, et al: Physical State and Biological Activity of Human Papillomavirus Genomes in Precancerous Lesions of the Female Genital Tract. *J Gen Virol* 69: 187-196, 1988.

Leiman G, Markowitz S, Margolius KA: Cytologic Detection of Cervical Granuloma Inguinale. *Diagn Cytopathol* 2: 138-143, 1986.

Lellé RJ, Heidenreich W, Schneider J: Cytologic Findings After Construction of a Neovagina Using Two Surgical Procedures. *Surg Gynecol Obstet* 170: 21-24, 1990.

Leman MH Jr, Benson WL, Kurman RJ, et al: Microinvasive Carcinoma of the Cervix. *Obstet Gynecol* 48: 571-578, 1976.

Leminen A, Paavonen J, Forss M, et al: Adenocarcinoma of the Uterine Cervix. *Cancer* 65: 53-59, 1990.

Leminen A, Paavonen J, Vesterinen E, et al: Human Papillomavirus Types 16 and 18 in Adenocarcinoma of the Uterine Cervix. *Am J Clin Pathol* 95: 647-652, 1991.

Lemoine NR, Hall PA: Epithelial Tumors Metastatic to the Uterine Cervix: A Study of 33 Cases and Review of the Literature. *Cancer* 57: 2002-2005, 1986.

Lencioni LJ, Martinez Amezaga LA, Lo Bianco VS: Urocytogram and Pregnancy. I. Methods and Normal Values. *Acta Cytol* 13: 279-287, 1969.

Lesack D, Wahab I, Gilks CB: Radiation-Induced Atypia of Endocervical Epithelium: A Histological, Immunohistochemical and Cytometric Study. *Int J Gynecol Pathol* 15: 242-247, 1996.

Leslie KO, Silverberg SG: Microglandular Hyperplasia of the Cervix: Unusual Clinical and Pathological Presentations and Their Differential Diagnosis. *Prog Surg Pathol* 5: 95-114, 1984.

Leung K-M, Chan W-Y, Hui P-K: Invasive Squamous Cell Carcinoma and Cervical Intraepithelial Neoplasia III of the Uterine Cervix. Morphologic Differences Other Than Stromal Invasion. *Am J Clin Pathol* 101: 508-513, 1994.

Leuschner I, Harms D, Mattke A, et al: Rhabdomyosarcoma of the Urinary Bladder and Vagina: A Clinicopathologic Study With Emphasis on Recurrent Disease—A Report From the Kiel Pediatric Tumour Registry and the German CWS Study. *Am J Surg Pathol* 25: 856-864, 2001.

Levi AW, Kelly DP, Rosenthal DL, et al: Atypical Squamous Cells of Undetermined Significance in Liquid-Based Cytologic Specimens: Results of Reflex Human Papillomavirus Testing and Histologic Follow-Up in Routine Practice With Comparison of Interpretive and Probabilistic Reporting Methods. *Cancer (Cancer Cytopathol)* 99: 191-197, 2003.

Levin ML, Kress LC, Goldstein H: Syphilis and Cancer: Reported Syphilis Prevalence Among 7,761 Cancer Patients. *NY State J Med* 42: 1737-1745, 1942.

Levine AJ, Harper J, Hilborne L, et al: HPV DNA and the Risk of Squamous Intraepithelial Lesions of the Uterine Cervix in Young Women. *Am J Clin Pathol* 100: 6-11, 1993.

Levine BB, Siraganian RP, Schenkein I: Allergy to Human Seminal Plasma. *N Engl J Med* 288: 894-896, 1973.

Levine L, Lucci JA III, Van Dinh T: Atypical Glandular Cells: New Bethesda Terminology and Management Guidelines. *Obstet Gynecol Surv* 58: 399-406, 2003.

Levine PH, Waisman J, Mittal K: Significance of the Cytologic Diagnosis of Endocervical Glandular Involvement in High-Grade Squamous Intraepithelial Lesions. *Diagn Cytopathol* 26: 217-221, 2002.

Levine PH, Elgert PA, Mittal K: False-Positive Squamous Cell Carcinoma in Cervical Smears: Cytologic-Histologic Correlation in 19 Cases. *Diagn Cytopathol* 28: 23-27, 2003.

Ley C, Bauer HM, Reingold A, et al: Determinants of Genital Human Papillomavirus Infection in Young Women. *J Natl Cancer Inst* 83: 997-1003, 1991.

Li H-q, Jin S-q, Xu H-x, et al: The Decline in the Mortality Rates of Cervical Cancer and a Plausible Explanation in Shandong, China. *Int J Epidemiol* 29: 398-404, 2000a.

Li H-q, Thomas DB and WHO (Collaborative Study of Neoplasia and Steroid Contraceptives): Tubal Ligation and Risk of Cervical Cancer. *Contraception* 61: 323-328, 2000b.

Li J-Y, Li FP, Blot WJ, et al: Correlation Between Cancers of the Uterine Cervix and Penis in China. *J Natl Cancer Inst* 69: 1063-1065, 1982.

Li S, Boudousquie AC, Baloch ZW, et al: Aluminum Silicate-Containing Psammoma Bodies in a Cervicovaginal Smear (Pap): Cytological, Ultrastructural, and Radiographic Microprobe Studies. *Diagn Cytopathol* 21: 122-124, 1999.

Liaw KL, Glass AG, Manos MM, et al: Detection of Human Papillomavirus DNA in Cytologically Normal Women and Subsequent Cervical Squamous Intraepithelial Lesions. *J Natl Cancer Inst* 91: 954-960, 1999.

Libcke JH: The Cytology of Cervical Pemphigus. *Acta Cytol* 14:42-44, 1970.

Licciardone JC, Wilkins JR III, Brownson RC, et al: Cigarette Smoking and Alcohol Consumption in the Aetiology of Uterine Cervical Cancer. *Int J Epidemiol* 18: 533-537, 1989.

Lickrish GM, Colgan TJ, Wright VC: Colposcopy of Adenocarcinoma In Situ and Invasive Adenocarcinoma of the Cervix. *Obstet Gynecol Clin North Am* 20: 111-122, 1993.

Limaye A, Connor AJ, Huang X, et al: Comparative Analysis of Conventional Papanicolaou Tests and a Fluid-Based Thin-Layer Method. *Arch Pathol Lab Med* 127: 200-204, 2003; erratum appears in *Arch Pathol Lab Med* 127: 923, 2003.

Lin C-T, Tseng C-J, Lai C-H, et al: High-Risk HPV DNA Detection by Hybrid Capture II: An Adjunctive Test for Mildly Abnormal Cytologic Smears in Women ? 50 Years of Age. *J Reprod Med* 45: 345-350, 2000.

Lin TJ, So-Bosita JL: Pitfalls in the Interpretation of Estrogenic Effect in Postmenopausal Women. *Am J Obstet Gynecol* 114: 929-931, 1972.

Lin WM, Ashfaq R, Michaelopulos EA, et al: Molecular Papanicolaou Tests in the Twenty-First Century: Molecular Analyses With Fluid-Based Papanicolaou Technology. *Am J Obstet Gynecol* 183: 39-45, 2000.

Lindheim SR, Smith-Nguyen G: Aggressive Evaluation for Atypical Squamous Cells in Papanicolaou Smears. *J Reprod Med* 35: 971-973, 1990.

Lindner JG, Plantema FH, Hoogkamp-Korstanje JA: Quantitative Studies of the Vaginal Flora of Healthy Women and of Obstetric and Gynaecological Patients. *J Med Microbiol* 11: 233-241, 1978.

Lindner LE, Geerling S, Nettum JA, et al: The Cytologic Features of Chlamydial Cervicitis. *Acta Cytol* 29: 676-682, 1985.

Lindner LE, Geerling S, Nettum JA, et al: Identification of Chlamydia in Cervical Smears by Immunofluorescence: Technic, Sensitivity, and Specificity. *Am J Clin Pathol* 85: 180-185, 1986.

Lindner LE, Nettum JA: The Diagnosis of Chlamydial Infection in a Cytology Laboratory: Ten Months' Experience Using Immunofluorescence With and Without Previous Cytologic Prediction. *Diagn Cytopathol* 4: 19-22, 1988.

Lininger RA, Ashfaq R, Albores-Saavedra J, et al: Transitional Cell Carcinoma of the Endometrium and Endometrial Carcinoma With Transitional Cell Differentiation. *Cancer* 79: 1933-1943, 1997.

Lininger RA, Wistuba I, Gazdar A, et al: Human Papillomavirus Type 16 Is Detected in Transitional Cell Carcinomas and Squamotransitional Cell Carcinomas of the Cervix and Endometrium. *Cancer* 83: 521-527, 1998.

Lippes J: Pelvic Actinomycosis: A Review and Preliminary Look at Prevalence. *Am J Obstet Gynecol* 180: 265-269, 1999.

Littell JT: Further Discussion on the Role of Pap Smear Screening (Letter). *Am Fam Physician* 62: 2232, 2000.

Little JB: Cellular Effects of Ionizing Radiation. *N Engl J Med* 278: 308-315, 1968.

Littman P, Clement PB, Henriksen B, et al: Glassy Cell Carcinoma of the Cervix. *Cancer* 37: 2238-2246, 1976.

Liu K, Marshall J, Shaw HS, et al: Effects of Chemotherapy and Tamoxifen on Cervical and Vaginal Smears in Bone Marrow Transplant Recipients. *Acta Cytol* 43: 1027-1033, 1999.

Liu S, Semenciw R, Probert A, et al: Cervical Cancer in Canada: Changing Patterns in Incidence and Mortality. *Int J Gynecol Cancer* 11: 24-31, 2001.

Liu T, Soong SJ, Wilson NP, et al: A Case Control Study of Nutritional Factors and Cervical Dysplasia. *Cancer Epidemiol Biomarkers Prev* 2: 525-530, 1993.

Liu W, Barrow MJ, Spitler MF, et al: Normal Exfoliation of Endometrial Cells in Premenopausal Women. *Acta Cytol* 7: 211-214, 1963.

Liu W: Positive Smears in Previously Screened Patients (Certain Cytologic Findings of Public Health Importance). *Acta Cytol* 11: 193-198, 1967a.

Liu W, Koebel L, Shipp J, et al: Cytologic Changes Following the Use of Oral Contraceptives. *Obstet Gynecol* 30: 228-232, 1967b.

Liu W: Hypoestrogenism and Endometrial Carcinoma. *Acta Cytol* 14: 583-585, 1970.

LiVolsi VA, Merino MJ, Schwartz PE: Coexistent Endocervical Adenocarcinoma and Mucinous Adenocarcinoma of Ovary: A Clinicopathologic Study of Four Cases. *Int J Gynecol Pathol* 1: 391-402, 1983.

LiVolsi VA: Cytologic Screening Intervals (Letter). *Am J Obstet Gynecol* 148: 833, 1984.

Lizano M, Berumen J, Guido MC, et al: Association Between Human Papillomavirus Type 18 Variants and Histopathology of Cervical Cancer. *J Natl Cancer Inst* 89: 1227-1231, 1997.

Llewellyn H: Observer Variation, Dysplasia Grading, and HPV Typing: A Review. *Am J Clin Pathol (Pathology Patterns Reviews)* 114: S21-S35, 2000.

Lobo TT, Feijo G, Carvalho SE, et al: A Comparative Evaluation of the Papanicolaou Test for the Diagnosis of Trichomoniasis. *Sex Transm Dis* 30: 694-699, 2003.

Lohe KJ: Early Squamous Cell Carcinoma of the Uterine Cervix. I. Definition and Histology. *Gynecol Oncol* 6: 10-30, 1978a.

Lohe KJ, Burghardt E, Hillemanns HG, et al: Early Squamous Cell Carcinoma of the Uterine Cervix. II. Clinical Results of a Cooperative Study in the Management of 419 Patients With Early Stromal Invasion and Microcarcinoma. *Gynecol Oncol* 6: 31-50, 1978b.

Lohe, KJ: Early Squamous Cell Carcinoma of the Uterine Cervix. III. Frequency of Lymph Node Metastases. *Gynecol Oncol* 6: 51-59, 1978c.

Lombard I, Vincent-Salomon A, Validire P, et al: Human Papillomavirus Genotype as a Major Determinant of the Course of Cervical Cancer. *J Clin Oncol* 16: 2613-2619, 1998.

Long ME, Doko F, Taylor HC Jr: Nucleoli and Nucleolar Ribonucleic Acid in Nonmalignant and Malignant Human Endometria. *Am J Obstet Gynecol* 75: 1002-1014, 1958.

Long SR, Cohen MB: Classics in Cytology. IV. Traut and the "Pap Smear." *Acta Cytol* 35: 140-142, 1991.

Longfield JC, Grimshaw RN, Monaghan JM: Simultaneous Sampling of the Endocervix and Ectocervix Using the Profile Brush. *Acta Cytol* 37: 472-476, 1993.

Lonky NM, Sadeghi M, Tsadik GW, et al: The Clinical Significance of the Poor Correlation of Cervical Dysplasia and Cervical Malignancy With Referral Cytologic Results. *Am J Obstet Gynecol* 181: 560-568, 1999.

Lonsdale RN, Gibbs S: Pemphigus Vulgaris With Involvement of the Cervix. *Br J Dermatol* 138: 363-365, 1998.

López-Rios F, San Miguel P, Bellas C, et al: Lymphoepithelioma-Like carcinoma of the Uterine Cervix. *Arch Pathol Lab Med* 124: 746-747, 2000.

Lörincz AT, Temple GF, Patterson JA, et al: Correlation of Cellular Atypia and Human Papillomavirus Deoxyribonucleic Acid Sequences in Exfoliated Cells of the Uterine Cervix. *Obstet Gynecol* 68: 508-512, 1986.

Lörincz AT, Temple GF, Kurman RJ, et al: Oncogenic Association of Specific Human Papillomavirus Types With Cervical Neoplasia. *J Natl Cancer Inst* 79: 671-677, 1987a.

Lörincz AT, Quinn AP, Lancaster WD, et al: A New Type of Papillomavirus Associated With Cancer of the Uterine Cervix. *Virology* 159: 187-190, 1987b.

Lörincz AT, Reid R, Jenson AB et al: Human Papillomavirus Infection of the Cervix: Relative Risk Associations of 15 Common Anogenital Types. Obstet Gynecol 79: 328-337, 1992.

Lörincz AT, Castle PE, Sherman ME: Viral Load of Human Papillomavirus and Risk of CIN3 or Cervical Cancer (Research Letter). *Lancet* 360: 228-229, 2002.

Lörincz AT, Richart RM: Human Papillomavirus DNA Testing as an Adjunct to Cytology in Cervical Screening Programs. *Arch Pathol Lab Med* 127: 959-968, 2003.

Lossick JG: The Diagnosis of Vaginal Trichomoniasis (Editorial). *JAMA* 259: 1230, 1988.

Lossick JG, Kent HL: Trichomoniasis: Trends in Diagnosis and Management. *Am J Obstet Gynecol* 165: 1217-1222, 1991.

Louro AP, Roberson J, Eltoum I, et al: Atypical Squamous Cells, Cannot Exclude High-Grade Squamous Intraepithelial Lesion: A Follow-Up Study of Conventional and Liquid-Based Preparations in a High-Risk Population. *Am J Clin Pathol* 120: 392-397, 2003.

Lousuebsakul V, Knutsen SMF, Gram IT, et al: Clinical Impact of Atypical Squamous Cells of Undetermined Significance: A Cytohistologic Comparison. *Acta Cytol* 44: 23-30, 2000.

Lousuebsakul V, Knutsen SM, Singh PN, et al: Variables Associated With Squamous Intraepithelial Lesions Among Women With a Cytologic Diagnosis of Atypical Squamous Cells of Undetermined Significance. *Anal Quant Cytol Histol* 23: 355-361, 2001.

Love RR, Kurtyca DF, Dumesic DA, et al: The Effect of Tamoxifen on the Vaginal Epithelium in Postmenopausal Women. *J Womens Health Gender-Based Med* 9: 559-563, 2000.

Lowe MP, Ault KA, Sood AK: Recurrent Carcinoma In Situ of a Neovagina. *Gynecol Oncol* 80: 403-404, 2001.

Lowry S, Harte R, Atkinson R: Cervical Cancer Deaths in Young Women (Letter). *Lancet* (i): 784, 1989.

Lowy DR, Schiller JT: Papillomaviruses: Prophylactic Vaccine Prospects. *Biochim Biophys Acta* 1423: M1-M8, 1998.

Lozowski MS, Mishriki Y, Talebian F, et al: The Combined Use of Cytology and Colposcopy in Enhancing Diagnostic Accuracy in Preclinical Lesions of the Uterine Cervix. *Acta Cytol* 26: 285-291, 1982.

Lozowski MS, Mishriki Y, Solitare GB: Factors Determining the Degree of Endometrial Exfoliation and Their Diagnostic Implications in Endometrial Adenocarcinoma. *Acta Cytol* 30: 623-627, 1986.

Lu DW, Pirog EC, Zhu X, et al: Prevalence and Typing of HPV DNA in Atypical Squamous Cells in Pregnant Women. *Acta Cytol* 47: 1008-1016, 2003.

Luboshitzky R, Shen-Orr Z, Herer P: Seminal Plasma Melatonin and Gonadal Steroids Concentrations in Normal Men. *Arch Androl* 48: 225-232, 2002.

Lucas WE, Benirschke K, Lebherz TB: Verrucous Carcinoma of the Female Genital Tract. *Am J Obstet Gynecol* 119: 435-440, 1974.

Luesley D, Blomfield P, Dunn J, et al: Cigarette Smoking and Histological Outcome in Women With Mildly Dyskaryotic Cervical Smears. *Br J Obstet Gynecol* 101: 49-52, 1994.

Luesley DM, Jordan JA, Woodman CBJ, et al: A Retrospective Review of Adenocarcinoma-In-Situ and Glandular Atypia of the Uterine Cervix. *Br J Obstet Gynaecol* 94: 699-703, 1987.

Luff RD, Gupta PK, Spence MR, et al: Pelvic Actinomycosis and the Intrauterine Contraceptive Device: A Cyto-Histomorphologic Study. *Am J Clin Pathol* 69: 581-586, 1978.

Lund CJ: An Epitaph for Cervical Carcinoma. *JAMA* 175: 98-99, 1961.

Lundberg GD: Quality Assurance in Cervical Cytology: The Papanicolaou Smear. *JAMA* 262: 1672-1679, 1989.

Lundeen SJ, Horzitz CA, Larson CJ, et al: Abnormal Cervicovaginal Smears Due to Endometriosis: A Continuing Problem. *Diagn Cytopathol* 26: 35-40, 2002.

Lundvall L: Comparison Between Abnormal Cytology, Colposcopy and Histopathology During Pregnancy. *Acta Obstet Gynecol Scand* 68: 447-452, 1989.

Lungu O, Sun XW, Felix J, et al: Relationship of Human Papillomavirus Type to Grade of Cervical Intraepithelial Neoplasia. *JAMA* 267: 2493-2496, 1992.

Luthy DA, Briggs RM, Buyco A, et al: Cervical Cytology. Increased Sensitivity With a Second Cervical Smear. *Obstet Gynecol* 51: 713-717, 1978.

Lutzner MA: The Human Papillomaviruses: A Review. *Arch Dermatol* 119: 631-635, 1983.

Luzzatto R, Brucker N: Benign Inclusion Cysts of the Ovary Associated With Psammoma Bodies in Vaginal Smears. *Acta Cytol* 25: 282-284, 1981.

Luzzatto R, Sisson G, Luzzatto L, et al: Psammoma Bodies and Cells from In Situ Fallopian Tube Carcinoma in Endometrial Smears: A Case Report. *Acta Cytol* 40: 295-298, 1996.

Luzzatto R, Poli M, Recktenvald M, et al: Human Papillomavirus Infection in Atrophic Smears: A Case Report. *Acta Cytol* 44: 420-422, 2000.

Lyall H, Duncan ID: Inaccuracy of Cytologic Diagnosis of High-Grade Squamous Intraepithelial Lesions (CIN 3). *Acta Cytol* 39: 50-54, 1995.

Lynch HT, Casey MJ, Shaw TG, et al: Hereditary Factors in Gynecologic Cancer. *Oncologist* 3: 319-338, 1998.

Lyon JL, Gardner JW, West DW, et al: Smoking and Carcinoma In Situ of the Uterine Cervix. *Am J Public Health* 73: 558-562, 1983.

M

Maccato M, Kaufman RH: Herpes Genitalis. *Dermatol Clin* 10: 415-422, 1992.

Macgregor JE: Evaluation of Mass Screening Programmes for Cervical Cancer in N.E. Scotland. *Tumori* 62: 287-295, 1976.

Macgregor JE, Teper S: Uterine Cervical Cytology and Young Women. *Lancet* (i): 1029-1031, 1978a.

Macgregor JE, Teper S: Mortality from Carcinoma of Cervix Uteri in Britain *Lancet* (ii): 774-776, 1978b.

Macgregor JE: Rapid Onset Cancer of the Cervix (Editorial). *Br Med J* 284: 441-442, 1982.

Macgregor JE: False Negative Cervical Smears. *Br J Obstet and Gynaecol* 100: 801-802, 1993.

Macgregor JE, Campbell MK, Mann EM, et al: Screening for Cervical Intraepithelial Neoplasia in North East Scotland Shows Fall in Incidence and Mortality from Invasive Cancer with Concomitant Rise in Preinvasive Disease. *Br Med J* 308: 1407-1411, 1994.

Mackay B, Osborne BM, Wharton JT: Small Cell Tumor of Cervix With Neuroepithelial Features: Ultrastructural Observations in Two Cases. *Cancer* 43: 1138-1145, 1979.

MacLean KS: Tubal Malignancy: A Method for Collecting Specimens for Cytologic Study. *Science* 114: 181, 1951.

MacMahon B: Risk Factors for Endometrial Cancer. *Gynecol Oncol* 2: 122-129, 1974.

Maddux HR, Varia MA, Spann CO, et al: Invasive Carcinoma of the Uterine Cervix in Women Age 25 or Less. *Int J Radiat Oncol Biol Physics* 19: 701-706, 1990.

Madeleine MM, Daling JR, Schwartz SM, et al: Human Papillomavirus and Long-Term Oral Contraceptive Use Increase the Risk of Adenocarcinoma In Situ of the Cervix. *Cancer Epidemiol Biomarkers Prev* 10: 171-177, 2001.

Madeleine MM, Cushing-Haugen KL, Daling JR, et al: Human Leukocyte Antigen Class II and Cervical Cancer Risk: A Population-Based Study. *J Infect Dis* 186: 1565-1574, 2002.

Maeda MYS, Filho AL, Shih LWS, et al: *Chlamydia trachomatis* in Cervical Uterine Irradiated Cancer Patients. *Diagn Cytopathol* 6: 86-88, 1990.

Maeda MYS, Di Loreto C, Shirata NK, et al: Image Analysis of Nuclear/Cytoplasmic Ratio in Cervical Smears to Discriminate Three Grades of Cervical Intraepithelial Neoplasia. *Acta Cytol* 41: 744-748, 1997.

Magnusson PKE, Sparen P, Gyllensten UB: Genetic Link to Cervical Tumours (Letter). *Nature* 400: 29-30, 1999.

Magnusson PKE, Gyllensten UB: Cervical Cancer Risk: Is There a Genetic Component? *Mol Med Today* 6: 145-148, 2000.

Maguire NC: Current Use of the Papanicolaou Class System in Gynecologic Cytology. *Diagn Cytopathol* 4: 169-176, 1988.

Maher CF, Haran MV, McLaughlin J: Abnormal Cervical Cytology Leading to the Diagnosis of a Primary Serous Adenocarcinoma of the Peritoneuum. *Aust NZ J Obstet Gynecol* 36: 100-101, 1996.

Maier RC, Norris HJ: Coexistence of Cervical Intraepithelial Neoplasia With Primary Adenocarcinoma of the Endocervix. *Obstet Gynecol* 56: 361-364, 1980.

Maiman M, Fruchter RG, Serur E, et al: Human Immunodeficiency Virus Infection and Cervical Neoplasia. *Gynecol Oncol* 38: 377-382, 1990.

Maiman M, Tarricone N, Vieira J, et al: Colposcopic Evaluation of Human Immunodeficiency Virus-Seropositive Women. *Obstet Gynecol* 78: 84-88, 1991.

Maiman M, Fruchter RG, Sedlis A, et al: Prevalence, Risk Factors, and Accuracy of Cytologic Screening for Cervical Intraepithelial Neoplasia in Women With the Human Immundeficiency Virus. *Gynecol Oncol* 68: 233-239, 1998.

Mainguené C, Clément N, Gabriel S: Urogenital *Schistosomiasis*: An Unusual Discovery on Cervical Smears from a Caucasian Female. *Acta Cytol* 42: 1045-1046, 1998.

Makino H, Sato S, Yajima A, et al: Evaluation of the Effectiveness of Cervical Cancer Screening: A Case-Control Study in Miyagi, Japan. *Tohoku J Exp Med* 175: 171-178, 1995.

Maksem JA: Ciliated Cell Adenocarcinoma of the Endometrium Diagnosed by Endometrial Brush Cytology and Confirmed by Hysterectomy: A Case Report Detailing a Highly Efficient Cytology Collection and Processing Technique. *Diagn Cytopathol* 16: 78-82, 1997.

Maksem JA: Performance Characteristics of the Indiana University Medical Center Endometrial Sampler (Tao Brush) in an Outpatient Office Setting, First Year's Outcomes: Recognizing Histological Patterns in Cytology Preparations of Endometrial Brushings. *Diagn Cytopathol* 22: 186-195, 2000.

Malamou-Mitsi VD, Agnantis NJ, Pappa LS, et al: Uterine Cervical Involvement in a Patient With Wegener's Granulomatosis (Letter). *Am J Med* 109: 74-75, 2000.

Mali BN, Joshi JV, Wagle U, et al: *Actinomyces* in Cervical Smears of Women Using Intrauterine Contraceptive Devices. *Acta Cytol* 30: 367-371, 1986.

Mali BN, Joshi JV: Vaginal Parasitosis: An Unusual Finding in Routine Cervical Smears. *Acta Cytol* 31: 866-868, 1987.

Mali BN, Joshi JV: Interpreting Inflammatory Changes in Cervical Smears (Letter). *Br Med J* 7: 383, 1993.

Malik SN, Wilkinson EJ, Drew PA, et al: Do Qualifiers of ASCUS Distinguish Between Low- and High-Risk Patients? *Acta Cytol* 43: 376-380, 1999.

Malik SN, Wilinson EJ, Drew PA, et al: Benign Cellular Changes in Pap Smears: Causes and Significance. *Acta Cytol* 45: 5-8, 2001.

Malle D, Pateinakis PA, Kapraki A, et al: Cytologic Diagnosis of an Ovarian Adenocarcinoma Metastatic to the Cervix in Cervicovaginal Smears (Letter). *Acta Cytol* 45: 490-492, 2001.

Mallow DW, Humphrey PA, Soper JT, et al: Metastatic Lobular Carcinoma of the Breast Diagnosed in Cervicovaginal Samples: A Case Report. *Acta Cytol* 41: 549-555, 1997.

Mancini R, Romano G, Sgambato A, et al: Polycyclic Aromatic Hydrocarbon-DNA Adducts in Cervical Smears of Smokers and Nonsmokers. *Gynecol Oncol* 75: 68-71, 1999.

Mandelblatt J, Gopaul I, Wistreich M: Gynecological Care of Elderly Women: Another Look at Papanicolaou Smear Testing. *JAMA* 256: 367-371, 1986.

Mandelblatt J, Richart R, Thomas L, et al: Is Human Papillomavirus Associated With Cervical Neoplasia in the Elderly? *Gynecol Oncol* 46: 6-12, 1992a.

Mandelblatt J, Fahs M, Garibaldi K, et al: Association Between HIV Infection and Cervical Neoplasia: Implications for Clinical Care of Women at Risk for Both Conditions. *AIDS* 6: 173-178, 1992b.

Mandelblatt J, Traxler M, Lakin P, et al: Breast and Cervical Cancer Screening of Poor, Elderly, Black Women: Clinical Results and Implications. *Am J Prev Med* 9: 133-138, 1993.

Mandelblatt JS, Lawrence WF, Womack SM, et al: Benefits and Costs of Using HPV Testing to Screen for Cervical Cancer. *JAMA* 287: 2372-2381, 2002.

Manetta A, Keefe K, Lin F, et al: Atypical Glandular Cells of Undetermined Significance in Cervical Cytologic Findings. *Am J Obstet Gynecol* 180: 883-888, 1999.

Manhart LE, Koutsky LA: Do Condoms Prevent Genital HPV Infection, External Genital Warts, or Cervical Neoplasia: A Meta-Analysis. *Sex Transm Dis* 29: 725-735, 2002.

Mann R, Roberts WS, Gunasakeran S, et al: Primary Lymphoma of the Uterine Cervix. *Gynecol Oncol* 26: 127-134, 1987.

Mannion C, Park W-S, Man YG, et al: Endocrine Tumors of the Cervix: Morphologic Assessment, Expression of Human Papillomavirus, and Evaluation for Loss of Heterozygosity on *1p, 3p 11q*, and *17p. Cancer* 83: 1391-1400, 1998.

Manos MM, Kinney WK, Hurley LB, et al: Identifying Women With Cervical Neoplasia: Using Human Papilloma Virus DNA Testing for Equivocal Papanicolaou Results. *JAMA* 281: 1605-1610, 1999.

Mao C, Hughes JP, Kiviat N, et al: Clinical Findings Among Young Women With Genital Human Papillomavirus Infection. *Am J Obstet Gynecol* 188: 677-684, 2003.

Mao K, Guillebaud J: Influence of Removal of Intrauterine Contraceptive Devices on Colonisation of the Cervix by *Actinomyces*-Like Organisms. *Contraception* 30: 535-544, 1984.

Marchetti AA: Biographic and Personal Recollections of George N. Papanicolaou. *Obstet Gynecol Surv* 24: 680-684, 1969.

Marcuse PM: Incipient Microinvasive Carcinoma of the Uterine Cervix: Morphology and Clinical Data of 22 Cases. *Obstet Gynecol* 37: 360-367, 1971.

Mårdh P-A, Stormby N, Westrom L: Mycoplasma and Vaginal Cytology. *Acta Cytol* 15: 310-315, 1971.

Mårdh P-A, Westtom L: Adherence of Bacterial to Vaginal Epithelial Cells. *Infect Immunol* 13: 661-666, 1976.

Mårdh P-A: The Vaginal Ecosystem. *Am J Obstet Gynecol* 165: 1163-1168, 1991.

Margolis KL, Carson LF, Setness PA, et al: Are Benign Cellular Changes on a Papanicolaou Smear Really Benign? A Prospective Cohort Study. *Arch Fam Med* 8: 433-439, 1999.

Marjoniemi V-M: Immunohistochemistry in Gynaecological Pathology: A Review. *Pathology* 36: 109-119, 2004.

Marques T, De Angelo Andrade LAL, Vassallo J: Endocervical Tubal Metaplasia and Adenocarcinoma In Situ: Role of Immunohistochemistry for Carcinoembryonic Antigen and Vimentin in Differential Diagnosis. *Histopathology* 28: 549-550, 1996.

Marsh MR: Papilloma of the Cervix: *Am J Obstet Gynecol* 64: 281-291, 1952.

Marshall LM, Cason Z, Cabaniss DE, et al: Reactive Cell Change in Cervicovaginal Smears. *Biomed Sci Instrum* 33: 298-304, 1997.

Martin CE: Epidemiology of Cancer of the Cervix. II. Marital and Coital Factors in Cervical Cancer. *Am J Public Health* 57: 803-814, 1967.

Martin DC, Khare VK, Miller BE: Association of *Chlamydia trachomatis* Immunoglobulin Gamma Titers With Dystrophic Peritoneal Calcification, Psammoma Bodies, Adhesions, and Hydrosalpinges. *Fertility Sterility* 63: 39-44, 1995.

Martin HE, Ellis EB: Biopsy by Needle Puncture and Aspiration. *Ann Surg* 92: 169-181, 1930.

Martin HL Jr, Nyange PM, Richardson BA, et al: Hormonal Contraception, Sexually Transmitted Diseases, and Risk of Heterosexual Transmission of Human Immunodeficiency Virus Type I. *J Infect Dis* 178: 1053-1059, 1998.

Martin HL, Richardson BA, Nyange PM, et al: Vaginal Lactobacilli, Microbial Flora, and Risk of Human Immunodeficiency Virus Type 1 and Sexually Transmitted Disease Acquisition. *J Infect Dis* 180: 1863-1868, 1999.

Martin PL: How Preventable Is Invasive Cervical Cancer? A Community Study of Preventable Factors. *Am J Obstet Gynecol* 113: 541-548, 1972.

Martin-Hirsch PL, Lilford R, Jarvis G, et al: Efficacy of Cervical-Smear Collection Devices: A Systematic Review and Meta-Analysis. *Lancet* 354: 1762-1770, 1999.

Martin-Hirsch PL, Koliopoulos G, Paraskevaidis E: Is it Now Time to Evaluate the True Accuracy of Cervical Cytology Screening? A Review of the Literature. *Eur J Gynaecol Oncol* 23: 363-365, 2002.

Martínez I: Relationship of Squamous Cell Carcinoma of the Cervix Uteri to Squamous Cell Carcinoma of the Penis Among Puerto Rican Women Married to Men With Penile Carcinoma. *Cancer* 24: 777-780, 1969.

Martínez-Girón R, Ribas-Barceló A: Algae in Cytologic Smears. *Acta Cytol* 45: 936-940, 2001.

Martínez-Girón R, Ribas-Barceló A, Garcia-Miralles MT, et al: Airborne Fungal Spores, Pollen Grains, and Vegetable Cells in Routine Papanicolaou Smears. *Diagn Cytopathol* 30: 381-385, 2004a.

Martínez-Girón R: Corpora Amylacea in Cervicovaginal Smears (Letter). *Diagn Cytopathol* 31: 68-69, 2004b.

Martius J, Krohn MA, Hillier SL, et al: Relationships of Vaginal Lactobacillus Species, Cervical *Chlamydia trachomatis*, and Bacterial Vaginosis to Preterm Birth. *Obstet Gynecol* 71: 89-95, 1988.

Martzloff KH: Cancer of the Cervix Uteri: Recognition of Early Manifestations. *JAMA* 111: 1921-1925, 1938.

Marx JL: The Annual Pap Smear: An Idea Whose Time Has Gone? *Science* 205: 177-178, 1979.

Mascarenhas L, van Beek A, Bennink HC, et al: A 2-Year Comparative Study of Endometrial Histology and Cervical Cytology of Contraceptive Implant Users in Birmingham, UK. *Hum Repro* 13: 3057-3060, 1998.

Masfari AN, Duerden BI, Kinghorn GR: Quantitative Studies of Vaginal Bacteria. *Genitourin Med* 62: 256-263, 1986.

Mass SB, Brennan JP, Silverman N, et al: Association Between a Shift in Vaginal Flora on Papanicolaou Smear and Acute Chorioamnionitis and Preterm Delivery. *Diagn Cytopathol* 21: 7-9, 1999.

Massad LS, Collins YC, Meyer PM: Biopsy Correlates of Abnormal Cervical Cytology Classified Using the Bethesda System. *Gynecol Oncol* 82: 516-522, 2001.

Massoni EA, Hajdu SI: Cytology of Primary and Metastatic Uterine Sarcomas. *Acta Cytol* 28: 93-100, 1984.

Masubuchi K, Kubo H, Tenjin Y, et al: Follow-Up Studies by Cytology on Cancer of the Cervix Uteri After Treatment. *Acta Cytol* 13: 323-326, 1969.

Masubuchi S Jr, Nagai I, Hirata M, et al: Cytological Studies of Malignant Melanoma of the Vagina. *Acta Cytol* 19: 527-532, 1975.

Masuda K, Yutani C, Akutagawa K, et al: Cytopathological Observations in a 27-Year-Old Female Patient With Endometrioid Adenocarcinoma Arising in the Lower Uterine Segment of the Uterus. *Diagn Cytopathol* 21: 117-121, 1999.

Matas AJ, Simmons RL, Kjellstrand CM, et al: Increased Incidence of Malignancy During Chronic Renal Failure. *Lancet* (i): 883-886, 1975.

Mathers ME, Johnson SJ, Wadehra V: How Predictive Is a Cervical Smear Suggesting Glandular Neoplasia? *Cytopathology* 13: 83-91, 2002.

Matlashewski G, Osborn K, Banks L, et al: Transformation of Primary Human Fibroblast Cells With Human Papillomavirus Type 16 and EJ-ras. *Int J Cancer* 42: 232-238, 1988.

Matsukuma K, Tsukamoto N, Kaku T, et al: Early Adenocarcinoma of the Uterine Cervix—Its Histologic and Immunohistologic Study. *Gynecol Oncol* 35: 38-43, 1989.

Matsukura T, Koi S, Sugase M: Both Episomal and Integrated Forms of Human Papillomavirus Type 16 Are Invoved in Invasive Cervical Cancers. *Virology* 172: 63-72, 1989.

Matsuura Y, Saito R, Kawagoe T, et al: Cytologic Analysis of Primary Stomach Adenocarcinoma Metastatic to the Uterine Cervix. *Acta Cytol* 41: 291-294, 1997.

Matsuura Y, Kashimura M, Hatanaka K, et al: Sarcoma Botryoides of the Cervix: Report of a Case With Cytopathologic Findings. *Acta Cytol* 43: 475-480, 1999.

Matsuyama T, Tsukamoto N, Kaku T, et al: Primary Malignant Lymphoma of the Uterine Corpus and Cervix: Report of a Case With Immunocytochemical Analysis. *Acta Cytol* 33: 228-232, 1989.

Matthews-Greer J, Dominguez-Malagon H, Herrera G, et al: Human Papillomavirus Typing of Rare Cervical Carcinomas. *Arch Pathol Lab Med* 128: 553-556, 2004.

Mattosinho de Castro Ferraz Mda G, Focchi J, Norberto J, et al: Atypical Glandular Cells of Undetermined Significance: Cytologic Predictive Value for Glandular Involvement in High-Grade Squamous Intraepithelial Lesions. *Acta Cytol* 47: 154-158, 2003.

Mauck CK, Callahan MM, Baker J, et al: The Effect of One Injection of Depo-Provera on the Human Vaginal Epithelium and Cervical Ectopy. *Contraception* 60: 15-24, 1999.

Mauney M, Eide D, Sotham J: Rates of Condyloma and Dysplasia in Papanicolaou Smears With and Without Endocervical Cells. *Diagn Cytopathol* 6: 18-21, 1990.

Mawad RM, Latour JPA: Primary Adenocarcinoma of the Vagina. *Obstet Gynecol* 44: 889-893, 1974.

May M, Dong XP, Beyer-Finkler E, et al: The E6/E7 Promoter of Extrachromosomal HPV 216 DNA in Cervical Cancers Escapes from Cellular Repression by Mutation of Target Sequences for YY1. *EMBO J* 13: 1460-1466, 1994.

Mayans MV, Maquire A, Miret M, et al: Disproportionate High Incidence of Invasive Cervical Cancer as an AIDS-Indicative Disease Among Young Women in Catalonia, Spain. *Sex Transm Dis* 26: 500-503, 1999.

Mayelo V, Garaud P, Renjard L, et al: Cell Abnormalities Associated With Human Papillomavirus-Induced Squamous Intraepithelial Cervical Lesions: Multivariate Data Analysis. *Am J Clin Pathol* 101: 13-18, 1994.

Mayer EG, Galindo J, Davis J, et al: Adenocarcinoma of the Uterine Cervix: Incidence and the Role of Radiation Therapy. *Radiology* 121: 725-729, 1976.

Mays RM, Zimet GD, Winston Y, et al: Human Papillomavirus, Genital Warts, Pap Smears, and Cervical Cancer: Knowledge and Beliefs of Adolescent and Adult Women. *Health Care Women Int* 21: 361-374, 2000.

Mazur MT, Battifora HA: Adenoid Cystic Carcinoma of the Uterine Cervix: Ultrastructure, Immunofluorescence, and Criteria for Diagnosis. *Am J Clin Pathol* 77: 494-500, 1982.

Mazur MT, Cloud GA: The Koilocyte and Cervical Intraepithelial Neoplasia: Time-Trend Analysis of a Recent Decade. *Am J Obstet Gynecol* 150: 354-358, 1984a.

Mazur MT, Hsueh S, Gersell DJ: Metastases to the Female Genital Tract: Analysis of 325 Cases. *Cancer* 53: 1978-1984, 1984b.

McArdle JP, Muller HK: Quantitative Assessment of Langerhans' Cells in Human Cervical Intraepithelial Neoplasia and Wart Virus Infection. *Am J Obstet Gynecol* 154: 509-515, 1986.

McCallum SM: New Observations on the Significance of Nipplelike Protrusions in the Nuclei of Endocervical Cells. *Acta Cytol* 32: 331-334, 1988.

McCance DJ, Campion MJ, Baram A, et al: Risk of Transmission of Human Papillomavirus by Vaginal Specula. *Lancet* (ii): 816-817, 1986.

McCance DJ: Human Papillomaviruses and Cervical Cancer (Editorial). *J Med Microbiol* 47: 371-373, 1998.

McCann MF, Irwin DE, Walton LA, et al: Nicotine and Cotinine in the Cervical Mucus of Smokers, Passive Smokers, and Nonsmokers. *Cancer Epidemiol Biomarkers Prev* 1: 125-129, 1992.

McCluggage WG: Lymphoepithelioma-Like Carcinoma of the Vagina. *J Clin Pathol* 54: 964-965, 2001a.

McCluggage WG, Price JH, Dobbs SP: Primary Adenocarcinoma of the Vagina Arising in Endocervicosis. *Int J Gynecol Pathol* 20: 399-402, 2001b.

McCluggage WG: Recent Advances in Immunohistochemistry in Gynaecological Pathology. *Histopathology* 40: 309-326, 2002.

McCormack JS: Cervical Smears: A Questionable Practice? *Lancet* (ii): 207-209, 1989.

McCormack WM, Braun P, Lee-Y-H, et al: The Genital Myoplasmas. *N Engl J Med* 288: 78-89, 1973.

McGough DA, Fothergill AW, Rinaldi MG: *Cockeromyces recurvatus* Poitras, a Distinctive Zygomycete and Potential Pathogen: Criteria for Identification. *Clin Microbiol Newsl* 12: 113-117, 1990.

McCoy DR: Defending the Pap Smear: A Proactive Approach to the Litigation Threat in Gynecologic Cytology. *Am J Clin Pathol (Pathology Patterns Reviews)* 114: S52-S58, 2000.

McCoy JP Jr, Haines HG: The Antigenicity and Immunology of Human Cervical Squamous Cell Carcinoma: A Review. *Am J Obstet Gynecol* 140: 329-336, 1981.

McCrory DC, Matchar DB, Bastian L et al: Evaluation of Cervical Cytology. Agency for Health Care Policy and Research, Publication NO 99-E010 [Duke Report] (Evidence Report/Technology Assessment #5), Rockville, MD, 1999.

McDonnell JM, Mylotte MJ, Gustafson RC: Colposcopy in Pregnancy. A Twelve Year Review. *Br J Obstet Gynaecol* 88: 414-420, 1981.

McDonnell JM, Emens JM, Jordan JA: The Congenital Cervicovaginal Transformation Zone in Young Women Exposed to Diethylstilbesterol *in utero. Br J Obstet Gynaecol* 91: 574-579, 1984.

McEndree B: Clinical Application of the Vaginal Maturation Index. *Nurse Practitioner* 48: 51-52, 55-56, 1999.

McGill F, Adachi A, Karimi N, et al: Abnormal Cervical Cytology Leading to the Diagnosis of Gastric Cancer. *Gynecol Oncol* 36: 101-105, 1990.

McGlennen RC: Human Papillomavirus Oncogenesis. *Clin Lab Med* 20: 383-405, 2000.

McGowan L: Cytologic Methods for the Detection of Endometrial Cancer. *Gynecol Oncol* 2: 272-278, 1974.

McGrath CM, Kurtis JD, Yu GH: Evaluation of Mild-to-Moderate Dysplasia on Cervical-Endocervical (Pap) Smear: A Subgroup of Patients Who Bridge LSIL and HSIL. *Diagn Cytopathol* 23: 245-248, 2000.

McGrath CM: ASCUS in Papanicolaou Smears: Problems, Controversies, and Potential Future Directions. *Am J Clin Pathol (Pathology Patterns Reviews)* 117: S62-S75, 2002.

McIndoe WA, Green GH: Vaginal Carcinoma In Situ Following Hysterectomy. *Acta Cytol* 13: 158-162, 1969.

McIndoe WA, McLean MR, Jones RW, et al: The Invasive Potential of Carcinoma In Situ of the Cervix. *Obstet Gynecol* 64: 451-458, 1984.

McIntyre-Seltman K: The Abnormal Papanicolaou Smear. *Med Clin North Am* 79: 1427-1442, 1995.

McKay DG, Terjanian B, Poschyachinda D, et al: Clinical and Pathologic Significance of Anaplasia (Atypical Hyperplasia) of the Cervix Uteri. *Obstet Gynecol* 13: 2-21, 1959.

McKee GT: The Cervical (Pap) Smear—Personal Experience on Both Sides of the Atlantic. *Cytopathology* 11: 82-90, 2000.

McKelvey JL, Goodlin RR: Adenoma Malignum: A Cancer of Deceptively Innocent Histologic Pattern. *Cancer* 16: 549-557, 1953.

McKenzie DC, Scurry JP, Planner RS, et al: Cytology in the Follow-Up of Cervical Cancer. *Acta Cytol* 40: 235-240, 1996.

McLachlan N, Patwardhan JR, Ayer B, et al: Management of Suboptimal Cytologic Smears: Persistent Inflammatory Atypia. *Acta Cytol* 38: 531-536, 1994.

McLachlin CM, Tate JE, Zitz JC, et al: Human Papillomavirus Type 18 and Intraepithelial Lesions of the Cervix. *Am J Pathol* 144: 141-147, 1994.

McLachlin CM, Shen LH, Sheets EE, et al: Disparities in Mean Age and Histopathologic Grade Between Human Papillomavirus Type-Specific Early Cervical Neoplasms. *Hum Pathol* 28: 1226-1229, 1997.

McLachlin CM: Human Papillomavirus in Cervical Neoplasia: Role, Risk Factors, and Implications. *Clin Lab Med* 20: 257-269, 2000.

McLellan R, Spence MR, Brockman M, et al: The Clinical Diagnosis of Trichomoniasis. *Obstet Gynecol* 60: 30-34, 1982.

McLennan MT, McLennan CE: Estrogenic Status of Menstruating and Menopausal Women Assessed by Cervicovaginal Smears. *J Obstet Gynecol* 37: 325-331, 1971.

McLennan MT, McLennan CE: Significance of Cervicovaginal Cytology After Radiation Therapy for Cervical Carcinoma. *Am J Obstet Gynecol* 121: 96-100, 1975a.

McLennan MT, McLennan CE: Hormonal Patterns in Vaginal Smears from Puerperal Women. *Acta Cytol* 19: 431-433, 1975b.

McMurray HR, Nguyen D, Westbook TF, et al: Biology of Human Papillomaviruses. *J Exp Pathol* 82: 15-33, 2001.

McNeill RE, de Moraes-Ruehsen M: Ameba Trophozoites in Cervico-Vaginal Smear of a Patient Using an Intrauterine Device. A Case Report. *Acta Cytol* 22: 91-92, 1978.

McPhee A: "Squeeze Therapy from Mars" (Martian Popping Thing™, Item #09500. Archie McPhee, PO Box 30852, Seattle WA 98113, ©Archie McPhee). [http://www.McPhee.com. 05/01/05]

Mead PB: Cervical-Vaginal Flora of Women With Invasive Cervical Cancer. *Obstet Gynecol* 52: 601-604, 1978.

Meanwell CA, Blackledge G, Cox MF, Maitland NJ: HPV 16 DNA in Normal and Malignant Cervical Epithelium: Implications for the Aetiology and Behaviour of Cervical Neoplasia. *Lancet* (i): 703-707, 1987.

Meanwell CA, Kelly KA, Wilson S, et al: Young Age as a Prognostic Factor in Cervical Cancer: Analysis of Population Based Data from 10,022 Cases. *Br Med J* 296: 386-391, 1988.

Meath AJ, Carley ME, Wilson TO: Atypical Glandular Cells of Undetermined Significance: Review of Final Histologic Diagnoses. *J Reprod Med* 47: 249-252, 2002.

Medley G, Surtees VM: Squamous Atypia in the Atrophic Cervical Vaginal Smear: A Plea for a More Painstaking Old Style Look Versus a New Look at the Old Problem (Editorial). *Cancer (Cancer Cytopathol)* 84: 200-201, 1998.

Mehal WZ, Lo YM, Herrington CS, et al: Role of Human Papillomavirus in Determining the HLA Associated Risk of Cervical Carcinogenesis. *J Clin Pathol* 47:1077-1081, 1994.

Mehrotra R, Gupta RK: Microfilaria of *Wuchereria bancrofti* Identified in a Cervicovaginal Smear (Letter). *Acta Cytol* 42: 840-841, 1998.

Meigs JV, Graham RM, Fremont-Smith M, et al: The Value of the Vaginal Smear in the Diagnosis of Uterine Cancer. *Surg Gynecol Obstet* 77: 449-461, 1943.

Meigs JV, Graham RM, Fremont-Smith M, et al: II. The Value of the Vaginal Smear in the Diagnosis of Uterine Cancer: A Report of 1015 Cases. *Surg Gynecol Obstet* 81: 337-345, 1945.

Meijer CJ, van den Brule AJ, Snijders PJ, et al: Detection of Human Papillomavirus in Cervical Scrapes by the Polymerase Chain Reaction in Relation to Cytology: Possible Implications for Cervical Cancer Screening. *IARC Science Publications* (119): 271-281, 1992.

Meisels A: The Menopause: A Cytohormonal Study. *Acta Cytol* 10: 49-55, 1966a.

Meisels A, Dubreuil-Charrois M: Hormonal Cytology During Pregnancy. *Acta Cytol* 10: 376-382, 1966b.

Meisels A: Hormonal Cytology of Pregnancy. *Clin Obstet Gynecol* 11: 1121-1142, 1968.

Meisels A, Fortin R: Genital Tuberculosis: Cytologic Detection. *Acta Cytol* 19: 79-81, 1975.

Meisels A, Ayotte D: Cells from the Seminal Vesicles: Contaminants of the V-C-E Smear. *Acta Cytol* 20: 211-219, 1976a.

Meisels A, Fortin R: Condylomatous Lesions of the Cervix and Vagina I. Cytologic Patterns. *Acta Cytol* 20: 505-509, 1976b.

Meisels A, Bégun R, Schneider V: Dysplasias of Uterine Cervix Epidemiological Aspects: Role of Age at First Coitus and Use of Oral Contraceptives. *Cancer* 40: 3076-3081, 1977a.

Meisels A, Fortin R, Roy M: Condylomatous Lesions of the Cervix II. Cytologic, Colposcopic and Histopathologic Study. *Acta Cytol* 21: 379-390, 1977b.

Meisels A, Roy M, Fortier M, et al: Condylomatous Lesions of the Cervix: Morphologic and Colposcopic Diagnosis. *Am J Diagn Gynecol Obstet* 1: 109-116, 1979.

Meisels A, Morin C: Human Papillomavirus and Cancer of the Uterine Cervix. *Gynecol Oncol* 12(2 Pt 2): S111-S123, 1981a.

Meisels A, Roy M, Fortier M, et al: Human Papillomavirus Infection of the Cervix: The Atypical Condyloma. *Acta Cytol* 25: 7-16, 1981b.

Meisels A, Morin C, Casas-Cordero M: Human Papillomavirus Infection of the Uterine Cervix. *Int J Gynecol Pathol* 1: 75-94, 1982.

Meisels A: The Story of a Cell: The George N. Papanicolaou Award Lecture. *Acta Cytol* 27: 584-596, 1983.

Meisels A: Cytologic Diagnosis of Human Papillomavirus. Influence of Age and Pregnancy Stage. *Acta Cytol* 36: 480-482, 1992.

Meisels A: *Cytopathology of the Uterus: ASCP Theory and Practice of Cytopathology, 1.* Chicago. ASCP Press, 1997.

Melamed MR, Koss LG, Flehinger BJ, et al: Prevalence Rates of Uterine Cervical Carcinoma In Situ for Women Using the Diaphragm or Contraceptive Oral Steroids. *Br Med J* 3: 195-200, 1969.

Melamed MR, Flehinger BJ: Non-Diagnostic Squamous Atypia in Cervico-Vaginal Cytology as a Risk Factor for Early Neoplasia. *Acta Cytol* 20: 108-110, 1976.

Melczer N: Über die ätilogische Identität der gewöhnlichen Warzen und Spitzen Kondylome. *Hautarzt* 16: 150-153, 1965.

Melkert PWJ, Hopman E, van den Brule AJC, et al: Prevalence of HPV in Cytomorphologically Normal Cervical Smears, as Determined by the Polymerase Chain Reaction, Is Age Dependent. *Int J Cancer* 53: 919-923, 1993.

Melnikow J, Nuovo J, Willan AR, et al: Natural History of Cervical Squamous Intraepithelial Lesions: A Meta-Analysis. *Obstet Gynecol* 92: 727-735, 1998.

Menezes GA, Wakely PE, Stripe DM, et al: Increased Incidence of Atypical Papanicolaou Tests from ThinPreps of Postmenopausal Women Receiving Hormone Replacement Therapy. *Cancer (Cancer Cytopathol)* 93: 357-363, 2001.

Meniru GI, Moore J, Thomlinson J: Aerosol Cap and Rectovaginal Fistula: Unusual Findings at Routine Cervical Smear (Letter). *Int J Gynecol Obstet* 52: 179-180, 1996.

Merki-Feld GS, Lebeda E, Hogg B, et al: The Incidence of *Actinomyces*-Like Organisms in Papanicolaou-Stained Smears of Copper- and Levonorgestrel-Releasing Intrauterine Devices. *Contraception* 61: 365-368, 2000.

Mestwerdt G: Pobeexzision und Kolposkopie in des Frühdiagnose des Portiokarcinom. *Zentralbl Gynäkol* 69: 326-332, 1947.

Mettlin C, Dodd GD: The American Cancer Society Guidelines for the Cancer-Related Checkup: An Update. *CA: Cancer J Clin* 41: 279-282, 1991.

Metzger GD: Laboratory Diagnosis of Vaginal Infections. *Clin Lab Sci* 11: 47-52, 1998.

Meyer R: The Histological Diagnosis of Early Cervical Carcinoma. *Surg Gynecol Obstet* 73: 129-139, 1941.

Mhawech P, Dellas A, Terracciano LM: Glassy Cell Carcinoma of the Endometrium: A Case Report and Review of the Literature. *Arch Pathol Lab Med* 125: 816-819, 2001.

Michael CW, Esfahani FM: Pregnancy-Related Changes: A Retrospective Review of 278 Cervical Smears. *Diagn Cytopathol* 17: 99-107, 1997.

Michael CW: The Papanicolaou Smear and the Obstetric Patient: A Simple Test With Great Benefits. *Diagn Cytopathol* 21: 1-3, 1999.

Michael H, Grawe L, Kraus FT: Minimal Deviation Endocervical Adenocarcinoma: Clinical and Histologic Features, Immunohistochemical Staining for Carcinoembryonic Antigen, and Differentiation from Confusing Benign Lesions. *Int J Gynecol Pathol* 3: 261-276, 1984.

Michaelis L, Gutmann C: Ueber Einschlüsse in Blasentumoren. *Zeitschrift f. Klin Medizin* 47: 208-215, 1902.

Michalas S: The Pap Test: George N. Papanicolaou (1883-1962): A Screening Test for the Prevention of Cancer of Uterine Cervix. *Eur J Obstet Gynecol Reprod Biol* 90: 135-138, 2000.

Miguel NL Jr, Lachowicz CM, Kline TS: *Candida*-Related Changes and ASCUS: A Potential Trap! *Diagn Cytopathol* 16: 83-86, 1997.

Mikami Y, Hata S, Fujiwara K, et al: Florid Endocervical Glandular Hyperplasia With Intestinal and Pyloric Gland Metaplasia: Worrisome Benign Mimic of "Adenoma Malignum". *Gynecol Oncol* 74: 504-511, 1999.

Mikami Y, Manabe T: Lobular Endocervical Glandular Hyperplasia Represents Pyloric Gland Metaplasia? (Letter) *Am J Surg Pathol* 24: 323-324, 2000; author reply 325-326.

Mikami Y, Hata S, Melamed J, et al: Lobular Endocervical Glandular Hyperplasia Is a Metaplastic Process With a Pyloric Gland Phenotype. *Histopathology* 39: 364-372, 2001.

Mikamo H, Sato Y, Hayasaki Y, et al: Vaginal Microflora in Healthy Women With *Gardnerella vaginalis*. *J Infect Chemother* 6: 173-177, 2000.

Mikhail GR, Drukker BH, Chow C: Pemphigus Vulgaris Involving the Cervix Uteri. *Arch Dermatol* 95: 496-498, 1967.

Mikhail MS, Runowicz CD, Kadish AS, et al: Colposcopic and Cytologic Detection of Chronic Lymphocytic Leukemia. *Gynecol Oncol* 34: 106-108, 1989.

Milde-Langosch K, Schreiber C, Becker G, et al: Human Papillomavirus Detection in Cervical Adenocarcinoma by Polymerase Chain Reaction. *Hum Pathol* 24: 590-594, 1993.

Milde-Langosch K, Riethdorf S, Löning T: Association of Human Papillomavirus Infection With Carcinoma of the Cervix Uteri and Its Precursor Lesions: Theoretical and Practical Implications. *Virchows Archiv (Path Anat)* 437: 227-233, 2000.

Miles PA, Herrera GA, Mena H, et al: Cytologic Findings in Primary Malignant Carcinoid Tumor of the Cervix: Including Immunohistochemistry and Electron Microscopy Performed on Cervical Smears. *Acta Cytol* 29: 1003-1008, 1985.

Miller AB, Linsay J, Hill GP: Mortality from Cancer of the Uterus in Canada and Its Relationship to Screening for Cancer of the Cervix. *Int J Cancer* 17: 602-612, 1976.

Miller AB: Failures of Cervical Cancer Screening (Editorial). *Am J Public Health* 85: 761-762, 1995.

Miller AB: Natural History of Cervical Human Papillomavirus Infections (Commentary). *Lancet* 357: 1816, 2001.

Miller BE, Flax SD, Arheart K, et al: The Presentation of Adenocarcinoma of the Uterine Cervix. *Cancer* 72: 1281-1285, 1993.

Miller JM, Chambers DC, Miller JM: The Need for Pap Tests After Hysterectomy for Benign Disease: Results of a Study of Black Patients. *Postgrad Med* 82: 200-203, 1987.

Miller KE, Losh DP, Folley A: Evaluation and Follow-Up of Abnormal Pap Smears. *Am Fam Physician* 45: 143-150, 1992.

Miller L, Patton DL, Meier A, et al: Depomedroxyprogesterone-Induced Hypoestrogenism and Changes in Vaginal Flora and Epithelium. *Obstet Gynecol* 96: 431-439, 2000.

Miller LG, Goldstein G, Murphy M, et al: Reversible Alterations in Immunoregulatory T Cells in Smoking: Analysis by Monoclonal Antibodies and Flow Cytometry. *Chest* 82: 526-529, 1982.

Miller MG, Sung H-Y, Sawaya GF, et al: Screening Interval and Risk of Invasive Squamous Cell Cervical Cancer. *Obstet Gynecol* 101: 29-37, 2003.

Milligan M, Carrow LA, Eggers V: A Source of False Positives in Cytologic Interpretation. *Am J Obstet Gynecol* 78: 599-603, 1959.

Mills SE, Austin MB, Randall ME: Lymphoepithelioma-Like Carcinoma of the Uterine Cervix: A Distinctive Undifferentiated Carcinoma With an Inflammatory Stroma. *Am J Surg Pathol* 9: 883-889, 1985.

Minassian H, Schinella R, Reilly JC: Crystalline Bodies in Cervical Smears: Clinicopathologic Correlation. *Acta Cytol* 37: 149-152, 1993.

Minato H, Shimizu M, Hirokawa M, et al: Adenocarcinoma In Situ of the Fallopian Tube: A Case Report. *Acta Cytol* 42: 1455-1457, 1998.

Mintzer M, Curtis P, Resnick JC, et al: The Effect of the Quality of Papanicolaou Smears on the Detection of Cytologic Abnormalities. *Cancer (Cancer Cytopathol)* 87: 113-117, 1999.

Mirhashemi R, Ganjei-Azar P, Nadji M, et al: Papillary Squamous Cell Carcinoma of the Uterine Cervix: An Immunophenotypic Appraisal of 12 Cases. *Gynecol Oncol* 90: 657-661, 2003.

Misch KA, Smithies A, Twomey D, et al: Tuberculosis of the Cervix: Cytology as an Aid to Diagnosis. *J Clin Pathol* 29: 313-316, 1976.

Mishell DR Jr, el-Habashy MA, Good RG, et al: Contraception With an Injectable Progestin: A Study of Its Use in Postpartum Women. *Am J Obstet Gynecol* 101: 1046-1053, 1968.

Mishell DR Jr: Pharmacokinetics of Depot Medroxyprogesterone Acetate Contraception. *J Reprod Med* 41: 381-390, 1996.

Misra JS, Engineer AD, Tandon P: Cytopathological Changes in Human Cervix and Endometrium Following Prolonged Retention of Copper-Bearing Intrauterine Contraceptive Devices. *Diagn Cytopathol* 5: 237-242, 1989.

Misra JS, Engineer AD, Das K, et al: Cervical Carcinogenesis and Contraception. *Diagn Cytopathol* 7: 346-352, 1991.

Misra JS, Engineer AD, Tandon P: Cervical Cytology Associated With Levonorgestrel Contraception. *Acta Cytol* 39: 45-49, 1995.

Misra JS, Tandon P, Srivastava A, et al: Cervical Cytological Studies in Women Inserted With Norplant-I Contraceptive. *Diagn Cytopathol* 29: 136-139, 2003.

Mitao M, Nagai N, Levine RU, et al: Human Papillomavirus Type 16 Infection: A Morphological Spectrum With Evidence for Late Gene Expression. *Int J Gynecol Pathol* 5: 287-296, 1986.

Mitchell H, Drake M, Medley G: Prospective Evaluation of Risk of Cervical Cancer After Cytological Evidence of Human Papillomavirus Infection. *Lancet* (i): 573-575, 1986.

Mitchell H, Medley G, Drake M: Quality Control Measures for Cervical Cytology Laboratories. *Acta Cytol* 32: 288-292, 1988.

Mitchell H, Medley G: Age and Time Trends in the Prevalence of Cervical Intraepithelial Neoplasia on Papanicolaou Smear Tests, 1970-1988. *Med J Aust* 152: 252-255, 1990a.

Mitchell H, Medley G, Giles G: Cervical Cancers Diagnosed After Negative Results on Cervical Cytology in the 1980s. *Br Med J* 300: 1622-1626, 1990b.

Mitchell H: Epidemiology of Cervical Cancer and Screening. *Cancer Forum* 14: 143-145, 1990c.

Mitchell H, Medley G: Longitudinal Study of Women With Negative Cervical Smears According to Endocervical Status. *Lancet* 337: 265-267, 1991.

Mitchell H, Medley G: Influence of Endocervical Status on the Cytologic Prediction of Cervical Intraepithelial Neoplasia. *Acta Cytol* 36: 875-880, 1992.

Mitchell H, Giles G, Medley G: Accuracy and Survival Benefit of Cytological Prediction of Endometrial Carcinoma on Routine Cervical Smears. *Int J Gynecol Pathol* 12: 34-40, 1993a.

Mitchell H: Improving Consistency in Cervical Cytology Reporting. *J Natl Cancer Inst* 85: 1592-1596, 1993b.

Mitchell H: Consistency of Reporting Endocervical Cells. An Intralaboratory and Interlaboratory Assessment. *Acta Cytol* 38: 310-314, 1994a.

Mitchell H, Higgins V: Recent Negative Cytology Prior to Histologically Confirmed Carcinoma In Situ of the Cervix. *Aust NZ J Obstet Gynecol* 34: 178-181, 1994b.

Mitchell H, Medley G, Gordon I, et al: Cervical Cytology Reported as Negative and Risk of Adenocarcinoma of the Cervix: No Strong Evidence of Benefit. *Br J Cancer* 71: 894-897, 1995a.

Mitchell H, Medley G: Differences Between Papanicolaou Smears With Correct and Incorrect Diagnoses. *Cytopathology* 6: 368-375, 1995b.

Mitchell H, Medley G: Abnormal Vaginal Bleeding Is Common, Malignancy Rare (Letter). *Med J Aust* 162: 164-166, 1995c.

Mitchell H, Giles GG: Cancer Diagnosis After a Report of Negative Cervical Cytology. *Med J Aust* 164: 270-273, 1996.

Mitchell H, Medley G: Differences Between False-Negative and True-Positive Papanicolaou Smears on Papnet-Assisted Review. *Diagn Cytopathol* 19: 138-140, 1998.

Mitchell H, Hocking J, Saville M: Improvement in Protection Against Adenocarcinoma of the Cervix Resulting from Participation in Cervical Screening. *Cancer (Cancer Cytopathol)* 99: 336-341, 2003.

Mitchell H: Longitudinal Analysis of Histologic High-Grade Disease After Negative Cervical Cytology According to Endocervical Status. *Cancer (Cancer Cytopathol)* 93: 237-240, 2001.

Mitchell H, Hocking, Saville M: Cervical Cytology Screening History of Women Diagnosed With Adenocarcinoma In Situ of the Cervix: A Case-Control Study. *Acta Cytol* 48: 595-600, 2004.

Mitchell MF, Hittelman WK, Lotan R, et al: Chemoprevention Trials and Surrogate End Point Biomarkers in the Cervix. *Cancer* 76(Suppl 10): 1956-1977, 1995.

Mitchell MF, Tortolero-Luna G, Wright T, et al: Cervical Human Papillomavirus Infection and Intraepithelial Neoplasia: A Review. *Monogr J Natl Cancer Inst* 21: 17-25, 1996.

Mitrani-Rosenbaum S, Tsvieli R, Tur-Kaspa R: Oestrogen Stimulates Differential Transcription of Human Papillomavirus Type 16 in SiHa Cervical Carcinoma Cells. *J Gen Virol* 70: 2227-2232, 1989.

Mittal K, Chan W, Demopoulos RL: Sensitivity and Specificity of Various Morphological Features of Cervical Condylomas. *Arch Pathol Lab Med* 114: 1038-1041, 1990.

Mittal K, Lin O, Chan W, et al: Cervical Squamous Dysplasias and Carcinomas With Immunodetectable p53 Frequently Contain HPV. *Gynecol Oncol* 58: 289-294, 1995.

Mittal K, Demopoulos RI, Tata M: A Comparison of Proliferative Activity and Atypical Mitoses in Cervical Condylomas With Various HPV Types. *Int J Gynecol Pathol* 17: 24-28, 1998.

Mittal K: Utility of Proliferation-Associated Marker MIB-1 in Evaluating Lesions of the Uterine Cervix. *Adv Anat Pathol* 6: 177-185, 1999a.

Mittal K, Mesia A, Demopoulos RI: MIB-1 Expression Is Useful in Distinguishing Dysplasia from Atrophy in Elderly Women. *Int J Gynecol Pathol* 18: 122-124, 1999b.

Mobiüs G: Cytological Early Detection of Cervical Carcinoma: Possibilities and Limitations: Analysis of Failures. *J Cancer Res Clin Oncol* 119: 513-521, 1993.

Mody DR: Agonizing Over AGUS (Editorial). *Cancer (Cancer Cytopathol)* 87: 243-244, 1999.

Mohammed DK, Lavie O, de B Lopes A, et al: A Clinical Review of Borderline Glandular Cells on Cervical Cytology. *Br J Obstet Gynaecol* 107: 605-609, 2000.

Moi H: Prevalence of Bacterial Vaginosis and Its Association With Genital Infections, Inflammation, and Contraceptive Methods in Women Attending Sexually Transmitted Disease and Primary Health Clinics. *Int J STD AIDS* 1: 86-94, 1990.

Mong K, Taylor D, Muzyka T, et al: Tricuspid Endocarditis Following a Papanicolaou Smear: Case Report. *Can J Cardiol* 13: 895-896, 1997.

Monk BJ, cogan M, Felix JC, et al: A Stiff Bristled, Spiral-Shaped Ectocervical Brush: A Device for Transepithelial Tissue Biopsy. *Obstet Gynecol* 100: 1276-1284, 2002.

Monk BJ, Wiley DJ: Human Papillomavirus Infections: Truth or Consequences (Editorial). *Cancer* 100: 225-227, 2004.

Monsonego J, Magdelenat H, Catalan F, et al: Estrogen and Progesterone Receptors in Cervical Human Papillomavirus Related Lesions. *Int J Cancer* 48: 533-539, 1991.

Montanari GD, Marconato A, Montanari GR. et al: Granulation Tissue on the Vault of the Vagina After Hysterectomy for Cancer: Diagnostic Problems. *Acta Cytol* 12: 25-29, 1968.

Montes MA, Cibas ES, DiNisco SA, et al: Cytologic Characteristics of Abnormal Cells in Prior "Normal" Cervical/Vaginal Papanicolaou Smears from Women With a High-Grade Squamous Intraepithelial Lesion. *Cancer (Cancer Cytopathol)* 87: 56-59, 1999.

Montgomery KD, Tedford KL, McDougall JK: Genetic Instability of Chromosome 3 in HPV-Immortalized and Tumorigenic Human Keratinocytes. *Genes Chromosomes Cancer* 14: 97-105, 1995.

Montone KT, Furth EE, Pietra GG, et al: Neonatal Adenovirus Infection: A Case Report With In Situ Hybridization Confirmation of Ascending Intrauterine Infection. *Diagn Cytopathol* 12: 341-344, 1995.

Montz FJ, Monk BJ, Fowler JM, et al: Natural History of the Minimally Abnormal Papanicolaou Smear. *Obstet Gynecol* 80: 385-388, 1992.

Montz FJ: Significance of "Normal" Endometrial Cells in Cervical Cytology from Asymptomatic Postmenopausal Women Receiving Hormone Replacement Therapy. *Gynecol Oncol* 81: 33-39, 2001.

Moodley M, Moodley J, Kleinschmidt I: Invasive Cervical Cancer and Human Immunodeficiency Virus (HIV) Infection: A South African Perspective. *Int J Gynecol Cancer* 11: 194-197, 2001.

Moore KL: The Sex Chromatin: Its Discovery and Variations in the Animal Kingdom. *Acta Cytol* 6: 1-12, 1962.

Moraes PS, Taketomi EA: Allergic Vulvovaginitis. *Ann Allergy Asthma Immunol* 85: 253-265, 2000.

Morell ND, Taylor JR, Snyder RN, et al: False-Negative Cytology Rates in Patients in Whom Invasive Cervical Cancer Subsequently Developed. *Obstet Gynecol* 60: 41-45, 1982.

Moreno V, Bosch FX, Muñoz N, et al: Effect of Oral Contraceptives on Risk of Cervical Cancer in Women With Human Papillomavirus Infection: The IARC Multicentric Case-Control Study. *Lancet* 359: 1085-1092, 2002.

Moriarty AT, Wilbur D: Those Gland Problems in Cervical Cytology: Faith or Fact? Observations from the Bethesda 2001 Terminology Conference. *Diagn Cytopathol* 28: 171-174, 2003a.

Moriarty AT, Young NA: The Four R's: Reactive/Repair, Reporting, and Regulations (Editorial). *Diagn Cytopathol* 29: 1-3, 2003b.

Morimoto N, Ozawa M, Kato Y, et al: Diagnostic Value of Mitotic Activity in Endometrial Stromal Sarcoma: Report of Two Cases. *Acta Cytol* 26: 695-698, 1982.

Morimura, Y, Nishiyama H, Hashimoto T, et al: Diagnosing Endometrial Carcinoma With Cervical Involvement by Cervical Cytology. *Acta Cytol* 46: 284-290, 2002.

Morin C, Bairati I, Bouchard C, et al: Cytologic Predictors of Cervical Intraepithelial Neoplasia in Women With an ASCUS Pap Smear. *Acta Cytol* 44: 576-586, 2000.

Moritani S, Ioffe OB, Sagae S, et al: Mitotic Activity and Apoptosis in Endocervical Glandular Lesions. *Int J Gynecol Pathol* 21: 125-133, 2002.

Morris CA, Morris DG: 'Normal' Vaginal Microbiology of Women of Childbearing Age in Relation to the Use of Oral Contraceptives and Vaginal Tampons. *J Clin Pathol* 20: 636-640, 1967.

Morris HHB, Gatter KC, Stein H, et al: Langerhans' Cells in Human Cervical Epithelium: An Immunohistological Study. *Br J Obstet Gynaecol* 90: 400-411, 1983a.

Morris HHB, Gatter KC, Sykes G, et al: Langerhans' Cells in Human Cervical Epithelium: Effects of Wart Virus Infection and Intraepithelial Neoplasia. *Br J Obstet Gynaecol* 90: 412-420, 1983b.

Morris M: Cervical Intraepithelial Neoplasia and Cervical Cancer. *Obstet Gynecol Clin North Am* 23: 347-410, 1996.

Morrison BJ, Coldman AJ, Boyes DA, et al: Forty Years of Repeated Screening: The Significance of Carcinoma In Situ. *Br J Cancer* 74: 814-819, 1996.

Morrison C, Catania F, Wakely P Jr: Highly Differentiated Keratinizing Squamous Cell Cancer of the Cervix: A Rare, Locally Aggressive Tumor Not Associated With Human Papillomavirus or Squamous Intraepithelial Lesions. *Am J Surg Pathol* 25: 1310-1315, 2001.

Morrison C, Prokorym P, Piquero C, et al: Oral Contraceptive Pills Are Associated With Artifacts in ThinPrep Pap Smears that Mimic Low-Grade Squamous Intraepithelial Lesions. *Cancer (Cancer Cytopathol)* 99: 75-82, 2003.

Morrison CS, Schwingl PJ, Cates W Jr, et al: Sexual Behavior and Cancer Prevention. *Cancer Causes Control* 8(Suppl 1): S21-S25, 1997.

Morrow CP, DiSaia PJ: Malignant Melanoma of the Female Genitalia: A Clinical Analysis. *Obstet Gynecol Surv* 31: 233-271, 1976.

Morrow CP, Cozen W: Perspective on Cervical Cancer: Why Prevent? *J Cell Biochem* Suppl 23: 61-70, 1995.

Morse AR, Coleman DV, Gardner SD: An Evaluation of Cytology in the Diagnosis of Herpes Simplex Virus Infection and Cytomegalovirus Infection of the Cervix Uteri. *J Obstet Gynaecol Br Commonw* 81: 393-398, 1974.

Moscicki A-B, Palefsky JM, Gonzales J, et al: The Association Between Human Papillomavirus Deoxyribonucleic Acid Status and the Results of Cytologic Rescreening Tests in Young, Sexually Active Women. *Am J Obstet Gynecol* 165: 67-71, 1991.

Moscicki A-B, Shiboski S, Broering J, et al: The Natural History of Human Papillomavirus Infection as Measured by Repeated DNA Testing in Adolescent and Young Women. *J Pediatr* 132: 277-284, 1998.

Moscicki A-B, Burt VG, Kanowitz S, et al: The Significance of Squamous Metaplasia in the Development of Low-Grade Squamous Intraepithelial Lesions in Young Women. *Cancer* 85: 1139-1144, 1999.

Moscicki A-B, Ellenberg JH, Vermund SH, et al: Prevalence of and Risks for Cervical Human Papillomavirus Infection and Squamous Intraepithelial Lesions in Adolescent Girls. *Arch Pediatr Adolesc Med* 154: 127-134, 2000.

Moscicki A-B, Hills N, Shiboski S, et al: Risks for Incident Human Papillomavirus Infection and Low-Grade Squamous Intraepithelial Lesion Development in Young Females. *JAMA* 285: 2995-3002, 2001.

Moscicki A-B, Shiboski S, Hills NK, et al: Regression of Low-Grade Squamous Intra-Epithelial Lesions in Young Women. *Lancet* 364: 1678-1683. 2004.

Moss GB, Clemetson D, D'Costa L, et al: Association of Cervical Ectopy With Heterosexual Transmission of Human Immunodeficiency Virus: Results of a Study of Couples in Nairobi, Kenya. *J Infect Dis* 164: 588-591, 1991.

Mount S, Papillo JL: A Study of 10296 Pediatric and Adolescent Papanicolaou Smear Diagnoses in Northern New England. *Pediatrics* 103: 539-545, 1999.

Mount S, Harmon M, Eltabbakh G, et al: False Positive Diagnosis in Conventional and Liquid-Based Cervical Specimens. *Acta Cytol* 48: 363-371, 2004.

Mounts P, Shah KV: Respiratory Papillomatosis: Etiological Relation to Genital Tract Papillomaviruses. *Prog Med Virol* 29: 90-114, 1984.

Mourits MJE, Pieters WJLM, Hollema H, et al: Three-Group Metaphase as a Morphologic Criterion of Progressive Cervical Intraepthelial Neoplasia. *Am J Obstet Gynecol* 167: 591-595, 1992.

Mravunac M, Verbeek DH, Sanders-Eras M, et al: Histologic Processing of Microbiopsies from Cervical Smears Is Diagnostically Useful in Selected Cases. *Am J Clin Pathol* 108: 191-196, 1997.

Mravunac M, Verbeek D, van Heusden C, et al: Applications of the Microbiopsy Technique in Non-Cervical Cytology: Where Cytology and Histology Meet. *Histopathology* 33: 174-182, 1998.

Mravunac M, Smedts F, Philippi A, et al: Interpreting Microbiopsies in Cervical Smears: A Cytohistologic Approach. *Acta Cytol* 44: 752-759, 2000.

Mudge TJ, Johnson J, MacFarlane A: Primary Malignant Melanoma of the Cervix: A Case Report. *Br J Obstet Gynaecol* 88: 1257-1259, 1981.

Mulford D, Rutkowski M, Sickel J: Unusual Cytologic Manifestations in Human Immunodeficiency Virus-Infected Patients: A Pot-Pourri of Cases (Abstract). *Acta Cytol* 35: 630, 1991.

Mulligan NJ, de las Morenas A, Soto-Wright V, et al: Percentages of Cervical Cytologic Diagnoses as a Quality Assurance Method. *Acta Cytol* 42: 928-932, 1998.

Mullins JD, Hilliard GD: Cervical Carcinoid ("Argyrophil Cell" Carcinoma) Associated With an Endocervical Adenocarcinoma: A Light and Ultrastructural Study. *Cancer* 47: 785-790, 1981.

Mulvany NJ, Khan A, Östör A: Arias-Stella Reaction Associated With Cervical Pregnancy: Report of a Case With a Cytologic Presentation. *Acta Cytol* 38: 218-222, 1994.

Mulvany NJ, Östör A: Microinvasive Adenocarcinoma of the Cervix: A Cytohistopathologic Study of 40 Cases. *Diagn Cytopathol* 16: 430-436, 1997.

Mulvany NJ, Surtees V: Cervical/Vaginal Endometriosis With Atypia: A Cytohistopathologic Study. *Diagn Cytopathol* 21: 188-193, 1999.

Münger K, Phelps WC, Bubb V, et al: The E6 and E7 Genes of the Human Papillomavirus Type 16 Together Are Necessary and Sufficient for Transformation of Primary Human Keratinocytes. *J Virol* 63: 4417-4423, 1989a.

Münger K, Werness BA, Dyson N, et al: Complex Formation of Human Papillomavirus E7 Proteins With the Retinoblastoma Tumor Suppressor Gene Product. *EMBO J* 8: 4099-4105, 1989b.

Münger K, Phelps WC: The Human Papillomavirus E7 Protein as a Transforming and Transactivating Factor. *Biochim Biophy Acta* 1155: 111-123, 1993.

Munguia H, Franco E, Valenzuela P: Diagnosis of Genital Amebiasis in Women by the Standard Papanicolaou Technique. *Am J Obstet Gynecol* 94: 181-188, 1966.

Munipalli B, Rinaldi MG, Greenberg SB: *Cokeromyces recuratus* Isolated from Pleural and Peritoneal Fluid: Case Report. *J Clin Microbiol* 34: 2601-2603, 1996.

Munk C, Svare EI, Poll P, et al: History of Genital Warts in 10,838 Women 20 to 29 Years of Age from the General Population: Risk Factors and Association With Papanicolaou Smear History. *Sex Transm Dis* 24: 567-572, 1997.

Munkarah A, Malone JM Jr, Budev HD, et al: Mucinous Adenocarcinoma Arising in a Neovagina. *Gynecol Oncol* 52: 272-275, 1994.

Muñoz N, Bosch FX, de Sanjosé S, et al: The Causal Link Between Human Papillomavirus and Invasive Cervical Cancer: A Population-Based Case-Control Study in Columbia and Spain. *Int J Cancer* 52: 743-749, 1992.

Muñoz N, Bosch FX, de Sanjosé S, et al: The Role of HPV in the Etiology of Cervical Cancer. *Mutation Res* 305: 293-301, 1994.,

Muñoz N, Bosch FX: The Causal Link between HPV and Cervical Cancer and Its Implications for Prevention of Cervical Cancer. *Bull Pan Am Health Org* 30: 362-377, 1996.

Muñoz N: Human Papillomavirus and Cancer: The Epidemiological Evidence. *J Clin Virol* 19: 1-5, 2000.

Muñoz N, Franceschi S, Bosetti C, et al: Role of Parity and Human Papillomavirus in Cervical Cancer: The IARC Multicentric Case-Control Study. *Lancet* 359: 1093-1101, 2002.

Muñoz N, Bosch FX, de Sanjosé S, et al: Epidemiologic Classification of Human Papillomavirus Types Associated With Cervical Cancer. *N Engl J Med* 348: 518-527, 2003.

Muntz HG, Ferry JA, Flynn D, et al: Stage IE Primary Malignant Lymphomas of the Uterine Cervix. *Cancer* 68: 2023-2032, 1991.

Muntz HG, Bell DA, Lage JM, et al: Adenocarcinoma In Situ of the Uterine Cervix. *Obstet Gynecol* 80: 935-939, 1992.

Murad TM, Terhart K, Flint A: Atypical Cells in Pregnancy and Postpartum Smears. *Acta Cytol* 25: 623-630, 1981.

Murad TM, August C: Radiation-Induced Atypia: A Review. *Diagn Cytopathol* 1: 137-152, 1985.

Muram D, Curry RH, Drouin P: Cytologic Follow-Up of Patients With Invasive Cervical Carcinoma Treated by Radiotherapy. *Am J Obstet Gynecol* 142: 350-354, 1982.

Murdoch JB, Cassidy LJ, Fletcher K, et al: Histological and Cytological Evidence of Viral Infection and Human Papillomavirus Type 16 DNA Sequences in Cervical Intraepithelial Neoplasia and Normal Tissue in the West of Scotland: Evaluation of Treatment Policy. *Br Med J* 296: 381-385, 1988.

Murphy JF, Allen JM, Jordan JA, et al: Scanning Electron Microscopy of Normal and Abnormal Exfoliated Cervical Squamous Cells. *Br J Obstet Gynaecol* 82: 44-51, 1975.

Murphy JF: The Origins of Cervical Cancer: A Scanning Electron Microscopy Study. *Irish J Med Sci* 146: 315-325, 1977.

Murphy N, Ring M, Killalea AG, et al: p16*INK4a* as a Marker for Cervical Dyskaryosis: CIN and cGIN in Cervical Biopsies and ThinPrep Smears. *J Clin Pathol* 56: 56-63, 2003.

Murthy NS, Mathew A: Risk Factors for Pre-Cancerous Lesions of the Cervix. *Eur J Cancer Prev* 9: 5-14, 2000.

Murty DA, Luthra UK, Sehgal K, et al: Cytologic Detection of *Strongyloides stercoralis* in a Routine Cervicovaginal Smear: A Case Report. *Acta Cytol* 38: 223-225, 1994.

N

Nagai Y, Maehama T, Asato T, et al: Detection of Human Papillomavirus DNA in Primary and Metastatic Lesions of Carcinoma of the Cervix in Women from Okinawa, Japan. *Am J Clin Oncol* 24: 160-166, 2001.

Nahhas WA, Lund CJ, Rudolph JH: Carcinoma of the Corpus Uteri: A 10-Year Review of 225 Patients. *Obstet Gynecol* 38: 564-570, 1971.

Nahmias AJ, Dowdle WR: Antigenic and Biologic Differences in *Herpesvirus hominis*. *Prog Med Virol* 10: 110-159, 1968.

Naib ZM: Single Trophoblastic Cells as a Source of Error in the Interpretation of Routine Vaginal Smears. *Cancer* 14: 1183-1185, 1961a.

Naib ZM, Masukawa N: Identification of *Condyloma acuminata* Cells in Routine Vaginal smears. *Obstet Gynecol* 18: 735-738, 1961b.

Naib ZM: Exfoliative Cytology of Viral Cervico-Vaginitis. *Acta Cytol* 10: 126-129, 1966a.

Naib ZM, Nahmias AJ, Josey WE: Cytology and Histopathology of Cervical Herpes Simplex Infection. *Cancer* 19: 1026-1031, 1966b.

Naib ZM: Cytology of TRIC Agent Infection of the Eye of Newborn Infants and Their Mothers' Genital Tracts. *Acta Cytol* 14: 390-395, 1970.

Nakagawa S, Yoshikawa H, Onda T, et al: Type of Human Papillomavirus Is Related to Clinical Features of Cervical Carcinoma. *Cancer* 78: 1935-1941, 1996.

Namiq AL, Fan F: Chronic Endometritis: An Added Diagnostic Value for Pap Smear (Images in Cytology). *Diagn Cytopathol* 31: 397-398, 2004.

Nand SL, Webster MA, Baber R, et al: Bleeding Pattern and Endometrial Changes During Continuous Combined Hormone Replacement Therapy: The Ogen/Provera Study Group. *Obstet Gynecol* 91: 678-684, 1998.

Nanda K, McCrory DC, Myers ER, et al: Accuracy of the Papanicolaou Test in Screening for and Follow-Up of Cervical Cytologic Abnormalities: A Systematic Review. *Ann Intern Med* 132: 810-819, 2000.

Narayansingh GV, Cumming GP, Dighe S, et al: Invasive Adenocarcinoma of the Vagina Following Surgery for Adenocarinoma In Situ of the Cervix—Recurrence or Implantation? *Int J Gynecol Cancer* 11: 493-495, 2001.

Naryshkin S, Davey DD: Terminology of False Negative and False Positive Pap Smears: "They're Just Worms" (Editorial). *Diagn Cytopathol* 14: 1-3, 1996.

Naryshkin S: Incredibly Low False-Negative Proportion: Watch Out! (Editorial) *Diagn Cytopathol* 22: 63-64, 2000.

Nasca PC, Ellish N, Caputo TA, et al: An Epidemiologic Study of Pap Screening Histories in Women With Invasive Carcinomas of the Uterine Cervix. *N Y State J Med* 91: 152-156, 1991.

Nash JD, Burke TW, Hoskins WJ: Biologic Course of Cervical Human Papillomavirus Infection. *Obstet Gynecol* 69: 160-162, 1987.

Nasiell K, Nasiell M, Vaclavinkova V: Behavior of Moderate Cervical Dysplasia During Long-Term Follow-up. *Obstet Gynecol* 61: 609-614, 1983.

Nasiell K, Roger V, Nasiell M: Behavior of Mild Cervical Dysplasia During Long-Term Follow-up. *Obstet Gynecol* 67: 665-669, 1986.

Nasiell M: Hodgkin's Disease Limited to the Uterine Cervix: A Case Report Including Cytological Findings in the Cervical and Vaginal Smears. *Acta Cytol* 8: 16-18, 1964.

Nassar A, Fleisher SR, Nasuti JF: Value of Histiocyte Detection in Pap Smears for Predicting Endometrial Pathology: An Institutional Experience. *Acta Cytol* 47: 762-767, 2003.

Nasser SM, Cibas ES, Crum CP, et al: The Significance of the Papanicolaou Smear Diagnosis of Low-Grade Squamous Intraepithelial Lesion Cannot Exclude High-Grade Squamous Intraepithelial Lesion. *Cancer (Cancer Cytopathol)* 99: 272-276, 2003.

Nasu I, Meurer W, Fu YS: Endocervical Glandular Atypia and Adenocarcinoma: A Correlation of Cytology and Histology. *Int J Gynecol Pathol* 12: 208-218, 1993.

Nasuti JF, Fleisher SR, Gupta PK: Atypical Glandular Cells of Undetermined Significance (AGUS): Clinical Considerations and Cytohistologic Correlation. *Diagn Cytopathol* 26: 186-190, 2002.

Nauth HF, Boon ME: Significance of the Morphology of Anucleated Squames in the Cytologic Diagnosis of Vulvar Lesions: A New Approach in Diagnostic Cytology. *Acta Cytol* 27: 230-236, 1983.

Navab A, Koss LG, LaDue JS: Estrogen-Like Activity of Digitalis: Its Effect on the Squamous Epithelium of the Female Genital Tract. *JAMA* 194: 142-144, 1965.

Navarro M, Furlani B, Songco L, et al: Cytological Correlates of Benign Versus Dysplastic Abnormal Keratinization. *Diagn Cytopathol* 17: 447-451, 1997.

Nayar M, Chandra M, Chitraratha K, et al: Incidence of Actinomycetes Infection in Women Using Intrauterine Contraceptive Devices. *Acta Cytol* 29: 111-116, 1985.

Nayar R, De Frias DVS: Upgrading ASCUS (Suggestive of HPV) to LSIL: Is There Enough Justification? (Abstract) *Acta Cytol* 43: 917, 1999.

Nayar R, Tabbara SO: Atypical Squamous Cells: Update on Current Concepts. *Clin Lab Med* 23: 605-632, 2003.

Naylor B: Regarding Cyanophilic Bodies, Toxoplasma Cysts and Ferruginous Bodies (Letter). *Acta Cytol* 21: 490-492, 1977.

Naylor B: Perspective in Cytology: From Battle Creek to New Orleans. *Acta Cytol* 32: 613-621, 1988.

Naylor B: Curschmann's Spirals in Pleural and Peritoneal Effusions. *Acta Cytol* 34: 474-478, 1990.

Naylor B, Tasca L, Bartziota E, et al: In Romania It's the *Méthode* Babes-*Papanicolaou. Acta Cytol* 46: 1-12, 2002.

[NCCLS]: *Papanicolaou Technique: Approved Guideline—Second Edition.* NCCLS Document GP15-A2. NCCLS, 940 West Valley Road, Suite 1400, Wayne, Pennsylvania 19087-1898, USA, 1-29, 2001.

[NCHS] National Center for Health Statistics: National Health Interview Survey: United States 1987. *Vital Health Statistics* Series 10: 118, 1987.

[NCI] National Cancer Institute: The 1988 Bethesda System for Reporting Cervical/Vaginal Cytologic Diagnoses. *Acta Cytol* 33: 567-574, 1989a.

[NCI] National Cancer Institute: The 1988 Bethesda System for Reporting Cervical/Vaginal Cytologic Diagnoses. *Diagn Cytopathol* 5: 331-334, 1989b.

[NCI] National Cancer Institute: The 1988 Bethesda System for Reporting Cervical/Vaginal Cytological Diagnoses. *JAMA* 262: 931-934, 1989c.

[NCI] National Cancer Institute: The Revised Bethesda System for Reporting Cervical/Vaginal Cytologic Diagnoses: Report of the 1991 Bethesda Workshop. *Acta Cytol* 36: 273-276, 1992.

[NCI] National Cancer Institute: The Bethesda System for Reporting Cervical/Vaginal Cytologic Diagnoses. *Acta Cytol* 37: 115-124, 1993a.

[NCI] National Cancer Institute: The Bethesda System for Reporting Cervical/Vaginal Cytologic Diagnoses. *Diagn Cytopathol* 9: 235-243, 1993b.

Neal MH, Kline TS: Distraction Index: Part I: The Elusive Trich (Editorial). *Diagn Cytopathol* 21: 367-369, 1999.

Negri G, Menia E, Egarter-Vigl E, et al: Thin Prep Versus Conventional Papanicolaou Smear in the Cytologic Follow-Up of Women With Equivocal Cervical Smears. *Cancer* 99: 342-345, 2003.

Nelson HD, Humphrey LL, Nygren P, et al: Postmenopausal Hormone Replacement Therapy: Scientific Review. *JAMA* 288: 872-881, 2002.

Nelson JH Jr, Averette HE, Richart RM: Cervical Intraepithelial Neoplasia (Dysplasia and Carcinoma In Situ) and Early Invasive Cervical Carcinoma. *Ca: Cancer J Clin* 39: 157-178, 1989.

Nelson RB, Hilberg AW: The Diagnosis of Unsuspected Cancer of the Cervix. *J Natl Cancer Inst* 11: 1081-1089, 1951.

Ness RB, Goodman MT, Shen C, et al: Serologic Evidence of Past Infection With *Chlamydia trachomatis*, in Relation to Ovarian Cancer. *J Infect Dis* 187: 1147-1152, 2003.

Neven P: Tamoxifen and Endometrial Lesions (Commentary). *Lancet* 342: 452, 1993.

Neven P, Vergote I: Controversies Regarding Tamoxifen and Uterine Carcinoma. *Curr Opin Obstet Gynecol* 10: 9-14, 1998.

Newfield L, Bradlow HL, Sepkovic DW, et al: Estrogen Metabolism and the Malignant Potential of Human Papillomavirus Immortalized Keratinocytes. *Proc Soc Exp Biol Med* 217: 322-326, 1998.

Newton ER, Piper JM, Shain RN, et al: Predictors of the Vaginal Microflora. *Am J Obstet Gynecol* 184: 845-855, 2001.

Ng ABP, Reagan JW: Microinvasive Carcinoma of the Uterine Cervix. *Am J Clin Pathol* 52: 511-529, 1969.

Ng ABP, Reagan JW, Lindner EA: The Cellular Manifestations of Primary and Recurrent Herpes Genitalis. *Acta Cytol* 14: 124-129, 1970a.

Ng ABP, Reagan JW, Yen SSC: Herpes Genitalis: Clinical and Cytopathologic Experience With 256 Patients. *Obstet Gynecol* 36: 645-651, 1970b.

Ng ABP, Reagan JW, Lindner EA: The Cellular Manifestation of Microinvasive Squamous Cell Carcinoma of the Uterine Cervix. *Acta Cytol* 16: 5-13, 1972.

Ng ABP, Reagan JW, Cechner RL: The Precursors of Endometrial Cancer: A Study of Their Cellular Manifestations. *Acta Cytol* 17: 439-448, 1973a.

Ng ABP, Reagan JW, Storaasli JP, et al: Mixed Adenosquamous Carcinoma of the Endometrium. *Am J Clin Pathol* 59: 765-781, 1973b.

Ng ABP: The Cellular Detection of Endometrial Carcinoma and Its Precursors. *Gynecol Oncol* 2: 162-179, 1974a.

Ng ABP, Reagan JW, Hawliczek S, Wentz BW: Significance of Endometrial Cells in the Detection of Endometrial Carcinoma and Its Precursors. *Acta Cytol* 18: 356-361, 1974b.

Ng ABP, Teeple D, Linder EA, et al: The Cellular Manifestations of Extrauterine Cancer. *Acta Cytol* 18: 108-117, 1974c.

Ng ABP, Reagan JW, Hawliczek S, et al: Cellular Detection of Vaginal Adenosis. *Obstet Gynecol* 46: 323-328, 1975.

Ng ABP, Reagan JW, Nadjii M, et al: Natural History of Vaginal Adenosis in Women Exposed to Diethylstilbestrol *in utero. J Reprod Med* 18: 1-13, 1977.

Ng W-K: Non-Small Cell Carcinoma of the Lung Metastatic to the Lower Female Genital Tract and Mimicking Glassy Cell Carcinoma (Letter). *Acta Cytol* 46: 438-440, 2002a.

Ng W-K, Cheung LKN, Li, ASM, et al: Transitional Cell Metaplasia of the Uterine Cervix Is Related to Human Papillomavirus: Molecular Analysis in Seven Patients With Cytohistologic Correlation. *Cancer (Cancer Cytopathol)* 96: 250-258, 2002b.

Ng W-K, Cheung LKN, Li ASM: Thin-Layer Cytology Findings of Small Cell Carcinoma of the Lower Female Genital Tract: Review of Three Cases With Molecular Analysis. *Acta Cytol* 47: 56-64, 2003a.

Ng W-K, Cheung LKN, Li ASM: Warty (Condylomatous) Carcinoma of the Cervix: A Review of 3 Cases With Emphasis on Thin-Layer Cytology and Molecular Analysis for HPV. *Acta Cytol* 47: 159-166, 2003b.

Ng W-K, Li ASM, Cheung LKN: Significance of Atypical Repair in Liquid-Based Gynecologic Cytology: A Follow-Up Study With Molecular Analysis for Human Papillomavirus. *Cancer (Cancer Cytopathol)* 99: 141-148, 2003c.

Ng W-K: Thin-Layer (Liquid-Based) Cytologic Findings of Papillary Squamotransitional Cell Carcinoma of the Cervix: Review of Cases Over a 4-Year Period With Emphasis on Potential Diagnostic Pitfalls. *Acta Cytol* 47: 141-148, 2003d.

Ng W-K: Thin-Layer Cytology Findings of Papillary Adenosquamous Carcinoma of the Cervix: Report of a Case With Histologic Correlation and Molecular Analysis. *Acta Cytol* 47: 649-656, 2003e.

Ng W-K, Cheung LK, Li AS: Liquid-Based Cytology Findings of Glassy Cell Carcinoma of the Cervix: Report of a Case With Histologic Correlation and Molecular Analysis. *Acta Cytol* 48: 99-106, 2004.

Ngadiman S, Yang GCH: Adenomyomatous, Lower Uterine Segment and Endocervical Polyps in Cervicovaginal Smears. *Acta Cytol* 39: 643-647, 1995.

Ngelangel C, Muñoz N, Bosch FX, et al: Causes of Cervical Cancer in the Philippines: A Case-Control Study *J Natl Cancer Inst* 90: 43-49, 1998.

Nguyen G-K: Exfoliative Cytology of Microinvasive Squamous-Cell Carcinoma of the Uterine Cervix: A Retrospective Study of 42 Cases. *Acta Cytol* 28: 457-460, 1984a.

Nguyen G-K, Jeannot AB: Exfoliative Cytology of In Situ and Microinvasive Adenocarcinoma of the Uterine Cervix. *Acta Cytol* 28: 461-467, 1984b.

Nguyen G-K, Daya DE: Cervical Adenocarcinoma and Related Lesions: Cytodiagnostic Criteria and Pitfalls. *Pathol Annu*(Pt 2) 28: 53-75, 1993.

Nguyen G-K, Nguyen-Ho P, Husain M, et al: Cervical Squamous Cell Carcinoma and Its Precursor Lesions: Cytodiagnostic Criteria and Pitfalls. *Anat Pathol* (Annual) 1: 139-164, 1996.

Nguyen G-K, Daya D: Exfoliative Cytology of Papillary Serous Adenocarcinomas of the Uterine Cervix (Letter). *Diagn Cytopathol* 16: 548-550, 1997.

Nguyen HN, Nordqvist SRB: The Bethesda System and Evaluation of Abnormal Pap Smears. *Semin Surg Oncol* 16: 217-221, 1999.

Nguyen TN, Bourdeau J-L, Ferenczy A, et al: Clinical Significance of Histiocytes in the Detection of Endometrial Adenocarcinoma and Hyperplasia. *Diagn Cytopathol* 19: 89-93, 1998.

Nichols GE, Williams ME, Gaffey MJ, et al: Cyclin *D1* Gene Expression in Human Cervical Neoplasia. *Mod Pathol* 9: 418-425, 1996.

Nichols TM, Boyes DA, Fidler HK: Advantages of Routine Step Serial Sectioning of Cervical Cone Biopsies. *Am J Clin Pathol* 49: 342-346, 1968.

Nichols TM, Fidler HK: Microglandular Hyperplasia in Cervical Cone Biopsies Taken for Suspicious and Positive Cytology. *Am J Clin Pathol* 56: 424-429, 1971.

Nicklin JL, Wright RG, Bell JR, et al: A Clinicopathological Study of Adenocarcinoma In Situ of the Cervix: The Influence of Cervical HPV Infection and Other Factors, and the Role of Conservative Surgery. *Aust NZ J Obstet Gynecol* 31: 179-183, 1991.

Nicklin JL, Perrin LC, Crandon AJ, et al: Microinvasive Adenocarcinoma of the Cervix. *Aust NZ J Obstet Gynecol* 39: 411-413, 1999.

Nicklin JL, Perrin L, Obermair A, et al: The Significance of Psammoma Bodies on Cervical Cytology Smears. *Gynecol Oncol* 83: 6-9, 2001.

Nieh S, Chen S-F, Chu T-Y, et al: Expression of p16^{INK4a} in Pap Smears Containing Atypical Glandular Cells From the Uterine Cervix. *Acta Cytol* 48: 173-180, 2004.

Nielsen AL: Human Papillomavirus Type 16/18 in Uterine Cervical Adenocarcinoma In Situ and Adenocarcinoma: A Study by In Situ Hybridization With Biotinylated DNA Probes. *Cancer* 65: 2588-2593, 1990.

Nielsen GP, Young RH: Mesenchymal Tumors and Tumor-Like Lesions of the Female Genital Tract: A Selective Review With Emphasis on Recently Described Entities. *Int J Gynecol Pathol* 20: 105-127, 2001.

Nielsen ML, Davey DD, Kline TS: Specimen Adequacy Evaluation in Gynecologic Cytopathology: Current Laboratory Practice in the College of American Pathologists Interlaboratory Comparison Program and Tentative Guidelines for Future Practice. *Diagn Cytopathol* 9: 394-403, 1993.

Niemann TH, Goetz SP, Benda JA, et al: Malignant Rhabdoid Tumor of the Uterus: Report of a Case With Findings in a Cervical Smear. *Diagn Cytopathol* 10: 54-59, 1994.

Nieminen P, Kallio M, Hakama M: The Effect of Mass Screening on Incidence and Mortality of Squamous and Adenocarcinoma of Cervix Uteri. *Obstet Gynecol* 85: 1017-1021, 1995.

Nilsson K, Risberg B, Heimer G: The Vaginal Epithelium in the Postmenopause—Cytology, Histology and pH as Methods of Assessment. *Maturitas* 21: 51-56, 1995.

Nobbenhuis MA, Walboomers JM, Helmerhort TJ, et al: Relation of Human Papillomavirus Status to Cervical Lesions and Consequences for Cervial Cancer Screening: A Prospective Study. *Lancet* 354: 20-25, 1999.

Nobbenhuis MAE, Helmerhorst TJM, van den Brule AJC, et al: Cytological Regression and Clearance of High-Risk Human Papillomavirus in Women With an Abnormal Cervical Smear (Research Letter). *Lancet* 358: 1782-1783, 2001.

Noda K, Kimura K, Ikeda M: Studies on the Histogenesis of Cervical Adenocarcinoma. *Int J Gynecol Pathol* 1: 336-346, 1983.

Noel J, Lespagnard L, Fayt I, et al: Evidence of Human Papilloma Virus Infection but Lack of Epstein-Barr Virus in Lymphoepithelioma-Like Carcinoma of Uterine Cervix: Report of Two Cases and Review of the Literature. *Hum Pathol* 32: 135-138, 2001.

Nold JL: Cervical Neoplasia: History—Screening—Diagnosis—Treatment. *So Dakota J Med* 51: 113-119, 1998.

Noller KL, O'Brien PC, Melton LJ III, et al: Coital Risk Factors for Cervical Cancer: Sexual Activity Among White Middle Class Women. *Am J Clin Oncol* 10: 222-226, 1987.

Noller KL: In Defense of the Pap Smear (Editorial). *Obstet Gynecol Surv* 53: 261, 1998.

Noller KL, Bibace R: The Centrality of the Clinician in the Evaluation of Patients With Abnormal Cervical Cytologic Studies. *Am J Obstet Gynecol* 187: 1533-1535, 2002.

Noller KL, Bettes B, Zinberg S, et al: Cervical Cytology Screening Practices Among Obstetrician-Gynecologists. *Obstet Gynecol* 102: 259-265, 2003.

Nonogaki H, Fujii S, Konishi I, et al: Estrogen Receptor Localization in Normal and Neoplastic Epithelium of the Uterine Cervix. *Cancer* 66: 2620-2627, 1990.

Norris HJ, Taylor HB: Postirradiation Sarcomas of the Uterus. *Obstet Gynecol* 26: 689-694, 1965.

Noumoff JS: Atypia in Cervical Cytology as a Risk Factor for Intraepithelial Neoplasia. *Am J Obstet Gynecol* 156: 628-631, 1987.

Novak PM, Kumar NB, Naylor B: Curschmann's Spirals in Cervicovaginal Smears: Prevalence, Morphology, Significance and Origin. *Acta Cytol* 28: 5-8, 1984.

Novotny DB, Maygarden SJ, Johnson DE, et al: Tubal Metaplasia: A Frequent Potential Pitfall in the Cytologic Diagnosis of Endocervical Glandular Dysplasia on Cervical Smears. *Acta Cytol* 36: 1-10, 1992.

Novotny DB, Ferlisi P: Villoglandular Adenocarcinoma of the Cervix: Cytologic Presentation. *Diagn Cytopathol* 17: 383-387, 1997.

Nowak JA: Telomerase, Cervical Cancer, and Human Papillomavirus. *Clin Lab Med* 20: 369-381, 2000.

Nucci MR: Symposium Part III: Tumor-Like Glandular Lesions of the Uterine Cervix. *Int J Gynecol Pathol* 21: 347-359, 2002.

Nugent RP, Krohn MA, Hillier SL: Reliability of Diagnosing Bacterial Vaginosis Is Improved by a Standardized Method of Gram Stain Interpretation. *J Clin Microbiol* 29: 297-301, 1991.

Nuñez C, Abdul-Karim FW, Somrak TM: Glassy-Cell Carcinoma of the Cervix: Cytopathologic and Histopathologic Study of Five Cases. *Acta Cytol* 29: 303-309, 1985.

Nuovo GJ, Nuovo MA, Cottral S, et al: Histological Correlates of Clinically Occult Human Papillomavirus Infection of the Uterine Cervix. *Am J Surg Pathol* 12: 198-204, 1988.

Nuovo GJ, Cottral S, Richart RM: Occult Human Papillomavirus Infection of the Uterine Cervix in Postmenopausal Women. *Am J Obstet Gynecol* 160: 340-344, 1989.

Nuovo GJ: Blanco JS, Leipzig S, et al: Human Papillomavirus Detection in Cervical Lesions Nondiagnostic for Cervical Intraepithelial Neoplasia: Correlation With Papanicolaou Smear, Colposcopy, and Occurrence of Cervical Intraepithelial Neoplasia. *Obstet Gynecol* 75: 1006-1011, 1990a.

Nuovo GJ, Pedemonte BM: Human Papillomavirus Types and Recurrent Cervical Warts. *JAMA* 263: 1223-1226, 1990b.

Nuovo GJ, Babury R, Calayag PT: Human Papillomavirus Types and Recurrent Cervical Warts in Immunocompromised Women. *Mod Pathol* 4: 632-636, 1991a.

Nuovo GJ, Walsh LL, Gentile JL, et al: Correlation of the Papanicolaou Smear and Human Papillomavirus Type in Women With Biopsy-Proven Cervical Squamous Intraepithelial Lesions. *Am J Clin Pathol* 96: 544-548, 1991b.

Nuovo GJ: Detection of Human Papillomavirus in Papanicolaou Smears: Correlation With Pathologic Findings and Clinical Outcome. *Diagn Mol Pathol* 7: 158-163, 1998.

Nuovo GJ: The Role of Human Papillomavirus in Gynecological Diseases. *Crit Rev Clin Lab Sci* 37: 183-215, 2000.

Nygard JF, Sauer T, Skjeldestad FE, et al: CIN 2/3 and Cervical Cancer After an ASCUS Pap Smear: A 7-Year, Prospective Study of the Norwegian Population-Based, Coordinated Screening Program. *Acta Cytol* 47: 991-1000, 2003.

Nyirjesy I: Atypical or Suspicious Cervical Smears: An Aggressive Diagnostic Approach. *JAMA* 222: 691-693, 1972.

Nyirjesy, I, Billingsley FS, Forman MR: Evaluation of Atypical and Low-Grade Cervical Cytology in Private Practice. *Obstet Gynecol* 92: 601-607, 1998.

Nyirjesy I: RE: Natural History of Dysplasia of the Uterine Cervix (Letter). *J Natl Cancer Inst* 91: 1420-1421, 1999.

O

Obenson K, Abreo F, Grafton WD: Cytophistologic Correlation Between AGUS and Biopsy-Detected Lesions in Postmenopausal Women. *Acta Cytol* 44: 41-45, 2000.

Ocana V, Nader-Macias ME: Adhesion of Lactobacillus Vaginal Strains With Probiotic Properties to Vaginal Epithelial Cells. *Biocell* 25: 265-273, 2001.

Oda H, Kumar S, Howley PM: Regulation of the Src Family Tyrosine Kinase Blk Through E6AP-Mediated Ubiquitination. *Proc Natl Acad Sci (USA)* 96: 9557-9562, 1999.

Oda K, Okada S, Nei T, et al: Cytodiagnostic Problems in Uterine Sarcoma: Analysis According to a Novel Classification of Tumor Growth Types. *Acta Cytol* 48: 181-186, 2004.

Ohwada M, Suzuki M, Ohno T, et al: Appearance of Primary Endometrial and Ovarian Clear Cell Adenocarcinoma 17 Months Postpartum: A Case Report. *Acta Cytol* 42: 765-768, 1998.

Ohwada M, Suzuki M, Onagawa T, et al: Primary Malignant Lymphoma of the Uterine Corpus Diagnosed by Endometrial Cytology: A Case Report. *Acta Cytol* 44: 1045-1049, 2000.

Okagaki T, Lerch V, Younge PA, et al: Diagnosis of Anaplasia and Carcinoma In Situ by Differential Cell Counts. *Acta Cytol* 6: 343-347, 1962.

Okagaki T, Meyer AA, Sciarra JJ: Prognosis of Irradiated Carcinoma of Cervix Uteri and Nuclear DNA in Cytologic Postirradiation Dysplasia. *Cancer* 33: 647-652, 1974.

Okagaki T, Clark BE, Zachow KR, et al: Presence of Human Papillomavirus in Verrucous Carcinoma (Ackerman) of the Vagina: Immunocytochemical, Ultrastructural and DNA Hybridization Studies. *Arch Pathol Lab Med* 108: 567-570, 1984.

Okagaki T, Tase T, Twiggs LB, et al: Histogenesis of Cervical Adenocarcinoma With Reference to Human Papillomavirus-18 as a Carcinogen. *J Reprod Med* 34: 639-644, 1989.

Okagaki T: Impact of Human Papillomavirus Research on the Histopathologic Concepts of Genital Neoplasms. *Curr Topics Pathol* 85: 273-307, 1992.

Okuyama T, Takahashi R, Mori M, et al: Polymerase Chain Reaction Amplification of *Trichomonas vaginalis* DNA from Papanicolaou-Stained Smears. *Diagn Cytopathol* 19: 437-440, 1998.

Olaharski AJ, Eastmond DA: Elevated Levels of Tetraploid Cervical Cells in Human Papillomavirus-Positive Papanicolaou Smears Diagnosed as Atypical Squamous Cells of Undetermined Significance. *Cancer (Cancer Cytopathol)* 102: 192-199, 2004.

Oliveira ERZM, Derchain SFM, Rabelo-Santos SH, et al: Detection of High-Risk Human Papillomavirus (HPV) DNA by Hybrid Capture II in Women Referred Due to Atypical Glandular Cells in the Primary Screening. *Diagn Cytopathol* 31: 19-22, 2004.

Ollayos CW: Update on the Papanicolaou Smear: New Issues for the 1990s. *Mil Med* 162: 521-523, 1997.

Olmsted SS, Dubin NH, Cone RA, et al: The Rate at Which Human Sperm Are Immobilized and Killed by Mild Acidity. *Fertility Sterility* 73: 687-693, 2000.

Olsen TG, Nycum LR, Graham L, et al: Primary Peritoneal Carcinoma Presenting on Routine Papanicolaou Smear. *Gynecol Oncol* 78: 71-73, 2000.

Ong C-K, Chan S-Y, Campo MS, et al: Evolution of Human Papillomavirus Type 18: An Ancient Phylogenetic Root in Africa and Intratype Diversity Reflect Coevolution With Human Ethnic Groups. *J Virol* 67: 6424-6431, 1993.

Opjorden SL, Caudill JL, Humphrey SK, et al: Small Cells in Cervical-Vaginal Smears of Patients Treated With Tamoxifen. *Cancer (Cancer Cytopathol)* 93: 23-28, 2001.

Ordóñez NG: Value of Thyroid Transcription Factor-1 Immunostaining in Distinguishing Small Cell Lung Carcinomas from Other Small Cell Carcinomas. *Am J Surg Pathol* 24: 1217-1223, 2000.

Oriel JD: Natural History of Genital Warts. *Br J Vener Dis* 47: 1-13, 1971.

Orr JW Jr, Shingleton HM, Gore H, et al: Cervical Intraepithelial Neoplasia Associated With Exposure to Diethylstilbestrol *in utero*: A Clinical and Pathologic Study. *Obstet Gynecol* 58: 75-82, 1981.

Orr JW Jr, Barrett JM, Orr PF, et al: The Efficacy and Safety of the Cytobrush During Pregnancy. *Gynecol Oncol* 44: 260-262, 1992.

Orr JW Jr: Cervical Cancer. *Surg Oncol Clin North Am* 7: 299-316, 1998.

Ortega-Gonzalez P, Chanona-Vilchis J, Dominguez-Malagon H: Transitional Cell Carcinoma of the Uterine Cervix: A Report of Six Cases With Clinical, Histologic and Cytologic Findings. *Acta Cytol* 46: 585-590, 2002.

Ortner A, Klammer J, Geir W: Cytology at the End of Pregnancy: Significance of Determinations of the Eosinophilic and Karyopyknotic Indices. *Acta Cytol* 21: 429-431, 1977.

Osborne NG, Grubin L, Pratson L: Vaginitis in Sexually Active Women: Relationship to Nine Sexually Transmitted Organisms. *Am J Obstet Gynecol* 142: 962-967, 1982.

Osset J, Bartolomé RM, Garcia E, et al: Assessment of the Capacity of *Lactobacillus* to Inhibit the Growth of Uropathogens and Block Their Adhesion to Vaginal Epithelial Cells. *J Infect Dis* 183: 485-491, 2001.

O'Sullivan JP, Ismail SM, Barnes WS, et al: Interobserver Variation in the Diagnosis and Grading of Dyskaryosis in Cervical Smears: Specialist Cytopathologists Compared With Non-Specialists. *J Clin Pathol* 47: 515-518, 1994.

O'Sullivan JP, Ismail SM, Barnes WS, et al: Inter- and Intra-Observer Variation in the Reporting of Cervical Smears: Specialist Cytopathologists Versus Histopathologists. *Cytopathology* 7: 78-89, 1996.

O'Sullivan JP: Observer Variation in Gynaecological Cytopathology. *Cytopathology* 9: 6-14, 1998a.

O'Sullivan JP, A'Hern RP, Chapman PA, et al: A Case Control Study of True Positive Versus False Negative Smears in Women With Cervical Intraepithelial Neoplasia (CIN) III. *Cytopathology* 9: 155-161, 1998b.

O'Sullivan JP, Chapman PA, Jenkins L, et al: Characteristics of High-Grade Dyskaryotic Cervical Smears Likely to Be Missed on Rapid Rescreening. *Acta Cytol* 44: 37-40, 2000.

Östör AG, Pagano R, Davoren RAM, et al: Adenocarcinoma In Situ of the Cervix. *Int J Gynecol Pathol* 3: 179-190, 1984.

Östör AG: Natural History of Cervical Intraepithelial Neoplasia: A Critical Review. *Int J Gynecol Pathol* 12: 186-192, 1993a.

Östör AG: Studies on 200 Cases of Early Squamous Cell Carcinoma of the Cervix. *Int J Gynecol Pathol* 12: 193-207, 1993b.

Östör AG, Rome R, Quinn M: Microinvasive Adenocarcinoma of the Cervix: A Clinicopathologic Study of 77 Women. *Obstet Gynecol* 89: 88-93, 1997.

Östör AG: Early Invasive Adenocarcinoma of the Uterine Cervix. *Int J Gynecol Pathol* 10: 29-38, 2000a.

Östör AG. Duncan A, Quinn M, et al: Adenocarcinoma In Situ of the Uterine Cervix: An Experience With 100 Cases. *Gynecol Oncol* 79: 207-210, 2000b.

Ou C-Y, Chang J-G, Tseng H-H, et al: Analysis of Microsatellite Instability in Cervical Cancer. *Int J Gynecol Cancer* 9: 67-71, 1999.

Ouwerkerk-Noordam E, Boon ME, Beck S: Computer-Assisted Primary Screening of Cervical Smears Using the PAPNET Method: Comparison With Conventional Screening and Evaluation of the Role of the Cytologist. *Cytopathology* 5: 211-218, 1994.

Ozkan F, Ramzy I, Mody DR: Glandular Lesions of the Cervix on Thin-Layer Pap Tests: Validity of Cytologic Criteria Used in Identifying Significant Lesions. *Acta Cytol* 48: 372-379, 2004.

Özsaran AA, Ates T, Dikmen Y, et al: Evaluation of the Risk of Cervical Intraepithelial Neoplasia and Human Papilloma Virus Infection in Renal Transplant Patients Receiving Immunosuppressive Therapy. *Eur J Gynaecol Oncol* 20: 127-130, 1999.

P

Paalman RJ. Counseller VS: Cylindroma of the Cervix With Procidentia. *Am J Obstet Gynecol* 58: 184-187, 1949.

Paavonen J, Vesterinen E, Meyer B, et al: Genital *Chlamydia trachomatis* Infections in Patients With Cervical Atypia. *Obstet Gynecol* 54: 289-291, 1979.

Paavonen J, Purola E: Cytologic Findings in Cervical Chlamydial Infection. *Med Biol* 58: 174-178, 1980.

Paavonen J, Vesterinen E, Meyer B, et al: Colposcopic and Histologic Findings in Cervical Chlamydial Infection. *Obstet Gynecol* 59: 712-715, 1982.

Paavonen J: Physiology and Ecology of the Vagina. *Scand J Infect Dis* Supplementum 40: 31-35, 1983.

Paavonen J, Kiviat NB, Wölner-Hanssen P, et al: Significance of Mild Cervical Cytologic Atypia in a Sexually Transmitted Disease Clinic Population. *Acta Cytol* 33: 831-838, 1989.

Paavonen J: Vulvodynia—A Complex Syndrome of Vulvar Pain. *Acta Obstet Gynecol Scand* 74: 243-247, 1995.

Pacey F, Ayer B, Greenberg M: The Cytologic Diagnosis of Adenocarcinoma In Situ of the Cervix Uteri and Related Lesions. III. Pitfalls in Diagnosis. *Acta Cytol* 32: 325-330, 1988.

Pacsa AS, Kummerländer L, Pejtsik B, et al: Herpesvirus Antibodies and Antigens in Patients With Cervical Anaplasia and in Controls. *J Natl Cancer Inst* 55: 775-781, 1975.

Pairwuti S: False Negative Papanicolaou Smears from Women With Cancerous and Precancerous Lesions of the Uterine Cervix. *Acta Cytol* 35: 40-46, 1991.

Pajtler M, Milojkovic M, Mrcela M: An Exophytic Lesion of the Vagina: Cytological Findings. *Cytopathology* 14: 150-152, 2003.

Pak HY, Yokota SB, Paladugu RR, et al: Glassy Cell Carcinoma of the Cervix: Cytologic and Clinicopathologic Analysis. *Cancer* 52: 307-312, 1983.

Palefsky J: Human Papillomavirus Infection Among HIV-Infected Individuals. Implications for Development of Malignant Tumors. *Hematol Oncol Clin North Am* 5: 357-370, 1991.

Paler RJ Jr, Simpson DR, Kaye AM, et al: The Relationship of Inflammation in the Papanicolaou Smear to *Chlamydia trachomatis* Infection in a High-Risk Population. *Contraception* 61: 231-234, 2000.

Pambuccian SE, Bachowski GJ, Twigs LB: Signet Ring Cell Lobular Carcinoma of the Breast Presenting in a Cervicovaginal Smear: A Case Report. *Acta Cytol* 44: 824-830, 2000.

Pan Q, Belinson JL, Li L, et al: A Thin-Layer, Liquid-Based Pap Test for Mass Screening in an Area of China With a High Incidence of Cervical Carcinoma: A Cross-Sectional, Comparative Study. *Acta Cytol* 47: 45-50, 2003.

Pandit AA, Klhilnani PH, Powar HS, et al: Value of Papanicolaou Smear in Detection of *Chlamydia trachomatis* Infection. *Diagn Cytopathol* 9: 164-167, 1993.

Panos JC, Jones BA, Mazzara PF: Usefulness of Concurrent Papanicolaou Smear at Time of Cervical Biopsy. *Diagn Cytopathol* 25: 270-273, 2001.

Pantanowitz L, Upton MP, Wang HH, et al: Cytomorphology of Verrucous Carcinoma of the Cervix: A Case Report. *Acta Cytol* 47: 1050-1054, 2003.

Pánuco CAB, Rodríguez ID, Méndez JTH, et al: Detection of *Chlamydia trachomatis* in Pregnant Women by the Papanicolaou Technique, Enzyme Immunoassay and Polymerase Chain Reaction. *Acta Cytol* 44: 114-123, 2000.

Pao CC, Tsai PL, Chang Y-L, et al: Non-Sexual Papillomavirus Transmission Routes (Letter). *Lancet* 339: 1479-1480, 1992.

Papanicolaou GN: The Diagnosis of Early Human Pregnancy by the Vaginal Smear Method. *Proc Soc Exp Biol Med* 22: 436-437, 1925.

Papanicolaou GN: New Cancer Diagnosis. *Proceedings of the Third Race Betterment Conference.* Battle Creek, Michigan, 528-534, 1928.

Papanicolaou GN: The Sexual Cycle in the Human Female as Revealed by Vaginal Smears. *Am J Anat* 52: 519-637, 1933.

Papanicolaou GN, Ripley HS, Shorr E: Suppressive Action of Testosterone Propionate on Menstruation and Its Effect on Vaginal Smears. *Endocrintology* 24: 339-346, 1939.

Papanicolaou GN, Traut HF: The Diagnostic Value of Vaginal Smears in Carcinoma of the Uterus. *Am J Obstet Gynecol* 42: 193-206, 1941.

Papanicolaou GN: A New Procedure for Staining Vaginal Smears. *Science* 95: 438-439, 1942.

Papanicolaou GN, Traut HF: *Diagnosis of Uterine Cancer by the Vaginal Smear.* New York. The Commonwealth Fund, 1943.

Papanicolaou GN: A General Survey of the Vaginal Smear and Its Use in Research and Diagnosis. *Am J Obstet Gynecol* 51: 316-328, 1946.

Papanicolaou GN: Diagnosis of Pregnancy by Cytologic Criteria in Catheterized Urine. *Proc Soc Exp Biol Med* 67: 247-249, 1948.

Papanicolaou GN: A Survey of the Actualities and Potentialities of Exfoliative Cytology in Cancer Diagnosis. *Ann Intern Med* 31: 661-674, 1949.

Papanicolaou GN: Observations on the Origin and Specific Function of the Histiocytes in the Female Genital Tract. *Fertility Sterility* 4: 472-478, 1953.

Papanicolaou GN: *Atlas of Exfoliative Cytology.* The Commonwealth Fund by Harvard University Press, Cambridge, MA, 1954.

Papanicolaou GN: The Evolutionary Dynamics and Trends of Exfoliative Cytology. *Texas Rep Biol Med* 13: 901-919, 1955a.

Papanicolaou GN, Wolinska WH: Vaginal Cytology in Trichomonas Infestation (Symposium on Trichomoniasis—Part I). *Intl Rec Med* 168: 551-556, 1955b.

Papanicolaou GN: Degenerative Changes in Ciliated Cells Exfoliating from the Bronchial Epithelium as a Cytologic Criterion in the Diagnosis of Diseases of the Lung. *NY State J Med* 56: 2647-2650, 1956.

Papanicolaou GN: Historical Development of Cytology as a Tool in Clinical Medicine and in Cancer Research. *Acta Unio Internat Cancr, Louvain* 14: 249-254, 1958.

Papillo JL, Zarka MA, St John TL: Evaluation of the ThinPrep Pap Test in Clinical Practice: A Seven-Month, 16,314-Case Experience in Northern Vermont. *Acta Cytol* 42: 203-208, 1998.

Paraiso MF, Brady K, Helmchen R, et al: Evaluation of the Endocervical Cytobrush and Cervex-Brush in Pregnant Women. *Obstet Gynecol* 84: 539-543, 1994.

Parashari A, Singh V, Gupta MM, et al: Significance of Inflammatory Cervical Smears. *APMIS* 103: 273-278, 1995.

Paraskevaidis E, Kitchener HC, Miller ID, et al: A Population-Based Study of Microinvasive Disease of the Cervix—A Colposcopic and Cytologic Analysis. *Gynecol Oncol* 45: 9-12, 1992.

Paraskevaidis E, Koliopoulos G, Alamanos Y, et al: Human Papillomavirus Testing and the Outcome of Treatment for Cervical Intraepithelial Neoplasia. *Obstet Gynecol* 98: 833-836, 2001.

Parazzini F, LaVecchia C, Negri E, et al: Risk Factors for Adenocarcinoma of the Cervix: A Case-Control Study. *Br J Cancer* 57: 201-204, 1988.

Parazzini F, LaVecchia C, Negri E, et al: Reproductive Factors and the Risk of Invasive and Intraepithelial Cervical Neoplasia. *Br J Cancer* 59: 805-809, 1989.

Parazzini F, LaVecchia C: Epidemiology of Adenocarcinoma of the Cervix. *Gynecol Oncol* 39: 40-46, 1990a.

Parazzini F, LaVecchia C, Negri E, et al: Oral Contraceptive Use and Invasive Cervical Cancer. *Int J Epidemiol* 19: 259-263, 1990b.

Parazzini F, Sideri M, Restelli S, et al: Determinants of High-Grade Dysplasia Among Women With Mild Dyskaryosis on Cervical Smear. *Obstet Gynecol* 86: 754-757, 1995.

Parellada CI, Schivartche PL, Pereyra EA, et al: Atypical Glandular Cells on Cervical Smears. *Int J Gynaecol Obstet* 78: 227-234, 2002.

Parham GP, Hicks ML: Race as a Factor in the Outcome of Patients With Cervical Cancer: Lift the Veil to Find the Wounded Spirit. *Gynecol Oncol* 71: 149-150, 1998.

Park JJ, Genest DR, Sun D, et al: Atypical Immature Metaplastic-Like Proliferations of the Cervix: Diagnostic Reproducibility and Viral (HPV) Correlates. *Hum Pathol* 30: 1161-1165, 1999.

Park JS, Namkoong SE, Lee HY, et al: Detection of Human Papillomavirus Genotypes in Cervical Neoplasia from Korean Women Using Polymerase Chain Reaction. *Gynecol Oncol* 41: 129-134, 1991.

Park TW, Fujiwara H, Wright TC: Molecular Biology of Cervical Cancer and Its Precursors. *Cancer* 76: 1902-1913, 1995.

Park TW, Richart RM, Sun X-W, et al: Association Between Human Papillomavirus Type and Clonal Status of Cervical Squamous Intraepithelial Lesions. *J Natl Cancer Inst* 88: 355-358, 1996.

Parkash V, Chacho MS: Psammoma Bodies in Cervicovaginal Smears: Incidence and Significance. *Diagn Cytopathol* 26: 81-86, 2002.

Parker JC, van Nagell JR, Bissig T: The Histomorphologic Spectrum of Endocervical (Müllerian) Adenocarcinoma—A Potential Prognostic Indicator. *J Surg Oncol* 9: 267-275, 1977.

Parker JE: Cytologic Findings Associated With Previous Uterine Malignancies of Mixed Cell Types (Malignant Mixed Müllerian Tumor). *Acta Cytol* 8: 316-320, 1964.

Parker MF, Arroyo GF, Geradts J, et al: Molecular Characterization of Adenocarcinoma of the Cervix. *Gynecol Oncol* 64: 242-251, 1997.

Parkin DM, Nguyen-Dinh X, Day NE: The Impact of Screening on the Incidence of Cervical Cancer in England and Wales. *Br J Obstet Gynaecol* 92: 150-157, 1985.

Parkin DM, Läärä E, Muir CS: Estimates of the Worldwide Frequency of Sixteen Major Cancers in 1980. *Int J Cancer* 41: 184-197, 1988.

Parkin DM, Pisani P, Ferlay J: Global Cancer Statistics. *CA: Cancer J Clin* 49: 33-64, 1999a.

Parkin DM, Pisani P, Ferlay J: Estimates of the Worldwide Incidence of 25 Major Cancers in 1990. *Int J Cancer* 80: 827-841, 1999b.

Parsons L, Taymor ML: Carcinoma of the Breast Metastatic to the Peritoneum as a Source of Positive Vaginal Smears. *Am J Obstet Gynecol* 66: 194-196, 1953.

Parsons WL, Godwin M, Robbins C, et al: Prevalence of Cervical Pathogens in Women With and Without Inflammatory Changes on Smear Testing. *Br Med J* 306: 1173-1174, 1993.

Partridge E: NCCN Practice Guidelines for Cervical Cancer Screening. *Oncology* 13: 550-574, 1999.

Pasetto N, Sesti F, De Santis L, et al: The Prevalence of HPV16 DNA in Normal and Pathological Cervical Scrapes Using the Polymerase Chain Reaction. *Gynecol Oncol* 46: 33-36, 1992.

Patel D, Gillespie B, Foxman B: Sexual Behavior of Older Women: Results of a Random-Digit-Dialing Survey of 2000 Women in the United States. *Sex Transm Dis* 30: 216-220, 2003.

Patel JK, Didolkar MS, Pickren JW, et al: Metastatic Pattern of Malignant Melanoma: A Study of 216 Autopsy Cases. *Am J Surg* 135: 807-810, 1978.

Pater A, Bayatpour M, Pater MM: Oncogenic Transformation by Human Papillomavirus Type 16 Deoxyribonucleic Acid in the Presence of Progesterone or Progestins from Oral Contraceptives. *Am J Obstet Gynecol* 162: 1099-1103, 1990.

Pater MM, Hughes GA, Hyslop DE, et al: Glucocorticoid-Dependent Oncogenic Transformation by Type 16 but Not Type 11 Human Papilloma Virus DNA. *Nature* 335: 832-835, 1988.

Paterson BA, Tabrizi SN, Garland SN, et al: The Tampon Test for Trichomoniasis: A Comparison Between Conventional Methods and a Polymerase Chain Reaction for *Trichomonas vaginalis* in Women. *Sex Transm Infect* 74: 136-139, 1998.

Paterson MEL, Peel KR, Joslin CAF: Cervical Smear Histories of 500 Women With Invasive Cervical Cancer in Yorkshire. *Br Med J* 289: 896-898, 1984.

Patsner B: Atypical (Favor Neoplastic) Glandular Cells of Undetermined Significance: Report of Two Cases of Occult Adnexal Malignancy in Patients With "Negative" Workups. *J Low Genital Tract Dis* 6: 1-3, 2002.

Patten SF Jr, Reagan JW, Obenauf M, et al: Postirradiation Dysplasia of Uterine Cervix and Vagina: An Analytical Study of the Cells. *Cancer* 16: 173-182, 1963.

Patten SF Jr: Diagnostic Cytopathology of the Uterine Cervix. In: Wied GL, ed. *Monographs in Clinical Cytology*, Vol 3, 2nd ed., rev. S. Karger, Basel, 1-209, 1978.

Patton DL, Thwin SS, Meier A, et al: Epithelial Cell Layer Thickness and Immune Cell Populations in the Normal Human Vagina at Different Stages of the Menstrual Cycle. *Am J Obstet Gynecol* 183: 967-973, 2000.

Paul C: The New Zealand Cervical Cancer Study: Could It Happen Again? *Br Med J* 297: 533-539, 1988.

Pavic N: Is There a Local Production of Nitrosamines by the Vaginal Microflora in Anaerobic Vaginosis/Trichomoniasis? *Med Hypotheses* 15: 433-436, 1984.

Pavlidis NA: Coexistence of Pregnancy and Malignancy. *Oncologist* 7: 279-287, 2002.

Pavlova SI, Kilic AO, Kilic SS, et al: Genetic Diversity of Vaginal Lactobacilli from Women in Different Countries Based on 16S rRNA Gene Sequences. *J Appl Microbiol* 92:451-459, 2002.

Payandeh F, Koss LG: Nuclear Grooves in Normal and Abnormal Cervical Smears. *Acta Cytol* 47: 421-425, 2003.

Payne S, Kernohan M, Walker F: Proliferation in the Normal Cervix and in Preinvasive Cervical Lesions. *J Clin Pathol* 49: 667-671, 1996.

Pearce KF, Haefner HK, Sarwar SF, et al: Cytopathological Findings on Vaginal Papanicolaou Smears After Hysterectomy for Benign Gynecologic Disease. *N Engl J Med* 335: 1559-1562, 1996.

Pearlstone AC, Grigsby PW, Mutch DG: High Rates of Atypical Cervical Cytology: Occurrence and Clinical Significance. *Obstet Gynecol* 80: 191-195, 1992.

Pedersen E, Hoeg K, Kolstad P: Mass Screening for Cancer of the Uterine Cervix in Ostfold County, Norway: An Experiment—Second Report of the Norwegian Cancer Society. *Acta Obstet Gynecol Scand* Supplement 11: 5-18, 1971.

Peete CH Jr, Carter FB, Cherry WB, et al: Follow-Up of Patients With Adenocarcinoma of the Cervix and Cervical Stump. *Am J Obstet Gynecol* 93: 343-356, 1965.

Peipert JF: Genital Chlamydial Infections. *N Engl J Med* 349: 2424-2430, 2003.

Pelehach L: Appraising the Pap Smear: Will Society, Insurers, Put Their Money Where the Value Is? *Laboratory Medicine* 28: 440-47, 449, 1997. (Comment: Tilting at Windmills? Moves in Washington). *Laboratory Medicine* 28: 448, 1997.

Perey R: Cervical Cancer and the Misdiagnosed Smear. *Acta Cytol* 42: 123-127, 1998.

Perkins CL, Morris CR, Wright WE: Cancer Incidence and Mortality in California by Race/Ethnicity, 1988-1993. California Cancer Registry (CCR, 1700 Tribute Road, Suite 100, Sacramento, CA, 95815-4405, USA), 1996.

Perlow JH, Yordan EL, Wool N, et al: Disseminated Pelvic Actinomycosis Presenting as Metastatic Carcinoma: Association With the Progestasert Intrauterine Device. *Rev Infect Dis* 13: 1115-1159, 1991.

Perren T, Farrant M, McCarthy K, et al: Lymphomas of the Cervix and Upper Vagina: A Report of Five Cases and a Review of the Literature. *Gynecol Oncol* 44: 87-95, 1992.

Peters AAW, Trimbos JB: The Absence of Human Papilloma Virus (HPV) Related Parameters in Sexually Non-Active Women. *Eur J Gynaecol Oncol* 15: 43-45, 1994.

Peters N, Van Leeuwen AM, Pieters WJ, et al: Bacterial Vaginosis Is Not Important in the Etiology of Cervical Neoplasia: A Survey on Women With Dyskaryotic Smears. *Sex Transm Dis* 22: 296-302, 1995.

Peters RK, Chao A, Mack TM, et al: Increased Frequency of Adenocarcinoma of the Uterine Cervix in Young Women in Los Angeles County. *J Natl Cancer Inst* 76: 423-428, 1986a.

Peters RK, Thomas D, Hagan DG, et al: Risk Factors for Invasive Cervical Cancer in Latinas and Non-Latinas in Los Angeles County. *J Natl Cancer Inst* 77: 1063-1077, 1986b.

Peters RK, Thomas D, Skultin G, et al: Invasive Squamous Cell Carcinoma of the Cervix After Recent Negative Cytologic Test Results—A Distinct Subgroup? *Am J Obstet Gynecol* 158: 926-935, 1988.

Petersen O: Precancerous Changes of the Cervical Epithelium in Relation to Manifest Cervical Carcinoma: Clinical and Histological Aspects. *Acta Radiol* Supplementum 127: 1-181, 1955.

Petersen O: Spontaneous Course of Cervical Precancerous Conditions. *Am J Obstet Gynecol* 72:1063-1071, 1956.

Peterson LS, Neumann AA: Cytologic Features of Adenoid Basal Carcinoma of the Uterine Cervix: A Case Report. *Acta Cytol* 39: 563-568, 1995.

Petitti DB, Yamamot D, Morgenstern N: Factors Associated With *Actinomyces*-Like Organisms on Papanicolaou Smear in Users of Intrauterine Contraceptive Devices. *Am J Obstet Gynecol* 145: 338-341, 1983.

Petrucco OM, Seamark RF, Holmes K, et al: Changes in Lymphocyte Function During Pregnancy. *Br J Obstet Gynaecol* 83: 245-250, 1976.

Petry KU, Scheffel D, Bode U, et al: Cellular Immunodeficiency Enhances the Progression of Human Papillomavirus-Associated Cervical Lesions. *Int J Cancer* 57: 836-840, 1994.

Petry KU, Böhmer G, Iftner T, et al: Human Papillomavirus Testing in Primary Screening for Cervical Cancer of Human Immunodeficiency Virus-Infected Women, 1990-1998. *Gynecol Oncol* 75: 427-431, 1999.

Pfeifer JD, Odem RR, Huettner PC: Menstrual Abnormalities in a Premenopausal Woman With Endometrial Malacoplakia (Case Report). *Obstet Gynecol* 93: 839, 1999.

Phillips AN, Smith GD. Smoking and Human Papillmavirus Infection: Causal Link Not Proved (Letter). *Br Med J* 306: 1268-1269, 1993.

Phillips B, Marshall ME, Brown S, et al: Effect of Smoking on Human Natural Killer Cell Activity. *Cancer* 56: 2789-2792, 1985.

Phillips RS, Hanff PA, Kauffman RS, et al: Use of a Direct Fluorescent Antibody Test for Detecting *Chlamydia trachomatis* Cervical Infection in Women Seeking Routine Gynecologic Care. *J Infect Dis* 156: 575-581, 1987.

Picoff RC, Meeker CI: Psammoma Bodies in the Cervicovaginal Smear in Association With Benign Papillary Structures of the Ovary. *Acta Cytol* 14: 45-47, 1970.

Pientong C, Ekalaksananan T, Swadpanich U, et al: Immunocytochemical Detection of p16^{INK4a} Protein in Scraped Cervical Cells. *Acta Cytol* 47: 616-623, 2003.

Pientong C, Ekalaksananan T, Kongyingyoes B, et al: Immunocytochemical Staining of p16^{INK4a} Protein From Conventional Pap Test and Its Association With Human Papillomavirus Infection. *Diagn Cytopathol* 31: 235-242, 2004.

Pinto ÁP, Crum CP: Natural History of Cervical Neoplasia: Defining Progression and Its Consequence. *Clin Obstet Gynecol* 43: 352-362, 2000.

Pinto ÁP, Tuon FFB, Bleggi LF, et al: Limiting Factors for Cytopathological Diagnosis of High-Grade Squamous Intraepithelial Lesions: A Cytohistological Correlation Between Findings in Cervical Smears and Loop Electrical Excision Procedure. *Diagn Cytopathol* 26: 15-18, 2002a.

Pinto ÁP, Tuon FFB, Tissot ELA, et al: Nonneoplastic Findings in Loop Electrical Excision Procedure Specimens from Patients With Persistent Atypical Squamous Cells of Uncertain Significance in Two Consecutive Pap Smears. *Diagn Cytopathol* 27: 123-127, 2002b.

Pirami L, Giache V, Becciolini A: Analysis of HPV 16, 18, 31, and 35 DNA in Pre-Invasive and Invasive Lesions of the Uterine Cervix. *J Clin Pathol* 50: 600-604, 1997.

Pirisi L, Yasumoto S, Feller M, et al: Transformation of Human Fibroblast and Keratinocytes With Human Papillomavirus Type 16 DNA. *J Virol* 61: 1061-1066, 1987.

Pirisi L, Creek KE, Doniger J, et al: Continuous Cell Lines With Altered Growth and Differentiation Properties Originate After Transfection of Human Keratinocytes With Human Papillomavirus Type 16 DNA. *Carcinogenesis* 9: 1573-1579, 1988.

Pirog EC, Kleter B, Olgac S, et al: Prevalence of Human Papillomavirus DNA in Different Histological Subtypes of Cervical Adenocarcinoma. *Am J Pathol* 157:1055-1062, 2000.

Pirog EC, Erroll M, Harigopal M, et al: Comparison of Human Papillomavirus DNA Prevalence in Atypical Squamous Cells of Undetermined Significance Subcategories as Defined by the Original Bethesda 1991 and the New Bethesda 2001 Systems. *Arch Pathol Lab Med* 128: 527-532, 2004.

Pisani P, Parkin DM, Muñoz N, et al: Cancer and Infection: Estimates of the Attributable Fraction in 1990. *Cancer Epidemiol Biomarkers Prev* 6: 387-400, 1997.

Pisani P, Parkin DM, Bray F, et al: Estimates of the Worldwide Mortality from 25 Cancers in 1990. *Int J Cancer* 83: 18-29, 1999.

Pisani P, Bray F, Parkin DM: Estimates of the World-Wide Prevalence of Cancer for 25 Sites in the Adult Population. *Int J Cancer* 97: 72-81, 2002.

Piscitelli JT, Bastian LA, Wilkes A, et al: Cytologic Screening After Hysterectomy for Benign Disease. *Am J Obstet Gynecol* 173: 424-430, 1995.

Pisharodi LR, Jovanoska S: Spectrum of Cytologic Changes in Pregnancy: A Review of 100 Abnormal Cervicovaginal Smears, With Emphasis on Diagnostic Pitfalls. *Acta Cytol* 39: 905-908, 1995.

Pitman MB, Cibas ES, Powers CN, et al: Reducing or Eliminating Use of the Category of Atypical Squamous Cells of Undetermined Significance Decreases the Diagnostic Accuracy of the Papanicolaou Smear. *Cancer (Cancer Cytopathol)* 96: 128-134, 2002.

Piver MS, Lele SB, Baker TR, et al: Cervical and Vaginal Cancer Detection at a Regional Diethylstilbestrol (DES) Screening Clinic. *Cancer Detect Prevent* 11: 197-202, 1988.

Piyathilake CJ, Macaluso M, Johanning GL, et al: Methylenetetrahydrofolate Reductase (MTHFR) Polymorphism Increases the Risk of Cervical Intraepithelial Neoplasia. *Anticancer Res* 20(3A): 1751-1757, 2000.

Platz-Christensen JJ, Larsson PG, Sundstrom E, et al: Detection of Bacterial Vaginosis in Papanicolaou Smears. *Am J Obstet Gynecol* 160: 132-133, 1989.

Platz-Christensen JJ, Sundstrom E, Larsson P-G: Bacterial Vaginosis and Cervical Intraepithelial Neoplasia. *Acta Obstet Gynecol Scand* 73: 586-588, 1994.

Platz-Christensen JJ, Larsson P-G, Sundstrom E, et al: Detection of Bacterial Vaginosis in Wet Mount, Papanicolaou Stained Vaginal Smears and in Gram Stained Smears. *Acta Obstet Gynecol Scand* 74: 67-70, 1995.

Plaut A: Historical and Cultural Aspects of the Uterus: Part I. Historical and Morphogenetic Considerations. *Ann NY Acad Sci* 75: 389-411, 1959.

Plaxe SC, Saltzstein SL: Estimation of the Duration of the Preclinical Phase of Cervical Adenocarcinoma Suggests That There Is Ample Opportunity for Screening. *Gynecol Oncol* 75: 55-61, 1999.

Plott AE, Martin FJ, Cheek SW, et al: Measuring Screening Skills in Gynecologic Cytology: Results of Voluntary Self-Assessment. *Acta Cytol* 31: 911-923, 1987.

Podczaski E, Abt A, Kaminski P, et al: Case Report: A Patient With Multiple Malignant Melanomas of the Lower Genital Tract. *Gynecol Oncol* 37: 422-426, 1990.

Podobnik M, Singer Z, Ciglar S, et al: Preoperative Diagnosis of Primary Fallopian Tube Carcinoma by Transvaginal Ultrasound, Cytological Finding and CA-125. *Ultrasound Med Bio* 19: 587-591, 1993.

Poggensee G, Saheball S, Van Marck E, et al: Diagnosis of Genital Cervical Schistosomiasis: Comparison of Cytological, Histopathological and Parasitological Examination. *Am J Trop Med Hyg* 65: 233-236, 2001.

Poindexter AN III, Levine H, Sangi-Haghpeykar S, et al: Comparison of Spermicides on Vulvar, Vaginal, and Cervical Mucosa. *Contraception* 53: 147-153, 1996.

Pollack RS, Taylor HC Jr: Carcinoma of the Cervix During the First Two Decades of Life. *Am J Obstet Gynecol* 53: 135-141, 1947.

Pomerance W, Mackles A: Adenocarcinoma of the Cervix. *Am J Obstet Gynecol* 84: 367-374, 1962.

Ponder TB, Easley KO, Dávila RM: Glandular Cells in Vaginal Smears from Posthysterectomy Patients. *Acta Cytol* 41: 1701-1704, 1997.

Pontén J, Adami H-O, Bergström R, et al: Strategies for Global Control of Cervical Cancer. *Int J Cancer* 60: 1-26, 1995.

Popescu NC, DiPaolo JA: Integration of Human Papillomavirus 16 DNA and Genomic Rearrangements in Immortalized Human Keratinocyte Lines. *Cancer Res* 50: 1316-1323, 1990a.

Popescu NC, Zimonjic D, DiPaolo JA: Viral Integration, Fragile Sites, and Proto-Oncogenes in Human Neoplasia. *Hum Genet* 84: 383-386, 1990b.

Poppe WA, Ide PS, Drijkoningen MP, et al: Tobacco Smoking Impairs the Local Immunosurveillence in the Uterine Cervix: An Immunohistochemical Study. *Gynecol Obstet Invest* 39: 34-38, 1995.

Pornthanakasem W, Shotelersuk K, Termrungruanglert W, et al: Human Papillomavirus DNA in Plasma of Patients With Cervical Cancer. *BMC Cancer* 1:2, 2001. [www. biomedcentral. com/1471-2407/1/2]

Porreco R, Penn I, Droegemueller W, et al: Gynecologic Malignancies in Immunosuppressed Organ Homograft Recipients. *Obstet Gynecol* 45: 359-364, 1975.

Potischman N: Nutritional Epidemiology of Cervical Neoplasia. *J Nutrition* 123(Suppl 2): 424-429, 1993.

Potishman N, Brinton LA: Nutrition and Cervical Neoplasia. *Cancer Causes Control* 7: 113-126, 1996.

Powell JL, Franklin EW III, Nickerson JF, et al: Verrucous Carcinoma of the Female Genital Tract. *Gynecol Oncol* 6: 565-573, 1978.

Powers CN: Radiation Treatment Effects in Cervical Cytology. *Diagn Cytopathol* 13: 75-80, 1995.

Powers CN, Stastny JF, Frable WJ: Adenoid Basal Carcinoma of the Cervix: A Potential Pitfall in Cervicovaginal Cytology. *Diagn Cytopathol* 14: 172-177, 1996.

Poynor EA, Barakat RR, Hoskins WJ: Management and Follow-Up of Patients With Adenocarcinoma In situ of the Uterine Cervix. *Gynecol Oncol* 57: 158-164, 1995.

Prade M, Gadenne C, Duvillard P, et al: Endometrial Carcinoma With Argyrophilic Cells. *Hum Pathol* 13: 870-871, 1982.

Prasad CJ, Sheets E, Selig AM, et al: The Binucleate Squamous Cell: Histologic Spectrum and Relationship to Low-Grade Squamous Intraepithelial Lesions. *Mod Pathol* 6: 313-317, 1993.

Prasad CJ, Genest DR, Crum CP: Nondiagnostic Squamous Atypia of the Cervix (Atypical Squamous Epithelium of Undetermined Significance): Histologic and Molecular Correlates. *Int J Gynecol Pathol* 13: 220-227, 1994.

Prasad CJ: Pathobiology of Human Papillomavirus. *Clin Lab Med* 15: 685-705, 1995.

Premoli-De-Percoco G, Ramírez JL, Galindo I: Correlation Between HPV Types Associated With Oral Squamous Cell Carcinoma and Cervicovaginal Cytology: An In Situ Hybridization Study. *Oral Surg Oral Med Oral Pathol Oral Radiol Endod* 86: 77-81, 1998.

Prempree T, Patanaphan V, Sewchand W, et al: The Influence of Patients' Age and Tumor Grade on the Prognosis of Carcinoma of the Cervix. *Cancer* 51: 1764-1771, 1983.

Prendiville W, Guillebaud J, Bamford P, et al: Carcinoma of Cervix With Recent Normal Papanicolaou Tests. *Lancet* (ii): 853-854, 1980.

Preti G, Huggins GR: Cyclical Changes in Volatile Acidic Metabolites of Human Vaginal Secretions and Their Relation to Ovulation. *J Chem Ecol* 1: 361-376, 1975.

Pretorius R, Semrad N, Watring W, et al: Presentation of Cervical Cancer. *Gynecol Oncol* 42: 48-53, 1991.

Pretorius R, Binstock M, Sadeghi M, et al: Cervical and Vaginal Cytologic Smears Suggestive of Adenocarcinoma. *J Reprod Med* 41: 478-482, 1996.

Prey M: Routine Pap Smears for the Diagnosis of Bacterial Vaginosis. *Diagn Cytopathol* 21: 10-13, 1999.

Pridan H, Lilienfeld AM: Carcinoma of the Cervix in Jewish Women in Israel, 1960-67: An Epidemiological Study. *Israel J Med Sci* 7: 1465-1470, 1971.

Priestley CJF, Jones BM, Dhar J, et al: What Is Normal Vaginal Flora? *Genitourin Med* 73: 23-28, 1997.

Pritchard KI: Screening for Endometrial Cancer: Is It Effective? (Editorial). *Ann Intern Med* 110: 177-179, 1989.

Proca DM, Keyhani-Rofagha S, Copeland LJ, et al: Exfoliatvie Cytology of Neuroendocrine Small Cell Carcinoma of the Endometrium: A Report of Two Cases. *Acta Cytol* 42: 978-982, 1998.

Proca DM, Hitchcock CL, Keyhani-Rofagha S: Exfoliative Cytology of Lymphoepithelioma-Like Carcinoma of the Uterine Cervix: A Report of Two Cases. *Acta Cytol* 44: 410-414, 2000.

Prokopczyk B, Cox JE, Hoffmann D, et al: Identification of Tobacco-Specific Carcinogen in the Cervical Mucus of Smokers and Nonsmokers. *J Natl Cancer Inst* 89: 868-873, 1997.

Prolla C; Curschmann Spirals in Cervical Mucus (Letter). *Ann Intern Med* 80: 674-675, 1974.

Pronai K: Zur Lehre von der Histogenese und dem Wachsthum des Uteruscarcinoms. *Arch f Gynaekol* 89: 596-607, 1909.

Provencher D, Valme B, Averette HE, et al: HIV Status and Positive Papanicolau [sic] Screening: Identification of a High-Risk Population. *Gynecol Oncol* 31: 184-188, 1988.

Przybora L, Plutowa A: Histological Topography of Carcinoma In Situ of the Cervix Uteri. *Cancer* 12: 263-277, 1959.

Pund ER, Niebrugs HE, Nettles JB, et al: Preinvasive Carcinoma of the Cervix Uteri. Seven Cases in Which It Was Detected by Examination of Routine Endocervical Smears. *Arch Pathol* 44: 571-577, 1947.

Puneet [ ], Khanna A, Khanna AK: Intravaginal Foreign Body—A Rare Cause of Large Bowel Obstruction (Case Note). *J Indian Med Assoc* 100: 671, 2002.

Purola E, Savia E: Cytology of Gynecologic *Condyloma acuminatum*. *Acta Cytol* 21: 26-31, 1977.

Purola E, Paavonen J: Routine Cytology as a Diagnostic Aid in Chlamydial Cervicitis. *Scand J Infect Dis* Supplementum 32: 55-58, 1982.

Puttarajurs BV, Taylor W: The Relationship Between Urinary Excretion of Ovarian Hormone Metabolites and Cornification of the Vaginal Epithelium During the Menstrual Cycle. *J Endocrinol* 18: 67-76, 1959.

Pybus V, Onderdonk AB: Microbial Interactions in the Vaginal Ecosystem, With Emphasis on the Pathogenesis of Bacterial Vaginosis. *Microbes Infect* 1: 285-292, 1999.

Q

Qazi FM, Geisinger KR, Barrett RJ, et al: Cervicovaginal Psammoma Bodies: The Initial Presentation of the Ovarian Borderline Tumor. *Arch Pathol Lab Med* 112: 564-566, 1988.

Qizilbash AH: Chronic Plasma Cell Cervicitis. A Rare Pitfall in Gynecological Cytology. *Acta Cytol* 18: 198-200, 1974a.

Qizilbash AH: Ovarian Carcinoma Identified by Psammoma Bodies in the Cervicovaginal and Endometrial Smears. *CMAJ* 110: 185-186, 1974b.

Qizilbash AH: Papillary Squamous Tumors of the Uterine Cervix: A Clinical and Pathological Study of 21 Cases. *Am J Clin Pathol* 61: 508-520, 1974c.

Qizilbash AH: In-Situ and Microinvasive Adenocarcinoma of the Uterine Cervix: A Clinical, Cytologic and Histologic Study of 14 Cases. *Am J Clin Pathol* 64: 155-170, 1975.

Quddus MR, Sung CJ, Steinhoff MM, et al: Atypical Squamous Metaplastic Cells: Reproducibility, Outcome, and Diagnostic Features on ThinPrep Pap Test. *Cancer* 93: 16-22, 2001.

Quddus MR, Sung J, Eklund CM, et al: ASC:SIL Ratio Following Implementation of the 2001 Bethesda System. *Diagn Cytopathol* 30: 240-242, 2004.

Queiroz C, Bacchi CE, Oliveira C, et al: Cytologic Diagnosis of Vaginal Metastasis from Renal Cell Carcinoma: A Case Report. *Acta Cytol* 43: 1098-1100, 1999.

Quinn M, Babb P, Jones J, et al: Effect of Screening on Incidence of and Morality from Cancer of Cervix in England: Evaluation Based on Routinely Collected Statistics. *Br Med J* 318: 904-908, 1999.

Quinn MA: Screening for Cervical Cancer—Where Are We Going Wrong? *Med J Aust* 150: 414-415, 1989.

Quinn TC, Gupta PK, Burkman RT, et al: Detection of *Chlamydia trachomatis* Cervical Infection: A Comparison of Papanicolaou and Immunofluorescent Staining With Cell Culture. *Am J Obstet Gynecol* 157: 394-399, 1987.

Quitllet FA, Morta MC, Cañas A, et al: Cytologic Atypia: Clinical Significance and Follow-Up Recommendations. *Acta Cytol* 41: 504-506, 1997.

Qureshi MN, Rudelli RD, Tubbs RR, et al: Role of HPV DNA Testing in Predicting Cervical Intraepithelial Lesions: Comparison of HC HPV and ISH HPV. *Diagn Cytopathol* 29: 149-155, 2003.

R

Raab SS: Diagnostic Accuracy in Cytopathology. *Diagn Cytopathol* 10: 68-75, 1994.

Raab SS, Isacson C, Layfield LJ, et al: Atypical Glandular Cells of Undetermined Significance: Cytologic Criteria to Separate Clinically Significant from Benign Lesions. *Am J Clin Pathol* 104: 574-582, 1995.

Raab SS, Snider TE, Potts SA, et al: Atypical Glandular Cells of Undetermined Significance: Diagnostic Accuracy and Interobserver Variability Using Select Cytologic Criteria. *Am J Clin Pathol* 107: 299-307, 1997.

Raab SS, Geisinger KR, Silverman JF, et al: Interobserver Variability of a Papanicolaou Smear Diagnosis of Atypical Glandular Cells of Undetermined Significance. *Am J Clin Pathol* 110: 653-659, 1998a.

Raab SS, Steiner AL, Hornberger J: The Cost-Effectiveness of Treating Women With a Cervical Vaginal Smear Diagnosis of Atypical Squamous Cells of Undetermined Significance. *Am J Obstet Gynecol* 179: 411-420, 1998b.

Raab SS: Low-Grade and ASCUS Lesions of the Cervix: Diagnostic Difficulties and Reproducibility. *Annales de Pathologie* 19(Suppl 5): S87-S89, 1999a.

Raab SS, Bishop NS, Zaleski MS: Effect of Cervical Disease History on Outcomes of Women Who Have a Pap Diagnosis of Atypical Glandular Cells of Undetermined Significance. *Gynecol Oncol* 74: 460-464, 1999b.

Raab SS, Bishop NS, Zaleski MS: Long-Term Outcome and Relative Risk in Women With Atypical Squamous Cells of Undetermined Significance. *Am J Clin Pathol* 112: 57-62, 1999c.

Raab SS: Can Glandular Lesions Be Diagnosed in Pap Smear Cytology? *Diagn Cytopathol* 23: 127-133, 2000.

Raab SS: Subcategorization of Papanicolaou Tests Diagnosed as Atypical Squamous Cells of Undetermined Significance. *Am J Clin Pathol* 116: 631-634, 2001a.

Raab SS, Hart AR, D'Antonio JA, et al: Clinical Perception of Disease Probability Associated With Bethesda System Diagnoses. *Am J Clin Pathol* 115: 681-688, 2001b.

Raab SS: Human Papillomavirus Reporting: Impact on Bethesda Cytology Reports. *Arch Pathol Lab Med* 127: 969-972, 2003.

Rader AE, Lazebnik R, Arora CD, et al: Atypical Squamous Cells of Undetermined Significance in the Pediatric Population: Implications for Management and Comparison With the Adult Population. *Acta Cytol* 41: 1073-1078, 1997.

Rader AE, Rose PG, Rodriguez M, et al: Atypical Squamous Cells of Undetermined Significance in Women Over 55: Comparison With the General Population and Implications for Management. *Acta Cytol* 43: 357-362, 1999.

Rader JS, Gerhard DS, O'Sullivan MJ, et al: Cervical Intraepithelial Neoplasia III Shows Frequent Allelic Loss in 3p and 6p. *Genes Chromosomes Cancer* 22: 57-65, 1988.

Rader JS, Rosenzweig BA, Spirtas R, et al: Atypical Squamous Cells: A Case-Series Study of the Association Between Papanicolaou Smear Results and Human Papillomavirus DNA Genotype. *J Reprod Med* 36: 291-297, 1991.

Rader JS, Kamarasova T, Huettner PC, et al: Allelotyping of All Chromosomal Arms in Invasive Cervical Cancer. *Oncogene* 13: 2737-2741, 1996.

Raffle AE, Alden B, Mackenzie EF: Detection Rates for Abnormal Cervical Smears: What Are We Screening For? *Lancet* 345: 1469-1473, 1995.

Rahilly MA, Williams ARW, Al-Nafussi A: Minimal Deviation Endometrioid Adenocarcinoma of Cervix: A Clinicopathological and Immunohistochemical Study of Two Cases. *Histopathology* 20: 351-354, 1992.

Rahimpanah F, Reid RI: Fallopian Tube Carcinoma Detected by ThinPrep Cytology Smear. *Med J Aust* 172: 38, 2000; errata, appear in *Med J Aust* 172: 283, and 374, 2000.

Raju GC, The M, Wee A: The Expression of HLA-DR Antigen in Cervical Neoplasia. *Cancer Detect Prevent* 18: 367-373, 1994.

Rakoff AE: Hormonal Cytology in Gynecology. *Clin Obstet Gynecol* 4: 1045-1061, 1961a.

Rakoff, AE: The Vaginal Cytology of Gynecologic Endocrinopathies. *Acta Cytol* 5: 153-167, 1961b.

Ramirez JE, Ramos DM, Clayton L, et al: Genital Human Papillomavirus Infections: Knowledge, Perception of Risk, and Actual Risk in a Nonclinic Population of Young Women. *J Womens Health* 6: 113-121, 1997.

Ramirez NC, Sastry KS, Pisharodi LR: Benign Glandular and Squamous Metaplastic-Like Cells Seen in Vaginal Pap Smears of Post Hysterectomy Patients: Incidence and Patient Profile. *Eur J Gynaecol Oncol* 21: 43-48, 2000.

Ramsamooj R, Doolin E, Greenberg G, et al: Real-Time, High-Definition, Three-Dimensional Microscopy for Evaluating Problematic Cervical Papanicolaou Smears Classified as Atypical Squamous Cells of Undetermined Significance. *Cancer (Cancer Cytopathol)* 96: 181-186, 2002.

Ramzy I, Yuzpe AA, Hendelman J: Adenoid Cystic Carcinoma of Uterine Cervix. *Obstet Gynecol* 45: 679-683, 1975.

Ramzy I, Smout MS, Collins JA: Verrucous Carcinoma of the Vagina. *Am J Clin Pathol* 65: 644-653, 1976.

Ramzy I, Vilos GA, Desrosiers PA: Antenatal Assessment of Fetal Age and Maturity Using Fetal Fat Staining Cells in Amniotic Fluid. *Acta Cytol* 22: 105-109, 1978.

Rand RJ, Lowe JW: Schistomsomiasis of the Uterine Cervix. *Br J Obstet Gynaecol* 105: 1329-1331, 1998.

Randall B: Persistence of Vaginal Spermatozoa as Assessed by Routine Cervicovaginal (Pap) Smears. *J Forensic Sci* 32: 678-683, 1987.

Randall ME, Andersen WA, Mills SE, et al: Papillary Squamous Cell Carcinoma of the Uterine Cervix: A Clinicopathologic Study of Nine Cases. *Int J Gynecol Pathol* 5: 1-10, 1986.

Ransdell JS, Davey DD, Zaleski S: Clinicopathologic Correlation of the Unsatisfactory Papanicolaou Smear. *Cancer (Cancer Cytopathol)* 81: 139-143, 1997.

Rarick TL, Tchabo J-G: Timing of the Postpartum Papanicolaou Smear. *Obstet Gynecol* 83: 761-765, 1994.

Rasbridge SA, Nayagam M: Discordance Between Cytologic and Histologic Reports in Cervical Intraepithelial Neoplasia: Results of a One-Year Audit. *Acta Cytol* 39: 648-653, 1995.

Raspollini MR, Baroni G, Taddei A, et al: Primary Cervical Adenocarcinoma With Intestinal Differentiation and Colonic Carcinoma Metastatic to Cervix: An Investigation Using Cdx-2 and a Limited Immunohistochemical Panel. *Arch Pathol Lab Med* 127: 1586-1590, 2003.

Rau AR, Saldanha P, Raghuveer CV: Metastatic Lobular Mammary Carcinoma Diagnosed in Cervicovaginal Smears: A Case Report. *Diagn Cytopathol* 29: 300-302, 2003.

Ravinsky E, Safneck JR, Chantziantoniou N: Cytologic Features of Primary Adenoid Cystic Carcinoma of the Uterine Cervix: A Case Report. *Acta Cytol* 40: 1304-1308, 1996.

Rawls WE, Tompkins WA, Melnick JL: The Association of Herpesvirus Type 2 and Carcinoma of the Uterine Cervix. *Am J Epidemiol* 89: 547-554, 1969.

Rawls WE, Lavery C, Marrett LD, et al: Comparison of Risk Factors for Cervical Cancer in Different Populations. *Int J Cancer* 37: 537-546, 1986.

Rayburn WF, van Nagell JR Jr: Cervicovaginal Cytology in the Diagnosis of Recurrent Carcinoma of the Cervix Uteri. *Surg Gynecol Obstet* 151: 15-16, 1980.

Raymond CA: For Women Infected With Papillomavirus, Close Watch Counseled. *JAMA* 257: 2398-2399, 1987.

Rayter Z, Gazet J-C, Trott PA, et al: Gynaecological Cytology and Pelvic Ultrasonography in Patients With Breast Cancer Taking Tamoxifen Compared With Controls. *Eur J Surg Oncol* 20: 134-140, 1994.

Reagan JW, Hicks DJ: A Study of In Situ and Squamous-Cell Cancer of the Uterine Cervix. *Cancer* 6: 1200-1214, 1953a.

Reagan JW, Seidemann IL, Saracusa Y: The Cellular Morphology of Carcinoma In Situ and Dysplasia or Atypical Hyperplasia of the Uterine Cervix. *Cancer* 6: 224-235, 1953b.

Reagan JW, Hicks DJ, Scott RB: Atypical Hyperplasia of Uterine Cervix. *Cancer* 8: 42-52, 1955.

Reagan JW, Hamonic MJ: Part IV. The Cytology of Early Cancer: Dysplasia of the Uterine Cervix. *Ann NY Acad Sci* 63: 1236-1244, 1956a.

Reagan JW, Hamonic MJ: The Cellular Pathology in Carcinoma In Situ. *Cancer* 9: 385-402, 1956b.

Reagan JW, Hamonic MJ, Wentz WB: Analytical Study of the Cells in Cervical Squamous-Cell Cancer. *Lab Invest* 6:241-250, 1957.

Reagan JW, Bell BA, Neuman JL, et al: Dysplasia in the Uterine Cervix During Pregnancy: An Analytical Study of the Cells. *Acta Cytol* 5: 17-29, 1961a.

Reagan JW, Patten SF Jr: Analytic Study of Cellular Changes in Carcinoma In Situ, Squamous-Cell Cancer, and Adenocarcinoma of Uterine Cervix. *Clin Obstet Gynecol* 4: 1097-1127, 1961b.

Reagan JW, Patten SF Jr: Dysplasia: A Basic Reaction to Injury in the Uterine Cervix. *Ann NY Acad Sci* 97: 662-682, 1962a.

Reagan JW, Seidemann IB, Patten SF Jr: Developmental Stages of In Situ Carcinoma in Uterine Cervix: An Analytical Study of the Cells. *Acta Cytol* 6: 538-546, 1962b.

Reagan JW: Presidential Address. *Acta Cytol* 9: 265-267, 1965.

Reagan JW, Wentz WB: Genesis of Carcinoma of the Uterine Cervix. *Clin Obstet Gynecol* 10: 883-921, 1967.

Reagan JW, Ng AB, Wentz WB: Concepts of Genesis and Development in Early Cervical Neoplasia. *Obstet Gynecol Surv* 24: 860-874, 1969.

Reagan JW, Ng ABP: The Cells of Uterine Adenocarcinoma. In: Wied GL, ed. *Monographs in Clinical Cytology*, Vol 1, 2nd ed. Rev. Basel, S. Karger, 1973.

Reagan JW: Cytologic Aspects of Endometrial Neoplasia [Proceedings]. *Acta Cytol* 24: 488-489, 1980.

Recher L, Srebnik E: Histopathologic Features of Koilocytotic Atypia: A Detailed Description. *Acta Cytol* 25: 377-382, 1981.

Redondo-Lopez V, Cook RL, Sobel JD: Emerging Role of Lactobacilli in the Control and Maintenance of the Vaginal Bacterial Microflora. *Rev Infect Dis* 12: 856-872, 1990.

Reeves WC, Brinton LA, Brenes MM, et al: Case Control Study of Cervical Cancer in Herrera Province, Republic of Panama. *Int J Cancer* 36: 55-60, 1985.

Reeves WC, Caussy D, Brinton LA, et al: Case-Control Study of Human Papillomaviruses and Cervical Cancer in Latin America. *Int J Cancer* 40: 450-454, 1987.

Reeves WC, Brinton LA, García M, et al: Human Papillomavirus Infection and Cervical Cancer in Latin America. *N Engl J Med* 320: 1437-1441, 1989.

Reich O, Pickel H, Pürstner P: Exfoliative Cytology of Invasive Neuroendocrine Small Cell Carcinoma in a Cervical Cytologic Smear: A Case Report. *Acta Cytol* 40: 980-984, 1996.

Reich O, Pickel H, Pürstner P: Exfoliative Cytology of a Lymphoepithelioma-Like Carcinoma in a Cervical Smear: A Case Report. *Acta Cytol* 43: 285-288, 1999.

Reich O, Tamussino K, Lahousen M, et al: Clear Cell Carcinoma of the Uterine Cervix: Pathology and Prognosis in Surgically Treated Stage IB-IIB Disease in Women Not Exposed *in utero* to Diethylstilbestrol. *Gynecol Oncol* 76: 331-335, 2000.

Reid BL, French PW, Singer A, et al: Sperm Basic Proteins in Cervical Carcinogenesis: Correlation with Socioeconomic Class. *Lancet* (ii): 60-62, 1978.

Reid G, Burton J: Use of *Lactobacillus* to Prevent Infection by Pathogenic Bacteria. *Microbes Infect* 4: 319-324, 2002.

Reid J: Women's Knowledge of Pap Smears, Risk Factors for Cervical Cancer, and Cervical Cancer. *J Obstet Gynecol Neonatal Nurs* 30: 299-305, 2001.

Reid R, Laverty CR, Coppleson M, et al: Noncondylomatous Cervical Wart Virus Infection. *Obstet Gynecol* 55: 476-483, 1980.

Reid R, Stanhope CR, Herschman BR et al: Genital Warts and Cervical Cancer. I. Evidence of an Association Between Subclinical Papillomavirus Infection and Cervical Malignancy. *Cancer* 50: 377-387, 1982.

Reid R: Genital Warts and Cervical Cancer. II. Is Human Papillomavirus Infection the Trigger to Cervical Carcinogenesis? *Gynecol Oncol* 15: 239-252, 1983.

Reid R, Crum CP, Herschman BR, et al: Genital Warts and Cervical Cancer. III. Subclinical Papillomaviral Infection and Cervical Neoplasia Are Linked by a Spectrum of Continuous Morphologic and Biologic Change. *Cancer* 53: 943-953, 1984a.

Reid R, Fu YS, Herschman BR, et al: Genital Warts and Cervical Cancer. IV. The Relationship Between Aneuploid and Polyploid Cervical Lesions. *Am J Obstet Gynecol* 150: 189-199, 1984b.

Reid R, Herschman BR, Crum CP, et al: Genital Warts and Cervical Cancer. V. The Tissue Basis of Colposcopic Change. *Am J Obstet Gynecol* 149: 293-303, 1984c.

Reid R, Scalzi P: Genital Warts and Cervical Cancer. VII. An Improved Colposcopic Index for Differentiating Benign Papillomaviral Infections from High-Grade Cervical Intraepithelial Neoplasia. *Am J Obstet Gynecol* 153: 611-618, 1985.

Reid R, Fu YS: *Viral Etiology of Cervical Cancer.* In: Petro R, ed. *Banbury Report 21.* Cold Spring Harbor Laboratory, NY, 1-362, 1986.

Reid R, Greenberg M, Jenson AB, et al: Sexually Transmitted Papillomaviral Infections. I. The Anatomic Distribution and Pathologic Grade of Neoplastic Lesions Associated With Different Viral Types. *Am J Obstet Gynecol* 156: 212-222, 1987.

Reid R, Campion MJ: HPV-Associated Lesions of the Cervix: Biology and Colposcopic Features. *Clin Obstet Gynecol* 32: 157-179, 1989.

Reis-Filho JS, Neto JF, Schonemann E, et al: Glassy Cell Carcinoma of the Uterine Cervix: Report of a Case With Cytohistologic and Immunohistochemical Study. *Acta Cytol* 45: 407-410, 2001.

Reissman SE: Comparison of Two Papanicolaou Smear Techniques in a Family Practice Setting. *J Fam Pract* 26: 525-529, 1988.

Reiter RC: Management of Initial Atypical Cervical Cytology: A Randomized Prospective Study. *Obstet Gynecol* 68: 237-240, 1986.

Remmink AJ, Walboomers JM, Helmerhorst TJ, et al: The Presence of Persistent High-Risk HPV Genotypes in Dysplastic Cervical Lesions Is Associated With Progressive Disease: Natural History Up to 36 Months. *Int J Cancer* 61: 306-311, 1995.

Renno SI, Moreland WS, Pettenati MJ, et al: Primary Malignant Lymphoma of Uterine Corpus: Case Report and Review of the Literature. *Ann Hematol* 81: 44-47, 2002.

Renshaw AA, Lee KR, Granter SR: Use of Statistical Analysis of Cytologic Interpretation to Determine the Causes of Interobserver Disagreement and in Quality Improvement. *Cancer (Cancer Cytopathol)* 81: 212-219, 1997.

Renshaw AA, Friedman MM, Rahemtulla A, et al: Accuracy and Reproducibility of Estimating the Adequacy of the Squamous Component of Cervicovaginal Smears. *Am J Clin Pathol* 111: 38-42, 1999.

Renshaw AA: Estimating the Percentage of Papanicolaou Smears That Can Be Reproducibly Identified: Modeling Papanicolaou Smear Interpretation Based on Multiple Blinded Rescreenings. *Cancer (Cancer Cytopathol)* 93: 241-245, 2001a.

Renshaw AA, Genest DR, Cibas ES: Should Atypical Squamous Cells of Undetermined Significance (ASCUS) Be Subcategorized? Accuracy Analysis of Papanicolaou Smears Using Receiver Operating Characteristic Curves and Implications for the ASCUS/ Squamous Intraepithelial Lesion Ratio. *Am J Clin Pathol* 116: 692-695, 2001b.

Renshaw AA: Déjà Vu in Pap Testing: Return of the 5% False-Negative Fraction and the Zero-Error Rate (Editorial). *Diagn Cytopathol* 26: 343-344, 2002a.

Renshaw AA: Measuring Sensitivity in Gynecologic Cytology: A Review. *Cancer (Cancer Cytopathol)* 96: 210-217, 2002b.

Renshaw AA, Davey DD, Birdsong GG, et al: Precision in Gynecologic Cytologic Interpretation: A Study from the College of American Pathologists Interlaboratory Comparison Program in Cervicovaginal Cytology. *Arch Pathol Lab Med* 127: 1413-1420, 2003.

Renshaw AA: Increased Cervical Cancer Screening Intervals: A Risky Investment? (Editorial) *Diagn Cytopathol* 30: 137-138, 2004a.

Renshaw AA, Young NA, Birdsong GG, et al: Comparison of Performance of Conventional and ThinPrep Gynecologic Preparations in the College of American Pathologists Gynecologic Cytology Program. *Arch Pathol Lab Med* 128: 17-22, 2004b.

Renshaw AA, Mody DR, Lozano RL, et al: Detection of Adenocarcinoma In Situ of the Cervix in Papanicolaou Tests: Comparison of Diagnostic Accuracy With Other high-Grade Lesions. *Arch Pathol Lab Med* 128: 153-157, 2004c.

Renshaw AA, Dubray-Benstein B, Dobb CJ, et al: Cytologic Features of Squamous Cell Carcinoma in ThinPrep Slides: Evaluation of Cases That Performed Poorly Versus Those That Performed Well in the College of American Pathologists Interlaboratory Comparison Program in Cervicovaginal Cytology. *Arch Pathol Lab Med* 128: 403-405, 2004d.

Renshaw AA, Schulte MA, Plott E, et al: Cytologic Features of High-Grade Squamous intraepithelial Lesion in ThinPrep Papanicolaou Test Slides: Comparison of Cases That performed poorly With Those That Operformed Well in the college of American pathologists interlaboratory Comparison program in Cervicovaginal Cytology. *Arch Pathol Lab Med* 128: 746-748, 2004e.

Renshaw AA, Young ML, Holladay EB: Blinded Review of papanicolaou Smears in the Context of Litigation: Using Statistical Analysis to Define Appropriate Thresholds. *Cancer (Cancer Cytopathol)* 102: 136-141, 2004f.

Repse-Fokter A, Fokter SK, Komadina R, et al: Morphological Analysis of Squamous Cells in Routine Pap Smears as a Predictor of Bone Mineral Density in Asymptomatic Women. *Eur J Obstet Gynecol Reprod Biol* 113: 221-225, 2004.

Reuss E, Price J, Koonings P: Atypical Glandular Cells of Undetermined Significance: Subtyping as a Predictor of Outcome. *J Reprod Med* 46: 701-705, 2001.

Reyniak V, Sedlis A, Stone D, et al: Cytohormonal Findings in Patients Using Various Forms of Contraception. *Acta Cytol* 13: 315-322, 1969.

Rha S-H, Dong SM, Jen J, et al: Molecular Detection of Cervical Intraepithelial Neoplasia and Cervical Carcinoma by Microsatellite Analysis of Papanicolaou Smears. *Int J Cancer* 93: 424-429, 2001.

Rhatigan RM: Endocervical Gland Atypia Secondary to Arias-Stella Change. *Arch Pathol Lab Med* 116: 943-946, 1992.

Rhemtula H, Grayson W, van Iddekinge B, et al: Large-Cell Neuroendocrine Carcinoma of the Uterine Cervix—A Clinicopathological Study of Five Cases. *S Afr Med J* 91: 525-528, 2001.

Rhoads JL, Wright DC, Redfield RR, et al: Chronic Vaginal Candidiasis in Women With Human Immunodeficiency Virus Infection. *JAMA* 257: 3105-3107, 1987.

Ribes JA, Vanover-Sams CL, Baker DJ: Zygomycetes in Human Disease. *Clin Microbiol Rev* 13: 236-301, 2000.

Rice PS, Cason J, Best JM, et al: High Risk Genital Papillomavirus Infections Are Spread Vertically. *Rev Med Virol* 9: 15-21, 1999.

Richard K, Dziura B, Hornish A: Cell Block Preparation as a Diagnostic Technique Complementary to Fluid-Based Monolayer Cervicovaginal Specimens. *Acta Cytol* 43: 69-73, 1999.

Richard L, Guranick M, Ferenczy A: Ultrastructure of Glassy Cell Carcinoma of Cervix. *Diagn Cytopathol* 3: 31-38, 1981.

Richards CJ, Furness PN: Basement Membrane Continuity in Benign, Premalignant and Malignant Epithelial Conditions of the Uterine Cervix. *Histopathology* 16: 47-52, 1990.

Richardson AC, Lyon JB: The Effect of Condom Use on Squamous Cell Cervical Intraepithelial Neoplasia. *Am J Obstet Gynecol* 140: 909-913, 1981.

Richart RM: A Radioautographic Analysis of Cellular Proliferation in Dysplasia and Carcinoma In Situ of the Uterine Cervix. *Am J Obstet Gynecol* 86: 925-930, 1963a.

Richart RM: Cervical Neoplasia in Pregnancy. *Am J Obstet Gynecol* 87: 474-477, 1963b.

Richart RM: Evaluation of the True False Negative Rate in Cytology. *Am J Obstet Gynecol* 89: 724-726, 1964a.

Richart RM: The Correlation of Schiller-Positive Areas on the Exposed Portion of the Cervix With Intraepithelial Neoplasia. *Am J Obstet Gynecol* 90: 697-701, 1964b.

Richart RM: Colpomicroscopic Studies of the Distribution of Dysplasia and Carcinoma In Situ on the Exposed Portion of the Human Uterine Cervix. *Cancer* 18: 950-954, 1965a.

Richart RM, Vaillant HW: Influence of Cell Collection Techniques Upon Cytological Diagnosis. *Cancer* 18: 1474-1478, 1965b.

Richart RM: Colpomicroscopic Studies of Cervical Intraepithelial Neoplasia. *Cancer* 19: 395-405, 1966a.

Richart RM: Influence of Diagnostic and Therapeutic Procedures on the Distribution of Cervical Intraepithelial Neoplasia. *Cancer* 19: 1635-1638, 1966b.

Richart RM, Lerch V, Baron B: A Time-Lapse Cinematographic Study In Vitro of Mitosis in Normal Human Cervical Epithelium, Dysplasia and Carcinoma In Situ. *J Natl Cancer Inst* 39: 571-577, 1967.

Richart RM: Natural History of Cervical Intraepithelial Neoplasia. *Clin Obstet Gynecol* 5: 748-784, 1968.

Richart RM: A Theory of Cervical Carcinogenesis. *Obstet Gynecol Surv* 24: 874-879, 1969a.

Richart RM, Barron BA: A Follow-Up Study of Patients With Cervical Dysplasia. *Am J Obstet Gynecol* 105: 386-393, 1969b.

Richart RM: Cervical Intraepithelial Neoplasia. *Pathol Annu* 8: 301-328, 1973.

Richart RM: Current Concepts in Obstetrics and Gynecology: The Patient With an Abnormal Pap Smear—Screening Techniques and Management. *N Engl J Med* 302: 332-334, 1980a.

Richart RM, Townsend DE, Crisp W, et al: An Analysis of "Long-Term" Follow-Up Results in Patients With Cervical Intraepithelial Neoplasia Treated by Cryotherapy. *Am J Obstet Gynecol* 137: 823-826, 1980b.

Richart RM: Screening Strategies for Cervical Cancer and Cervical Intraepithelial Neoplasia. *Cancer* 47: 1176-1181, 1981a.

Richart RM, Crum CP, Townsend DE: Workup of the Patient With an Abnormal Papanicolaou Smear. *Gynecol Oncol* 12(2 Pt2): S265-S276, 1981b.

Richart RM: Causes and Management of Cervical Intraepithelial Neoplasia. *Cancer* 60: 1951-1959, 1987.

Richart RM: A Modified Terminology for Cervical Intraepithelial Neoplasia. *Obstet Gynecol* 75: 131-133, 1990.

Richart RM, Wright TC: Controversies in the Management of Low-Grade Cervical Intraepithelial Neoplasia. *Cancer* 71: 1413-1421, 1993.

Richart RM: Screening: The Next Century. *Cancer* 76: 1919-1927, 1995.

Richart RM, Masood S, Syrjänen KJ, et al: Human Papillomavirus: IAC Task Force Summary. *Acta Cytol* 42: 50-58, 1998.

Richart RM: "Current Understanding and Management of Glandular Lesions of the Cervix 'Problems in Detection and Identification'; 'Problems with AGUS'." *Contemporary OB/GYN* (April 15, Suppl): 7-13, 2000.

Riethdorf L, Riethdorf S, Lee KR, et al: Human Papillomaviruses, Expression of p16^{INK4a}, and Early Endocervical Gandular Neoplasia. *Hum Pathol* 33: 899-904, 2002.

Riethdorf S, Riethdorf L, Schulz G, et al: Relationship Between Telomerase Activation and HPV 16/18 Oncogene Expression in Squamous Intraepithelial Lesions and Squamous Cell Carcinomas of the Uterine Cervix. *Int J Gynecol Pathol* 20: 177-185, 2001.

Rietveld WJ, Boon ME, Meulman JJ: Seasonal Fluctuations in the Cervical Smear Detection Rates for (Pre)Malignant Changes and for Infections. *Diagn Cytopathol* 17: 452-455, 1997.

Rigoni-Stern D: Fatti statistici relativi alle malattie cancerose che servirono di base alle poche cose dal dette Dott. Giornale Servire. *Prog Pathol Ter Ser* 2: 507-517, 1842.

Rilke F, Alasio L: Detached Ciliary Tufts in Cervico-Vaginal Smears (Letter). *Acta Cytol* 20: 189-190, 1976.

Rimm DL, Gmitro S, Frable WJ: Atypical Reparative Change on Cervical/Vaginal Smears May Be Associated With Dysplasia. *Diagn Cytopathol* 14: 374-379, 1996.

Rinas AC: The Gynecological Pap Test. *Clin Lab Sci* 12: 239-245, 1999.

Rincón-Arano H, Rosales R, Mora N, et al: R-Ras Promotes Tumor Growth of Cervical Epithelial Cells. *Cancer* 97: 575-585, 2003.

Rintala MA, Rantanen VT, Salmi TA, et al: Pap Smear After Radiation Therapy for Cervical Carcinoma. *Anticancer Res* 17: 3747-3750, 1997.

Rintala MA, Greenman SE, Pollanen PP, et al: Detection of High-Risk HPV DNA in Semen and Its Association With the Quality of Semen. *Int J STD AIDS* 15: 740-743, 2004.

Riotton G, Christopherson WM, eds: World Health Organization. International Classification of Tumors. No. 8. Cytology of the Female Genital Tract. Geneva: World Health Organization. 1973.

Riou G, Favre M, Jeannel D, et al: Association Between Poor Prognosis in Early-Stage Invasive Cervical Carcinomas and Non-Detection of HPV DNA. *Lancet* 335: 1171-1174, 1990.

Rippon JW, Dolan CT: Colonization of the Vagina by Fungi of the Genus *Mucor*. *Clin Microbiol Newsl* 1: 4-5, 1979.

Rippon JW, Dolan CT: Mucorales: Colonization of the Human Vagina and Colon. In: Kuttin ES, Baum GL, eds. *Human and Animal Mycology* (Proceedings of the VII Congress of ISHAM, Jerusalem, Israel, 11-16 March 1979). Elsevier North-Holland, Amsterdam, The Netherlands, 39-42, 1980.

Risse EK, Beerthuizen RJ, Vooijs GP: Cytologic and Histologic Findings in Women Using an IUD. *Obstet Gynecol* 58: 569-573, 1981.

Ritchie DA: The Vaginal Maturation Index and Endometrial Carcinoma. *Am J Obstet Gynecol* 91: 578-579, 1965.

Ritter DB, Kadish AS, Vermund SH, et al: Detection of Human Papillomavirus Deoxyribonucleic Acid in Exfoliated Cervicovaginal Cells as a Predictor of Cervical Neoplasia in a High-Risk Population. *Am J Obstet Gynecol* 159: 1517-1525, 1988.

Rizzo T, Linker G, Schumann GB: Cytologic Pitfalls Associated With Microglandular Hyperplasia (Abstract). *Acta Cytol* 33: 738, 1989.

Roa PN, Collins LA, Geisinger KR, et al: Identification of Male Epithelial Cells in Routine Postcoital Cervicovaginal Smears Using Fluorescence In Situ Hybridization: Application in Sexual Assault and Molestation. *Am J Clin Pathol* 104: 32-35, 1995.

Roach N: Delivering Human Papillomavirus Testing to the Public: One Patient Advocate's Perspective. *Arch Pathol Lab Med* 127: 995-996, 2003.

Robb J: The Pap Smear Is a Cancer Screening Test: Why Not Put the Screening Error Rate in the Report? *Diagn Cytopathol* 9: 485-486, 1993.

Robb JA: The "ASCUS" Swamp (Editorial). *Diagn Cytopathol* 11: 319-320, 1994.

Robboy SJ, Friedlander LM, Welch WR, et al: Cytology of 575 Young Women With Prenatal Exposure to Diethylstilbestrol. *Obstet Gynecol* 48: 511-515, 1976.

Robboy SJ, Scully RE, Welch WR, et al: Intrauterine Diethylstilbestrol Exposure and Its Consequences: Pathologic Characteristics of Vaginal Adenosis, Clear Cell Adenocarcinoma, and Related Lesions. *Arch Pathol Lab Med* 101: 1-5, 1977.

Robboy SJ, Keh PC, Nickerson RJ, et al: Squamous Cell Dysplasia and Carcinoma In Situ of the Cervix and Vagina After Prenatal Exposure to Diethylstilbestrol. *Obstet Gynecol* 51: 528-535, 1978.

Robboy SJ, Bradley R: Changing Trends and Prognostic Features in Endometrial Cancer Associated With Exogenous Estrogen Therapy. *Obstet Gynecol* 54: 269-277, 1979a.

Robboy SJ, Kaufman RH, Prat J, et al: Pathologic Findings in Young Women Enrolled in the National Cooperative Diethystilbesterol Adenosis (DESAD) Project. *Obstet Gynecol* 53: 309-317, 1979b.

Robboy SJ, Truslow GY, Anton J, et al: Role of Hormones Including Diethylstilbestrol (DES) in the Pathogenesis of Cervical and Vaginal Intraepithelial Neoplasia. *Gynecol Oncol* 12(2 Pt 2): S98-S110, 1981.

Robboy SJ, Noller KL, O'Brien P, et al: Increased Incidence of Cervical and Vaginal Dysplasia in 3,980 Diethylstilbestrol-Exposed Young Women: Experience of the National Collaborative Diethylstilbestrol Adenosis Project. *JAMA* 252: 2979-2983, 1984.

Robboy SJ, Hill EC, Sandberg EC, et al: Vaginal Adenosis in Women Born Prior to the Diethylstilbestrol Era. *Hum Pathol* 17: 488-492, 1986.

Robboy SJ, Anderson MC, Morse A, et al: Cervical Precancer (Intraepithelial Neoplasia). In: Robboy SJ, Anderson MC, Russell P, eds. *Pathology of the Female Reproductive Tract.* Churchill Livingstone, London, 165-193, 2002.

Robert ME, Fu YS: Squamous Cell Carcinoma of the Uterine Cervix—A Review With Emphasis on Prognostic Factors and Unusual Variants. *Semin Diagn Pathol* 7: 173-189, 1990.

Roberts ADG, Denholm RB, Cordiner JW: Cervical Intraepithelial Neoplasia in Postmenopausal Women With Negative Cervical Cytology (Short Report). *Br Med J* 290: 281, 1985.

Roberts CM, Pfister JR, Spear SJ: Increasing Proportion of Herpes Simplex Virus Type1 as a Cause of Genital Herpes Infection in College Students. *Sex Transm Dis* 30: 797-800, 2003.

Roberts JM, Thurloe JK, Bowditch RC, et al: Comparison of ThinPrep and Pap Smear in Relation to Prediction of Adenocarcinoma In Situ. *Acta Cytol* 43: 74-80, 1999.

Roberts JM, Thurloe JK, Bowditch RC, et al: Subdividing Atypical Glandular Cells of Undetermined Significance According to the Australian Modified Bethesda System. *Cancer (Cancer Cytopathol)* 90: 87-95, 2000.

Roberts TH, Ng ABP: Chronic Lymphocytic Cervicitis: Cytologic and Histopathologic Manifestations. *Acta Cytol* 19: 235-243, 1975.

Robertson AJ: Histopathological Grading of Cervical Intraepithelial Neoplasia (CIN)—Is There a Need for Change? *J Pathol* 159: 273-275, 1989a.

Robertson AJ, Anderson JM, Beck JS, et al: Observer Variability in Histopathological Reporting of Cervical Biopsy Specimens. *J Clin Pathol* 42: 231-238, 1989b.

Robertson JH, Woodend BE, Hutchinson J: Risk of Cervical Cancer Associated With Mild Dyskaryosis. *Br Med J* 297: 18-21, 1988.

Robertson JH, Woodend B: Negative Cytology Preceding Cervical Cancer: Causes and Prevention. *J Clin Pathol* 46: 700-702, 1993.

Robertson JH, Woodend B, Elliott H: Cytological Changes Preceding Cervical Cancer. *J Clin Pathol* 47: 278-279, 1994.

Robin CP: Sur quelques hypertrophies glandulaire. *Gaz d hôp* (Paris) 25: 41, 1852.

Robinson W III: Invasive and Preinvasive Cervical Neoplasia in Human Immunodeficiency Virus-Infected Women. *Semin Oncol* 27: 463-470, 2000.

Robinson WR, Morris CB: Cervical Neoplasia: Pathogenesis, Diagnosis, and Management. *Hematol/Oncol Clin North Am* 10: 1163-1176, 1996.

Robinson WR, Barnes SE, Adams S, et al: Histology/Cytology Discrepancies in HIV-Infected Obstetric Patients With Normal Pap Smears. *Gynecol Oncol* 65: 430-433, 1997.

Robles SC, White F, Peruga A: Trends in Cervical Cancer Mortality in the Americas. *Bull Pan Am Health Org* 20: 290-302, 1996.

Rock CL, Michael CW, Reynolds RK, et al: Prevention of Cervix Cancer. *Crit Rev Oncol/Hematol* 33: 169-185, 2000.

Roden RBS, Lowry DR, Schiller JT: Papillomavirus Is Resistent to Dessication. *J Infect Dis* 176: 1076-1079, 1997.

Rodney P, Rodney ZK, Nu S, et al: Cervical Cancer and Black Women: An Analysis of the Disparity in Prevalence of Cervical Cancer. *J Health Care Poor Underserved* 13: 24-37, 2002.

Rogo KO, Linge K: Human Immunodeficiency Virus Seroprevalence Among Cervical Cancer Patients. *Gynecol Oncol* 37: 87-92, 1990.

Rohr LR: Quality Assurance in Gynecologic Cytology. What Is Practical? *Am J Clin Pathol* 94: 754-758, 1990.

Rojansky N, Anteby SO: Gynecologic Neoplasias in the Patient With HIV Infection. *Obstet Gynecol Surv* 51: 679-683, 1996.

Rollason TP, Cullimore J, Bradgate MG: A Suggested Columnar Cell Morphological Equivalent of Squamous Carcinoma In Situ With Early Stromal Invasion. *Int J Gynecol Pathol* 8: 230-236, 1989.

Roman A, Fife K: Human Papillomavirus DNA Associated With Foreskins of Normal Newborns. *J Infect Dis* 153: 855-61, 1986.

Romney SL, Palan PR, Duttagupta C, et al: Retinoids and the Prevention of Cervical Dysplasias. *Am J Obstet Gynecol* 141: 890-894, 1981.

Romney SL, Duttagupta C, Basu J, et al: Plasma Vitamin C and Uterine Cervical Dysplasia. *Am J Obstet Gynecol* 151: 976-980, 1985.

Ronnett BM, Manos MM, Ransley JE, et al: Atypical Glandular Cells of Undetermined Signficance (AGUS): Cytopathologic Features, Histopathologic Results, and Human Papillomavirus DNA Detection. *Hum Pathol* 30: 816-825, 1999.

Roongpisuthipong A, Grimes DA, Hadgu A: Is the Papanicolaou Smear Useful for Diagnosing Sexually Transmitted Diseases? *Obstet Gynecol* 69: 820-824, 1987.

Rorat E, Benjamin F, Richart RM: Verrucous Carcinoma of the Cervix: A Problem in Diagnosis and Management. *Am J Obstet Gynecol* 130: 851-853, 1978.

Rosati LA, Jarzynski DJ: Clear Cell (Mesonephric) Adenocarcinoma of the Vagina: A Case Report. *Acta Cytol* 17: 493-497, 1973.

Rose BR, Thompson CH, Simpson JM, et al: Human Papillomavirus Deoxyribonucleic Acid as a Prognostic Indicator in Early-Stage Cervical Cancer: A Possible Role for Type 18. *Am J Obstet Gynecol* 173: 1461-1468, 1995.

Rosen T: Update on Genital Lesions. *JAMA* 290: 1001-1005, 2003.

Rosenfeld WD, Vermund SH, Wentz SJ, et al: High Prevalence Rate of Human Papillomavirus Infection and Association With Abnormal Papanicolaou Smears in Sexually Active Adolescents. *Am J Dis Child* 143: 1443-1447, 1989.

Rosenfeld WD, Rose E, Vermund SH, et al: Follow-Up Evaluation of Cervicovaginal Human Papillomavirus Infection in Adolescents. *J Pediatr* 121: 307-311, 1992.

Rosenthal DL, McLatchie C, Stern E, et al: Endocervical Columnar Cell Atypia Coincident With Cervical Neoplasia Characterized by Digital Image Analysis. *Acta Cytol* 26: 115-120, 1982.

Roteli-Martins CM, Panetta K, Alves VAF, et al: Cigarette Smoking and High-Risk HPV DNA as Predisposing Factors for High-Grade Cervical Intraepithelial Neoplasia (CIN) in Young Brazilian Women. *Acta Obstet Gynecol Scand* 77: 678-682, 1998.

Rotkin ID: Relation of Adolescent Coitus to Cervical Cancer Risk. *JAMA* 179: 486-491, 1962.

Rotkin ID: Adolescent Coitus and Cervical Cancer: Associations of Related Events With Increased Risk. *Cancer Res* 27: 603-617, 1967a.

Rotkin ID: Epidemiology of Cancer of the Cervix. III. Sexual Characteristics of a Cervical Cancer Population. *Am J Public Health* 5: 815-829, 1967b.

Rotkin ID, Cameron JR: Clusters of Variables Influencing Risk of Cervical Cancer. *Cancer* 21: 663-671, 1968.

Rotkin ID: A Comparison Review of Key Epidemiological Studies in Cervical Cancer Related to Current Searches for Transmissible Agents. *Cancer Res* 33: 1353-1367, 1973.

Rotmensch J, Rosenshein N, Dillon M, et al: Carcinoma Arising in the Neovagina: A Case Report and Review of the Literuture. *Obstet Gynecol* 61: 534-536, 1983.

Rous P: Transmission of a Malignant New Growth by Means of a Cell-free Filtrate (Brief Report). *JAMA* 56: 198, 1911.

Rous P, Beard JW: Carcinomatous Changes in Virus-Induced Papillomas of the Skin of Rabbits. *Proc Soc Exp Biol Med* 32: 578-580, 1934.

Rous P, Beard JW: The Progression to Carcinoma of Virus-Induced Rabbit Papillomas (Shope). *J Exp Med* 62: 523-554, 1935.

Rousseau MC, Villa LL, Costa MC, et al: Occurrence of Cervical Infection With Multiple Human Papillomavirus Types Is Associated With Age and Cytologic Abnormalities. *Sex Transm Dis* 30:581-587, 2003.

Rowe LR, Marshall CJ, Bentz JS: Cell Block Preparation as an Adjunctive Diagnostic Technique in ThinPrep® Monolayer Preparations: A Case Report. *Diagn Cytopathol* 24: 142-144, 2001.

Rowe LR, Aldeen W, Bentz JS: Prevalence and Typing of HPV DNA by Hybrid Capture II in Women With ASCUS, ASC-H, LSIL, and AGC on ThinPrep® Pap Tests. *Diagn Cytopathol* 30: 426-432, 2004.

Rozendaal L, Walboomers JM, van der Linden JC, et al: PCR-Based High-Risk HPV Test in Cervical Cancer Screening Gives Objective Risk Assessment of Women With Cytomorphologically Normal Cervical Smears. *Int J Cancer* 68: 766-769, 1996.

Ruba S, Schoolland M, Allpress S, et al: Adenocarcinoma In Situ of the Uterine Cervix: Screening and Diagnostic Errors in Papanicolaou Smears. *Cancer (Cancer Cytopathol)* 102: 280-287, 2004.

Rubin DK, Frost JK: The Cytologic Detection of Ovarian Cancer. *Acta Cytol* 7: 191-195, 1963.

Rubin IC: The Pathological Diagnosis of Incipient Carcinoma of the Uterus. *Am J Obstet* 62: 668-676, 1910.

Rubin IC: Julius Schottlænder, Pioneer Pathologist in Obstetrics and Gynecology: With Personal Recollections and Notes on Early Contributions to Histopathology of Incipient Uterine Cancer. *J Mount Sinai Hosp NY* 24: 1173-1185, 1957.

Rubin SC: Cervical Cancer: Successes and Failures. *CA: Cancer J Clin* 51: 89-91, 2001.

Rubio CA: Prognostic Value of the Karyopyknotic Index in Carcinoma of the Cervix. *Obstet Gynecol* 28: 383-393, 1966.

Rubio CA: Estrogenic Effect in Vaginal Smears in Cases of Carcinoma In Situ and Microinvasive Carcinoma of the Uterine Cervix. *Acta Cytol* 17: 361-365, 1973.

Rubio CA, Söderbertg G, Einhorn N: Histolgcial and Follow-Up Studies in Cases of Micro-Invasive Carcinoma of the Uterine Cervix *Acta Pathol Microbiol Scand* 82A: 397-410, 1974.

Rubio CA: The False Positive Smear. *Acta Cytol* 19: 212-213, 1975a.

Rubio CA, Lagerlof B: Who Is Responsible for the False Negative Smear? (Letter). *Acta Cytol* 19: 319, 1975b.

Rubio CA, Kranz I: The Exfoliating Cervical Epithelial Surface in Dysplasia, Carcinoma In Situ and Invasive Squamous Carcinoma. I. Scanning Electron Microscopic Study. *Acta Cytol* 20: 144-150, 1976.

Rubio CA: The False Negative Smear. II. The Trapping Effect of Collecting Instruments. *Obstet Gynecol* 49: 576-580, 1977a.

Rubio CA, Einhorn N: The Exfoliating Epithelial Surface of the Uterine Cervix. IV. Scanning Electron Microscopical Study in Invasive Squamous Carcinoma of Human Subjects. *Beitr Pathol* 161: 72-81, 1977b.

Rubio CA, Kock Y, Berglund K: Studies of the Distribution of Abnormal Cells in Cytologic Preparations. I. Making the Smear With a Wooden Spatula. *Acta Cytol* 24: 49-53, 1980a.

Rubio CA, Kock Y, Berglund K, et al: Studies on the Distribution of Abnormal Cells in Cytological Preparations. II. Making the Smear With the Cotton Swab. *Gynecol Oncol* 9: 127-134, 1980b.

Rubio CA, Berglund K, Kock Y, et al: Studies on the Distribution of Abnormal Cells in Cytologic Preparations. III. Making the Smear With a Plastic Spatula. *Am J Obstet Gynecol* 137: 843-846, 1980c.

Rubio CA: Cellular Changes Preceding Slight Dysplasia of the Uterine Cervix. *Acta Cytol* 25: 193-194, 1981a.

Rubio CA: False Negatives in Cervical Cytology: Can They Be Avoided? *Acta Cytol* 25: 199-202, 1981b.

Rubio CA, Kock Y: Studies on the Distribution of Abnormal Cells in Cytologic Preparations: V. The Gradient of Cell Deposition on Slides. *Obstet Gynecol* 57: 754-758, 1981c.

Rubio CA, Stormby N, Kock Y, et al: Studies on the Distribution of Abnormal Cells in Cytologic Preparations: VI. Pressure Exerted by the Gynecologist While Smearing. *Gynecol Oncol* 15: 391-395, 1983.

Rubio CA: Review of Negative Papanicolaou Tests: Is the Retrospective 5-Year Review Necessary? (Letter) *Am J Clin Pathol* 102: 266, 1994.

Ruiter DJ, Mauw BJ, Beyer-Boon ME: Ultrastructure of Normal Epithelial Cells in Papanicolaou-Stained Cervical Smears. An Application of a Modified Open-Face Embedding Technique for Transmission Electron Microscopy. *Acta Cytol* 23: 507-515, 1979.

Rushing L, Cibas ES: Frequency of Tumor Diathesis in Smears from Women With Squamous Cell Carcinoma of the Cervix. *Acta Cytol* 41: 781-785, 1997.

Russell JM, Blair V, Hunter RD: Cervical Carcinoma: Prognosis in Younger Patients. *Br Med J (Clin Res Ed)* 295: 300-303, 1987.

Russin V, Valente PT, Hanjani P: Psammoma Bodies in Neuroendocrine Carcinoma of the Uterine Cervix. *Acta Cytol* 31: 791-795, 1987.

Rutledge CE, Christopherson WM, Parker JE: Cervical Dysplasia and Carcinoma in Pregnancy. *Obstet Gynecol* 19: 351-354, 1962.

Rylander E: Cervical Cancer in Women Belonging to a Cytologically Screened Population. *Acta Obstet Gynecol Scand* 55: 361-366, 1976.

Rylander E: Negative Smears in Women Developing Invasive Cervical Cancer. *Acta Obstet Gynecol Scand* 56: 115-118, 1977.

Rylander E, Ruusuvaara L, Almstromer MW, et al: The Absence of Vaginal Human Papillomavirus 16 DNA in Women Who Have Not Experienced Sexual Intercourse. *Obstet Gynecol* 83: 735-737, 1994.

Ryu JS, Chung HL, Min DY, et al: Diagnosis of Trichomoniasis by Polymerase Chain Reaction. *Yonsei Med J* 40: 56-60, 1999.

S

Saad AJ, Donovan TM, Truong LD: Malakoplakia of the Vagina Diagnosed by Fine-Needle Aspiration Cytology. *Diagn Cytopathol* 9: 559-561, 1993.

Sadeghi SB, Hsieh EW, Gunn SW: Prevalence of Cervical Intraepithelial Neoplasia in Sexually Active Teenagers and Young Adults: Results of Data Analysis of Mass Papanicolaou Screening of 796,337 Women in the United States in 1981. *Am J Obstet Gynecol* 148: 726-729, 1984.

Sadeghi SB, Sadeghi A, Robboy SJ: Prevalence of Dysplasia and Cancer of the Cervix in a Nationwide, Planned Parenthood Population. *Cancer* 61: 2359-2361, 1988.

Sadeghi SB, Sadeghi A, Cosby M, et al: Human Papillomavirus Infection: Frequency and Association With Cervical Neoplasia in a Young Population. *Acta Cytol* 33: 319-323, 1989.

Safall H, Azar HA: Keratin Granulomas in Irradiated Squamous Cell Carcinoma of Various Sites. *Cancer Res* 26: 500-508, 1966.

Safret A, Bösch B, Bannwart F, et al: Carcinoma In Situ of the Fallopian Tube Presenting as a Positive Pap Smear (Letter). *Acta Cytol* 48: 462-464, 2004.

Sagebiel RW, Gates EA, Hill LC: Cytologic Detection of Recurrent Vaginal Melanoma. *Acta Cytol* 22: 353-357, 1978.

Sagher F, Bercovici B, Romem R: Nikolsk Sign on Cervix Uteri in Pemphigus. *Br J Dermatol* 90: 407-411, 1974.

Sagiroglu N: Progression and Regression Studies of Precancer (Anaplastic or Dysplastic) Cells, and the Halo Test. *Am J Obstet Gynecol* 85: 454-469, 1963.

Sagiroglu N, Sagiroglu E: The Cytology of Intrauterine Contraceptive Devices. *Acta Cytol* 58-64, 1970.

Sagiroglu N: Phagocytosis of Spermatozoa in the Uterine Cavity of Woman Using Intrauterine Device. *Int J Fertility* 16: 1-14, 1971.

Sahebali S, Depuydt CE, Segers K, et al: P16^{INK4a} as an Adjunct Marker in Liquid-Based Cervical Cytology. *Int J Cancer* 108: 871-876, 2004.

Sahoo S, DeMay RM: Collagen Balls in Cervical Smears: A Previously Undescribed Finding. *Acta Cytol* : 48: 161-164, 2004.

Saigo PE, Wolinska WH, Kim WS, et al: The Role of Cytology in the Diagnosis and Follow-Up of Patients With Cervical Adenocarcinoma. *Acta Cytol* 29: 785-794, 1985.

Saigo PE: Cytology of Condyloma of the Uterine Cervix. *Semin Diagn Pathol* 3: 204-210, 1986a.

Saigo PE, Cain JM, Kim WS, et al: Prognostic Factors in Adenocarcinoma of the Uterine Cervix. *Cancer* 57: 1584-1593, 1986b.

Saito K, Saito A, Fu YS, et al: Topographic Study of Cervical Condyloma and Intraepithelial Neoplasia. *Cancer* 59: 2064-2070, 1987.

Salomão DR, Hughes JH, Raab SS: Atypical Glandular Cells of Undetermined Significance Favor Endometrial Origin: Criteria for Separating Low-Grade Endometrial Adenocarcinoma from Benign Endometrial Lesions. *Acta Cytol* 46: 458-464, 2002.

Samaratunga H, Cox N, Wright RG: Human Papillomavirus DNA in Glandular Lesions of the Uterine Cervix. *J Clin Pathol* 46: 718-721, 1993.

Saminathan T, Lahoti C, Kannan V, et al: Postmenopausal Squamous-Cell Atypias: A Diagnostic Challenge. *Diagn Cytopathol* 11: 226-230, 1994.

Samra Z, Scherf E, Dan M: Herpes Simplex Virus Type 1 Is the Prevailing Cause of Genital Herpes in the Tel Aviv Area, Israel. *Sex Transm Dis* 30: 794-796, 2003.

Sanclemente G, Gill DK: Human Papillomavirus Molecular Biology and Pathogenesis. *JEADV* (European Academy Dermatology Venereology) 16: 231-240, 2002.

San Cristobal A, deMundi A: *Enterobius vermicularis* Larvae in Vaginal Smears. *Acta Cytol* 20: 190-192, 1976.

Sand PK, Bowen LW, Blischke SO: Evaluation of Male Consorts of Women With Genital Human Papilloma Virus Infection. *Obstet Gynecol* 68: 679-681, 1986.

Sandberg EC: The Incidence and Distribution of Occult Vaginal Adenosis. *Am J Obstet Gynecol* 101: 322-333; discussion 333-334, 1968.

Sandmire HF, Austin SD, Bechtel RC: Experience With 40,000 Papanicolaou Smears. *Obstet Gynecol* 48: 56-60, 1976.

Sankar KN, Tayal SC: Cervical Smear: Is Screening of Teenagers Justified? (Audit Report) *Int J STD AIDS* 9: 303, 1998; comment: *Int J STD AIDS*, 556-557, 1998.

Santo T, Ueki M: Stromal Reactions to Squamous Cell Carcinoma of the Cervix. *Am J Obstet Gynecol* 156: 906-910, 1987.

Sano T, Oyama T, Kashiwabara K, et al: Expression Status of p16 Protein Is Associated With Human Papillomavirus Oncogenic Potential in Cervical and Genital Lesions. *Am J Pathol* 153: 1741-1748, 1998.

Santoso JT, Kucera PR, Ray J: Primary Malignant Melanoma of the Uterine Cervix: Two Case Reports and a Century's Review. *Obstet Gynecol Surv* 45: 733-740, 1990.

Saqi A, Pasha TL, McGrath CM et al: Overexpression of p16^{INK4a} in Liquid-Based Specimens (SurePath) as Marker of Cervical Dysplasia and Neoplasia. *Diagn Cytopathol* 27: 365-370, 2002.

Sardana S, Sohani P, Agarwal SS, et al: Epidemiologic Analysis of *Trichomonas vaginalis* Infection in Inflammatory Smears. *Acta Cytol* 38: 693-697, 1994.

Sarode VR, Rader AE, Rose PG, et al: Significance of Cytologically Normal Endometrial Cells in Cervical Smears from Postmenopausal Women. *Acta Cytol* 45: 153-156, 2001.

Sarode VR, Werner C, Gander R, et al: Reflex Human Papillomavirus DNA Testing on Residual Liquid-Based (TPPT) Cervical Samples: Focus on Age-Stratified Clinical Performance. *Cancer* 99: 149-155, 2003.

Sasadeusz J, Kelly H, Szer J, et al: Post-Transplant Complications: Abnormal Cervical Cytology in Bone Marrow Transplant Recipients. *Bone Marrow Transplantation* 28: 393-397, 2001.

Sasagawa M, Nishino K, Honma S, et al: Origin of Adenocarcinoma Cells Observed on Cervical Cytology. *Acta Cytol* 47: 410-414, 2003.

Sasagawa T, Shimakage M, Nakamura M, et al: Epstein-Barr Virus (EBV) Genes Expression in Cervical Intraepithelial Neoplasia and Invasive Cervical Cancer: A Comparative Study With Human Papillomavirus (HPV) Infection. *Hum Pathol* 31:318-326, 2000.

Sasieni P, Adams J: Effect of Screening on Cervical Cancer Mortality in England and Wales: Analysis of Trends With an Age Period Cohort Model. *Br Med J* 318: 1244-1245, 1999.

Sasieni P, Adams J: Changing Rates of Adenocarcinoma and Adenosquamous Carcinoma of the Cervix in England. *Lancet* 357: 1490-1493, 2001.

Saslow D, Runowicz, CD, Solomon D, et al: American Cancer Society Guideline for the Early Detection of Cervical Neoplasia and Cancer. *CA: Cancer J Clin* 52: 342-362, 2002.

Sass MA: Use of a Liquid-Based, Thin-Layer Pap Test in a Community Hospital: Impact on Cytology Performance and Productivity. *Acta Cytol* 48: 17-22, 2004.

Sasson IM, Haley NJ, Hoffmann D, et al: Cigarette Smoking and Neoplasia of the Uterine Cervix: Smoke Constituents in Cervical Mucus. *N Engl J Med* 312: 315-316, 1985.

Sato S, Okagaki T, Clark BA, et al: Sensitivity of Koilocytosis, Immunocytochemistry, and Electron Microscopy as Compared to DNA Hybridization in Detecting Human Papillomavirus in Cervical and Vaginal Condyloma and Intraepithelial Neoplasia. *Int J Gynecol Pathol* 5: 297-307, 1986.

Sato S, Ito K, Konno R, et al: Adenoma Malignum: Report of a Case With Cytologic and Colposcopic Findings and Immunohistochemical Staining With Antimucin Monoclonal Antibody HIK-1083. *Acta Cytol* 44: 389-392, 2000.

Sato Y, Shimamoto T, Amada S, et al: Large Cell Neuroendocrine Carcinoma of the Uterine Cervix: A Clinicopathological Study of Six Cases. *Int J Gynecol Pathol* 22: 226-230, 2003.

Savargaonkar PR, Hale RJ, Mutton A, et al: Neuroendocrine Differentiation in Cervical Carcinoma. *J Clin Pathol* 49: 139-141, 1996.

Saw H-S, Lee J-K, Lee H-L, et al: Natural History of Low-Grade Squamous Intraepithelial Lesion. *J Low Genital Tract Dis* 5: 153-158, 2001.

Sawaya GF, Kerlikowske K, Lee NC, et al: Frequency of Cervical Smear Abnormalities Within 3 Years of Normal Cytology. *Obstet Gynecol* 96: 219-223, 2000.

Sawaya GF, Brown AD, Washington AE, et al: Current Approaches to Cervical-Cancer Screening. *N Engl J Med* 344: 1603-1607, 2001.

Sawaya GF, McConnell KJ, Kulasingam SL, et al: Risk of Cervical Cancer Associated With Extending the Interval Between Cervical-Cancer Screenings. *N Engl J Med* 349: 1501-1509, 2003.

Schachter A, Beckerman A, Bahary C, et al: The Value of Cytology in the Diagnosis of Endometrial Pathology. *Acta Cytol* 24: 149-152, 1980.

Schachter A, Kopmar A, Avram E, et al: Hormonal and Cytopathological Changes in Vaginal and Cervical Smears from Women Undergoing Chemotherapy for Extragenital Malignant Diseases. *Acta Obstet Gynecol Scand* 62: 621-624, 1983.

Schachter J, Hill EC, King EB, et al: Chlamydial Infection in Women With Cervical Dysplasia. *Am J Obstet Gynecol* 123: 753-757, 1975.

Schachter J, Hill EC, King EB, et al: *Chlamydia trachomatis* and Cervical Neoplasia. *JAMA* 248: 2134-2138, 1982.

Scharpe K, McCarthy J, Padwick M, et al: Ovarian Carcinoma Detected by Routine Cervical Smear. *J Obstet Gynecol* 23: 91-92, 2003.

Schauenstein W: Histologische Untersuchungen über atypisches Plattenepithel an der Portio und an der Innenfläche der Cervic uteri. *Arch Gynak* 85: 576-616, 1908.

Scheiden R, Wagener C, Knolle U, et al: Atypical Squamous Cells of Undetermined Significance: Audit and the Impact of Potential Litigation. Retrospective Review of 682 Cases. *Cytopathology* 14: 257-262, 2003.

Schenck U, Herbert A, Solomon D, et al: Terminology: IAC Task Force Summary (Cytology Towards the 21st Century: An International Expert Conference and Tutorial). *Acta Cytol* 42: 5-15, 1998.

Schiffman MH, Bauer HM, Lorincz AT, et al: Comparison of Southern Blot Hybridization and Polymerase Chain Reaction Methods for the Detection of Human Papillomavirus DNA. *J Clin Microbiol* 29: 573-577, 1991.

Schiffman MH: Recent Progress in Defining the Epidemiology of Human Papillomavirus Infection and Cervical Neoplasia (Commentary). *J Natl Cancer Inst* 84: 394-398, 1992.

Schiffman MH, Bauer HM, Hoover RN, et al: Epidemiologic Evidence Showing That Human Papillomavirus Infection Causes Most Cervical Intraepithelial Neoplasia. *J Natl Cancer Inst* 85: 958-964, 1993.

Schiffman MH, Brinton LA: The Epidemiology of Cervical Carcinogensis. *Cancer* 76: 1888-1901, 1995a.

Schiffman MH: New Epidemiology of Human Papillomavirus Infection and Cervical Neoplasia. *J Natl Cancer Inst* 87: 1345-1347, 1995b.

Schiffman MH, Adrianza ME: ASCUS-LSIL Triage Study: Design, Methods and Characteristics of Trial Participants. *Acta Cytol* 44: 726-742, 2000a.

Schiffman MH, Herrero R, Hildesheim A, et al: HPV DNA Testing in Cervical Cancer Screening: Results from Women in a High-Risk Province of Costa Rica. *JAMA* 283: 87-93, 2000b.

Schiffman MH, Castle PE: Human Papillomavirus: Epidemiology and Public Health. *Arch Pathol Lab Med* 127: 930-934, 2003a.

Schiffman MH, Solomon D: Findings to Date from the ASCUS-LSIL Triage Study (ALTS). *Arch Pathol Lab Med* 127: 946-949, 2003b.

Schiller W: Untersuchungen zur Entstehung der Geschwülste. I. Teil: Collumcarcinom des Uterus. *Virchows Archiv (Path Anat)* 263: 279-367, 1927.

Schiller W: Early Diagnosis of Carcinoma of the Cervix. *Surg Gynecol Obstet* 56: 210-222, 1933.

Schiller W: Pathology of the Cervix. *Am J Obstet Gynecol* 34: 430-438, 1937.

Schiller W: Leucoplakia, Leucokeratosis, and Carcinoma of the Cervix. *Am J Obstet Gynecol* 35: 17-38, 1938.

Schindler S, Pooley RJ, De Frias DVS, et al: Follow-Up of Atypical Glandular Cells in Cervical-Endocervical Smears. *Ann Diagn Pathol* 2: 312-317, 1998.

Schlaen I, Gonzalez Garcia MR, Weismann EA: Predictive Value of Phenotypic Cytologic Characteristics in Early Dysplastic Cervical Lesions. *Acta Cytol* 32: 298-302, 1988.

Schlecht NF, Kulaga S, Robitaille J, et al: Persistent Human Papillomavirus Infection as a Predictor of Cervical Intraepithelial Neoplasia. *JAMA* 286: 3106-3114, 2001.

Schlesinger C, Silverberg SG: Endocervical Adenocarcinoma In Situ of Tubal Type and Its Relation to Atypical Tubal Metaplasia. *Int J Gynecol Pathol* 18: 1-4, 1999.

Schlosshauer PW, Heller DS, Koulos JP: Malignant Melanoma of the Uterine Cervix Diagnosed on a Cervical Cytologic Smear (Letter). *Acta Cytol* 42: 1043-1045, 1998.

Schmauz R, Okong P, de Villiers EM, et al: Multiple Infections in Cases of Cervical Cancer from a High-Incidence Area in Tropical Africa. *Int J Cancer* 43: 805-809, 1989.

Schmidt WA, Bedrossian CW, Ali V, et al: Actinomycins and Intrauterine Contraceptive Devices: The Clinicopathologic Study. *Diagn Gynecol Obstet* 2: 165-177, 1980.

Schmidt WA: IUDs, Inflammation, and Infection. *Hum Pathol* 13: 878-881, 1982.

Schnadig VJ, Davie KD, Shafer SK, et al: The Cytologist and Bacterioses of the Vaginal-Ectocervical Area: Clues, Commas and Confusion. *Acta Cytol* 33: 287-297, 1989.

Schneider A, Kraus H: The "Suspicious" Gynecologic Smear. *Acta Cytol* 29: 795-799, 1985.

Schneider A, Hotz M, Gissmann L: Increased Prevalence of Human Papillomaviruses in the Lower Genital Tract of Pregnant Women. *Int J Cancer* 40: 198-201, 1987a.

Schneider A, Meinhardt G, De-Villiers E-M, et al: Sensitivity of the Cytologic Diagnosis of Cervical Condyloma in Comparison With HPV-DNA Hybridization Studies. *Diagn Cytopathol* 3: 250-255, 1987b.

Schneider A, Oltersdorf T, Schneider V, et al: Distribution Pattern of Human Papilloma Virus 16 Genome in Cervical Neoplasia by Molecular In Situ Hybridization of Tissue Sections. *Int J Cancer* 39: 717-721, 1987c.

Schneider A, Sawada E, Gissman L, et al: Human Papillomaviruses in Women With a History of Abnormal Papanicolaou Smears and in Their Male Partners. *Obstet Gynecol* 69: 554-562, 1987d.

Schneider A, Kirchmayr R, De Villiers E-M, et al: Subclinical Human Papillomavirus Infections in Male Sexual Partners of Female Carriers. *J Urol* 140: 1431-1434, 1988a.

Schneider A, Sterzik K, Buck G, et al: Colposcopy Is Superior to Cytology for the Detection of Early Genital Human Papillomavirus Infection. *Obstet Gynecol* 71: 236-241, 1988b.

Schneider A: What Are the Various Methods for HPV Detection? *Diagn Cytopathol* 5: 339-341, 1989a.

Schneider A, Shah K: The Role of Vitamins in the Etiology of Cervical Neoplasia: An Epidemiological Review. *Arch Gynecol Obstet* 246: 1-13, 1989b.

Schneider A, Meinhardt G, Kirchmayr R, et al: Prevalence of Human Papillomavirus Genomes in Tissues from the Lower Genital Tract as Detected by Molecular In Situ Hybridization. *Int J Gynecol Pathol* 10: 1-14, 1991.

Schneider A, Kirchhoff T, Meinhardt G, et al: Repeated Evaluation of Human Papillomavirus 16 Status in Cervical Swabs of Young Women With a History of Normal Pap Smears. *Obstet Gynecol* 79: 683-688, 1992a.

Schneider A, Koutsky LA: Natural History and Epidemiological Features of Genital HPV Infection. *IARC Sci Publ* (119): 25-52, 1992b.

Schneider C, Wright E, Perucchini D, et al: Primary Carcinoma of the Fallopian Tube. A Report of 19 Cases With Literature Review. *Eur J Gynaecol Oncol* 21: 578-582, 2000.

Schneider ML, Wortmann, Weigel A: Influence of the Histologic and Cytologic Grade and the Clinical and Postsurgical Stage on the Rate of Endometrial Carcinoma Detection by Cervical Cytology. *Acta Cytol* 30: 616-622, 1986.

Schneider V: Arias-Stella Reaction of the Endocervix: Frequency and Location. *Acta Cytol* 25: 224-228, 1981a.

Schneider V, Barnes LA: Ectopic Decidual Reaction of the Uterine Cervix: Frequency and Cytologic Presentation. *Acta Cytol* 25: 616-622, 1981b.

Schneider V, Kay S, Lee HM: Immunosuppression as a High-Risk Factor in the Development of *Condyloma acuminatum* and Squamous Neoplasia of the Cervix. *Acta Cytol* 27: 220-224, 1983.

Schneider V: Microscopic Diagnosis of HPV Infection. *Clin Obstet Gynecol* 32: 148-156, 1989.

Schneider V: Hormonal Cytology: When and Why. *Diagn Cytopathol* 13: 163-165, 1995.

Schneider V, Henry MR, Jimenez-Ayala M, et al: Cervical Cancer Screening, Screening Errors and Reporting. *Acta Cytol* 45: 493-498, 2001.

Schneider V: Symposium Part 2: Should the Bethesda System Terminology Be Used in Diagnostic Surgical Pathology?: Counterpoint. *Int J Gynecol Oncol* 22: 13-17, 2003a.

Schneider V: CIN Prognostication: Will Molecular Techniques Do the Trick? *Acta Cytol* 47: 115-116, 2003b.

Schoolland M, Sterrett GF, Knowles SA, et al: The "Inconclusive—Possible High-Grade Epithelial Abnormality" Category in Papanicolaou Smear Reporting. *Cancer (Cancer Cytopathol)* 84: 208-217, 1998.

Schoolland M, Allpress S, Sterrett GF: Adenocarcinoma of the Cervix: Sensitivity of Diagnosis by Cervical Smear and Cytologic Patterns and Pitfalls in 24 Cases. *Cancer (Cancer Cytopathol)* 96: 5-13, 2002a.

Schoolland M, Segal A, Allpress S, et al: Adenocarcinoma In Situ of the Cervix: Sensitivity of Detection by Cervical Smear. *Cancer (Cytopathol)* 96: 330-337, 2002b.

Schorge JO, Lee KR, Flynn CE, et al: Stage IA1 Cervical Adenocarcinoma: Definition and Treatment. *Obstet Gynecol* 93: 219-222, 1999.

Schorge JO, Saboorian MH, Hynan L, et al: ThinPrep Detection of Cervical and Endometrial Adenocarcinoma: A Retrospective Cohort Study. *Cancer (Cancer Cytopathol)* 96: 338-343, 2002.

Schorzman CM, Sucato GS: Sexually Transmitted Infections in Adolescents: A Treatment Update. *J Pediatr Adolesc Gynecol* 17: 205-213, 2004.

Schottlaender J, Kermauner F: *Zur Kenntnis des Uteruskarzinoms*: Monographische Studie über Morphologie, Enticklung, Wachstum, nebst Beiträgen zur Klinik der erkrankung. Karger, Berlin, 1912.

Schramm G: Development of Severe Cervical Dysplasia Under Treatment With Azathiprine (Imuran). *Acta Cytol* 14: 507-509, 1970.

Schulze A, Mannhardt B, Zerfass-Thome K, et al: Anchorage-Independent Transcription of the Cyclin A Gene Induced by the E7 Oncoprotein of Human Papillomavirus Type 16. *J Virol* 72: 2323-2334, 1998.

Schwarz E, Freese UK, Gissmann L et al: Structure and Transcription of Human Papillomavirus Sequences in Cervical Carcinoma Cells. *Nature* 314: 111-114, 1985.

Schwartz PE, Merino MJ, Curnen MGM: Clinical Management of Patients With Invasive Cervical Cancer Following a Negative Pap Smear. *Yale J Biol Med* 61: 327-338, 1988.

Schwartz PE, Hadjimichael O, Lowell MJ, et al: Rapidly Progressive Cervical Cancer: The Connecticut Experience. *Am J Obstet Gynecol* 175: 1105-1109, 1996.

Schwartz SM, Weiss NS: Increased Incidence of Adenocarcinoma of the Cervix in Young Women in the United States. *Am J Epidemiol* 124: 1045-1047, 1986.

Schwartz SM, Daling JR, Doody DR, et al: Oral Cancer Risk in Relation to Sexual History and Evidence of Human Papillomavirus Infection. *J Natl Cancer Inst* 90: 1626-1636, 1998.

Schwebke JR, Zajackowski ME: Effect of Concurrent Lower Genital Tract Infections on Cervical Cancer Screening. *Genitourin Med* 73: 383-386, 1997.

Schwebke JR, Richey CM, Weiss HL: Correlation of Behaviors With Microbiological Changes in Vaginal Flora. *J Infect Dis* 180: 1632-1636, 1999.

Scott DR, Hagmar B, Maddox P, et al: Use of Human Papillomavirus DNA Testing to Compare Equivocal Cervical Cytologic Interpretations in the United States, Scandinavia, and the United Kingdom. *Cancer (Cancer Cytopathol)* 96: 14-20, 2002.

Scott RB, Ballard LA: Cytology and Its Office Application as Viewed by the Clinician. *Clin Obstet Gynecol* 5: 175-195, 1962.

Scotto J, Bailar JC III: Rigoni-Stern and Medical Statistics: A Nineteenth-Century Approach to Cancer Research. *J Hist Med Allied Sci* 24: 65-75, 1969.

Scully RE, Aguirre P, DeLellis RA: Argyrophilia, Serotonin, and Peptide Hormones in the Female Genial Tract and Its Tumors. *Int J Gynecol Pathol* 3: 51-70, 1984.

Scurry J, Planner R, Grant P: Unusual Variants of Vaginal Adenosis: A Challenge for Diagnosis and Treatment. *Gynecol Oncol* 41: 172-177, 1991.

Sebastião AP, de Noronha L, Pinheiro DL, et al: Influence of Specimen Adequacy on the Diagnosis of ASCUS. *Diagn Cytopathol* 31: 155-158, 2004.

Seckin NC, Turhan NO, Ozmen S, et al: Routine Colposcopic Evaluation of Patients With Persistent Inflammatory Cellular Changes on Pap Smear. *Int J Gynaecol Obstet* 59: 25-29, 1997.

Secor RM: Cytolytic Vaginosis: A Common Cause of Cyclic Vulvovaginitis. *Nurse Pract Forum* 3: 145-148, 1992.

Sedlacek TV, Cunnane M, Carpiniello V: Colposcopy in the Diagnosis of Penile Condyloma. *Am J Obstet Gynecol* 154: 494-496, 1986.

Sedlacek TV, Lindheim S, Eder C, et al: Mechanism for Human Papillomavirus Transmission at Birth. *Am J Obstet Gynecol* 161: 55-59, 1989.

Sedlacek TV, Riva JM, Magen AB, et al: Vaginal and Vulvar Adenosis: An Unsuspected Side Effect of CO_2 Laser Vaporization. *J Reprod Med* 35: 995-1001, 1990.

Sedlacek TV, Sedlacek AE, Neff DK, et al: The Clinical Role of Human Papilloma Virus Typing. *Gynecol Oncol* 42: 222-226, 1991.

Sedlacek TV: Advances in the Diagnosis and Treatment of Human Papillomavirus Infections. *Clin Obstet Gynecol* 42: 206-220, 1999.

Sedlis A: Primary Carcinoma of the Fallopian Tube. *Obstet Gynecol Surv* 16: 209-226, 1961.

Sedlis A, Walters AT, Balin H, et al: Evaluation of Two Simultaneously Obtained Cervical Cytological Smears: A Comparison Study. *Acta Cytol* 18: 291-296, 1974.

Seguin RE, Ingram K: Cervicovaginal Psammoma Bodies in Endosalpiniosis: A Case Report. *J Reprod Med* 45: 526-528, 2000.

Seidman J, Tavassoli FA: Mesonephric Hyperplasia of the Uterine Cervix: A Clinicopathologic Study of 51 Cases. *Int J Gynecol Pathol* 14: 293-299, 1995.

Seidman J, Kurman RJ: Tamoxifen and the Endometrium (Editorial). *Int J Gynecol Pathol* 18: 293-296, 1999.

Seidman SN, Rieder RO: A Review of Sexual Behavior in the United States. *Am J Psychiatry* 151: 330-341, 1994.

Sekhon HS, Press RD, Schmidt WA, et al: Identifcation of Cytomegalovirus in a Liquid-Based Gynecologic Sample Using Morphology, Immunohistochemistry, and DNA Real-Time PCR Detection. *Diagn Cytopathol* 30: 411-417, 2004.

Sekhri A, Le Faou AE. Tardieu J-C, et al: What Can Be Expected from the Cytologic Examination of Cervicovaginal Smears for the Diagnosis of *Chlamydia trachomatis* Infections? *Acta Cytol* 32: 805-810, 1988.

Sellors JW, Mahony JB, Kaczorowski J, et al: Prevalence and Predictors of Human Papillomavirus Infection in Women in Ontario, Canada. *CMAJ* 163: 503-508, 2000a.

Sellors JW, Lorincz AT, Mahony JB, et al: Comparison of Self-Collected Vaginal, Vulvar and Urine Samples With Physician-Collected Cervical Samples for Human Papillomavirus Testing to Detect High-Grade Squamous Intraepithelial Lesions. *CMAJ* 163: 513-518, 2000b.

Sellors JW, Karwalajtys TL, Kaczorowski JA, et al: Prevalence of Infection With Carcinogenic Human Papillomavirus Among Old Women. *CMAJ* 167: 871-873, 2002.

Seltzer V, Spitzer M: Psammoma Bodies in Papillary Adenocarcinoma of the Endocervix. *Int J Gynecol Pathol* 2: 216-221, 1983.

Selvaggi SM: Cytologic Detection of Condylomas and Cervical Intraepithelial Neoplasia of the Uterine Cervix With Histologic Correlation. *Cancer* 58: 2076-2081, 1986.

Selvaggi SM: Cytologic Features of Squamous Cell Carcinoma In Situ Involving Endocervical Glands in Endocervical Cytobrush Specimens. *Acta Cytol* 38: 687-692, 1994.

Selvaggi SM, Haefner HK, Lelle RJ, et al: Neovaginal Cytology After Total Pelvic Exenteration for Gynecological Malignancies. *Diagn Cytopathol* 13: 22-25, 1995a.

Selvaggi SM, Haefner HK: Reporting of Atypical Squamous Cells of Undetermined Significance on Cervical Smears: Is It Significant? *Diagn Cytopathol* 13: 352-356, 1995b.

Selvaggi SM, Haefner HK: Microglandular Endocervical Hyperplasia and Tubal Metaplasia: Pitfalls in the Diagnosis of Adenocarcinoma on Cervical Smears. *Diagn Cytopathol* 16: 168-173, 1997.

Selvaggi SM: Please! No "AGUS" Swamp (Editorial). *Diagn Cytopathol* 21: 157-158, 1999a.

Selvaggi SM: Is It Time to Revisit the Classification System for Cervicovaginal Cytology? *Arch Pathol Lab Med* 123: 993-994, 1999b.

Selvaggi SM: Microglandular Hyperplasia of the Uterine Cervix: Cytological Diagnosis in Cervical Smears (Letter). *Acta Cytol* 44: 480-481, 2000.

Selvaggi SM: Implications of Low Diagnostic Reproducibility of Cervical Cytologic and Histologic Diagnoses (Commentary). *JAMA* 285: 1506-1508, 2001.

Selvaggi SM: Cytologic Features of High-Grade Squamous Intraepithelial Lesions Involving Endocervical Glands on ThinPrep Cytology. *Diagn Cytopathol* 26: 181-185, 2002a; erratum appears in *Diagn Cytopathol* 26: 409.

Selvaggi SM: Atrophic Vaginitis Versus Invasive Squamous Cell Carcinoma on ThinPrep® Cytology: Can the Background Be Reliably Distinguished? *Diagn Cytopathol* 27: 362-364, 2002b.

Selvaggi SM, Guidos BJ: Endocervical Component: Is It a Determinant of Specimen Adequacy? *Diagn Cytopathol* 26: 53-55, 2002c.

Selvaggi SM: Reporting of Atypical Squamous Cells, Cannot Exclude a High-Grade Squamous Intraepithelial Lesion (ASC-H) on Cervical Samples: Is It Significant? *Diagn Cytopathol* 29: 38-41, 2003.

Sen DK, Langley FA: Vaginal Cytology as a Monitor of Fetal Wellbeing in Early Pregnancy. *Acta Cytol* 16: 116-119, 1972.

Sen SK, Talley P, Zua M: Blastomycosis: Report of a Case With Noninvasive, Rapid Diagnosis of Dermal Lesions by the Papanicolaou Technique. *Acta Cytol* 41(Suppl 4): 1399-1401, 1997.

Seski JC, Abell MR, Morley GW: Microinvasive Squamous Carcinoma of the Cervix: Definition, Histologic Analysis, Late Results of Treatment. *Obstet Gynecol* 50: 410-414, 1977.

Sewankambo N, Gray RH, Wawer MJ, et al: HIV-1 Infection Associated With Abnormal Vaginal Flora Morphology and Bacterial Vaginosis. *Lancet* 350: 546-550, 1997.

Seybolt JF, Johnson WD: Cervical Cytodiagnostic Problems: A Survey. *Am J Obstet Gynecol* 109: 1089-1103, 1971.

Shafer M-A, Chew KL, Kromhout LK, et al: Chlamydial Endocervical Infections and Cytologic Findings in Sexually Active Female Adolescents. *Am J Obstet Gynecol* 151: 765-771, 1985.

Shah KV, Kessis TD, Shah F, et al: Human Papillomavirus Investigation of Patients With Cervical Intraepithelial Neoplasia 3, Some of Whom Progressed to Invasive Cancer. *Int J Gynecol Pathol* 15: 127-130, 1996.

Shah KV: Human Papillomaviruses and Anogenital Cancer. *N Engl J Med* 337: 1386-1388, 1997.

Shapiro S, Carrara H, Allan BR, et al: Hypothesis: The Act of Taking a Papanicolaou Smear Reduces the Prevalence of Human Papillomavirus Infection—A Potential Impact on the Risk of Cervical Cancer. *Cancer Causes Control* 14: 953-957, 2003.

Shapiro SP, Nunez C: Psammoma Bodies in the Cervicovaginal Smear in Association With a Papillary Tumor of the Peritoneum. *Obstet Gynecol* 61: 130-134, 1983.

Sharma S, Boyle D, Wansbrough-Jones MH, et al: Cervical Schistosomiasis (Correspondence and Case Report). *Int J Gynecol Cancer* 11: 491-492, 2002.

Sharma SD, Zeigler O, Trussell RR: A Cytologic Study of Dipetolenema [sic] Perstans in Cervical Smears. *Acta Cytol* 15: 479-481, 1971.

Sharp GLM, Cordiner JW, Murray EL, et al: Healing of Cervical Epithelium After Laser Ablation of Cervical Intraepithelial Neoplasia. *J Clin Pathol* 37: 611-615, 1984.

Sheffield MV, Simsir A, Talley L, et al: Interobserver Variability in Assessing Adequacy of the Squamous Component in Conventional Cervicovaginal Smears. *Am J Clin Pathol* 119: 367-373, 2003.

Sheils LA, Wilbur DC: Atypical Squamous Cells of Undetermined Significance: Stratification of the Risk of Association With, or Progression to, Squamous Intraepithelial Lesions Based on Morphologic Subcategorization. *Acta Cytol* 41: 1065-1072, 1997.

Shepherd J, Peersman G, Weston R, et al: Cervical Cancer and Sexual Lifestyle: A Systematic Review of Health Education Interventions Targeted at Women. *Health Educ Res* 15: 681-694, 2000a.

Shepherd J, Weston R, Peersman G, et al: Interventions for Encouraging Sexual Lifestyles and Behaviours Intended to Prevent Cervical Cancer. *Cochrane Database Syst Rev.* (2): CD001035, 2000b.

Sherlaw-Johnson C, Gallivan S, Jenkins D, et al: Cytological Screening and Management of Abnormalities in Prevention of Cervical Cancer: An Overview With Stochastic Modelling. *J Clin Pathol* 47: 430-435, 1994.

Sherman ME, Bitterman P, Rosenshein NB, et al: Uterine Serous Carcinoma: A Morphologically Diverse Neoplasm With Unifying Clinical Features. *Am J Surg Pathol* 16: 600-610, 1992a.

Sherman ME, Kelly D: High-Grade Squamous Intraepithelial Lesions and Invasive Carcinoma Following the Report of Three Negative Papanicolaou Smears: Screening Failures or Rapid Progression? *Mod Pathol* 5: 337-342, 1992b.

Sherman ME, Schiffman MH, Erozan YS, et al: The Bethesda System. A Proposal for Reporting Abnormal Cervical Smears Based on the Reproducibility of Cytopathologic Diagnoses. *Arch Pathol Lab Med* 116: 1155-1158, 1992c.

Sherman ME, Weinstein M, Sughayer M, et al: The Bethesda System. Impact on Reporting Cervicovaginal Specimens and Reproducibility of Criteria for Assessing Endocervical Sampling. *Acta Cytol* 37: 55-60, 1993.

Sherman ME, Schiffman MH, Lorincz AT, et al: Toward Objective Quality Assurance in Cervical Cytopathology: Correlation of Cytopathologic Diagnoses With Detection of High-Risk Human Papillomavirus Types. *Am J Clin Pathol* 102: 182-187, 1994.

Sherman ME, Sturgeon S, Brinton LA, et al: Risk Factors and Hormone Levels in Patients With Serous and Endometrioid Uterine Carcinomas. *Mod Pathol* 10: 963-968, 1997.

Sherman ME, Schiffman MH, Strickler H, et al: Prospects for a Prophylactic HPV Vaccine: Rationale and Future Implications for Cervical Cancer Screening. *Diagn Cytopathol* 18: 5-9, 1998.

Sherman ME, Tabbara SO, Scott DR, et al: "ASCUS, Rule Out HSIL": Cytologic Features, Histologic Correlates, and Human Papillomavirus Detection. *Mod Pathol* 12: 335-342, 1999.

Sherman ME: Theories of Endometrial Carcinogenesis: A Multidisciplinary Approach. *Mod Pathol* 13: 295-308, 2000.

Sherman ME, Solomon D, Schiffman M: Qualification of ASCUS: A Comparison of Equivocal LSIL and Equivocal HSIL Cervical Cytology in the ASCUS LSIL Triage Study. *Am J Clin Pathol* 116: 386-394, 2001.

Sherman ME, Schiffman M, Cox JT: Effects of Age and Human Papilloma Viral Load on Colposcopy Triage: Data from the Randomized Atypical Squamous Cells of Undetermined Significance/Low-Grade Squamous Intraepithelial Lesion Triage Study (ALTS). *J Natl Cancer Inst* 94: 102-107, 2002.

Sherman ME, Lorincz AT, Scott DR, et al: Baseline Cytology, Human Papillomavirus Testing, and Risk for Cervical Neoplasia: A 10-Year Cohort Analysis. *J Natl Cancer Inst* 95: 46-52, 2003.

Shew ML, Fortenberry JD, Miles P, et al: Interval Between Menarche and First Sexual Intercourse, Related to Risk of Human Papillomavirus Infection. *J Pediatr* 125: 661-666, 1994.

Sheyn I, Mira JL, Thompson MB: *Paracoccidioides brasiliensis* in a Postpartum Pap Smear: A Case Report. *Acta Cytol* 45: 79-81, 2001.

Shidham VB, Dayer AM, Basir Z, et al: Cervical Cytology and Immunohistochemical Features in Endometrial Adenocarcinoma Simulating Microglandular Hyperplasia: A Case Report. *Acta Cytol* 44: 661-666, 2000.

Shidham VB, Rao RN, Machhi J, et al: Microglandular Hyperplasia Has a Cytomorphological Spectrum Overlapping With Atypical Squamous Cells—Cannot Exclude High-Grade Squamous Intraepithelial Lesion (ASC-H). *Diagn Cytopathol* 30: 57-61, 2004.

Shield PW, Wright RG, Free K, et al: The Accuracy of Cervicovaginal Cytology in the Detection of Recurrent Cervical Carcinoma Following Radiotherapy. *Gynecol Oncol* 41: 223-229, 1991.

Shield PW, Daunter B, Wright RG: Post-Irradiation Cytology of Cervical Cancer Patients. *Cytopathology* 3: 167-182, 1992.

Shield PW: Chronic Radiation Effects: A Correlative Study of Smears and Biopsies from the Cervix and Vagina. *Diagn Cytopathol* 13: 107-119, 1995.

Shiffer JD, Sandweiss L, Bos S: The 'Polka Dot' Cell (Letter). *Acta Cytol* 45: 903-905, 2001.

Shiina Y: Cytomorphologic and Immunocytochemical Studies of Chlamydial Infections in Cervical Smears. *Acta Cytol* 29: 683-691, 1985.

Shiina Y, Kobayashi TK: Detection of *Chlamydia trachomatis* by Papanicolaou-Stained Smear and Its Limitations (Letter). *Diagn Cytopathol* 6: 148-151, 1990.

Shin CH, Schorge JO, Lee KR, et al: Conservative Management of Adenocarcinoma In Situ of the Cervix. *Gynecol Oncol* 79: 6-10, 2000.

Shin CH, Schorge JO, Lee KR, et al: Cytologic and Biopsy Findings Leading to Conization in Adenocarcinoma In Situ of the Cervix. *Obstet Gynecol* 100: 271-276. 2002.

Shingleton HM, Richart RM, Wiener J, et al: Human Cervical Intraepithelial Neoplasia: Fine Structure of Dysplasia and Carcinoma In Situ. *Cancer Res* 28: 695-706, 1968.

Shingleton HM, Wilbanks GD: Fine Structure of Human Cervical Intraepithelial Neoplasia In Vivo and In Vitro. *Cancer* 33: 981-989, 1974.

Shingleton HM, Gore H, Straughn JM, et al: The Contribution of Endocervical Smears to Cervical Cancer Detection. *Acta Cytol* 19: 261-264, 1975.

Shingleton HM, Bone H, Bradley DH, et al: Adenocarcinoma of the Cervix. I: Clinical Evaluation and Pathological Features. *Am J Obstet Gynecol* 139: 799-814, 1981.

Shingleton HM, Bell MC, Fremgen A, et al: Is There Really a Difference in Survival of Women With Squamous Cell Carcinoma, Adenocarcinoma, and Adenosquamous Cell Carcinoma of the Cervix? *Cancer* 76(Suppl 10): 1948-1955, 1995.

Shiota A, Igarashi T, Kurose T, et al: Reciprocal Effects of Tamoxifen on Hormonal Cytology in Postmenopausal Women. *Acta Cytol* 46: 499-506, 2002.

Shipman SD, Bristow RE: Adenocarcinoma In Situ and Early Invasive Adenocarcinoma of the Uterine Cervix. *Curr Opin Oncol* 13: 394-398, 2001.

Shokri-Tabibzadeh S, Koss LG, Molnar J, et al: Association of Human Papillomavirus With Neoplastic Processes in the Genital Tract of Four Women With Impaired Immunity. *Gynecol Oncol* 12(2 Pt 2): S129-S140, 1981.

Shorrock K, Johnson J, Johnson IR: Epidemiological Changes in Cervical Carcinoma With Particular Reference to Mucin-Secreting Subtypes. *Histopathology* 17: 53-57, 1990.

Shrago SS: The Arias Stella Reaction: A Case Report of a Cytologic Presentation. *Acta Cytol* 21: 310-313, 1977.

Shroyer KR, Hosey J, Swanson LE, et al: Cytologic Diagnosis of Human Papillomavirus Infection: Spindled Nuclei. *Diagn Cytopathol* 6: 178-183, 1990.

Shulman JJ, Leyton M, Hamilton R: The Papanicolaou Smear: An Insensitive Case-Finding Procedure. *Am J Obstet Gynecol* 120: 446-451, 1974.

Shurbaji MJ, Burja IT, Sawyer WL Jr: Clinical Significance of Identifying Candida on Cervicovaginal (Pap) Smears. *Diagn Cytopathol* 21: 14-17, 1999.

Shy K, Chu J, Mandelson M, et al: Papanicolaou Smear Screening Interval and Risk of Cervical Cancer. *Obstet Gynecol* 74: 838-843, 1989.

Siapco BJ, Kaplan BJ, Bernstein GS, et al: Cytodiagnosis of *Candida* Organisms in Cervical Smears. *Acta Cytol* 30: 477-480, 1986.

Sickel J, Rutkowski M, Bonfiglio T: Cytomegalovirus Inclusions in Routine Cervical Papanicolaou Smears: A Clinicopathologic Study of Three Cases (Abstract). *Acta Cytol* 35: 646, 1991.

Sidawy MK: Cytology in Gynecological Disorders. *Curr Topics Pathol* 85: 233-272, 1992.

Sidawy MK, Tabbara SO: Reactive Change and Atypical Squamous Cells of Undetermined Significance in Papanicolaou Smears: A Cytohistologic Correlation. *Diagn Cytopathol* 9: 423-429, 1993.

Sidawy MK, Siriaunkgul S, Frost AR: Retrospective Analysis of Non-Correlating Cervical Smears and Colposcopically Directed Biopsies. *Diagn Cytopathol* 11: 343-347, 1994.

Sidawy MK, Solomon D: Pitfalls in Diagnostic Cervicovaginal Cytology. *Monogr Pathol* 39: 1-15, 1997.

Siddiqui G, Kurzel RB, Lampley EC, et al: Cervical Dysplasia in Pregnancy: Progression Versus Regression Post-Partum. *Int J Fertil Womens Med* 46: 278-280, 2001.

Siebers AG, de Leeuw H, Verbeek ALM, et al: Prevalence of Squamous Abnormalities in Women With a Recent Smear Without Endocervical Cells Is Lower as Compared to Women With Smears With Endocervical Cells. *Cytopathology* 14: 58-65, 2003.

Siegler EE: Microdiagnosis of Carcinoma In Situ of the Uterine Cervix: A Comparison Study of Pathologists' Diagnoses. *Cancer* 9: 463-469, 1956.

Siegler EE: Cervical Carcinoma in the Aged. *Am J Obstet Gynecol* 103: 1093-1097, 1969.

Silcocks PBS, Moss SM: Rapidly Progressive Cervical Cancer: Is It a Real Problem? *Br J Obstet Gynaecol* 95: 1111-1116, 1988.

Silva CS, Souza MAH, Ângelo AG, et al: Increased Frequency of Abnormal Papanicolaou Smears in Adolescents. *Arch Gynecol Obstet* 266: 154-156, 2002.

Silverberg SG, Boring C: Annual Cancer Statistics. *CA: Cancer J Clin* Volumes 20 to 43, years 1970-1994.

Silverberg SG, DeGiorgi LS: Clear Cell Carcinoma of the Vagina: A Clinical, Pathologic, and Electron Microscopic Study. *Cancer* 29: 1680-1690, 1972.

Silverberg SG, Frable WJ: Prolapse of Fallopian Tube Into Vaginal Vault After Hysterectomy: Histopathology, Cytopathology, and Differential Diagnosis. *Arch Pathol* 97: 100-103, 1974.

Silverberg SG, Hurt WG: Minimal Deviation Adenocarcinoma ("Adenoma Malignum") of the Cervix: A Reappraisal. *Am J Obstet Gynecol* 121: 971-975, 1975.

Silverberg SG, Mullen D, Faraci JA, et al: Endometrial Carcinoma: Clinical-Pathologic Comparison of Cases in Postmenopausal Women Receiving and Not Receiving Exogenous Estrogens. *Cancer* 45: 3018-3026, 1980.

Silverberg SG, Major FJ, Blessing JA, et al: Carcinosarcoma (Malignant Mixed Mesodermal Tumor) of the Uterus. A Gynecologic Oncology Group Pathologic Study of 203 Cases. *Int J Gynecol Pathol* 9: 1-19, 1990.

Silverberg SG: Molecular Diagnosis and Prognosis in Gynecologic Oncology. *Arch Pathol Lab Med* 123: 1035-1040, 1999.

Silverman EM, Silverman AG: Persistence of Spermatozoa in the Lower Genital Tracts of Women. *JAMA* 240: 1875-1877, 1978.

Simon A, Kopolovic J, Beyth Y: Primary Squamous Cell Carcinoma of the Endometrium. *Gynecol Oncol* 31: 454-461, 1988.

Simons AM, Phillips DH, Coleman DV: Damage to DNA in Cervical Epithelium Related to Tobacco Smoking. *Br Med J* 306: 1444-1448, 1993.

Simons AM, Phillips DH, Coleman DV: DNA Adduct Assay in Cervical Epithelium. *Diagn Cytopathol* 10: 284-288, 1994.

Simons AM, Mugica van Herckenrode C, Rodriguez JA, et al: Demonstration of Smoking-Related DNA Damage in Cervical Epithelium and Correlation With Human Papillomavirus Type 16, Using Exfoliated Cervical Cells. *Br J Cancer* 71: 246-249, 1995; erratum appears in *Br J Cancer* 74: 1152, 1996.

Simsir A, Ioffe OB, Bourquin P, et al: Repeat Cervical Cytology at the Time of Colposcopy: Is There an Added Benefit? *Acta Cytol* 45: 23-27, 2001.

Simsir A, Brooks S, Cochran L, et al: Cervicovaginal Smear Abnormalities in Sexually Active Adolescents: Implications for Management. *Acta Cytol* 46: 271-276, 2002.

Simsir A, Hwang S, Cangiarella J, et al: Glandular Cell Atypia on Papanicolaou Smears: Interobserver Variability in the Diagnosis and Prediction of the Cell of Origin. *Cancer (Cancer Cytopathol)* 99: 323-330, 2003.

Singer A: The Uterine Cervix from Adolescence to the Menopause. *Br J Obstet Gynaecol* 82: 81-99, 1975.

Singer A, Reid BL, Coppleson M: A Hypothesis—The Role of a High-Risk Male in the Etiology of Cervical Carcinoma: A Correlation of Epidemiology and Molecular Biology. *Am J Obstet Gynecol* 126: 110-115, 1976.

Singer A, Walker P, Tay SK, et al: Impact of Introduction of Colpscopy to a District General Hospital. *Br Med J Clin Res Ed* 289: 1049-1051, 1984.

Singh V, Gupta MM, Satyanarayana L, et al: Association Between Reproductive Tract Infections and Cervical Inflammatory Epithelial Changes. *Sex Transm Dis* 22: 25-30, 1995.

Singh V, Parashari A, Satyanarayana L: Biological Behavior and Etiology of Inflammatory Cervical Smears. *Diagn Cytopathol* 20: 199-202, 1999.

Singh V, Rastogi S, Garg S, et al: Polymerase Chain Reaction for Detection of Endocervical *Chlamydia trachomatis* Infection in Women Attending a Gynecology Outpatient Department in India. *Acta Cytol* 46: 540-544, 2002.

Sirovich BE, Welch HG: The Frequency of Pap Smear Screening in the United States. *J Gen Intern Med* 19: 243-250, 2004a.

Sirovich BE, Welsch HG: Cervical Cancer Screening Among Women Without a Cervix. *JAMA* 291: 2990-2993, 2004b.

Sivanesaratnam V, Jayalakshmi P, Loo C: Surgical Management of Early Invasive Cancer of the Cervix Associated With Pregnancy. *Gynecol Oncol* 48: 68-75, 1993.

Sividis E, Fox H, Buckley CH: Endometrial Carcinoma: Two or Three Entities? *Int J Gynecol Cancer* 8: 1525-1539, 1998.

Siziopikou KP, Wang HH, Abu-Jawdeh G: Cytologic Features of Neoplastic Lesions in Endocervical Glands. *Diagn Cytopathol* 17: 1-7, 1997.

Sjolin KE: Cytological Findings and Their Significance in Gynaecology: Clinico-Pathologic and Cytologic Correlation. *Acta Obstet Gynecol Scand* 49: 7-12, 1970.

Skaarland E: Nuclear Size and Shape of Epithelial Cells from the Endometrium: Lack of Value as a Criterion for Differentiation Between Normal, Hyperplastic, and Malignant Conditions. *J Clin Pathol* 38: 502-506, 1985.

Skegg DC, Corwin PA, Paul C, et al: Importance of the Male Factor in Cancer of the Cervix. *Lancet* (ii): 581-583, 1982.

Skoumal SM, Maygarden SJ: Malpractice in Gynecologic Cytology: A Need for Expert Witness Guidelines. *Mod Pathol* 10: 267-269, 1997.

Skrabanek P: Cervical Cancer in Nuns and Prostitutes: A Plea for Scientific Continence. *J Clin Epidemiol* 41: 577-582, 1988.

Slater DN, Milner PC, Radley H: Audit of Deaths from Cervical Cancer: Proposal for an Essential Component of the National Screening Program. *J Clin Pathol* 47: 27-28, 1994.

Slattery ML, Robison LM, Schuman KL, et al: Cigarette Smoking and Exposure to Passive Smoke are Risk Factors for Cervical Cancer. *JAMA* 261: 1593-1598, 1989a.

Slattery ML, Overall JC Jr, Abbott TM, et al: Sexual Activity, Contraception, Genital Infections, and Cervical Cancer: Support for a Sexually Transmitted Disease Hypothesis. *Am J Epidemiol* 130: 248-258, 1989b.

Slavin HB, Gavett E: Primary Herpetic Vulvovaginitis. *Proc Soc Exp Biol Med* 63: 343-345, 1946.

Smedts F, Troyanovsky S, Pruszczynski M: Keratin Expression in Cervical Cancer. *Am J Pathol* 141: 497-511, 1992.

Smedts F: Efficacy of Ki-67 Antigen Staining in Papanicolaou (PAP) Smears in Postmenopausal Women With Atypia: An Audit (Letter). *Cytopathology* 12: 130-132, 2001.

Smith AE, Sherman ME, Scott DR, et al: Review of the Bethesda System Atlas Does Not Improve Reproducibility or Accuracy in the Classification of Atypical Squamous Cells of Undetermined Significance Smears. *Cancer (Cancer Cytopathol)* 90: 201-206, 2000.

Smith EM, Johnson SR, Figuerres EJ, et al: The Frequency of Human Papillomavirus Detection in Postmenopausal Women on Hormone Replacement Therapy. *Gynecol Oncol* 65: 441-446, 1997.

Smith EM, Johnson SR, Ritchie JM, et al: Persistent HPV Infection in Postmenopausal Age Women. *Int J Gynecol Obstet* 87: 131-137, 2004.

Smith HO, Tiffany MF, Qualls CR et al: The Rising Incidence of Adenocarcinoma Relative to Squamous Cell Carcinoma: A 24-Year Population-Based Study. *Gynecol Oncol* 78: 97-105, 2000.

Smith HO, Padilla LA: Adenocarcinoma In Situ of the Cervix: Sensitivity of Detection by Cervical Smear (Editorial). *Cancer Cytopathol* 96: 319-322, 2002.

Smith J, Coleman DV: Electron Microscopy of Cells Showing Viral Cytopathic Effects in Papanicolaou Smears. *Acta Cytol* 27: 605-613, 1983.

Smith JH: Cervical Cytology Through the Looking Glass. *Cytopathology* 11: 53-56, 2000.

Smith JW, Townsend DE, Sparkes RS: Genetic Variants of Glucose-6-Phosphate Dehydrogenase in the Study of Carcinoma of the Cervix. *Cancer* 28: 529-532, 1971.

Smith MR, Figge DC, Bennington JL: The Diagnosis of Cervical Cancer During Pregnancy. *Obstet Gynecol* 31: 193-197, 1968.

Smith PA, Turnbull LS: Small Cell and "Pale" Dyskaryosis. *Cytopathology* 8: 3-8, 1997.

Smith PG, Kinlen LJ, White GC, et al: Mortality of Wives of Men Dying With Cancer of the Penis. *Br J Cancer* 41: 422-428, 1980.

Smith-McCune K, Mancuso V, Contant T, et al: Management of Women With Atypical Papanicolaou Tests of Undetermined Significance by Board-Certified Gynecologists: Discrepancies With Published Guidelines. *Am J Obstet Gynecol* 185: 551-556, 2001.

Smolensky MH, Reinberg A, Bicakove-Rocher A, et al: Chronoepidermiological Search for Circannual Changes in the Sexual Activity of Human Males. *Chronobiologia* 8: 217-230, 1981.

Smotkin D, Berek JS, Fu YS, et al: Human Papillomavirus Deoxyribonucleic Acid in Adenocarcinoma and Adenosquamous Carcinoma of the Uterine Cervix. *Obstet Gynecol* 68: 241-244, 1986.

Snyder RN, Ortiz Y, Willie S, et al: Dysplasia and Carcinoma In Situ of the Uterine Cervix: Prevalence in Very Young Women (Under Age 22). *Am J Obstet Gynecol* 124: 751-756, 1976.

Sobel JD: Vaginitis. *N Engl J Med* 337: 1896-1903, 1997.

Sobel JD: Bacterial Vaginosis. *Annu Rev Med* 51: 349-356, 2000.

Sodhani P, Murthy NS, Sardana S, et al: Seasonal Variation in Genital Tract Infections as Detected on Papanicolaou's Smear Examination. *Diagn Cytopathol* 10: 98-99, 1994.

Sodhani P, Gupta S, Prakash S, et al: Columnar and Metaplastic Cells in Vault Smears: Cytologic and Colposcopic Study. *Cytopathology* 10: 122-126, 1999.

Sodhani P, Gupta S, Singh V, et al: Eliminating the Diagnosis Atypical Squamous Cells of Undetermined Significance: Impact on the Accuracy of the Papanicolaou Test. *Acta Cytol* 48: 783-787, 2004.

Soh LT, Heng D, Lee, IW, et al: The Relevance of Oncogenes as Prognostic Markers in Cervical Cancer. *Int J Gynecol Cancer* 12: 465-474, 2002.

Soler ME, Blumenthal PD: New Technologies in Cervical Cancer Precursor Detection. *Curr Opin Oncol* 12: 460-465, 2000.

Solomon D, Frable WJ, Vooijs GP, et al: ASCUS and AGUS Criteria: IAC Task Force Summary. *Acta Cytol* 42: 16-24, 1998.

Solomon D, Schiffman M, Tarrone R: Comparison of Three Management Strategies for Patients With Atypical Squamous Cells of Undetermined Signficance: Baseline Results from a Randomized Trail. *J Natl Cancer Inst* 93: 293-299, 2001.

Solomon D, Davey D, Kurman R, et al: Consensus Statement. The 2001 Bethesda System: Terminology for Reporting Results of Cervical Cytology. *JAMA* 287: 2114-2119, 2002.

Soloway HB: Vaginal and Cervical Cytology of the Early Puerperium. *Acta Cytol* 13: 136-138, 1969.

Sonek M: Vaginal Cytology in Childhood and Puberty. Part I: Newborn through Prepuberty. *J Reprod Med* 11: 39-56, 1969.

Song S, Liem A, Miller JA, et al: Human Papillomavirus Types 16 E6 and E7 Contribute Differently to Carcinogenesis. *Virology* 267: 141-150, 2000.

Song Y-L, Kato N, Matsumiya Y, et al: Identification of, and Hydrogen Peroxide Production by Fecal and Vaginal Lactobacilli Isolated from Japanese Women and Newborn Infants. *J Clin Microbiol* 37: 3062-3064, 1999.

Song YS: The Cytological Diagnosis of Carcinoma of the Fallopian Tube. *Am J Obstet Gynecol* 70: 29-33, 1955.

Song YS: The Significance of Positive Vaginal Smears in Extrauterine Carcinomas. *Am J Obstet Gynecol* 73: 341-348, 1957.

Sonnex C: Human Papillomavirus Infection With Particular Reference to Genital Disease. *J Clin Pathol* 51: 643-648, 1998.

Soofer SB, Sidawy MK: Reactive Cellular Change: Is There an Increased Risk for Squamous Intraepithelial Lesions? *Cancer (Cancer Cytopathol)*: 81: 144-147, 1997.

Soofer SB, Sidawy MK: Atypical Glandular Cells of Undetermined Significance: Clinically Significant Lesions and Means of Patient Follow-Up. *Cancer (Cancer Cytopathol)* 90: 207-214, 2000.

Soost H-J, Bockmühl B, Zock H: Results of Cytologic Mass Screening in the Federal Republic of Germany. *Acta Cytol* 26: 445-452, 1982.

Soost H-J, Lange H-J, Lehmacher W, et al: The Validation of Cervical Cytology. Sensitivity, Specificity and Predictive Value. *Acta Cytol* 35: 8-14, 1991.

Soper DE: The Normal Vaginal Microbial Ecosystem: Importance of the Diagnosis and Treatment of Bacterial Vaginosis. *OB/GYN Special Edition* 5: 9-11, 2002.

Sörensen HM, Petersen O, Nielsen J, et al: The Spontaneous Course of Premalignant Lesions of the Vaginal Portion of the Uterus. *Acta Obstet Gynecol Scand* 43: 103-104, 1964.

Sorosky JI, Kaminski PF, Wheelock JB, et al: Clinical Significance of Hyperkeratosis and Parakeratosis in Otherwise Negative Papanicolaou Smears. *Gynecol Oncol* 39: 132-134, 1990.

Southern EM: Detection of Specific Sequences Among DNA Fragments Separated by Gel Electrophoresis. *J Mol Biol* 98: 503-517, 1975.

Southern SA, Herrington CS: Molecular Events in Uterine Cervical Cancer. *Sex Transm Infect* 74: 101-109, 1998.

Soutter WP, Wisdom S, Brough AK, et al: Should Patients With Mild Atypia in a Cervical Smear Be Referred for Colposcopy? *Br J Obstet Gynaecol* 93: 70-74, 1986.

Spahr J, Behm FG, Schneider V: Preleukemic Granulocytic Sarcoma of Cervix and Vagina: Initial Manifestation by Cytology. *Acta Cytol* 26: 55-60, 1982.

Spanos WJ Jr, King A, Keeney E, et al: Age as a Prognostic Factor in Carcinoma of the Cervix. *Gynecol Oncol* 35: 66-68, 1989.

Speers WC, Picaso LG, Silverberg SG: Immunohistochemical Localization of Carcinoembryonic Antigen in Microglandular Hyperplasia and Adenocarcinoma of the Endocervix. *Am J Clin Pathol* 79: 105-107, 1983.

Spence MR, Gupta PK, Frost JK, et al: Cytologic Detection and Clinical Significance of *Actinomyces israelii* in Women Using Intrauterine Contraceptive Devices. *Am J Obstet Gynecol* 131: 295-298, 1978.

Spence MR, Hollander DH, Smith J, et al: The Clinical and Laboratory Diagnosis of *Trichomonas vaginalis* Infection. *Sex Transm Dis* 7: 168-171, 1980.

Spence MR, Barbacci M, Kappus E, et al: A Correlative Study of Papanicolaou Smear, Fluorescent Antibody, and Culture for the Diagnosis of *Chlamydia trachomatis*. *Obstet Gynecol* 68: 691-695, 1986.

Spencer CP, Cooper AJ, Whitehead MI: Management of Abnormal Bleeding in Women Receiving Hormone Replacement Therapy. *Br Med J* 315: 37-42, 1997.

Spiegel CA, Eschenbach DA, Amsel R, et al: Curved Anerobic Bacteria in Bacterial (Nonspecific) Vaginosis and Their Response to Antimicrobial Therapy. *J Infect Dis* 148: 817-822, 1983.

Spiegel CA: Bacterial Vaginosis. *Clin Microbiol Rev* 4: 485-502, 1991.

Spiegel GW: Endometrial Carcinoma In Situ in Postmenopausal Women. *Am J Surg Pathol* 19: 417-432, 1995.

Spiegel GW, Ashraff M, Brooks JJ: Eosinophils as a Marker for Invasion in Cervical Squamous Neoplastic Lesions. *Int J Gynecol Pathol* 21: 117-124, 2002.

Spinillo A, Capuzzo E, Tenti P, et al: Adequacy of Screening Cervical Cytology Among Human Immunodeficiency Virus-Seropositive Women. *Gynecol Oncol* 69: 109-113, 1998.

Spires SE, Banks ER, Weeks JA, et al: Assessment of Cervicovaginal Smear Adequacy. The Bethesda System Guidelines and Reproducibility. *Am J Clin Pathol* 102: 354-359, 1995.

Spitzer M, Krumholz BA, Chernys AE, et al: Comparative Utility of Repeat Papanicolaou Smears, Cervicography, and Colposcopy in the Evaluation of Atypical Papanicolaou Smears. *Obstet Gynecol* 69: 731-735, 1987.

Spitzer M, Chernys AE, Hirschfield L, et al: Assessment of Criteria Used in the Histologic Diagnosis of Human Papillomavirus-Related Disease of the Female Lower Genital Tract. *Gynecol Oncol* 38: 105-109, 1990.

Spitzer M, Ryskin M, Chernys AE, et al: The Value of Repeat Pap Smear at the Time of Initial Colposcopy. *Gynecol Oncol* 67: 3-7, 1997.

Spjut HJ, Kaufman RH, Carrig SS: Psammoma Bodies in the Cervicovaginal Smear. *Acta Cytol* 8: 352-355, 1964.

Spratt DW, Lee SC: Verrucous Carcinoma of the Cervix. *Am J Obstet Gynecol* 129: 699-700, 1977.

Spriggs AI: Follow-Up of Untreated Carcinoma-In-Situ of the Cervix Uteri (Letter). *Lancet* (ii): 599-600, 1971a.

Spriggs AI, Bowley CE, Cowdell RH: Chromosomes of Precancerous Lesions of the Cervix Uteri: New Data and a Review. *Cancer* 27: 1239-1254, 1971b.

Staebler A, Sherman ME, Zaino RJ, et al: Hormone Receptor Immunohistochemistry and Human Papillomavirus In Situ Hybridization Are Useful for Distinguishing Endocervical and Endometrial Adenocarcinomas. *Am J Surg Pathol* 26: 998-1006, 2002.

Stafl A, Mattingly RF: Colposcopic Diagnosis of Cervical Neoplasia. *Obstet Gynecol* 41: 168-176, 1973.

Stafl A, Mattingly RF: Vaginal Adenosis: A Precancerous Lesion? *Am J Obstet Gynecol* 120: 666-675; discussion 675-677, 1974.

Stafl A, Mattingly RF: Angiogenesis of Cervical Neoplasia. *Am J Obstet Gynecol* 121: 845-852, 1975.

Stahl R, Demopoulos RI, Bigelow B: Carcinoid Tumor Within a Squamous Cell Carcinoma of the Cervix. *Gynecol Oncol* 11: 387-392, 1981.

Stanbridge CM, Butler EB, Langley FA: Problems in Cervicovaginal Cytology: Fine Structure as an Aid to Diagnosis. *Acta Cytol* 24: 335-343, 1980.

Stanbridge CM, Suleman BA, Persad RV, et al: A Cervical Smear Review in Women Developing Cervical Carcinoma With Particular Reference to Age, False Negative Cytology and the Histologic Type of Carcinoma. *Int J Gynecol Cancer* 2: 92-100, 1992.

Stanhope CR, Smith JP, Wharton JT, et al: Carcinoma of the Cervix: The Effect of Age on Survival. *Gynecol Oncol* 10: 188-193, 1980.

Stanley DE, Plowden K, Sherman ME: Reclassification of Negative Smears as Atypical Squamous Cells of Undetermined Significance in Quality Assurance Reviews. *Cancer (Cancer Cytopathol)* 87: 346-350, 1999.

Stanley MA: Human Papillomavirus and Cervical Carcinogenesis. *Best Pract Res Clin Obstet Gynaecol* 15: 663-676, 2001a.

Stanley MA: Immunobiology of Papillomavirus Infections. *J Reprod Immunol* 32: 45-59, 2001b.

Stastny JF, Remmers RE, London WB, et al: Atypical Squamous Cells of Undetermined Significance: A Comparative Review of Original and Automated Rescreen Diagnosis of Cervicovaginal Smears With Long Term Follow-Up. *Cancer (Cancer Cytopathol)* 81: 348-353, 1997.

Stavola BD: Statistical Facts About Cancers on Which Doctor Rigoni-Stern Based His Contribution to the Surgeons' Subgroup of the IV Congress of the Italian Scientists on 23 September 1842. *Stat Med* 6: 881-884, 1987.

Stearns V, Gelmann EP: Does Tamoxifen Cause Cancer in Humans? *J Clin Oncol* 16: 779-792, 1998.

Steeper TA, Wick MR: Minimal Deviation Adenocarcinoma of the Uterine Cervix ("Adenoma Malignum"): An Immunohistochemical Comparison With Microglandular Endocervical Hyperplasia and Conventional Endocervical Adenocarcinoma. *Cancer* 58: 1131-1138, 1986.

Steiner E, Woernle F, Kuhn W, et al: Carcinoma of the Neovagina: Case Report and Review of the Literature. *Gynecol Oncol* 84: 171-175, 2002.

Steinmetz KA, Potter JD: Vegetables, Fruit, and Cancer: I. Epidemiology. *Cancer Causes Control* 2: 325-327, 1991a.

Steinmetz KA, Potter JD: Vegetables, Fruit, and Cancer: II. Mechanisms. *Cancer Causes Control* 2: 427-442, 1991b.

Stelow EB, Pambuccian SE, Bardales R, et al: *Loa loa* Presenting in a ThinPrep® PapTest™: Case Report and Review of Parasites in Cervicovaginal Cytology Specimens. *Diagn Cytopathol* 29: 167-171, 2003.

Stelow EB, Gulbahce HE, Kjeldahl K, et al: Interpretive Yields of Screening Pap Tests and Diagnostic Pap Tests. *Diagn Cytopathol* 31: 427-429, 2004.

Stemmermann GN: Extrapelvic Carcinoma Metastatic to the Uterus. *Am J Obstet Gynecol* 82: 1261-1266, 1961.

Stenzel A, Semczuk A, Rozynskal K, et al: "Low-Risk" and "High Risk" HPV-Infection and K-*ras* Gene Point Mutations in Human Cervical Cancer: A Study of 31 Cases. *Pathol Res Pract* 197: 597-603, 2001.

Steppeler Y, Shaikh H: A Rare Presentation of a Rare Disease (Letter). *J Clin Pathol* 56: 78, 2003.

Stern E, Neely PM: Cancer of the Cervix in Reference to Circumcision and Marital History. *J Am Med Womens Assoc* 17: 739-740, 1962.

Stern E, Neely PM: Carcinoma and Dysplasia of the Cervix: A Comparison of Rates for New and Returning Populations. *Acta Cytol* 7: 357-361, 1963.

Stern E, Neely PM: Dysplasia of the Uterine Cervix: Incidence of Regression, Recurrence, and Cancer. *Cancer* 17: 508-512, 1964.

Stern E: Epidemiology of Dysplasia. *Obstet Gynecol Surv* 24: 711-723, 1969.

Stern E, Clark VA, Coffelt CF: Contraceptives and Dysplasia: Higher Rate for Pill Choosers. *Science* 169: 497-498, 1970.

Stern E: Cytohisopathology of Cervical Cancer. *Cancer Res* 33:1368-1378, 1973.

Stern PL, Faulkner R, Veranes EC, et al: The Role of Human Papillomavirus Vaccines in Cervical Neoplasia. *Best Pract Res Clin Obstet Gynecol* 15: 783-799, 2001.

Stevenson CS, Scipiades E Jr: Non-Invasive Potential "Carcinoma" of the Cervix. *Surg Gynecol Obstet* 66: 822-835, 1938.

Stewart CJ, Thomas MA: Malacoplakia of the Uterine Cervix and Endometrium. *Cytopathology* 2: 271-275, 1991.

Stewart CJ, Livingstone D, Mutch AF: Borderline Nuclear Abnormality in Cervical Smears: A Cytological Review of 200 Cases With Histological Correlation. *Cytopathology* 4: 339-345, 1993a.

Stewart CJ, Taggart CR. Brett F, et al: Mesonephric Adenocarcinoma of the Uterine Cervix With Focal Endocrine Cell Differentiation. *Int J Gynecol Pathol* 12: 264-269, 1993b.

Stockard CR, Papanicolaou GN: A Rhythmical "Heat Period" in the Guinea-Pig. *Science* 46(n.s.): 42-44, 1917a.

Stockard CR, Papanicolaou GN: The Existence of a Typical Oestrous Cycle in the Guinea-Pig—With a Study of Its Histological and Physiological Changes. *Am J Anat* 22: 225-285, 1917b.

Stockdale AD, Leader M, Phillips RH, et al: The Carcinoid Syndrome and Multiple Hormone Secretion Associated With a Carcinoid Tumour of the Uterine Cervix: Case Report. *Br J Obstet Gynaecol* 93: 397-401, 1986.

Stocks P: Cancer of the Uterine Cervix and Social Conditions. *Br J Cancer* 9: 487-494, 1955.

Stockton D, Cooper P, Lonsdale RN: Changing Incidence of Invasive Adenocarcinoma of the Uterine Cervix in East Anglia. *J Med Screen* 4: 40-43, 1997.

Stoler MH, Broker TR: In Situ Hybridization Detection of Human Papillomavirus DNAs and Messenger RNAs in Genital Condylomas and a Cervical Carcinoma. *Hum Pathol* 17: 1250-1258, 1986.

Stoler MH, Mills SE, Gersell DJ, et al: Small-Cell Neuroendocrine Carcinoma of the Cervix: A Human Papillomavirus Type 18-Associated Cancer. *Am J Surg Pathol* 15: 28-32, 1991.

Stoler MH, Steinetz C, Shick, HE, et al: The Association of Human Papillomaviruses With Nonendocervical Types of Cervical Adenocarcinoma Has Carcinogenic Implications (Abstract). *Lab Invest* 70: 96A, 1994.

Stoler MH: A Brief Synopsis of the Role of Human Papillomaviruses in Cervical Carcinogenesis. *Am J Obstet Gynecol* 175: 1091-1098, 1996.

Stoler MH: Does Every Little Cell Count? Don't "ASCUS" (Editorial). *Cancer (Cancer Cytopathol)* 87: 45-47, 1999.

Stoler MH: Human Papillomaviruses and Cervical Neoplasia: A Model for Carcinogenesis. *Int J Gynecol Pathol* 19: 16-28, 2000a.

Stoler MH: HPV Testing Is Not Useful for LSIL Triage—But Stay Tuned. *Adv Anat Pathol* 8: 160-164, 2000b.

Stoler MH: Advances in Cervical Screening Technology. *Mod Pathol* 13: 275-284, 2000c.

Stoler MH: HPV for Cervical Cancer Screening: Is the Era of the Molecular Pap Smear Upon Us? *J Histochem Cytochem* 49: 1197-1198, 2001a.

Stoler MH, Schiffman M: Interobserver Reproducibility of Cervical Cytologic and Histologic Interpretations: Realistic Estimates from the ASCUS-LSIL Triage Study (Toward Optimal Laboratory Use). *JAMA* 285: 1500-1505, 2001b.

Stoler MH: Toward Objective Quality Assurance: The Eyes Don't Have It. *Am J Clin Pathol* 117: 520-522, 2002.

Stoler MH: Human Papillomavirus Biology and Cervical Neoplasia: Implications for Diagnostic Criteria and Testing. *Arch Pathol Lab Med* 127: 935-939, 2003a.

Stoler MH: Testing for Human Papillomavirus: Data Driven Implications for Cervical Neoplasia Management. *Clin Lab Med* 23: 569-583, 2003b.

Storey A, Thomas M, Kalita A, et al: Role of a p53 Polymorphism in the Development of Human Papillomavirus-Associated Cancer. *Nature* 393: 229-234, 1998.

Stowell SB, Wiley CM, Powers CN: Herpesvirus Mimics. A Potential Pitfall in Endocervical Brush Specimens. *Acta Cytol* 38: 43-50, 1994.

Stransky GC, Acosta A, Kaplan AL, et al: Reticulum Cell Sarcoma of the Cervix. *Obstet Gynecol* 41: 183-187, 1973.

Strauss MJ, Shaw EW, Bunting H: "Crystalline" Virus-Like Particles from Skin Papillomas Characterized by Intranuclear Inclusion Bodies. *Proc Soc Exp Biol Med* 72: 46-50, 1949.

Strauss S, Sastry P, Sonnex C, et al: Contamination of Environmental Surfaces by Genital Human Papillomaviruses. *Sex Transm Infect* 78: 135-138, 2002.

Studeman KD, Ioffe OB, Puszkiewicz J, et al: Effect of Cellularity on the Sensitivity of Detecting Squamous Lesions in Liquid-Based Cervical Cytology. *Acta Cytol* 47: 605-610, 2003.

Sugimori H, Kashimura Y, Kashimura M, et al: Analytical Study of Repair Cells. *Acta Cytol* 26: 439-444, 1982.

Sugimori H, Iwasak T, Yoshimura T: Cytology of Microinvasive Squamous-Cell Carcinoma of the Uterine Cervix. *Acta Cytol* 31: 412-416, 1987.

Suh K-S, Silverberg SG: Tubal Metaplasia of the Uterine Cervix. *Int J Gynecol Pathol* 9: 122-128, 1990.

Suh-Burgmann E, Darragh T, Smith-McCune K: Atypical Squamous Cells of Undetermined Significance: Management Patterns at an Academic Medical Center. *Am J Obstet Gynecol* 178: 991-995, 1998.

Suh-Burgmann EJ, Goodman A: Surveillance for Endometrial Cancer in Women Receiving Tamoxifen. *Ann Intern Med* 131: 127-135, 1999.

Sulik S, Kroeger K, Schultz J, et al: Are Fluid-Based Cytologies Superior to the Conventional Papanicolaou Test? A Systematic Review. *J Fam Pract* 50: 1040-1046, 2001.

Sullivan Å, Edlund C, Nord CE: Effect of Antimicrobial Agents on the Ecological Balance of Human Microflora. *Lancet (Infect Dis)* 1: 101-114, 2001.

Sun W, Grafton WD: Litigation Cells: Their Incidence and Classification in Gynecologic Smears. *Diagn Cytopathol* 26: 345-348, 2002.

Sun X-W, Kuhn L, Ellerbrock V, et al: Human Papillomavirus Infection in Women Infected With the Human Immunodeficiency Virus. *N Engl J Med* 337: 1343-1349, 1997.

Sung H-Y, Kearney KA, Miller M, et al: Papanicolaou Smear History and Diagnosis of Invasive Cervical Carcinoma Among Members of a Large Prepaid Health Plan. *Cancer* 88: 2283-2289, 2000.

Surís JC, Dexeus S, López-Marín L: Epidemiology of Preinvasive Lesions. *Eur J Gynaecol Oncol* 20: 302-305, 1999.

Suurmeijer AJ: A Pubic Louse in a Pap Smear (Images in Pathology). *Int J Surg Pathol* 10: 296, 2002.

Suzich JA, Ghim S-J, Palmer-Hill FJ, et al: Systemic Immunization With Papillomavirus L1 Protein Completely Prevents the Development of Viral Mucosal Papillomas. *Proc Natl Acad Sci (USA)* 92: 11553-11557, 1995.

Suzuki M, Sugiura Y, Machida S, et al: Pale Cells in a Cervical Smear. *Cytopathology* 13: 171-174, 2002.

Svitil KA: Killer Cancer in the Cretaceous. (Ancient Life Section). *Discover* November 03, 2003. [http://www.discover.com/web-exclusives/killer-cancer1102 01/07/04].

Swan DC, Tucker RA, Tortolero-Luma G, et al: Human Papillomavirus (HPV) DNA Copy Number Is Dependent on Grade of Cervical Disease and HPV Type. *J Clin Microbiol* 37: 1030-1034, 1999.

Swan SH, Brown WL: Vasectomy and Cancer of the Cervix (Letter). *N Engl J Med* 301: 46, 1979.

Swan SH, Petitti DB: A Review of Problems of Bias and Confounding in Epidemiologic Studies of Cervical Neoplasia and Oral Contraceptive Use. *Am J Epidemiol* 115: 10-18, 1982.

Swanson J, Eschenbach DA, Alexander ER, et al: Light and Electron Microscopic Study of *Chlamydia trachomatis* Infection of the Uterine Cervix. *J Infect Dis* 131: 678-687, 1975.

Swerdloff RS, Wang C, Kandeel FR: Evaluation of the Infertile Couple. *Endocrinol Metab Clin North Am* 17: 301-337, 1988.

Swinker M, Cutlip AC, Ogle D: A Comparison of Uterine Cervical Cytology and Biopsy Results: Indications and Outcomes for Colposcopy. *J Fam Pract* 38: 40-44, 1994.

Symmans F, Mechanic L, MacConnell P, et al: Correlation of Cervical Cytology and Human Papillomavirus DNA Detection in Postmenopausal Women. *Int J Gynecol Pathol* 11: 204-209, 1992.

Symonds DA, Reed TP, Didolkar SM, et al: AGUS in Cervical Endometriosis. *J Reprod Med* 42: 39-43, 1997.

Symonds P, Bolger B, Hole D, et al: Advanced-Stage Cervix Cancer: Rapid Tumour Growth Rather than Late Diagnosis. *Br J Cancer* 83: 566-568, 2000.

Symons J, Kempfert N, Speroff L: Vaginal Bleeding in Postmenopausal Women Taking Low-Dose Norethindrone Acetate and Ethinyl Estradiol Combinations. The FemHRT Study Investigators. *Obstet Gynecol* 96: 366-372, 2000.

Syrjänen K: Morphologic Survey of the Condylomatous Lesions in Dysplastic and Neoplastic Epithelium of the Uterine Cervix. *Arch Gynecol* 227: 153-161, 1979.

Syrjänen K: Condylomatous Lesions in Dysplastic and Neoplastic Epithelium of the Uterine Cervix. *Surg Gynecol Obstet* 150: 372-376, 1980.

Syrjänen K, Heinonen U-M, Kauraniemi T: Cytologic Evidence of the Association of Condylomatous Lesions With Dysplastic and Neoplastic Changes in the Uterine Cervix. *Acta Cytol* 25: 17-22, 1981.

Syrjänen K: Human Papillomavirus Lesions in Association With Cervical Dysplasias and Neoplasias. *Obstet Gynecol* 62: 617-624, 1983.

Syrjänen K, Väyrynen M, Castrén O, et al: Sexual Behavior of Women With Human Papillomavirus (HPV) Lesions of the Uterine Cervix. *Br J Vener Dis* 60: 243-248, 1984.

Syrjänen K: Human Papillomavirus (HPV) Infections of the Female Genital Tract and Their Associations With Intraepithelial Neoplasia and Squamous Cell Carcinoma. *Pathol Annu* 21: 53-89, 1986a.

Syrjänen K, Mäntyjärvi R, Väyrynen M, et al: Coexistent Chlamydial Infections Related to Natural History of Human Papillomavirus Lesions in Uterine Cervix. *Genitourin Med* 62: 345-351, 1986b.

Syrjänen K, Mäntyjärvi R, Saarikoski S, et al: Factors Associated With Progression of Cervical Human Papillomavirus (HPV) Infections Into Carcinoma In Situ During a Long-Term Prospective Follow-up. *Br J Obstet Gynecol* 95: 1096-1102, 1988.

Syrjänen K, Hakama M, Saarikoski S, et al: Prevalence, Incidence, and Estimated Life-Time Risk of Cervical Human Papillomavirus Infections in a Nonselected Finnish Female Population. *Sex Transm Dis* 17: 15-19, 1990.

Syrjänen K, Kataja V, Yliskoski M, et al: Natural History of Cervical Human Papillomavirus Lesions Does Not Substantiate the Biologic Relevance of the Bethesda System. *Obstet Gynecol* 79: 675-682, 1992.

Syrjänen K: Human Papillomavirus in Genital Carcinogenesis. *Sex Transm Dis* 21(S2): S86-S89, 1994.

Syrjänen K: Is Improved Detection of Adenocarcinoma In Situ by Screening a Key to Reducing the Incidence of Cervical Adenocarcinoma? *Acta Cytol* 48: 591-594, 2004.

Syrjänen SM: Basic Concepts and Practical Applications of Recombinant DNA Techniques in Detection of Human Papillomavirus (HPV) Infections. *APMIS* 98: 95-110, 1990.

Syrjänen SM, Syrjänen KJ: New Concepts on the Role of Human Papillomavirus in Cell Cycle Regulation. *Ann Med* 31: 175-187, 1999.

Syrjänen K: Is Improved Detection of Adenocarcinoma In Situ by Screening a Key to Reducing the Incidence of Cervical Adenocarcinoma? (Editorial) *Acta Cytol* 48: 591-594, 2004.

Szarewski A, Cuzick J, Nayagam M, et al: A Comparison of Four Cytological Sampling Techniques in a Genitourinary Medicine Clinic. *Genitourin Med* 66: 439-443, 1990.

Szarewski A, Cuzick J, Edwards R, et al: The Use of Cervicography in a Primary Screening Service. *Br J Obstet Gynaecol* 98: 313-317, 1991.

Szarewski A, Curran G, Edwards R, et al: Comparison of Four Cytologic Sampling Techniques in a Large Family Planning Center. *Acta Cytol* 37: 457-460, 1993.

Szarewski A, Jarvis MJ, Sasieni P, et al: Effect of Smoking Cessation on Cervical Lesion Size. *Lancet* 347: 941-943, 1996.

Szarewski A, Cuzick J: Smoking and Cervical Neoplasia: A Review of the Evidence. *J Epidemiol Biostat* 3: 229-256, 1998.

Szarewski A, Sasieni, P: Cervical Screening in Adolescents—At Least Do No Harm. *Lancet* 364: 1642-1644, 2004.

Szyfelbein WM, Young RH, Scully RE: Adenoma Malignum of the Cervix: Cytologic Findings. *Acta Cytol* 28: 691-698, 1984.

Szyfelbein WM, Baker PM, Bell DA: Superficial Endometriosis of the Cervix: A Source of Abnormal Glandular Cells on Cervicovaginal Smears. *Diagn Cytopathol* 30: 88-91, 2004.

T

Tabatabai ZL, Krishnamurthy S: Radiation-Induced Atypical Glandular Cells Mimicking Recurrent Adenocarcinoma in a Posthysterectomy Vaginal Smear (Letter). *Acta Cytol* 47: 106-107, 2003.

Tabbara SO, Saleh AM, Andersen WA, et al: The Bethesda Classification for Squamous Intraepithelial Lesions: Histologic, Cytologic, and Viral Correlates. *Obstet Gynecol* 79: 338-346, 1992.

Tabbara SO, Horbach N, Sidawy MK: The Adequacy of the One-Slide Cervical Smear in the Detection of Squamous Intraepithelial Lesions. *Am J Clin Pathol* 101: 647-650, 1994.

Tabbara SO, Sidawy MK: Evaluation of the 5-Year Review of Negative Cervical Smears in Patients With High-Grade Squamous Intraepithelial Lesions. *Diagn Cytopathol* 15: 7-10; discussion 10-11 1996.

Tabrizi SN, Fairley CK, Chen S, et al: Epidemiological Characteristics of Women with High-Grade CIN Who Do and Do Not Have Human Papillomavirus. *Br J Obstet Gynaecol* 106: 252-257, 1999.

Tachezy R, Salakova M, Hamiskova E, et al: Prospective Study on Cervical Neoplasia: Presence of HPV DNA in Cytological Smears Preceeds the Development of Cervical Neoplastic Lesions. *Sex Transm Infect* 79: 191-196, 2003.

Taft PD, Robboy SJ, Herbst AL, et al: Cytology of Clear-Cell Adenocarcinoma of Genital Tract in Young Females: Review of 95 Cases from the Registry. *Acta Cytol* 18: 279-290, 1974.

Tahlan A, Dey P: Nuclear Grooves: How Specific Are They? *Acta Cytol* 45: 48-50, 2001.

Tajima M, Inamura M, Nakamura M, et al: The Accuracy of Endometrial Cytology in the Diagnosis of Endometrial Adenocarcinoma. *Cytopathology* 9: 369-380, 1998.

Takamizawa H, Wong K: Effect of Anticancer Drugs on Uterine Carcinogenesis. *Obstet Gynecol* 41: 701-706, 1973.

Takashi T, Ito E, Kudo R: Cytologic Diagnosis of Primary Tubal Cancer. *Acta Cytol* 29: 367-372, 1985.

Takashina T, Kanda Y, Tsumura N: Postoperative Changes in Vaginal Smears After Vaginal Reconstruction With a Free Skin Graft. *Acta Cytol* 32: 109-112, 1988a.

Takashina T, Ono M, Kanda Y, et al: Cervicovaginal and Endometrial Cytology in Ovarian Cancer. *Acta Cytol* 32: 159-162, 1988b.

Takeda M, Diamond SM, DeMarco M, et al: Cytologic Diagnosis of Malignant Melanoma Metastatic to the Endometrium. *Acta Cytol* 22: 503-506, 1978.

Takehara M, Ito E, Saito T, et al: Primary Malignant Melanoma of the Uterine Cervix: A Case Report. *J Obstet Gynaecol Res* 25: 129-132, 1999.

Takehara M, Ito E, Saito T, et al: HMB-45 Staining for Cytology of Primary Melanoma of the Vagina: A Case Report. *Acta Cytol* 44: 1077-1080, 2000.

Takeshima N, Hirai Y, Yamauchi K, et al: Clinical Usefulness of Endometrial Aspiration Cytology and CA-125 in the Detection of Fallopian Tube Carcinoma. *Acta Cytol* 41: 1445-1450, 1997.

Takeshima N, Tabata T, Nishida H, et al: Müllerian Adenosarcoma of the Uterus: Report of a Case With Imprint Cytology. *Acta Cytol* 45: 613-616, 2001.

Takeuchi T, Fujii A, Okumiya T, et al: The Study of Cytopathological Aspects Induced by Human Cytomegalovirus Infection. *Diagn Cytopathol* 31: 289-293, 2004.

Taki I, Aozasa K, Kurokawa K: Malignant Lymphoma of the Uterine Cervix: Cytologic Diagnosis of a Case With Immunocytochemical Corroboration. *Acta Cytol* 29: 607-611, 1985.

Talerman A, Alenghat E, Okagaki T: Glassy Cell Carcinoma of the Uterine Cervix. *Acta Pathol Microbiol Immunol Scand* Supplementum 23: 119-125, 1991.

Tam MR, Stamm WE, Handfield HH, et al: Culture-Independent Diagnosis of *Chlamydia trachomatis* Using Monoclonal Antibodies. *N Engl J Med* 310: 1146-1150, 1984.

Tambouret R, Pitman MB, Bell DA: Benign Glandular Cells in Posthysterectomy Vaginal Smears. *Acta Cytol* 42: 1403-1408, 1998.

Tambouret R, Bell DA, Centeno BA: Significance of Histocytes in Cervical Smears from Peri/Postmenopausal Women. *Diagn Cytopathol* 24: 271-275, 2001.

Tambouret RH, Wilbur DC: The Many Faces of Atrophy in Gynecologic Cytology. *Clin Lab Med* 23: 659-679, 2003.

Tamimi HK, Figge DC: Adenocarcinoma of the Uterine Cervix. *Gynecol Oncol* 13: 335-344, 1982.

Tamiolakis D, Anastasiadis P, Karamanidis D, et al: K Statistic as a Measure of Quality Control in Cervicovaginal Cytology. *Clin Exp Obstet Gynecol* 28: 229-231, 2001.

Tanaka H, Chua KL, Lindh E, et al: Patients With Various Types of Human Papillomavirus: Covariation and Diagnostic Relevance of Cytological Findings in Papanicolaou Smears. *Cytopathology* 4: 273-283, 1993.

Tardio JC, Salas C: Vaginal Papillary Carcinomas with Transitional Cell Differentiation: A Morphological Variant of Squamous Cell Carcinoma? (Case Reports, Letter) *Histopathology* 39: 433-438, 2001.

Tarnberg M, Jakobsson T, Jonasson J, et al: Identification of Randomly Selected Colonics of Lactobacilli from Normal Vaginal Fluid by Pyrosequencing of the 16S rDNA Variable V1 and V3 Regions. *APMIS* 110: 802-810, 2002.

Tasca L, Östör AG, Babes' V: History of Gynecologic Pathology. XII. Aurel Babes'. *Int J Gynecol Pathol* 21: 198-202, 2002.

Tase T, Okagaki T, Clark BA, et al: Human Papillomavirus Types and Localization in Adenocarcinoma and Adenosquamous Carcinoma of the Uterine Cervix: A Study by In Situ DNA Hybridization. *Cancer Res* 48: 993-998, 1988.

Tase T, Okagaki T, Clark BA, et al: Human Papillomavirus DNA in Adenocarcinoma In Situ, Microinvasive Adenocarcinoma of the Uterine Cervix, and Coexisting Cervical Squamous Intraepithelial Neoplasia. *Int J Gynecol Pathol* 8: 8-17, 1989a.

Tase T, Okagaki T, Clark BA, et al: Human Papillomavirus DNA in Glandular Dysplasia and Microglandular Hyperplasia: Presumed Precursors of Adenocarcinoma of the Uterine Cervix. *Obstet Gynecol* 73: 1005-1008, 1989b.

Tasker JT, Collins JA: Adenocarcinoma of the Uterine Cervix. *Am J Obstet Gynecol* 118: 344-348, 1974.

Tateishi R, Wada A, Hayakawa K, et al: Argyrophil Cell Carcinomas (Apudomas) of the Uterine Cervix: Light and Electron Microscopic Observations of 5 Cases. *Virchows Archiv (Path Anat)* 366: 257-274, 1975.

Tavernier LA, Connor PD, Gates D: Water Versus Gel Lubricant for Cervical Cytology Specimens. *J Family Pract* 52: 701-704, 2003.

Taxy JB, Trujillo YP: Breast Cancer Metastatic to the Uterus: Clinical Manifestations of a Rare Event. *Arch Pathol Lab Med* 118: 819-821, 1994.

Tay SK, Jenkins D, Maddox P, et al: Subpopulations of Langerhans' Cells in Cervical Neoplasia. *Br J Obstet Gynaecol* 94: 10-15, 1987a.

Tay SK, Jenkins D, Maddox P, et al: Lymphocyte Phenotypes in Cervical Intraepithelial Neoplasia and Human Papillomavirus Infection. *Br J Obstet Gynaecol* 94: 16-21, 1987b.

Tay SK, Jenkins D, Singer A: Natural Killer Cells in Cervical Intraepithelial Neoplasia and Human Papillomavirus Infection. *Br J Obstet Gynaecol* 94: 901-906, 1987c.

Tay SK, Jenkins D, Maddox P, et al: Tissue Macrophage Response in Human Papillomavirus Infection and Cervical Intraepithelial Neoplasia. *Br J Obstet Gynaecol* 94: 1094-1097, 1987d.

Tay SK, Jenkins D, Singer A: Management of Squamous Atypia (Borderline Nuclear Abnormalities): Repeat Cytology or Colposcopy? *Aust N Z J Obstet Gynaecol* 27: 140-141, 1987e.

Tay SK, Tay K-J: Passive Cigarette Smoking Is a Risk Factor in Cervical Neoplasia. *Gynecol Oncol* 93: 116-120, 2004.

Taylor HB, Irey NS, Norris HJ: Atypical Endocervical Hyperplasia in Women Taking Oral Contraceptives. *JAMA* 202: 185-187, 1967.

Taylor PT Jr, Andersen WA, Barber SR, et al: The Screening Papanicolaou Smear: Contribution of the Endocervical Brush. *Obstet Gynecol* 70: 734-738, 1987.

Taylor RR, Guerrieri JP, Nash JD, et al: Atypical Cervical Cytology: Colposcopic Follow-Up Using the Bethesda System. *J Reprod Med* 38: 443-447, 1993.

Taylor RS: Nippling of Endocervical Cell Nuclei (Letter). *Acta Cytol* 28: 86-88, 1984.

Taylor S, Drake SM, Dedicoat M, et al: Genital Ulcers Associated With Acute Epstein-Barr Virus Infection. *Sex Transm Infect* 74: 296-297, 1998.

Taylor Y, Melvin WT, Flannelly G, et al: Prevalence of Epstein-Barr Virus in the Cervix. *J Clin Pathol* 47: 92-93, 1994.

Taylor-Robinson D, Thomas BJ: The Role of *Chlamydia trachomatis* in Genital-Tract and Associated Diseases. *J Clin Pathol* 33: 205-233, 1980.

Teaff NL, Malone JM Jr, Ginsburg KA, et al: Cervical Dysplasia in the Postmenopausal Female: Diagnosis and Treatment. *Int J Gynecol Obstet* 34: 145-149, 1990.

Telang NT, Suto A, Wong GY, et al: Induction by Estrogen Metabolite 16 Alpha-Hydroxyestrone of Genotopic Damage and Aberrant Proliferation in Mouse Mammary Epithelial Cells. *J Natl Cancer Inst* 84:634-638, 1992.

Te Linde RW: Demonstration of the Relationship of Carcinoma In Situ to Invasive Carcinoma of the Cervix. *Am J Obstet Gynecol* 115: 1022-1024, 1973.

Tenti P, Romagnoli S, Silini E, et al: Human Papillomavirus Types 16 and 18 Infection in Infiltrating Adenocarcinoma of the Cervix: PCR Analysis of 138 Cases and Correlation With Histologic Type and Grade. *Am J Clin Pathol* 106: 52-56, 1996.

ter Meulen J, Eberhardt HC, Luande J, et al: Human Papillomavirus (HPV) Infection, HIV Infection and Cervical Cancer in Tanzania, East Africa. *Int J Cancer* 51: 515-521, 1992.

Terris M, Oalmann MC: Carcinoma of the Cervix: An Epidemiologic Study. *JAMA* 174: 1847-1851, 1960.

Terris M, Wilson F, Nelson JH Jr: Relation of Circumcision to Cancer of the Cervix. *Am J Obstet Gynecol* 117: 1056-1066, 1973.

Terris M, Wilson F, Nelson JH Jr: Comparative Epidemiology of Invasive Carcinoma of the Cervix, Carcinoma In Situ, and Cervical Dysplasia. *Am J Epidemiol* 112: 253-257, 1980.

Teshima S, Shimosato Y, Kishi K, et al: Early Stage Adenocarcinoma of the Uterine Cervix: Histopathologic Analysis With Consideration of Histogenesis. *Cancer* 56: 167-172, 1985.

Tevi-Bénissan C, Bélec L, Lévy M, et al: In Vivo Semen-Associated pH Neutralization of Cervicovaginal Secretions. *Clin Diagn Lab Immunol* 4: 367-374, 1997.

Tewari KS, DiSaia PJ: Primary Prevention of Uterine Cervix Cancer: Focus on Vaccine History and Current Strategy. *Obstet Gynecol Clin North Am* 29: 843-868, 2002.

Teyssier JR: The Chromosomal Analysis of Human Solid Tumors: A Triple Challenge. *Cancer Genet Cytogenet* 37: 103-125, 1989.

Thar TL, Million RR, Daly JW: Radiation Treatment of Carcinoma of the Cervix. *Semin Oncol* 9: 299-311, 1982.

Thomas DB: Relationship of Oral Contraceptives to Cervical Carcinogenesis. *Obstet Gynecol* 40: 508-518, 1972.

Thomas DB: The WHO Collaborative Study of Neoplasia and Steroid Contraceptives: The Influence of Combined Oral Contraceptives on Risk of Neoplasms in Developing and Developed Countries. *Contraception* 43: 695-710, 1991.

Thomas DB, Ray RM: Oral Contraceptives and Invasive Adenocarcinomas and Adenosquamous Carcinomas of the Uterine Cervix: The World Health Organization Collaborative Study of Neoplasia and Steroid Contraceptives. *Am J Epidemiol* 144: 281-289, 1996a.

Thomas DB, Ray RM, Pardthaisong T, et al: Prostitution, Condom Use, and Invasive Squamous Cell Cervical Cancer in Thailand. *Am J Epidemiol* 143: 779-786, 1996b.

Thomas M, Banks L: Inhibition of BAK-Induced Apoptosis by HPV-18 E6. *Oncogene* 17: 2943-2954, 1998.

Thomas PA, Zaleski MS, Ohlhausen WW, et al: Cytomorphologic Characteristics of Thermal Injury Related to Endocervical Brushing Following Loop Electrosurgical Excision Procedure (LEEP). *Diagn Cytopathol* 14: 212-215, 1996.

Thomason JL, Gelbart SM, Sobun JF, et al: Comparison of Four Methods to Detect *Trichomonas vaginalis*. *J Clin Microbiol* 26: 1869-1870, 1988.

Thompson FE, Patterson BH, Weinstein SJ, et al: Serum Selenium and the Risk of Cervical Cancer Among Women in the United States. *Cancer Causes Control* 13: 517-526, 2002.

Thorsen P, Jensen IP, Jeune B, et al: Few Microorganisms Associated With Bacterial Vaginosis May Constitute the Pathologic Core: A Population-Based Microbiologic Study Among 3596 Pregnant Women. *Am J Obstet Gynecol* 178: 580-587, 1998.

Tidbury P, Singer A, Jenkins D: CIN 3: The Role of Lesion Size in Invasion. *Br J Obstet Gynaecol* 99: 583-586, 1992.

Tidy J, Parry GCN, Ward P, et al: High Rate of Human Papillomavirus Type 16 Infection in Cytologically Normal Cervices (Letter). *Lancet* (i): 434, 1989; erratum appears in *Lancet* (ii): 996; retraction in Tidy J, Farrell PJ, *Lancet* (2): 1535, 1989a.

Tidy J, Vousden KH, Mason KH, et al: A Novel Deletion Within the Upstream Regulatory Region of Episomal Human Papillomavirus Type 16. *J Gen Virol* 70: 999-1004, 1989b.

Tindle RW: Human Papillomavirus Vaccines for Cervical Cancer. *Curr Opin Immunol* 8: 643-650, 1996.

Titus K: HPV Test: Antidote to ASCUS Headache? *CAP Today* 10: 52-54, 56-58, 1996.

Tobón H, Dave H: Adenocarcinoma In Situ of the Cervix. Clinicopathologic Observations of 11 Cases. *Int J Gynecol Pathol* 7: 139-151, 1988.

Toki T, Shiozawa T, Hosaka N, et al: Minimal Deviation Adenocarcinoma of the Uterine Cervix Has Abnormal Expression of Sex Steroid Receptors, CA125, and Gastric Mucin. *Int J Gynecol Pathol* 16: 111-116, 1997.

Toki T, Zhai YL, Park JS, et al: Infrequent Occurrence of High-Risk Human Papillomavirus and of p53 Mutation in Minimal Deviation Adenocarcinoma of the Cervix. *Int J Gynecol Pathol* 18: 215-219, 1999.

Tokyol C, Aktepe OC, Cevrioglu AS, et al: Bacterial Vaginosis: Comparison of Pap Smear and Microbiological Test Results. *Mod Pathol* 17: 857-860, 2004.

Tomé A, Puig-Tintoré LM, Ordi J, et al: Effect of Smoking Cessation on Cervical Lesion Size (Letter). *Lancet* 347: 1619-1620, 1996.

Tong TR, Chan OWH, Chow T-C, et al: Detection of Human Papillomavirus in Sanitary Napkins: A New Paradigm in Cervical Cancer Screening. *Diagn Cytopathol* 28: 140-141, 2003.

Toolenaar TA, Freundt I, Huikeshoven FJ, et al: The Occurrence of Diversion Colitis in Patients With a Sigmoid Neovagina. *Hum Pathol* 24: 846-849, 1993.

Toon PG, Arrand JR, Wilson LP: Human Papillomavirus Infection of the Uterine Cervix of Women Without Cytological Signs of Neoplasia. *Br Med J* 293: 1261-1264, 1986.

Torres LM, Cabrera T, Concha A, et al: HLA Class I Expression and HPV-16 Sequences in Premalignant and Malignant Lesions of the Cervix. *Tissue Antigens* 41: 65-71, 1993.

Tortolero-Luna G: Epidemiology of Genital Human Papillomavirus. *Hematol/Oncol Clin North Amer* 13: 245-257, 1999.

Towne JE: Carcinoma of the Cervix in Nulliparous and Celibate Women. *Am J Obstet Gynecol* 69: 606-613, 1955.

Traynor RM, Parratt D, Duguid HL, et al: Isolation of Actinomycetes from Cervical Specimens. *J Clin Pathol* 34: 914-916, 1981.

Trevathan E, Layde P, Webster LA, et al: Cigarette Smoking and Dysplasia and Carcinoma In Situ of the Uterine Cervix. *JAMA* 250: 499-502, 1983.

Tritz DM, Weeks JA, Spires SE, et al: Etiologies for Non-Correlating Cervical Cytologies and Biopsies. *Am J Clin Pathol* 103: 594-597, 1995.

Trivijitsilp P, Mosher R, Sheets EE: Papillary Immature Metaplasia (Immature Condyloma) of the Cervix: A Clinicopathologic Analysis and Comparison With Papillary Squamous Carcinoma. *Hum Pathol* 29: 641-648, 1998.

Trofatter KF Jr: Diagnosis of Human Papillomavirus Genital Tract Infection. *Am J Med* 102(5A): 21-27, 1997.

Trowell JE: Intestinal Metaplasia With Argentaffin Cells in the Uterine Cervix. *Histopathology* 9: 551-559, 1985.

Trunk MJ, Dallenbach-Hellweg G, Ridder R, et al: Morphologic Characteristics of p16*INK4a*-Positive Cells in Cervical Cytology Samples. *Acta Cytol* 48: 771-782, 2004.

Tseng C-J, Pao C-C, Tseng L-H, et al: Lymphoepithelioma-Like Carcinoma of the Uterine Cervix: Association With Epstein-Barr Virus and Human Papillomavirus. *Cancer* 80: 91-97, 1997.

Tsuda H, Hashiguchi Y, Nishimura S, et al: Relationship Between HPV Typing and Abnormality of G1 Cell Cycle Regulators in Cervical Neoplasm. *Gynecol Oncol* 91: 476-485, 2003.

Tsutsui F, et al: Carcinosarcoma of the Uterus: Cytologic and Ultrastructural Features. *Acta Cytol* 29: 602-606, 1985.

Tunca JC, Reddi PR, Shah SH, et al: Malignant Non-Hodgkin's-Type Lymphoma of the Cervix Uteri Occurring During Pregnancy. *Gynecol Oncol* 7: 385-393, 1979.

Tuncer M, Graham R, Graham J: Diagnostic Efficiency in Invasive Cervical Cancer. *N Y State J Med* 11: 2317-2319, 1967.

Turner CF, Rogers SM, Miller WC, et al: Prevalence of Untreated Sexually Transmitted Disease. *JAMA* 287: 2362-2363, 2002.

Tutschka BG, Lauchlan SC: Psammoma Bodies in Cervico-Vaginal Smears: Case Report and Review of the Literature. *Acta Cytol* 22: 507-509, 1978.

Tweddel G, Heller P, Cunnane M, et al: The Correlation Between HIV Seropositivity, Cervical Dysplasia, and HPV Subtypes 6/11, 16/18, 31/33/35. *Gynecol Oncol* 52: 161-164, 1994.

Tweeddale DN, Scott RC, Fields MJ, et al: Giant Cells in Cervico-Vaginal Smears. *Acta Cytol* 12: 298-304, 1968.

Tweeddale DN, Langenbach SR, Roddick JW Jr, et al: The Cytopathology of Microinvasive Squamous Cancer of the Cervix Uteri. *Acta Cytol* 13: 447-454, 1969.

Twombly R: Guidelines Recommended Less Frequent Screening Interval for Cervical Cancer. *J Natl Cancer Inst* 95: 424-425, 2003.

U

Ueda G, Shimizu C, Shimizu H, et al: An Immunohistochemical Study of Small-Cell and Poorly Differentiated Carcinomas of the Cervix Using Neuroendocrine Markers. *Gynecol Oncol* 34: 164-169, 1989.

Ueki M, Ueda M, Kurokawa A, et al: Cytologic Study of the Tissue Repair Cells of the Uterine Cervix: With Special Reference to Their Origin. *Acta Cytol* 36: 310-318, 1992.

Ulbright TM, Gersell DJ: Glassy Cell Carcinoma of the Uterine Cervix: A Light and Electron Microscopic Study of Five Cases. *Cancer* 51: 2255-2263, 1983.

Umezaki K, Sanezumi M, Okada H, et al: Distribution of Epithelial-Specific Antigen in Uterine Cervix With Endocervical Glandular Dysplasia. *Gynecol Oncol* 66: 393-398, 1997.

Unger ER: In Situ Diagnosis of Human Papillomaviruses. *Clin Lab Med* 20: 289-299, 2000.

Unger ER, Duarte-Franco E: Human Papillomaviruses: Into the New Millennium. *Obstet Gynecol Clin North Am* 28: 653-666, 2001.

Ursin G, Peters RK, Henderson BE, et al: Oral Contraceptive Use and Adenocarcinoma of Cervix. *Lancet* 344: 1390-1394, 1994.

Ursin G, Pike MC, Preston-Martin S, et al: Sexual, Reproductive, and Other Risk Factors for Adenocarcinoma of the Cervix: Results from a Population-Based Case-Control Study (California, United States). *Cancer Causes Control* 7: 391-401, 1996.

[USHHS] United States Department of Health and Human Services: *The National Strategic Plan for the Early Detection and Control of Breast and Cervical Cancers.* GPO Item #0504. US Dept. of Health and Human Services, Atlanta, GA, 1993.

Uyar DS, Eltbbakh GH, Mount SL: Positive Predictive Value of Liquid-Based and Conventional Cervical Papanicolaou Smears Reported as Malignant. *Gynecol Oncol* 89: 227-232, 2003.

Uyeda CK, Stephens SR, Bridger WM: Cervical Smear Diagnosis of Hodgkin's Disease: Report of a Case. *Acta Cytol* 11: 652-655, 1969.

V

Vadmal M, Brones C, Hajdu SI: Metastatic Lobular Carcinoma of the Breast in a Cervical-Vaginal Smear (Letter). *Acta Cytol* 42: 1236-1237, 1997.

Vaghese R, Raghuveer CV, Muktha R, et al: Microfilariae in Cytologic Smears: A Report of Six Cases. *Acta Cytol* 40: 299-301, 1996.

Vail-Smith K, White DM: Risk Level, Knowledge, and Preventive Behavior for Human Papillomaviruses Among Sexually Active College Women. *J Am Coll Health* 40: 277-230, 1992.

Valdivieso M, Luna M, Bodey GP, et al: Fungemia Due to *Torulopsis glabrata* in the Compromised Host. *Cancer* 38: 1750-1756, 1976.

Valente PT, Ernst CS, Atkinson BF: Pemphigus Vulgaris With Subclinical Involvement of the Uterine Cervix: Report of a Case With Persistence of Abnormal Papanicolaou Smears Posthysterectomy. *Acta Cytol* 28: 681-683, 1984.

Valente PT, Hanjani P: Endocervical Neoplasia in Long-Term Users of Oral Contraceptives: Clinical and Pathologic Observations. *Obstet Gynecol* 67: 695-704, 1986.

Valente PT, Schantz HD, Tribal JF: The Determination of Papanicolaou Smear Adequacy Using a Semiquantitative Method to Evaluate Cellularity. *Diagn Cytopathol* 7: 576-580, 1991.

Valente PT: Government Mandated Cytology Proficiency Testing: Time for Reality Testing. *Diagn Cytopathol* 10: 105-106, 1994a.

Valente PT: Cytologic Atypia Associated With Microglandular Hyperplasia. *Diagn Cytopathol* 10: 326-331, 1994b.

Valente PT, Schantz HD: The Diagnosis of Glandular Abnormalities in Cervical Smears. In: Schmidt WA, Katz RL, Miller TR, et al, eds. *Cytopathology 1996*, Vol. I (ASCP Reviews in Pathology). American Society of Clinical Pathologists, Chicago, IL, 39-68, 1996.

Valente PT, Schantz HD, Trabal JF: Cytologic Changes in Cervical Smears Associated With Prolonged Use of Depot-Medroxyprogesterone Acetate. *Cancer (Cancer Cytopathol)* 84: 328-334, 1998.

Valente PT: The Life of George N. Papanicolaou and the Origins of Cytology. *Cyto Paths* 6(Suppl to 43, 1, *Acta Cytologica*): 3-10, 1999 [http://www.cytology-iac.org/cytopaths/1999/CytoSpring99.htm].

Valente PT: Squamous and Glandular Lesions of the Cervix: Can They Be Reliably Distinguished in Cervical Smears? *Laboratory Medicine* 32: 35-38, 2001.

Valicenti JF, Priester SK: Psammoma Bodies of Benign Endometrial Origin in Cervicovaginal Cytology. *Acta Cytol* 21: 550-552, 1977.

Valicenti JF Jr, Pappas AA, Graber CD, et al: Detection and Prevalence of IUD-Associated *Actinomyces* Colonization and Related Morbidity: A Prospective Study of 69,925 Cervical Smears. *JAMA* 247: 1149-1152, 1982.

Vallor AC, Antonio MAD, Hawes SE, et al: Factors Associated with Acquisition of, or Persistent Colonization by, Vaginal Lactobacilli: Role of Hydrogen Peroxide Production. *J Infect Dis* 184: 1431-1436, 2001.

Valore EV, Park CH, Igreti SL, et al: Antimicrobial Components of Vaginal Fluid. *Am J Obstet Gynecol* 187: 561-568, 2002.

van Aspert-van Erp AJM, van't Hof-Grottenboer AB, Brugal G, et al : Endocervical Columnar Cell Intraepithelial Neoplasia. I. Discriminating Cytomorphologic Criteria. *Acta Cytol* 39: 1199-1215, 1995a.

van Aspert-van Erp AJM, van't Hof-Grottenboer AB, Brugal G, et al: Endocervical Columnar Cell Intraepithelial Neoplasia. II. Grades of Expression of Cytomorphologic Criteria. *Acta Cytol* 39: 1216-1232, 1995b.

van Aspert-van Erp AJM, van't Hof-Grottenboer BE, Brugal G, et al: Endocervical Columnar Cell Intraepithelial Neoplasia (ECCIN), 3. Interobserver Variability in Feature Use. *Anal Cell Pathol* 10: 115-135, 1996a.

van Aspert-van Erp AJM, van't Hof-Grottenboer BE, Brugal G, et al: Individual Use of Cytomorphologic Characteristics in the Diagnosis of Endocervical Columnar Cell Abnormalities: Selection of Preferred Features With Help of the 'NAVIGATOR' Microscope. *Analy Cell Pathol* 11: 73-95, 1996b.

van Aspert-van Erp AJM, van't Hof-Grottenboer BE, Vooijs GP: Identifying Cytologic Characteristics and Grading Endocervical Columnar Cell Abnormalities: A Study Aided by High-Definition Television. *Acta Cytol* 41: 1659-1670, 1997.

van Aspert-van Erp, AJM, Smedts FMM, Vooijs GP: Severe Cervical Glandular Cell Lesions and Severe Cervical Combined Lesions: Predictive Value of the Papanicolaou Smear. *Cancer (Cancer Cytopathol)* 102: 210-217, 2004a.

van Aspert-van Erp, AJM, Smedts FMM, Vooijs GP: Severe Cervical Glandular Cell Lesions With Coexisting Squamous Cell Lesions: A Reevaluation of Cytologic (and Histologic) Specimens. *Cancer (Cancer Cytopathol)* 102: 218-227, 2004 b.

van den Akker-van Marle ME, van Balleggoijen M, van Oortmarssen GJ: Cost-Effectiveness of Cervical Cancer Screening: Comparison of Screening Policies. *J Natl Cancer Inst* 94: 193-203, 2002.

van den Bosch T, Vandendael A, Wranz PA, et al: Cervical Cytology in Menopausal Women at High Risk for Endometrial Disease. *Eur J Cancer Prev* 7: 149-152, 1998.

van der Graaf Y, Vooijs GP: False Negative Rate in Cervical Cytology. *J Clin Pathol* 40: 438-442, 1987a.

van der Graaf Y, Vooijs GP, Gaillard HLJ, et al: Screening Errors in Cervical Cytologic Screening. *Acta Cytol* 31: 434-438, 1987b.

van der Graaf Y, Vooijs GP, Zielhuis GA: Cervical Screening Revisited. *Acta Cytol* 34: 366-372, 1990.

van der Voort PHJ, ten Velden JJAM, Wassenaar RP, et al: Malakoplakia: Two Case Reports and a Comparison of Treatment Modalities Based on a Literature Review. *Arch Intern Med* 156: 577-583, 1996.

van Diest PJ, Holzel H: Cervical Cancer (Editorial). *J Clin Pathol* 55: 241-242, 2002.

van Driel WJ, Kievit-Tyson P, Lambert CJM, et al: Presence of an Eosinophilic Infiltrate in Cervical Squamous Carcinoma Results from a Type 2 Immune Response. *Gynecol Oncol* 74: 188-195, 1999.

VanEenwyk J, Davis FG, Colman N: Folate, Vitamin C, and Cervical Intraepithelial Neoplasia. *Cancer Epidemiol Biomarkers Prev* 1: 119-124, 1992.

Vang R, Medeiros LJ, Ha CS, et al: Non-Hodgkin's Lymphomas Involving the Uterus: A Clinicopathologic Analysis of 26 Cases. *Mod Pathol* 13: 19-28, 2000.

van Helvoort T: A Century of Research into the Cause of Cancer: Is the New Oncogene Paradigm Revolutionary? *Hist Philos Life Sci* 21: 291-330, 1999.

van Hoeven KH, Bertolini PK: Prevalence. Identification and Significance of Fiber Contaminants in Cervical Smears. *Acta Cytol* 40: 489-495, 1996a.

van Hoeven KH, Hanau CA, Hudock JA: The Detection of Endocervical Gland Involvement by High-Grade Squamous Intraepithelial Lesions in Smears Prepared from Endocervical Brush Specimens. *Cytopathology* 7: 310-315, 1996b.

Van Le L, Novotny D, Dotters DJ: Distinguishing Tubal Metaplasia from Endocervical Dysplasia on Cervical Papanicolaou Smears. *Obstet Gynecol* 78: 974-976, 1991.

van Muyden RC, ter Harmsel BW, Smedts FM, et al: Detection and Typing of Human Papillomavirus in Cervical Carcinomas in Russian Women: A Prognostic Study. *Cancer* 85: 2011-2016, 1999.

van Nagell JR Jr, Rayburn W, Donaldson ES, et al: Therapeutic Implications of Patterns of Recurrence in Cancer of the Uterine Cervix. *Cancer* 44: 2354-2361, 1979.

van Nagell JR Jr, Greenwell N, Powell DF, et al: Microinvasive Carcinoma of the Cervix. *Am J Obstet Gynecol* 145: 981-991, 1983.

van Nagell JR Jr, Powell DE, Gallion HH, et al: Small Cell Carcinoma of the Uterine Cervix. *Cancer* 62: 1586-1593, 1988.

van Niekerk WA: Cervical Cytological Abnormalities Caused by Folic Acid Deficiency. *Acta Cytol* 10: 67-73, 1966.

van Oortmarssen GJ, Habbema JDF: Epidemiologic Evidence for Age-Dependent Regression of Pre-Invasive Cervical Cancer. *Br J Cancer* 64: 559-565, 1991.

van Oortmarssen GJ, Habbema JDF: Duration of Preclinical Cervical Cancer and Reduction in Incidence of Invasive Cancer Following Negative Pap Smears. *Int J Epidemiol* 24: 300-307, 1995.

Van Peenen HJ, Bickerstaff LK: Clinical Insignificance of a "Dirty" Background in Cervicovaginal Smears (Letter). *Acta Cytol* 27: 380, 1983.

van Roon, E, Boon ME, Kurver PJH, et al: The Association Between Precancerous-Columnar and Squamous Lesions of the Cervix: A Morphometric Study. *Histopathology* 7: 887-896, 1983.

Varma VA, Sanchez-Lanier M, Unger ER, et al: Association of Human Papillomavirus With Penile Carcinoma: A Study Using Polymerase Chain Reaction and In Situ Hybridization. *Hum Pathol* 22: 908-913, 1991.

Varras M, Polyzos D, Akrivis Ch: Effects of Tamoxifen on the Human Female Genital Tract: Review of the Literature. *Eur J Gynaecol Oncol* 24: 258-268, 2003.

Vásquez A, Jakobsson T, Ahrné S, et al: Vaginal *Lactobacillus* Flora of Healthy Swedish Women. *J Clin Microbiol* 40: 2746-2749, 2002.

Vecchione A, Zanesi N, Trombetta G, et al: Cervical Dysplasia, Ploidy, and Human Papillomavirus Status Correlate With Loss of *FHIT* Expression. *Clin Cancer Res* 7: 1306-1312, 2001.

Vela C, Mendoza N, Otiniano L: Cytologic Diagnosis of Chlamydia in Cervicovaginal Secretions: Use of a Papanicolaou Stain Modification With Buffered Wright Solution. *Acta Cytol* 42: 954-958, 1998.

Vela Velasquez CTV: "Atypical Parakeratosis" Cells in Cervical Carcinoma Cytology (Letter). *Acta Cytol* 41: 614-616, 1997.

Veldman T, Horikawa I, Barrett JC, et al: Transcriptional Activation of the Telomerase hTERT Gene by Human Papillomavirus Type 16 E6 Oncoprotein. *J Virol* 75: 4467-4472, 2001.

Veljovich DS, Stoler MH, Andersen WA, et al: Atypical Glandular Cells of Undetermined Significance: A Five-Year Retrospective Histopathologic Study. *Am J Obstet Gynecol* 179: 382-390, 1998.

Verloop J, Rookus MA, van Leeuwen FE: Prevalence of Gynecologic Cancer in Women Exposed to Diethylstilbestrol *in utero*. *N Engl J Med* 342: 1838-1839, 2000.

Vermund SH, Kelley KF, Klein RS, et al: High Risk of Human Papillomavirus Infection and Cervical Squamous Intraepithelial Lesions Among Women With Symptomatic Human Immunodeficiency Virus Infection. *Am J Obstet Gynecol* 165: 392-400, 1991.

Vernon SD, Unger ER, Reeves WC: Human Papillomavirus and Cervical Cancer. *Curr Prob Obstet Gynecol Fert* 21: 104, 1998.

Vesoulis Z, Erhardt CA: Cytologic Diagnosis of Vaginal Papillary Squamotransitional Cell Carcinoma: A Case Report. *Acta Cytol* 45: 465-469, 2001.

Vessey MP, McPherson K, Lawless M, et al: Neoplasia of the Cervix Uteri and Contraception: A Possible Adverse Effect of the Pill. *Lancet* (i): 930-934, 1983.

Vessey MP: Epidemiological Studies of the Effects of Diethylstilbesterol. *IARC Scientific Publications* 96: 335-348, 1989a.

Vessey MP, Villard-Mackintosh L, McPherson K, et al: Mortality Among Oral Contraceptive Users: 20 Year Follow Up of Women in a Cohort Study. *Br Med J* 299: 1487-1491, 1989b.

Vesterinen E, Leinikki P, Saksela E: Cytopathogenicity of Cytomegalovirus to Human Ecto- and Endocervical Epithelial Cell In Vitro. *Acta Cytol* 19: 473-481, 1975.

Vesterinen E, Purola E, Saksela E, et al: Clinical and Virological Findings in Patients With Cytologically Diagnosed Gynecologic Herpes Simplex Infections. *Acta Cytol* 21: 199-205, 1977.

Vesterinen E, Forss M, Nieminen U: Increase of Cervical Adenocarcinomas: A Report of 520 Cases of Cervical Carcinomas Including 112 Tumors With Glandular Elements. *Gynecol Oncol* 33: 49-53, 1989.

Viac J, Guerin-Reverchon J, Chardonnet Y, et al: Langerhans' Cells and Epithelial Cell Modifications in Cervical Intraepithelial Neoplasia: Correlation With Human Papillomavirus Infection. *Immunobiology* 180: 328-338, 1990.

Viana O: La diagnosi precoce del cancro uterino mediante lo striscio. [The Early Diagnosis of Uterine Cancer by Smears.] *La Clinica Ostetrica* 30: 781-793, 1928.

Viana O, Vozza F: L'Ostetricia e la Ginecologia in Italia. Societá Italiana di Ostetricia e Ginecologia, Milano, p. 606, 1933.

Villa LL, Lopes A: Human Papillomavirus DNA Sequences in Penile Carcinomas in Brazil. *Int J Cancer* 37: 853-855, 1986.

Villa LL, Franco ELF: Epidemiologic Correlates of Cervical Neoplasia and Risk of Human Papillomavirus Infection in Asymptomatic Women in Brazil. *J Natl Cancer Inst* 81: 332-340, 1989.

Villa LL: Human Papillomaviruses and Cervical Cancer. *Adv Cancer Res* 71: 321-341, 1997.

Vilos GA: The History of the Papanicolaou Smear and the Odyssey of George and Andromache Papanicolaou. *Obstet Gynecol* 91: 479-483, 1998.

Vinette-Leduc D, Yazdi HM, Jessamine P, et al: Reliability of Cytology to Detect Chlamydial Infection in Asymptomatic Women. *Diagn Cytopathol* 17: 258-261, 1997.

Vinette-Leduc D, Yazdi HM, Payn G, et al: Metastatic Salivary Duct Carcinoma to the Uterus: Report of a Case Diagnosed by Cervical Smear. *Diagn Cytopathol* 21: 271-275, 1999.

Visvalingam S, Blumenthal N, Clarke A, et al: Vaginal Melanoma Masquerading as Adenocarcinoma Based on Cervical Cytology: A Case Report and Review of the Literature. *Aust NZ J Obstet Gynaecol* 40: 466-467, 2000.

Viswanathan AN, Deavers MT, Jhingran A, et al: Small Cell Neuroendocrine Carcinoma of the Cervix: Outcome and Patterns of Recurrence. *Gynecol Oncol* 93: 27-33, 2004.

Vizcaino P, Moreno V, Bosch FX, et al: International Trends in the Incidence of Cervical Cancer: I. Adenocarcinoma and Adenosquamous Cell Carcinomas. *Int J Cancer* 75: 536-545, 1998.

Vlahos NP, Dragisic KG, Wallach EE, et al: Clinical Significance of the Qualification of Atypical Squamous Cells of Undetermined Significance: An Analysis on the Basis of Histological Diagnoses. *Am J Obstet Gynecol* 182: 885-890, 2000.

Voelker R: Milwaukee Deaths Reignite Critical Issues in Cervical Cancer Screening (News & Perspectives). *JAMA* 273: 1559-1560, 1995.

Vogelsang PJ, Nguyen G-K, Honoré LH: Exfoliative Cytology of Adenoma Malignum (Minimal Deviation Adenocarcinoma) of the Uterine Cervix. *Diagn Cytopathol* 13: 146-150, 1995.

Vogt B, Zerfass-Thome K, Schulze A, et al: Regulation of Cyclin E Gene Expresssion by the Human Papillomavirus Type 16 E7 Oncoprotein. *J Gen Virol* 80: 2103-2113, 1999.

Volk EE, Jax JM, Kuntzman TJ: Cytologic Findings in Cervical Smears in Patients Using Intramuscular Medroxyprogesterone Acetate (Depo-Provera) for Contraception. *Diagn Cytopathol* 23: 161-164, 2000.

von Haam E: Some Observations in the Field of Exfoliative Cytology. *Am J Clin Pathol* 24: 652-662, 1954.

von Haam E: The Cytology of Pregnancy. *Acta Cytol* 5: 320-329, 1961.

von Haam E: A Comparative Study of the Accuracy of Cancer Cell Detection by Cytological Methods. *Acta Cytol* 6: 508-518, 1962.

von Hansemann D: Über Malakoplakie der Harnblase. *Virchows Archiv (Path Anat)* 173: 302-308, 1903.

Vonka V, Kanka J, Hirsch I, et al: Prospective Study on the Relationship Between Cervical Neoplasia and Herpes Simplex Type 2 Virus. II. Herpes Simplex Type 2 Antibody Presence in Sera Taken at Enrollment. *Int J Cancer* 33: 61-66, 1984.

von Knebel Doeberitz M, Oltersdorf T, Schwarz E, et al: Correlation of Modified Human Papilloma Virus Early Gene Expression With Altered Growth Properties in C4-1 Cervical Carcinoma Cells. *Cancer Res* 48: 3780-3786, 1988.

von Knebel Doebertiz M, Rittmüller C, zur Hausen H, et al: Inhibition of Tumorigenicity of Cervical Cancer Cells in Nude Mice by HPV E6-E7 Anti-Sense RNA (Letter). *Int J Cancer* 81: 831-834, 1992.

von Ludinghausen M, Anastasiadis P: Anatomic Basis of Endometrial Cytology. *Acta Cytol* 28: 555-562, 1984.

von Preuschen [ ]: Ueber Cystenbildung in der Vagina. *Virchows Archiv (Path Anat)* 70: 111-128, 1877.

Vooijs GP, Ng ABP, Wentz WB: The Detection of Vaginal Adenosis and Clear Cell Carcinoma. *Acta Cytol* 17: 59-63, 1973.

Vooijs GP, Elias A, van der Graaf Y, et al: Relationship Between the Diagnosis of Epithelial Abnormalities and the Composition of Cervical Smears. *Acta Cytol* 29: 323-328, 1985.

Vooijs GP, Elias A, van der Graaf Y, et al: The Influence of Sample Takers on the Cellular Composition of Cervical Smears. *Acta Cytol* 30: 251-257, 1986.

Vooijs GP, van der Graaf Y, Elias AG: Cellular Composition of Cervical Smears in Relation to the Day of the Menstrual Cycle and Method of Contraception. *Acta Cytol* 31: 417-426, 1987a.

Vooijs GP, van der Graaf Y, Vooijs MA: The Presence of Endometrial Cells in Cervical Smears in Relation to the Day of the Menstrual Cycle and the Method of Contraception. *Acta Cytol* 31: 427-433, 1987b.

Voytek TM, Kannan V, Kline TS: Atypical Parakeratosis: A Marker of Dysplasia? *Diagn Cytopathol* 15: 288-291, 1996.

Voytek TM: A Kinder and Gentler CLIA? (Editorial) *Diagn Cytopathol* 29: 123-124, 2003.

Vrscaj MU, Kovacic J, Bebar S, et al: Endometrial and Other Primary Cancer After Tamoxifen Treatment of Breast Cancer—Results of Retrospective Cohort Study. *Eur J Obstet Gynecol Reprod Biol* 95: 105-110, 2001.

Vuong PN, Neveux Y, Schoonaert M-F, et al: Adenoid Cystic (Cylindromatous) Carcinoma Associated With Squamous Cell Carcinoma of the Cervix Uteri: Cytologic Presentation of a Case With Histologic and Ultrastructural Correlations. *Acta Cytol* 40: 289-294, 1996.

Vuopala S: Diagnostic Accuracy and Clinical Applicability of Cytological and Histological Methods for Investigating Endometrial Carcinoma. *Acta Obstet Gynecol Scand* Supplementum 70: 1-72, 1977.

W

Wachtel E: The Cytology of Tumors of the Ovary and Fallopian Tubes. *Clin Obstet Gynecol* 4: 1159-1171, 1961.

Wachtel E: The Cytology of Amenorrhoea. *Acta Cytol* 10: 56-61, 1966.

Wachtel MS, Dahm PF: The ASCUS: SIL Ratio and the Reference Laboratory Pathologist. *Cytopathology* 14: 249-256, 2003.

Waddell CA: Glandular Abnormalities: Dilemmas in Cytological Prediction and Clinical Management. *Cytopathology* 8: 27-30, 1997.

Wadehra V, Johnson SJ: An Audit of the Positivie Predictive Value of High-Grade Dyskaryosis in Cervical Smears: 2001-2002. *Cytopathology* 14: 107-114, 2003.

Waggoner SE, Woodworth CD, Stoler MH, et al: Human Cervical Cells Immortalized In Vitro With Oncogenic Human Papillomavirus DNA Differentiate Dysplastically In Vivo. *Gynecol Oncol* 38: 407-412, 1990.

Waggoner SE, Anderson SM, Van Eyck S, et al: Human Papillomavirus Detection and p53 Expression in Clear-Cell Adenocarcinoma of the Vagina and Cervix. *Obstet Gynecol* 84: 404-408, 1994.

Waggoner SE: Cervical Cancer. *Lancet* 361: 2217-2225, 2003.

Wagner D: Trophoblastic Cells in the Blood Stream in Normal and Abnormal Pregnancy. *Acta Cytol* 12: 137-139, 1968.

Wagner D, Ikenberg H, Boehm N, et al: Identification of Human Papillomavirus in Cervical Swabs by Deoxyribonucleic Acid In Situ Hybridization. *Obstet Gynecol* 64: 767-772, 1984.

Wagner D, de Villiers E-M, Gissmann L: Der Nachweis verschiedener Papillomvirustypen in zytologischen Abstrichen von Präkanzerosen und Karzinomen der Cervix Uteri. [Identification of Different Types of Cytological Smears of Precanceroses [sic] and Carcinomas of the Cervix Uteri.] *Geburtsh u Frauenheilk* 45: 226-231, 1985.

Wahl RW: Malakoplakia of the Uterine Cervix: Report of Two Cases. *Acta Cytol* 26: 691-694, 1982.

Wahlström T, Lindgren J, Korhonen M, et al: Distinction Between Endocervical and Endometrial Adenocarcinoma With Immunoperoxidase Staining of Carcinoembryonic Antigen in Routine Histological Tissue Specimens. *Lancet* (ii): 1159-1160, 1979.

Wain GV, Farnsworth A, Hacker NF: Cervical Carcinoma After Negative Pap Smears: Evidence Against Rapid-Onset Cancers. *Int J Gynecol Cancer* 2: 318-322, 1992.

Walboomers JM, Fokke HE, Polak M, et al: In Situ Localization of Human Papilloma Virus Type 16 DNA in a Metastasis of an Endocervical Adenocarcinoma. *Intervirology* 27: 81-85, 1987.

Walboomers JM, Meijer CJLM: Do HPV-Negative Cervical Carcinomas Exist? (Editorial). *J Pathol* 181: 253-254, 1997.

Walboomers JM, Jacobs MV, Manos MM, et al: Human Papillomavirus Is a Necessary Cause of Invasive Cervical Cancer Worldwide. *J Pathol* 189: 12-19, 1999.

Wald A: Herpes: Transmission and Viral Shedding. *Dermatol Clin* 16: 795-797, 1998.

Walker AN, Mills SE, Taylor PT: Cervical Neuroendocrine Carcinoma: A Clinical and Light Microscopic Study of 14 Cases. *Int J Gynecol Pathol* 7: 64-74, 1988.

Walker EM, Hare MJ, Cooper P: A Retrospective Review of Cervical Cytology in Women Developing Invasive Squamous Cell Carcinoma. *Br J Obstet Gynaecol* 90: 1087-1091, 1983.

Walker EM, Dodgson J, Duncan ID: Does Mild Atypia on a Cervical Smear Warrant Further Investigation? *Lancet* (ii): 672-673, 1986.

Walker J, Bloss JD, Liao S-Y, et al: Human Papillomavirus Genotype as a Prognostic Indicator in Carcinoma of the Uterine Cervix. *Obstet Gynecol* 74: 781-785, 1989.

Wallace DL, Slankard JE: Teenage Cervical Carcinoma In Situ. *Obstet Gynecol* 41: 697-700, 1973.

Wallin K-L, Wiklund F, Angstrom T, et al: Type-Specific Persistence of Human Papillomavirus DNA Before the Development of Invasive Cervical Cancer. *N Engl J Med* 341: 1633-1638, 1999.

Wallin K-L, Wiklund F, Luostarinen T, et al: A Population-Based Prospective Study of *Chlamydia trachomatis* Infection and Cervical Carcinoma. *Int J Cancer* 101: 371-374, 2002.

Walsh CB, Kay EW, Leader MB: The Pathology of Cervical Cancer. *Clin Obstet Gynecol* 38: 653-661, 1995.

Walsh JM: Cervical Cancer: Developments in Screening and Evaluation of the Abnormal Pap Smear. *West J Med* 169: 304-310, 1998.

Walton RJ: Cervical Cancer Screening Programs. I. Epidemiology and Natural History of Carcinoma of the Cervix. (Report of the task force appointed by the Conference of Deputy Ministers of Health) *CMAJ* 114: 1003-1033, 1976.

Walton RJ: Cervical Cancer Screening Programs: Summary of the 1982 Canadian Task Force Report. *CMAJ* 127: 581-589, 1982.

Wang N, Emancipator SN, Rose P, et al: Histological Follow-Up of Atypical Endocervical Cells: Liquid-Based, Thin-Layer Preparation Vs. Conventional Pap Smear. *Acta Cytol* 46: 453-457, 2002.

Wang P-H, Liu Y-C, Lai C-R, et al: Small Cell Carcinoma of the Cervix: Analysis of Clinical and Pathological Findings. *Eur J Gynaecol Oncol* 19: 189-192, 1998.

Wang P-H, Chao K-C, Lin G, et al: Primary Malignant Lymphoma of the Cervix in Pregnancy: A Case Report. *J Reprod Med* 44: 630-632, 1999a.

Wang P-H, Yuan C-C, Lai C-R: Detecting Abnormal Cells from Primary Serous Peritoneal Carcinoma by Pap Smear (Letter). *Acta Cytol* 43: 1200-1202, 1999b.

Wang SE: The Consequences of Public Disclosure: An Opinion from Newport Hospital, Newport, Rhode Island. *Diagn Cytopathol* 11: 211-212, 1994.

Wang SS, Sherman ME, Hildesheim A, et al: Cervical Adenocarcinoma and Squamous Cell Carcinoma Incidence Trends Among White Women and Black Women in the United States for 1976-2000. *Cancer* 100: 1035-1044, 2004.

Wang X, Khoo U-S, Xue W-C, et al: Cervical and Peritoneal Fluid Cytology of Uterine Sarcomas. *Acta Cytol* 46: 465-469, 2002.

Wang-Johanning F, Lu DW, Wang Y, et al: Quantiation of Human Papillomavirus 16E6 and E7 DNA and RNA in Residual Material from ThinPrep Papanicolaou Tests Using Real-Time Polymerase Chain Reaction Analysis. *Cancer* 94: 2199-2210, 2002.

Wank R, Thomssen C: High Risk of Squmaous Cell Carcinoma of the Cervix for Women With HLA-DQw3 (Letter). *Nature* 352: 723-725, 1991.

Ward BE, Burkett B, Petersen C, et al: Cytologic Correlates of Cervical Papillomavirus Infection. *Int J Gynecol Pathol* 9: 297-305, 1990.

Ward BG, Shepherd JH, Monaghan JM: Occult Advanced Cervical Cancer. *Br Med J* 290: 1301-1302, 1985.

Ward BS, Hitchcock C, Keyhani S: Primitive Neuroectodermal Tumor of the Uterus: A Case Report. *Acta Cytol* 44: 667-672, 2000.

Ward P, Parry GN, Yule R, et al: Comparison Between the Polymerase Chain Reaction and Slot Blot Hybridization for the Detection of HPV Sequences in Cervical Scrapes. *Cytopathology* 1: 19-23, 1990.

Ward RM, Bristow RE: Cancer and Pregnancy: Recent Developments. *Curr Opin Obstet Gynecol* 14: 613-617, 2002.

Warner TF: Carcinoid Tumour of the Uterine Cervix. *J Clin Pathol* 31: 990-995, 1978.

Warshal DP, Burgelson ER, Aikins JK, et al: Post-Hysterectomy Fallopian Tube Carcinoma Presenting With a Positive Papanicolaou Smear. *Obstet Gynecol* 94: 834-836, 1999.

Wassertheil-Smoller S, Romney SL, Wylie-Rosett J, et al: Dietary Vitamin C and Uterine Cervical Dysplasia. *Am J Epidemiol* 114: 714-724, 1981.

Watanabe A, Wachi T, Omi H, et al: Granulocyte Colony-Stimulating Factor-Producing Small-Cell Carcinoma of the Uterine Cervix: Report of a Case. *Diagn Cytopathol* 23: 269-274, 2000.

Watanabe Y, Ueda H, Nozaki K, et al: Advanced Primary Clear Cell Carcinoma of the Vagina Not Asssociated With Diethylstilbestrol. *Acta Cytol* 46: 577-581, 2002.

Waters EG: Carcinoma of the Cervix in a Seven Months Old Infant. *Am J Obstet Gynecol* 39: 1055-1057, 1940.

Waters SA, Sterrett GF: Intracytoplasmic Vacuoles in Cervical Smears: Relationship to Chlamydial Inclusions-Morphology, Mucin Histochemistry, and Immunocytochemistry. *Diagn Cytopathol* 7: 252-260, 1991.

Wathne B, Holst E, Hovelius B, et al: Vaginal Discharge—Comparison of Clinical, Laboratory and Microbiological Findings. *Acta Obstet Gynecol Scand* 73: 802-808, 1994.

Watts KC, Campion MJ, Butler EB, et al: Quantitative Deoxyribonucleic Acid Analysis of Patients With Mild Cervical Atypia: A Potentially Malignant Lesion? *Obstet Gynecol* 70: 205-207, 1987.

Way S: Carcinoma Metastatic in the Cervix. *Gynecol Oncol* 9: 298-302, 1980.

Weaver EJ, Kovatich AJ, Bibbo M: Cyclin E Expression and Early Cervical Neoplasia in ThinPrep Specimens: A Feasibility Study. *Acta Cytol* 44: 301-304, 2000.

Weaver RJ, Wilson R: Endometrial Carcinoma With Psammoma Bodies in the Vaginal Smear. *Am J Obstet Gynecol* 97: 869-870, 1967.

Webb JC, Key CR, Qualls CR, et al: Population-Based Study of Microinvasive Adenocarcinoma of the Uterine Cervix. *Obstet Gynecol* 97: 701-706, 2001a.

Webb, JC, Wharton GG, Hawley-Bowland C, et al: Efficacy of Treatment of Inflammatory Cytologic Abnormalities Detected by Papanicolaou Smears: A Pilot Study. *J Low Genital Tract Dis* 5: 82-84, 2001b.

Webster SD, Cason Z, Lemos LB, et al: Cytohistologic Correlation in Patients With Clinical Symptoms of Postmenopausal Bleeding. *Biomed Sci Instrum* 36: 367-372, 2000.

Weed JC Jr, Graff AT, Shoup B, et al: Small Cell Undifferentiated (Neuroendocrine) Carcinoma of the Uterine Cervix. *J Am Coll Surg* 197: 44-51, 2003.

Weiderpass E, Ye W, Tamimi R, et al: Alcoholism and Risk for Cancer of the Cervix Uteri, Vagina, and Vulva. *Cancer Epidemiol Biomarkers Prev* 10: 899-901, 2001.

Weinberg E, Hoisington S, Eastman AY, et al: Uterine Cervical Lymphoepithelial-Like Carcinoma: Absence of Epstein-Barr Virus Genomes. *Am J Clin Pathol* 99: 195-199, 1993.

Weinberger MW, Harger JH: Accuracy of the Papanicolaou Smear in the Diagnosis of Asymptomatic Infection With *Trichomonas vaginalis*. *Obstet Gynecol* 82: 425-429, 1993.

Weintraub NT, Violi E, Freedman ML: Cervical Cancer Screening in Women Aged 65 and Over. *J Am Geriatr Soc* 35: 870-875, 1987.

Weir MM, Bell DA, Young RH: Transitional Cell Metaplasia of the Uterine Cervix and Vagina: An Underrecognized Lesion that May Be Confused With High-Grade Dysplasia. A Report of 59 Cases. *Am J Surg Pathol* 21: 510-517, 1997.

Weir MM, Bell DA: Transitional Cell Metaplasia of the Cervix: A Newly Described Entity in Cervicovaginal Smears. *Diagn Cytopathol* 18: 222-226, 1998.

Weisbrot IM, Stabinsky C, Davis AM: Adenocarcinoma In Situ of the Uterine Cervix. *Cancer* 29: 1179-1187, 1972.

Weisenberg E, Froula E: *Chlamydia trachomatis* in a Thin-Prep Papanicolaou Test (Brief Article). *Arch Pathol Lab Med* 125: 981, 2001.

Weiss LK, Kau T-Y, Sparks BT, et al: Trends in Cervical Cancer Incidence Among Young Black and White Women in Metropolitan Detroit. *Cancer* 73: 1849-1854, 1994.

Weiss NS, Szekely DR, Austin DF: Increasing Incidence of Endometrial Cancer in the United States. *N Engl J Med* 294: 1259-1262, 1976.

Weiss RJ, Lucas WE: Adenocarcinoma of the Uterine Cervix. *Cancer* 57: 1996-2001, 1986.

Weitzman GA, Korhonen MO, Reeves KO, et al: Endocervical Brush Cytology. An Alternative to Endocervical Curettage? *J Reprod Med* 33: 677-683, 1988.

Welch JM, Ciesla MC, Selvaggi SM: Serous Papillary Cystadenocarcinoma of the Ovary Diagnosed With the ThinPrep Pap Test. *Acta Cytol* 44: 1122-1124, 2000.

Welch JW, Hellwig CA: Reticulum Cell Sarcoma of the Uterine Cervix: Report of a Case. *Obstet Gynecol* 22: 293-294, 1963.

Wells M, Brown LJR: Glandular Lesions of the Uterine Cervix: The Present State of Our Knowledge. *Histopathology* 10: 777-792, 1986.

Wells M, Brown LJR: Symposium Part IV: Investigative Approaches to Endocervical Pathology. *Int J Gynecol Pathol* 21: 360-367, 2002.

Welsh T, Fu YS, Chan J, et al: Mesonephric Remnants or Hyperplasia Can Cause Abnormal Pap Smears: A Study of Three Cases. *Int J Gynecol Pathol* 22: 121-126, 2003.

Wen P, Abramovich CM, Wang N, et al: Significance of Histocytes on Otherwise-Normal Cervical Smears from Postmenopausal Women: A Retrospective Study of 108 Cases. *Acta Cytol* 47: 135-140, 2003.

Wende GW: Keratosis Follicularis Resulting in Multiple Epithelioma: Report of a Case. *J Cutaneous Dis* 26: 531-551, 1908.

Wentz WB, Reagan JW: Survival in Cervical Cancer With Respect to Cell Type. *Cancer* 12: 384-388, 1959.

Wentz WB: The Significance of Mucosal Lesions Antedating Mouse Cervical Cancer. *Am J Obstet Gynecol* 84: 1506-1511, 1962.

Wentz WB, Lewis GC: Correlation of Histologic Morphology and Survival in Cervical Cancer Following Radiation Therapy. *Obstet Gynecol* 26: 228-232, 1965.

Wentz WB, Reagan JW: Clinical Significance of Postirradiation Dysplasia of the Uterine Cervix. *Am J Obstet Gynecol* 106: 812-817, 1970.

Werness BA, Levine AJ, Howley PM: Association of Human Papillomavirus Types 16 and 18 E6 Proteins With p53. *Science* 248: 76-79, 1990.

Wheeler CM, Greer CE, Becker TM, et al: Short-Term Fluctuations in the Detection of Cervical Human Papillomavirus DNA. *Obstet Gynecol* 88: 261-268, 1996.

Wheeler DT, Bell KA, Kurman RJ, et al: Minimal Uterine Serous Carcinoma: Diagnosis and Clinicopathologic Correlation. *Am J Surg Pathol* 24: 797-806, 2000.

Wheelock JB, Schneider V, Goplerud DR: Malignancy Arising in the Transplanted Vagina. *South Med J* 79: 1585-1587, 1986.

Wheelock JB, Kaminski PF: Value of Repeat Cytology at the Time of Colposcopy for the Evaluation of Cervical Intraepithelial Neoplasia on Papanicolaou Smears. *J Reprod Med* 34: 815-817, 1989.

Whitaker D: The Role of Cytology in the Detection of Malignant Lymphoma of the Uterine Cervix. *Acta Cytol* 20: 510-513, 1976.

Whitaker SJ, Blake PR, Trott PA: The Value of Cervical Cytology in Detecting Recurrent Squamous Carcinoma of the Cervix Postradiotherapy. *Clin Oncol* 2: 254-259, 1990.

White AJ, Buchsbaum HJ, Macasaet MA: Primary Squamous Cell Carcinoma of the Endometrium. *Obstet Gynecol* 41: 912-919, 1973.

Whitehead N, Reyner F, Lindenbaum J: Megaloblastic Changes in the Cervical Epithelium: Association With Oral Contraceptive Therapy and Reversal With Folic Acid. *JAMA* 226: 1421-1424, 1973.

[WHO] World Health Organization Collaborative Study of Neoplasia and Steroid Contraceptives. Invasive Cervical Cancer and Combined Oral Contraceptives. *Br Med J* 290: 961-965, 1985.

[WHO] World Health Organization Collaborative Study of Neoplasia and Steriod Contraceptives. Invasive Squamous-Cell Cervical Carcinoma and Combined Oral Contraceptives: Results From a Multinational Study. *Int J Cancer* 55: 228-236, 1993.

Wick MJ: Diagnosis of Human Papillomavirus Gynecologic Infections. *Clin Lab Med* 20: 271-287, 2000.

Wideroff L, Potischman N, Glass AG, et al: A Nested Case-Control Study of Dietary Factors and the Risk of Incident Cytological Abnormalities of the Cervix. *Nutrition Cancer* 30: 130-136, 1998.

Widrich T, Kennedy AW, Myers TM, et al: Adenocarcinoma In Situ of the Uterine Cervix: Management and Outcome. *Gynecol Oncol* 61: 304-308, 1996.

Wied GL: Suggested Standard for Karyopyknosis: Use in Hormonal Reading of Vaginal Smears. *Fertility Sterility* 6: 61-65, 1955a.

Wied GL: The Cytolytic Changes of the Vaginal Epithelial Cells and the Leukorrhea Following Estrogenic Therapy. *Am J Obstet Gynecol* 70: 51-59, 1955b.

Wied GL: Importance of the Site from Which Vaginal Cytologic Smears Are Taken. *Am J Clin Pathol* 25: 742-750, 1955c.

Wied GL, Bahr GF: Vaginal, Cervical and Endocervical Cytologic Smears on a Single Slide. *Obstet Gynecol* 14: 362-367, 1959.

Wied GL: An International Agreement on Histological Terminology for Lesions of the Uterine Cervix. *Acta Cytol* 6: 235-236, 1962a.

Wied GL: Cytology of Invasive Cervical Carcinoma and Carcinoma In Situ. *Ann NY Acad Sci* 97: 759-766, 1962b.

Wied GL, Davis ME: Cytologic Screening During Pregnancy. *Clin Obstet Gynecol* 6: 573-603, 1963.

Wied GL: Pap-Test or Babès Method? *Acta Cytol* 8: 173-174, 1964.

Wied GL, Keebler CM: Vaginal Cytology of Female Children. *Ann NY Acad Sci* 142: 646-653, 1967.

Wied GL (Moderator): Symposium on Hormonal Cytology. *Acta Cytol* 12: 87-91, 1968.

Wied GL, Bartels PH, Bibbo M, et al: Frequency and Reliability of Diagnostic Cytology of the Female Genital Tract. *Acta Cytol* 25: 543-549, 1981.

Wied GL: Tutorial on Clinical Cytology. Universal City, CA, February 25, 1995.

Wiese W, Patel SR, Patel SC, et al: A Meta-Analysis of the Papanicolaou Smear and Wet Mount for the Diagnosis of Vaginal Trichomoniasis. *Am J Med* 108: 301-308, 2000.

Wilbanks GD, Richart RM, Terner JY: DNA Content of Cervical Intraepithelial Neoplasia Studied by Two-Wavelength Feulgen Cytophotometry. *Am J Obstet Gynecol* 98: 792-799, 1967.

Wilbur DC, Maurer S, Smith NJ: Behçet's Disease in a Vaginal Smear. Report of a Case With Cytologic Features and Their Distinction from Squamous Cell Carcinoma. *Acta Cytol* 37: 525-530, 1993.

Wilbur DC, Mulford DK, Sickel JZ, et al: The Problem of Endocervical Atypia: New Cytologic Presentations of Normal Endocervical Cells and Squamous Neoplasia (Abstract). Acta Cytol 38: 808, 1994.

Wilbur DC: Endocervical Glandular Atypia: A "New" Problem for the Cytologist. *Diagn Cytopathol* 13: 463-469, 1995.

Wilbur DC: Atypical Squamous Cells of Undetermined Significance: Is Help on the Way? (Editorial). *Am J Clin Pathol* 105: 661-664, 1996a.

Wilbur DC, Dubeshter B, Angel C, et al: Use of Thin-Layer Preparations for Gynecologic Smears With Emphasis on the Cytomorphology of High-Grade Intraepithelial Lesions and Carcinomas. *Diagn Cytopathol* 14: 201-211, 1996b.

Wilbur DC: Stanley F. Patten Jr., M.D., Ph.D., and Atypical Cells of Squamous Type (Patten Tribute). *Cancer* 81: 327-331, 1997a.

Wilbur DC, Dressel DM: Metaplastic Variants of Atypical Squamous Cells of Undetermined Significance. *Pathol Case Rev* 2: 53-57, 1997b.

Wilbur DC, Parker EM, Foti JA: Location-Guided Screening of Liquid-Based Cervical Cytology Specimens: A Potential Improvement in Accuracy and Productivity Is Demonstrated in a Preclinical Feasibility Trial. *Am J Clin Pathol* 118: 399-407, 2002.

Wilczynski SP, Bergen S, Walker J, et al: Human Papillomaviruses and Cervical Cancer: Analysis of Histopathologic Features Associated With Different Viral Types. *Hum Pathol* 19: 697-704, 1988a.

Wilczynski SP, Walker J, Liao S-Y, et al: Adenocarcinoma of the Cervix Associated With Human Papillomavirus. *Cancer* 62: 1331-1336, 1988b.

Willcox F, de Somer ML, Van Roy J: Classification of Cervical Smears With Discordance Between the Cytologic and/or Histologic Ratings. *Acta Cytol* 31: 883-886, 1987.

Willett GD, Kurman RJ, Reid R, et al: Correlation of the Histologic Appearance of Intraepithelial Neoplasia of the Cervix With Human Papillomavirus Types: Emphasis on Low-Grade Lesions Including So-Called Flat Condyloma. *Int J Gynecol Pathol* 8: 18-25, 1989.

Willett WC, MacMahon B: Diet and Cancer—An Overview, Part I. *N Engl J Med* 310: 633-638. 1984a.

Willett WC, MacMahon B: Diet and Cancer—An Overview, Part II. *N Engl J Med* 310: 697-703, 1984b.

Williams AB, Darragh TM, Vranizan K, et al: Anal and Cervical Human Papillomavirus Infection and Risk of Anal and Cervical Epithelial Abnormalities in Human Immunodeficiency Virus-Infected Women. *Obstet Gynecol* 83: 205-211, 1994.

Williams AE, Jordan JA, Allen JM, et al: The Surface Ultrastructure of Normal and Metaplastic Cervical Epithelia and of Carcinoma In Situ. *Cancer Res* 33: 504-513, 1973.

Williams J: *On Cancer of the Uterus: Being the Harveian Lectures for 1886.* HK Lewis: London, 1888.

Williams ML, Rimm DL, Pedigo MA, et al: Atypical Squamous Cells of Undetermined Significance: Correlative Histologic and Follow-Up Studies from an Academic Medical Center. *Diagn Cytopathol* 16: 1-7, 1997.

Williamson BA, DeFrias D, Gunn R, et al: Significance of Extensive Hyperkeratosis on Cervical/Vaginal Smears. *Acta Cytol* 47: 749-752, 2003.

Wilson JD, Robinson AJ, Kinghorn SA, et al: Implications of Inflammatory Changes on Cervical Cytology. *Br Med J* 300: 638-640, 1990.

Wilson SH, Johnson J: An Audit of Cervical Cancer Deaths in Nottingham. *Cytopathology* 3: 79-83, 1992.

Winer RL, Lee S-K, Hughes JP, et al: Genital Human Papillomavirus Infection: Incidence and Risk factors in a Cohort of Female University Students. *Am J Epidemiol* 157: 218-226, 2003.

Wingfield M: The Daughters of Stilboestrol (Editorial). *Br Med J* 302: 1414-1415, 1991.

Wingo PA, Tong T, Bolden S: Cancer Statistics, 1995. *CA: Cancer J Clin* 45: 8-30, 1995.

Winkelstein W Jr: Smoking and Cancer of the Uterine Cervix: Hypothesis. *Am J Epidemiol* 106: 257-259, 1977.

Winkelstein W Jr, Shillitoe EJ, Brand R, et al: Further Comments on Cancer of the Uterine Cervix, Smoking, and Herpesvirus Infection. *Am J Epidemiol* 119: 1-8, 1984.

Winkelstein W Jr: Smoking and Cervical Cancer—Current Status: A Review. *Am J Epidemiol* 131: 945-957, 1990.

Winkler B, Crum CP, Fujii T, et al: Koilocytotic Lesions of the Cervix: The Relationship of Mitotic Abnormalities to the Presence of Papillomavirus Antigens and Nuclear DNA Content. *Cancer* 53: 1081-1087, 1984.

Winkler B, Crum CP: *Chlamydia trachomatis* Infection of the Female Genital Tract: Pathogenic and Clinicopathologic Correlations. *Pathol Annu* 22(Pt 1): 193-223, 1987.

Winston RML: The Relation Between Size and Pathogenicity of *Trichomonas vaginalis*. *J Obstet Gynaecol Br Commonw* 81: 399-404, 1974.

Wistuba II, Montellano FD, Milchgrub S, et al: Deletions of Chromosome 3p Are Frequent and Early Events in the Pathogenesis of Uterine Cervical Carcinoma. *Cancer Res* 57: 3154-3158, 1997.

Wistuba II, Thomas B, Behrens C, et al: Molecular Abnormalities Associated With Endocrine Tumors of the Uterine Cervix. *Gynecol Oncol* 72: 3-9, 1999.

Witkin SS, Jeremias J, Ledger WJ: Vaginal Eosinophils and IgE Antibodies to *Candida albicans* in Women With Recurrent Vaginitis. *J Med Vet Mycol* 27: 57-58, 1989.

Wolf JK, Levenback C, Malpica A, et al: Adenocarcinoma In Situ of the Cervix: Significance of Cone Biopsy Margins. *Obstet Gynecol* 88: 82-86, 1996.

Wolf JK, Ramierez PT: The Molecular Biology of Cervical Cancer. *Cancer Invest* 19: 621-629, 2001.

Wolf JK, Franco EL, Arbeit JM, et al: Innovations in Understanding the Biology of Cervical Cancer. *Cancer* 98(Suppl 9): 2064-2069, 2003.

Wolfendale MR: Exfoliative Cytology in a Case of Prolapsed Fallopian Tube. *Acta Cytol* 24: 545-548, 1980.

Wolfendale MR, King S, Usherwood MM: Abnormal Cervical Smears: Are We in for an Epidemic? *Br Med J* 287: 526-528, 1983.

Wolfendale MR: Cervical Samplers (Editorial). *Br Med J* 302: 1554-1555, 1991.

Wolfson WL: Histologic and Cytologic Correlation in Endometrial Wreaths. *Acta Cytol* 27: 63-64, 1983.

Wolinska WH. Melamed MR, de las Heras P, et al: Clear Cell Endometrial Adenocarcinoma in a Young Woman: Report of a Case Detected by Cytology. *Gynecol Oncol* 8: 119-120, 1979.

Wollner A: The Early Diagnosis of Cervical Carcinoma. *Surg Gynecol Obstet* 68: 147-154, 1939.

Wolner-Hanssen P, Krieger JN, Stevens CE, et al: Clinical Manifestations of Vaginal Trichomoniasis. *JAMA* 261: 571-576, 1989.

Wolner-Hanssen P, Eschenbach DA, Paavonen J, et al: Association Between Vaginal Douching and Acute Pelvic Inflammatory Disease. *JAMA* 263: 1936-1941, 1990.

Wolrath H, Borén H, Hallén A, et al: Trimethylamine Content in Vaginal Secretion and Its Relation to Bacterial Vaginosis. *APMIS* 110: 819-824, 2002.

Womack SD, Chirenje M, Gaffikin L, et al: HPV-Based Cervical Cancer Screening in a Population at High Risk for HIV Infection. *Int J Cancer* 85: 206-210, 2000.

Wood WG, Giustini FG, Sohn S, et al: Verrucous Carcinoma of the Vagina. *South Med J* 71: 368-371, 1978.

Woodhouse SL, Stastny JF, Styer P, et al: Interobserver Variability in Subclassification of Squamous Intraepithelial Lesions. *Arch Pathol Lab Med* 123: 1079-1084, 1999.

Woodman CB, Yates M, Ward K, et al: Indicators of Effective Cytological Sampling of the Uterine Cervix. *Lancet* (ii): 88-90, 1989.

Woodman CB, Collins S, Winter H, et al: Natural History of Cervical Human Papillomavirus Infection in Young Women: A Longitudinal Cohort Study. *Lancet* 357: 1831-1836, 2001.

Woodman CB, Collins S, Rollason TP, et al: Human Papillomavirus Type 18 and Rapidly Progressing Cervical Intraepithelial Neoplasia. *Lancet* 361: 40-43, 2003.

Woodman CL: What Is Informed? What Is Consent? What the Cytopathlogist Needs to Know (Editorial). *Diagn Cytopathol* 19: 1-3, 1998.

Woodruff JD, Peterson WF: *Condyloma acuminata* of the Cervix. *Am J Obstet Gynecol* 75: 1354-1362, 1958.

Woodruff JD: Carcinoma In Situ of the Vagina. *Clin Obstet Gynecol* 24: 485-501, 1981.

Woodworth CD, Bowden PE, Doniger J, et al: Characterization of Normal Human Exocervical Epithelial Cells Immortalized In Vitro by Papillomavirus Types 16 and 18 DNA. *Cancer Res* 48: 4620-4628, 1988.

Workman L, Schwartz MR, McCullough LB: Qualitative Analysis of Value Judgments in Interpreting Cervicovaginal Smears Using The Bethesda System. *Arch Pathol Lab Med* 124: 556-562, 2000.

Worth AJ, Boyes DA: A Case Control Study into the Possible Effects of Birth Control Pills on Pre-Clinical Carcinoma of the Cervix. *J Obstet Gyaecol Br Commonw* 79: 673-679, 1972.

Wosnitzer M: Use of Office Colposcope to Diagnose Subclinical Papillomaviral and Other Infections of Male and Female Genitalia. *Urology* 31: 340-341, 1988.

Wright C, Pipingas A, Grayson W, et al: Pemphigus Vulgaris of the Uterine Cervix Revisited: Case Report and Review of the Literature. *Diagn Cytopathol* 22: 304-307, 2000.

Wright CA, Leiman G, Burgess SM: The Cytomorphology of Papillary Serous Carcinoma of the Endometrium in Cervical Smears. *Cancer (Cancer Cytopathol)* 87: 12-18, 1999.

Wright CJE: Solitary Malignant Lymphoma of the Uterus. *Am J Obstet Gynecol* 117: 114-120, 1973.

Wright JD, Horowitz NS, Rader JS: Primary Peritoneal Carcinoma Presenting as Adenocarcinoma on a Pap Smear: A Case Report. *J Reprod Med* 47: 933-935, 2002.

Wright JD, Heroz TJ, Mutch DG, et al: Liquid-Based Cytology for the Postirradiation Surveillance of Women With Gynecologic Malignancies. *Gynecol Oncol* 91: 134-138, 2003.

Wright NH, Vessey MP, Kenward B, et al: Neoplasia and Dysplasia of the Cervix Uteri and Contraception: A Possible Protective Effect of the Diaphragm. *Br J Cancer* 38: 273-279, 1978.

Wright TC, Richart RM: Role of Human Papillomavirus in the Pathogenesis of Genital Tract Warts and Cancer. *Gynecol Oncol* 37: 151-164, 1990.

Wright TC, Ellerbrock TV, Chiasson MA, et al: Cervical Intraepithelial Neoplasia in Women Infected With Human Immunodeficiency Virus: Prevalence, Risk Factors, and Validity of Papanicolaou Smears. *Obstet Gynecol* 84: 591-597, 1994a.

Wright TC, Kurman RJ: A Critical Review of the Morphologic Classification Systems of Preinvasive Lesions of the Cervix: The Scientific Basis for Shifting the Paradigm. *Papillomavirus Rep* 5: 175-182, 1994b.

Wright TC, Koulos J, Schnoll F, et al: Cervical Intraepithelial Neoplasia in Women Infected With the Human Immunodeficiency Virus: Outcome After Loop Electrosurgical Excision. *Gynecol Oncol* 55: 253-258, 1994c.

Wright TC, Moscarelli RD, Dole P, et al: Significance of Mild Cytologic Atypia in Women Infected With Human Immunodeficiency Virus. *Obstet Gynecol* 87: 515-519, 1996.

Wright TC, Lorincz AT, Ferris DG, et al: Reflex HPV DNA Testing in Women With Abnormal Papanicolaou Smears. *Am J Obstet Gynecol* 178: 962-966, 1998.

Wright TC, Denny L, Kuhn L, et al: HPV DNA Testing of Self-Collected Vaginal Samples Compared With Cytologic Screening to Detect Cervical Cancer. *JAMA* 283: 81-86, 2000a.

Wright TC, Goldie SJ: Screening for Cervical Cancer (Letter). *Science* 290: 1651. 2000b.

Wright TC, Cox JT, Massad LS, et al: 2001 Consensus Guidelines for the Management of Women With Cervical Cytological Abnormalities. *JAMA* 287: 2120-2129, 2002a.

Wright TC, Kurman RJ, Ferenczy A: Precancerous Lesions of the Cervix. In: Kurman RJ, ed. *Blaustein's Pathology of the Female Genital Tract*. 5th ed. New York: Springer-Verlag NY Inc, New York, 253-324, 2002b.

Wright TC, Cox JT, Massad S, et al: 2001 Consensus Guidelines for the Management of Women With Cervical Intraepithelial Neoplasia. *Am J Obstet Gynecol* 189: 295-304, 2003a.

Wright TC, Schiffman M: Adding a Test for Human Papillomavirus DNA to Cervical Cancer Screening. *N Engl J Med* 348: 489-490, 2003b.

Wright TC Jr, Schiffman M, Solomon D, et al: Interim Guidance for the Use of Human Papillomavirus DNA Testing as an Adjunct to Cervical Cytology for Screening. *Obstet Gynecol* 103: 304-309, 2004.

Wright VC, Riopelle MA: Age at Beginning of Coitus Versus Chronologic Age as a Basis for Papanicolaou Smear Screening: An Analysis of 747 Cases of Preinvasive Disease. *Am J Obstet Gynecol* 149: 824-830, 1984.

Wu HH, Harshbarger KE, Berner HW, et al: Endometrial Brush Biopsy (Tao Brush)— Histologic Diagnosis of 200 Cases With Complemetary Cytology: An Accurate Sampling Technique for the Detection of Endometrial Abnormalities. *Am J Clin Pathol* 114: 412-418, 2000.

Wu HH-J, Schuetz MJ, Cramer H: Significance of Benign Endometrial Cells in Pap Smears from Postmenopausal Women. *J Reprod Med* 46: 795-798, 2001.

Wylie JG, Henderson A: Identity and Glycogen-Fermenting Ability of Lactobacilli Isolated from the Vagina of Pregnant Women. *J Med Microbiol* 2: 363-366, 1969.

Wynder EL. Cornfield J, Schroff PD, et al: A Study of Environmental Factors in Carcinoma of the Cervix. *Am J Obstet Gynecol* 68: 1016-1052, 1954.

X

Xi LF, Koutsky LA, Galloway DA, et al: Genomic Variation of Human Papillomavirus Type 16 and Risk for High-Grade Cervical Intraepithelial Neoplasia. *J Natl Cancer Inst* 89: 796-802, 1997.

Xi LF, Carter JJ, Galloway DA, et al: Acquisition and Natural History of Human Papillomavirus Type 16 Variant Infection Among a Cohort of Female University Students. *Cancer Epidemiol Biomarkers Prev* 11: 343-351, 2002.

Y

Yacobi E, Tennant C, Ferrante J, et al: University Student's Knowledge and Awareness of HPV. *Prev Med* 28: 535-541, 1999.

Yahr LJ, Lee KR: Cytologic Findings in Microglandular Hyperplasia of the Cervix. *Diagn Cytopathol* 7: 248-251, 1991.

Yamada T, Itou U, Watanabe Y, et al: Cytologic Diagnosis of Malignant Melanoma. *Acta Cytol* 16: 70-76, 1972.

Yamakawa Y, Forslund O, Teshima H, et al: Human Papillomavirus DNA in Adenocarcinoma and Adenosquamous Carcinoma of the Uterine Cervix Detected by Polymerase Chain Reaction (PCR). *Gynecol Oncol* 53: 190-195, 1994.

Yamazawa K, Matsui H, Seki K, et al: Human Papillomavirus-Positive Well-Differentiated Villoglandular Adenocarcinoma of the Uterine Cervix: A Case Report and Review of the Literature. *Gynecologic Oncol* 77: 473-477, 2000.

Yancey M, Magelssen D, Demaurez A, et al: Classification of Endometrial Cells on Cervical Cytology. *Obstet Gynecol* 76: 1000-1005, 1990.

Yang M, Zachariah S: ASCUS on Cervical Cytologic Smears: Clinical Significance. *J Reprod Med* 42: 329-331. 1997.

Yang X, Jin G, Nakao Y, et al: Malignant Transformation of HPV 16-Immortalized Human Endocervical Cells by Cigarette Smoke Condensate and Characterization of Multistage Carcinogenesis. *Int J Cancer* 65: 338-344, 1996.

Yang Y-C, Chang C-L, Chen M-L: Effect of p53 Polymorphism on the Susceptibility of Cervical Cancer. *Gynecol Obstet Invest* 51: 197-201, 2001.

Yang YJ, Trapkin LK, Demoski RK, et al: The Small Blue Cell Dilemma Associated With Tamoxifen Therapy. *Arch Pathol Lab Med* 125: 1047-1050, 2001.

Yap EH, Ho TH, Chan YC, et al: Serum Antibodies to *Trichomonas vaginalis* in Invasive Cervical Cancer Patients. *Genitourin Med* 71: 402-404, 1995.

Yates WA, Persad RV, Stanbridge CM: The Arias-Stella Reaction in the Cervix: A Case Report With Cervical Cytology. *Cytopathology* 8: 40-44, 1997.

Yeh I-T, LiVolsi VA, Noumoff JS: Endocervical Carcinoma. *Pathol Res Pract* 187: 129-144, 1991.

Yelverton CL, Bentley RC, Olenick S, et al: Epithelial Repair of the Uterine Cervix: Assessment of Morphologic Features and Correlations With Cytologic Diagnosis. *Int J Gynecol Pathol* 15: 338-344, 1996.

Ylinen K, Nieminen U, Forss M, et al: Changing Pattern of Cervical Carcinoma: A Report of 709 Cases of Invasive Carcinoma Treated in 1970-1974. *Gynecol Oncol* 20: 378-386, 1985.

Ylitalo N, Sorensen P, Josefsson A, et al: Smoking and Oral Contraceptives as Risk Factors for Cervical Carcinoma In Situ. *Int J Cancer* 81: 357-365, 1999.

Ylitalo N, Josefsson A, Melbye M, et al: A Prospective Study Showing Long-Term Infection With Human Papillomavirus 16 Before the Development of Cervical Carcinoma In Situ. *Cancer Res* 60: 6027-6032, 2000a.

Ylitalo N, Sorensen P, Josefsson AM, et al: Consistent High Viral Load of Human Papillomavirus 16 and Risk of Cervical Carcinoma In Situ: A Nested Case-Control Study. *Lancet* 355: 2194-2198, 2000b.

Yobs AR, Swanson RA, Lamotte LC: Laboratory Reliability of the Papanicolaou Smear. *Obstet Gynecol* 65: 235-244, 1985.

Yobs AR, Plott AE, Hicklin MD, et al: Retrospective Evaluation of Gynecologic Cytodiagnosis. II. Interlaboratory Reproducibility as Shown in Rescreening Large Consecutive Samples of Reported Cases. *Acta Cytol* 31: 900-910, 1987.

Yokoyama M, Tsutsumi K, Pater A, et al: Human Papillomavirus 18-Immortalized Endocervical Cells With In Vitro Cytokeratin Expression Characteristics of Adenocarcinoma. *Obstet Gynecol* 83: 197-204, 1994.

Yoonessi M: Carcinoma of the Fallopian Tube. *Obstet Gynecol Surv* 34: 257-270, 1979.

Yoonessi M, Wieckowska W, Mariniello D, et al: Cervical Intra-Epithelial Neoplasia in Pregnancy. *Int J Gynaecol Obstet* 20: 111-118, 1982.

Yoshida T, Fukuda T, Sano T, et al: Usefulness of Liquid-Based Cytology Specimens for the Immunocytochemical Study of p16 Expression and Human Papillomavirus Testing: A Comparative Study Using Simultaneously Sampled Histology Materials. *Cancer (Cancer Cytopathol)* 102: 100-108, 2004.

Younes MS: Electron Microscope Observations on Carcinoma In Situ of the Cervix. *Obstet Gynecol Surv* 24: 768-784, 1969.

Young LS, Bevan IS, Johnson MA, et al: The Polymerase Chain Reaction: A New Epidemiological Tool for Investigating Cervical Human Papillomavirus Infection. *Br Med J* 298: 14-18, 1989.

Young NA, Kline TS: Benign Cellular Changes: Allied Ambiguity in CLIA '88 And The Bethesda System. *Diagn Cytopathol* 10: 307-308, 1994a.

Young NA, Naryshkin S, Atkinson BF, et al: Interobserver Variability of Cervical Smears With Squamous-Cell Abnormalities: A Philadelphia Study. *Diagn Cytopathol* 11: 352-357, 1994b.

Young NA: Back to the Negative Pap Test: Behind the Scenes at Bethesda 2001 (Editorial). *Diagn Cytopathol* 26: 207-208, 2002.

Young QA, Pacey NF: The Cytologic Diagnosis of Clear Cell Adenocarcinoma of the Cervix Uteri. *Acta Cytol* 22: 3-6, 1978.

Young RH, William R, Welch WR, et al: Ovarian Sex Cord Tumor With Annular Tubules: Review of 74 Cases Including 27 With Peutz-Jeghers Syndrome and Four With Adenoma Malignum of the Cervix. *Cancer* 50: 1384-1402, 1982.

Young RH, Scully RE: Villoglandular Papillary Adenocarcinoma of the Uterine Cervix. A Clinicopathologic Analysis of 13 Cases. *Cancer* 63: 1773-1779, 1989a.

Young RH, Scully RE: Atypical Forms of Microglandular Endocervical Hyperplasia of the Cervix Simulating Adenocarcinoma. A Report of Five Cases and Review of the Literature. *Am J Surg Pathol* 13: 50-56, 1989b.

Young RH, Scully RE: Invasive Adenocarcinoma and Related Tumors of the Uterine Cervix. *Semin Diagn Pathol* 7: 205-227, 1990.

Young RH, Scully RE: Uterine Carcinomas Simulating Microglandular Hyperplasia: A Report of Six Cases. *Am J Surg Pathol* 16: 1092-1097, 1992.

Young RH, Scully RE: Minimal-Deviation Endometrioid Adenocarinoma of the Uterine Cervix. A Report of Five Cases of a Distinctive Neoplasm that May Be Misinterpreted as Benign. *Am J Surg Pathol* 17: 660-665, 1993.

Young RH, Clement PB: Endocervical Adenocarcinoma and Its Variants: Their Morphology and Differential Diagnosis. *Histopathology* 41: 185-207, 2002.

Youseff AF, Fayad MM: The Post-Partum Vaginal Smear. *J Obstet Gynaecol Br Commonw* 70: 32-38, 1963.

Yu HC, Ketabchi M: Detection of Malignant Melanoma of the Uterine Cervix from Papanicolaou Smears: A Case Report. *Acta Cytol* 31: 73-76, 1987.

Yule R: The Frequency of Cytology Testing (Abstract). *Acta Cytol* 16: 389-390, 1972.

Yule R: Mortality from Carcinoma of the Cervix. *Lancet* (i): 1031-1032, 1978.

Yun K, Cho NP, Glassford GN: Large Cell Neuroendocrine Carcinoma of the Uterine Cervix: A Report of a Case With Coexisting Cervical Intraepithelial Neoplasia and Human Papillomavirus 16. *Pathology* 31: 158-161, 1999.

Yunis JJ, Soreng AL: Constitutive Fragile Sites and Cancer. *Science* 226: 1199-1204, 1984.

Z

Zachariadou-Veneti S: George Papanicolaou (1882-1962): A Tribute. *Cytopathology* 11: 152-157, 2000.

Zaharopoulos P, Wong JY, Keagy N: Hematoidin Crystals in Cervicovaginal Smears: Report of Two Cases. *Acta Cytol* 29: 1029-1034, 1985a.

Zaharopoulos P, Wong JY, Edmonston G, et al: Crystalline Bodies in Cervicovaginal Smears: A Cytochemical and Immunochemical Study. *Acta Cytol* 29: 1035-1042, 1985b.

Zahn CM, Askew AW, Hall KL, et al: The Significance of Hyperkeratosis/Parakeratosis on Otherwise Normal Papanicolaou Smears. *Am J Obstet Gynecol* 187: 997-1001, 2002.

Zaino RJ, Nahhas WA, Mortel R: Glassy Cell Carcinoma of the Uterine Cervix: An Ultrastructural Study and Review. *Arch Pathol Lab Med* 106: 250-254, 1982.

Zaino RJ, Kurman R, Herbold D, et al: The Significance of Squamous Differentiation in Endometrial Carcinoma: Data from a Gynecologic Oncology Group Study. *Cancer* 68: 2293-2302, 1991.

Zaino RJ: Glandular Lesions of the Uterine Cervix. *Mod Pathol* 13: 261-274, 2000.

Zaino RJ: Symposium Part I: Adenocarcinoma In Situ, Glandular Dysplasia, and Early Invasive Adenocarcinoma of the Uterine Cervix. *Int J Gynecol Pathol* 21: 314-326, 2002.

Zaleski S, Setum C, Benda J: Cytologic Presentation of Alveolar Soft-Part Sarcoma of the Vagina: A Case Report. *Acta Cytol* 30: 655-670, 1986.

Zaneveld LJD, Tauber PF, Port C, et al: Scanning Electron Microscopy of Cervical Mucus Crystallization. *Obstet Gynecol* 46: 419-428, 1975.

Zappa M, Visioli CB, Ciatto S, et al: Lower Protection of Cytological Screening for Adenocarcinomas and Shorter Protection for Younger Women: The Results of a Case-Control Study in Florence. *Br J Cancer* 90: 1784-1786, 2004.

Zardawi IM, Rode JW: Clinical Value of Repeat Pap Smear at the Time of Colposcopy. *Acta Cytol* 46: 495-498, 2002.

Zehbe I, Wilander E: Human Papillomavirus Infection and Invasive Cervical Neoplasia: A Study of Prevalence and Morphology. *J Pathol* 101: 270-275, 1997.

Zehbe I, Wilander E, Delius H, et al: Human Papillomavirus 16 E6 Variants Are More Prevalent in Invasive Cervical Carcinoma than the Prototype. *Cancer Res* 58: 829-833, 1998.

Zenilman JM: Chlamydia and Cervical Cancer. *JAMA* 285: 81-83, 2001.

Zerfass K, Schulze A, Spitkovsky D, et al: Sequential Activation of Cyclin E and Cyclin A Gene Expression by Human Papillomavirus Type 16 E7 Through Sequences Necessary for Transformation. *J Virol* 69: 6389-6399, 1995.

Zerfass-Thome K, Zwerscgje W, Mannhardt B et al: Inactivation of the cdk Inhibitor p27[KIP1] by the Human Papillomavirus Type 16 E7 Oncoprotein. *Oncogene* 13: 2323-2330, 1996.

Zhang J, Thomas AG, Leybovich E: Vaginal Douching and Adverse Health Effects: A Meta-Analysis. *Am J Public Health* 87: 1207-1211, 1997.

Zhang Y, Selvaggi SM: Significance of Psammoma Bodies on a Cervical Sample from an Asymptomatic Woman. *Diagn Cytopathol* 29: 339-340, 2003.

Zhang Z-F, Begg CB: Is *Trichomonas vaginalis* a Cause of Cervical Neoplasia? Results from a Combined Analysis of 24 Studies. *Int J Epidemiol* 23: 682-690, 1994.

Zhang Z-F: Epidemiology of *Trichomonas vaginalis*: A Prospective Study in China. *Sex Transm Dis* 23: 415-424, 1996.

Zheng P-S, Iwasaka T, Zhang Z-M, et al: Telomerase Activity in Papanicolaou Smear-Negative Exfoliated Cervical Cells and Its Association With Lesions and Oncogenic Human Papillomaviruses. *Gynecol Oncol* 77: 394-398, 2000.

Zheng T, Holford TR, Ma Z, et al: The Continuing Increase in Adenocarcinoma of the Uterine Cervix: A Birth Cohort Phenomenon. *Int J Epidemiol* 25: 252-258, 1996.

Zhou C, Matisic JP, Clement PB, et al: Cytologic Features of Papillary Serous Adenocarcinoma of the Uterine Cervix. *Cancer (Cancer Cytopathol)* 81: 98-104, 1997.

Zhou C, Gilks CB, Hayes M, et al: Papillary Serous Carcinoma of the Uterine Cervix: A Clinicopathologic Study of 17 Cases. *Am J Surg Pathol* 22: 113-120, 1998a.

Zhou C, Hayes MM, Clement PB, et al: Small Cell Carcinoma of the Uterine Cervix: Cytologic Findings in 13 Cases. *Cancer* 84: 281-288, 1998b.

Ziabkowski TA, Naylor B: Cyanophilic Bodies in Cervico-Vaginal Smears. *Acta Cytol* 20: 340-342, 1976.

Ziegler RG, Brinton LA, Hamman RF, et al: Diet and the Risk of Invasive Cervical Cancer Among White Women in the United States. *Am J Epidemiol* 132: 432-445, 1990.

Zielinski GD, Snijders PJF, Rozendaal L, et al: HPV Presence Precedes Abnormal Cytology in Women Developing Cervical Cancer and Signals False Negative Smears. *Br J Cancer* 85: 398-404, 2001.

Zimmer TS: Late Irradiation Changes: A Cytological Study of Cervical and Vaginal Smears. *Cancer* 12: 193-196, 1959.

Ziol M, Di Tomaso C, Biaggi A, et al: Virological and Biological Characteristics of Cervical Intra-epithelial Neoplasia Grade I With Marked Koilocytotic Atypia. *Hum Pathol* 29: 1068-1073, 1998.

Zondervan KT, Carpenter LM, Painter R, et al: Oral Contraceptives and Cervical Cancer—Further Findings from the Oxford Family Planning Association Contraceptive Study. *Br J Cancer* 73: 1291-1297, 1996.

Zreik TG, Rutherford TJ: Psammoma Bodies in Cervicovaginal Smears. *Obstet Gynecol* 97: 693-695, 2001.

Zucker PK, Kasdon EJ, Feldstein ML: The Validity of Pap Smear Parameters as Predictors of Endometrial Pathology in Menopausal Women. *Cancer* 56: 2256-2263, 1985.

Zucker PK, Kasdon EJ: Normal Endometrial Cells in Papanicolaou Smears: Prevalence in Women With and Without Endometrial Disease (Letter). *Obstet Gynecol* 97: 798, 2001.

Zuna RE: Association of Condylomas With Intraepithelial and Microinvasive Cervical Neoplasia: Histopathology of Conization and Hysterectomy Specimens. *Int J Gynecol Pathol* 2: 364-372, 1984. Zuna RE, Erroll M: Utility of the Cervical Cytologic Smear in Assessing Endocervical Involvement by Endometrial Carcinoma. *Acta Cytol* 40: 878-884, 1996.

Zuna RE, Slenko A, Lightfoot S, et al: Cervical Smear Interpretations in Women With a Histological Diagnosis of Severe Dysplasia: Factors Associated With Discrepant Interpretations. *Cancer (Cancer Cytopathol)* 96: 218-224, 2002.

Zuna RE, Allen RA, Moore WE, et al: Comparison of Human Papillomavirus Genotypes in High-Grade Squamous Intraepithelial Lesions and Invasive Cervical Carcinoma: Evidence for Differences in Biologic Potential of Precursor Lesions. *Mod Pathol* 17: 1314-1322, 2004.

Zunzunegui MV, King M-C, Coria CF, et al: Male Influences on Cervical Cancer Risk. *Am J Epidemiol* 123: 302-307, 1986.

zur Hausen H, Meinhof W, Scheiber W, et al: Attempts to Detect Virus-Specific DNA in Human Tumors. I. Nucleic Acid Hybridizations With Complementary RNA of Human Wart Virus. *Int J Cancer* 13: 650-656, 1974.

zur Hausen H: Condylomata Acuminata and Human Genital Cancer. [Symposium: Approaches to Immunological Control of Virus-Associated Tumors in Man: Prospects and Problems. Cervical Cancer Program] *Cancer Res* 36: 794, 1976. zur Hausen H: Human Papillomaviruses and Their Possible Role in Squamous Cell Carcinomas. *Curr Top Microbiol Immunol* 78: 1-30, 1977.

zur Hausen H, de Villiers E-M, Gissmann L: Papillomavirus Infections and Human Genital Cancer. *Gynecol Oncol* 12(2 Pt 2): S124-S128, 1981.

zur Hausen H: Human Genital Cancer: Synergism Between Two Virus Infections for Synergism Between a Virus Infection and Initiating Events? *Lancet* (ii): 1370-1372, 1982.

zur Hausen H: Herpes Simplex Virs in Human Genital Cancer. *Int Rev Exp Pathol* 25: 307-326, 1983.

zur Hausen H: Papillomaviruses in Human Cancer. *Appl Pathol* 5: 19-24, 1987.

zur Hausen H: Papillomaviruses in Human Cancers. *Proc Assoc Am Physicians* 111: 581-587, 1999.

zur Hausen H: Papillomaviruses Causing Cancer: Evasion from Host-Cell Control in Early Events in Carcinogenesis. *J Natl Cancer Inst* 92: 690-698, 2000.

zur Hausen H: Papillomaviruses and Cancer: From Basic Studies to Clinical Application. *Nature Rev (Cancer)* 2: 342-350, 2002.

Zweizig S, Noller K, Reale F, et al: Neoplasia Associated With Atypical Glandular Cells of Undetermined Significance on Cervical Cytology. *Gynecol Oncol* 65: 314-318, 1977.

Index

I

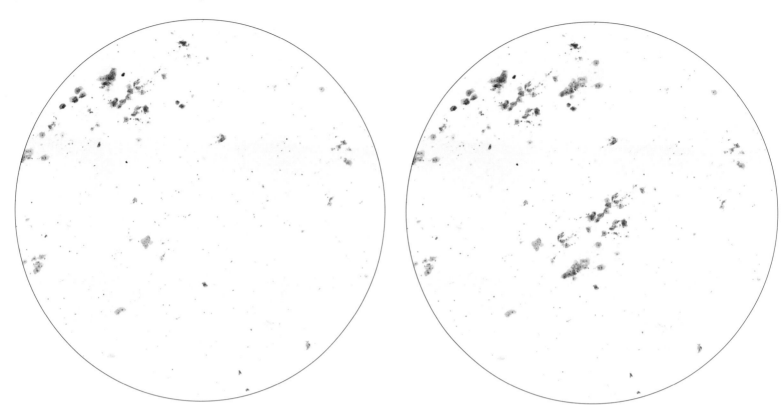

~100 cells. Inadequate if all fields have no more than this cellularity. (4× field, CPS) [Courtesy of Dr. George Birdsong, Atlanta]

~150 cells. Barely adequate if all fields have similar cellularity. (4× field, CPS) [Courtesy of Dr. George Birdsong, Atlanta]

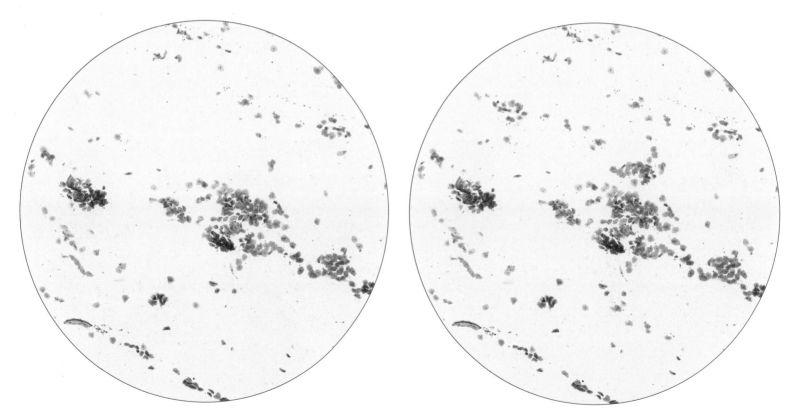

~370 cells. Adequate if at least 22 fields have similar (or greater) cellularity. (4× field, CPS) [Courtesy of Dr. George Birdsong, Atlanta]

~400 cells. Adequate if at least 20 fields have similar (or greater) cellularity. (4× field, CPS) [Courtesy of Dr. George Birdsong, Atlanta]